Essentials of Clinical Pharmacology in Nursing

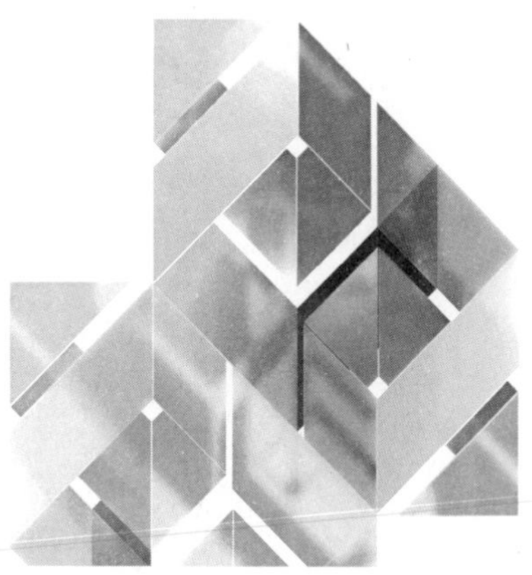

THIRD EDITION

Essentials of Clinical Pharmacology in Nursing

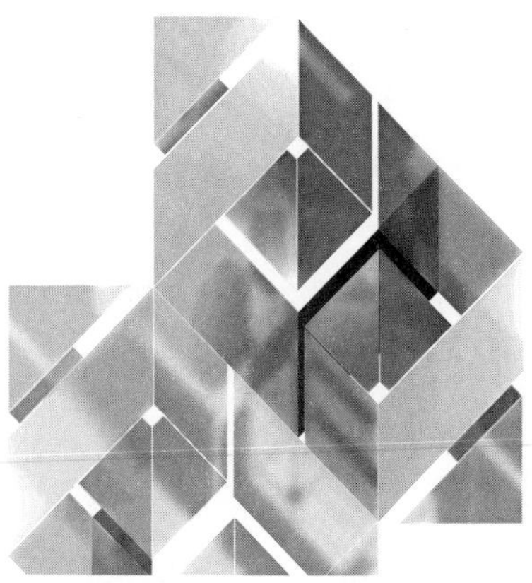

THIRD EDITION

Bradley R. Williams, PharmD
Associate Professor of Clinical Pharmacy and Clinical Gerontology
School of Pharmacy and Andrus Gerontology Center
University of Southern California
Los Angeles

Charold L. Baer, RN, PhD, FCCM, CCRN
Professor and Director of the Acute Care Nurse Practitioner Program
School of Nursing
Oregon Health Sciences University
Portland

Springhouse Corporation
Springhouse, Pennsylvania

Staff

Vice President, Planning and Development
Minnie Bowen Rose, RN, BSN, MEd

Executive Director
Patricia Dwyer Schull, RN, MSN

Art Director
John Hubbard

Editorial Manager
A. T. McPhee, RN, BSN

Clinical Manager
Ann M. Barrow, RN, MSN, CCRN

Editors
Laini Berlin, Naina Chohan, Bernice Heller, Peter Johnson, Ann Lenkiewicz, Suzanne McHugh, Nancy Priff, Michelle Stephenson

Clinical Editors
Deborah Becker, RN, MSN, CCRN; V. Jane Bliss-Holtz, RN,C, DNSC; Mary Christian, RN,C, MSN, OCN; Colleen M. Fries, RN, BSN, CCRN; Collette Bishop Hendler, RN, CCRN; Lori Musolf Neri, RN, MSN, CCRN; Kimberly Zalewski, RN, MSN, CEN

Associate Acquisitions Editor
Betsy K. Snyder

Copy Editors
Cynthia C. Breuninger (manager), Karen C. Comerford, Stacey A. Follin, Linda Gundersen, Brenna H. Mayer, Beth Pitcher, Pamela Wingrod

Designers
Arlene Putterman (associate art director), Elaine Ezrow, Joseph John Clark, Jacalyn B. Facciolo, Donald G. Knauss, Matie Anne Patterson

Illustrators
Jacalyn B. Facciolo, Dan Fione, Will Davidson, Julie Devito, BJ Krim, Bob Neumann, Judy Newhouse, Gary B. Welch

Typographers
Diane Paluba (manager), Joyce Rossi Biletz, Valerie Rosenberger

Manufacturing
Deborah Meiris (director), Pat Dorshaw, Otto Mezei

Editorial Assistants
Carol A. Caputo, Mary Madden, Margaret A. Rastiello

Indexer
Barbara Hodgson

The clinical procedures described and recommended in this publication are based on research and consultation with nursing, medical, and legal authorities. To the best of our knowledge, these procedures reflect currently accepted practice; nevertheless, they can't be considered absolute and universal recommendations. For individual application, all recommendations must be considered in light of the patient's clinical condition and, before the administration of new or infrequently used drugs, in light of the latest package-insert information. The authors and publisher disclaim responsibility for adverse effects resulting directly or indirectly from the suggested procedures, from undetected errors, or from the reader's misunderstanding of the text.

ESS3-010298
Printed in the United States of America

 A member of the Reed Elsevier plc group

Library of Congress Cataloging-in-Publication Data
Essentials of clinical pharmacology in nursing/[edited by]
Bradley R. Williams, Charold L. Baer—3rd ed.
p.cm.
Includes bibliographical references and index.
1. Pharmacology. 2. Nursing. I. Williams, Bradley R.
II. Baer, Charold Lee Morris
[DNLM: 1. Pharmacology. Clinical—nurses' instruction.
2. Drug Therapy—nurses' instruction. QV 38 E7774 1998]
RM300.E82 1998
615.5'8—dc21
DNLM/DLC 97-34614
ISBN 0-87434-931-1 CIP

Contents

UNIT IV
DRUGS TO TREAT NEUROLOGIC AND NEUROMUSCULAR SYSTEM DISORDERS

UNIT V
DRUGS TO PREVENT AND TREAT PAIN

UNIT VI
DRUGS TO IMPROVE CARDIOVASCULAR FUNCTION

APPENDICES

Advisory board

Kathleen G. Andreoli, RN, DSN, FAAN
Vice President, Nursing Affairs and the John L. and Helen Kellogg Dean, College of Nursing
Rush–Presbyterian–St. Luke's Medical Center
Rush University
Chicago

Marie Scott Brown, RN, PhD, CNM, PNP
Pediatric Nurse Practitioner, Professor of Family Nursing
School of Nursing
Oregon Health Sciences University
Portland

Kathleen Dracup, RN, MN, DNSc, FAAN
L.W. Hassenplug Professor, School of Nursing
University of California
Los Angeles

Elizabeth Grossman, RN, EdD, FAAN
Dean and Professor of Nursing Emeritus
Indiana University School of Nursing
Indianapolis

Evelyn R. Hayes, RN, PhD
Associate Professor, College of Nursing
University of Delaware
Newark

Mary D. Naylor, RN, PhD, FAAN
Associate Dean and Director of Undergraduate Studies
School of Nursing
University of Pennsylvania
Philadelphia

Contributors and consultants

Steven R. Abel, BS, PharmD, FASHP, Professor and Head, Department of Pharmacy Practice, Purdue University, School of Pharmacy and Pharmacal Sciences, Wishard Memorial Hospital, Indianapolis

Gary J. Arnold, MD, FACS, Assistant Professor, University of Southwestern Louisiana, College of Nursing, Lafayette

Charold L. Baer, RN, PhD, FCCM, CCRN, Professor and Director of the Acute Care Nurse Practitioner Program, Oregon Health Sciences University, School of Nursing, Portland

Carol L. Beck, RPh, PharmD, PhD, Post-doctoral Research Fellow, Vanderbilt University, Department of Medicine, Division of Nephrology, Nashville, Tenn.

Deborah Becker, RN, MSN, CCRN, Lecturer, University of Pennsylvania, School of Nursing, Philadelphia

V. Jane Bliss-Holtz RN,C, DNSc, Executive Director, JBH Logical Enterprises, Rocky Hill, N.J.

Rebecca E. Boehne, RN, PhD, Patient and Family Education Coordinator, Portland (Ore.) Veterans Administration Medical Center

Mary E. Bowen, RN, DNS, CNAA, Assistant Professor, Thomas Jefferson University, Philadelphia

Karna J. Bramble, RN, PhD, C-GNP, Section Chief, Non-Physician Services, Medical Service, Long Beach (Calif.) Veterans Administration Medical Center

Barbara Braverman, RN,CS, MSN, Geropsychiatric Clinical Nurse Specialist, Abington (Pa.) Memorial Hospital

Linda P. Brown, RN, PhD, FAAN, Associate Professor, University of Pennsylvania, School of Nursing, Philadelphia

Karen T. Bruchak, RN, MSN, MBA, Assistant Administrator, Cancer Clinical Programs, University of Pennsylvania, Philadelphia

Kathleen C. Byington, RN,CS, MSN, Pediatric Clinical Nurse Specialist and Case Manager, Vanderbilt University, Nashville, Tenn.

James Camamo, PharmD, Clinical Pharmacist for Medication Information and Policy Development, University Medical Center, Tucson, Ariz.

Lawrence P. Carey, PharmD, Clinical Pharmacist Coordinator, Jefferson Home Infusion Service, Thomas Jefferson University Hospital, Philadelphia

James D. Carlson, PharmD, President, PRACS Institute, Ltd., Fargo, N.D.

Bruce C. Carlstedt, RPh, PhD, Associate Professor of Clinical Pharmacy, Purdue University, Department of Pharmacy Practice, Wishard Memorial Hospital, Indianapolis

Vivian Hayes Churness, RN, DNSc, Assistant Clinical Professor, University of Southern California, Department of Nursing, Los Angeles

Marlene Ciranowicz, RN, MSN, CDE, Independent Consultant, Philadelphia

Rachel Clark-Vetri, PharmD, Clinical Assistant Professor of Pharmacy Practice, Temple University, Philadelphia

Barbara Ann Costa, RN, MS, Professor Emeritus, Syracuse (N.Y.) University, College of Nursing

N. Michael Davis, RPh, MS, Clinical Coordinator, Pharmacy Information and Research, Jackson Memorial Hospital, Miami

Cathi Dennehy, PharmD, Assistant Clinical Professor, University of California at San Francisco

Robin Donohoe Dennison, RN,CS, MSN, CCRN, Critical Care Consultant, Lexington, Ky.

Laura D. D'Oria, RPh, PharmD, Pharmacist, Community Medical Center, Toms River, N.J.

Teresa S. Dunsworth, PharmD, BCPS, Associate Professor of Clinical Pharmacy, West Virginia University School of Pharmacy, Morgantown

Patricia L. Eltz, RN, MSN, CEN, Community Health Educator, Pottstown (Pa.) Memorial Medical Center

Belle Erickson, RN,C, PhD, Assistant Professor, Villanova (Pa.) University, College of Nursing

Carmel A. Esposito, RN, MSN, EdD, Coordinator, Continuing Education and Nurse Educator, Trinity Health System School of Nursing, Steubenville, Ohio

Janet M. Farahmand, RN,C, MSN, EdD, Associate Professor of Nursing, Neumann College, Division of Nursing and Health Services, Aston, Pa.

Latrell P. Fowler, RN, PhD, Assistant Professor, Medical University of South Carolina, Florence

Colleen M. Fries, RN, BSN, CCRN, Clinical Leader, Abington (Pa.) Memorial Hospital

Joan Parker Frizzell, RN, MSN, PhD, Assistant Professor, La Salle University, Philadelphia

Douglas R. Geraets, RPh, PharmD, FCCP, Clinical Pharmacy Specialist, Ambulatory Care, Veterans Administration Medical Center, Iowa City

Mary Jo M. Gerlach, RN, MSNEd, Assistant Professor, Adult Nursing, Medical College of Georgia, School of Nursing, Athens

Martin R. Giannamore, RPh, PharmD, Assistant Professor of Clinical Pharmacy Practice, Ohio State University, College of Pharmacy, Columbus

Richard K. Gibson, RN,CS, MN, JD, CCRN, Clinical Nurse Specialist, San Diego Veterans Administration Medical Center

Mary Beth Gross, PharmD, FASCP, Manager, Pharmacy, Mercy Hospital Medical Center; Associate Professor of Pharmacy, Drake University, Des Moines, Iowa

Anne Myers Gudmundsen, RN, PhD, FNPC, Family Nurse Practitioner, John Peter Smith South Campus Clinic, Fort Worth, Tex.

Bridget A. Haupt, BS, PharmD, Director of Pharmacy Services, Children's Seashore House, Philadelphia

David W. Hawkins, PharmD, Professor and Assistant Dean of Pharmacy, University of Georgia, Athens

Marcia Jo Hill, RN, MSN, Assistant Clinical Professor, Baylor College of Medicine, Department of Dermatology, Houston, Tex.

Sande Jones, RN,C, MSN, MSEd, Clinical Specialist, Medical-Surgical and Immunology, Mount Sinai Medical Center, Miami Beach, Fla.

Lynne Kreutzer-Baraglia, RN, MS, Administrative Dean, Concordia University, West Suburban College of Nursing, Oak Park, Ill.

Eileen Hayes Lantier, RN, PhD, Assistant Professor, Director for Learning Resources, Syracuse (N.Y.) University, College of Nursing

Brenda L. Lyon, RN, DNS, FAAN, Associate Professor, Adult Health Nursing, Indiana University, School of Nursing, Indianapolis

Mary Y. Ma, PharmD, FASHP, Infectious Disease Pharmacy Specialist, Veterans Administration Medical Center, West Los Angeles

Sara Lynn Machowsky, RN, MS, Clinical Administrator, Donald E. Willard, M.D. and Associates, Easton, Pa.

Catherine Todd Magel, RN,C, EdD, Assistant Professor, Villanova (Pa.) University, College of Nursing

Marie Maloney, PharmD, Clinical Pharmacist, University Medical Center, Tucson, Ariz.

Dawna Martich, RN, MSN, Clinical Manager, University Family Practice Associates, Inc., Moon Township, Pa.

Carol Lynn Maxwell-Thompson, RN, MSN, CCRN, Nursing Faculty, University of Virginia, School of Nursing, Charlottesville

Carrie A. McCoy, RN, MSN, CEN, Associate Professor of Nursing, Northern Kentucky University, Department of Nursing, Highland Heights

Gary Milavetz, RPh, PharmD, Associate Professor of Pharmacy, University of Iowa, College of Pharmacy, Iowa City

Michaelene P. Mirr, RN,CS, PhD, Professor and Gerontological Nurse Practitioner, University of Wisconsin, Eau Claire

John J. Nagelhout, RN, PhD, Director, Kaiser Permanente School of Anesthesia, Pasadena, Calif.

Jean M. Nappi, PharmD, FCCP, BCPS, Professor and Vice Chair for Academic Affairs, Medical University of South Carolina, Charleston

Patricia Ann O'Leary, RN, DSN, Associate Professor, Middle Tennessee State University, School of Nursing, Murfreesboro

Nina Olesinski, RN, PhD, Clinical Nurse Specialist, Critical Care, University of Illinois at Chicago Medical Center

C. Lynne Ostrow, RN, MSN, EdD, Associate Professor, West Virginia University, School of Nursing, Morgantown

Andrew M. Peterson, PharmD, BCPS, Assistant Professor of Clinical Pharmacy, Philadelphia College of Pharmacy and Science

Larry A. Pfeifer, RPh, MApSt, Chief, Pharmacy Services, Gillis W. Long Hansen's Disease Center, Carville, La.

David R. Pipher, RPh, PharmD, Director of Pharmacy, Forbes Regional Hospital, Monroeville, Pa.

Frances W. Quinless, RN, PhD, Dean, University of Medicine and Dentistry of New Jersey, School of Nursing, Newark

Ann E. Rogers, RN, PhD, Associate Professor, University of Michigan, School of Nursing, Ann Arbor

Gary Smith, PharmD, RPh, Clinical Manager, Asthma Disease Management, Value Rx, Plymouth, Minn.

Dawn M. Specht, RN, MSN, CEN, CCRN, PHRN, Clinical Nurse Specialist, Cooper Health System, Camden, N.J.; Nursing Instructor, Episcopal Hospital, School of Nursing, Philadelphia

Joseph F. Steiner, RPh, PharmD, Professor and Director of Pharmacy Practice, University of Wyoming, School of Pharmacy, Laramie

Margot T. Stock, RN, CNRN, DPhil, Assistant Professor, East Carolina University, School of Nursing, Greenville, N.C.

Candy Tsourounis, RPh, PharmD, Assistant Clinical Professor, University of California, School of Nursing, Drug Information Analysis Service, San Francisco

Paul J. Vitale, PharmD, FASCP, Assistant Director of Pharmacy Services, Anne Arundel Medical Center, Annapolis, Md.; Director, Clinical Services, Technicare Pharmaceutical Services, Washington, D.C.

Margaret Wallhagen, RN, PhD, Assistant Professor, University of California, Department of Physiological Nursing, San Francisco

Rosemarie C. Westberg, RN, MSN, CPN, Professor, Nursing, Northern Virginia Community College, Annandale

Kenneth K. Wieland, PharmD, Director of Pharmacy, Chestnut Hill Hospital, Department of Pharmacy, Philadelphia

Bradley R. Williams, PharmD, Associate Professor, Clinical Pharmacy and Clinical Gerontology, University of Southern California, School of Pharmacy and Andrus Gerontology Center, Los Angeles

Foreword

For almost 30 years, I've watched and listened as nursing students tackled the overwhelming task of learning pharmacology, a vast, complex topic typically presented early in the curriculum. I know how hard it can be to learn how to think critically about pharmacology — about possible drug interactions or patient conditions that may require a different drug, route, or dosage.

Yet all nurses need to do just that — every day in every area. They're accountable for the safe, effective administration and monitoring of drug therapy. All nurses need to understand that clinical pharmacology is a science that integrates chemistry, anatomy, physiology, pathophysiology, and cellular and molecular biology into the art of nursing. By learning how pharmacology relates to nursing, the nurse can more readily and clearly understand why, when, and how drugs manage diseases and maintain health.

This textbook, *Essentials of Clinical Pharmacology in Nursing,* now in its third edition, can help nurses gain that understanding. The book provides a refreshing and useful framework for learning pharmacologic concepts and applying them to clinical situations. Its logical flow of complex information offers an innovative approach to learning, which makes the task of studying pharmacology far more rewarding. The book integrates key information and highlights the connections between drugs' actions and the effects of those actions on patients — and on the nursing care given to those patients.

This newest edition of *Essentials of Clinical Pharmacology in Nursing* retains the best features of earlier editions — and then adds to them. It continues the consistent format built on: (1) learning objectives for each chapter, (2) recurring and comprehensive charts and tables offering the latest in drug information, (3) a detailed nursing-process approach, (4) clear and concise chapter summaries, and (5) study questions for students to consider after reviewing the chapter. These valuable features help the reader understand, recall, and use pharmacologic information as it relates to nursing care.

Throughout its 16 units and 61 chapters, *Essentials of Clinical Pharmacology in Nursing,* Third Edition, relates the fundamental principles of pharmacology to vital aspects of nursing practice. Unit I introduces pharmacology and its fundamental principles, including pharmacokinetics, pharmacodynamics, pharmacotherapeutics, and adverse drug reactions. Unit II presents the nursing process as it relates to the nurse's responsibilities in drug administration, information about dosage measurements and calculations, and explanations of routes and techniques of administration. Units III through XVI offer comprehensive coverage of major drugs, grouped by therapeutic categories to enhance recall of related information. Each chapter in those units covers:

- objectives and an introduction that clearly prioritize the content for learning
- a selected major drug chart that lists up-to-date dosages, contraindications, and precautions for all major drugs of that class
- pharmacokinetics, pharmacodynamics, and pharmacotherapeutics
- drug interactions, often with charts that highlight drug-drug and drug-food interactions
- adverse drug reactions
- nursing-process information that covers nursing care — including patient teaching — specific to each drug class
- common nursing diagnoses related to each drug class and based on the latest NANDA taxonomy
- a chapter summary and questions to consider to reinforce learning and test understanding of the content.

The book also contains many new features designed to enhance learning and increase interest in drug information. Those new features include:

- more than 25 recently approved drugs
- colorful, cellular-level illustrations of the mechanisms of action of a dozen commonly used drugs
- geriatric considerations and cultural considerations, sections marked by eye-catching logos and designed to help the reader gain extra understanding of patients with unique needs
- at-a-glance charts that summarize onset, peak, and duration information for each drug class
- critical-thinking exercises to help students apply their knowledge to simulated clinical situations
- a free computer disk that contains a test bank with more than 300 study questions, written in a style similar to that used in national certification examinations.

This third edition of *Essentials of Clinical Pharmacology in Nursing* also includes:

- two new chapters: one covering the antitubercular drugs and one covering the wide range of drugs used to treat skin disorders and diseases
- two new appendices — "Drugs that should not be crushed," a real timesaver when administering drugs in a clinical situation, and "Complementary therapies," an invaluable look at alternative treatment methods and how they apply to today's clinical environments.

Essentials in Clinical Pharmacology in Nursing, Third Edition, is clearly a must for students, instructors, and clinicians. For students, the text provides dynamic, up-to-date information in a user-friendly format that can help them learn pharmacologic principles more easily and apply them to nursing practice.

For instructors, it's a valuable, authoritative teaching tool. Its authors and contributors are accomplished teachers, clinicians, and researchers whose knowledge of pharmacotherapeutics brings vital information to students clearly and concisely.

For clinicians, it can serve as a trusted reference for years to come, a text that busy practicing nurses will return to again and again for its clear-cut explanations and comprehensive content.

For everyone who uses it, *Essentials of Clinical Pharmacology in Nursing,* Third Edition, can serve as an experienced colleague, helping to ensure error-free medication administration and the highest quality health care possible.

Gail P. Poirrier, RN, DNS
Acting Dean and Associate Professor
University of Southwestern Louisiana
College of Nursing
Lafayette

Preface

The nurse is responsible for administering prescribed drugs, evaluating their effects, and teaching patients about their particular drug therapies. To fulfill these crucial roles, the nurse needs to be confident, safe, and thoroughly informed when carrying out pharmacological responsibilities.

Essentials of Clinical Pharmacology in Nursing, Third Edition, prepares the reader for all of these responsibilities. It provides the needed data, guidelines, and instructions for mastering pharmacologic information, administering drugs, and applying the nursing process to provide related care. Specifically, it includes:

- detailed coverage of all drug classes and of more than 1,000 generic drugs
- complete information on numerous newly approved drugs
- updated information of drugs included in all earlier editions
- a chapter on antitubercular agents, to address the growing health threat of tuberculosis, especially among immunocompromised patients
- a chapter on dermatologic agents, to meet the needs of patients with a wide variety of skin conditions
- descriptions of nursing care for each drug class, using the steps of the nursing process
- identification of critical aspects of nursing care in ***boldfaced italic*** type, which the nurse can use to prioritize care
- new multiple-choice questions to consider at the end of each chapter for the reader to use as a self-test.

Each chapter begins with learning objectives that focus the reader's attention and an introduction that provides a context for the information that follows. The text promotes critical thinking by presenting its data systematically and by adding critical thinking exercises (with analyses) that give students a chance to assess their learning and get instant feedback.

Terms defined in the Master Glossary are printed in **boldfaced** type. A chapter summary pulls together vital information and reinforces learning and recall. Questions to Consider also allow self-assessment. Drug-entry chapters each include the following recurring features:

- *Selected major drugs,* a reference chart that presents the most current generic and trade names, major indications, usual adult and (where applicable) pediatric dosages, contraindications, and precautions for each major drug in clinical use.
- *Drug interactions,* a chart including drugs and foods that may interact with the prescribed medication, possible effects from this interaction, and related nursing implications.
- *Patient teaching,* a list that highlights key points for the nurse to teach the patient.

The drug chapters also include these features:

- *Onset, peak, duration,* a new chart that allows the reader to quickly compare pharmacokinetic data for different administration routes of drugs within a specific drug class
- *Geriatric considerations,* special information that prepares the student to meet the pharmacological needs of an aging population
- *Cultural considerations,* a boxed text highlight that alerts the student to the pharmacological needs of patients from diverse cultures
- *Critical thinking* exercises that pose thought-provoking questions about clinical scenarios and provide analyses and possible answers.

The back of the book includes:

- new appendices covering complementary therapies and drugs that should not be crushed
- updated appendices on substance abuse and drugs used to treat poisoning
- a master glossary that defines **boldfaced terms** from the text.
- an updated master list of selected references organized by general and unit-specific references.

Supplementary materials promote learning and teaching. With the text, a free computer disk provides more than 300 pharmacology self-test questions, with answers and rationales so students can receive immediate feedback.

The instructor's manual presents a chapter overview, suggested lecture topics, and a test bank for each chapter. The test bank is designed to be photocopied for in-class use and is also available on the accompanying computer disk. With this disk, the instructor can create customized examinations, automatically generate a blank answer sheet for copying and distributing to students and a correct-answer template for easy scoring of tests and quizzes.

Each chapter in the instructor's manual also includes:

- suggested teaching-learning strategies to help the instructor plan lessons
- critical thinking exercises to help promote student learning.

To provide the most current, accurate, and clinically appropriate information, *Essentials of Clinical Pharmacology in Nursing,* Third Edition, and its supplements were written by practicing clinicians, instructors, and pharmacists — all of whom possess at least a master's degree. All materials were reviewed extensively by nurses and pharmacists from appropriate specialty areas. *Essentials of Clinical Pharmacology in Nursing,* Third Edition, can enhance any nurse's ability to provide safe, therapeutic care.

UNIT I

Overview of pharmacology

Just about everyone uses a prescription or nonprescription **drug** (pharmaceutical agent) at some point. Because of that, the nurse should consider routine drug use — and the accompanying **drug interactions** and toxic effects — as a major potential health problem for patients. The nurse must know the physiologic and psychological alterations produced by specific drugs and their interactions. The nurse must also know how certain patient traits influence **pharmacokinetics, pharmacodynamics,** and **pharmacotherapeutics**. Such information is as necessary for providing the best possible patient care as knowing the name, classification, onset and duration of action, dosage range, route of classification, contraindications, potential **adverse drug reactions,** drug interactions, and predicted outcomes of a specific drug.

The information in unit one provides a framework for understanding all of the aspects of pharmacology. Its chapters introduce fundamental concepts basic to understanding the drugs discussed later in the text.

Chapter 1 defines pharmacology, describes its scope, and provides an overview of its five branches: pharmacokinetics, pharmacodynamics, pharmacotherapeutics, **toxicology,** and **pharmacognosy.** It introduces terminology and drug nomenclature that the nurse needs to know to make drug therapy decisions. It concludes with an overview of the development process for a new drug and the legal regulations and standards governing the uniform quality of drugs.

The second chapter presents the fundamental principles of pharmacology: pharmacokinetics, pharmacodynamics, pharmacotherapeutics, and adverse drug reactions. It begins with the pharmacokinetic properties of a drug, including drug **absorption, distribution, metabolism,** and **excretion,** onset of action, **peak concentration level,** duration of action, drug **bioavailability,** and blood concentration levels. Understanding these principles helps the nurse determine the proper drug and dosage form required to produce the desired therapeutic effect.

The chapter continues with a discussion of pharmacodynamics, or the mechanisms by which drugs produce biochemical or physiologic changes in the body. It also includes an introduction to the **therapeutic index,** a concept vital to safe drug therapy. By learning about a drug's action (interaction at the cellular level between a drug and cell components) and a drug's effect (the response resulting from the drug action), the nurse gains a fuller understanding of the interaction between drugs and receptors and the outcomes of drug therapy.

Chapter Two also explores the pharmacotherapeutics of drugs, or the use of drugs to treat disease. After describing different types of therapy, it describes the factors that influence the choice of therapy and the patient's response to the administered drugs. It includes an overview of drug interactions with other drugs, food, and diagnostic tests. This information helps the nurse accurately interpret a patient's response to drug therapy and differentiate drug interactions from adverse reactions or signs of disease.

Key concepts related to adverse drug reactions are also discussed in Chapter 2. It presents information about predisposing factors related to patient characteristics, drug characteristics, and exogenous factors. Then it describes the two classifications of adverse drug reactions: dose-related and patient sensitivity–related adverse drug reactions. With this information, the nurse can monitor patients for predictable reactions and can identify unpredictable reactions that might occur.

The chapter concludes with an exploration of developmental considerations related to variations in pharmacokinetics, pharmacodynamics, pharmacotherapeutics, and adverse drug reactions. Its information assists the nurse in providing appropriate drug therapy for pediatric, geriatric, pregnant, and breast-feeding patients.

Introduction to pharmacology

OBJECTIVES

After reading and studying this chapter, the student should be able to:

1. differentiate among the five branches of pharmacology: pharmacokinetics, pharmacodynamics, pharmacotherapeutics, toxicology, and pharmacognosy.
2. briefly define prescription, nonprescription, controlled, and recreational drugs.
3. explain the differences among a drug's chemical, generic, and trade names.
4. describe the four phases required by the Food and Drug Administration (FDA) for approval and marketing of a new drug.
5. explain why orphan drugs can be unprofitable, even though they may be needed.
6. describe two consequences of the Federal Food, Drug, and Cosmetic Act (FFDCA) of 1906.
7. define the five schedules of controlled drugs.
8. explain these six drug properties: purity, bioavailability, potency, efficacy, safety, and toxicity.

INTRODUCTION

Chapter 1 begins by defining **pharmacology** and describing its scope. Then it presents important terminology and drug nomenclature (names), sources, types, development, regulations, and standards. Throughout, it covers all the vital information that nurses must have to fulfill major responsibilities.

The increasing numbers, kinds, and complexities of new drugs require that every clinician's knowledge of pharmacology be updated continually.

Definition and scope

Pharmacology — one of the most dynamic aspects of nursing — represents the scientific study of the origin, nature, chemistry, effects, and uses of drugs. (See *Five branches of pharmacology.*)

Pharmacokinetics refers to the absorption, distribution, metabolism, and excretion of a drug in a living organism. **Pharmacodynamics** is the study of the biochemical and physical effects of drugs and the mechanisms of drug actions in living organisms. **Pharmacotherapeutics** (clinical pharmacology) is a general term covering the use of drugs (clinical indications) to prevent and treat diseases. Most of a nurse's drug-related functions fall under this heading. **Toxicology** represents the study of poisons, including the adverse effects of drugs on living organisms. Detailed discussions of pharmacokinetics, pharmacodynamics, pharmacotherapeutics, and toxicology appear in chapter 2, Fundamental principles of pharmacology. A discussion of poisons (a branch of toxicology) appears in the Appendix. **Pharmacognosy** deals with natural drug sources — that is, plants, animals, or minerals and their products. It is discussed later in this chapter.

Pharmacology is an interdisciplinary science. Although most students traditionally associate chemistry with pharmacology, the physical, biological, and social sciences also contribute information on using drugs to achieve and maintain optimum health without causing toxicity or patient dependence.

TERMINOLOGY

Nurses must know the following terminology to enhance their own understanding and to enable them to interpret information for patients.

A **drug** (medication) is a pharmacologic agent that is capable of interacting with living organisms to produce biological effects.

A **prescription drug** can be used safely — and legally — only under the supervision of a health care professional who is licensed to prescribe or dispense drugs according to state laws.

A **nonprescription drug** (over-the-counter, or OTC, drug) can be used by consumers safely without the supervision of a licensed health care practitioner, provided consumers follow the directions.

A **controlled drug** may lead to drug abuse or drug dependence and therefore its use is controlled by federal, state, and local laws.

Drug abuse describes the self-directed use of drugs for nontherapeutic purposes, a practice that does not comply with a culture's sociocultural norms.

Five branches of pharmacology

An extensive science, pharmacology includes absorption, distribution, metabolism, and excretion (pharmacokinetics); biochemical and physical effects and mechanism of action (pharmacodynamics); clinical indications or uses (pharmacotherapeutics); toxicity and adverse effects (toxicology); and natural sources of drugs (pharmacognosy).

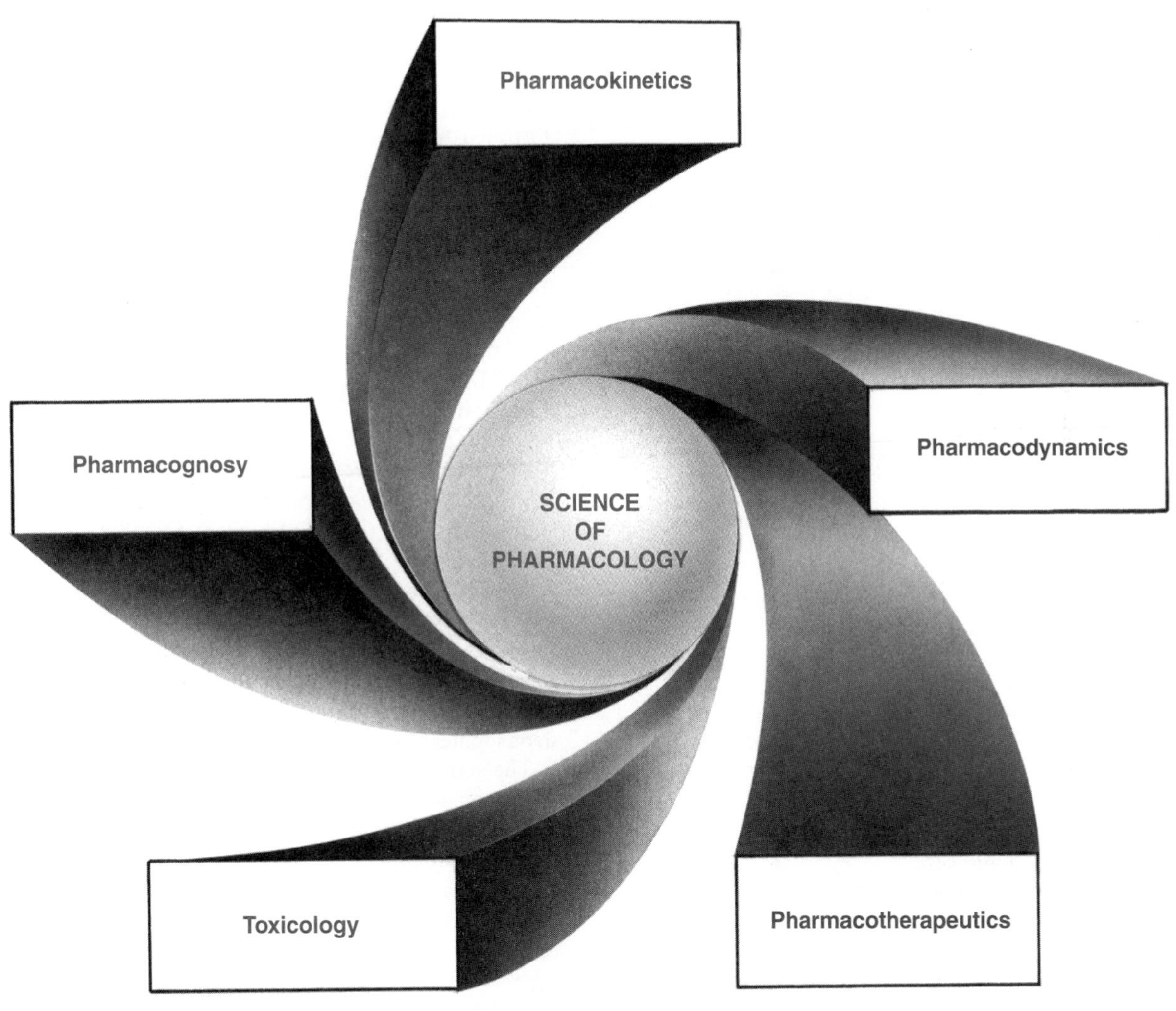

Drug dependence results when a person cannot control drug intake. Drug dependence may be physiologic, psychological, or both.

Drug misuse, the improper use of common drugs, can lead to acute and chronic toxicity with such problems as gastrointestinal bleeding, kidney damage, or liver damage.

A **recreational drug** is one used for its pleasant psychological or physical effects with no therapeutic intent.

DRUG NOMENCLATURE

A drug's **chemical name** precisely describes its atomic and molecular structure. When a manufacturer wishes to market a promising new drug, the United States Adopted Names (USAN) Council selects a **generic name.** (The USAN is sponsored by the American Medical Association, the American Pharmaceutical Association, and the United States Pharmacopeial Convention.) Typically derived from a drug's chemical name, its generic name usually is shorter — abbreviated for simplicity. The drug company selling the product selects its **trade name** (also known as the brand name or proprietary name). Trade names are protected by copyright. The symbol ® after the trade name indicates that the name is registered by and restricted to the drug manufacturer. Because pharmacies stock various trade-name drugs, nurses can avoid confusion by always using the

Sources of drug information

Many types of publications help fulfill the need of physicians, nurses, and pharmacists for up-to-date and detailed drug information. The nurse in a clinical situation may need to consult various references to obtain all of the necessary information. The following are reliable sources.

Pharmacopeia — Official
- The United States Pharmacopeia (USP) and National Formulary (NF)
- The British Pharmacopoeia (BP)
- The British National Formulary (BF)

Compendia — Nonofficial
- Martindale: The Extra Pharmacopoeia
- Drug Information — American Hospital Formulary Service, published by authority of American Society of Hospital Pharmacists
- Facts and Comparisons
- USP Dispensing Information

Pharmaceutical Companies
- Physicians' Desk Reference (PDR)
- Package inserts — brochures required by law. Content is approved by the Food and Drug Administration.

Journal
- The Medical Letter on Drugs and Therapeutics

generic name when speaking or writing about a drug. In 1962, the federal government mandated the use of **official names** so that only one official name would represent each drug. The official names are listed in the United States Pharmacopeia (USP) and National Formulary (NF). (See *Sources of drug information.*)

Drugs that share similar characteristics are grouped together as a pharmacologic class (family), such as beta blockers. A second grouping is the therapeutic classification, which groups drugs by therapeutic use, such as antihypertensives. Thiazides and beta blockers are both antihypertensives, but they share few characteristics, as the discussions in later chapters show.

Pharmacognosy

Traditionally, **pharmacognosy** refers to the study of natural drug sources, such as plants, animals, or minerals and their products. Today, however, chemicals developed and used in the laboratory allow researchers to increase the number of drug sources. For example, oral contraceptives, which are synthetic analogues of human sex hormones, are manufactured chemically. Chemically developed drugs are free of the impurities found in natural substances.

Researchers and drug developers also can now manipulate the molecular structure of substances, such as antibiotics, so that a slight change in the chemical structure makes the drug effective against different organisms. The first-generation cephalosporins, produced by an organism cultured in seawater, were effective against the organisms *Streptococcus, Staphylococcus, Escherichia coli, Proteus mirabilis,* and *Shigella.* Subsequent chemically altered structures of cephalosporins (second and third generation) effectively treat infections caused by *Bacteroides fragilis* and *Haemophilus influenzae* (second generation) and *Pseudomonas* (third generation).

The hormone insulin, used to treat diabetes mellitus, was customarily obtained from the pancreata of slaughtered animals, mainly cattle and pigs. Although animal insulin is not chemically identical to human insulin, it is physiologically active in humans. Porcine insulin (derived from pigs) most nearly resembles human insulin. The chemical alteration of three amino acids in porcine insulin makes it identical to human endogenous insulin. The chemically altered porcine insulin is marketed and usually referred to as "human insulin." Drug developers also can manufacture human insulin from bacteria.

Plant sources of drugs

In most cases, the earliest concoctions using plants as drug sources consisted of the entire plant, including leaves, roots, bulb, stem, seeds, buds, and blossoms. Much extraneous material, some of it harmful to human tissues, found its way into the mixture. The active components in the crude mixture caused the drug's effect. As the understanding of plants as drug sources became more sophisticated, researchers sought to isolate the active components and avoid the extraneous material.

The active components consist of several types and vary in character and effect. The most important are alkaloids (one of the largest groups of active components), which act as alkali. The organic alkaloids react with acids to form a salt. This salt, a neutralized or partially neutralized form, is more readily soluble in body fluids. The names of alkaloids and their salts usually end in *-ine;* examples include atropine, caffeine, and nicotine.

Other active components include glycosides, gums, resins, and oils. As glycosides decompose, they yield sugars and an aglycon, or the noncarbohydrate group of a glycoside molecule. Names of glycosides usually end in *-in,* as in digitoxin and digoxin. Gums, usually polysaccharides producing viscous solutions, constitute another group of active components. Gums give products the ability to attract and hold water. Examples include seaweed extractions and seeds with starch. Resins, of which the chief source is pine tree sap, commonly act as local irritants or as laxatives and caustic agents. Oils, thick and sometimes greasy liquids, are classified as volatile or fixed. Examples of volatile oils include peppermint, spearmint, and juniper. Fixed oils, not easily evaporated, include castor oil and olive oil.

Animal sources of drugs

The body fluids or glands of animals can act as sources of drugs. The drugs obtained from animal sources include hormones, such as insulin; oils and fats (usually fixed), such as cod-liver oil; and enzymes, produced by living cells, which act as catalysts. Enzymes include pancreatin and pepsin. Vaccines (suspensions of killed, modified, or attenuated microorganisms) also are obtained from animal sources.

Mineral sources of drugs

Metallic and nonmetallic minerals provide various inorganic materials not available from plants or animals. The mineral sources are used as they occur in nature or are combined with other ingredients to yield acids, bases, or salts. For example, when mixed with other substances, the acid coal tar yields salicylic acid, aluminum hydroxide (a base), and sodium chloride (a salt).

Laboratory-produced sources of drugs

Today's researchers produce an ever-increasing number of drugs in the laboratory. The new drugs may be natural (from animal or plant sources), synthetic, or a combination of the two. Examples of drugs produced in the laboratory include thyroid hormone (natural), cimetidine (synthetic), and anistreplase (combination of natural and synthetic). Recombinant deoxyribonucleic acid (DNA) research has led to another chemical source of organic compounds: the reordering of genetic information enables scientists to develop bacteria that produce insulin for humans.

CRITICAL THINKING: To enhance your critical thinking about pharmacology, consider the following situation and its analysis.
Situation: Janet Larson, age 55, tells the nurse she wants to treat her menopausal symptoms (hot flashes, sweating, and mood changes) with medicinal herbs and plants supplied by a Doctor of Naturology who grows and packages them. This practice falls under the branch of pharmacology known as *pharmacognosy,* which deals with the study of natural drug sources.

What health promotion information should the nurse discuss with Ms. Larson to ensure that she makes an informed choice about this nontraditional treatment?
Analysis: The nurse could begin by discussing the use of traditional and nontraditional treatments for menopausal symptoms. Then the nurse could encourage her to consider the advantages and disadvantages of each. To obtain this information, the nurse may suggest checking various sources, such as menopause seminars, libraries, Internet sites, and the patient's primary health care provider. The nurse also could help Ms. Larson evaluate research about the use of drugs to treat menopausal symptoms. If the patient chooses a nontraditional drug, the nurse may suggest a reputable health food store that may offer a safer, higher quality medications.

The nurse should inform the patient that:
- extraneous materials may reduce the purity of the compound and may be harmful to human tissues.
- the strength of the drugs in the compound may vary, so the results may be hard to control.
- the compound's exact ingredients — and their effects and adverse effects — may not be known.
- she should monitor her reaction to the compound to detect allergic or toxic reactions and prevent them from becoming severe.

New drug development

In the past, drugs were found by trial and error. Now, they are developed primarily by systematic scientific research. Scientists still search for new organic and inorganic sources; however, they now focus most of their attention on the laboratory to discover needed drugs.

The Food and Drug Administration (FDA) carefully monitors new drug development, which can take many years to complete. Testing of new drugs begins with animals to evaluate the drug's pharmacologic use, dosage ranges, and possible toxic effects. Only after reviewing extensive animal studies and data on the safety and effectiveness of the proposed drug will the FDA approve the application for an Investigational New Drug (IND). (See *Unlabeled uses of drugs,* page 6.)

Four phases of clinical evaluation involving human subjects follow approval of the IND. The clinical studies are intended to provide information on purity, **bioavailability,** potency, efficacy, safety, and **toxicity.** Depending on the results of testing, the studies can be stopped at any phase.

Phase I

In phase I, a clinical pharmacologist supervises studies involving a small number of healthy volunteers. All effects of the drug on the volunteers are recorded. The recorded clinical data determine the need for further testing.

Phase II

A small number of individuals who have the disease for which the drug is purported to be diagnostic or therapeutic are then given the drug. Supervisors carefully document toxic effects and adverse reactions to determine the drug's proper dosage. Researchers then review and compare data from the animal studies and human studies, closely monitoring drug effects on animal and human fertility and reproduction.

Phase III

In phase III, large numbers of patients in medical research centers receive the drug. This larger sampling provides information about infrequent or rare adverse effects. Information collected during this phase helps determine risks associated with the new drug. Researchers also must perform

Unlabeled uses of drugs

When approving a new drug, the Food and Drug Administration (FDA) accepts it *only* for the indications for which phase II and III clinical studies have shown it to be safe and effective. These indications are approved (labeled); all others are not approved (unlabeled).

For example, the FDA may approve a new drug to treat hypertension if phase II and III studies showed that it was safe and effective in patients with hypertension. If the drug also works well as an antianginal agent, the FDA cannot approve it for this indication unless formal studies in patients with angina pectoris are completed successfully. Such a drug is unapproved for treatment of angina pectoris, yet it may be used for this unlabeled indication, based on empirical evidence. Here is how this may occur.

After prescribing a new drug approved to treat hypertension, a physician may discover that it also decreases the patient's angina. Then the physician may share this finding with colleagues in medical journals or at meetings, and they may prescribe it for unlabeled uses, too.

The FDA recognizes that a drug's labeling does not always contain the most current information about its usage. Therefore, after the FDA approves a drug for one indication, a physician legally may prescribe it, a pharmacist may dispense it, and a nurse may administer it for any labeled — or unlabeled — indication.

Although clinicians are *not* prohibited from prescribing, dispensing, or administering a drug for an unlabeled use, the FDA forbids the manufacturer from promoting a drug for any unlabeled indications. That's why drug package inserts and the *Physicians' Desk Reference* (a collection of drug manufacturers' product labeling) contain no information about unlabeled uses, and pharmaceutical sales representatives cannot discuss such uses.

Nevertheless, many drugs commonly are prescribed for unlabeled uses. One famous example is tretinoin (Retin-A), which is approved to treat acne — its only labeled use. However, because independent studies have shown that tretinoin helps eliminate skin wrinkles, many dermatologists prescribe it for this unlabeled use.

various tests that take into account those patients who are so emotionally involved that they experience relief of symptoms based on suggestion. The administration of a placebo, a medically inert substance, to some patients provides control for such psychological responses. In one frequently used procedure, one-half of the patients receive the drug and one-half receive the placebo. To remove all bias, neither the patients nor the physician knows who has received the drug and who has received the placebo until completion of the study, known as a double-blind study. In another type of study (crossover study), patients receive the drug for part of the time and a placebo for the rest of the time.

After the first three phases, the FDA evaluates the results. If the FDA announces a favorable evaluation, the company developing the drug then completes a New Drug Application (NDA). FDA approval of the company's NDA means that the new drug has been accepted and can be marketed exclusively by its sponsoring company.

Phase IV

Phase IV is voluntary. After the NDA is approved, the drug company begins surveillance or post-market surveillance. It receives from physicians reports about the therapeutic results of the drug. The company must communicate adequately with the FDA and with the public during the drug's use. Some medications, such as benoxaprofen (Oraflex), have been found to be toxic and have been removed from the market after their initial release. At times, manufacturers have contended that a drug's benefits for a certain segment of the population outweigh its risks. Such was the manufacturer's response when the antidepressant tranylcypromine was withdrawn from the market. Eventually, but with certain restrictions, the FDA reinstated tranylcypromine in the market for use by severely depressed patients.

Expedited drug approval

Although most INDs undergo all four phases of clinical evaluation, a few can receive expedited approval. For example, because of the public health threat posed by acquired immunodeficiency syndrome (AIDS), the FDA and drug companies have agreed to shorten the IND approval process, allowing physicians to give qualified AIDS patients so-called Treatment INDs not yet approved by the FDA. Sponsors of drugs that reach Phase II or III clinical trials can apply for FDA approval of Treatment IND status. When the IND is approved, the sponsor supplies the drug to physicians whose patients meet appropriate criteria.

ORPHAN DRUGS

Some drugs useful to treat various diseases never reach the market. Drug companies do not adopt and develop these medications, appropriately referred to as **orphan drugs.** The reasons vary. Some orphan drugs useful for rare diseases have a limited market; others produce high-risk adverse drug reactions that make insurance costs prohibitive. Many useful drugs remain orphans because manufacturers cannot hope to recover the huge amounts of money spent in developing a new drug.

In 1983, Congress signed the Orphan Drug Act, which offers substantial tax credits to companies that develop orphan drugs. Small companies may receive federal financial grants to help them research and develop orphan drugs. As a result, thousands of patients now may use drugs that until recently were unavailable. Despite the legislation, many orphan drugs remain without developers.

LEGAL REGULATIONS AND STANDARDS

As a society develops and uses drugs, it needs to establish controls regulating the manufacture, distribution, and use of those drugs. Religious and social mores may provide informal controls on drug use. In most cases, a society's attitudes and values more strictly determine the acceptable limits of drug use than formal controls. Formal drug controls

Federal drug legislation

Since 1906, when Congress passed the Federal Food, Drug, and Cosmetic Act, the federal government has legislated drug manufacture, sales, and use. The following list gives the major legislative acts and their significance.

YEAR	LEGISLATION	SIGNIFICANCE TO THE PUBLIC
1906	Federal Food, Drug, and Cosmetic Act (FFDCA)	Designated official standards for drugs (United States Pharmacopeia and National Formulary)
1912	Federal Food, Drug, and Cosmetic Act — Sherley Amendment	Prohibited drug companies from making fraudulent claims about their products
1914	Harrison Narcotic Act	Classified certain habit-forming drugs as narcotics and regulated their importation, manufacture, sale, and use
1938	Federal Food, Drug, and Cosmetic Act — Amendment	Provided for governmental approval of new drugs before they enter interstate commerce; defined labeling requirements
1945	Federal Food, Drug, and Cosmetic Act — Amendment	Provided for certification of certain drugs through testing by the Food and Drug Administration
1952	Federal Food, Drug, and Cosmetic Act — Durham-Humphrey Amendment	Distinguished between prescription and over-the-counter drugs; specified procedures for the distribution of prescription drugs
1962	Federal Food, Drug, and Cosmetic Act — Kefauver-Harris Amendment	Provided assurance of the safety and effectiveness of drugs and improved communication about drugs
1970	Comprehensive Drug Abuse Prevention and Control Act (Controlled Substances Act)	Outlined controls on habit-forming drugs; established governmental programs to prevent and treat drug abuse; assisted with the campaign against drug abuse by developing a classification that categorized drugs according to their abuse liability; placed drugs into schedules
1973	Executive Order of the President under Title 21 of the U.S. Code	Created Drug Enforcement Administration to enforce the laws against illegal drug use
1983	Orphan Drug Act	Offered substantial tax credits to companies to develop drugs that are used to treat rare diseases or that have a limited market

range from individual institutional policies to governmental legislation.

International controls

The United Nations, through its World Health Organization, attempts to influence international health by providing technical assistance and encouraging research for drug use. One committee has been established to cope with the problems associated with habit-forming drugs. Drug enforcement agencies in various nations cooperate, but no administrative or judicial structures enforce controls. As a result, control of international drug trade depends largely on the voluntary cooperation of nations.

Controls in the United States

Legislative drug control in the United States began in 1906 with the passage of the Federal Food, Drug, and Cosmetic Act (FFDCA). Although the FFDCA primarily addressed the issue of food purity, it also designated the USP and the NF as the official standards for drugs. (See *Federal drug legislation.*)

In the 1930s, the need for stringent drug regulations became apparent when more than 100 people died from ingesting sulfanilamide, an antibacterial drug. Researchers discovered that the sulfanilamide had been prepared with a previously uninvestigated toxic substance called diethylene glycol. After the sulfanilamide incident, Congress passed the 1938 amendment to the FFDCA that established regulations for approval by the federal government of all new drugs and specified requirements for drug labeling. According to the amendment, drug labels were to consist of the following elements before the products could enter interstate commerce:

- a statement accurately describing the package's contents
- the usual names of the drugs, for official drugs (preparations listed in the pharmacopeia and adopted by the government as meeting pharmaceutical standards) and nonofficial drugs (those drugs not listed in the pharmacopeia)
- indication of the presence, quantity, and proportion of certain drugs (such as alcohol, atropine, and bromides) in the product

Schedules of controlled drugs

In the United States, the Comprehensive Drug Abuse Prevention and Control Act of 1970 classified drugs into categories (schedules) according to their abuse potential. In Canada, the Food and Drugs Act (amended yearly) and Narcotic Control Act of 1965 provide similar classifications, although the specific drugs in each class may differ. Health care professionals must be aware of these schedules to ensure the proper handling of controlled substances. The following list provides examples of representative controlled drugs in the United States and Canada.

UNITED STATES

Category	Examples
Schedule I No recognized medical use. High abuse potential. Research use only.	**Opiates** • Heroin **Hallucinogens** • LSD • Mescaline **Depressants** • Methaqualone
Schedule II Written prescriptions required. No telephone renewals. In an emergency, a prescription may be renewed by telephone, but a written prescription must follow within 72 hours.	**Opiates** • Codeine • Morphine • Meperidine **Stimulants** • Amphetamines • Phenmetrazine **Depressants** • Secobarbital
Schedule III Prescriptions required to be rewritten after 6 months or 5 refills. Prescriptions may be ordered by telephone.	**Opiates** • Codeine of less than 1.8 g/dl • Opium 25 mg/5 ml **Stimulants** • Benzphetamine • Mazindol **Depressants** • Butabarbital • Glutethimide • Talbutal **Anabolic steroids** • Ethylestrenol • Fluoxymesterone • Methyltestosterone • Nandrolone decanoate
Schedule IV Prescriptions required to be rewritten after 6 months or 5 refills.	**Opiates** • Pentazocine • Propoxyphene **Stimulants** • Fenfluramine • Phentermine **Depressants** • Benzodiazepines • Chloral hydrate
Schedule V Dispensed as any (nonnarcotic) prescription. Some may be dispensed without prescription unless additional state regulations apply.	Primarily small amounts of opiates, such as opium, dihydrocodeine, and diphenoxylate, when used as antitussives or antidiarrheals in combination products.

CANADA

Category	Examples
Schedule H Restricted drugs. No recognized medicinal properties.	**Hallucinogens** • Peyote • LSD • Mescaline
Narcotics Schedule Stringently restricted drugs. The letter *N* must appear on all labels and professional advertisements.	**Coca leaf derivatives** • Cocaine **Opiates and opiate derivatives** • Morphine • Codeine • Methadone • Hydromorphone • Meperidine **Other drugs** • Phencyclidine • Cannabis
Schedule G Controlled drugs. Prescriptions are controlled because of the abuse potential of these drugs.	**Narcotic analgesics** • Nalbuphine • Butorphanol **Stimulants** • Amphetamines **Barbiturates** • Phenobarbital • Amobarbital • Secobarbital
Schedule F Prescription drugs. Although not controlled drugs, agents in this category include some with a relatively low abuse potential. The symbol *Pr* must appear on their labels.	**Anxiolytics** • Benzodiazepines
Nonprescription Drug Schedule (Group 3) Drugs available only in the pharmacy and used only on the physician's recommendation. Limited public access.	**Analgesics** • Low-dose codeine preparations **Other drugs** • Insulin • Nitroglycerin • Muscle relaxants

• a warning of habit-forming drugs in the product and of their effects
• the names of the manufacturer, packager, and distributor
• directions for use and warnings against unsafe use, including recommendations for dosage levels and frequency
• a statement on all new drugs not yet approved for interstate commerce; for example, "Caution: New Drug — Limited by Federal Law to Investigational Use." Finally, no false or misleading statements were to appear on the label.

In 1970, Congress passed the Comprehensive Drug Abuse Prevention and Control Act (Controlled Substances Act or CSA), designed to contain the rapidly increasing problem of drug abuse. The CSA promoted drug education programs and research into the prevention and treatment of drug dependence. It also provided for the establishment of treatment and rehabilitation centers and strengthened drug enforcement authority. Further, the act designated categories, or schedules, that classified controlled drugs according to their abuse potential. (See *Schedules of controlled drugs.*)

State, local, and institutional controls

Although state drug controls must conform to federal laws, states usually impose additional regulations, such as those determining the legal age for drinking alcohol. Local drug regulations imposed by counties or municipalities usually involve restrictions on the sale or use of alcohol or tobacco.

Institutional drug controls must conform to federal, state, and local regulations. Public and private institutions adopt and impose drug controls primarily to prevent health problems and legal violations by people within the institution.

Legislation in Canada

Drug control in Canada falls under the direct supervision of the Department of National Health and Welfare. The 1953 Canadian Food and Drugs Act (amended yearly) provides regulations for drug manufacture and sale. In 1965, the Canadian Narcotic Control Act restricted the sale, possession, and use of narcotics. It further restricts narcotic possession to authorized personnel. Under the law, legal possession of narcotics by a nurse is limited to occasions when the nurse administers the drug to a patient under a physician's order, when the nurse serves as a custodian of narcotics in a health care agency, or when the nurse personally uses the narcotic as part of a prescribed treatment.)

DRUG STANDARDS

The federal government establishes and enforces drug standards to ensure the uniform quality of drugs. The standards pertain to the following drug properties:

• *Purity* refers to the uncontaminated state of a drug containing only one active component. In reality, a drug consisting of only one active component rarely exists because manufacturers usually must add other ingredients to facilitate drug formation and to determine absorption rate. Extraneous substances from the manufacturing plant also may contaminate the pure drug. As a result, standards of purity do not demand 100% pure active ingredients but specify the type and acceptable amount of extraneous material.
• *Bioavailability* describes the degree to which a drug becomes absorbed and reaches the general circulation. Factors affecting bioavailability include the particle size, crystalline structure, solubility, and polarity of the compound. The blood or tissue concentration of a drug at a specified time after administration usually determines bioavailability.
• *Potency* of a drug refers to its strength or its power to produce the desired effect. Potency standards are set by testing laboratory animals to determine the definite measurable effect of an administered drug.
• *Efficacy* refers to the effectiveness of a drug used in treatment. Objective clinical trials attempt to determine efficacy, but absolute measurement remains difficult.
• *Safety and toxicity* are determined by the incidence and severity of reported adverse reactions to the use of a drug. Some harmful effects may not appear for a considerable time. Safety and toxicity standards are being refined constantly as past experiences illuminate deficiencies in the standards.

The modern laboratory testing procedures of bioassay significantly help to determine drug standards and assure adherence to the standards. Still, much remains to be improved in testing procedures, some of which remain expensive and unreliable.

CHAPTER SUMMARY

Chapter 1 defined the science of pharmacology and identified and explained its five branches: pharmacokinetics, pharmacodynamics, pharmacotherapeutics, toxicology, and pharmacognosy. Here are the chapter highlights.

Nurses must know drug terminology to enhance their own understanding and to help them interpret information for patients.

Based on drug nomenclature, each drug has at least three names: a chemical name, a generic name, and a trade name.

Drugs that share similar characteristics can be categorized by families or pharmacologic classes, such as beta blockers. Drugs also can be categorized by therapeutic classification, such as antihypertensives.

Pharmacognosy is the study of the natural sources of drugs. Active components in drugs traditionally were found in plants, animals, and minerals. Today, chemical sources produced in laboratories provide active components in most drugs. Laboratory methods also provide means to purify, alter, or synthesize active components found in nature.

Sources of drug information for physicians, nurses, and pharmacists who need current data include pharmacopeias (official), compendia (nonofficial), pharmaceutical companies, and journals.

A newly developed drug must go through an approval process before it reaches the market. The FDA approves an application for an Investigational New Drug (IND). After the manufacturer has conducted extensive animal studies, phase I of the new drug development involves testing the drug on healthy volunteers. Phase II involves trials with human subjects who have the disease for which the drug is thought to be effective. The tests determine the proper dosage as well as effects of the drug on fertility and reproduction. Phase III involves large numbers of patients in medical research centers, using unbiased research methods to detect infrequent or rare adverse reactions. The FDA will approve a New Drug Application (NDA) if phase III studies are satisfactory. Phase IV involves postmarket surveillance of the drug's therapeutic effects at the completion of phase III.

Drugs sometimes become orphan drugs because of difficulties in researching and developing them and the prospect of little financial gain. The Orphan Drug Act of 1983 has helped, providing tax incentives and monies for research to drug companies.

Drug regulations and standards have been developed to control drug use and promote public safety. The 1938 amendment to the Federal Food, Drug, and Cosmetic Act (FFDCA) of 1906 established the elements of drug labeling. Labels had to give the package contents and the usual names of the drugs, as well as the presence, quantity, and proportion of certain drugs (such as alcohol, atropine, digitalis, and bromides). Labels also had to include a warning of habit-forming drugs in the product and their effects; names of manufacturer, packager, and distributor; directions for use, including recommended dosages; and a warning statement on all new drugs not approved for interstate commerce. No false or misleading statements could appear on the label.

In 1970, the Comprehensive Drug Abuse Prevention and Control Act (the Controlled Substances Act or CSA) attempted to control drug abuse. The CSA aided drug education, research, treatment, and enforcement. It also classified controlled drugs (Schedules I through V) according to their abuse potential.

Drug control in Canada falls under the direct supervision of the Department of National Health and Welfare. Canadian laws mandate that nurses legally may possess narcotics only when administering a narcotic to a patient under a physician's order, acting as custodians of narcotics in a health care agency, or receiving the narcotic as prescribed treatment for themselves.

Drug standards help achieve uniform quality with respect to purity, bioavailability, potency, efficacy, safety, and toxicity.

Questions to consider

See Appendix 1 for answers.

1. Robert Evans, age 60, carefully follows the diabetic diet and exercise program prescribed by his physician. Because his blood glucose level remains elevated, his physician prescribes glipizide (Glucotrol) 2.5 mg P.O. daily. The nurse wants to learn more about this drug's absorption, distribution, metabolism, and excretion. Which branch of pharmacology provides this information?
   (a) Pharmacognosy
   (b) Pharmacokinetics
   (c) Pharmacodynamics
   (d) Pharmacotherapeutics

2. Which branch of pharmacology studies the biochemical and physical effects of drugs and their mechanisms of action in living organisms?
   (a) Pharmacognosy
   (b) Pharmacokinetics
   (c) Pharmacodynamics
   (d) Pharmacotherapeutics

3. Marjorie Ewing, age 52, has just received a prescription for glipizide. This drug may be called by various names. Which of the following names should the nurse use to minimize confusion?
   (a) Brand name
   (b) Generic name
   (c) Chemical name
   (d) Proprietary name

4. The federal government has established drug standards to ensure uniform quality of drugs. Which of the following standards refer to the drug's effectiveness in treatment?
   (a) Bioavailability
   (b) Potency
   (c) Efficacy
   (d) Purity

5. After extensive oral surgery, Jane Preston, age 36, receives a prescription for meperidine hydrochloride (Demerol), 50 mg P.O. every 3 to 4 hours p.r.n. for pain. In the United States, this drug requires a written prescription because it is a controlled drug. According to the Comprehensive Drug Abuse Prevention and Control Act of 1970, meperidine belongs to which schedule?
   (a) Schedule I
   (b) Schedule II
   (c) Schedule III
   (d) Schedule V

6. John Marks, age 43, takes diazepam (Valium) 5 mg P.O. b.i.d. for anxiety. A controlled substance, diazepam is classified as a Schedule IV drug. Which classification includes drugs that can be used only for research?
   (a) Schedule I
   (b) Schedule II
   (c) Schedule III
   (d) Schedule V

Fundamental principles of pharmacology

OBJECTIVES

After reading and studying this chapter, the student should be able to:

1. differentiate among pharmacokinetics, pharmacodynamics, pharmacotherapeutics, and adverse drug reactions.
2. describe the processes involved in drug absorption, distribution, metabolism, and excretion.
3. explain how a drug's onset of action, peak concentration, and duration of action affect its pharmacokinetics.
4. describe the relationship between a drug's pharmacodynamic properties and the patient's response to the drug.
5. differentiate between drug action and drug effect and between drug potency and drug efficacy.
6. describe factors that may alter a patient's response to drug therapy.
7. compare the three kinds of drug interactions and their effects on the patient.
8. differentiate between dose-related and patient sensitivity–related adverse reactions.
9. identify differences in pharmacokinetics, pharmaodynamics, pharmacotherapeutics, and adverse effects of drugs in pediatric, geriatric, pregnant, and breast-feeding patients.

INTRODUCTION

Chapter 2 focuses on the fundamental principles of **pharmacology: pharmacokinetics, pharmacodynamics, pharmacotherapeutics,** and **adverse drug reactions.** It begins by discussing the pharmacokinetic properties of a **drug,** including drug **absorption, distribution, metabolism,** and **excretion.** It also describes several clinically relevant properties of drugs, such as a drug's onset of action, **peak concentration level,** and duration of action as well as **bioavailability** and blood concentration levels.

Next, the chapter describes pharmacodynamics, or the mechanisms by which drugs produce biochemical or physiologic changes in the body. It describes the interaction between drugs and **receptors** as well as **drug action** and **drug effect.** It also explores the **therapeutic index,** a concept vital to safe drug therapy.

The chapter continues by discussing the pharmacotherapeutic aspects of drug therapy. After describing the different types of therapy, it identifies factors that influence the choice of therapy and the patient's response to drugs during therapy. An overview of **drug interactions** with other drugs, food, and laboratory tests follows.

Then the chapter presents key concepts related to adverse drug reactions, identifying predisposing factors related to patient characteristics, drug characteristics, and exogenous factors. This portion of the chapter also describes the two classifications of adverse drug reactions: dose-related and patient sensitivity–related reactions.

Chapter 2 concludes with a discussion of the potential developmental variations in these fundamental principles of pharmacology for pediatric, geriatric, pregnant, and breast-feeding patients.

Pharmacokinetics

Pharmacokinetics deals with a drug's actions as it is absorbed into, distributed to, metabolized within, and excreted from a living organism. This branch of pharmacology also reflects the drug's onset of action, peak concentration level, and duration of action.

DRUG ABSORPTION

Drug absorption encompasses a drug's progress from its pharmaceutical dosage form to a biologically available substance that can then pass through or across tissues. The transformation from dosage form to a biologically available substance must occur before the active drug ingredient reaches the systemic circulation. After a tablet or capsule disintegrates in the stomach or small intestine, enough liquid must be available for the active drug ingredients to dissolve before systemic absorption can occur. The body requires a solution of the drug's active ingredients because tissues cannot absorb dry powders or dry crystals. (**Pinocytosis,** the exception to the rule, is explained on page 12.) Because syrups and suspensions occur in dosage form as solutions, their progress from drug administration to drug absorption is more rapid, leading to a quicker onset of drug action.

Oral drug absorption

A brief account of the most common types of drug formulations and their components provides a useful basis for the study of drug absorption. A discussion of commonly used formulations also will help the student understand why certain tablets and capsules may not provide the anticipated response in selected situations.

Formulations. A *compressed tablet,* the most frequently dispensed form of a drug, provides a readily administered, standard dosage form. Compressed tablets, which may be engraved with a company symbol and code number for identification, usually have a thin, shiny coating that reduces dust during manufacturing and helps the patient swallow by decreasing the tablet's tendency to stick to the mouth or throat. The tablet may or may not be scored for dividing the dose. An unscored tablet should not be broken. Leaving an unscored tablet intact can protect the patient's stomach from a potentially irritating drug and protect the drug from stomach acid. Leaving the tablet intact also prevents too-rapid release of the drug from an otherwise sustained-release tablet.

Sustained-release formulations release drugs in a controlled, predictable manner, providing safe and effective drug absorption throughout the entire alimentary tract. Under normal circumstances, the nurse should never break or divide a sustained-release tablet or capsule formulation to provide a lower dose for a patient.

Repeat-action tablets carry an initial dose in an outer shell and a second dose within an inner shell. The inner shell of a repeat-action tablet disintegrates later in the intestinal tract.

The newest process for manufacturing sustained-release formulations produces the *osmotic pump.* Osmotic pumps usually are tablets with special semipermeable membrane coverings. The tablet's covering allows water to enter. The drug in solution can then leave the tablet, but only through a single small hole made by a laser beam during formulation. The osmotic pump formulation provides controlled release of a drug for several hours.

Other novel formulations can improve patient compliance with oral tablets. Chewable tablets were developed for a few products, such as children's aspirin and acetaminophen, to simplify administering the products to children. Cardiac patients can take sublingual or buccal tablets. The soft compression of sublingual and buccal tablets combined with a sufficient lactose content causes rapid, almost instantaneous disintegration of the drug when the patient places the tablet sublingually or buccally.

Inert ingredients. Tablets and capsules contain multiple inert ingredients, including diluents, lubricants, disintegrating agents, binders, and coloring agents. The inert ingredients assist the pharmaceutical manufacturer by (1) forming a powder that readily flows through the manufacturer's tableting equipment, (2) increasing the dimensions of a finished tablet to a manageable size for the patient, (3) binding the tablet to avoid crumbling in shipment, (4) enhancing the tablet's disintegration in the stomach or small intestine, and (5) providing an aesthetically pleasing product. Furthermore, combinations of inert ingredients in a tablet or capsule stimulate disintegration, dissolution, and drug availability in the body. Although inert ingredients normally do not produce a biological effect, some patients experience allergic reactions to them.

Parenteral drug absorption

Fewer formulation variables affect the release of a parenteral drug into the system. Clear liquid solutions for direct entry into the venous or arterial circulatory system usually pose no absorption problems because they rapidly become available to the appropriate target tissue. Differences in absorption occur, however, depending on the parenteral route selected. For example, intravenous (I.V.) administration requires no absorption time, whereas intramuscular (I.M.) and subcutaneous (S.C.) injections do.

Parenteral drugs indicated for any route other than I.V. or intrathecal, however, can pose absorption problems, although such problems rarely occur. For example, I.M. injections that provide a "long-acting" effect may be formulated in an oil or as microfine crystals. The nurse should never administer either formulation into a vein or an artery because the crystals or oil diluent may create emboli. The general principle regarding formulations is: *If the formulation looks cloudy or "thick," do not inject it into a vein or an artery.*

Physiochemical basis of drug absorption

Drug absorption varies, depending on the absorptive surface. Damaged, impaired, or surgically removed absorptive surfaces can increase or decrease the amount of drug absorbed into the body and alter a patient's response. To predict the result of drug activity accurately, the health care professional should consider the drug absorption site, whether it is the intestinal lumen or a target cell wall. Drug absorption may occur by **passive transport, active transport,** or **pinocytosis.**

Passive transport requires no cellular energy because the drug moves from an area of higher concentration to one of lower concentration. It occurs when small molecules diffuse across membranes or, to a lesser degree, through pores. Diffusion ceases when drug concentration on both sides of the membrane is equal.

Active transport requires cellular energy to move the drug from an area of lower concentration to one of higher concentration. Active transport is the cellular mechanism used during the absorption of the electrolytes sodium and potassium as well as some drugs, such as levodopa.

Pinocytosis is a unique form of active transport that occurs when a cell engulfs a drug particle in a manner comparable to phagocytosis. During pinocytosis, the drug need not be dissolved because the cell forms a vacuole or vesicle for drug transport across the cell membrane and into the inner cell. Cells commonly employ pinocytosis to transport fat-soluble vitamins (vitamins A, D, E, and K).

Other variables affecting drug absorption

Besides the type of drug formulation, the condition of the absorptive surface, and the mechanism of absorption, other variables affect the rate of absorption as well as the amount of drug absorbed.

Surface area. Most absorption of orally administered drugs occurs in the small intestine, where the mucosal villi provide extensive surface area. If large sections of the small intestine have been surgically resected, drug absorption decreases because of the reduced surface area. In some cases, the shortened intestine reduces intestinal transit time, which in turn diminishes the time that a drug is exposed to the intestinal lumen for absorption. Furthermore, not all areas of the intestine absorb drugs well. For example, the decreased number of villi in the distal small intestine and the absence of villi throughout the large intestine reduce the amount of absorption possible in these locations.

Blood flow. Drug absorption also depends on blood flow to the absorption site. During normal oral drug absorption, the drug moves rapidly from the blood capillary side of the intestinal lumen. A slow rate of oral drug absorption probably indicates a low availability of the drug at the intestinal lumen wall. Food stimulates blood flow (splanchnic blood flow) to the gastrointestinal (GI) viscera and may enhance drug absorption. Strenuous physical exercise diminishes splanchnic blood flow by diverting blood to the muscles and, therefore, slows drug absorption.

With I.M. drug absorption, drugs administered in the deltoid muscle are absorbed faster than drugs administered in the larger gluteal muscle because of the increased blood flow in the deltoid muscle. The more rapid absorption leads to a quicker onset of drug action.

Pain and stress. Pain, such as that with a migraine headache, can decrease the total amount of drug absorbed. Although the exact cause of the decreased absorption remains unknown, it probably results from a change in blood flow, reduced GI motility, or gastric retention triggered by autonomic nervous system activity that causes pyloric sphincter contraction. Decreased drug absorption also can occur during periods of stress, possibly from similar causes.

First-pass effect. Orally administered drugs do not go directly into the systemic circulation after absorption. They move from the intestinal lumen to the mesenteric vascular system to the portal vein and into the liver with its elaborate enzyme system before passing into the general circulation. During this passage, part of a drug dose may be metabolized.

Enzymes in the intestinal wall, liver, and terminal portal vein may metabolize a significant portion of the drug to an inactive form before it passes into the circulatory system and to the site of action.

The metabolic change of a drug before it reaches the systemic circulation is referred to as the **first-pass effect.** Many orally administered drugs may undergo some metabolism during the first pass through the liver. For drugs undergoing a significant first-pass effect, the orally administered dose required for a therapeutic response is much greater than the dose for a route that bypasses the portal circulation (such as the vaginal, parenteral, and sublingual routes). Although such routes avoid the first-pass effect, they are not always preferred.

Propranolol hydrochloride represents a classic example of a first-pass effect drug. The usual recommended *oral* antiarrhythmic dose is 40 to 120 mg; the *I.V.* dose, 1 to 3 mg. The disparity between these dose ranges points out how knowing which drugs are susceptible to the first-pass effect can help the nurse avoid drug administration errors.

Enterohepatic recycling. After absorption, a drug moves through the bloodstream and eventually reaches the liver. From there, such drugs as digoxin and digitoxin leave the circulation and enter the biliary tract. The drug is excreted in bile intact and travels along the biliary tract, eventually returning to the intestine. From there, the drug is reabsorbed into the bloodstream. This process is known as enterohepatic recycling.

Drug solubility. To facilitate drug absorption, the solubility of the administered drug must match the cellular constituents of the absorption site. Lipid-soluble (fat-soluble) drugs can penetrate lipoid (fat-containing) cells; water-soluble drugs cannot. For example, a water-soluble drug, such as penicillin, cannot penetrate the highly lipoid cells that act as barriers between the blood and brain. However, a highly lipid-soluble drug, such as thiopental, can penetrate the lipoid cells, cross into the brain, and induce an effect such as anesthesia.

GI motility. High-fat meals and solid food affect alimentary transit time by delaying gastric emptying, which in turn delays initial drug delivery to intestinal absorption surfaces. The administration of anticholinergics, such as atropine, scopolamine, and the belladonna alkaloids, may slow intestinal motility and prolong intestinal transit time. The prolonged intestinal transit time may increase total drug absorption. Cathartics and diarrhea shorten a drug's contact time with small intestine mucosa, and this shortened contact time may decrease drug and nutrient absorption.

Dosage form. The drug absorption rate and the time needed to reach peak blood concentration levels depend on the dosage form used. Tablets and capsules dissolve at different rates. The time needed to reach peak effect for sublingual tablets is less than that needed for compressed tablets and sustained-release tablets.

Drug interactions. Combining one drug with another drug or with food can cause interactions that affect drug absorption. For instance, administering tetracycline with an antacid reduces the amount of tetracycline available for absorption. Similarly, tetracycline administered with milk undergoes reduced availability.

Routes for drug absorption

The three routes of drug administration discussed here are the enteral, parenteral, and topical. The enteral route is used when drugs are administered by mouth or rectum or directly into the intestinal system (such as through a gastrostomy tube). The parenteral route is used for drugs administered as injections into a vein, an artery, a muscle, a joint, or a skin layer or into the spinal column. The topical route is used for drugs administered onto the skin or the mucous membranes. Each drug administration route presents advantages and disadvantages that affect the drug's pharmacokinetics.

Enteral route. Drug absorption after enteral administration can occur in the oral mucosa, gastric mucosa, small and large intestine, or rectum. Drug administration for absorption through the oral mucosa usually is restricted to small quantities of sublingual and buccal preparations. The preparations themselves also are restricted to nonirritating drugs with little flavor and drugs requiring a rapid onset of action.

The gastric mucosa usually is not important to drug absorption because of the small gastric surface area (1 m^2) and the unremarkable capillary blood flow (150 ml/minute). The gastric region is, however, an important site for disintegrating and dissolving tablets or capsules in preparation for their absorption in the small intestine.

The major site of absorption for drugs administered by enteral routes is the small intestine. From there, the active drug passes into the systemic circulation. The large intestine primarily reabsorbs water and electrolytes rather than drugs.

Rectal drug absorption advantageously circumvents the first-pass effect, but only if the drug is administered in the lower rectum. Administration in the lower rectum is an alternative enteral route if oral administration poses a problem because of potential emesis or mechanical obstacles. Rectal absorption may be erratic because of varied retention of the dosage form by the patient. Furthermore, the lack of fluid in the rectum can inhibit a drug's disintegration and dissolution and retard its transfer across the intestinal mucosal layer, further delaying absorption.

Parenteral route. The administration routes for parenteral drugs include intradermal, S.C., I.M., intrathecal, intra-articular, and I.V. The nurse usually does not administer drugs by the intrathecal and intra-articular routes. Compared with orally administered drugs, parenteral drugs must overcome fewer barriers between the sites of drug administration and drug action. Parenteral drugs, however, still must be absorbed into the tissues or cells to exert an effect on the system.

Using the intradermal route usually involves administering parenteral drugs between the skin layers just below the surface (stratum corneum). The drugs diffuse slowly from the injection site into the local microcapillary system. In most cases, the intradermal route is limited to allergens of various strengths used in diagnostic allergy testing.

Using the S.C. route involves administering drugs in the region below the epidermis. S.C. administration facilitates drug diffusion to the capillary vascular system at a much faster rate than that achieved by the intradermal route. Adding vasoconstrictors will slow the uptake of the drug by the circulation. The administration of mixtures, such as a combination of epinephrine (a vasoconstrictor) and lidocaine hydrochloride (a local anesthetic), prolongs the local anesthetic effect of lidocaine by slowing the removal of the drug from the local area. In contrast, gently massaging the area or applying warm compresses increases drug uptake by improving the blood flow and facilitating drug absorption from the injection site.

Parenteral drug absorption from I.M. sites depends on whether an I.M. solution, suspension, or emulsion is used. Solutions, which are clear preparations containing one or more substances dissolved in a fluid, provide a rapid therapeutic effect. Suspensions, which contain crystalline particles causing a cloudy appearance, and emulsions, which have an oil-like base, prolong drug activity by slowing active drug absorption from the I.M. injection site. The muscle area selected for I.M. administration also may make a difference in the drug absorption rate. For example, blood flows faster through the deltoid muscle than through the gluteal muscle; however, the gluteal muscle can accommodate a larger volume of drug than can the deltoid muscle.

Administering drugs by the I.V. route bypasses the absorption barriers and provides an immediate systemic response. I.V. administration is prescribed for an immediate response or for drugs not tolerated or absorbed by other administration routes.

Topical route. Using topical routes of drug administration involves applying drugs to various body surfaces. In recent years, the transdermal drug delivery system (TDDS) has gained popularity. With this system, the nurse usually applies a multilayered laminate to the skin, covering an area about the diameter of a U.S. quarter. A protective film from the contact adhesive is removed and applied to an unshaven, preferably hairless, skin area. (Shaving alters the skin's integrity and allows the drug to penetrate faster.) The drug used for TDDS is available as a gel solution in a reservoir and migrates from the reservoir across the skin. Some TDDS formulations rely on intact skin to help slow drug entry into the body.

The chief advantage of the TDDS is that it provides continuous drug delivery to achieve a constant, steady blood concentration level. A disadvantage of TDDS application, however, is the slow onset of drug action from initiation until a steady blood concentration level is attained (up to several hours).

Topical ointments, creams, and gels typically provide local rather than systemic effects. Ointments, usually occlusive-type topical preparations, are used to treat chronic dry skin conditions. They resist removal by water and readily attain and maintain hydrated skin; however, systemic absorption from ointments usually is poor. Creams, sometimes called "vanishing creams," are easier to apply and remove with water than ointments. Gels contain large amounts of water for easy spreading of the drug. Topical preparations can cause some systemic adverse reactions, and adequate skin hydration for optimal drug absorption may be difficult to maintain without a protective covering over the applied ointment, cream, or gel. Because drug absorption from topical ointments, creams, and gels is unreliable, the topical route seldom is used to treat systemic disorders.

Ophthalmic preparations administered in solution usually are absorbed rapidly. However, ophthalmic drugs can be administered as solutions, suspensions, ointments, or inserts (small elliptic disks placed directly on the eyeball behind the lower eyelid). Ophthalmic solutions and ointments usually are applied two to four times a day. However, ophthalmic inserts provide a sustained-release preparation for drug absorption; some can remain on the eye for several days.

Drugs instilled into the ears usually result in negligible absorption. An otic preparation is used primarily for its local effect, to soften and solubilize earwax and ease its removal or to treat a superficial ear canal rash or infection.

The skin behind the ear (postauricular) provides an area for rapid drug absorption. Used to prevent motion sickness, a scopolamine patch for transdermal administration is an example of a drug that is absorbed rapidly from the postauricular area.

Drug absorption from nasal instillation or inhalation may cause local or systemic effects. Although nasal decongestant drops and sprays act locally to induce vasoconstriction, excessive use or abuse may result in systemic absorption.

Drug administration by inhalation demands the delivery of micron-size particles that can navigate the bronchial tree and reach the affected portions of the lung. The small particle size also enhances drug absorption because only a thin membrane separates the air and the drug in each pulmonary alveolus from the capillary blood flow. Drug administration by inhalation provides local effect in the bronchial tree (albuterol administered by oral inhalation to asthmatics) or systemic effect (vasopressin administered by nasal inhalation to treat diabetes insipidus).

Rate of drug absorption

Absorption rate determines when peak concentration levels of a drug will be reached. Although a dosage form (such as a solution) may make a drug immediately available, the onset of drug activity may be rapid, intermediate, or slow, depending on the administration route and the number of barriers between the drug and the site of action. If only one or a few cells separate the active drug from the systemic circulation, rapid absorption will occur. Hence, a predicted rapid onset of action usually means that drug absorption occurs within seconds or minutes of administration via the sublingual, I.V., or inhalation route. Drugs with an intermediate absorption rate usually demonstrate an onset of action within 1 to 2 hours. In most cases, they are administered by the oral, I.M., or S.C. route. The onset of action occurs at a slower rate by the oral, I.M., or S.C. route because the complex membrane systems of GI mucosal layers, muscle, and skin delay drug passage. The slowest absorption rate may cause the drug to take several hours or days to reach peak concentration levels. A slow rate usually occurs with rectally administered or sustained-release drugs. Using a solution to disperse a rectally administered drug to the intestinal mucosae can accelerate onset of action. With sustained-release drugs, onset usually depends on the release rate from the system used, not on the drug.

DRUG DISTRIBUTION

Distribution of an absorbed drug within the body depends on several factors: blood flow, the drug's affinity for lipoid or aqueous tissue, and protein binding. How efficiently a drug is distributed throughout the body affects the concentration level of the drug remaining in the circulatory system and at the site of action. Evaluating the blood concentration level of a drug helps determine the efficiency of drug absorption, the achievement of therapeutic blood concentration levels, and the time that the drug will remain in the body.

In the body, a drug may be stored in various sites. During drug distribution through the vascular or lymphatic system, the drug comes in contact with proteins and remains free or binds to plasma carrier protein, storage tissue protein, or receptor protein. As soon as a drug binds to plasma carrier protein or storage tissue protein, it becomes inactive, rendering it unavailable for binding to a receptor protein and incapable of exerting therapeutic activity. However, a bound drug can free itself rapidly to maintain a balance between the amounts of free and bound drug. Only the free, or unbound, percentage of the drug remains active.

The percentage of drug that remains free and available for activity depends on the amount of plasma protein available for binding. The major intravascular source for carrier protein binding is plasma albumin.

The percentage of free drug usually is constant for a single drug but differs between drugs. The amount of free drug in the plasma also differs among patients, depending on their medical conditions. For example, malnutrition, which directly affects the liver, deprives the body of protein building blocks and decreases plasma albumin production. This decrease in plasma albumin and the consequent decrease in protein-binding sites boosts the amount of free drug in the plasma, which may be undesirable. The nurse must note any changes in the patient's status that could alter the percentage of free drug in the patient's plasma.

A drug's volume of distribution refers to the body areas or compartments (such as blood, total body water, or fat) in which it distributes and localizes. Volume of distribution is not actual volume, but a measure of the size of a compartment that would be filled by the amount of drug in the same concentration as that found in the blood or plasma. The nurse must keep in mind, however, that a drug's volume of distribution is unrelated to its effectiveness or duration of action.

A highly water-soluble drug possesses a small volume of distribution and has a high blood concentration level, whereas a highly fat-soluble drug possesses a large volume of distribution and has a low blood concentration level. Factors that tend to keep a drug in the circulatory system, such as high water solubility and high serum protein binding, result in a lower volume of distribution and a higher blood concentration level. Conversely, factors that promote the movement of a drug from the blood to other compartments, such as high lipid solubility (promoting storage of the drug in fat) or high degrees of binding to body tissues, result in a higher volume of distribution and lower blood concentration levels.

Other factors also can influence a drug's volume of distribution, such as blood flow through different types of tissues that absorb a drug or a drug's ability to cross different barriers, such as the blood-brain barrier. The blood-brain barrier refers to a network of capillary endothelial cells in the brain. These cells have no pores and are surrounded by a sheath of glial connective tissue that makes them impermeable to water-soluble drugs. The network excludes most ionized drug molecules, such as dopamine, from the brain. However, it allows nonionized, unbound drug molecules, such as barbiturates, to pass readily and enter the brain.

The nurse never should assume that a drug distributes well throughout the body. Abscesses, exudates, glands, and tumors can adversely affect drug distribution. For example, antibiotics typically do not distribute to abscesses and exudates. Glands, such as the prostate, tend to be impermeable to most antibiotics, rendering a prostatic infection difficult to treat effectively.

Variable drug concentrations among different organs and sometimes different tissues within a single organ also can complicate drug distribution. The differences in tissue drug concentration levels result from such variables as tissue affinity for the drug, blood flow, and protein-binding sites.

DRUG METABOLISM

Drug metabolism, or biotransformation, refers to the body's ability to change a drug biologically from its dosage or parent form to a more water-soluble form. The resulting metabolite usually is an inactive form of the parent drug; however, the metabolism of some drugs results in the ability of one or all of the metabolites to demonstrate some degree of drug activity.

Through metabolism, the body detoxifies and disposes of foreign substances. Because drugs are unnatural to the body, they are disposed of as are other toxins. In most cases, the enzyme system increases the water solubility of a drug so that the renal system can excrete it. The lipid solubility of some drugs may be altered enzymatically so that the end products enter into and are excreted through the biliary system. Using the renal or the biliary pathway for disposal, the body usually transforms the drug into a readily eliminated, pharmacologically inactive product.

The metabolism of some parent drugs may, however, result in metabolites capable of drug activity. In a few cases, the body metabolizes an inactive parent drug to an active metabolite.

Not all drugs are metabolized to the same extent or by the same mechanisms. Some drugs, such as the aminoglycosides, are not metabolized; they pass through the body and are excreted in unchanged form. Other drugs, such as barbiturates, stimulate or induce enzyme metabolic activity, thus reducing the amount of active drug in the body.

In contrast, some drugs inhibit or compete for enzyme metabolism, which may cause the accumulation of concurrently administered drugs. The accumulation increases the potential for an adverse reaction or drug **toxicity.** Before interpreting a drug response or altering therapy because of an inappropriate blood concentration level of an active drug, the physician usually investigates the possibility of drug-induced changes in drug metabolism.

Disease-induced physiologic changes can affect drug metabolism negatively. When end-stage cirrhosis damages the liver enough to reduce or alter liver blood flow, the supply of a drug to liver enzyme metabolic sites decreases. When congestive heart failure decreases the patient's cardiac output, drug metabolism decreases because the drug delivery to liver metabolic sites becomes inefficient. Genetics also may affect the efficiency of drug metabolism, as evidenced by the ability of some individuals to metabolize drugs rapidly while others metabolize them more slowly. Slowed metabolism of a drug may cause it to accumulate to toxic levels. Environment, too, may alter drug metabolism. For example, cigarette smokers metabolize theophylline much more rapidly than nonsmokers do. Developmental changes, particularly during infancy and old age, also can affect drug metabolism.

DRUG EXCRETION

The body eliminates drugs by metabolism (usually hepatic) and excretion (usually renal). Drug excretion refers to movement of a drug or its metabolites from the tissues back into the circulation and from the circulation into the organs of excretion. Physiologically, drugs can be eliminated via the lungs, exocrine glands (sweat, salivary, or mammary glands), kidneys, liver, skin, and intestinal tract. Drugs also may be removed artificially by direct interventions, such as peritoneal dialysis or hemodialysis.

Half-life

To predict the frequency of the drug dosage schedule, the physician must determine how long a drug will remain in the body. Usually, the rate of drug loss from the body can be estimated by determining the drug's **half-life.** Drug half-life represents the time required for the total amount of a drug in the body to diminish by one half. The half-life of a drug can be determined from a drug concentration-time curve, which plots the drug's concentration level on the vertical axis and the elapsed time (in hours) on the horizontal axis.

If a patient receives a single dose of a drug with a half-life of 5 hours, the total amount of the drug in the patient's body would diminish by one half after 5 hours. The drug amount would continue to decrease accordingly with each subsequent half-life. Most drugs essentially are eliminated after five half-lives because the amount remaining is too low to exert any beneficial or adverse effect. This concept is useful in many situations. For example, if a drug overdose occurs and the excretion rate of the drug is not compromised, about 97% of the original dose will be eliminated after five half-lives.

Accumulation

Drug half-life also proves to be a useful tool when assessing drug accumulation. A drug that is not readministered is eliminated almost completely after five half-lives, but a regularly administered drug reaches a "constant" total body amount, or steady state, after about five half-lives.

Having once reached a steady state, the blood concentration levels of the drug will fluctuate above and below the "average" concentration level. This means that, although the drug was once at steady state, its concentration levels do not remain uniform; rather, they increase, peak, and decline, although within a constant range.

For some drugs, the time required to reach therapeutic blood concentration levels may be too long. For example, when using digoxin, with a half-life of about 1.6 days, the physician would not be able to wait 8 days (1.6 days times 5 half-lives) to achieve steady-state blood concentration levels to control a life-threatening arrhythmia, such as atrial fibrillation. Therefore, an initial large dose, called a loading dose, would be rapidly administered to reach the desired therapeutic blood concentration level. Subsequently, smaller "maintenance dosages" would be given daily to replace the amount of drug eliminated since the last dose. These dosages maintain a therapeutic blood concentration level in the body at all times.

Clearance

Drug clearance refers to removal of a drug from the body. A drug with a low clearance rate is removed from the body slowly; one with a high clearance rate is removed rapidly. A drug with a high clearance may require more frequent administration and higher doses than a comparable drug with a low clearance. A drug with a low clearance can accumulate to toxic concentration levels in the body unless it is administered less frequently or at lower doses.

ONSET, PEAK, AND DURATION

Besides absorption, distribution, metabolism, and excretion, three other factors play an important role in a drug's pharmacokinetics: onset of action, peak concentration, and duration of action.

The onset of action refers to the time when the drug is sufficiently absorbed to reach an effective blood level and sufficiently distributed to its site of action to elicit a therapeutic response.

As the body absorbs more drug, the blood concentration level rises, more drug reaches the site of action, and the therapeutic response increases. These occurrences characterize the peak concentration level for the drug dose administered.

As soon as the drug begins to circulate in the blood, it also begins to be eliminated. Eventually, drug elimination exceeds its absorption rate because less of the dose remains to be absorbed. At this point, the blood concentration level, and the drug's effect, begin to decline. When the blood concentration falls below the minimum needed to produce an effect, drug action ceases although some drug remains in the blood. Therefore, the duration of action is the length of time that drug concentration is sufficient in the blood to produce a therapeutic response.

A drug's onset, peak, and duration are determined primarily by its bioavailability (the extent to which a drug's active ingredient is absorbed and transported to its site of action) and blood concentration level.

Pharmacodynamics

Pharmacodynamics is the study of the mechanisms by which specific drug dosages act to produce biochemical or physiologic changes in the body. The pharmacodynamic phase is one of the four phases involved in the disposition of a drug and progresses concurrently with the pharmacokinetic processes of (1) drug absorption from the administration site; (2) drug distribution throughout the body via body fluids; (3) metabolism of the parent drug to inactive, active, or more active metabolites; and (4) drug excretion.

MECHANISMS OF ACTION

To understand pharmacodynamics, the nurse must differentiate between drug action and drug effect. The interaction at the cellular level between a drug and cellular components, such as the complex proteins that make up the cell membrane, enzymes, or target receptors, represents *drug action.* The response resulting from drug action represents the *drug effect,* which may affect total body function. For example, when insulin is administered, the expected drug action is glucose transport across the cell membrane. The lowering of the blood glucose level represents the expected drug effect.

Drug-receptor interaction

The two receptors in the cell surface at left are structurally compatible with drug A. Drug B will not interact with these receptors.

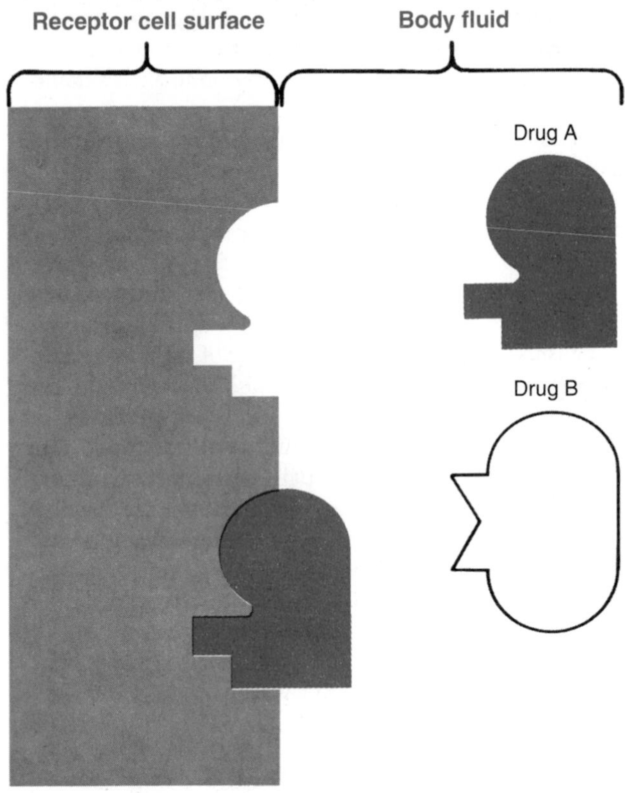

By modifying cell function, a drug causes a response that may lead to a positive therapeutic outcome or an adverse drug reaction. Remember that a drug may modify cell function or the rate of function, but *a drug cannot impart a new function to a cell or target tissue.* Therefore, the drug effect or response depends on what the cell should be capable of accomplishing.

An alteration in cell function to cause a response in the target tissue may be initiated by one of two mechanisms of action. A drug may alter the target cell's function by modifying the cell environment or the cell function.

A modification of the cell environment results from drugs that produce their therapeutic responses by affecting the cells externally. The mechanism of drug action occurs through a physical or chemical change in the cell environment.

By contrast, modification in cell function occurs when a drug molecule interacts with macromolecules within the target tissue. These macromolecules consist of a receptive substance or a configuration of molecules that acts as a receptor. Regardless of the target area, the process, referred to as a drug-receptor interaction, may accelerate or slow cell function in the target tissue. (See *Drug-receptor interaction.*)

DRUG RECEPTORS

Several basic concepts help explain the action of drugs at receptor sites. A drug attracted to a receptor displays an affinity for that receptor. The drug's ability to initiate a response after binding with the receptor is referred to as intrinsic activity. When a drug displays an affinity for a receptor and then enhances or stimulates the functional properties of the receptor, the drug acts as an **agonist.** A drug that is not an agonist can compete with an agonist for a receptor by occupying the receptor, thereby preventing the action of the agonist. Such a drug, called an **antagonist,** does not initiate an effect. Instead, the antagonist prevents a response from occurring.

Antagonists consist of two types. The first, a competitive antagonist, competes with the agonist for receptor sites. For example, naloxone is a competitive antagonist with an affinity for opioid receptors. Because naloxone competes with opioids for these receptors, parenteral administration of naloxone reverses opioid-induced respiratory depression in 1 to 2 minutes, thereby reversing the effects of opioid overdose.

The second type of antagonist, the noncompetitive antagonist, inhibits agonist response regardless of agonist concentration. For example, the noncompetitive antagonist phenoxybenzamine protects the patient from the intermittent release of large amounts of catecholamines from adrenal tumors.

Classification of receptors

Drug receptors usually are classified by the effects produced. However, a nonselective drug may interact with more than one receptor type, thereby causing multiple effects. Also, some receptors are classified further by their specific effects. For example, the *beta receptors* usually produce increased heart rate and bronchial relaxation, besides other systemic effects.

Beta receptors, however, can be subdivided into $beta_1$ receptors (which act primarily on cardiac tissue) and $beta_2$ receptors (which act primarily on smooth muscles and gland cells). $Beta_1$ receptors predominate in the heart; $beta_2$ receptors, in the lungs. Administering a nonselective beta antagonist, or beta blocker, such as propranolol, to a patient with tachycardia will decrease the heart rate. Unfortunately, the nonselectivity of propranolol also will block $beta_2$ receptors, which could precipitate an asthmatic attack in a susceptible patient. Administering a selective $beta_1$ antagonist, such as metoprolol or atenolol, will reduce the risk of receptor nonselectivity and specifically will decrease heart rate, but should not affect pulmonary function.

Epinephrine is a nonselective beta agonist used to treat acute asthmatic disorders. Unfortunately, when administered S.C., epinephrine will interact with $beta_1$ and $beta_2$ receptors and further increase the asthmatic patient's accelerated heart rate. Therefore, terbutaline, administered parenterally, is a preferred drug: it is more selective for $beta_2$ receptors.

OUTCOME OF DRUG ACTION

The major factors determining the outcome of drug action include the location and function of the receptors with which the drug interacts and the drug concentration at the receptor site. If the drug interacts with common receptors located throughout the body, the drug effects will be widespread. The use of drugs exhibiting such widespread response can be particularly dangerous because potential toxicity may affect many organ systems. The margin of safety for such drugs can be narrow, as in chemotherapeutic drugs.

If the drug interacts with specific receptors that are unique for highly differentiated cells, the response should be quite predictable. For example, the careful use of controlled doses of radioactive iodine, which has a strong affinity for receptor sites within the thyroid gland, effectively treats hyperthyroidism.

Outcome also depends on the drug concentration at the receptor site. The amount of drug at the site usually affects the intensity of the drug-induced response. The effect of drug concentration at the receptor site on outcome is best reflected in the dose-response curve.

DOSE-RESPONSE CURVE

As its name implies, a dose-response curve graphically represents the relationship between the dose of a drug and the response elicited.

On a dose-response curve, an initial low dose usually corresponds with a low response. A high correlation between the dose and the response indicates that the dose regimen can be increased to reach a point where receptor sites are saturated without causing adverse reactions. At this point, further increase in dose will not increase response. In short, the maximal response to the drug has been attained.

All drugs elicit more than one response. Morphine at low doses may calm an irritable bowel; higher doses of the drug can serve as a narcotic analgesic. Unfortunately, some adverse reactions commonly occur at normal therapeutic doses. On a dose-response curve, the curve representing the doses of morphine used as a narcotic analgesic would overlap the curve representing the drug's adverse effects. In the case of morphine, respiratory depression may preclude the continual increase in dose to achieve pain relief. Ideally, a drug will possess a low-dose-response curve, a high-dose-response curve, and an adverse effect–dose-response curve, none of which overlaps the other.

DRUG POTENCY AND EFFICACY

Drug potency, a frequently used and misunderstood term, refers to the relative amount of a drug required to produce the desired response. Comparing the drug potency of one drug with that of another drug can reveal the more potent drug. For example, comparing the usual doses of two diuretics shows that chlorothiazide requires 500 to 1,000 mg daily to achieve a therapeutic effect, whereas hydrochlorothiazide requires only 50 to 100 mg daily. Because hydrochlorothiazide achieves comparable effects at a lower dose, it is the more potent of the two diuretics.

Drug efficacy differs from drug potency in that it relates to the maximal response or effect achieved when the dose-response curve reaches its plateau. For example, compare the use of morphine and aspirin to treat pain. Aspirin is effective for mild to moderate pain only; morphine is effective for all pain levels.

THERAPEUTIC INDEX

Most drugs produce multiple effects. For example, morphine acts as an analgesic, cough suppressant, and sedative, and also causes respiratory depression, constipation, and other adverse reactions. The relationship between a drug's desired therapeutic effects and its adverse effects is termed the drug's therapeutic index, its selectivity, or its margin of safety.

In humans, the therapeutic index usually represents a measure of the difference between an effective dose for 50% of the patients treated and the minimal dose at which adverse reactions occur. All drugs with a narrow therapeutic index should be monitored frequently and thoroughly.

Pharmacotherapeutics

Pharmacotherapeutics is the use of drugs to treat disease. The therapeutic steps include assessing the problem, assessing the options, selecting the therapy, implementing the therapy, monitoring the therapy, and reassessing the problem. Specifically, it begins with the assessment of the nature and extent of the patient's health problem. This assessment is based on a patient history obtained by the health care professional, as well as on a careful clinical examination, diagnostic procedures, and laboratory tests. Assessing the options and selecting appropriate therapies are based on a knowledge of the patient, related socioeconomic factors, and the risks and benefits of the applicable therapies.

After the treatment has been implemented, the nurse monitors the patient for adverse and therapeutic drug effects, recording expected and unexpected reactions. Therapy is adjusted if the patient's problem resolves or progresses, if unacceptable adverse reactions occur, or if the therapy proves unsuccessful.

TYPES OF THERAPY

The required therapy depends on the severity, urgency, and prognosis of the patient's condition. The patient's therapy may be acute, empiric, supportive, palliative, maintenance, supplemental, or replacement.

Critically ill patients require acute intensive therapy. For example, a trauma patient may require antibiotics to prevent or treat infection, pressor agents to treat hypotension, volume expanders to treat blood loss, and analgesics to relieve pain.

Empiric therapy is based on practical experience rather than on pure scientific data. Fever spikes in hospitalized patients commonly are treated initially with empiric antibiotic therapy, using broad-spectrum antibiotics. A broad spectrum antibiotic will treat most commonly occuring microorganisms. Treatment may be a adjusted after results of culture and sensitivity tests.

Some diseases require supportive therapy, which does not treat the cause of the disease but maintains other threatened body systems until the patient's condition resolves. For example, no antiviral agents are available to treat acute viral gastroenteritis, which causes nausea, vomiting, and diarrhea. Instead, patients with this virus receive fluid and electrolyte replacements to prevent dehydration until the condition resolves.

Palliative therapy typically is used for patients with end-stage or terminal diseases, to make the patient as comfortable as possible. For example, high-dose continuous infusions of narcotic analgesics may be used to manage pain in a terminal cancer patient, or home oxygen may be supplied for a patient with end-stage pulmonary disease.

Maintenance therapy is used for patients with chronic conditions that do not resolve. This therapy seeks to maintain the patient's level of well-being while preventing further progression of the disease, if possible. An example is hypertension, in which the long-term effects can include decreased renal function, impaired vision, cerebrovascular accident, myocardial infarction, cardiac enlargement, and cardiac failure if maintenance therapy is not instituted.

Supplemental or replacement therapy may be short- or long-term. A patient with iron-deficiency anemia, for example, may receive iron supplements until hemoglobin and hematocrit levels are corrected and the body stores of iron are replenished, which may take about 6 months. However, a patient with diabetes mellitus who cannot produce adequate amounts of insulin may require lifelong injections that substitute for the missing hormone.

Other medical conditions may require continual supplemental or replacement therapies. A patient taking a potassium-depleting diuretic, such as furosemide, usually requires daily potassium replacement, and a patient with a hypoactive thyroid gland needs daily replacement of thyroid hormones.

CLINICAL RESPONSE TO DRUGS

Several drug-related factors, including adverse and cumulative effects, influence the patient's response to drugs during therapy. The nurse must consider these factors when planning and implementing the patient's care.

A drug is prescribed to benefit the patient; however, adverse reactions do occur. Recognizing them and knowing their effects on the patient are integral components of monitoring drug therapy. (A drug also may produce undesirable responses because of cumulative effects, sometimes resulting in toxicity. Cumulative effects may occur when the drug is excreted more slowly than it is absorbed or when another dose of the drug is administered before the previous dose is metabolized or cleared from the body.

The therapeutic index of a drug represents the ratio between its effective and toxic plasma concentrations. The therapeutic index is a quantitative measure of a drug's safety. A low therapeutic index indicates a narrow range between a therapeutically active dose and a toxic dose. A drug with a low therapeutic index has a higher risk of adverse reactions and requires close monitoring.

Toxic drug concentration levels may result when standard drug doses normally eliminated by the kidneys are administered to patients with decreased renal function. Because diseased or damaged kidneys cannot effectively remove the drug from the body, the drug accumulates and leads to toxicity.

Drugs that undergo extensive hepatic metabolism may become toxic in patients with impaired or immature hepatic function. Neonates, for example, must receive reduced doses of the antibiotic chloramphenicol.

Although a new drug undergoes extensive testing before receiving Food and Drug Administration (FDA) approval, its adverse effects cannot be predicted reliably until it has received widespread exposure in the general population. In recent years, some new FDA-approved drugs have been withdrawn from the market after some unpredicted, serious adverse effects had become evident.

Other factors, many related to the patient's overall health, can alter the patient's response to a drug. As a result, a physician must consider a patient's concurrent diseases and other medical conditions when selecting an appropriate drug therapy. (See *Factors affecting a patient's response to a drug.*)

Diseases and disorders

A patient's response to drugs can be altered by diseases and disorders of the major body systems, such as the GI, renal, hepatic, and circulatory systems, or of the glands, such as the thyroid gland. Altered absorption, distribution, metabolism, and excretion can influence a drug's effect and necessitate alterations in its dosage.

Physiologic factors also may determine and modify drug activity in a patient. The most influential factors are the patient's age, genetically determined rate of drug metabolism, sex, body build (muscle mass and fat content), and variations caused by circadian or daily variations.

Drug administration

The route and timing of drug administration affect drug activity. The timing of drug administration is an important nursing responsibility, whether the nurse administers the drug or teaches the patient to self-administer it.

The dosing schedule of a drug can significantly influence the patient's response to therapy. Therapeutic serum levels of antibiotics, antiarrhythmics, and anticonvulsants must be maintained to achieve therapeutic effects. When these drugs are prescribed four times a day, the nurse should administer doses every 6 hours to maintain therapeutic levels. If more time separates the last dose of the day from the first dose of the next day, the patient may experience breakthrough effects during the night. Evenly spaced dosing intervals are not as essential for a drug with an extremely long half-life, such as digoxin or levothyroxine; however, the nurse should encourage the patient on long-term therapy with such a drug to take the dose at the same time each day. Observing a regular dosing schedule also improves patient compliance.

Onset and duration of action. A drug's onset and duration of action depend largely on the drug's pharmacologic characteristics, such as lipid solubility. The drug's formulation and route of administration can, however, alter the onset of action.

Stability of pharmaceutical preparations

To ensure that a drug is as potent and therapeutically effective as intended, the nurse must carefully observe expiration dates and follow storage recommendations provided by the manufacturer or pharmacy.

Federal regulations require that expiration dates appear on all drug containers. The regulations stipulate that at least 90% of the active ingredient must be available up to the expiration date, ensuring that a patient does not receive a drug that is no longer therapeutically active or that has degraded to toxic compounds. Hospital pharmacists relabel expiration dates on oral drugs that are repackaged for hospital administration. Parenteral drugs are given new expiration dates after being reconstituted or mixed with I.V. fluids.

Drug storage can affect stability and, ultimately, therapeutic effectiveness. Drugs degrade more rapidly in warm, humid conditions. Tablets and capsules usually can be stored safely at room temperature, unless otherwise specified. Liquid dosage forms and injectable drugs sometimes require refrigeration. Some drugs also must be protected from light. For example, nitroglycerin should be stored in light-resistant bottles. The nurse should always check the label for storage requirements.

Psychological and emotional factors

Psychological and emotional factors can also affect drug activity. These factors include the placebo effect, patient compliance, and health beliefs. The nurse must consider these factors during drug therapy.

A *placebo* is an inert or inactive substance sometimes administered in place of a drug. Because it can satisfy the patient's psychological need for a drug, a placebo may elicit a therapeutic response.

Factors affecting a patient's response to a drug

Because no two people are alike physiologically or psychologically, patient response to a drug may vary greatly, depending upon the factors listed here.

- disease
- infection
- immunization
- occupational exposure
- drug interactions
- circadian variations
- diet
- cardiovascular function
- GI function
- immunologic function
- hepatic function
- renal function
- albumin concentration
- genetic constitution
- enzyme induction
- stress
- fever
- starvation
- alcohol intake
- age
- sex
- pregnancy
- lactation
- exercise
- sunlight
- barometric pressure
- smoking
- hypersensitivity
- trauma

The nurse must monitor *patient compliance* carefully, particularly in the ambulatory adult patient with little supervision. Many factors influence a patient's conscious or unconscious decision to take drugs as prescribed. Patient education about drug therapy (preferably by the nurse, pharmacist, *and* physician) can promote patient compliance significantly.

A patient's *health beliefs* reflect what the patient considers a normal healthy state and what the patient believes can be accomplished by medical care. (See Cultural Considerations: *Cultural health beliefs,* page 22.) A patient who does not perceive abdominal upset and cramping after every meal as abnormal probably will not seek medical attention. Health beliefs vary among cultures, age-groups, and regions of the country and affect compliance, especially in patients with long-term diseases like hypertension who may never feel sick. The nurse should consider health beliefs when assessing a patient's condition and counseling the patient and family members.

Tolerance and dependence

Tolerance, a patient's decreased response to a repeated drug dose, differs from **drug dependence.** A drug-dependent patient displays a physical or psychological need for the drug. For example, an alcohol-dependent patient not only needs increasing quantities of alcohol to achieve the same effects, but also risks physical and psychological withdrawal symptoms if alcohol use is discontinued.

A cancer patient using a narcotic analgesic for severe pain can display tolerance and dependence. However, the psychological aspects differ from those of the substance abuser. The cancer patient usually is concerned with maintaining a

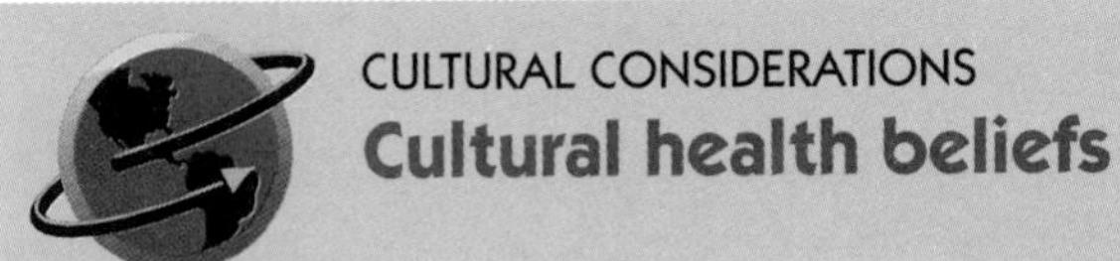

CULTURAL CONSIDERATIONS

Cultural health beliefs

The table below provides examples of common health beliefs held by patients from different cultures. Understanding how these groups historically view diseases and their treatments can help the nurse offer more deliberative, compassionate care.

CULTURAL GROUP	HEALTH BELIEFS
Latin American	• Four humors (fluids) exist in the body: blood, phlegm, black bile, and yellow bile. Health depends on the presence, temperature, and moisture of these fluids.
East Indian	• The balance of three humors (phlegm, bile, and wind) determines an individual's health and well-being.
Hispanic (traditional)	• Illness is a punishment from God.
Black (traditional)	• Disease represents a disharmony with spirits and demons.
Chinese	• Health is a gift from one's ancestors and is maintained through a balance of Yin and Yang.

reasonable level of pain relief; the substance abuser desires the euphoric effects of the drug.

DRUG INTERACTIONS

Drug interactions may occur between drugs or between drugs and foods. They may interfere with the results of a laboratory test or produce physical or chemical incompatibilities. The more drugs a patient receives, the greater the probability of a drug interaction. The nurse particularly should monitor a geriatric patient, who typically has increased sensitivity to drug effects and receives several medications.

Interactions between drugs

Interactions involving two drugs can produce a combined effect equal to the single most active component of the mixture. Such an interaction, called indifference, does not alter the therapeutic effects of either drug, nor does it produce any unpredictable adverse reactions.

Two or more drugs administered to a patient also can produce additive effects that usually are equivalent to the sum of the effects of either drug administered alone in higher doses. The concept of additive pharmacologic response is illustrated by the two analgesics acetaminophen and codeine. Acetaminophen 325 mg and codeine 30 mg are equal in analgesic effect. When combined, as in Codeine #3, their analgesic effect is the same as either acetaminophen 650 mg or codeine 60 mg. Giving the combination drug has these advantages: lower doses of each drug, decreased probability of adverse effects, and greater decrease in pain intensity than from one of these drugs alone (probably because of different mechanisms of action).

A synergistic effect occurs when two drugs producing the same qualitative effect together produce a greater response than either drug alone. For example, ethanol depresses the central nervous system (CNS), leading to sedation and drowsiness. When ethanol and other drugs that have a CNS-depressant effect are combined, the sedative effect is enhanced and psychomotor skills are impaired. Therefore, a patient taking a barbiturate, benzodiazepine, or other drug that causes drowsiness or sedation is cautioned against ingesting moderate to heavy amounts of ethanol.

An antagonistic drug interaction occurs when the combined response of two drugs is less than the response produced by either drug singly. For example, a physician who prescribes levodopa to decrease a patient's stiffness, rigidity, and other symptoms of Parkinson's disease must know that pyridoxine (vitamin B_6) combined with levodopa reverses (or antagonizes) levodopa's effects. Pyridoxine may enhance the metabolism of levodopa, making less drug available to action sites within the brain.

Pharmacokinetic interactions. Many drug interactions alter the pharmacokinetic characteristics of the drugs involved, including absorption, distribution, metabolism, and excretion.

Two drugs given concurrently may change the rate or extent of absorption of one or both of the drugs. For example, the combination of an antacid and the nonsteroidal anti-inflammatory drug naproxen slows the absorption rate of naproxen, but produces no effect on the total amount absorbed. This interaction does not require any dosage adjustments. In contrast, an antacid administered with the antibiotic tetracycline will decrease the extent, or total amount, of tetracycline absorbed. To prevent this interaction, the nurse should space doses and avoid giving tetracycline within 1 to 2 hours of an antacid.

Concurrent administration of two drugs can alter the volume of distribution by changes in protein binding. For example, the oral anticoagulant warfarin is highly protein-bound (greater than 97%), and the anticonvulsant drug phenytoin successfully competes with warfarin for protein-binding sites. Combining these two drugs increases the amount of active warfarin available, which significantly increases the risk of bleeding in a patient receiving both drugs.

Drug interactions can alter the metabolism and excretion of the drugs. For example, in the antagonistic interaction between pyridoxine and levodopa, pyridoxine increases the metabolism of levodopa. Drug interactions affecting metabolism and excretion commonly lead to toxic levels of the inhibited drug. For example, the antibiotic erythromycin may decrease hepatic metabolism of terfenadine, resulting in high blood levels of terfenadine and leading to arrhythmias. Alterations in hepatic blood flow resulting from drug interactions and disease also affect drug metabolism and excretion. Decreased hepatic blood flow affects drugs, such as propranolol, whose metabolism and excretion depend more on blood flow than on enzyme activity. Conversely, drugs whose metabolism and excretion depend on intrinsic enzyme activity generally are not affected by changes in hepatic blood flow.

Some drug interactions affect excretion only. For example, the interaction between the uricosuric drug probenecid and penicillin can produce therapeutic effects. Combining probenecid and penicillin decreases the renal excretion of penicillin and increases the drug's half-life and blood concentration levels.

Pharmacodynamic interactions. Drug interactions also produce pharmacodynamic alterations. The synergistic interaction and the enhanced sedation produced by combining ethanol and a barbiturate is an example of such a pharmacodynamic alteration.

Drug interactions and laboratory tests

Drug interactions can alter laboratory tests. Health care professionals assess renal function by using a laboratory test that measures serum creatinine levels. The test uses a colorimetric method. Many cephalosporins, such as cefazolin and cefoxitin, contain noncreatinine chromogens that cannot be differentiated by the colorimetric method. As a result, the laboratory test may overestimate the creatinine levels, possibly leading to inadequate drug dosages.

Guaiac tests of feces for the presence of occult, or unseen, blood can show false-positive results in a patient who takes large amounts of iron supplements.

Blood glucose testing is the preferred method of monitoring diabetes. However, some stable diabetic patients monitor their diabetes using urine testing for glucose. Drugs that interfere with urine glucose testing include cephalothin, isoniazid, levodopa, probenecid, and large amounts (1 to 2 g/day) of ascorbic acid. False-positive results indicating high glucose levels could cause a patient to decrease food intake or to increase insulin doses when, in fact, the blood glucose level is stable.

Drug effects on the ECG. Some drugs, particularly cardiac drugs, produce visible effects on the electrocardiogram (ECG) that can lead to misinterpreted results. For example, the antiarrhythmic drug quinidine can widen the QRS complex and prolong the QT interval. The prolongation of the QT interval can be up to 35% greater than the baseline value without representing toxicity. ECG changes of this significance require medical attention in a patient not taking quinidine. The ECG also provides information about electrolyte imbalances that may be related to drug therapy.

Drug and food interactions

Interactions between drugs and food can produce alterations in the therapeutic effects of the drug or in the use of nutrients.

Alterations in bioavailability. Food can alter the rate and amount of drug absorbed from the GI tract, affecting bioavailability — that is, the amount of a drug dose available to the systemic circulation. For example, the bioavailability of the antifungal drug griseofulvin increases when the drug is administered with a high-fat meal, and the bioavailability of theophylline increases with a low-protein, high-carbohydrate diet. Drugs also can bind with foods and impair vitamin and mineral absorption.

Induction of enzymes. Some drugs induce, or stimulate, enzyme production, and this induction increases metabolic rates and the demand for vitamins that are enzyme cofactors. For example, in an alcoholic patient, the increased demand for thiamine, a cofactor in alcohol metabolism, decreases serum levels and places the patient at high risk for thiamine deficiency and associated neurologic complications.

Alterations in sites of action. Broad-spectrum antibiotics interfere with vitamin K synthesis by altering the GI flora. Microorganisms in the colon are the normal sites for the GI production of vitamin K, important for coagulation. Prolonged use of a broad-spectrum antibiotic kills the synthesizing microorganisms and can result in bleeding problems, especially in a debilitated or geriatric patient, if not accompanied by vitamin K supplements.

Increased toxicity. The antiacne drug isotretinoin is a structural isomer of vitamin A. Therefore, a patient taking isotretinoin must avoid taking vitamin A supplements or increasing dietary vitamin A because vitamin A overdose is a risk.

Many foods also produce pharmacologic activities. For example, aged cheddar cheese and wine contain tyramine. A patient taking a monoamine oxidase inhibitor (an antidepressant) should avoid foods containing tyramine because they could cause a release of catecholamines that are present in large amounts in nerve endings and the adrenal medulla, precipitating a hypertensive crisis.

Parenteral drug incompatibilities

The nurse must carefully consider drug incompatibilities when administering drugs via parenteral (I.V., I.M., or S.C.) routes. Drug incompatibility can produce a physical reaction or a chemical inactivation.

Physically incompatible drugs interact before the drugs reach the site of action, usually interfering with the pharmacologic activity of one or both drugs. Mixing incompatible drugs can form precipitates or change a drug's color. Precipitate formation is especially dangerous for the patient if the solution is to be infused I.V.

Some light-sensitive drugs may change color if they are not protected. Whether the changed color indicates decreased drug activity is not known. Usually, the nurse should not administer drugs that have changed color.

Monitoring response

The nurse can maintain an effective therapeutic drug regimen by understanding the prescribed drug and closely monitoring the patient. Knowing the biological half-life of a drug and the physiologic factors that may alter the half-life enables the nurse to understand the appropriate dosing interval for a patient.

When developing a drug therapy that will not interfere with the patient's lifestyle, the nurse also must consider the drug's adverse effects, which can lead to noncompliance. For example, a hypertensive patient who operates a vehicle or heavy machinery on the job may choose not to take an antihypertensive that causes drowsiness and CNS disturbances. Knowledge of adverse reactions also is necessary for accurate patient monitoring and effective patient education.

Therapeutic drug monitoring. For drugs with low therapeutic indices, toxic and therapeutic levels are close. When the therapeutic response and toxicity of a drug can be related to blood concentration levels, the nurse uses those levels to monitor drug therapy.

Drug level analysis

When samples need to be drawn for monitoring drug concentration levels, the nurse should refer to a current laboratory manual for appropriate procedures and therapeutic levels.

Adverse drug reactions

A drug's desired effect is the expected therapeutic response. An adverse drug reaction, also called a side effect or adverse effect, is a harmful, undesirable response, which may result from any clinically useful drug. Adverse drug reactions can range from mild ones that disappear when the drug is discontinued to debilitating diseases that become chronic. Some adverse reactions are related to the drug dose and may be preventable with careful prescription and administration or may be inseparable from the drug's primary therapeutic effects. Others are related to patient sensitivity and may not be predictable.

FACTORS THAT LEAD TO ADVERSE DRUG REACTIONS

A patient's therapeutic responses to a drug result from the interplay among patient characteristics, drug characteristics, and exogenous (external) factors. Patient, drug, and exogenous factors can alter that interplay to produce adverse drug reactions.

Patient factors include extremes of age, extremes of body weight, genetic variations, the patient's temperament and attitudes, circadian rhythms, changes associated with disease, and changes associated with pregnancy. Drug factors that influence adverse reactions may include bioavailability, additives, degradation, dosage, administration, and the number of drugs administered. Diet and environment are exogenous factors that also may influence a patient's predisposition to adverse drug reactions.

CLASSIFICATION OF ADVERSE DRUG REACTIONS

Adverse drug reactions can be classified as dose-related or patient sensitivity–related.

Dose-related adverse reactions. Most adverse drug reactions result from the known pharmacologic effects of a drug and typically are dose-related. Therefore, they can be predicted in most cases.

Excessive therapeutic effects occur most commonly from miscalculations and overdose of a drug that requires precise, individualized dosage calculation. For example, a diabetic patient being treated with insulin may experience hypoglycemia from even a slight miscalculation of the insulin dose.

A drug typically produces not only a major therapeutic effect, but also additional and inseparable *secondary pharmacologic actions* that can be adverse. For example, morphine for pain control may lead to two undesirable secondary effects: constipation and respiratory depression. A physician may prescribe a drug for its secondary pharmacologic effects. For example, the physician may prescribe an antihistamine, typically used for allergies, to induce sleep because the secondary action of an antihistamine is drowsiness from CNS depression.

A patient may be *hypersusceptible* to the primary or secondary pharmacologic actions of a drug. Even when given a usual therapeutic dose, a hypersusceptible patient can experience an excessive therapeutic response or augmented secondary effects. Hypersusceptibility typically results from altered pharmacokinetics, which leads to higher-than-expected blood concentration levels. Increased receptor sensitivity also may increase the patient's response to therapeutic or adverse effects.

Most drugs produce *toxicity* if given in large enough doses, or when drug concentration levels exceed the threshold needed for therapeutic effect. Dose-related toxic effects may result from the local accumulation of a drug, as when chemotherapeutic agents accumulate in and damage hair follicle cells, which leads to alopecia (hair loss). Systemic drug effects also can produce toxicity. For example, rapid I.V. administration of aminophylline can precipitate severe hypotension and circulatory collapse.

Toxic effects may seriously damage tissues and organs and precipitate drug-induced diseases. Such conditions result from treatment with various drugs and can lead to serious, chronic health problems. Toxic effects may cause only

Drug allergies

Drug allergies are categorized into four basic groups: types I, II, III, and IV.

TYPE	RESPONSE	EXAMPLES
I	Immediate reactions to stings and drugs	Anaphylaxis, urticaria, angioedema
II	Drug-induced autoimmune disorders	Sulfonamide-induced granulocytopenia, quinidine-induced thrombocytopenic purpura, hydralazine-induced systemic lupus erythematosus
III	Reactions to penicillins, sulfonamides, iodides; antibody targeted against tissue antigens	Urticarial skin eruptions, arthralgia, lymphadenopathy, fever
IV	Reexposure to an antigen	Poison ivy and its resulting contact dermatitis

transient changes in affected organs or more serious, irreversible changes, such as the tardive dyskinesias associated with antipsychotic therapy. Such effects can be more serious than the original illness.

Some adverse drug effects induced by the prescribed drug, known as *iatrogenic effects*, may mimic pathologic disorders. For example, some drugs, such as antineoplastics, aspirin, corticosteroids, and indomethacin, commonly cause GI irritation and bleeding. Other examples of iatrogenic effects include propranolol-induced asthma, methicillin-induced nephritis, gentamicin-induced deafness, and thiazide-induced dizziness. Obtaining complete medical and drug histories from the patient helps reduce the risk of iatrogenic effects.

Patient sensitivity–related adverse reactions. A less common type of adverse reaction is unrelated to dosage and results from a patient's unusual and extreme sensitivity to a drug or its components. These adverse reactions arise from unique tissue response rather than from an extension or alteration of the expected pharmacologic action. Extreme patient sensitivity may be manifested as a drug allergy or as an idiosyncratic response.

A *drug allergy* occurs when a patient's immune system identifies a drug, a drug metabolite, or a drug contaminant as a dangerous foreign substance that must be neutralized or destroyed. Previous exposure to the drug or to one with similar chemical characteristics sensitizes the patient's immune system, and subsequent exposure mobilizes the system and causes an allergic reaction (hypersensitivity). An allergic reaction not only directly injures cells and tissues, but also produces broader systemic damage by initiating cellular release of vasoactive and inflammatory substances.

A drug allergy can be categorized according to the underlying immunologic mechanism it provokes. The adverse reaction may vary in intensity from an immediate, life-threatening anaphylactic reaction to penicillin, to a contact dermatitis secondary to topical application of neomycin cream. (See *Drug allergies.*)

Patient sensitivity-related adverse reactions that do not result from known pharmacologic properties of a drug or from patient allergy but are peculiar to the patient are called *idiosyncratic responses.* For example, a patient may experience nervousness and excitability after ingesting phenobarbital, normally a tranquilizing agent. A patient's idiosyncratic response sometimes has a genetic cause.

Developmental considerations

The pharmacokinetics, pharmacodynamics, pharmacotherapeutics, and adverse effects of drugs in pediatric, geriatric, pregnant, and breast-feeding patients may vary substantially from those in the general adult population. Developmental differences or immature or declining body systems can exaggerate these variations and make medication effects less predictable — sometimes even risky. The nurse must keep these variations in mind when administering a drug to a patient with these developmental considerations.

PEDIATRIC PATIENTS

In a pediatric patient, many factors can influence the pharmacokinetic, pharmacodynamic, and pharmacotherapeutic processes that occur in the body.

Pharmacokinetics

A child's age, physiologic state, body composition, immature organ function, and other factors can affect the absorption, distribution, metabolism, and excretion of a drug.

Absorption. After a drug is administered orally, its absorption depends on the child's age, the underlying disease, the dosage form, and the presence of other drugs or foods taken concurrently.

In a young child, the gastric pH is higher, or less acidic, than in an adult. As the child develops, gastric pH decreases, acidity increases, and drug absorption is altered. For example, nafcillin and penicillin G are better absorbed by an infant than an adult because of low gastric acidity. Milk and formula also can affect gastric pH and may alter absorption. Therefore, most pediatric medications are administered when the child's stomach is empty.

Several other factors can influence drug absorption from the GI tract and make it less predictable and less efficient in a child under age 2. The shortness of the intestine and the presence of diarrhea can reduce the amount of time a drug is available for absorption. Decreased transit time through the GI tract also can decrease drug absorption.

Absorption of I.M. medications in infants may be unpredictable because of vasomotor instability and decreased muscle tone. Percutaneous absorption of S.C. medications in infants is increased because of an underdeveloped epidermal barrier and increased skin hydration.

A child will absorb a topical drug at about the same rate as an adult, but will absorb it more completely because of a greater body-surface area relative to total body mass.

Distribution. A drug's distribution is affected by its dilution in the body. The higher percentage of water in neonates and infants dilutes water-soluble drugs, reducing their blood concentration levels. That is why neonates and infants often require higher mg/kg dosages to achieve therapeutic drug concentration levels in the blood.

Extracellular fluid volume also influences a water-soluble drug's concentration and effect because most drugs travel through extracellular fluid to reach their receptors. Children have a larger proportion of fluid to solid body weight, so their distribution area is proportionately greater.

Body composition affects the distribution of fat-soluble drugs, although to a lesser degree than water-soluble ones. As the percentage of fat increases with age, so does the distribution of fat-soluble drugs. Therefore, distribution of these drugs is more limited in children than in adults.

In a neonate, the immature liver also may affect drug distribution by decreasing formation of plasma proteins, which results in lower serum protein levels and higher fluid volume than in an adult. This reduces the number of plasma proteins for drugs to bind to. Because only unbound, or free, drugs produce a pharmacologic effect, the infant's decreased protein binding can intensify drug effects and possibly cause toxicity.

Several diseases and disorders, such as nephrotic syndrome and malnutrition, also can decrease plasma protein and increase the the concentration of an unbound drug, intensifying the drug's effect or producing toxicity.

Metabolism. In an infant, the immature liver may metabolize drugs inefficiently. As the liver matures during the first year of life, drug metabolism improves.

Dosage and choice of therapeutic agent may be altered for an infant with immature liver function or liver disease. The immature liver function increases the risk of toxicity with some drugs, such as chloramphenicol. When the liver fails to inactivate this drug, toxic levels can accumulate in the blood and produce gray syndrome of the neonate, characterized by rapid respirations; ashen gray cyanosis; vomiting; loose, green stools; progressive abdominal distention; vasomotor collapse; and possibly death. Fortunately, drug discontinuation can reverse the syndrome if discontinuation occurs as soon as symptoms appear.

Conversely, intrauterine exposure to drugs may induce precocious development of hepatic enzyme mechanisms, increasing the infant's capacity to metabolize potentially harmful substances.

Children typically metabolize drugs that require oxidation, such as theophylline, caffeine, phenobarbital, and phenytoin, more rapidly than adults. The rate of metabolism for drugs such as aspirin and the sulfonamides that are catalyzed by microsomal or nonmicrosomal enzymes can vary among individuals and may be genetically determined.

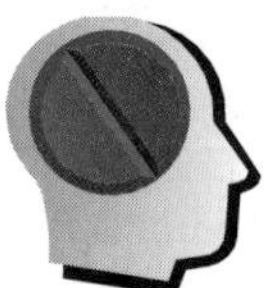

CRITICAL THINKING: To enhance your critical thinking about pharmacologic principles, consider the following situation and its analysis.
Situation: Brenda Lane, age 4 months, has biliary atresia, which compromises her liver function. The nurse plans to closely monitor Brenda's response to her prescribed medications. Why?
Analysis: Many drugs undergo a first-pass effect in the liver, where metabolic changes occur. In any infant, the immature liver may metabolize drugs inefficiently. In this infant, however, liver dysfunction may produce even greater effects on drug metabolism.

Excretion. Because most drug excretion occurs in the urine, the degree of renal development can affect drug excretion and, ultimately, dosage requirements for a pediatric patient.

At birth, the kidneys are immature, renal excretion is slow, and drug dosages must be adjusted carefully. As the kidneys mature during the first few months after birth, renal excretion of drugs increases, although the rate of increase is slow for a premature neonate.

Some drugs, such as nafcillin, are excreted by the biliary tract into the intestinal tract. In the first few days after birth, however, biliary blood flow is low, which can prolong the effects.

Pharmacodynamics

Biochemically, a drug will display the same mechanism of action in all individuals. The response to a drug, however, can be affected by the maturity of the target organ and may require a dosage adjustment for a neonate, infant, or child. In addition, receptor sensitivity varies in infants and young children; it may be increased or decreased for certain drugs. Therefore, an infant or child may require a lower or higher dosage of a drug than expected.

Pharmacotherapeutics

The goal of medication administration is to achieve and maintain a therapeutic drug level without producing toxicity. To maintain therapeutic levels, the patient must receive repeated doses at intervals that may vary according to age. Also, the child may need higher doses more frequently or may need sustained-release preparations to achieve therapeutic drug levels.

Adverse drug reactions

Some drugs can have an adverse effect on a child's growth and development. For example, long-term treatment with glucocorticosteroids, which may be necessary for a child with an organ transplant or asthma, may stunt growth. In these cases, the benefits of drug therapy must be evaluated against the effects on growth.

GERIATRIC PATIENTS

Aging usually is accompanied by a decline in organ function, which can profoundly affect drug distribution and clearance, among other things. This physiologic decline is likely to be exacerbated by a disease or chronic disorder. Such a combination can significantly increase the geriatric patient's risk of drug toxicity and adverse reactions.

Pharmacokinetics

Many physiologic changes of aging affect drug absorption, distribution, metabolism, and excretion. The nurse must be especially aware of these changes when administering medications to a geriatric patient and when observing for adverse drug reactions.

Absorption. Several age-related changes in the GI system can alter drug absorption patterns. Decreased gastric acidity may affect drug solubility and alter drug absorption. Reduced blood flow to the GI tract and the decreased number of cells available for absorption also can delay drug absorption. However, because the GI transit time is slowed, drugs remain in the system longer, which increases absorption. Overall, the effects of aging slow the absorption rate, but allow absorption to be as complete as in a younger patient.

Distribution. Total body mass and body water decrease with age. These changes in body composition lead to a relative increase in body fat and decrease in body water, which changes the distribution patterns for most drugs. A highly fat-soluble drug, such as diazepam, will have an increased volume of distribution and a prolonged distribution phase, leading to a prolonged half-life and duration of action. A highly water-soluble drug, such as gentamicin, will have a decreased volume of distribution.

Aging also reduces plasma levels of albumin, a blood protein that binds with and transports many drugs. As a result, more unbound drug may circulate, which typically increases the pharmacologic action of drugs that are extensively protein-bound.

Other factors that alter drug distribution in geriatric patients include declining cardiac output, poor nutrition, extremes of body weight, dehydration, electrolyte and mineral imbalances, inactivity, and prolonged bed rest. Perhaps the most significant factor is size: Geriatric patients typically are smaller than younger patients. So if a geriatric patient receives the same drug dose as a younger patient, the geriatric patient's typically smaller volume can result in higher blood concentrations of the drug.

Metabolism. Aging reduces the liver's ability to metabolize drugs. Liver disease may further compromise its functioning as may other diseases that reduce hepatic blood flow, such as heart failure.

Drug metabolism by the liver depends primarily on two processes: hepatic blood flow and metabolic enzyme action. Because aging decreases blood flow to the liver, less drug is delivered for metabolism to inactive compounds. The hepatic enzymes metabolize drugs in two major phases. Aging reduces the efficiency of both phases, but phase I reactions (oxidation, reduction, or hydrolysis of drug molecules) are affected more than phase II reactions (coupling of the drug or its metabolite with an acid to produce an inactive compound). Aging leads to different clinical effects, depending on whether a drug is metabolized in phase I, phase II, or both.

Excretion. With aging, glomerular filtration and tubular secretion decline progressively. Also, dehydration and cardiovascular and renal diseases may impair renal function. The nurse should keep in mind that the geriatric patient has a smaller renal reserve than a younger patient, even if the blood urea nitrogen and serum creatinine levels appear normal.

The kidneys excrete many drugs. When the geriatric patient receives drugs that do not undergo metabolism, the nurse must monitor for signs of toxicity because drug clearance and excretion may be delayed. Potentially nephrotoxic drugs, such as the aminoglycoside gentamicin, are of particular concern because they may cause severe nephrotoxicity faster in a geriatric patient.

Pharmacodynamics

Many changes in drug effect in geriatric patients do not result from pharmacokinetic factors. Instead, they may be caused by the aging organ system and its role in drug-receptor or drug-organ interactions.

Aging causes many receptors to function less efficiently and reduces the density of beta-adrenergic receptors. As a result, geriatric patients show diminished response to drugs such as isoproterenol and increased toxicity to beta-adrenergic blockers such as propranolol. Aging produces a decline in parasympathetic control, which enhances the effects of anticholinergic agents. It also reduces the number of neurotransmitters, particularly dopamine and acetylcholine.

Adverse drug reactions

Geriatric patients experience adverse drug reactions two to seven times more frequently than younger patients. Age-related physiologic changes account for many of these adverse reactions. For example, reduced dopamine in the brain makes the geriatric patient more susceptible to the adverse extrapyramidal effects of neuroleptics, metoclopramide, and other drugs.

Physiologic changes in the CNS may cause drug-related problems. These changes include increased sensitivity to depressants and decreased cerebral blood flow, which increase susceptibility to sedation and diminished cognitive function during drug therapy. Other CNS changes may include deterioration of the blood-brain barrier, which may allow a greater CNS concentration of some drugs and may account for the high incidence of drug-induced behavioral changes in geriatric patients. One such change, paradoxical excitement, commonly occurs with the use of sedatives and anxiolytics.

Age-related cardiovascular changes that may alter drug response include decreased cardiac output, increased total peripheral resistance, increased circulating norepinephrine, and decreased sensitivity and function of baroreceptors. These changes may cause such common adverse drug reactions as orthostatic hypotension and heart failure.

Several endocrine changes may influence drug therapy. For example, the age-related decline in glucose tolerance may cause greater hyperglycemia in response to a thiazide diuretic. Reduced response to hypoglycemia may cause a geriatric patient to delay seeking treatment until the hypoglycemia worsens. Reduced thyroid function may decrease body metabolism, which can slow drug metabolism.

Age-related changes in the respiratory, GI, urinary, and musculoskeletal systems also can predispose a geriatric patient to adverse drug reactions. For example, decreased respiratory function may lead to increased sensitivity to respiratory depressants, such as narcotics and barbiturates. Decreased GI motility and activity may cause constipation and greater sensitivity to the effects of anticholinergic drugs.

Several risk factors help identify geriatric patients who are prone to adverse drug reactions. Identification of high-risk geriatric patients can allow the nurse to protect them by monitoring closely, preventing errors, identifying drug-related problems promptly, and intervening as needed. The risk factors include advanced age, small physique, multiple illnesses, multiple medications, type of drugs prescribed (such as CNS depressants), previous adverse drug reactions, living alone, and malnutrition.

PREGNANT PATIENTS

Most drugs ingested by a pregnant patient cross the placenta to the fetus. In 1979, the FDA established six categories (A, B, C, D, X, NR) to indicate the level of risk to a fetus posed by drugs. Although these categories are helpful, they may not be entirely accurate. (See *Pregnancy drug risk categories.*)

Pharmacokinetics

A number of pregnancy-related changes and structures can alter the absorption, distribution, metabolism, and excretion of a drug ingested by the pregnant patient. The fetus also significantly influences drug distribution and disposition.

Absorption. During pregnancy, the tone and motility of the GI tract decrease, probably from increased progesterone production and decreased levels of motilin (an intestinal hormone that causes increased intestinal motility and also stimulates pepsin secretion). These effects prolong the gastric emptying and intestinal transit times. The formation of hydrochloric acid in the stomach also decreases. All these factors delay absorption of drugs that require an acidic environment or that are absorbed in the small intestine.

Absorption of drugs administered parenterally also may be altered during pregnancy. Because of peripheral vasodilation, drugs administered S.C., I.M., or intradermally may be absorbed more rapidly.

Distribution. The physiologic changes of pregnancy also alter drug distribution. Influencing factors include increased interstitial and cellular water and increased blood volume, elevated nearly 45% by the end of gestation. These increases change the ratios of blood constituents that affect drug distribution. For example, the ratio of albumin to water decreases during pregnancy, altering protein-binding capacity.

During pregnancy, estrogen and progesterone levels also rise, as do those of free fatty acids (triglycerides, cholesterol, and phospholipids) from increased fatty tissue metabolism. These effects are accompanied by increased competition for protein-binding sites. With fewer binding sites, a larger percentage of drug remains free to move to receptor sites or across the placenta.

The term "placental barrier" can be misleading because it implies that the placenta protects the fetus from drug effects. In fact, many drugs ingested by the pregnant patient will cross the placenta and reach the fetus. Although some drugs, such as insulin, do not cross the placenta, most do when administered at therapeutic levels. Placental transport of substances to and from the fetus begins at approximately the 5th week of gestation. Later in pregnancy when the placenta thins, drugs with high lipid solubility or low protein-binding ability pass more easily through the placenta.

The fetus also significantly may affect drug distribution and disposition by fetal circulation, binding of plasma and tissue proteins, and excretory activity.

Metabolism. Because the placenta is metabolically active, it can affect drug disposition. The placenta appears to be capable of several enzymatic reactions that can reduce the potency of a drug's metabolites. Conversely, these reactions may produce a more potent and toxic metabolite, thereby increasing fetal danger.

Excretion. Numerous changes in the urinary system occur during pregnancy and can affect drug excretion. The glomerular filtration rate and renal plasma flow increase early in pregnancy, and the former persists to delivery. Because of the increased renal plasma flow, drugs that normally are excreted easily may be eliminated even more rapidly.

The fetus has slower drug clearance than the adult, and drugs persist longer in the fetus's tissues and blood than in the mother's.

Pharmacotherapeutics

When counseling the pregnant patient, the physician should evaluate each drug to determine whether equivalent benefits can be obtained through alternative measures. The patient should participate actively in these decisions. If a drug must be used, the physician should prescribe one that has been used during pregnancy for many years rather than a recently introduced drug with inadequately established effects.

The physician will substitute alternative measures, if possible, during the trimester when a drug may produce teratogenic effects (those that cause fetal anomalies). For example, a patient with diabetes mellitus that was controlled with oral hypoglycemic agents before pregnancy may receive insulin instead during pregnancy.

The physician and nurse should teach pregnant and nonpregnant patients of childbearing age about the use of drugs, including over-the-counter medications. The pregnant patient should never self-medicate without consulting her physician.

Adverse drug reactions

Drug effects on the fetus depend on the timing of drug administration in relation to gestational age. The fetus is most susceptible to the adverse effects of drugs from the time of implantation to the embryonic period, with limb formation defects potentially occurring through the end of the first trimester. During conception and implantation, the ovum is bathed in fallopian tube fluid. At that time, any damage to the ovum from drug exposure usually is lethal; however, the ovum can recover completely from damage inflicted by a sublethal dose. During the embryonic period, major structural anomalies may occur after only a single exposure to a toxic drug. Teratogenic drug exposure during the fetal period may slow cell growth and retard growth of the exposed part or of the entire fetus. Such an effect is called intrauterine growth retardation.

The care with which a drug is administered to the mother and fetus during pregnancy is critical to the safety of the fetus. Maternal-fetal equilibrium of drug levels usually is reached within 40 minutes after drug ingestion and more rapidly with parenteral or I.V. administration.

BREAST-FEEDING PATIENTS

A woman who breast-feeds during drug therapy may subject her infant to the effects of the drug. Unlike the fetus, the infant cannot depend on the placenta for the metabolism and excretion of maternally ingested drugs.

Infant sucking behavior, the amount consumed per feeding, and the frequency of breast-feeding affect the amount of drug the infant ingests. Low gastric acidity and slower absorption rates in the infant affect the amount of drug absorbed by the infant. Changes in plasma protein binding in the infant may alter drug concentration levels at receptor sites. Further, drugs that are metabolized insufficiently and excreted by immature neonatal systems may accumulate, increasing the risk of toxicity.

Because most drugs and chemicals ingested by a mother appear in breast milk, physicians must evaluate drug effects on the breast-feeding mother and the infant.

Pregnancy drug risk categories

The following summarizes the Food and Drug Administration (FDA) risk-factor categories for drugs used during pregnancy.

Category A: Controlled studies in women fail to demonstrate a risk to the fetus in the first trimester (no evidence of a risk in later trimesters); the possibility of fetal harm appears remote.

Category B: Either animal reproduction studies have not demonstrated a fetal risk (no controlled studies in pregnant women), or animal reproduction studies have shown an adverse effect other than decreased fertility that was not confirmed in controlled studies with women in the first trimester; no evidence of a risk in later trimesters.

Category C: Either animal studies have revealed teratogenic, embryocidal, or other adverse effects on the fetus (no controlled studies in women are available), or no studies in women or animals are available. Drugs should be administered only if the potential benefit to the woman justifies the potential risk to the fetus.

Category D: Positive evidence of human fetal risk exists, but the benefits from use in pregnant women may be acceptable despite the risk (for example, if the drug is needed in a life-threatening situation or for a serious disease for which safer drugs cannot be used or are ineffective).

Category X: Studies in animals or women have demonstrated fetal abnormalities, or evidence of fetal risk exists based on human experience, or both, and the risk in pregnant women clearly outweighs any possible benefit. The drug is contraindicated in women who are or may become pregnant.

Category NR: No rating available.

CHAPTER SUMMARY

Chapter 2 explored the fundamental principles of pharmacology: pharmacokinetics, pharmacodynamics, pharmacotherapeutics, and adverse drug reactions. It also investigated variations in these fundamental principles for pediatric, geriatric, pregnant, and breast-feeding patients. Here are the chapter highlights.

Pharmacokinetics deals with a drug's actions as it is absorbed into, distributed to, metabolized within, and excreted from a living organism.

Pharmacodynamics refers to the mechanisms of action by which drugs produce biochemical or physiologic changes in the body.

Pharmacotherapeutics is the use of drugs to treat disease. The therapeutic steps include assessing the problem, assessing the options, selecting the therapy, implementing the therapy, monitoring the therapy, and reassessing the problem.

Adverse drug reactions can be classified as dose-related or patient sensitivity–related. Most dose-related adverse reactions result from excessive therapeutic effect, secondary reactions, hypersusceptibility to pharmacologic actions, toxicity, or iatrogenic drug effects. Patient sensitivity–related adverse reactions stem from drug allergy or idiosyncratic response.

The pharmacokinetics, pharmacodynamics, pharmacotherapeutics, and adverse effects of drugs in pediatric, geriatric, pregnant, and breast-feeding patients may vary substantially from those in the general adult population.

A child's age, physiologic state, body composition, immature organ function, and other factors can affect the absorption, distribution, metabolism, and excretion of a drug.

Maternal, placental, and fetal factors alter the pharmacokinetics of a drug. Maternal factors include decreased tone and motility of the GI tract, increased blood volume, altered fat metabolism, increased glomerular filtration rate, and increased renal plasma flow. Placental factors include drug transport across the placenta and several enzymatic reactions. Fetal factors include fetal circulation, binding of plasma and tissue proteins, and excretory activity.

Because most drugs and chemicals ingested by a mother appear in breast milk, physicians must evaluate drug effects on the breast-feeding mother and her infant.

Questions to consider

See Appendix 1 for answers.

1. Leonard Becchetti, age 65, has recently learned that he has diabetes mellitus. His care includes attending classes about the disorder. During the class on drug therapy for diabetes, the nurse briefly reviews the absorption, distribution, metabolism, and excretion of insulin and oral hypoglycemic agents. What is the purpose of drug metabolism?
   (a) To initiate a physiologic response
   (b) To break down the drug for absorption throughout the body
   (c) To transform the drug for renal and biliary elimination
   (d) To break down the drug for distribution throughout the body

2. The nurse is teaching Rita Randolph, age 47, about her newly prescribed antihypertensive agent. During the session, the nurse explains the difference between drug potency and drug efficacy. Which of the following statements best describes drug efficacy?
   (a) The relationship between a drug's therapeutic effects and its adverse effects
   (b) The amount of drug at which adverse reactions occur
   (c) The amount of drug needed to produce the desired response
   (d) The amount of drug needed to reach the plateau of the dose-response curve

3. Which of the following types of drug therapy is used for patients who have a chronic condition that can't be cured?
   (a) Empiric therapy
   (b) Supportive therapy
   (c) Palliative therapy
   (d) Maintenance therapy

4. When teaching Robert Harman, age 32, about anticonvulsant drug therapy, the nurse informs him that patient characteristics, drug characteristics, and exogenous factors may predispose him to adverse reactions to his prescribed drug. Which of the following is a patient factor?
   (a) Drug dosage
   (b) Dietary factors
   (c) Genetic variation
   (d) Number of drugs taken

5. At age 6 months, Shannon Carter is recovering from a bowel resection that was performed to correct an obstruction. Shortening of the bowel is most likely to affect which of the following aspects of a drug's pharmacokinetics?
   (a) Absorption
   (b) Distribution
   (c) Metabolism
   (d) Excretion

6. Mary Hemphill, age 4 months, has diarrhea and must receive an antibiotic. To ensure that she receives therapeutic levels of the antibiotic, which of the following routes should be used for administration?
   (a) Oral route
   (b) S.C. route
   (c) I.M. route
   (d) I.V. route

7. The physician prescribes an oral hypoglycemic agent for a diabetic patient, Sylvia Cohen, age 72. In a geriatric patient, such as Ms. Cohen, absorption of oral medication may be altered. What accounts for this alteration?
   (a) Decreased gastric acid secretion
   (b) Decreased total body mass
   (c) Increased total body fat
   (d) Decreased cardiac output

UNIT II

The nursing process and drug administration

Nurses near and far would agree that medication administration is the most challenging, and sometimes most frightening, new experience for a nursing student. It is challenging because safe, therapeutic administration requires technical competence, sound judgment, and meticulous attention to detail. It can be frightening because giving medications is a complex activity that can harm the patient if not implemented properly.

Nurses are legally responsible for maintaining patient safety, ethically responsible for making moral nursing decisions, and professionally responsible for facilitating the therapeutic effects of medications. To meet these responsibilities, the nurse must apply a broad knowledge base to all aspects of care and must be aware of the related legal and ethical implications of nursing care.

Although learning to administer medications is a complex task, the information contained in unit 2 should help the nurse successfully meet the challenge. The unit provides the basic information necessary for the nurse to become knowledgeable and competent in safe, therapeutic drug administration. It presents the nursing process, nursing responsibilities in drug administration, dosage measurements and calculations, and routes and techniques of administration. The information in this unit serves as a foundation for chapters 6 through 61, which illustrate specific nursing care (in the nursing process framework) related to each drug class.

NURSING PROCESS AND DRUG THERAPY

The **nursing process,** a framework that aids in the development, implementation, and evaluation of patient care, consists of five essential steps: **assessment,** formulation of a **nursing diagnosis** (identifying a patient's health need), **planning, implementation** of the nursing plan of care, and **evaluation.** Because it is dynamic, the nursing process allows the nurse to develop and modify a total plan of care in a logical sequence for a particular patient.

Assessment

During the assessment step, the nurse gathers information that helps guide the patient's drug therapy. One important information source is the patient's drug history, which the nurse obtains from data given by the patient, spouse or partner, parent, or others who know that patient well. The nurse also obtains information by performing a physical assessment, consulting medical records, and reviewing laboratory or diagnostic test findings to detect adverse reactions or document drug efficacy.

Components of a drug history. The nurse must obtain a thorough drug history upon the patient's admission to the health care facility. When compiling a comprehensive drug history, the nurse should ask specific questions that cover the patient's general information and use of prescription and over-the-counter (OTC) drugs. (See *Critical components of a drug history,* page 32.)

Clinical behaviors. During assessment, the nurse also needs to consider these two important factors that affect drug administration: the patient's cognitive abilities and the body systems that may be affected by the prescribed drugs.

A patient with intact cognitive abilities should be able to understand and implement the actions necessary for **compliance.** If the patient's cognitive abilities are impaired, the nurse may need to teach a family member or friend to administer the drug, obtain a visiting nurse referral, use a daycare setting, or consider consulting the physician about admitting the patient to an extended-care facility.

Every drug produces a particular effect on a specific body system or systems. Some of the effects may represent the desired action of the drug. However, every drug potentially can affect other body systems in adverse ways. For instance, chemotherapeutic drugs destroy cancerous cells, yet they also destroy normal cells and lead to nausea, loss of appetite, hair loss, and diarrhea. The nurse must closely monitor a drug's adverse effects to ensure that the patient does not become seriously compromised.

Critical components of a drug history

When obtaining the patient's drug history, the nurse gathers general information about certain components essential to proper nursing practice as well as specific information about prescription and over-the-counter (OTC) drugs. The following list serves as a guide for obtaining a drug history.

GENERAL INFORMATION

Allergies
- Drugs
- Food

Medical history
- Associated illnesses and diseases

Habits
- Dietary
- Recreational drug use
  - alcohol
  - tobacco
  - stimulants, such as caffeine
  - illegal drugs

Socioeconomic status
- Age
- Educational level
- Occupation
- Health insurance coverage
- Lifestyle and beliefs
- Support systems
- Marital status
- Childbearing status
- Attitudes toward health and health care
- Use of the health care system
- Daily activities pattern

Sensory deficits

PRESCRIPTION AND O.T.C. DRUGS

- Reason for use
- Knowledge of drugs
- Frequency or dosage
- Effectiveness or reactions
- Pattern and route of administration

Nursing diagnoses

Analysis of essential assessment data and identification of the specific signs or symptoms (defining characteristics) and probable cause (etiology) helps the nurse formulate a particular nursing diagnosis.

Nursing diagnoses provide a common language to convey the nursing management needed for each patient among the many nurses involved in that patient's care. To help ensure standardized nursing diagnosis terminology and use, the North American Nursing Diagnosis Association (NANDA) has formulated and classified a series of nursing diagnosis categories based on nine human response patterns. (See *NANDA taxonomy of nursing diagnoses.*)

Knowledge deficit and *noncompliance* are the two most common diagnostic labels used by the nurse to develop care plans for managing a patient's drug regimen. The nurse also may identify other nursing diagnoses depending on the potential risks or adverse effects of drug therapy.

Defining characteristics of *knowledge deficit* may include:
- statement of misconception
- verbalization of the problem
- request for information
- inaccurate follow-up of instructions
- inadequate test performance
- inappropriate or exaggerated behaviors.

Etiologies associated with *knowledge deficit* may include lack of exposure, information misinterpretation, unfamiliarity with information resources, lack of recall, cognitive limitation, and lack of interest in learning or obtaining information.

Some defining characteristics of *noncompliance* include:
- behavior indicating failure to follow a regimen, supported by direct observation or statement by the patient or an informed observer
- failure on objective tests
- evidence of the development of complications
- exacerbations of the symptoms
- failure to keep appointments
- failure to progress
- inability to set or maintain mutual goals.

Etiologies associated with *noncompliance* may include lack of knowledge, lack of necessary resources, denial of a health problem, information misinterpretation, and belief that treatment measures are ineffective or unnecessary.

The nurse may formulate and use many other nursing diagnoses, depending on the adverse effects of drugs, such as *risk for injury related to anticoagulant therapy, impaired skin integrity related to a reaction to the prescribed medication,* and *altered oral mucous membrane related to a superimposed infection from antibiotic use.*

Planning

Once the nursing diagnosis is formulated, the nurse can proceed to the planning step of the nursing process, determining the nursing plan of care for the patient. This consists of two major components: **outcome criteria** (patient **goals**) and **nursing interventions.**

Outcome criteria. Outcome criteria represent patient goals and state the desired patient behaviors or responses that should result from the nursing care. Each criterion should be measurable and objective, concise, realistic for the patient, and attainable by nursing management. Furthermore, each criterion should include only one behavior, express that behavior in terms of patient expectations, and indicate a time frame.

All outcome criteria should have three major components:
- *content area,* which describes the subject that the patient will focus on or the physiologic or psychological response to be elicited
- *action verb,* which describes how the patient will achieve the goal of the content area
- *time frame,* which is a target date for completion of the expected outcome criterion.

Each criterion also may have criterion modifiers, which add significant details that delineate specified limits for a specific action.

Nursing interventions. After developing the outcome criteria, the nurse determines the interventions needed to help the patient reach the desired behavior or response

NANDA Taxonomy of nursing diagnoses

The currently accepted classification system for nursing diagnoses is that of the North American Nursing Diagnosis Association (NANDA), as shown in *NANDA nursing diagnoses: Definitions and classification 1997-1998.*

Pattern 1. Exchanging: A human response pattern involving mutual giving and receiving

1.1.2.1	Altered nutrition: More than body requirements
1.1.2.2	Altered nutrition: Less than body requirements
1.1.2.3	Altered nutrition: Risk for more than body requirements
1.2.1.1	Risk for infection
1.2.2.1	Risk for altered body temperature
1.2.2.2	Hypothermia
1.2.2.3	Hyperthermia
1.2.2.4	Ineffective thermoregulation
1.2.3.1	Dysreflexia
1.3.1.1	Constipation
1.3.1.1.1	Perceived constipation
1.3.1.1.2	Colonic constipation
1.3.1.2	Diarrhea
1.3.1.3	Bowel incontinence
1.3.2	Altered urinary elimination
1.3.2.1.1	Stress incontinence
1.3.2.1.2	Reflex incontinence
1.3.2.1.3	Urge incontinence
1.3.2.1.4	Functional incontinence
1.3.2.1.5	Total incontinence
1.3.2.2	Urinary retention
1.4.1.1	Altered (specify type) tissue perfusion (renal, cerebral, cardiopulmonary, gastrointestinal, peripheral)
1.4.1.2.1	Fluid volume excess
1.4.1.2.2.1	Fluid volume deficit
1.4.1.2.2.2	Risk for fluid volume deficit
1.4.2.1	Decreased cardiac output
1.5.1.1	Impaired gas exchange
1.5.1.2	Ineffective airway clearance
1.5.1.3	Ineffective breathing pattern
1.5.1.3.1	Inability to sustain spontaneous ventilation
1.5.1.3.2	Dysfunctional ventilatory weaning response
1.6.1	Risk for injury
1.6.1.1	Risk for suffocation
1.6.1.2	Risk for poisoning
1.6.1.3	Risk for trauma
1.6.1.4	Risk for aspiration
1.6.1.5	Risk for disuse syndrome
1.6.2	Altered protection
1.6.2.1	Impaired tissue integrity
1.6.2.1.1	Altered oral mucous membrane
1.6.2.1.2.1	Impaired skin integrity
1.6.2.1.2.2	Risk for impaired skin integrity
1.7.1	Decreased adaptive capacity: Intracranial
1.8	Energy field disturbance

Pattern 2. Communicating: A human response pattern involving sending messages

2.1.1.1	Impaired verbal communication

Pattern 3. Relating: A human response pattern involving establishing bonds

3.1.1	Impaired social interaction
3.1.2	Social isolation
3.1.3	Risk for loneliness
3.2.1	Altered role performance
3.2.1.1.1	Altered parenting
3.2.1.1.2	Risk for altered parenting
3.2.1.1.2.1	Risk for altered parent/infant/child attachment
3.2.1.2.1	Sexual dysfunction
3.2.2	Altered family processes
3.2.2.1	Caregiver role strain
3.2.2.2	Risk for caregiver role strain
3.2.2.3.1	Altered family process: Alcoholism
3.2.3.1	Parental role conflict
3.3	Altered sexuality patterns

Pattern 4. Valuing: A human response pattern involving the assigning of relative worth

4.1.1	Spiritual distress (distress of the human spirit)
4.2	Potential for enhanced spiritual well-being

Pattern 5. Choosing: A human response pattern involving the selection of alternatives

5.1.1.1	Ineffective individual coping
5.1.1.1.1	Impaired adjustment
5.1.1.1.2	Defensive coping
5.1.1.1.3	Ineffective denial
5.1.2.1.1	Ineffective family coping: Disabling
5.1.2.1.2	Ineffective family coping: Compromised
5.1.2.2	Family coping: Potential for growth
5.1.3.1	Potential for enhanced community coping
5.1.3.2	Ineffective community coping
5.2.1	Ineffective management of therapeutic regimen: (individual)
5.2.1.1	Noncompliance (specify)
5.2.2	Ineffective management of therapeutic regimen: (families)
5.2.3	Ineffective management of therapeutic regimen: (community)
5.2.4	Effective management of therapeutic regimen: (individual)
5.3.1.1	Decisional conflict (specify)
5.4	Health-seeking behaviors

Pattern 6. Moving: A human response pattern involving activity

6.1.1.1	Impaired physical mobility
6.1.1.1.1	Risk for peripheral neurovascular dysfunction
6.1.1.1.2	Risk for perioperative postioning injury
6.1.1.2	Activity intolerance
6.1.1.2.1	Fatigue
6.1.1.3	Risk for activity intolerance
6.2.1	Sleep pattern disturbance
6.3.1.1	Diversional activity deficit
6.4.1.1	Impaired home maintenance management
6.4.2	Altered health maintenance
6.5.1	Feeding self-care deficit
6.5.1.1	Impaired swallowing

(continued)

NANDA Taxonomy of nursing diagnoses *(continued)*

Pattern 6. Moving: A human response pattern involving activity *(continued)*

6.5.1.2	Ineffective breast-feeding
6.5.1.2.1	Interrupted breast-feeding
6.5.1.3	Effective breast-feeding
6.5.1.4	Ineffective infant feeding pattern
6.5.2	Bathing or hygiene self-care deficit
6.5.3	Dressing or grooming self-care deficit
6.5.4	Toileting self-care deficit
6.6	Altered growth and development
6.7	Relocation stress syndrome
6.8.1	Risk for disorganized infant behavior
6.8.2	Disorganized infant behavior
6.8.3	Potential for enhanced organized infant behavior

Pattern 7. Perceiving: A human response pattern involving the reception of information

7.1.1	Body image disturbance
7.1.2	Self-esteem disturbance
7.1.2.1	Chronic low self-esteem
7.1.2.2	Situational low self-esteem
7.1.3	Personal identity disturbance
7.2	Sensory or perceptual alterations (specify—visual, auditory, kinesthetic, gustatory, tactile, olfactory)
7.2.1.1	Unilateral neglect
7.3.1	Hopelessness
7.3.2	Powerlessness

Pattern 8. Knowing: A human response pattern involving the meaning associated with information

8.1.1	Knowledge deficit (specify)
8.2.1	Impaired environmental interpretation syndrome
8.2.2	Acute confusion
8.2.3	Chronic confusion
8.3	Altered thought processes
8.3.1	Impaired memory

Pattern 9. Feeling: A human response pattern involving the subjective awareness of information

9.1.1	Pain
9.1.1.1	Chronic pain
9.2.1.1	Dysfunctional grieving
9.2.1.2	Anticipatory grieving
9.2.2	Risk for violence: self-directed or directed at others
9.2.2.1	Risk for self-mutilation
9.2.3	Post-trauma response
9.2.3.1	Rape-trauma syndrome
9.2.3.1.1	Rape-trauma syndrome: Compound reaction
9.2.3.1.2	Rape-trauma syndrome: Silent reaction
9.3.1	Anxiety
9.3.2	Fear

goals. Interventions are the actions that the nurse implements to help the patient meet the identified outcome criteria.

When developing interventions for effective drug therapy, the nurse must include patient teaching. The patient must understand the prescribed drug regimen to enhance compliance and receive maximum therapeutic effect.

Development of an effective patient teaching program parallels the steps of the nursing process. The nurse uses the nursing process to assess patient learning needs, to develop a nursing diagnosis, to develop a teaching plan, to implement the plan, and to evaluate the teaching and learning that occurred. (See *Nursing process and patient teaching.*)

To achieve the optimal effects from drug therapy, the patient must comply with the prescribed regimen. Many factors, categorized as patient characteristics or clinical characteristics, can affect patient compliance. Patient characteristics include demographic, physiologic, drug knowledge, and psychosocial factors. Clinical characteristics include the nurse-patient relationship and the therapeutic regimen.

Implementation

During the implementation step of the nursing process, the nurse puts interventions into action and provides care as described in the **nursing care plan.** By following the care plan and gearing actions toward the outcome criteria, the nurse can implement proposed interventions effectively.

In drug therapy, implementation includes all aspects of medication administration: working with the physician, administering drugs as prescribed, calculating dosages, preparing drugs, using appropriate administration techniques, and modifying techniques for patients with special needs, such as pediatric, geriatric, pregnant, and breast-feeding patients. Other aspects of implementation include staying alert for medication errors, documenting drugs given, and teaching patients about drugs. Implementation also includes monitoring the patient to evaluate the effectiveness of drug therapy.

Evaluation

Integral to the nursing process, evaluation is a formal and systematic procedure for determining the effectiveness of nursing care. Evaluation provides descriptive data that enable the nurse to understand the patient's status and thereby make better-informed decisions about what to change and what to maintain.

The nurse evaluates the care to determine whether the outcome criteria have been met. For example, the nurse might ask the patient if headache relief was achieved within 1 hour after administering a p.r.n. analgesic. If the headache was relieved, the outcome criterion was met. If the headache was better but not completely relieved, the outcome criterion was partially met. If the headache was the same or worse, the outcome criterion was not met. Evaluation enables the

Nursing process and patient teaching

This flow chart demonstrates the steps of the nursing process as they relate to patient teaching.

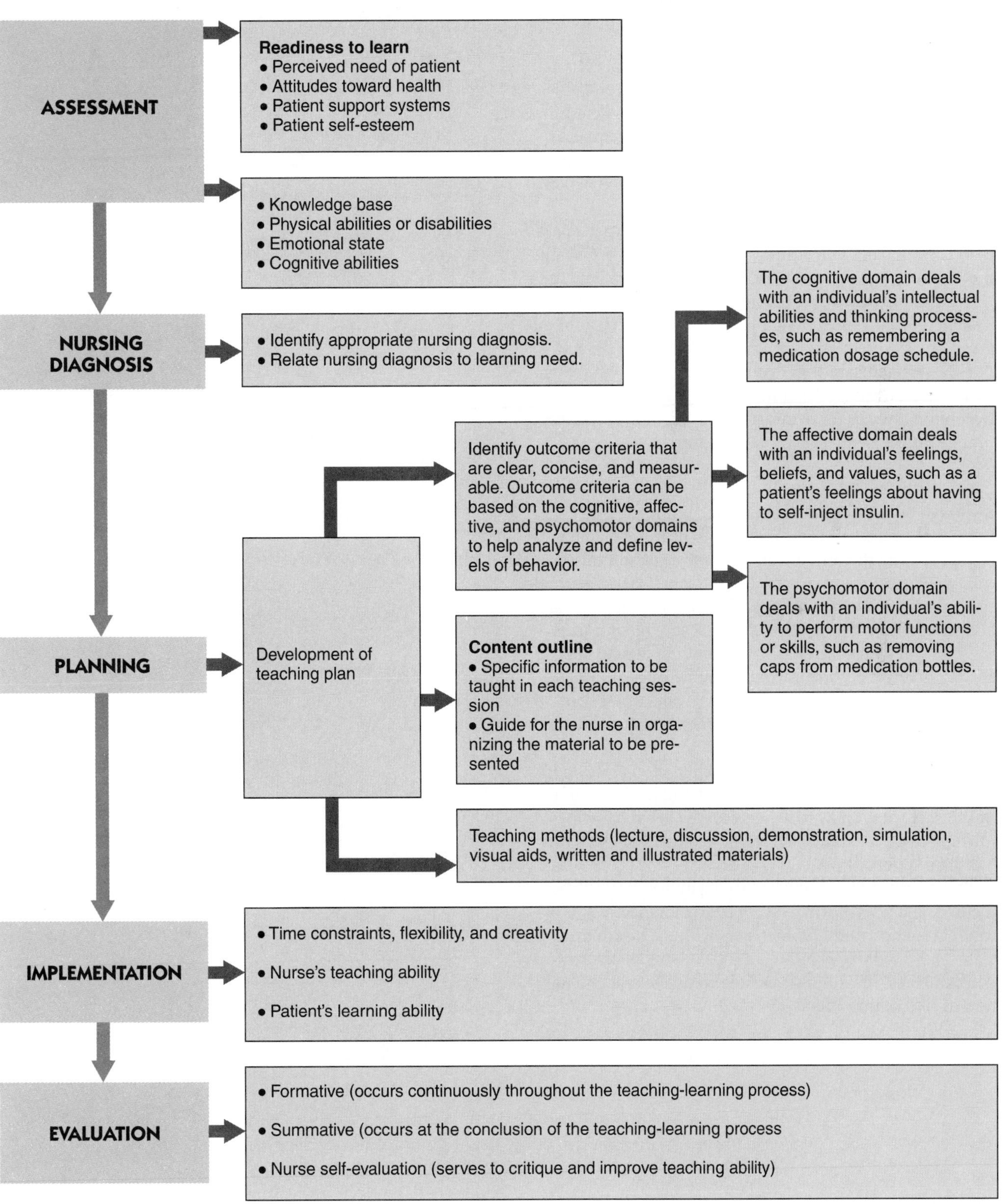

nurse to design and implement a revised nursing care plan, reevaluating outcome criteria continually and replanning until each nursing diagnosis is resolved.

The nurse also can use evaluation to determine whether nursing interventions for drug administration have been effective. To do so, the nurse reassesses for therapeutic effects, adverse drug reactions, and drug interactions.

In addition, the nurse evaluates what the learner has accomplished based on outcome criteria or behavioral objectives. Behaviors specified in the outcome criteria determine how the evaluation should be conducted. For example, if the patient was to *state the action of digoxin at the end of the session,* the evaluation would be based on what the patient said.

Evaluation can help the nurse determine whether a patient is compliant with a prescribed drug regimen. Current methods used to evaluate patient compliance can help the nurse minimize factors that might lead to noncompliance. The methods include physiologic assessment, such as blood pressure measurements, serum or urine drug levels, and other assessments; ratings by health care professionals; patient self-reporting; pill counts; and direct observation. Combining two or more measurement methods produces more accurate evaluation of patient compliance.

Documentation

Although documentation is not a step in the nursing process, the nurse is legally required to document activities related to drug therapy, including the time of administration, the quantity administered, and the patient's reaction to the drug. To deliver the best possible patient care, the nurse also should record evaluation data. Because other nurses must be able to read the evaluation and implement appropriate nursing care, documentation must be clear, concise, and complete. It should begin with an evaluation of outcome criteria and proceed to a reassessment of specific interventions.

The nurse also must document each teaching session in the patient's chart so that other nurses and members of the health care team know what was covered, what patient learning resulted, and which areas need refinement or further instruction.

The chart is one method of sharing information. Other methods include informal health care team meetings, educational rounds, family conferences with the health care team, and discharge planning rounds. Above all, the patient's medical record must include complete documentation of all teaching efforts.

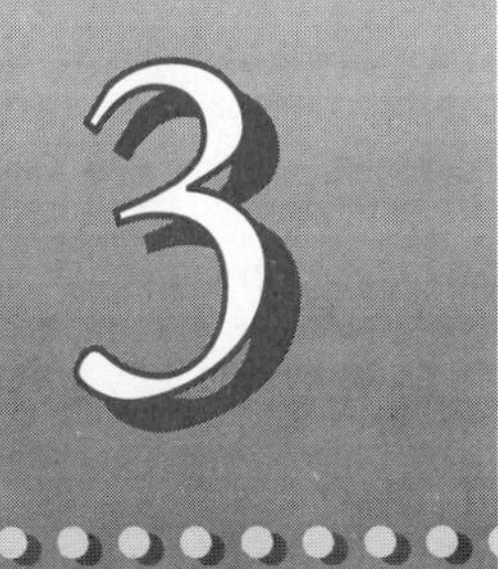

Responsibilities in drug administration

OBJECTIVES

After reading and studying this chapter, the student should be able to:

1. identify the essential components of a properly written medication order.
2. describe the purposes of the seven types of medication orders routinely used in the hospital.
3. describe standard nursing practices that help the nurse achieve the five "rights" of drug administration.
4. define malpractice and describe how it relates to the administration of medications.
5. explain how the nurse applies the principles of autonomy, paternalism, truthfulness, beneficence, fidelity, and respect for property to professional practice.

INTRODUCTION

Chapter 3 discusses the nurse's role in drug administration. It presents essential background information about requirements for medication orders, the nurse's responsibilities in receiving and transcribing medication orders, and the proper procedures for preventing errors during drug administration. It also explores various **legal responsibilities,** such as what the nurse should know and do to administer medications safely, the components that constitute **malpractice,** and the special nursing responsibilities related to controlled drugs. The chapter concludes with a discussion of some of the fundamental values and moral principles that guide nursing practice in medication administration.

Medication orders

Under the law, as outlined in the medical practice act of each state, licensed physicians as well as dentists, podiatrists, and in some states optometrists and nurse practitioners may prescribe, dispense, and administer drugs. In selected circumstances and within certain protocols, other health care professionals, such as nurses, pharmacists, or physician's assistants, may legally prescribe and dispense drugs. Nevertheless, physicians write the vast majority of medication orders. Usually, pharmacists dispense the drugs, and nurses administer them to patients.

REQUIREMENTS FOR MEDICATION ORDERS

A medication order may take one of two forms, depending on whether the prescriber is treating a hospitalized patient or an outpatient. For the hospitalized patient, the prescriber can order medications — along with all other orders, such as those for diet, X-rays, and laboratory work — on the order sheet in the patient's chart. The prescriber also can use a separate medication order sheet. For outpatients, the prescriber usually writes the medication order on a prescription pad sheet and gives it directly to the patient. The patient takes the medication order to a hospital or community pharmacy to be filled. (See *Components of a medication order,* page 38.)

The prescriber's order sheet lists the patient's full name for identification purposes, the generic or trade name of the drug, and its dosage form, if more than one form of the drug is available. The prescriber should also express the dose to be given at each administration, preferably in metric measures, and should state the administration route.

The prescriber usually states the time schedule for administration as the number of times per day that the medication is to be administered. Upon noting the time schedule, the nurse then schedules the specific hours according to how quickly a supply of the medication can be procured, the medication's characteristics, and institutional policies. The medication's characteristics, including its nature and onset and duration of action, primarily determine the schedule. For instance, if regular, intermittent peak blood concentration levels of antibiotics must be maintained to combat infections, the prescriber will schedule the drug administration at regular intervals around the clock.

To a lesser extent, institutional policy determines the schedule, such as a 10 a.m. administration for all drugs given only once a day. Sometimes, the specific responses of the patient to the illness and treatment determine the administration schedule. For example, the nurse may receive an order to administer 5 units of regular insulin to a diabetic patient whenever the blood glucose level exceeds 210 mg/dl.

The prescriber's signature, along with the date and time of day the order was written, also should appear. The date

Components of a medication order

The prescriber writes medication orders for hospitalized patients on an order sheet in the patient's chart. As shown in the sample below, the medication order should give the patient's full name, the name of the drug, the dosage form, the dose amount, the administration route, the time schedule, the prescriber's signature, and the date and time of the order. (*Note:* Prescriber's order sheets vary from one health care facility to another.)

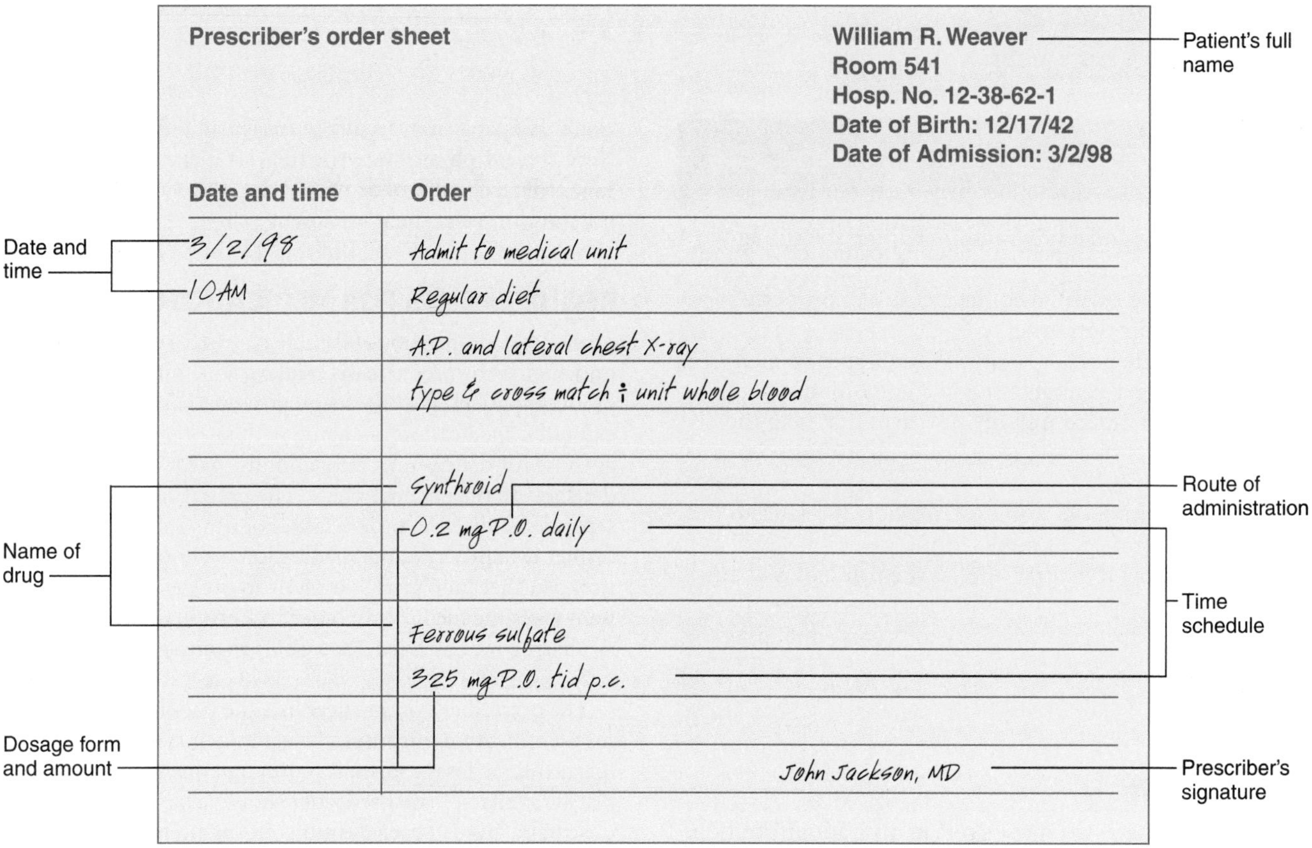

Prescriber's order sheet

William R. Weaver
Room 541
Hosp. No. 12-38-62-1
Date of Birth: 12/17/42
Date of Admission: 3/2/98

Date and time	Order
3/2/98	Admit to medical unit
10 AM	Regular diet
	A.P. and lateral chest X-ray
	type & cross match ī unit whole blood
	Synthroid
	0.2 mg P.O. daily
	Ferrous sulfate
	325 mg P.O. tid p.c.
	John Jackson, MD

and time are often referred to when the order has an expiration date. For example, a narcotic order valid for 72 hours, written at noon on August 21, will expire three days later, at noon on August 24.

Outpatient medication orders usually are written as **prescriptions.** Before the patient leaves the outpatient setting, the nurse should clarify for the patient any abbreviations used in the prescription. By clarifying any doubtful abbreviations, the nurse can help avoid subsequent misinterpretation of the prescription by the patient.

Outpatients must fill most prescriptions for controlled substances within 6 months of the date written and cannot refill the prescription more than five times. Many prescriptions also will indicate whether the pharmacist should fill the prescription with generic or trade name products. If unspecified, most states allow the pharmacist to dispense the generic form of the drug, which may reduce the patient's expense. Patients should be aware that they have the right to ask the prescriber to write the prescription for the generic drug.

Besides the previously mentioned prescription requirements, all states now require the pharmacist to label each prescription container with the name, strength, and drug amount dispensed. These requirements contribute significantly to the patient's knowledge and understanding of the treatment regimen.

TYPES OF MEDICATION ORDERS

The following seven types of medication orders are routine in the hospital: standard written orders, single orders, stat orders, p.r.n. orders, standing orders, verbal (or oral) orders, and telephone orders.

Standard written orders

These orders apply indefinitely until the prescriber writes another order to alter or discontinue the first one. In some cases, the prescriber may specify on the standard written order a particular termination date. In many cases, hospitals establish policies that indicate how long orders for certain classes of drugs remain valid. Examples of drugs with controlled termination dates include narcotic orders for 3 days and antibiotic orders for 7 days. If the patient still needs the drug after the expiration date, the prescriber must rewrite the order. The prescriber also must rewrite standard written orders postoperatively if the medications are to be continued.

Single orders

These orders are written for medications that are given only once. For example, a prescriber may order one tetanus toxoid injection for a patient with a laceration or puncture wound who received a primary tetanus toxoid series more than 10 years earlier.

Stat orders

Calls for medications that are to be administered immediately for an urgent patient problem are known as stat orders. For instance, a prescriber may order a single dose of an antianxiety drug to calm an acutely agitated patient.

p.r.n. orders

Orders called p.r.n. orders derive their name from a Latin phrase that means "as the occasion arises." Prescribers write p.r.n. orders for medications that are to be given when needed. The administration time results from the collaborative judgments of the nurse and the patient. Sometimes a p.r.n. order delineates the reason for giving the drug. For example, the prescriber may write "Tylenol 650 mg P.O. p.r.n. for a temperature above 101.3° F (38.5° C)." If an ordered drug such as acetaminophen (Tylenol) serves multiple purposes, some hospital policies state that the nurse administer the drug only for the specific condition mentioned in the order. Under such a policy, the nurse would not give Tylenol ordered only for fever if the patient complained of a headache but had no fever. Other institutions allow the nurse to determine when to administer a p.r.n. drug. When administering a p.r.n. medication, the nurse should describe in the patient's record the reason for its use and its degree of subsequent effectiveness.

Standing orders

Also known as protocols, standing orders establish guidelines for treating a particular disease or set of symptoms. These orders require considerable judgment and expertise in assessing the patient's need for the medication and any dose-related adverse drug reactions that might occur.

Special care areas of the hospital, such as the coronary care unit, routinely establish standing orders that apply to such drug therapies as morphine sulfate for chest pain and anxiety, lidocaine (Xylocaine) for ventricular tachycardia, and furosemide (Lasix) for pulmonary congestion. Hospitals also may institute medication protocols that specifically designate drugs that a nurse may *not* give. For example, a nurse who is not certified in cardiac care but "floats" to a cardiac stepdown unit, may not be permitted to administer metoprolol (Lopressor) by intravenous (I.V.) push.

Verbal orders

Medication orders given orally rather than in writing are known as verbal orders. Health care professionals try to avoid using verbal orders because such orders can lead to miscommunication. In urgent situations, the nurse should write and sign the order dictated by the prescriber. Then the nurse should repeat the order aloud for the prescriber's verification and request the prescriber to spell the drug name if necessary. The prescriber should sign the verbal order that the nurse has written as soon as possible. The institution should have a policy that dictates the time period in which the prescriber must sign a verbal order. If the prescriber will administer the medication but verbally requests it, the nurse should show the prescriber the label on the medication container while simultaneously stating the drug's name and handing the drug to the prescriber. Such actions allow the prescriber to confirm the accuracy of the drug and its dose.

Telephone orders

Verbal orders given to a nurse by a prescriber over the telephone may result in dangerous errors from mechanical problems involving the telephone and from the lack of nonverbal communication cues between the prescriber and nurse. Nurses should avoid telephone orders whenever possible. When a nurse must take a telephone order, the nurse should ask another nurse to monitor the call on an extension telephone. By monitoring the call, the second nurse can confirm the order. Besides verifying the drug name given during a telephone order, the nurse should repeat orally the individual digits of the dose. Repeating the order gives the prescriber the opportunity to confirm or correct the order. The nurse then writes the order, indicating that it was a telephone order. Later, the prescriber must cosign the order within the time period established by institutional policy.

Unusual circumstances

The nurse will encounter situations related to the standard written order that require considerable nursing judgment in deciding whether and how to give the drug. On some occasions, the nurse may omit or at least delay a dose. This frequently occurs for patients prohibited from ingesting anything in preparation for certain diagnostic tests. In such cases, the nurse should confer with the prescriber. The nurse and prescriber may decide to omit the drug, give the drug orally with a very small amount of water, administer the drug by another route, or give the drug orally after completion of the test. Other circumstances may arise in which the nurse intentionally omits a dose of medication because the patient no longer needs it. For example, the nurse may omit a laxative dose if the patient has had a bowel movement since the medication order. The nurse sometimes omits medications because the patient refuses to take them.

In all instances in which patients do not receive an ordered medication, the nurse should indicate the omission on the medication administration record, describe the reason for the omission, and notify the patient's prescriber immediately if appropriate to do so.

Preventing medication errors

The safe, accurate administration of medications demands that the nurse possess current, pertinent drug knowledge and follow safe procedures. From the beginning of a nursing student's professional preparation, educators make every effort to ensure the progressive accumulation of adequate knowledge about drug therapy.

Knowing about drugs as well as the factors to observe when preparing and administering each drug helps the nurse avoid medication errors. So does preparing medications in a quiet area, conducive to concentration.

After receiving a written order, the nurse transcribes it onto the appropriate working document approved by the hospital. The working document may be a medication administration record (MAR), a medication Kardex, medication cards or tickets, or a computer printout. Because the chance for error increases with the repeated copying of orders, the nurse must read each order carefully and prepare the medications directly from the approved document. The nurse must never rely on memory or personal worksheet notations. As a precaution against omitted orders, the established practices of many hospitals require the nurse to check periodically all MARs against the original order sheet. Also, the nurse preparing the change-of-shift report usually alerts the oncoming staff to any new medication orders.

THE FIVE "RIGHTS" OF MEDICATION ADMINISTRATION

Classic safeguards, known as the five "rights," exist to ensure accurate medication administration. Although the five "rights" — the right drug, dose, patient, time, and route — address various issues, health care professionals generally regard the safeguards as the minimum requirements for safety. Much additional forethought is required before any medication is administered.

Right drug

While working with the vast number of today's available drugs, the nurse must discriminate carefully among similar-sounding names. For example, digoxin (Lanoxin), digitoxin (Crystodigin), and Desoxyn (methamphetamine) all have similar-sounding names but are very different drugs. Digoxin and digitoxin represent different forms of the cardiac drug digitalis; Desoxyn is a drug used for weight reduction. The nurse always should compare the name of the drug on the container label to the medication order. For medications that are individually wrapped in single doses, the nurse should check the name when removing the drug from the drawer and again when unwrapping and giving the drug to the patient.

Before administering any drug, the nurse should tell the patient its name and action or use. Anytime a patient comments that the medication seems unusual, the nurse should recheck the drug name and strength. For example, a patient may say, "Nurse, this can't be my medication. I always take one pink pill, but you've given me two yellow pills." As a result, the nurse may discover a medication error or need to explain to the patient that the pink pill contains 10 mg of the drug whereas one yellow pill contains 5 mg of the same drug. Any patient comment mandates that the nurse explore the situation before administering the drug.

Right dose

The widespread use of unit-dose medications, individually wrapped and labeled single doses, has alleviated many problems related to drug dosage. Also, the many commercially prepared medications, available in various size tablets, decreases the number of calculations that the nurse must make to determine the dosage. The nurse should develop the standard practice of first mentally calculating the approximate dose, then calculating the actual dose in writing, using the correct formulas. For example, when giving 75 mg of a drug labeled 50 mg/ml, the nurse can mentally estimate the dosage to be 1.5 ml. Then the nurse can calculate the definitive dose by using the following formula:

$$50 : 1 :: 75 : X$$
$$50X = 75$$
$$X = 1.5 \text{ ml}$$

The nurse should recheck all calculations with another nurse or the pharmacist when possible. Many hospitals require double checks of dosage calculations for children's medications and for all drugs with narrow safety margins, such as heparin and insulin. Because more than one or two dosage units rarely are needed to prepare a prescribed dose, the nurse always should recheck the dosage if the calculations call for more than one tablet for a single dose or for a very small fraction of a dosage. The nurse also must be especially careful using decimal points because a misplaced or obscured decimal point can increase the dose many times or decrease it to a fraction of the intended dose. The nurse always should write a zero in front of a decimal point so that no one misreads a figure, such as 0.25 mg as 25 mg. Likewise, a zero should never follow a dosage that includes a decimal point because it easily could be misread and could increase the dosage tenfold. For example, the nurse should not write 0.250 for a dosage of 0.25 mg.

Occasionally, the nurse encounters unusual situations that cause difficulty in measuring the precise dose because of the supplied drug's form. The nurse should not break unscored tablets because the resulting doses will not be exact. The nurse should confer with the pharmacist to have an inconvenient form of a drug changed into a form that can be measured accurately.

The nurse must never alter the dosage specified in the prescriber's order. For example, at the time of surgery, a physician orders 75 mg of meperidine (Demerol) for pain for the postoperative patient. The nurse later observes that the patient remains in excruciating pain and that the 75 mg of Demerol does not seem to be sufficient. The nurse may believe that 100 mg of Demerol would alleviate the patient's pain, but the nurse does *not* have the prerogative to change the dose. The nurse should consult with the physician and obtain a new written order. In many instances, prescribers now write medication orders with dosage ranges so that the nurse can decide the appropriate dose within the specified range.

Right patient

The nurse always should check the patient's identification bracelet carefully against the MAR before giving any medication. As a further check, the nurse should ask the patient to state his or her name. The nurse should not suggest the patient's name because a patient may misunderstand the name or become confused and answer to the wrong name. Furthermore, the nurse should never assume that the patient in a correctly labeled bed is the right patient. A confused patient may get into the wrong bed.

Right time

Most hospitals establish routine times for drug administration. When administering a drug for which a consistent blood concentration level must be maintained to achieve therapeutic effects, the nurse observes equal time intervals around the clock. The nurse also may have to measure certain patient responses to a therapy before administering another dose. For instance, the nurse should check the patient's apical pulse rate before giving a digitalis preparation and assess the patient's respiratory rate before administering a drug such as morphine.

For a drug with no dictating features, the nurse may space the divided doses over the patient's waking hours. Spacing the daily dosage serves to prevent adverse effects, which might be caused by a too-high concentration of the drug in the bloodstream at any given time. Sometimes, the nurse must consider other events, such as mealtime, when administering a drug.

By administering all drugs at evenly spaced intervals and at consistent times each day, the nurse can prevent errors and accommodate the patient's daily schedule. Routine administration schedules also help the patient develop the habit of taking the drug at a regular time. As a result, the patient is less likely to forget the drug after returning home.

The nurse should avoid scheduling medication administration at busy hours on the nursing unit, such as during a shift change. Instead of scheduling a twice-daily (b.i.d.) medication for 8 a.m. and 6 p.m., the nurse could schedule the administration for 9 a.m. and 7 p.m. to avoid the busy 8 a.m. hour after the shift change. Regardless of the exact schedule, the nurse should follow standard practice and allow a half hour before and after the designated time for medication administration. In many institutions, medications given beyond these time limits are considered errors.

Sustained-action drugs

Nurses increasingly encounter drugs designed to achieve an extended action over many hours. Prepared to dissolve at different rates, the drugs are released gradually but continuously into the bloodstream. Convenient for the patient, sustained-action drugs require fewer doses per day and provide more even control of symptoms.

Sustained-action drugs are supplied as plain tablets, coated tablets, and capsules filled with tiny granules. These drugs may be identified by "SA" after the drug name or by many prefixes used in the drug name to indicate prolonged effect. Common examples include Quinaglute *Dura-Tabs,* Dimetapp *Extentabs,* Chlor-Trimeton *Repetabs,* and Desoxyn *Gradumet.* Other names sometimes used include spansules, gyrocaps, and plateau caps.

The nurse must know that sustained-action tablets should never be split, crushed, or chewed and that capsules should never be emptied into foods or beverages because doing so may alter the absorption rates, causing adverse reactions or a subtherapeutic level of activity. The nurse must be certain that the patient understands the importance of taking the sustained-action drug in its supplied form.

Right route

The nurse must pay careful attention to the administration route specified in the medication order and on the product label. Some drugs must be given in certain manufactured forms to be appropriate for particular entry routes into the body. For example, the eye, with its delicate nature, requires special preparations. Also, the nurse should never inject a solution anywhere into the body unless the label clearly indicates that the solution is *for injection.*

The administration route also may affect the amount of the medication given. If given intramuscularly (I.M.), 10 mg of morphine sulfate, a frequently used adult dose, relieves pain. If the drug is given I.V., the equivalent dose would decrease to 2 to 4 mg. If given orally, the morphine sulfate dose would need to be greater than 10 mg.

The procedure used to administer a drug also may affect the rate of drug absorption into the bloodstream. Some topical ointments, such as nitroglycerin paste, enter the bloodstream more rapidly and completely if spread over a large surface area and covered with plastic wrap or special paper supplied with the medication. On the other hand, crushing enteric-coated tablets or opening sustained-action capsules and dissolving the drug in liquid will result in improper absorption of the drug into the bloodstream and possibly unintended effects. (See *Sustained-action drugs.*)

PROCEDURAL SAFEGUARDS

Besides acknowledging the minimum requirements of the five "rights," the nurse practices other procedural safeguards

Nursing responsibilities associated with medication administration

When giving medication to any patient, the nurse must:

1. Assess the patient's physiologic and psychosocial status.
2. Form nursing diagnoses that identify actual or potential responses requiring nursing intervention.
3. Administer the right drug in the right dose to the right patient at the right time by the right route.
4. Assess the patient's responses to drug therapy and determine if the drug is producing therapeutic or adverse effects.
5. Question medication orders that are not clear or that appear to be inappropriate for the patient.
6. Inform the prescriber of necessary deviations in medication administration and of adverse patient reactions to drug therapy.
7. Teach the patient about the safe, therapeutic self-administration of drugs.
8. Evaluate the effectiveness of nursing interventions.

to prevent errors. (See *Nursing responsibilities associated with medication administration.*) This section discusses several special precautions, but the list is not all-inclusive. The nurse always should think of safety and analyze situations that could lead to medication errors.

• Health care professionals should handle and store drugs carefully to maintain the drugs' stability and strength. Because temperature, air, moisture, and light may affect a drug's stability, the nurse should follow drug-specific precautions. The nurse always should keep drugs in the containers in which the pharmacy dispensed them. Bottles should be capped tightly and stored away from sources of heat, light, and moisture. Ordinarily, drugs are stored at room temperature. Only those drugs that require cool temperatures are refrigerated because refrigeration causes moisture formation through condensation. Usually, the nurse allows refrigerated drugs to reach room temperature before administration.

• The law requires that narcotics and controlled substances be kept under lock and key.

• The nurse always should note a drug's expiration date — the date after which the original potency of the drug is believed to change. The nurse should never administer an outdated drug or one that looks or smells unusual. If the manufacturer's drug package appears to have been tampered with, the nurse should not administer the drug but should return the package to the pharmacy for investigation. Drugs to be dispensed as powders may be reconstituted at administration time. Any unused medication should be labeled with the date, time, strength, and the nurse's initials or signature. The nurse should discard any drug that will remain stable for only a short time and will reach its expiration date before another dose is scheduled. The nurse should never administer a drug that has not been labeled properly after reconstitution. If the nurse finds an unlabeled syringe containing a medication, the nurse should discard it.

• When delivering drugs to a patient's room, the nurse should stay with the medication cart or tray. The nurse should never leave without locking the cart and taking it or the tray back to the medication room or to the usual storage place. The nurse should remain until the patient takes the medication to verify that it was taken as directed and should never leave medication doses at the patient's bedside unless a specific order to do so exists.

• The nurse should administer only medications prepared personally or by the pharmacist, unwrapping individual doses (unit doses) at the patient's bedside just before administration.

• Before administering a medication based on new orders, the nurse should review the patient's medication history to detect any known allergies or other idiosyncracies. The chart of any patient who has allergies should be labeled clearly.

• When administering an oral drug, the nurse should encourage the patient to drink a full glass of water, if appropriate. The water helps to move the medication through the esophagus and into the stomach and dilutes the drug, reducing the chance of gastric irritation.

• The prescriber must order drugs that are to be left at the patient's bedside for self-administration. Such drugs should be marked with the patient's name, the drug name and dose, and instructions. The nurse remains responsible for supervising a patient whose drugs are left at the bedside. For example, the nurse must know how many nitroglycerin tablets the patient took, the exact times of self-administration, whether the patient obtained relief, and any unusual reactions to the drug. The nurse must record the information in the chart and report it to the prescriber.

• The nurse should chart drugs immediately after administering them. Delayed charting, especially of p.r.n. medications, can result in an error of repeated doses; early charting (charting before giving the medication) may result in omitted doses.

• The nurse should record observations of the patient's positive and negative responses to the medication. Severe adverse reactions may prompt the prescriber to substitute another drug.

Legal responsibilities

Chapter 1 discussed the sources and types of laws governing drug administration. This section covers specific nursing responsibilities imposed by the law. Practice acts passed by the legislature of each state govern the practice of each of the major health professions. Therefore, the **nurse practice act,** medical practice act, and pharmacy practice act of each state represent statutory laws and determine the scope of practice for those professionals. Essentially, practice acts allow physicians to prescribe, dispense, and administer drugs; pharmacists to prepare, dispense, and furnish drugs to the patient; and nurses to administer medications and, if licensed to do so, prescribe. Also, the Controlled Substances

Act, a federal legislation, regulates the manner in which narcotics and other controlled substances are dispensed and administered, thus directly affecting nursing practice.

EXPECTATIONS OF THE LAW

The law expects nurses who administer drugs to patients to know about those drugs. The nurse should know the goals of the drug therapy, the drug's mechanism of action, expected and unusual effects, dosage, proper administration methods, and any contraindications. The nurse also should assess the patient's medication responses and teach the patient about self-administration. The nurse practice acts in some states specifically include patient teaching as a legal expectation.

On receiving a medication order, the nurse should consider it carefully. If any part of the order seems unusual, the nurse should not implement it until clarifying the problem with the prescriber. Under no circumstances should the nurse *ignore* the medication order and fail to carry it out. The nurse has an obligation to seek clarification of any questions concerning the order. Sometimes nurses are reluctant to approach a prescriber and question an order for fear of being rebuked. Questioning a medication order requires assertiveness and tact on the nurse's part. Frequently, nurses consult pharmacists or approved published drug references to confirm their knowledge of the drug before approaching a prescriber. When questioning an order, the nurse should discuss the matter with the prescriber privately, professionally, and with an attitude of objective scientific inquiry. If the prescriber's explanation is unacceptable, the nurse must notify the supervisor and withhold the medication until further clarification of the order is received.

CRITICAL THINKING: To enhance your critical thinking about responsibilities in drug administration, consider the following situation and its analysis.

Situation: Mildred Brown, age 78, has just been admitted to the floor from the emergency department with heart failure and renal failure. For the past year, she has been taking the following medications as prescribed: digoxin 0.25 mg P.O. daily, Lasix 20 mg P.O. daily, Colace 100 mg P.O. daily, and potassium chloride 10 mEq P.O. b.i.d.

When assessing Mrs. Brown, the nurse discovers these findings: recent loss of appetite and onset of nausea, vomiting, and diarrhea; reports of blurred vision with yellow-green halos; apical and radial pulses of 50 beats/minute; and blood pressure of 96/70 mm Hg. Written admission orders for this patient include digoxin 0.25 mg I.V. stat. Should the nurse administer the drug as ordered?

Analysis: Because Mrs. Brown displays signs of digitalis toxicity (bradycardia and GI symptoms), the nurse should withhold the digoxin dose and call the physician, despite the written orders. Digoxin administration is contraindicated in patients with digitalis-induced toxicity and requires extreme caution in geriatric patients and those with renal failure, such as Mrs. Brown. After consulting together, the nurse and physician may decide to omit this dose of digoxin.

MALPRACTICE

Malpractice refers to a professional's wrongful conduct, improper discharge of duties, or failure to meet standards of care that causes harm to another. **Negligence** is a form of malpractice. Negligence refers to the failure to do something that reasonably could be expected to be done by an individual in a given situation or the performance of an act that a reasonable and prudent person would not do.

Under the law, nurses are judged to be responsible for their own actions. Thus, upon the implementation of an incorrect order, the nurse as well as the prescriber and the hospital may be held legally liable. Medication errors resulting in malpractice may take two forms: errors of omission and errors of commission. An error of omission occurs when the nurse omits an important part of care. For example, a nurse who overlooks a patient's 2 p.m. dose of cimetidine (Tagamet) makes an error of omission. An error of commission occurs when the nurse performs a procedure improperly. For example, a nurse administers 3 ml (0.15 mg) of digoxin (Lanoxin) to an infant I.M. rather than orally, and the infant suffers cardiac arrest. The nurse has made an error of commission.

Although malpractice may sound harsh, especially to the beginning nursing student, the student may feel reassured by learning that the law does not expect the nurse to be infallible. The law does expect sound knowledge, good judgment, and due care. Because medication errors, along with falls, rank at the top of the list of causes of malpractice suits, the nurse must safeguard against medication errors by carefully considering and following the five "rights" of medication administration.

Further legal expectations of the nurse arise when an error occurs. Upon discovery of the error, the nurse should (1) immediately notify the prescriber, the nursing supervisor, and the pharmacist — that is, *only* those personnel who can do something to rectify the error; (2) carefully assess the patient's condition and render care as necessary; and (3) complete a medication error incident report.

Medication error incident reports

Most hospitals include medication error incident reports among their unusual incident forms. The medication error incident report typically requires a clear description of the event, including the time and date of the error and what the nurse did about it. The prescriber completes a section describing the patient's condition and any medical action taken. The nurse should not neglect to fill out a medication error incident report for fear that the report will be used in disciplinary action. Administrative personnel can use medication error incident reports to help improve patient care by implementing policies or procedures to prevent similar errors from occurring in the future.

Circulation of a medication error incident report should be limited to administrative personnel who need to know the facts about a specific incident. The medication error incident report usually is not placed in the patient's chart, but the nurse's charting on the patient's record should explain what happened and what actions subsequently were taken.

CONTROLLED SUBSTANCES

The Controlled Substances Act of the federal government imposes a few special responsibilities on the nurse. Under its provisions, the nurse must account for the proper use of controlled drugs with specific patients. Thus, when administering a narcotic, a barbiturate, or another controlled drug, the nurse must sign for the drug on a special narcotics record. Every dose that the pharmacy dispenses must be accounted for, whether the dose was used for a particular patient or was discarded accidentally. Most hospitals require change-of-shift controlled substance or narcotics counts to assure that the supply on hand correlates exactly with the records.

The law also requires that controlled drugs be stored in locked cabinets. The nurse maintains the narcotics supply under lock and key. The nurse always should carry the narcotics keys, never leaving them in a drawer or hung on a hook where unauthorized persons could have access to them.

Ethical obligations

Nursing ethics represent the application of moral principles and values to professional practice. Whereas legal affairs concern rights and correlated responsibilities, **ethical responsibility** deals with the duties and obligations that the nurse has to self, patients, and professional colleagues. Conflicts of value can occur when the nurse, patient, and physician express differences of opinion about what actions to take in a particular situation.

Ethical conflicts always have existed in nursing but have become prominent today because of the quality-of-life issue. Rapidly advancing technology often prolongs life, resulting in conditions that some people may want to avoid.

Moral principles

The nurse applies six moral principles when considering all types of patient care, including medication administration. These principles are autonomy, paternalism, truthfulness, beneficence, fidelity, and respect for property. In analyzing ethical issues involving these principles, the nurse emphasizes:

- What is morally right and therefore ought to be done?
- What benefits and harms would result from this action?
- Who would be benefited or harmed?

Autonomy refers to the right of every person to make rational decisions about one's life. The nurse's belief in autonomy leads to a respect for the patient's decisions. The nurse must assess each patient and consider the patient's decision regarding medication administration.

Paternalism results when someone decides what is best for another person and acts without consulting the person. Anyone acting paternalistically toward a patient must consider whether the action is justifiable.

The nurse may practice justified paternalism when administering pain medication to a terminally ill patient who may refuse medication because the drug causes drowsiness. The nurse knows the positive and negative consequences of the medication and convinces the patient to take the medication by deemphasizing the drug's sedative effects. In such a situation, the nurse's justified paternalism benefits the patient.

Truthfulness refers to being honest. The nurse displays truthfulness by not withholding information. The nurse must answer all questions honestly and provide or seek further information if necessary.

Beneficence refers to the concept that nursing actions always should cause beneficial effects, never harmful ones. All nursing procedures are based on the principle of beneficence. The nurse always should plan and implement actions that assure safe outcomes for the patient and avoid negative consequences, which might cause harm. Hence, the nurse reads drug labels repeatedly, double-checks dosage calculations, and compares the patient's identification band to the name on the medication order.

Fidelity requires the nurse to be faithful and truthful and to keep promises made to self, patients, families, coworkers, and employers. A nurse should not make a promise to a patient without absolute certainty that the promise can be kept.

Respect for property refers to the safekeeping of the patient's personal possessions. If a patient brings medications to the hospital, most hospitals require that the nurse take the medications from the patient upon admission and store them to prevent double dosing or undesirable drug interactions. The patient, however, must consent to the storage, and the nurse must return the medications to the patient upon discharge. Medications ordered from the pharmacy become the patient's personal property even though the nurse keeps the drugs in the medication cart and administers them.

Placebos

Placebos (substances such as glucose pills and saline solution injections, used for nonspecific, psychological effects without the patient's immediate knowledge that a placebo is being given) create certain ethical quandaries. Placebo use requires the nurse to withhold information, which violates the moral principle of truthfulness. Traditionally, physicians and nurses have not told patients about placebos because doing so usually diminishes the chance of the placebo producing the desired effect. The success of placebo use seems to depend on a patient's susceptibility.

Health care professionals who administer placebos should acknowledge the extenuating circumstances and comply with the following guidelines:

- Use a placebo only after careful diagnosis.
- Use only an inert substance.
- Answer questions as truthfully as possible.
- Honor the patient's request if the patient specifically asks not to receive a placebo.
- Never give a placebo when other treatment is indicated or before exploring all treatment options.

CHAPTER SUMMARY

Chapter 3 presented the nurse's role in medication administration. Here are the chapter highlights.

Medication orders usually originate with the physician or other prescriber and vary in form, depending on whether they apply to a hospitalized patient or to an outpatient. Prescribers write medication orders for hospitalized patients along with or in addition to all other medical orders.

Requirements of the medication order include the patient's full name; the name, dose, and dosage form of the drug; the administration route; the schedule; the prescriber's signature; and the date and time. Prescribers write medication orders for outpatients as prescriptions.

Seven types of medication orders are routine in the hospital: standard written, single, stat, p.r.n., standing, verbal, and telephone.

Classic safeguards, known as the five "rights," exist to ensure accurate medication administration. Nurses ensure that they are giving the right drug and the right dose of the drug. Nurses also should check the patient's identification to ensure that they are giving the drug to the right patient. They also must establish and verify the right time for drug administration. Finally, nurses must be sure that they use the right administration route when giving a drug to a patient. The medication order and the drug product label specify the administration route.

Other procedural safeguards, such as checking expiration dates, staying with the patient until the patient has taken the medication, and recording observations of patient responses to the medication, can help the nurse prevent medication errors.

The law expects the nurse administering medications to possess sound knowledge and good judgment and to exercise due care in executing procedures. The nurse is obligated to clarify any unusual or unclear medication orders with the prescriber before implementing them. The nurse cannot ignore a medication order, but can refuse to administer a medication if the prescriber cannot explain the order satisfactorily.

Causes of malpractice include errors of omission, in which the nurse fails to give necessary care, and errors of commission, in which the nurse renders necessary care in an improper way. The nurse can be held liable for a patient's injury if the injury directly results from the nurse's action.

The nurse must apply fundamental values and moral principles to professional nursing practice. Moral principles that the nurse applies when considering patient care include autonomy, paternalism, truthfulness, beneficence, fidelity, and respect for property.

Questions to consider

See Appendix 1 for answers.

1. Stephen Phillips, age 22, is admitted to the hospital with uncontrolled diabetes mellitus. The physician prescribes 5 units of regular insulin S.C. stat. When should the nurse administer this medication?
   (a) At bedtime
   (b) Immediately
   (c) As the occasion arises
   (d) When the patient requests it

2. Sandra Dillon, age 39, is scheduled to receive codeine sulfate, 15 mg P.O. at 7 a.m. Before administering this medication, the nurse must ensure that the drug is being given to the right patient. What is the best way to do this?
   (a) Check the identification bracelet against the name on the bed.
   (b) Check the identification bracelet against the name on the chart.
   (c) Check the identification bracelet and ask the patient her name.
   (d) Check the identification bracelet and call the patient by name.

3. The nurse receives a medication order for Jack Germaine, age 68, with a dosage that seems unusually high. How should the nurse proceed?
   (a) Administer the drug exactly as prescribed.
   (b) Question the physician about the dosage.
   (c) Ignore the medication order.
   (d) Have another nurse double-check the order.

4. John Green, RN, has just realized that he gave Dora Platt, age 62, 1.25 mg of digoxin I.V., rather than 0.125 mg as prescribed. Which of the following nursing responses is *not* appropriate?
   (a) Immediately notify the physician and the nursing supervisor.
   (b) Immediately notify the physician and fill out a medication error incident report and place it on the patient's chart.
   (c) Assess the patient's condition and provide care as necessary.
   (d) Complete a medication error incident report and submit it to administrative personnel.

5. After the physician tells Ellen Hurst, age 58, that she will need to take insulin daily at home, she refuses to do it. When the nurse explains what will happen to her if she does not take the insulin, Ms. Hurst reluctantly consents to regular insulin therapy. In this situation, the nurse is demonstrating a belief in which of the following moral principles?

(a) Beneficence
(b) Paternalism
(c) Truthfulness
(d) Fidelity

6. Neil Johnson, age 41, has chronic back pain. His physician has ordered Demerol 50 mg I.M. q 3 hours p.r.n. The physician's order also states, "may give normal saline 1 ml I.M. as a placebo p.r.n." Mr. Johnson's last Demerol dose was 1½ hours ago, yet he is already reporting pain. Which of the following nursing actions is *most* appropriate?

(a) Give Mr. Johnson 1 ml of normal saline I.M. and tell him it is his regular dose of Demerol.
(b) Increase the Demerol dose to 75 mg I.M. and give it to Mr. Johnson early.
(c) Carefully reassess Mr. Johnson's condition and consult with the physician about his pain management.
(d) Give Mr. Johnson 25 mg of Demerol and 1 ml of normal saline, telling him that it is a larger dose of pain medication.

4 Dosage measurements and calculations

OBJECTIVES

After reading and studying this chapter, the student should be able to:

1. explain the advantages of the metric system over the apothecaries' and household systems of measurement.
2. give at least two clinical examples of how the metric, apothecaries', and household systems of measurement are used in medication administration.
3. identify two drugs that use special systems of measurement developed by the manufacturers.
4. use the fraction and ratio methods to calculate the dosage of a drug ordered in one system of measurement but available only in another system of measurement.
5. perform the calculations for reconstituting a powdered drug for injection, an intravenous (I.V.) infusion rate, and a percentage solution, using the fraction and ratio methods.

INTRODUCTION

This chapter contains information related to administering safe, accurate dosages of drugs — a major responsibility for nurses. It begins by discussing the major systems of drug weights and measures, including their characteristics and units for liquid and solid measures. It also provides examples of physicians' orders for drugs measured in each system. Then the chapter explains conversions between the systems of measurement and presents methods for calculating drug dosages within each system of drug weights and measures. Sample problems and their solutions appear throughout the chapter to assist in the step-by-step approach needed to calculate correct dosages. The chapter concludes with a discussion of special considerations related to dosage calculations for pediatric and geriatric patients.

Systems of drug weights and measures

Physicians use several systems of measurement when ordering drugs. The three systems of measurement most often used in clinical situations are the **metric system,** the **apothecaries' system,** and the **household system.** These systems are so widely used that the medication cup for liquid measurements may be calibrated in all three systems. A fourth system, the **avoirdupois system,** is used for ordering and purchasing pharmaceutical products and for weighing patients.

METRIC SYSTEM

The metric system, the most widely used and international system of measurement, is also the system used by the U.S. Pharmacopoeia. Among its many advantages, the metric system affords a way to achieve accuracy in calculating small drug dosages. Furthermore, the metric system uses Arabic numerals, which commonly are used by health care professionals throughout the world. Finally, most manufacturers calibrate newly developed drugs in the metric system.

Unfortunately, the general population in the United States has shown little eagerness to adopt the metric system. As a consequence, nurses and nursing students commonly view the metric system as a new and complicated concept. However, when they understand the general principles of this system, nurses easily can perform drug calculations and conversions within it. Nurses can use the metric system to measure liquids and solids. (See *Metric measures,* page 48.)

Liquid measures

The liter (L) of the metric system approximates 1 quart in volume. A milliliter (ml) equals one one-thousandth of a liter. Liters commonly are used when ordering and administering I.V. solutions. Milliliters are used in the administration of parenteral and some oral drugs.

Solid measures

In the metric system, the gram (g) serves as the basis for solid measures or units of weight. A milligram (mg) equals one one-thousandth of a gram. Many drugs are ordered in

Metric measures

This table shows the relationships among some commonly used metric measures. Several less commonly used measures, such as the hectogram, also appear.

LIQUIDS

1 milliliter (ml)	= 1 cubic centimeter (cc)
1 deciliter (dl)	= 100 milliliters
1,000 milliliters	= 1 liter (L)
100 centiliters (cl)	= 1 liter
10 deciliters	= 1 liter
10 liters	= 1 dekaliter (dkl)
100 liters	= 1 hectoliter (hl)
1,000 liters	= 1 kiloliter (kl)

SOLIDS

1,000 milligrams (mg)	= 1 gram (g)
1,000 grams	= 1 kilogram (kg)
100 centigrams (cg)	= 1 gram
10 decigrams (dg)	= 1 gram
10 grams	= 1 dekagram (dkg)
100 grams	= 1 hectogram (hg)

milligrams. Body weight is recorded in kilograms (kg). A kilogram equals 1,000 g.

The following examples represent possible orders using the metric system:

- 1 L 5% dextrose solution I.V. per 8 hours
- 30 ml Milk of Magnesia orally (P.O.) at bedtime (h.s.)
- Ancef 1 g I.V.P.B. every 6 hours (q6h)
- Lanoxin 0.125 mg P.O. daily
- Maintain 10 kg continuous traction.

APOTHECARIES' SYSTEM

The apothecaries' system is slowly being phased out. In January 1995, the United States Pharmacopeial Convention changed its standards to require that prescriptions state the quantity and strength in metric units. It also stipulated that, if any other units are used to express strength or quantity, only the metric equivalent is to be dispensed. This change is particularly significant to the nurse because, if a health care professional writes a prescription using the apothecaries' system, the nurse will need to know how to convert the dosage into the metric system in which the drug will be dispensed.

The apothecaries' system possesses two unique features: the use of Roman numerals and the placement of the unit of measurement before the Roman numeral. For example, *5 grains* would be written as *grains v*. In the apothecaries' system, the equivalents among the various units of measure are close approximations. When using equivalents for calculations and conversions, keep in mind that the calculations, though not precise, will fall within acceptable standards. The apothecaries' system is the only system of measurement that uses symbols besides abbreviations to represent several of the units of measure. The nurse may use the apothecaries' system to measure liquids or solids. (See *Apothecaries' measures.*)

Liquid measures

Visualize the minim (♏), the smallest of the units, as the approximate size of a drop of water. Fifteen to sixteen minims comprise about 1 ml. (Note the approximation of the measure.)

Solid measures

The grain (gr) represents the solid measure or unit of weight in the apothecaries' system. Historians claim that the weight of an average grain of wheat originally determined the grain of the apothecaries' system.

The following examples represent possible orders using the apothecaries' system:

- multivitamin elixir ♏ xii P.O.
- Robitussin f℥ (fluidrams) iv P.O. q6h
- Mylanta f℥ (fluidounce) i P.O. 1 hour after meals (p.c.)
- Tylenol gr (grains) x P.O. q4h as needed (p.r.n) headache.

HOUSEHOLD SYSTEM

Most people in the United States are familiar with the household system of weights and measures. In most cases, food products, recipes, over-the-counter drugs, and home remedies use the household system. Although the units of measure in the household system may be the most familiar, discrepancies exist about quantities attributed to each measure and conversions between the measures. In the clinical setting, health care professionals seldom use the household system for drug administration; however, some household measures may prove useful.

Liquid measures

Liquid measurements in the household system most often used in the clinical setting are teaspoons (tsp) and tablespoons (tbs). The clinically used teaspoon and tablespoon have been standardized to equal 5 ml and 15 ml, respectively. Thus, 3 tsp equal 1 tbs, and 6 tsp equal 1 ounce (oz). Patients with prescribed medications to be taken in dosages of teaspoons or tablespoons should obtain clinical equipment calibrated in these measures to receive the exact prescribed dosage.

The following examples represent possible orders using the household system:

- 2 tsp elixir of terpin hydrate P.O. twice a day (b.i.d.)
- Riopan 2 tbs P.O. 1 hour before meals (a.c.) and at bedtime (h.s.)

AVOIRDUPOIS SYSTEM

The solid measures or units of weight in the avoirdupois system include the ounce (437.5 gr) and the pound (16 oz or 7,000 gr). Note that the apothecaries' pound equals 12 oz in contrast to the 16-oz pound of the avoirdupois system.

MIXED SYSTEMS

Several units of measure may appear arbitrarily in the apothecaries', household, or avoirdupois systems. Two such units of measure, the drop and ounce, appear in the apothecaries' and household systems. The drop, traditionally considered equal to a drop of water, is an inexact measure that varies in size depending on the physical characteristics of the liquid being measured and the equipment used to form the drop. The drop is the unit of measure used when instilling liquid medication into such areas as the ear, nose, or conjunctival sac of the eye. When held vertically, a standard medication dropper usually is calibrated to deliver 20 drops of liquid/ml. Nurses also use the drop as the unit of measure when monitoring I.V. solutions. Standard I.V. administration sets usually deliver 10 to 20 drops/ml; microdrip sets deliver 60 drops/ml.

The pound and the ounce appear in the apothecaries' and avoirdupois systems. The determination of which system to place the pound and ounce within may vary from authority to authority, but the size and equivalents of the measures remain consistent within systems.

OTHER MEASURES

Some drugs require special systems developed by the manufacturers for measuring their quantities. The following discussion addresses special systems of measurement.

Units

Insulin, a drug used by many diabetic patients to assist in controlling blood sugar, is measured in units (U). Many types of insulin exist; however, all are measured in units. The international standard of U-100 insulin means that 1 ml of insulin solution contains 100 U of insulin regardless of type. Heparin, an anticoagulant, also is measured in units.

Several antibiotics, available in liquid, solid, and **powder** forms for oral or parenteral use, also have units as their basis of measure. Each drug manufacturer provides information about measurement of its drugs. For example, nystatin, an oral liquid preparation, contains 100,000 U/ml, but penicillin G benzathine **suspension** is available in two strengths (300,000 U/ml and 600,000 U/ml). The antibiotic penicillin also is manufactured in powdered form for later reconstitution for parenteral or oral administration, as **tablets** for oral use, and liquid form prepackaged in syringes for intramuscular (I.M.) injection.

The following examples represent possible orders using units:

- 14 U NPH insulin subcutaneous (S.C.) this a.m.
- heparin 5,000 U S.C. b.i.d.
- nystatin 200,000 U P.O. q6h
- 300,000 U procaine penicillin intramuscular (I.M.) q4h.

The nurse should keep in mind that the unit is not a standard measure. This means that different drugs measured in units may have no relationship to each other in quality or activity.

Apothecaries' measures

This table displays the relationships between measures, both liquid and solid, within the apothecaries' system.

LIQUIDS

60 minims (♏)	= 1 fluidram (f℥)
8 fluidrams	= 1 fluidounce (f℥)
16 fluidounces	= 1 pint (pt)
2 pints	= 1 quart (qt)
4 quarts	= 1 gallon (gal)

SOLIDS

20 grains (gr)	= 1 scruple (℈)
3 scruples	= 1 dram (ʒ)
8 drams	= 1 ounce (℥)
12 ounces	= 1 pound (lb)

International units

International units (IU) represent the unit of measurement of biologicals, such as vitamins, enzymes, and hormones. For instance, the activity of calcitonin (Calcimar), a synthetic hormone used in calcium regulation, is expressed in international units.

Milliequivalents

Electrolytes may be measured in **milliequivalents** (mEq). The drug manufacturers provide information about the number of metric units required to provide the prescribed number of milliequivalents. The electrolyte potassium chloride usually is ordered in milliequivalents. Potassium preparations for I.V., oral, or other use come in liquid (elixir and parenteral) and solid (powder and tablet) forms.

The following examples represent possible orders using milliequivalents:

- 30 mEq KCl P.O. b.i.d.
- 1 L dextrose 5% in normal saline solution with 40 mEq KCl to run at 125 ml/hour.

Conversions between systems of measurement

Nurses sometimes must make conversions from one system of drug measurement to another. Conversions are necessary when a drug is ordered in one system of measurement but is available only in another system. To perform conversion calculations, the nurse must know the equivalents among the different systems of measurement. (See *Units of exchange among systems of drug measurement,* page 50.)

Several methods can be used to convert a drug measurement from one unit to another. Use the method that feels

Units of exchange among systems of drug measurement

The following shows some approximate liquid equivalents among the household, apothecaries', and metric systems.

HOUSEHOLD	APOTHECARIES'	METRIC
1 teaspoonful (tsp)	1 fluidram (f℥)	5 ml
1 tablespoonful (tbs)	½ fluidounce (f℥)	15 ml
2 tbs	1 f℥	30 ml
1 measuring cupful	8 f℥	240 ml
1 pint (pt)	16 f℥	473 ml
1 quart (qt)	32 f℥	946 ml (1 L)
1 gallon (gal)	128 f℥	3,785 m

The following shows some approximate solid equivalents between the apothecaries' system and the metric system.

APOTHECARIES'	METRIC
15 grains (gr)	1 gram (g) (1,000 mg)
10 gr	0.6 g (600 mg)
7½ gr	0.5 g (500 mg)
5 gr	0.3 g (300 mg)
3 gr	0.2 g (200 mg)
1½ gr	0.1 g (100 mg)
1 gr	0.06 g (60 mg) or 0.065 g (65 mg)
¾ gr	0.05 g (50 mg)
½ gr	0.03 g (30 mg)
¼ gr	0.015 g (15 mg)
1/60 gr	0.001 g (1 mg)
1/100 gr	0.6 mg
1/120 gr	0.5 mg
1/150 gr	0.4 mg

The following lists some approximate solid equivalents among the avoirdupois, apothecaries', and metric systems.

AVOIRDUPOIS	APOTHECARIES'	METRIC
1 gr	1 gr	0.065 g
15.4 gr	15 gr	1 g
1 ounce (oz)	480 gr	28.35 g
437.5 gr	1f℥	31 g
0.75 pound (lb)	1 lb	373 g
1 lb	1.33 lb	454 g
2.2 lb	2.7 lb	1 kilogram (kg)

most comfortable. Remember, dosage calculations may require converting measurements from one measure to another within the same system, or from one system to the equivalent measurement in another system. Making conversions associated with drug administration is a skill nurses use frequently.

Fraction method for conversions

The fraction method for conversions requires an equation consisting of two fractions. Set up the first fraction by placing the ordered dosage needed to convert over *X* units of the available dosage. For example, the physician orders 300 mg of aspirin. The bottle is labeled *aspirin gr v per tablet.* The milligram dosage represents the ordered dosage, and the grain dosage represents the available dosage. Because the amount of the available dosage is unknown, it is represented by an *X*. The first fraction of the equation appears as:

$$\frac{300 \text{ mg}}{\text{X gr}}$$

Then set up the second fraction of the equation. The second fraction consists of the standard equivalents between the ordered and available measures. Because milligrams must be converted to grains, the second fraction appears as:

$$\frac{60 \text{ mg}}{1 \text{ gr}}$$

because 60 mg equal 1 gr. Remember, the same unit of measure appears in the numerator of both fractions. Likewise, the same unit of measure appears in both denominators. The entire equation should appear as:

$$\frac{300 \text{ mg}}{\text{X gr}} = \frac{60 \text{ mg}}{1 \text{ gr}}$$

To solve for X, cross multiply:

$$300 \text{ mg} \times 1 \text{ gr} = 60 \text{ mg} \times \text{X gr}$$
$$300 = 60\text{X}$$
$$\frac{300}{60} = \frac{60\text{X}}{60}$$
$$5 \text{ gr} = \text{X}$$

The patient should receive 5 gr (gr v) of aspirin, which in this case equal 1 tablet.

Ratio method for conversions

When using the ratio method to make conversions, first express the ordered dosage and available dosage as a ratio. For example, a physician's order calls for ASA (aspirin) gr x, but the aspirin is available in tablets measured in milligrams. As a result, the first ratio appears as 10 gr : X mg. The *X* represents the unknown dosage of milligrams. The second ratio represents the standard equivalents between the ordered and available measures. Because 60 mg equal 1 gr, the second ratio appears as 1 gr : 60 mg. Note that the same unit of measure (gr) appears in the first half of each ratio, and the same unit (mg) appears in the second half. The equation should appear as:

$$10 \text{ gr} : \text{X mg} :: 1 \text{ gr} : 60 \text{ mg}$$

To solve for X, set up an equation in which the product of the means (inner portions of the ratio) equals the product of the extremes (outer portions):

$$\text{X mg} \times 1 \text{ gr} = 10 \text{ gr} \times 60 \text{ mg}$$
$$\text{X} = 600 \text{ mg}$$

Ten grains equal 600 mg.

Computation of drug dosages

Determining the drug dosage to be administered occurs after verification of the physician's order. Computing drug dosages is a two-step process. During the first step, ascertain if the drug ordered is available in units within the same system of measurement. If the ordered drug is available only in another system of measurement, perform the conversion between the two systems. Use the fraction method or the ratio method explained in the previous section. If the physician orders the drug in units that are available, proceed directly to the next step.

If the ordered units of measurement are available, calculate the quantity of a particular dosage form to be administered. For example, if the prescribed dose is 250 mg, determine the quantity of tablets, powder, or liquid equal to 250 mg. To determine the quantity, use the fraction or ratio method, similar to the methods used for converting units of measure. Explanations of the fraction and ratio methods follow.

Fraction method

When using the fraction method to compute drug dosage, write an equation consisting of two fractions. First, set up a fraction showing the number of units to be given over *X*, which represents the quantity of the dosage form, or the number of tablets or milliliters. On the other side of the equation, form a fraction showing the number of units of the drug in its dosage form over the quantity of dosage forms that contain the measure stated in the numerator. (Information provided on the drug label should supply the details needed to form the second fraction. The number of units and the quantity of dosage form are specific for each drug. In most cases, the stated quantity equals 1 ml or 1 tablet.)

Here is an example of the fraction method for computation. If the number of units to be administered equals 250 mg, the first fraction in the equation is:

$$\frac{250 \text{ mg}}{\text{X tab}}$$

The drug label states that each tablet contains 125 mg. The second fraction is:

$$\frac{125 \text{ mg}}{1 \text{ tab}}$$

The same units of measure must appear in the numerator of each fraction. Likewise, each denominator should show the same units of measure. The units of measure in the denominators will differ from the units in the numerators. The entire equation should appear as:

$$\frac{250 \text{ mg}}{\text{X tab}} = \frac{125 \text{ mg}}{1 \text{ tab}}$$

Solving for *X* determines the quantity of the dosage form (number of tablets, in this example) to give to the patient. In this case, the patient should receive 2 tablets.

Ratio method

First, write the amount of the drug to be given and the quantity of the dosage (*X*) as a ratio. Using the example shown for the fraction method, in which the drug ordered equaled 250 mg, write the ratio as 250 mg : X tab. Next, complete the equation by forming a second ratio consisting of the number of units of the drug in the dosage form and the stated quantity of the dosage form. If, for example, each tablet contained 125 mg, write the second ratio as 125 mg : 1 tab. The entire equation is:

$$250 \text{ mg} : \text{X tab} :: 125 \text{ mg} : 1 \text{ tab}$$

Solving for X determines the quantity of the dosage form.

The following example uses the ratio method to convert between systems of measurement, then uses the fraction method to compute drug dosage. The physician orders 15 mg of phenobarbital for a patient. The drug is available in scored tablets containing gr $\overline{ss}$ (½ gr). How many tablets should the patient be given?

First, convert the milligrams of the metric system into grains of the apothecaries' system. The standard conversion is 60 mg = 1 gr. Using the ratio method, the equation is:

$$15 \text{ mg} : \text{X gr} :: 60 \text{ mg} : 1 \text{ gr}$$

To solve for *X*, multiply the means and the extremes:

$$\text{X gr} \times 60 \text{ mg} = 15 \text{ mg} \times 1 \text{ gr}$$

$$60 \text{ X} = 15$$

$$\text{X} = \frac{15}{60}$$

$$\text{X} = \frac{1}{4} = 0.25 \text{ gr}$$

Next, determine the drug dosage, in this case the number of tablets to administer. The drug label states that each tablet contains $\overline{ss}$ or ½ (0.5) gr of phenobarbital. The patient is to receive ¼ (0.25) gr or ½ tablet of phenobarbital. Using the fraction method, the equation is:

$$\frac{0.25 \text{ gr}}{\text{X tab}} = \frac{0.5 \text{ gr}}{1 \text{ tab}}$$

To solve for X, cross multiply:

$$0.25 \text{ gr} \times 1 \text{ tab} = 0.5 \text{ gr} \times \text{X tab}$$

$$0.25 = 0.5 \text{ X}$$

$$\frac{0.25}{0.5} = \text{X}$$

$$0.5 = \text{X}$$

The patient should receive ½ tablet of phenobarbital.

"Desired-available" method

The "desired (ordered)-available" method, also known as the dose over on-hand (D/H) method, represents a third way to compute drug dosages. The desired-available method combines the conversion of ordered units into available units and the computation of drug dosage into one step. The equation for doing this is:

$$\text{ordered units} \times \text{conversion fraction} \times \frac{\text{quantity of dosage form}}{\text{stated quantity of drug within each dosage form}} = \text{X quantity to give}$$

The following situation shows how the equation works. The physician orders 10 gr of a drug. The drug is available only in 300-mg tablets. To determine the drug dosage, or the number of tablets to give the patient, substitute 10 gr (the ordered number of units) for the first element of the equation. Then use the conversion fraction

$$\frac{60 \text{ mg}}{1 \text{ gr}}$$

as the second portion of the formula. The measure in the denominator of the conversion fraction must be the same as the measure in the ordered units. In this instance, the physician ordered 10 gr. As a result, grains appear in the denominator of the conversion fraction.

The third element of the equation shows the dosage form over the stated drug quantity within each dosage form. Because the drug is available in 300-mg tablets, the equation is:

$$\frac{1 \text{ tab}}{300 \text{ mg}}$$

The dosage form, in this case tablets, always should appear in the numerator, and the quantity of drug in each dosage form always should appear in the denominator. The completed equation is:

$$10 \text{ gr} \times \frac{60 \text{ mg}}{1 \text{ gr}} \times \frac{1 \text{ tab}}{300 \text{ mg}} = \text{X tab}$$

Solving for *X* shows that the patient should receive 2 tablets.

The desired-available method has the advantage of requiring only one equation. However, it requires memorizing an equation more elaborate than the one used in the fraction or ratio method. Having to memorize a more complicated equation may increase the chance of error.

SPECIAL COMPUTATIONS

The fraction, ratio, and desired-available methods can be used to compute drug dosage when the ordered drug and available form of the drug occur in the same units of measure. The three methods also can be used when the quantity of the particular dosage form differs from the units in which the dosage form will be administered. For example, if a patient is to receive 1,000 mg of a drug available in liquid form and measured in milligrams, with 100 mg contained in 6 ml, how many milliliters would the patient receive? Because the ordered and the available doses occur in milligrams, no initial conversion calculations need to be made. Simply use the ratio or fraction method to determine the number of milliliters of drug the patient should receive. The ratio method would be 1,000 mg : X ml :: 100 mg : 6 ml. Solving for *X* determines that 60 ml of the drug should be given.

Next, because the drug is to be administered in ounce form, determine the number of ounces needed, using a conversion method. For the fraction method for conversion, the equation is:

$$\frac{60 \text{ ml}}{\text{X oz}} = \frac{30 \text{ ml}}{1 \text{ oz}}$$

Solving for *X* indicates that the patient should receive 2 oz of the drug.

To use the desired-available method, simply change the order of the elements in the equation to correspond with the situation. The revised equation is:

$$\text{ordered units} \times \frac{\text{quantity of dosage form}}{\text{stated quantity of drug within each dosage form}} \times \text{conversion fraction} = \text{X quantity to give}$$

Placing the given information into the equation results in:

$$1{,}000 \text{ mg} \times \frac{6 \text{ ml}}{100 \text{ mg}} \times \frac{1 \text{ oz}}{30 \text{ ml}} = \text{X}$$

Solving for *X* indicates that the patient should receive 2 oz of the drug.

Computing drug dosages in special systems

The three methods for drug dosage calculation may be used to calculate dosages of drugs measured in special systems. For example, the physician orders 3,000,000 U of penicillin for a patient. The penicillin is available in liquid form for I.M. use, with 5,000,000 U/ml; however, the dosage is to be administered in minims. When determining the number of minims to administer, first write the dosages as 5 m.U and 3 m.U instead of 5,000,000 and 3,000,000 U. The shorter notation eliminates the need for all the zeros in each dosage and makes the computation appear more manageable. The shorter notation also reduces the chance of error in miscopying the number of zeros during the calculation.

Using the fraction method, set up the initial equation as:

$$\frac{3 \text{ m.U}}{\text{X ml}} = \frac{5 \text{ m.U}}{1 \text{ ml}}$$

Solving for *X* indicates that the patient should receive 0.6 ml of penicillin.

Using the ratio method to determine the number of minims to administer, set up the equation as:

0.6 ml : X ♏ :: 1 ml :15 ♏

Solving for *X* determines that the patient should receive 9 ♏ of penicillin.

Using the desired-available method, the equation is:

$$3 \text{ m.U} \times \frac{1 \text{ ml}}{5 \text{ m.U}} \times \frac{15 \text{ ♏}}{1 \text{ ml}} = 9 \text{ ♏}$$

Solving the equation results in the same number of minims (9). (See *Computing dosages of heparin.*)

CRITICAL THINKING: To enhance your critical thinking about dosage measurements and calculations, consider the following situation and its analysis.

Situation: The nurse is caring for Ida Chang, a 56-year-old diabetic patient. At 11 a.m., a fingerstick test

shows Mrs. Chang's blood glucose level is 250 mg/dl. In response, the physician orders regular insulin 200 U S.C. stat. The insulin is available in 100 U/ml, and the U-100 syringe is designed to hold a maximum of 100 U. Should the nurse prepare and administer the dose as ordered?
Analysis: Because the nurse is responsible for safe medication administration and should be familiar with dosages of common medications, the nurse should question this order after calculating the dosage. For Mrs. Chang, the prescribed dose would require two syringes filled with U-100 insulin (100 U in each syringe). More than one syringe rarely is needed to administer a common dosage. This unusually high dosage should alert the nurse to a possible error in the drug order.

Inexact nature of conversions and computations

Converting drug measurements from one system to another and then determining the amount of a dosage form to give easily can produce inexact dosages. A rounding error during computation or discrepancies in the dosage to give may occur, depending on the conversion standard used in calculation. The nurse may determine a precise drug amount to be given, only to find that administering that amount is impossible. The nurse may determine, for example, that a patient should receive 0.97 tablet. Administering such an amount is impossible. The following general rule helps avoid calculation errors and discrepancies between theoretical and real dosages: *No more than 10% variation should exist between the dosage ordered and the dosage to be given.* Following the rule, a nurse who determined that the patient should receive 0.97 tablet could give 1 tablet permissibly.

The nurse often encounters such discrepancies when administering aspirin and acetaminophen (Tylenol). Physicians may order aspirin and acetaminophen in grains (gr x being the usual adult dose); however, both drugs usually are available in 325-mg tablets. Converting gr x to milligrams indicates that 600 mg should be given, but 2 tablets would equal 650 mg, not 600 mg. To apply the rule concerning such discrepancies, first calculate 10% of 600 mg, which equals 60 mg. Adding 60 mg to 600 mg indicates that giving up to 660 mg is permissible. Because 2 tablets equal only 650 mg, the dosage would be safe to administer.

COMPUTATION OF DRUGS FOR PARENTERAL ADMINISTRATION

The methods for computing drug dosages can be used for oral or parenteral routes. The following example shows how to determine drug dosages to be given via the parenteral route.

The physician orders 75 mg of Demerol. The package label reads: meperidine (Demerol), 100 mg/ml. Using the fraction method to determine the number of milliliters the patient should receive, the equation is:

$$\frac{75 \text{ mg}}{\text{X ml}} = \frac{100 \text{ mg}}{1 \text{ ml}}$$

Computing dosages of heparin

The physician orders 5,000 U of heparin S.C. for a patient. On hand is heparin 10,000 U/ml. How many milliliters should the patient receive?

Use the fraction method to set up the equation:

$$\frac{10{,}000 \text{ U}}{1 \text{ ml}} = \frac{5{,}000 \text{ U}}{\text{X ml}}$$

Cross multiply:

$$10{,}000 \text{ X} = 5{,}000$$

Solve for X:

$$\text{X} = \frac{5{,}000}{10{,}000} = 0.5 \text{ ml}$$

The patient should receive 0.5 or ½ ml of heparin.

To solve for *X*, cross multiply:

$$75 \text{ mg} \times 1 \text{ ml} = \text{X ml} \times 100 \text{ mg}$$
$$75 = 100 \text{ X}$$
$$\frac{75}{100} = \text{X}$$
$$0.75 \text{ or } 3/4 \text{ ml} = \text{X}$$

The patient should receive 0.75 or 3/4 ml.

The nurse might need to know the number of minims that would deliver the same dosage. The equation for the ratio method is:

$$0.75 \text{ ml} : \text{X} \text{ ♏} :: 1 \text{ ml} : 15 \text{ ♏}$$

To solve for *X*, multiply the means and the extremes:

$$\text{X ♏} \times 1 \text{ ml} = 0.75 \text{ ml} \times 15 \text{ ♏}$$
$$\text{X} = 12 \text{ ♏}$$

Twelve minims equal 0.75 ml, which would contain the 75 mg of Demerol ordered by the physician.

RECONSTITUTION OF POWDERS FOR INJECTION

Although the pharmacist usually reconstitutes powders for parenteral use, nurses sometimes perform the function. The nurse also often computes I.V. fluid rates. The following discussion addresses the reconstitution of powders for injection and the computation of I.V. drip rates.

When reconstituting powders for injection, consult the drug label for the needed information. The label gives the total quantity of drug in the **vial** or **ampule,** the amount and type of diluent to add to the powder, and the strength and shelf life (expiration date) of the resulting solution. When diluent is added to a powder, the powder increases the fluid volume. Therefore, the label calls for less diluent than the total volume of the prepared solution. For example, the nurse may have to add 1.7 ml of diluent to a vial of powdered drug to obtain a 2-ml total volume of prepared solution. Reconstituting a powdered drug simply requires following the directions on the drug label.

I.V. flow rates

The number of drops (gtt) required to deliver 1 ml of I.V. solution varies with the type of administration set used and the manufacturer. To calculate the flow rate, the nurse must know the calibration of the drip rate for each manufacturer's product. The chart below provides a quick reference guide.

MANUFACTURER	DROPS/ML	DROPS/MINUTE TO INFUSE					
		500 ml/ 24 hr	1,000 ml/ 24 hr	1,000 ml/ 20 hr	1,000 ml/ 10 hr	1,000 ml/ 8 hr	1,000 ml/ 6 hr
		21 ml/hr	42 ml/hr	50 ml/hr	100 ml/hr	125 ml/hr	166 ml/hr
Abbott	15	5 gtt	10 gtt	12 gtt	25 gtt	31 gtt	42 gtt
Baxter-Healthcare	10	3 gtt	7 gtt	8 gtt	17 gtt	21 gtt	28 gtt
Cutter	20	7 gtt	14 gtt	17 gtt	34 gtt	42 gtt	56 gtt
IVAC	20	7 gtt	14 gtt	17 gtt	34 gtt	42 gtt	56 gtt
McGaw	15	5 gtt	10 gtt	12 gtt	25 gtt	31 gtt	42 gtt

To determine the amount of solution to administer, use the manufacturer's information about the concentration of the solution. For example, if the nurse wants to administer 500 mg of a drug, and the concentration of the prepared solution is 1 g (1,000 mg)/10 ml, the nurse can set up a fraction or ratio equation as follows:

Fraction method

$$\frac{500 \text{ mg}}{\text{X ml}} = \frac{1{,}000 \text{ mg}}{10 \text{ ml}}$$

Ratio method

$$500 \text{ mg} : \text{X ml} :: 1{,}000 \text{ mg} : 10 \text{ ml}$$

The patient should receive 5 ml of the prepared solution.

I.V. drip rates and flow rates

For these special computations, first set up a fraction showing the volume of solution to be delivered over the number of minutes in which that volume is to be infused. For example, if a patient is to receive 100 ml of solution within 1 hour, the fraction would be written as

$$\frac{100 \text{ ml}}{60 \text{ min}}$$

Next, multiply the fraction by the drip factor (the number of drops contained in 1 ml) to determine the drip rate (the number of drops per minute to be infused). The drip factor varies among different I.V. sets and appears on the package containing the I.V. tubing administration set. Following the manufacturer's directions for drip factor is a crucial step. (See *I.V. flow rates.*) Standard administration sets have drip factors of 10, 15, or 20 drops/ml. A microdrip (minidrip) set has a drip factor of 60 drops/ml.

Use the following equation to determine the drip rate of an I.V. solution:

$$\frac{\text{Total no. of ml}}{\text{total no. of min.}} \times \text{drip factor} = \text{drops per minute}$$

The equation applies to I.V. solutions that infuse over many hours or to such small-volume infusions as those used for antibiotics, which are administered in less than 1 hour. (See *Calculating I.V. drip rate.*)

The nurse can modify the equation by first determining the number of milliliters to be infused over 1 hour (the flow rate). The nurse then divides the flow rate by 60 minutes. The resulting calculation is then multiplied by the drip factor to determine the number of drops per minute. The nurse also will use the flow rate when working with I.V. infusion pumps to set the number of milliliters to be delivered in 1 hour.

Quick methods for calculating drip rates

Besides the equation and its modified version, quicker methods exist for computing I.V. solution administration rates. To administer I.V. solutions via a microdrip set, adjust the flow rate (number of milliliters per hour) to equal the drip rate (number of drops per minute). Using the equation, divide the flow rate by 60 minutes and then multiply by the drip factor, which also equals 60. Because the flow rate and drip factor are equal, the two arithmetic operations "cancel out" each other. For example, if 125 ml of fluid/hour represented the ordered flow rate, the equation would be:

$$\frac{125 \text{ ml}}{60 \text{ min}} \times 60 = \text{drip rate (125)}$$

Rather than spend time calculating the equation, the nurse simply can use the number assigned to the flow rate as the drip rate.

For I.V. solution administration sets that deliver 15 drops/ml, the flow rate divided by 4 equals the drip rate. For sets with a drip factor of 10, the flow rate divided by 6 equals the drip rate.

PERCENTAGE SOLUTIONS

In most clinical settings, the pharmacy department or pharmaceutical companies prepare solutions containing drugs for topical use (for example, wound irrigation and the soaking of infected or inflamed body parts). Nurses, however, must prepare special **percentage solutions** for emergencies, such as resuscitation attempts after cardiac arrest. Furthermore, home care nurses may need to prepare large-volume solutions if prepared solutions are not accessible to the patient.

Calculation of percentage solutions

An example of a percentage solution is 0.9% saline, which indicates that every 100 ml of solution contain 0.9 g of sodium chloride. Expressed as a fraction, the figures would appear as:

$$\frac{0.9}{100}$$

The ratio form would appear as 0.9 : 100. A liter of 0.9% saline would contain 9 g of sodium chloride. The figures for 1 L would be

$$\frac{9}{1{,}000}$$

in fraction form, and 9 : 1,000 in ratio form.

The nurse may prepare percentage solutions by adding solutes (solid or liquid forms of drugs) to solvents (diluents). The solvents usually used include sterile water, normal saline solution, and dextrose 5% in water (D_5W). As a general rule when preparing solutions, the nurse should consider the solid form, whether crystals, powders, or tablets, to be 100% strength. The liquid form, also known as the stock solution, may vary in strength.

The nurse may use the following formulas to calculate the strength of percentage solutions. The fraction method offers two usable formulas:

$$\frac{\text{weaker solution}}{\text{stronger solution}} = \frac{\text{solute}}{\text{solvent}}$$

$$\frac{\text{small \% strength}}{\text{large \% strength}} = \frac{\text{small volume}}{\text{large volume}}$$

The ratio method also offers two formulas:

weaker : stronger :: solute : solvent

small % strength : large % strength :: small volume : large volume

Although a solid combined with a diluent will increase the total volume of the prepared solution, the increase usually is insignificant and may not need to be calculated. The increase, however, will prove significant and should be considered when adding a large amount of solid or a small amount of diluent. When adding a liquid, subtract the amount of the liquid from the total volume desired. This calculation tells the amount of diluent to add. For example, if the preparation of 1 L of solution requires 50 ml of a liquid drug, add the 50 ml of liquid drug to 950 ml of diluent.

As an example, the nurse must prepare 500 ml of a 0.5% lidocaine (Xylocaine) solution and finds on hand a 2% Xylocaine solution and D_5W, which is the diluent. The nurse must determine the number of milliliters of Xylocaine solution to use, and the number of milliliters of dextrose solution to use. Using the ratio method, the nurse sets up the following equation:

0.5% : 2% :: X ml : 500 ml

Multiplying the means and the extremes gives $2\chi = 250$. The nurse then divides to solve for χ:

$$X = \frac{250}{2}$$

X = 125 ml of 2% Xylocaine solution

Because the nurse wants a total volume of 500 ml and must use 125 ml of Xylocaine solution, the nurse next must determine the amount of dextrose solution to use as the diluent. Subtracting 125 from 500 yields the amount of dextrose solution to use:

500 ml − 125 ml = 375 ml of dextrose solution

Calculating I.V. drip rate

The physician's order states: *1,000 ml dextrose 5% in 0.45% sodium chloride to infuse over 12 hours.* The administration set delivers 15 drops per milliliter. What should the drip rate be?

Use the equation:

$$\frac{\text{Total no. of ml}}{\text{Total no. of min}} \times \text{drip factor} = \text{drip rate}$$

Set up the equation using the given data:

$$\frac{1{,}000 \text{ ml}}{12 \text{ hr} \times 60 \text{ min}} \times 15 \text{ gtt/ml} = X \text{ gtt/min}$$

Multiply the elements in the denominator:

$$\frac{1{,}000 \text{ ml}}{720 \text{ min}} \times 15 \text{ gtt/ml} = X \text{ gtt/smin}$$

Divide the fraction:

1.39 ml/min × 15 gtt/ml = X gtt/min

The final answer is 20.85 gtt/min, which can be rounded to 21 gtt/min. The drip rate is 21 drops per minute.

SPECIAL CONSIDERATIONS

Dosage determinations for pediatric and geriatric patients may need to be handled differently. Calculations of pediatric dosages require the use of special rules. Dosages for geriatric patients require the nurse to be aware of special considerations. (See Geriatric considerations: *Individualized dosages,* page 56.)

Pediatric dosage considerations

To determine the correct pediatric dosage of a medication, physicians, pharmacists, and nurses usually use two computation methods. One is based on the child's weight in kilo-

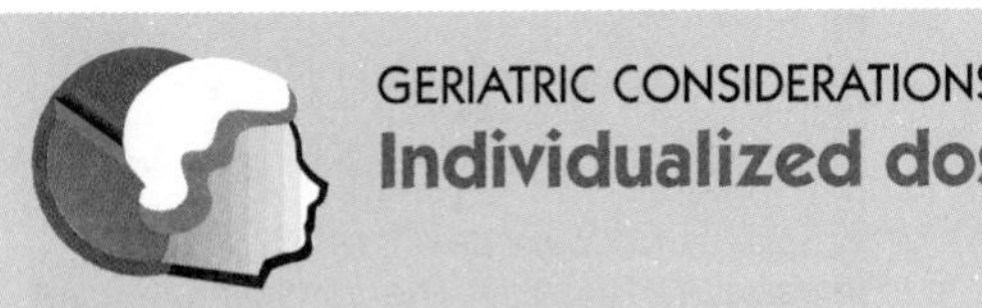

GERIATRIC CONSIDERATIONS

Individualized dosages

Geriatric patients may require drug dosages that differ from the usual adult dosages because of chronic illnesses or the physiologic effects of aging, which may alter a drug's pharmacokinetics. As a result, the physician determines dosages for individual geriatric patients. No general rules exist. Because of the individual nature of aging and the unique medical history of each geriatric patient, the nurse in a gerontologic setting consistently must assess each patient's response to drugs. Although a patient may receive an average adult dosage, such a dosage does not account for individual differences.

grams; the other uses the child's body-surface area. Other methods are less accurate and are not recommended.

Dosage range per kilogram of body weight. Currently, many pharmaceutical companies provide information on the safe dosage ranges for drugs given to children. The companies usually provide the dosage ranges in milligrams per kilogram of body weight and in many cases give similar information for adult dosage ranges. The following example and explanation indicate how to calculate the safe pediatric dosage range for a drug, using the company's suggested safe dosage range provided in milligrams per kilogram.

For a pediatric patient, a physician orders a drug with a suggested dosage range of 10 to 12 mg/kg of body weight/day. The child weighs 12 kg. What is the safe daily dosage range for the child?

The nurse must calculate the lower and upper limits of the dosage range provided by the manufacturer. The nurse first calculates the dosage based on 10 mg/kg of body weight, then calculates the dosage based on 12 mg/kg of body weight. The answers represent the lower and upper limits of the daily dosage range, expressed in mg/kg of the child's weight. (See *Calculating pediatric dosages.*)

Body-surface area. A second method for calculating safe pediatric dosages uses the child's body-surface area as a factor. This method may provide a more accurate calculation because the child's body-surface area is thought to parallel the child's organ growth and maturation and metabolic rate.

The nurse determines the body-surface area of a child by using a three-columned chart called a nomogram. (See *Calculating pediatric dosages by body-surface area.*) The nurse marks the child's height in the first column and the child's weight in the third column, then draws a line between the two marks. The point at which the line intersects the vertical scale in the second column indicates the estimated body-surface area of the child in square meters. To calculate the child's approximate dose, the nurse uses the body-surface area measurement in the following equation:

$$\frac{\text{body-surface area of child}}{\text{average adult body-surface area (1.73 m}^2\text{)}} \times \begin{matrix}\text{average}\\\text{adult}\\\text{dose}\end{matrix} = \begin{matrix}\text{child's}\\\text{dose}\end{matrix}$$

The following example illustrates the use of the equation. Using a nomogram, the nurse finds that a 25-lb (11.3-kg) child 33″ (84 cm) tall has a body-surface area of 0.52 m^2. The nurse needs to determine the child's dose of a drug with an average adult dose of 100 mg. The equation would appear as:

$$\frac{0.52\text{ m}^2}{1.73\text{ m}^2} \times 100\text{ mg} = 30.06\text{ mg (child's dose)}$$

The child should receive 30 mg of the drug.

Other rules. Clark's rule, Fried's rule, and Young's rule are other rules used to calculate a pediatric dosage. They are based on the average adult dose, and their results are approximate. Because of this, calculating with equations other than those involving dosage ranges per kilogram of body weight or body-surface area is *not* recommended for determining dosages.

Many facilities have guidelines that determine the acceptable calculation method. Nurses in pediatric settings must familiarize themselves with the particular facility's policy about pediatric dosages.

Calculating pediatric dosages

The physician orders 150 mg of a drug to be given q6h to an 18-kg child. (Remember that 1 kg equals 2.2 lb). The literature provided by the manufacturer indicates that the safe dosage range for the drug is 30 mg/kg to 35 mg/kg per day, to be given in divided doses. Can the nurse safely administer the ordered dosage?

Use the ratio method to determine the lower limit of the safe dosage range:

$$30\text{ mg} : X\text{ mg} :: 1\text{ kg} : 18\text{ kg}$$

Cross multiply the means and the extremes to find that $X = 540$ mg, which represents the low dosage.

Use the same method to calculate the upper limit of the safe dosage range:

$$35\text{ mg} : X\text{ mg} :: 1\text{ kg} : 18\text{ kg}$$

Cross multiply the means and the extremes to find that $X = 630$ mg, the high dosage.

The safe dosage range for the child is 540 to 630 mg per day. Because the physician ordered 150 mg to be given every 6 hours, the child would receive four doses per day, or a total daily dosage of 150 mg × four doses per day = 600 mg per day. This daily dosage falls within the safe range, so the nurse can safely administer 150 mg q6h.

Calculating pediatric dosages by body-surface area

The nurse can determine a correct pediatric drug dosage by estimating the child's body-surface area. If the child is average size, find the child's weight and corresponding surface area on the first, boxed scale. Otherwise, use the nomogram to the right. To do this, mark the child's height in the first column and weight in the third column; then draw a line between the two marks. Where the line intersects the scale in the second column indicates the estimated body-surface area of the child in square meters.

To calculate the child's dosage, complete this equation:

$$\frac{\text{body-surface area of child}}{\text{average adult body-surface area } (1.73 \text{ m}^2)} \times \text{adult average dose} = \text{child's dose}$$

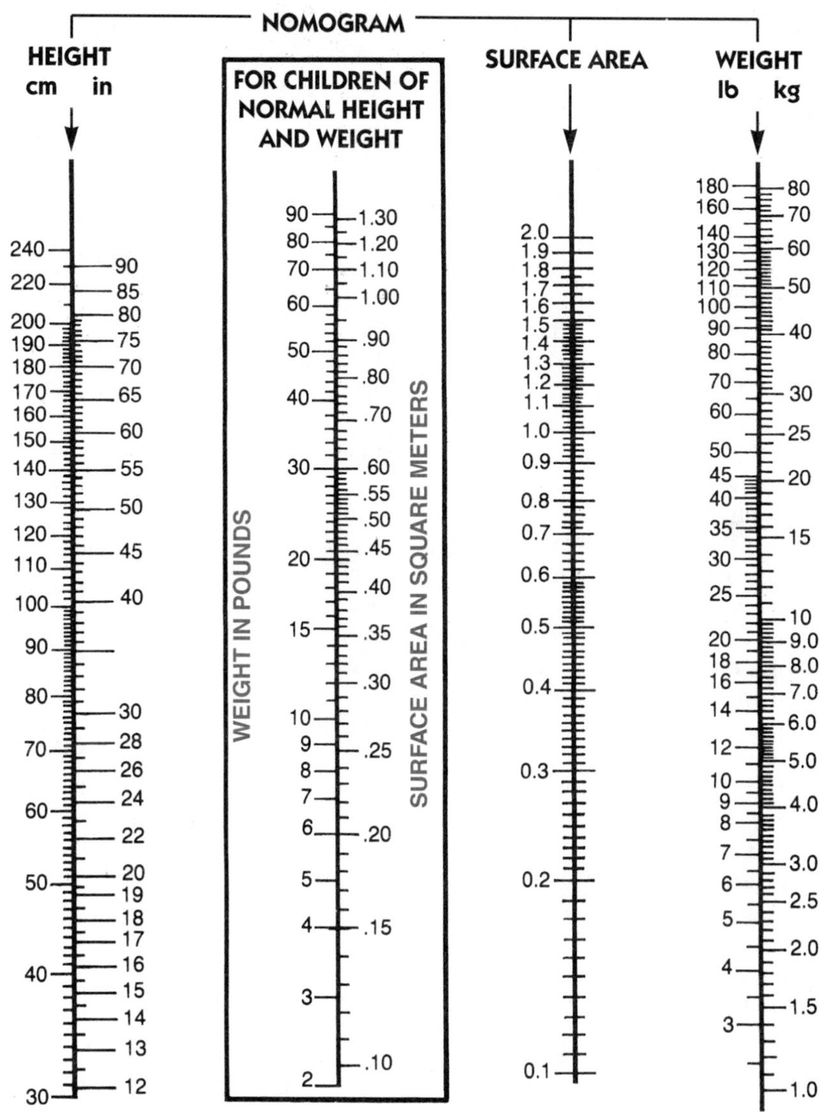

Reprinted with permission from Richard E. Behrman (Ed.). (1996). *Nelson textbook of pediatrics* (15th ed.). Philadelphia: W.B. Saunders Co.

CHAPTER SUMMARY

To help the student nurse achieve the goal of safe, accurate drug administration, chapter 4 presented various ways to calculate drug dosages. Here are the chapter highlights.

The metric system is used internationally for ordering drugs, and most new drugs are measured in metric units. Use of the metric system is advantageous because it allows accurate calculation of small drug dosages. This system uses liquid measures based on the liter and solid measures based on the gram. Drugs measured in the metric system frequently are available in liters, milliliters, grams, and milligrams.

The apothecaries' system, older and less precise than the metric system, is used less often. Equivalents in the apothecaries' system are approximate rather than exact. Liquids are measured in minims, fluidrams, fluidounces, pints, quarts, and gallons; solids are measured in grains, scruples, drams, ounces, and pounds.

The household system, familiar because of its use in food measurement, is the least used system of measurement in the clinical area. In many cases, over-the-counter medications are measured in the household system. Commonly used liquid measurements in the household system are teaspoons and tablespoons.

Some drugs are measured in special systems developed by the manufacturer. Units and milliequivalents represent special drug measures. The labels of products manufactured in special measures give information on the size of the measures. Some drugs, such as insulin, require special equipment for measuring dosages.

The nurse must make conversions from one system of drug measurement to another when a drug is ordered in one system but is available only in another system. The nurse must know the equivalents among the systems of measurement to make the conversion calculations.

The fraction method for conversion uses an equation made up of two fractions. The first fraction shows the ordered dosage to be converted over *X* units of the available dosage. The second fraction consists of the standard equivalents between the ordered and available measures. The ratio method for conversion uses the same information; however, it is set up as ratios.

If the physician orders the drug in available units, the nurse proceeds directly to computing the drug dosage. The nurse may use the fraction method, the ratio method, or the desired-available method to perform the calculation.

When reconstituting powdered drugs before parenteral administration, the nurse should consult the drug label for needed information.

The nurse calculates I.V. fluid rates regulated manually or by an I.V. fluid pump. The nurse must know how to calculate the hourly rate, or flow rate, as well as the drip rate, or number of drops per minute. Intravenous administration sets vary in the size of the drop produced. Therefore, the nurse must be familiar with the equipment in use and aware of the drip factor, or number of drops per milliliter that the equipment delivers.

Sometimes the nurse must prepare special percentage solutions for emergencies. To prepare such solutions, the nurse adds solutes (solid or liquid forms of drugs) to solvents, such as normal saline solution. The nurse can use the fraction method or ratio method to calculate the amount of drug, or solute, and the volume of the solvent to use when preparing a solution of desired concentration.

The nurse must be aware of special considerations related to pediatric and geriatric dosage determinations.

Questions to consider

See Appendix 1 for answers.

1. George Williams, age 69, is admitted to the coronary unit with heart failure. The physician prescribes digoxin 0.25 mg I.V. daily. Which system of measurement does this prescription represent?
   (a) Metric system
   (b) Household system
   (c) Avoirdupois system
   (d) Apothecaries' system

2. When preparing to administer I.V. digoxin to Norma Miller, age 73, the nurse notes that the drug comes in an ampule that contains 0.5 mg of digoxin/2 ml. To administer a dose of 0.25 mg, how much should the nurse draw up?
   (a) 4 ml
   (b) 2 ml
   (c) 1 ml
   (d) 0.5 ml

3. For Samuel McDonald, age 35, the physician orders 200 mg of a drug available in an elixir that contains 100 mg/30 ml. How many ounces of the drug should the nurse administer?
   (a) ½ oz
   (b) 1 oz
   (c) 2 oz
   (d) 3 oz

4. The physician prescribes aspirin gr v P.O. q4h p.r.n. for mild pain for Bonita Perez, age 47. When calculating a conversion between the apothecaries' and metric systems, the nurse finds that the dosage is inexact. How much variation is allowed between dosage ordered and dosage delivered?
   (a) No more than 5%
   (b) No more than 10%
   (c) No more than 15%
   (d) No more than 20%

5. For Arthur Grant, age 56, the nurse must administer heparin 5,000 U S.C. The vial of heparin contains 20,000 U/ml. How many milliliters of heparin should the nurse administer?
   (a) 0.25
   (b) 0.5
   (c) 1.0
   (d) 4.0

6. After a car accident, Mark Lumley, age 29, is admitted to the intensive care unit. The physician prescribes 1,000 ml of normal saline solution to be infused over 6 hours. Which equation would the nurse use to determine the I.V. drip rate?
   (a) $\frac{\text{Total no. of minutes}}{\text{Total no. of ml}} \times \text{drip factor} = \text{drip rate}$
   (b) $\frac{\text{Total no. of minutes}}{\text{Drip factor}} \times \text{total no. of ml} = \text{drip rate}$
   (c) $\frac{\text{Total no. of ml}}{\text{Total no. of minutes}} \times \text{drip factor} = \text{drip rate}$
   (d) $\frac{\text{Total no. of minutes}}{\text{Drip factor}} \times \text{total no. of ml} = \text{drip rate}$

7. The nurse must calculate the correct dosage of a medication for Beth Cleary, age 4. Which of the following methods yields the most accurate calculation?
   (a) Clark's rule
   (b) Fried's rule
   (c) Young's rule
   (d) Body-surface area

5 Routes and techniques of administration

OBJECTIVES

After reading and studying this chapter, the student should be able to:

1. differentiate among the following solid drug forms in terms of their disintegration and absorption sites: tablets, capsules, enteric-coated tablets, and wax matrix tablets.
2. dentify the composition of each of the following oral liquid drug forms: syrups, suspensions, tinctures, and elixirs.
3. describe how suppository and inhalant drug forms are absorbed.
4. identify the procedure for administering the following drug forms using the oral route: tablets, capsules, and liquids.
5. explain how to administer a drug using a nasogastric or gastrostomy tube.
6. describe how to administer sublingual and buccal medications.
7. describe how to insert a rectal suppository and administer a retention enema.
8. describe how to reconstitute a powdered medication from a vial.
9. differentiate among the techniques for administering medications by these parenteral routes: intradermal, subcutaneous, intramuscular, and intravenous.
10. explain the rationales for using the intrathecal and epidural routes of drug administration.
11. explain how to administer urethral and vaginal medications.
12. describe how to administer medication to a pediatric patient by the oral, intramuscular, subcutaneous, intravenous, topical, rectal, ophthalmic, otic, and nasal routes.

INTRODUCTION

The complexity and variety of available medications make proper administration a task requiring knowledge and skill. Before administering a medication, the nurse must know the pharmacokinetics, pharmacodynamics, pharmacotherapeutics, dosage range, drug interactions, adverse drug reactions, and nursing implications related to the specific drug. Also, the nurse must ensure that the five rights of medication administration are observed: the right patient, right drug, right route, right dose, and right time.

Chapter 5 presents techniques as well as rationales for administering medications in the clinical setting. It presents drug administration for adult patients and then discusses pediatric variations.

Drug packaging and forms

Drugs are packaged in numerous styles. When administering drugs, the nurse must consider packaging differences. Drugs may be packaged in unit-dose format, in which one dose of a drug comes in a labeled container or wrapper. They also can be packaged in bulk format, in which multiple doses of a drug are packaged in a container, bottle, or wrapper. The nurse always should remember to *read the label.* Valuable information appears on the label, and reading it helps the nurse administer medications properly. Other important information may appear in the package insert. For example, the insert may include information about changes in drug actions related to the consumption of food or alcohol with the drug.

Drugs are manufactured in many different forms, including solids, liquids, **suppositories, inhalants,** sprays, **creams, lotions, patches,** and **lozenges.** To administer drugs safely, the nurse must be knowledgeable about the different effects of the many drug forms. For example, nitroglycerin administered sublingually (allowing it to dissolve under the tongue) can relieve anginal pain in less than 1 minute. The same drug administered as an **ointment** applied to the chest wall may not relieve acute pain at all; however, it may be used prophylactically for anginal pain.

SOLIDS

The solid drug forms include **tablets, capsules, enteric-coated tablets, osmotic pump tablets,** and **wax matrix tablets.** A tablet is the result of compressing a drug, usually combined with inert ingredients, into one of many different shapes. Chewable tablets offer several advantages over other types of drug formulations: palatable taste, enhanced absorption, and easier ingestion for patients who have difficulty swallowing large tablets. Disintegration and some dissolution of chewed tablets take place in the mouth, and some absorption occurs in the stomach. Most drug absorption, however, occurs in the small intestine.

When swallowed, uncoated tablets disintegrate and dissolve in the stomach. They usually are absorbed in the small intestine. Sublingual tablets disintegrate in the mouth and are absorbed directly into the bloodstream by the blood vessels under the tongue; buccal tablets also disintegrate in the mouth, but are absorbed by blood vessels in the cheek.

A capsule is a hard or soft gelatin shell that contains a drug in a **powder,** in sustained-released beads, or in liquid form. Usually, solid drugs are contained in hard gelatin shells and liquid medications are contained in soft gelatin shells. Swallowed capsules disintegrate and dissolve in the stomach; absorption occurs in the small intestine. The precise degree of dissolution and absorption as well as the site of those activities depends on the specific drug.

Enteric-coated tablets have a thin coating that allows the tablet to pass through the stomach and disintegrate and dissolve in the small intestine, where the drug is absorbed. Because the enteric-coated drug form delivers a concentrated dose of drug to the intestinal mucosa, irritation or ulceration of the intestinal mucosa may result.

Unscored tablets, enteric-coated tablets, and capsules should *never* be divided. Each of these products may contain inert or other ingredients along with the drug, and dividing the drug form could result in incorrect dosage administration or damage to the stomach mucosa. Also, dividing an enteric-coated tablet destroys the enteric barrier, allowing stomach secretions to act on the medication and alter its absorption.

Osmotic pump tablets release the drug through a single, tiny hole. Drug movement is driven by moisture and concentration, which gives the tablets the name *osmotic pump.*

In the wax matrix form of an orally administered drug, the drug is deposited throughout a honeycomb-like structure made of a wax material. Many of these tablets are covered with an enteric-coated shell, allowing disintegration and absorption to occur in the small intestine. The wax matrix allows for the sustained release of a drug, which in turn provides a more constant blood level of the drug. The nurse should inform the patient taking a wax matrix preparation that the indigestible casing may be expelled in the feces.

LIQUIDS

Liquid medications usually are given parenterally or orally. The nurse also may administer liquid medications as irrigations, soaks, enemas, or gargles. Orally administered liquids, which contain the drug mixed with some type of fluid, are classified as **syrups, suspensions, tinctures,** or **elixirs.**

Syrups are drugs mixed in a sugar-water solution. Cough syrup frequently is given in this form.

Suspensions consist of finely divided drug particles suspended in a suitable liquid medium. The nurse or patient administering a suspension should shake the preparation thoroughly before using it. Shaking the suspension ensures that the drug particles are dispersed uniformly throughout the liquid. Antacids commonly are manufactured in suspension form.

Tinctures and elixirs are two types of alcoholic solutions. Tinctures are hydroalcoholic drug solutions; elixirs are hydroalcoholic solutions plus glycerin, sorbitol, or another sweetener. The nurse or patient should consult a pharmacist before mixing an alcoholic solution with any liquid because some alcohol-soluble drugs may form a precipitate when mixed with any solution — even water. The nurse should never give an alcoholic solution to a patient who also takes the drug disulfiram (Antabuse) or any other drug that can cause disulfiram-like effects when taken with alcohol, such as metronidazole.

Liquids given parenterally are available in three packaging styles: **vials, ampules,** and self-contained systems or prefilled syringes.

Vials, which are bottles sealed with a rubber diaphragm, can contain a single dose or several doses. Multidose vials contain preservatives that enable them to be used for more than one dose, whereas single-dose vials do not contain such agents. The nurse must discard single-dose vials after one use or dose. The medication in vials may come in a liquid form or in a powder that the nurse must reconstitute before use.

An ampule contains a single dose of medication. The ampule is a glass container with a thin neck, which usually is scored so it can be snapped off. Ampules usually contain liquid medications.

Self-contained systems, or prefilled parenteral medications, contain a single dose of a drug in a plastic bag or in a prefilled syringe with an attached needle. Nurses and physicians use prefilled syringes for narcotics and other analgesics as well as for drugs used during cardiopulmonary resuscitation or advanced life-support activities. Prefilled syringes also are used in unit-dose drug administration systems.

SUPPOSITORIES

Administered rectally and vaginally, suppositories carry medications in a solid base that melts at body temperature. Suppositories produce local (analgesic, laxative, and anti-infective) and systemic (antiemetic, antipyretic, and analgesic) effects. Usually bullet-shaped, most suppositories are about 1" (2.5 cm) long and require lubrication for insertion. Because they melt at body temperature, suppositories usually require refrigeration until administration.

INHALANTS

Inhalants are powdered or liquid forms of a drug that are given using the respiratory route and are absorbed rapidly by the rich supply of capillaries in the lungs. Powdered forms must be broken into fine particles by means of a mechanical device before inhalation. Several frequently used methods of inhalation include ultrasonic nebulizers, metered-dose aerosol or turbo inhalers, and vaporizers.

OTHER DRUG FORMS

Other drug forms described in this chapter include sprays, which are used with several administration routes; creams, lotions, and patches, which are administered topically; and lozenges, which are used for local effects with the oral route.

Gastrointestinal tract administration techniques

The gastrointestinal (GI) tract provides a fairly safe but relatively slow-acting site for drug absorption. Oral, sublingual, buccal, and rectal preparations are given by the GI tract.

ORAL

Orally routed drug forms include tablets, capsules, liquids, and lozenges. As long as the patient is alert and able to swallow, oral administration is relatively simple and safe.

After checking the five rights of medication administration, the nurse must gather the necessary equipment. To administer tablets or capsules, the nurse needs a souffle cup (medicine cup), a glass of water or other suitable liquid, and the medication container. (If the facility uses the unit-dose system, the nurse should not need a souffle cup or separate medication container because the exact dose should be provided.) When using a bottle, the nurse should follow these instructions: (1) Shake the correct number of tablets or capsules comprising a dose into the lid, then transfer them to the souffle cup. Do not touch the medication directly, to avoid contamination of other tablets or capsules. (2) Take the souffle cup containing the appropriate number of tablets or capsules and the glass of water to the patient. If the tablets or capsules come in a unit-dose form, take the appropriate dose to the patient's bedside. (If the patient has difficulty handling the medication, the nurse may open the unit-dose packaging at the patient's bedside and place the dose in a souffle cup.) (3) Identify the patient by checking the armband and name tag and asking the patient to state his or her name. State the name of the drug and its action or use; then instruct the patient to place the tablets or capsules in the mouth and swallow them with the water. The patient may take the tablets or capsules one at a time or all at once. For the patient who has difficulty swallowing medications, suggest sitting in an upright position and drinking liquid before and while swallowing the capsules or tablets. The patient should drink at least 3 oz (90 ml) of liquid after swallowing the medication to ensure that it travels down the esophagus and to decrease the risk of local irritation by the medication, particularly in an elderly patient. (4) Remain at the bedside until the patient swallows all of the medication, thus ensuring that the medication has not been aspirated and that it has entered the GI tract. Never leave the medication at the patient's bedside. This precaution ensures that the medication is not hoarded, lost, discarded, or ingested by someone other than the intended patient.

Special techniques for oral administration

Giving medications through a gastric tube, such as a nasogastric (NG) tube or a gastrostomy tube, involves special techniques. Drugs administered through a gastric tube enter the stomach directly, thus bypassing the mouth and esophagus and the disintegration and dissolution processes that occur there. To administer a drug appropriately via an NG or gastrostomy tube, the nurse must reproduce the disintegration and dissolution processes by crushing a tablet and preparing a liquid form. When using an NG or gastrostomy tube, the nurse must know how the action of a medication changes when a tablet is crushed. A crushed tablet disintegrates immediately, and absorption from the GI tract occurs rapidly. These changes may not produce significant differences in blood levels and absorption rate if the tablet was designed for rapid disintegration and absorption. If, however, the tablet was designed for slow release and absorption, crushing can alter the drug's effect significantly. In some cases, the nurse may consult the physician or pharmacist about using a different form of the drug or a different route to achieve the intended effect.

The nurse must never place an intact tablet or capsule in a gastrostomy or NG tube. The small diameter of most tubes prevents tablets and capsules from passing through the lumen.

To determine which drugs can be crushed or should not be crushed, the nurse should read the label, consult a pharmacist, or check the package insert information. Uncoated tablets or those with sugar coatings designed only to camouflage a bitter taste usually can be crushed. Enteric-coated tablets should not be crushed because the coating is designed to protect the drug from stomach acids and ensure that it reaches and dissolves in the small intestine. When these tablets are crushed, gastric or esophageal irritation as well as altered drug action can result. Wax matrix tablets should not be crushed because the drug would dissolve faster, thereby increasing the serum level of the drug and causing it to be excreted more rapidly. The intended sustained-release action of the wax matrix tablet would become unpredictable.

The beads in sustained-release capsules should not be crushed because all of the drug would be released at once; the sustained-release action of the drug would be altered in much the same way as in crushing a wax matrix tablet. The nurse who must administer a sustained-release drug through a gastric tube should obtain and use a liquid form of the drug if possible. Otherwise, the patient may require more frequent doses, which may result in toxic effects. Capsules that contain a powder can be emptied for easy administration by gastric tube.

Administering medication through an NG tube

Before administering medication, the nurse identifies the patient by checking the armband and name tag and asking the patient to state his or her name, if appropriate. Then the nurse should state the name and action or use of the drug. To administer medication through a nasogastric (NG) or gastrostomy tube, the nurse will need these supplies: a 50-ml syringe with a catheter tip that fits snugly into the gastric tube, a plastic medicine cup (containing the medication), a tissue or washcloth, a stethoscope, and a glass of tap water.

1. Check for NG tube displacement as shown below for the Salem Sump tube. To do this, connect the NG tube to the syringe and aspirate a small amount of stomach contents into the syringe. If stomach contents do not return upon aspiration, or if the diameter of the feeding tube is too small, insert a bolus of 10 cc of air into the tube while auscultating the abdomen midline, just below the xiphoid process. The stomach will emit a loud gurgle when the bolus of air enters. A patient with a gastrostomy tube will not require this procedure because the gastrostomy tube is placed directly into the stomach through a surgical incision.

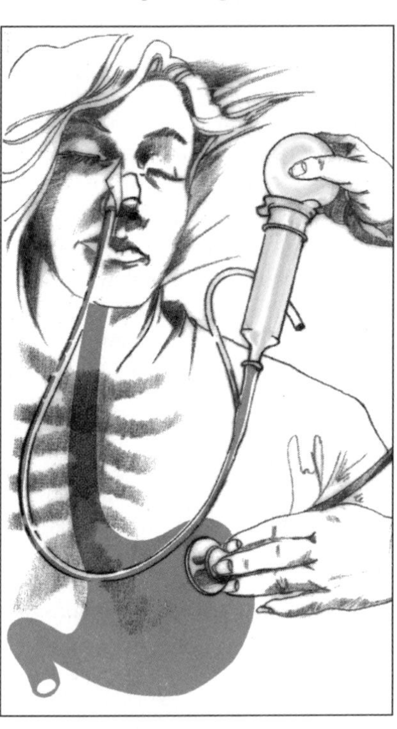

2. Remove the syringe from the tube. Then remove the plunger or bulb from the syringe and place the syringe back into the NG tube, making sure that it fits snugly.

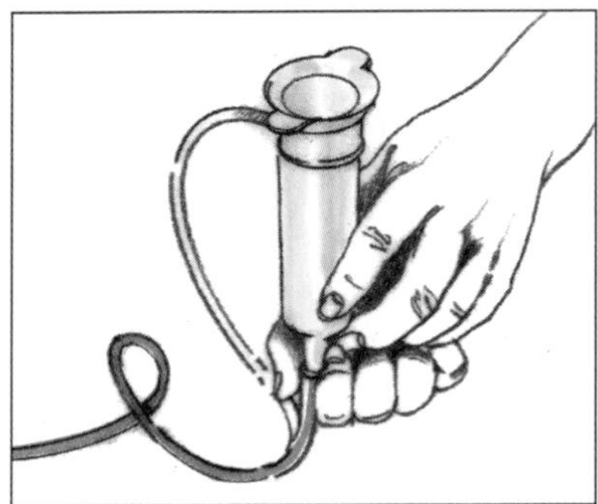

3. Slowly pour the medication into the syringe, which acts as a funnel.

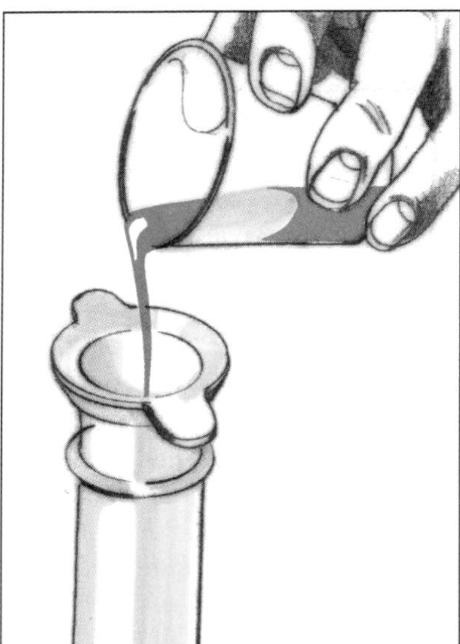

4. After the medication enters the gastric tube, measure 30 to 50 ml of room-temperature water in the medicine cup and pour it into the syringe. The amount of water needed depends on the length and diameter of the tube. Usually a large-bore tube requires 30 to 50 ml and a small-bore tube requires 15 to 25 ml. Flow into the gastric tube should occur by gravity. The water will help ensure that all medication is rinsed from the sides of the syringe, the gastric tube, and the medicine cup. This additional fluid also assists in maintaining tube patency. Any residue in the tube lumen may occlude the tube.

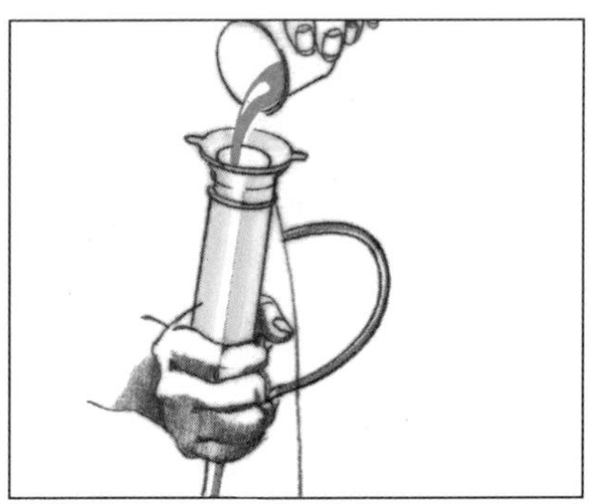

5. Remove the syringe from the tube while keeping a tissue or washcloth below the connection to catch any excess liquid. Then recap or clamp the gastric tube.

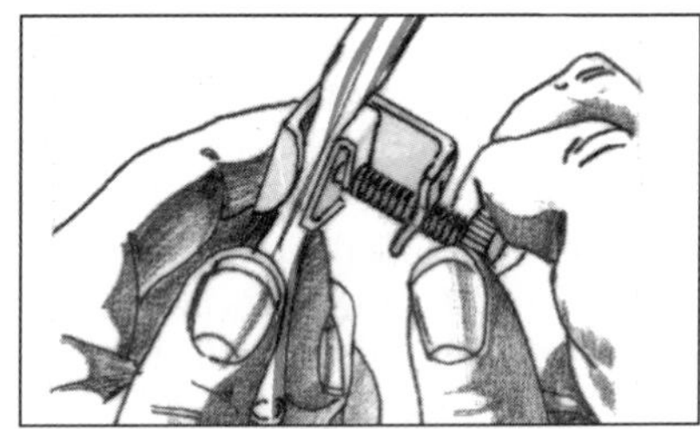

If crushing the tablet is necessary, the nurse should use a glass mortar and pestle or a special pill-crushing device. The pharmacy may perform this service for patients who cannot take medications orally. Ideally, the tablet would be available in a unit-dose package and the nurse would crush it without opening the package. When a unit-dose package is not available, the nurse crushes the tablet using a clean, dry mortar and pestle or places the tablet in a souffle cup and uses the pill-crushing device. The nurse then removes the uniformly crushed powder from the unit-dose package, mortar, or souffle cup, mixes it with a liquid, and administers the dose to the patient through the NG or gastrostomy tube. Then the nurse washes the mortar and pestle with soap and water.

Powders can be dissolved in lukewarm water. For capsules containing a liquid, the nurse can prick the capsule in one end with a needle and squeeze the contents into the gastric tube. The nurse also can dissolve the whole capsule in a small amount of lukewarm water and then administer the dose. Dissolving the capsule ensures administration of the entire dose, but the dissolution process can take a long time.

Many medications that require administration through a gastric tube are available in liquid form, the use of which always is preferable to crushing tablets. Some of these medications also may be given parenterally. When using a gastric tube, the nurse should administer only room-temperature liquids. Liquids going through a gastric tube bypass the mouth and esophagus, which normally help warm or cool fluid entering the stomach. A burning or cramping sensation can occur in the patient's stomach if a liquid that is too hot or too cold is administered through a gastric tube. (See *Administering medication through an NG tube.*)

SUBLINGUAL AND BUCCAL

Uncoated tablets are used for the **sublingual route** and **buccal route**. The tablets disintegrate and dissolve in the mouth, under the tongue (sublingual), or between the cheek and gum (buccal). Sublingual and buccal drugs are absorbed directly into the bloodstream from the oral mucosa, thus bypassing the GI and hepatic systems.

When a drug bypasses the liver, first-pass metabolism cannot reduce significantly the percentage of drug that reaches the systemic circulation. The time required for a drug to begin therapeutic action also greatly diminishes when the drug bypasses the GI tract. The reduced time needed for therapeutic action can be advantageous in certain circumstances. For example, nitroglycerin given sublingually for acute anginal pain dissolves under the tongue, where it enters the bloodstream directly. The onset of action can occur in seconds. The same drug orally routed via a gastrostomy tube takes up to 30 minutes to produce effective action.

The time difference produced by sublingual and buccal routing also influences peak serum levels and the duration of action. For example, the duration of action of sublingual nitroglycerin for acute anginal pain is approximately 5 minutes. A patient experiencing acute anginal pain lasting longer than 5 minutes may need another dose of sublingual nitroglycerin.

To administer drugs using the sublingual route, the nurse follows these steps: (1) Place the tablet in a souffle cup. (2) Identify the patient by checking the armband and name tag and asking the patient to state his or her name. (3) State the name of the drug and its action or use. (4) Ask the patient to open the mouth and touch the tip of the tongue to the roof of the mouth. (5) Place the tablet on the floor of the mouth and have the patient close the mouth. Instruct the patient not to swallow the tablet, but rather to hold it in place until it has been absorbed.

Another drug form used for sublingual administration is the spray. The nurse should identify the patient by using the standard procedures and then administer the spray according to the manufacturer's instructions. For example, the nurse dispenses nitroglycerin spray by completely depressing the plunger once on the pressurized aerosol container. Doing so provides the patient with a metered dose of the drug. The nurse should deliver the dose while the patient maintains an open mouth with or without the tongue raised toward the roof of the mouth. The spray is deposited on the floor of the mouth, in the same location as a sublingual tablet. The patient then closes the mouth and resumes normal activity.

For drug administration using the buccal route, the nurse follows these steps: (1) Place the medication in a souffle cup. (2) Identify the patient by using the standard procedure. (3) State the name of the drug and its action or use. (4) Have the patient open the mouth. (5) Place the tablet between the gum and cheek near the back of the mouth, and instruct the patient to close the mouth and keep the tablet against the cheek until it is absorbed.

Sublingual and buccal medications typically are kept at the patient's bedside for immediate use. In those instances, the medications are self-administered. Self-administration necessitates that the nurse provide adequate patient teaching and supervision and document it properly.

RECTAL

Nurses administer medications using the **rectal route** for various reasons. This route may be used when the oral route is prohibited, such as in a postoperative patient with an NG tube connected to continuous suction or in a patient with nausea or vomiting. The rectal route is the route of choice when certain local and systemic effects are desired. For example, bisacodyl suppositories are given to treat constipation. The rectal route also may represent the route of choice for unconscious patients because they cannot swallow.

Using the rectal route for administering medications poses several disadvantages. Receiving drugs rectally may embarrass the patient. Using the rectal route also can result in incomplete drug absorption if the patient cannot retain the medication or if the rectum contains feces. Also, pain can result if the patient has hemorrhoids or if the drug is irritating.

A drug may be administered using the rectal route in the form of a suppository or enema. (See *Inserting a rectal suppository*, page 64.)

The technique used for administering medications by enema depends on the time the patient must retain the fluid in the rectum. Medicated fluid that requires retention for at least 30 minutes is called a retention enema. In most cases, a retention enema contains 100 to 200 ml of fluid for adults and 75 to 150 ml of fluid for children ages 6 and over. Children under age 6 should not receive retention enemas because they cannot voluntarily retain the fluid.

The equipment that the nurse needs to administer a retention enema includes a rectal tube (14 or 20 French for adults and 12 to 14 French for children), water-soluble lubricant, a bedsaver pad, a 4" × 4" gauze pad or tissue, a rubber-tipped hemostat, a bedpan, a 200-ml catheter tip or bulb syringe with the plunger or bulb removed, and a paper

Inserting a rectal suppository

Before administering the medication, the nurse identifies the patient by checking the armband and name tag and asking the patient to state his or her name. Then the nurse states the name and action or use of the drug. To administer a suppository, the nurse will need these supplies: a finger cot or nonsterile disposable examination glove, a water-soluble lubricant, the foil-wrapped or unwrapped suppository, and a tissue or clean 4"×4" gauze pad. The nurse should draw the curtains or close the door to ensure the patient's privacy.

1. After helping the patient into a comfortable position in which the anus is exposed, place the glove or finger cot on the index finger of the dominant hand. Then remove the foil wrapper, if present. Holding the suppository in the gloved hand, lubricate the tapered end of the suppository with approximately 1 tsp (5 ml) of lubricant.

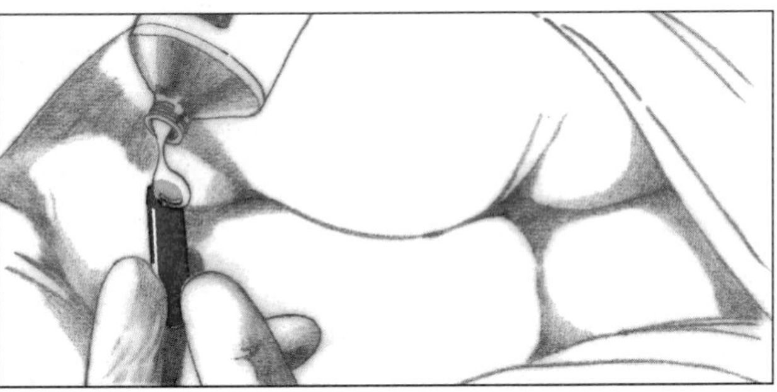

2. Spread the patient's buttocks and insert the suppository, tapered end first, into the anal opening, gently advancing the suppository past the anal sphincter. Use the index finger with the glove or the finger cot to advance the suppository far enough to pass the internal anal sphincter. In an adult, this distance is about 3" (7 cm); in a child, it may be considerably less depending on the child's size and age. Clean the excess lubricant from the anal area with the 4"×4" gauze pad or tissue, and encourage the patient to retain the suppository for at least 20 minutes. If the suppository is not a cathartic, the patient may feel little or no urge to expel it. If, however, the suppository is intended to relieve constipation, the patient may want to expel it as soon as an urge to defecate occurs.

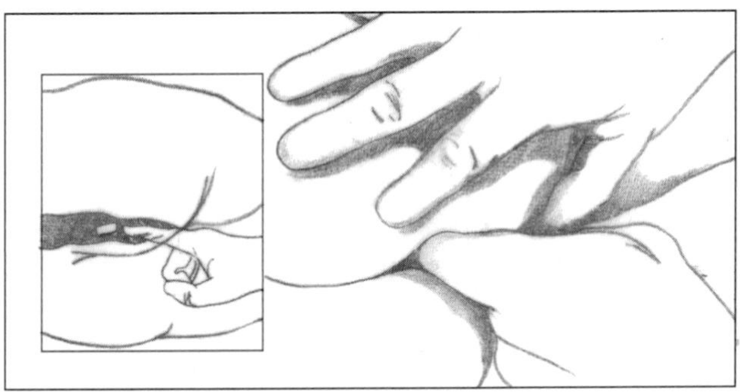

towel. To administer the retention enema, the nurse follows these steps: (1) After identifying the patient and explaining the purpose of the medication and the procedure, ensure the patient's privacy by closing the door or drawing the curtains. (2) With the bed flat, assist the patient onto the left side with the right knee flexed. This position allows the medication to flow from the rectum into the colon. If the patient cannot assume this position, help the patient lie on the right side or the back. (3) Place the bedsaver pad well under the patient's buttocks to protect the bed linen. (4) Insert the tip of the syringe into the rectal tube. (The syringe will act as a funnel.) Purge the air from the rectal tube by first turning the tip of the tube upward and pinching it off with the fingers. (5) Pour a small amount of the medicated solution into the syringe, slowly lowering the tip of the tube until the solution flows out. Immediately turn the tip upward and attach the hemostat, or close the clamp, about 8" (20 cm) from the tip. *Do not* lay down the syringe and tube from this point until the medication is instilled and the tube removed from the patient. Laying these items down would allow the fluid to flow out, and the procedure would need to begin again. (6) After purging the air from the tube, lubricate the tip of the tube with the water-soluble lubricant. Place approximately 1 tbs (15 ml) of lubricant on the paper towel and roll the distal 2" (5 cm) of the tip of the tube in the lubricant. (7) Separate the patient's buttocks and insert the tube into the anus. Advance the tube about 4" (10 cm) in an adult and 2" to 3" (5 to 7 cm) in a child, directing it toward the umbilicus. This technique can be awkward because the tube must be inserted with the same hand that is holding the syringe. To help alleviate awkwardness, hold the tube and syringe in the dominant hand and spread the patient's buttocks with the nondominant hand. (8) Slowly pour the prescribed solution into the syringe, holding the tip of the syringe about 4" to 5" (10 to 13 cm) above the anus. Release the clamp and allow the fluid to flow into the patient by gravity. If the fluid level rises too far above the anus, the patient may experience cramping or a strong urge to defecate. Instruct the patient to take deep breaths during the insertion and instillation to aid relaxation and avoid the urge to defecate. After instilling all of the solution, clamp the tubing. Inform the patient that you are going to remove the tube. (9) Instruct the patient to take a deep breath. As the patient inhales, quickly remove the tube. Firmly apply pressure against the anus with the 4"× 4" gauze pad or tissue for 10 to 20 seconds or until the urge to defecate passes. (10) Clean the area of any solution or lubricant, and encourage the patient to wait the prescribed length of time (usually at least 30 minutes) before evacuating the enema. Leave the bedsaver pad in place and the bedpan near the patient until the patient has defecated.

For patients who require a retention enema but cannot retain the fluid, the nurse may need to use a catheter with an inflatable balloon for administration. The nurse inserts the catheter into the rectum, inflates the balloon with the appropriate amount of air or saline solution, and administers the medication. After administration, the nurse clamps the catheter, thereby helping the patient retain the fluid. After the retention period, the nurse unclamps and removes the catheter. Expulsion of the retained fluid usually occurs simultaneously with catheter removal.

Nonretention enemas, which may be medicated or unmedicated, are given to evacuate the lower bowel. Nonretention enemas contain 750 to 1,000 ml of fluid for adults and lesser amounts for children and infants. Ideally, the adult and older child retain the fluid for 10 minutes. To administer the nonretention enema, the nurse uses an enema bag.

Parenteral administration techniques

Administration by the **parenteral route** can involve all routes other than the GI tract. The discussion in this chapter, however, concentrates on those medications given by **injection.** Nurses use the parenteral route to provide a rapid onset of action and to ensure high blood levels of the drug. The parenteral route also is used when the GI route would inactivate the drug, in unconscious patients, and in unstable or seriously ill patients who require precise administration and monitoring.

PREPARATION

Medications can be injected into several body spaces, and the type of injection depends on the body space that is used. The techniques and equipment used for each injection type vary. All injections require a liquid form of the prescribed drug and some type of syringe and needle; the nurse must know and use the correct type of needle and syringe for the different kinds of injections. For example, an intramuscular (I.M.) injection requires a long I.M. needle. A short subcutaneous (S.C.) needle would not reach the muscle, and pain or tissue damage could result. Using an incorrect needle also could alter the drug action and decrease the efficacy of the drug. (See *Syringes and needles,* pages 66 and 67.)

Dead space

After selecting the correct needle and syringe, the nurse must prepare the syringe. Part of this preparation may include consideration of the dead space in the syringe. Dead space refers to the volume of fluid in a syringe and needle that remains after the plunger has been depressed completely. Manufacturers calibrate syringes so that dead space compensation is not necessary.

However, the package inserts of iron dextran and aluminum-adsorbed toxoids and vaccines recommend use of the dead space to create an air bubble. With iron dextran, an air bubble and the Z-track method of injection help prevent permanent staining of the patient's skin should the solution leak into the subcutaneous tissue. To create an air bubble, the nurse may withdraw 0.2 cc of air after drawing up the correct dose of a medication into the syringe. (See *Z-track method for I.M. injections,* page 68.) Tracking of aluminum toxoids can cause abscesses and tissue necrosis, and the sealing action of the air bubble technique helps prevent these problems.

The nurse should not use the air bubble method with other types of I.M. injections or with any S.C. injections. No scientific evidence supports the use of an air bubble to prevent bruising after S.C. heparin injections, nor does the air bubble decrease the pain associated with I.M. injections.

Reconstitution and withdrawal from a vial

Liquid and powdered medications for parenteral administration are packaged in sterile vials. The nurse can withdraw liquid medication into the syringe, but powdered forms must be reconstituted first. (See *Reconstituting and withdrawing medications,* page 69.) The nurse must use sterile technique during all medication preparation and injection procedures to decrease the risk of infection.

Small air bubbles may adhere to the interior surface of the syringe when medication is withdrawn from a vial. This small amount of air would not harm the patient if injected; however, it could change the dose of medication actually administered. Therefore, the nurse should remove the air bubbles. To do so, hold the syringe with the needle pointed upward, tap the side of the syringe until the bubbles accumulate at the hub, then slowly push the plunger until the air is expelled. If the amount of medication is not accurate after this procedure, withdraw more of the drug to complete the prescribed dose.

Withdrawal from an ampule

Liquid medications for parenteral administration also can be packaged in sterile ampules. Powdered ones rarely are packaged in ampules. Before administering medication from an ampule, the nurse must withdraw it carefully. (See *Withdrawing solution from an ampule,* page 70.)

Mixing drugs

The nurse frequently must mix drugs in one syringe. Probably the most commonly mixed drugs are insulin preparations. Because the onset of action, peak concentration level, and duration of action of insulin preparations vary, the nurse may have to combine a rapid-acting and a longer-acting type to manage a patient's diabetes. Rather than administer two injections, the nurse mixes the two insulins together and administers a single injection. For example, the nurse might mix 10 U of regular insulin with 33 U of NPH insulin.

Before mixing 10 U of regular insulin and 33 U of NPH insulin in one syringe, the nurse should gather these supplies: an insulin syringe calibrated in units equal to the insulin concentration, two alcohol swabs, a vial of NPH insulin, and a vial of regular insulin. To mix the drugs, the nurse may use the following technique: (1) Gently roll the NPH insulin vial between the hands to mix the particles into suspension. This action is not necessary for regular insulin. (2) Clean the tops of the vials with the alcohol swabs. (3) Remove the needle cap and withdraw the plunger until 43 U of air, which equals the total insulin dose, are in the sy-

Syringes and needles

For every injection, the nurse must know and use the correct type of needle and syringe, as described below.

SYRINGES

Standard syringes are available in 3-, 5-, 10-, 20-, 25-, 30-, 35-, and 50-ml sizes. They are used to administer a wide variety of medications in numerous settings. Each one consists of a plunger, barrel, hub, needle, and dead space. The dead space in a syringe is the volume of fluid remaining in the syringe and needle when the plunger is depressed completely. Some syringes, such as insulin syringes, do not have dead space areas.

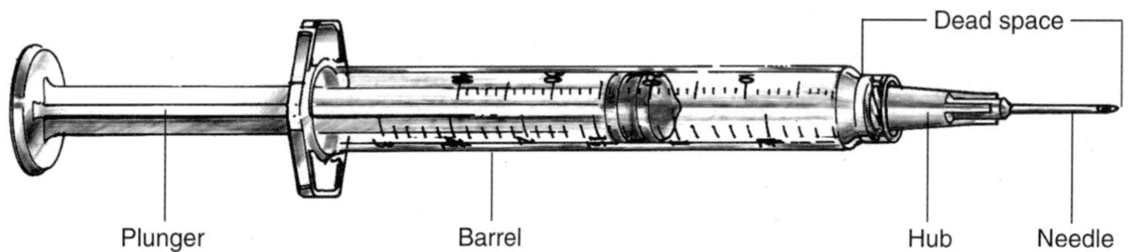

The **insulin syringe** has an attached 25-gauge (25G) needle and no dead space. The syringe is divided into units rather than milliliters for measurement. This syringe should be used only for insulin administration.

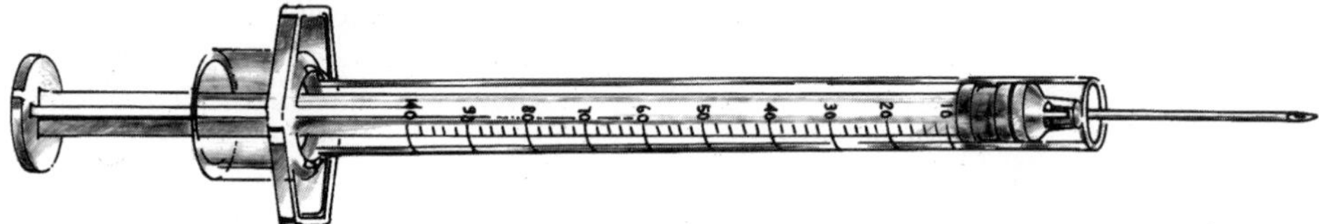

The **tuberculin syringe** holds up to 1 ml of medication. Used most commonly for intradermal injections, it also is used to administer small volumes of medication, such as might be required in pediatric and intensive care units.

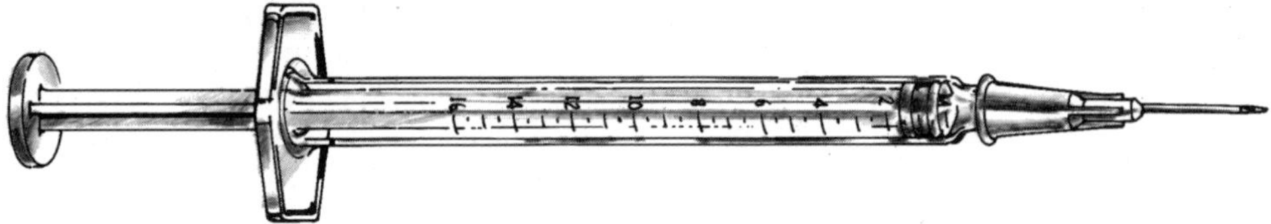

NEEDLES

When choosing a needle, the nurse must consider the needle gauge, bevel, and length. Gauge refers to the inside diameter of the needle. The smaller the gauge, the larger the diameter. Bevel refers to the angle at which the needle tip is opened, and length is the distance from the tip to the hub of the needle.

Needles usually used for **intradermal** injections are ⅜" to ⅝" (1 to 1.5 cm) long and are 25G. Such needles usually have short bevels.

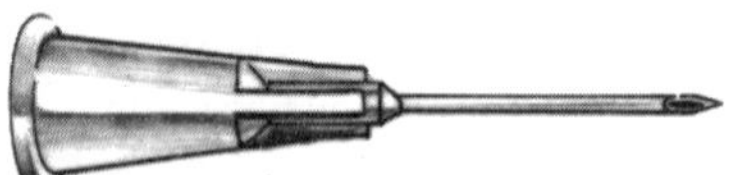

Needles for **subcutaneous** injections are ⅝" to ⅞" (1.5 to 2 cm) long, have medium bevels, and are 25G to 23G.

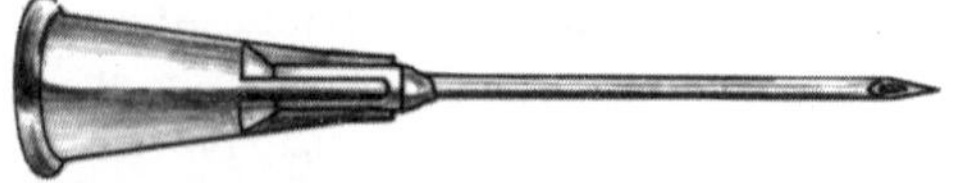

Needles for **intramuscular** use are 1" to 3" (2.5 to 7.5 cm) long, have medium bevels, and are 23G to 18G.

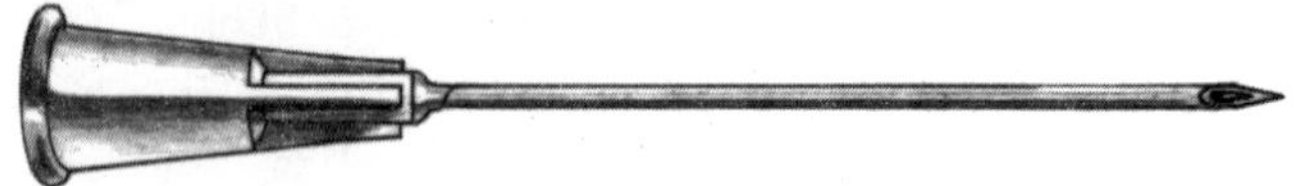

Syringes and needles *(continued)*

NEEDLES *(continued)*

Needles for **intravenous** use are 1" to 3" long, have long bevels, and are 25G to 14G.

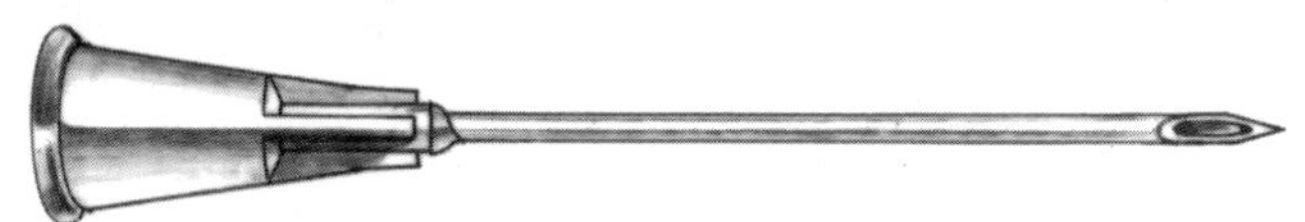

Microscopic pieces of rubber or glass may enter the solution when the nurse punctures the diaphragm of a vial with a needle or snaps open an ampule. The nurse can use a **filter needle** with a screening device contained within the hub to remove minute particles of foreign material from a liquid solution. Filter needles should not be used for injection. Filter needles are 1½" (4 cm) long, have medium bevels, and are 20G.

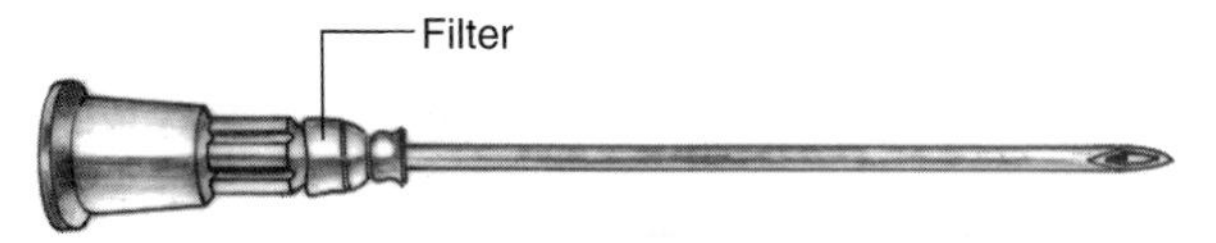

A **closed system device** comes with the needle in place. These devices come with the plunger attached (prefilled syringe) or as a cartridge to be inserted into a barrel with a plunger attached (cartridge-needle unit). Emergency drugs, such as atropine and lidocaine, are manufactured in prefilled syringes. Narcotic analgesics, heparin, and injectable vitamins are manufactured in cartridge-needle units.

To prepare a prefilled syringe, shown here, flip the protective caps off both ends. Remove the needle cap and expel any air in the system. To prepare a cartridge-needle unit, insert a cartridge into the reusable syringe. Twist the barrel until it is engaged. Then insert the plunger and twist until the barrel rotates in the reusable syringe. Remove the needle cap and purge the device of air and any extra medication.

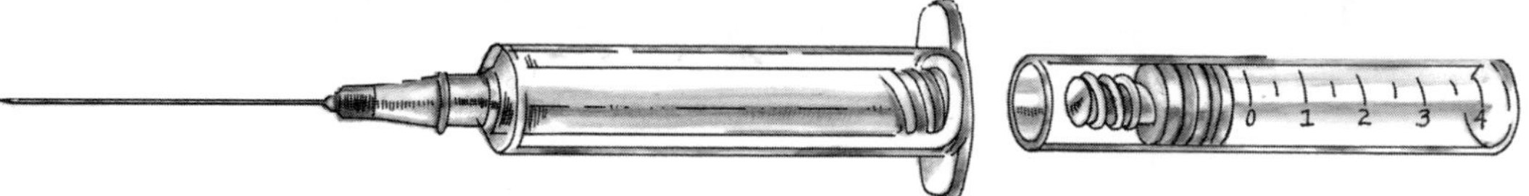

ringe. (4) Carefully inject 33 U of air into the NPH insulin vial and then inject the remaining 10 U into the regular insulin vial. Do not inject air into the solution itself because doing so may produce air bubbles that can alter the dose. Without removing the needle, invert the vial of regular insulin and withdraw exactly 10 U of regular insulin. (5) Insert the needle into the vial of NPH insulin. Invert the vial, and withdraw 33 U of NPH insulin. The plunger should be at the 43-U calibration. The medications now are mixed in one syringe and are ready for injection.

As in this example, regular insulin should be drawn up first to avoid the risk of contamination with the longer-acting insulin, which can cause potentially serious adverse reactions. However, if accidental mixing is suspected in either vial, the nurse should discard it because the contents have been altered.

Skin preparation

After filling the syringe, the nurse must prepare the patient's skin for injection. If the injection site is soiled, wash and dry the site thoroughly. Then use one of several antiseptic agents to disinfect the skin; ethyl alcohol and iodophor are two of the most commonly used. Use alcohol with intradermal injections because iodophor discolors the skin and can interfere with interpretation of skin test results. Also use alcohol with patients who are allergic to iodine.

Take care not to touch the patient's skin with anything except the sterile swab, cotton, or gauze impregnated with the disinfectant. When using a disinfectant, always begin at the point where the needle will be inserted and wipe in a spiral pattern from the center outward. Cleaning from the puncture site outward carries bacteria away from the site.

Before injecting the medication, allow the disinfected area to dry for about 1 minute. Do not blow on or fan the area to hasten the drying process because these activities increase the risk of contamination. Injecting while the skin is still moist can introduce alcohol or iodophor into the tissues and causes irritation. Allowing the skin to dry before injection in many cases reduces injection pain.

For a diabetic patient in a hospital or clinic, prepare the skin as described above. For a diabetic patient who self-administers insulin at home, teach the patient to simply wash the injection site with soap and water.

ADMINISTRATION

Common administration techniques for parenteral drugs include injections via the **intradermal, subcutaneous,** and **intramuscular routes** as well as administration via the **intravenous (I.V.) route.**

Z-track method for I.M. injections

The Z-track method for I.M. injections involves pulling the skin in such a way that subcutaneous layers are staggered, causing the needle track to be sealed off after the injection, minimizing subcutaneous irritation and discoloration. Following an injection, never massage the site or allow the patient to wear tight-fitting clothing over the site immediately after an injection. Either action could force the medication into the subcutaneous tissue and cause irritation. To increase the patient's absorption rate, encourage physical activity such as walking. For subsequent injections, remember to rotate the sites.

1. After withdrawing the appropriate amount of medication, draw 0.2 cc of air into the syringe. Then replace the needle with a sterile 3" (7.5-cm) needle.

Pull the skin laterally away from the intended injection site to ensure the needle's proper entry into the muscle tissue.

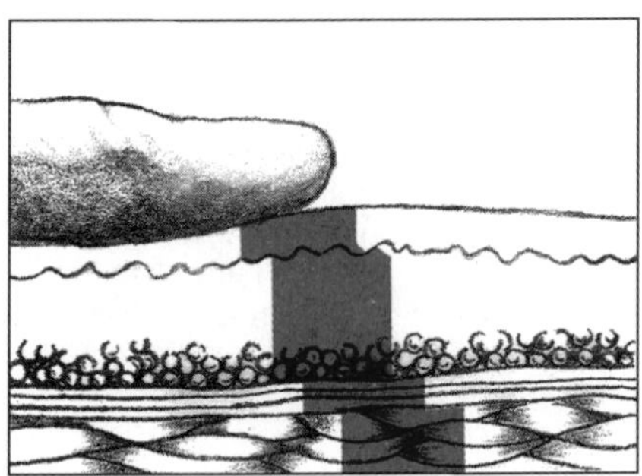

2. After cleaning the site, insert the needle, and inject the medication slowly.

When the injection is completed, wait 10 seconds before withdrawing the needle. Waiting prevents medication seepage from the site.

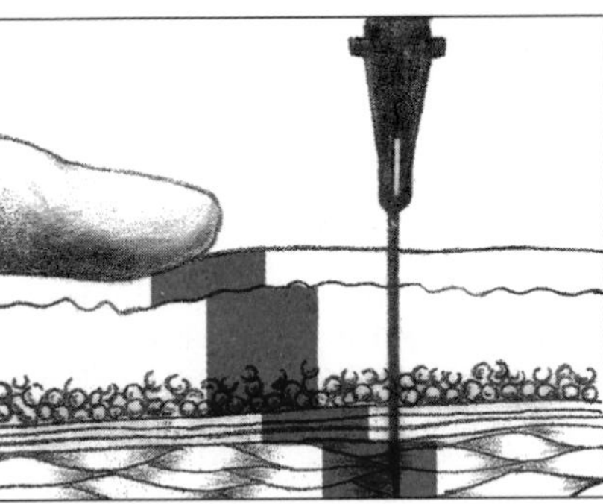

3. Withdraw the needle and syringe, and allow the retracted skin to resume its normal position, which effectively seals the needle track.

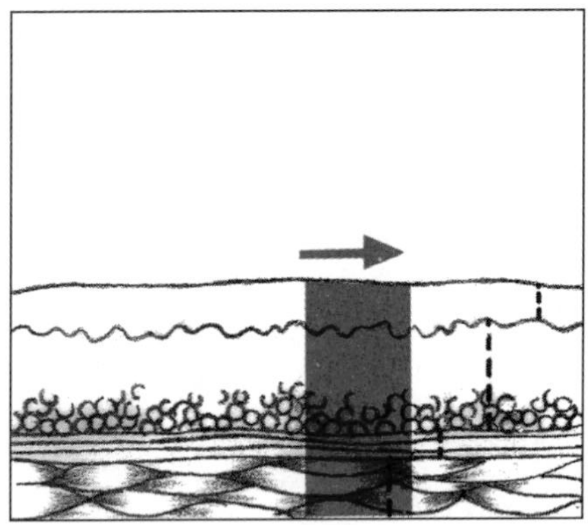

Intradermal

Intradermal injections are used for skin tests, such as the tuberculin or histoplasmin test. Most nurses seldom give intradermal injections. However, when they do, they should administer the injection in the area of the scapula, upper chest, dorsal upper arm, or the ventral forearm. The ventral forearm is the site of choice. Any area with scars, blemishes, or abundant hair should not be used because it could hamper interpretation of the test results. Identify the patient by checking the armband and asking his name. Then explain the medication and the procedure to the patient. (See *Injection sites and techniques,* pages 71 through 75.)

Subcutaneous

Subcutaneous (S.C.) injections provide a slow, sustained release of medication and a longer duration of action and are used when the total volume injected is no more than 1 ml of liquid. Many medications, including insulin, heparin, and epinephrine, are given by the S.C. route.

S.C. injection sites, all areas relatively distant from bones and major blood vessels, include the area over the scapula, the lateral aspects of the upper arm and thigh, and the abdomen. At least a 1" (2.5-cm) pinched fold of skin and tissue is necessary for administering an S.C. injection. Burned, edematous, or scarred skin should not be used as an S.C. injection site, nor should the area 2" (5 cm) in diameter around the umbilicus or the belt line.

The nurse should ensure that injection sites are rotated and that a rotation pattern is established for patients who receive frequent S.C. injections. Site rotation helps promote adequate absorption of the medication and prevents the formation of hard nodules in the subcutaneous tissue. Because site rotation is especially critical for diabetic patients, the nurse must include it as part of the teaching plan for self-care. One effective method of rotating sites is to use a diagram to represent the patient's pattern.

When a patient does not self-administer injections, the rotation pattern being used must be communicated to other nurses. Most facilities have special flow sheets available to record the rotation patterns used for a specific patient. Notations also can be made on medication sheets.

In many cases, heparin and insulin are administered by the S.C. route using the abdominal sites. The administration technique for these sites resembles that used for the general S.C. injection, and the nurse or patient usually gives the injection holding the needle at a 90-degree angle. Grasping a skin fold, however, is not always necessary at the abdominal site. Furthermore, if the patient is dehydrated, cachectic, or frail, the abdominal site may not provide adequate subcutaneous tissue for injections.

Aspiration is not necessary with S.C. injection because subcutaneous tissue usually contains only small blood vessels. Therefore, the danger of unintended I.V. injection is minimal. In fact, aspirating S.C. injections may cause tissue damage that could affect drug absorption adversely and in the case of insulin injection may lead to nodule formation in the subcutaneous tissue.

Reconstituting and withdrawing medications

To reconstitute and withdraw medication from a vial, the nurse will need these supplies: the medication vial, a vial or ampule of an appropriate diluent, an iodophor or ethyl alcohol swab, a syringe, two needles of appropriate size, and a filter needle, if available, to screen particulate matter that may accumulate from reconstitution.

1. Place the medication vial on a countertop. Wipe the rubber diaphragm with the alcohol or iodophor swab. Do not rub the diaphragm vigorously because doing so can introduce bacteria from the nonsterile rim of the vial. Repeat the process with the vial of diluent.

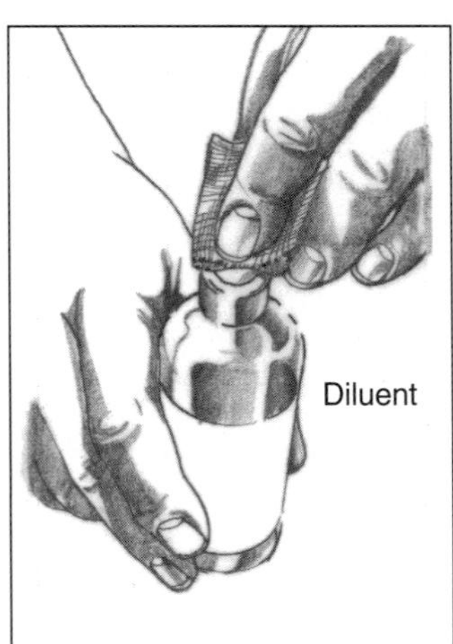

2. Pick up the syringe, uncap the needle, and pull back on the plunger until the space inside the syringe equals the amount of diluent desired. Puncture the rubber diaphragm of the diluent vial with the needle, and inject the air, as shown. Injecting the air counters the fluid volume and creates a positive pressure. The positive pressure allows the fluid to be easily withdrawn from the vial and prevents a vacuum from forming after the contents are withdrawn. Invert the vial, and withdraw the desired amount of diluent.

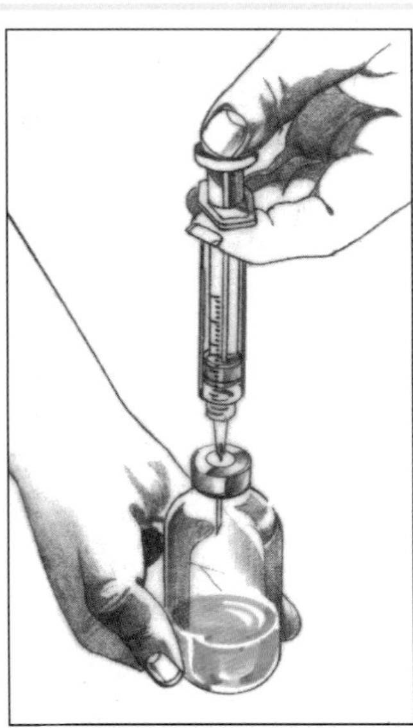

3. Inject the diluent into the medication vial, and withdraw the needle. Roll or shake the vial to mix the medication thoroughly. If a filter needle is available, remove the first needle, and attach the filter needle to the syringe and uncap it. If a filter needle is not available, leave the first needle attached to the syringe.

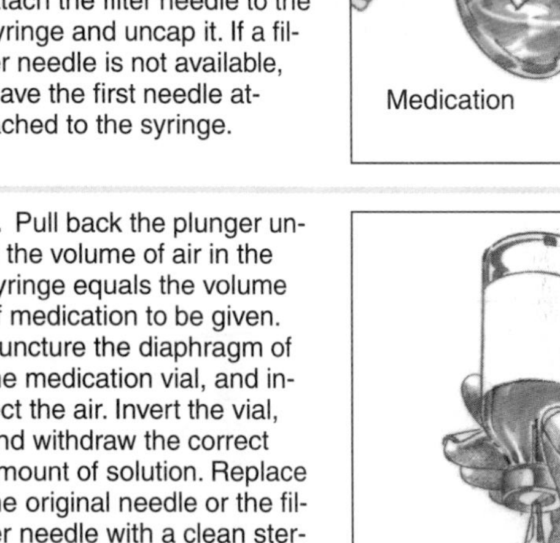

4. Pull back the plunger until the volume of air in the syringe equals the volume of medication to be given. Puncture the diaphragm of the medication vial, and inject the air. Invert the vial, and withdraw the correct amount of solution. Replace the original needle or the filter needle with a clean sterile needle because medication that may have adhered to the needle when the solution was withdrawn from the vial can irritate the patient's tissues. The syringe filled with medication is now ready to label and administer to the patient. If the medication is already in a liquid form, withdrawing it from a vial involves the same steps as previously described in handling a medication after reconstitution.

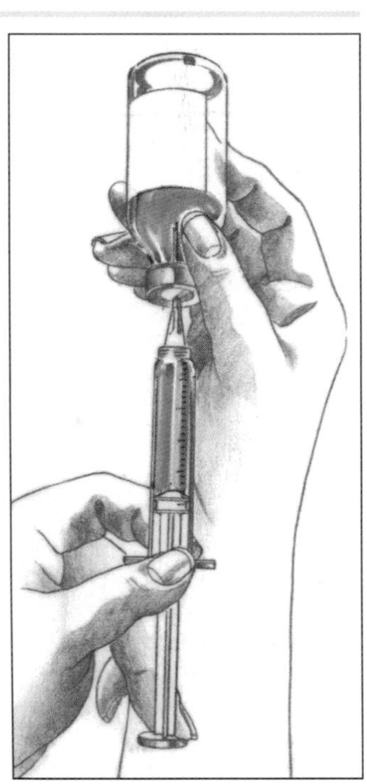

Insulin pumps. An insulin pump is a device that delivers a continuous infusion of insulin into a selected subcutaneous site, commonly the abdomen. The patient places the day's supply of insulin in a syringe and inserts the syringe into the pump. A length of special tubing is connected to the hub of the syringe, and a subcutaneous needle is attached to the distal end. The patient inserts the special needle into the abdomen at a 45-degree angle. Then the patient tapes the needle in place and begins the infusion.

The nurse must instruct the patient to change the insertion site every 2 days and keep the site dry to prevent bacterial contamination. The nurse also must teach the patient how to operate the insulin pump and where to seek help if a problem arises at home.

Intramuscular

Intramuscular (I.M.) injections are given for various reasons, especially when the rapid absorption of medication is desired. The onset of action usually occurs within 10 to 15 minutes after an I.M. injection. However, the blood flow to the injection site affects the absorption rate. I.M. injections of drugs that irritate subcutaneous tissues cause less pain than S.C. injections. Also, a larger amount of fluid can be administered in an I.M. injection. The recommended maximum volume for a single I.M. injection for an adult is 5 ml.

Commonly used I.M. injection sites include the dorsogluteal, ventrogluteal, vastus lateralis, rectus femoris, and deltoid muscles. The nurse needs to identify I.M. injection sites accurately. Major blood vessels and nerves traverse the

Withdrawing solution from an ampule

To withdraw medication from an ampule, the nurse will need these supplies: an ampule with the medication, a syringe, two needles of appropriate size, and a dry 2" × 2" gauze pad. These illustrations show the steps involved.

Make sure that all of the fluid is located in the base of the ampule; if any remains in the stem, or top portion, gently tap the stem to cause the liquid to flow through the thin neck to the base. If tapping the stem does not work, grasp the stem of the ampule, raise it to approximately eye level, and then quickly swing it down at arm's length.

Wrap the ampule stem with the 2" × 2" gauze pad to protect your fingers from cuts as the neck is snapped (below). Hold the body of the ampule in one hand and the tip between the thumb and finger of the other hand. While pointing the ampule away from you and others, snap off the top. Inspect the solution for small particles of glass. Discard the solution if any are present.

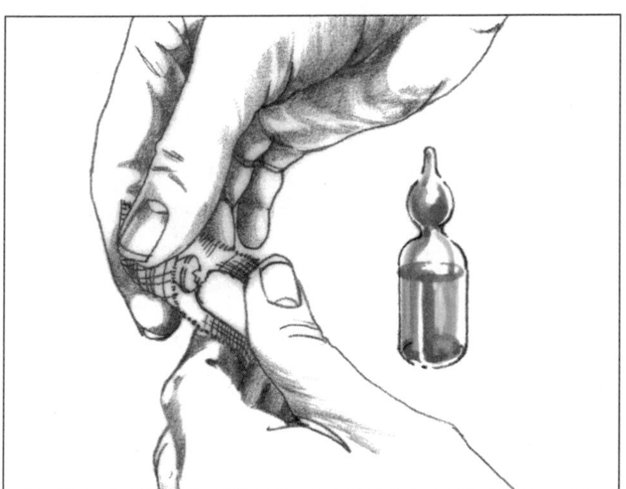

Place the first needle, such as a filter needle, on the syringe. Insert the needle into the fluid, and withdraw the appropriate amount of medication (below). Finally, replace this needle with the second needle for administering the medication. (By changing needles, the nurse prevents irritation that results from medication that remains on the outside of the first needle.) The medication is now ready for injection.

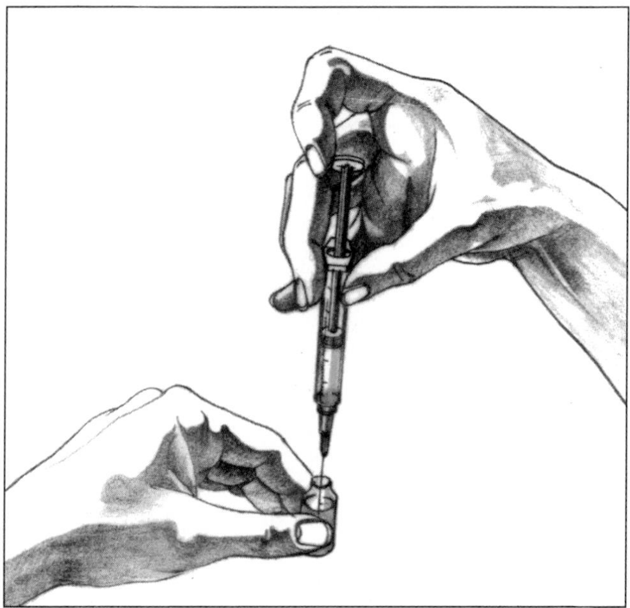

muscle groups used for I.M. injection. Therefore, using an inappropriate injection site could result in permanent damage to the patient.

Damage to a muscle also can occur if the muscle group is overused for injections, which can be avoided by rotating sites. For example, if the nurse gives an injection in the left ventrogluteal muscle, the next injection might be in the left dorsogluteal or right ventrogluteal site, and a third injection might be given in the right dorsogluteal site. The nurse should record on the medication sheet each I.M. site used.

The technique for administering an I.M. injection is the same for an adult or a pediatric patient. The nurse should use the Z-track method for I.M. injection when a medication, such as iron dextran (Imferon), can irritate or discolor subcutaneous tissue.

CRITICAL THINKING: To enhance your critical thinking about routes and techniques of administration, consider the following situation and its analysis.

Situation: During the second day after a total hip replacement, Mabel Ennis, age 82 and 105 lb (47.6 kg), asks the nurse not to use her thigh to inject her pain medication because she's already had two I.M. injections there today. Mrs. Ennis is now positioned on her back. What should the nurse do?

Analysis: The nurse should consider other I.M. sites. The volume of most I.M. injections for pain medication would be too large for such a small person's deltoid muscle. The nurse would want to rotate the site (and not use the vastus lateralis muscle again), but the dorsal gluteal muscle isn't an option because of the patient's current positioning. The nurse may use the ventrogluteal site because it is easily accessible and can absorb a larger amount of medication than the deltoid.

Intravenous

Medications are administered intravenously (I.V.) to obtain an immediate onset of action, to attain the highest possible blood concentration level of a drug, and to treat conditions that require the constant titration of medication. In many cases, life-threatening situations, such as shock, require such constant titration. I.V. administration also is used when the

(Text continues on page 75.)

Injection sites and techniques

Before giving an intradermal, subcutaneous (S.C.), intramuscular (I.M.), or intravenous (I.V.) injection, the nurse should be familiar with the appropriate injection sites and techniques, as described here. The nurse should always identify the patient according to standard procedure and state the drug's name and action or use.

Intradermal injection sites and techniques

Common sites for intradermal injections include the scapula, upper chest, dorsal upper arm, and ventral forearm (the site of choice).

1. To identify the injection site on the ventral forearm, have the patient extend the forearm and rest it on a table with the palm up. Measure two to three finger-widths distal from the antecubital space. Then measure a hand-width proximal from the wrist. The space between these measures represents the area available for injection. Prepare the injection site with an alcohol swab. Expel any air in the syringe.

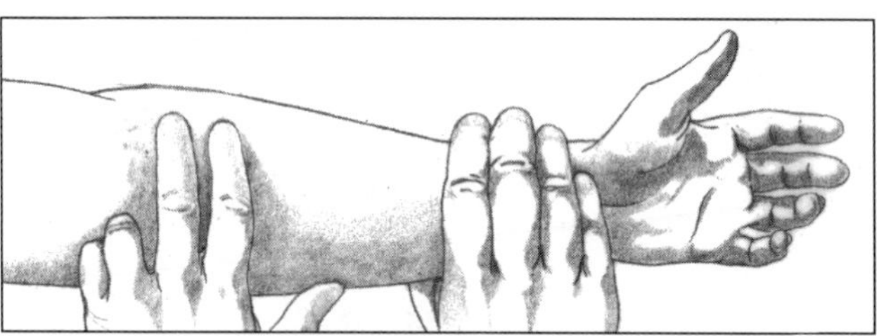

2. With the nondominant hand, retract the patient's skin proximal to the injection site until the skin over the site is taut. To prevent contamination, do not touch the injection site. With the other hand, place the syringe almost flat against the patient's skin (approximately at a 15-degree angle) with the bevel up. Insert the needle by pressing it slowly against the skin.

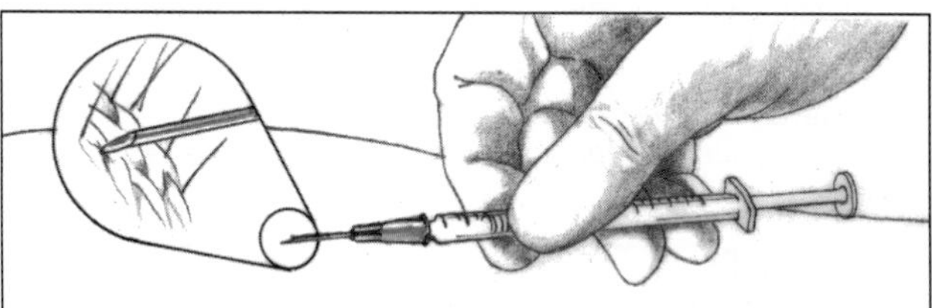

3. Inject the drug slowly and gently. During injection, the needle should be visible through the skin, and resistance should be felt. The area should display blanching and formation of a wheal about 6 mm in diameter.

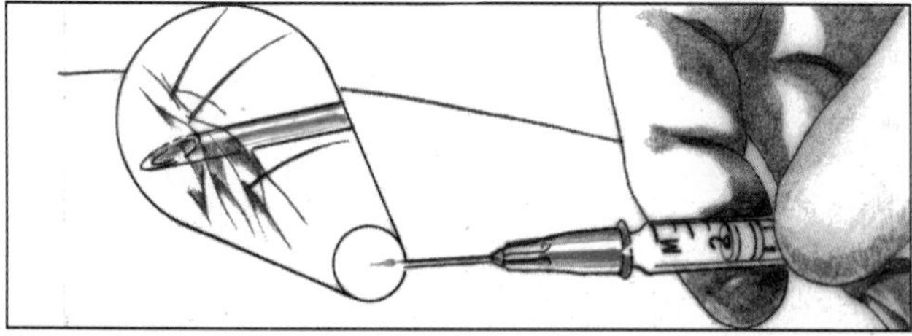

4. When the injection is completed, withdraw the needle and apply gentle pressure to the site. Do not massage the area because massage can irritate the site and interfere with results.

Subcutaneous injection sites

The nurse or patient can use a number of administration sites in several areas for S.C. injections. Systematic rotation of injections helps maintain those sites. In documenting a patient's site rotation pattern, the nurse frequently uses a diagram similar to the one below.

In a typical patient, the nurse would administer the first injection in the site represented by a dot on the upper right quadrant and administer the next injection in the area represented by the second dot in that row. This continues until the sites represented by the top row of dots have been used once, then proceeds with the site represented by the dot on the figure's right side in the center row. When each of the sites on the abdomen have been used once, injections may begin in the right leg and follow a similar pattern. When all right leg sites have been used, injections can begin in another area.

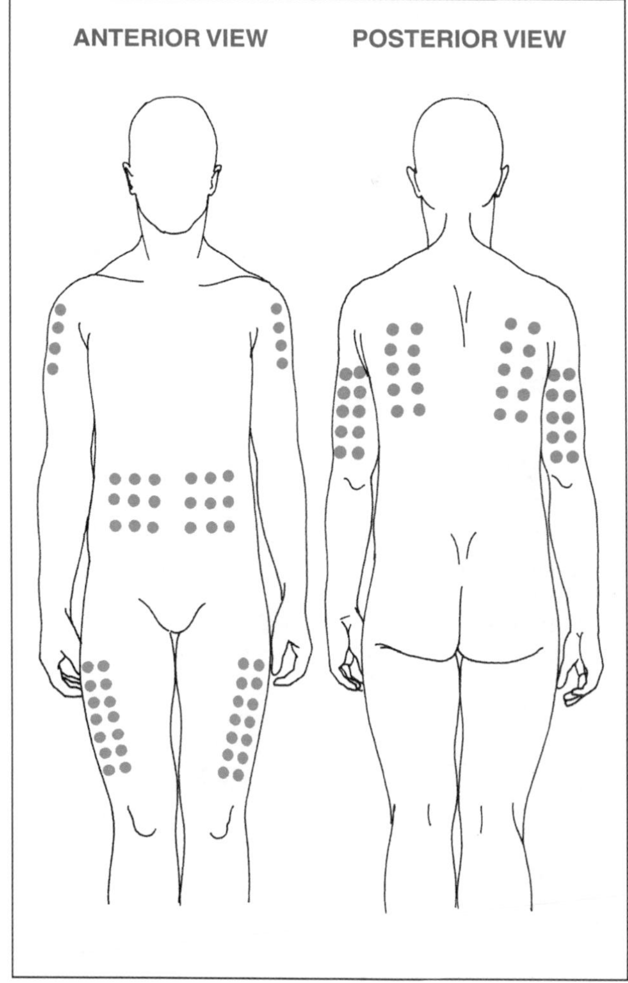

(continued)

Injection sites and techniques *(continued)*

Subcutaneous injection techniques

To administer an S.C. injection, the nurse will need a syringe with a 25G to 23G needle, the medication, and two alcohol or iodophor swabs.

1. Gather the necessary equipment. Then, identify and prepare the injection site using an alcohol swab.

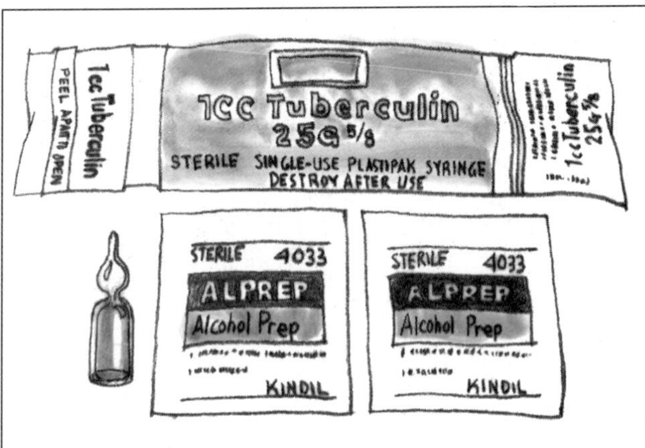

2. Open a second alcohol swab. To keep the swap accessible and maintain sterility of the portion that will contact the insertion site, remove the swab from the wrapper while touching only a corner. Place that same corner between the index and middle finger of the nondominant hand while administering the injection. Grasp at least a 1" (2.5-cm) skin fold of the prepared skin area between the thumb and first two fingers of the nondominant hand. Remember, the swab is also in this hand.

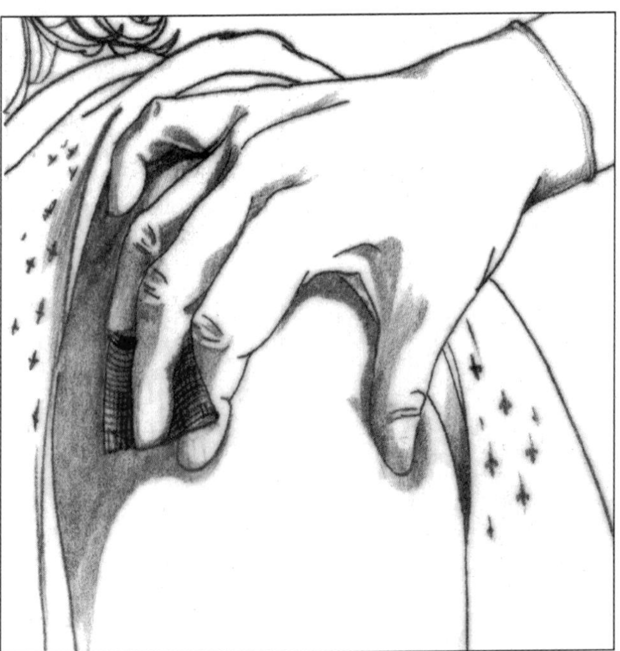

3. In the dominant hand, hold the syringe like a pencil with the bevel of the needle up. If the needle is ½" or shorter, hold it at a 90-degree angle to the skin fold. If the needle is ⅝", as in the illustration, hold it at a 45-degree angle.

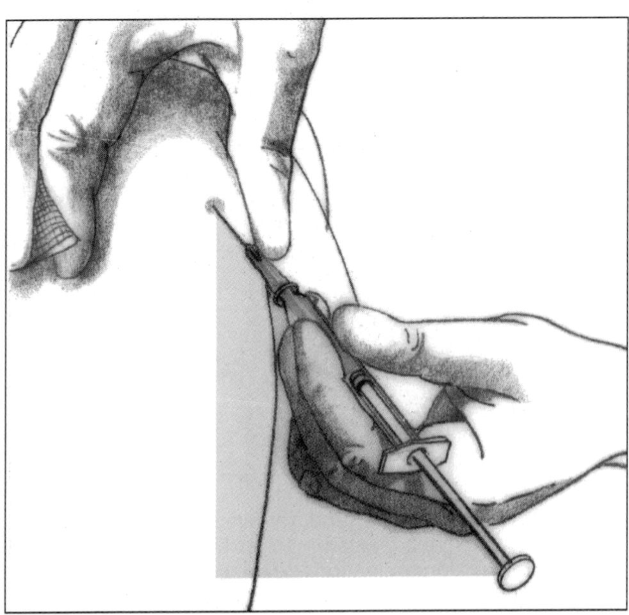

4. Insert the needle using a quick, dartlike motion. Then release the skin fold, and slowly inject the medication. When the plunger is completely depressed and all medication has been injected, place the sterile portion of the second alcohol swab over the insertion site. While gently applying downward pressure, quickly withdraw the needle and syringe. Continue to apply gentle pressure to the site for several seconds.

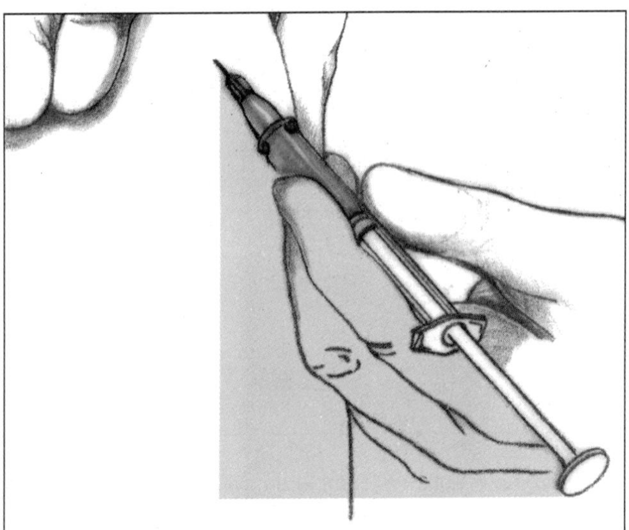

Injection sites and techniques *(continued)*

Intramuscular injection sites

In adult patients, the most commonly used I.M. injection sites are the ventrogluteal, dorsogluteal, deltoid, vastus lateralis, and rectus femoris muscles. The following illustrations identify each injection site and its anatomic landmarks.

Ventrogluteal

Used for all patients, this site is desirable because it is not only relatively free of large nerves and adipose tissue, but is also remote from the rectum (which minimizes the risk of contamination).

For this site, position the patient on the back or side.

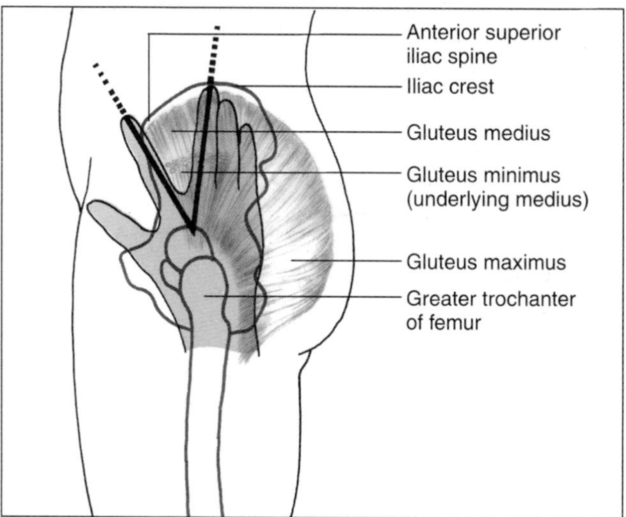

Deltoid

This muscle is small, is near the radial nerve, and can accommodate only small doses of medications.

For this site, seat the patient upright or have the patient lie flat with the arms apart.

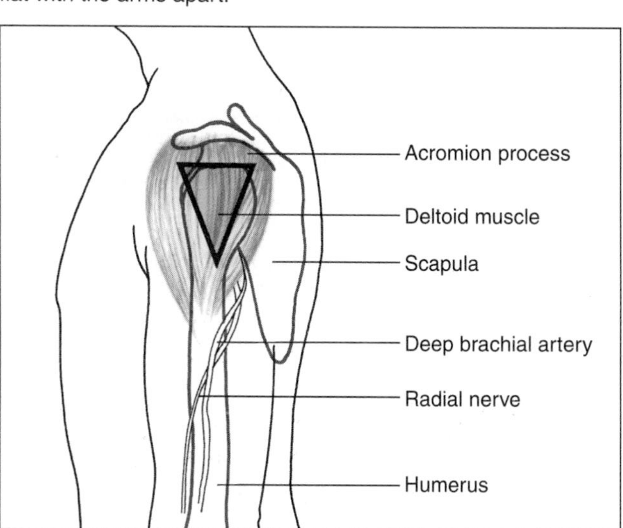

Dorsogluteal

Commonly used for adults, the dorsogluteal site is not used for infants and children under age 3 because these muscles are not well developed.

Position the patient flat on the stomach with the toes pointed inward and the arms apart and flexed toward the head.

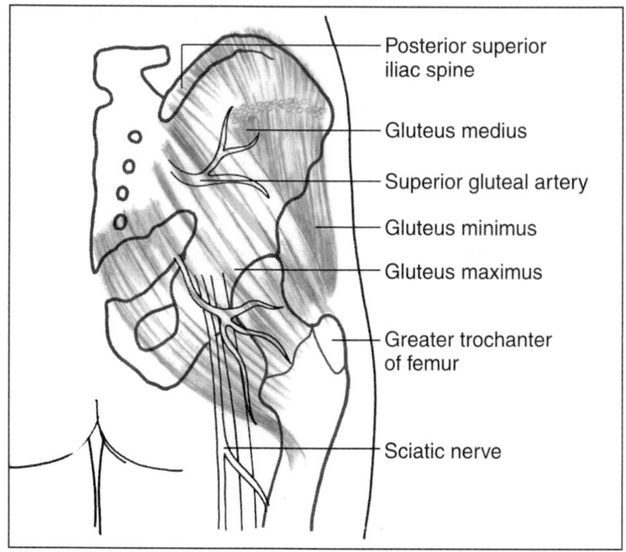

Vastus lateralis and rectus femoris

The vastus lateralis is used for all patients, especially children. It is well developed and has few major blood vessels and nerves. The rectus femoris is used most commonly for self-injection because of its accessibility.

For this site, position the patient sitting up or lying flat.

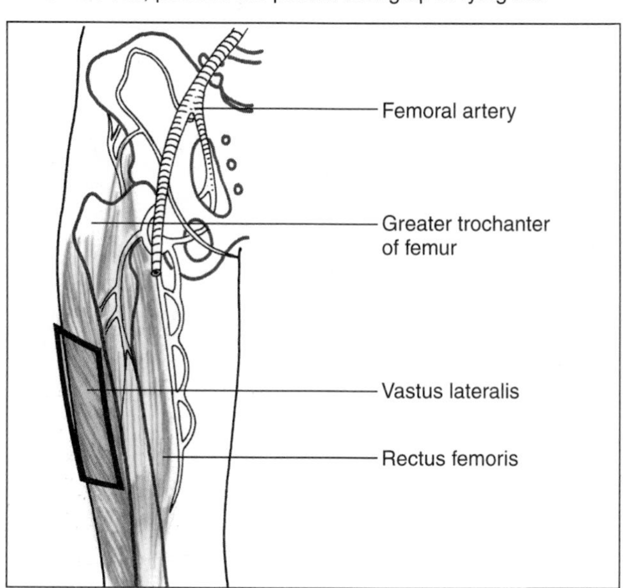

(continued)

Injection sites and techniques *(continued)*

Intramuscular injection techniques

To administer a medication by an I.M. injection, the nurse will need two alcohol swabs, a syringe containing the medication to be injected, and a needle of appropriate size.

1. Expose the area where the injection will be administered. Remember to provide privacy for the patient if any site other than the deltoid muscle is being used. Palpate the appropriate anatomic landmarks, and identify the exact site for the injection. In this illustration, the vastus lateralis muscle is being used.

Prepare a 2" (5-cm) diameter area of skin around the injection site using an alcohol swab. Open a second alcohol swab and place it between the index and second finger of the nondominant hand.

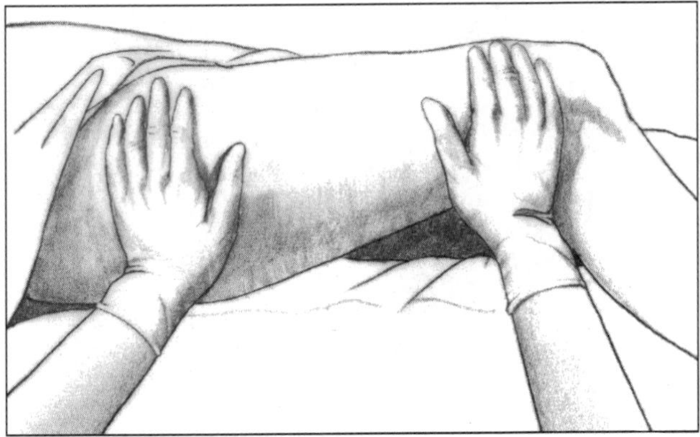

2. Grasp the syringe like a pencil in the dominant hand, and remove the needle cap. With the nondominant hand, spread the skin surrounding the injection site until it is taut. This action helps displace the subcutaneous tissue and brings the muscle closer to the surface.

With a quick, dartlike motion, insert the needle at a 90-degree angle into the muscle. Release the skin surrounding the injection site and use the nondominant hand to steady the syringe for aspiration.

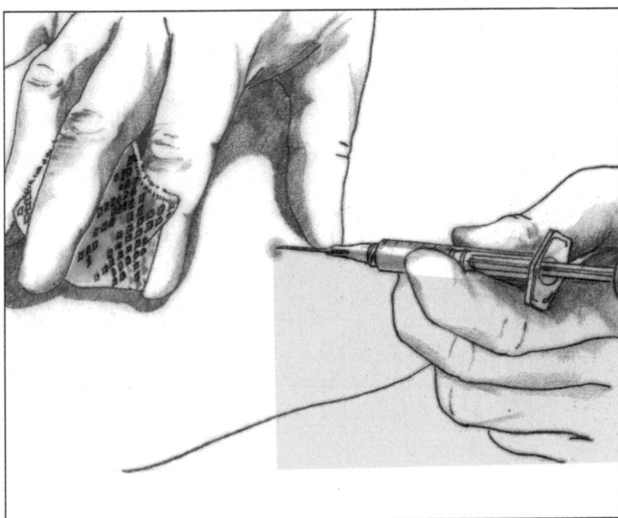

3. Gently aspirate; aspiration is used to determine if the inserted needle has entered a vessel. Pull back slightly on the plunger after inserting the needle into the injection site. If the needle has entered a vessel, blood will flow into the syringe. If blood is aspirated, remove and discard the syringe. Then start the procedure again. If no blood is aspirated, *slowly* inject the medication. Steady the syringe with the nondominant hand during aspiration and injection.

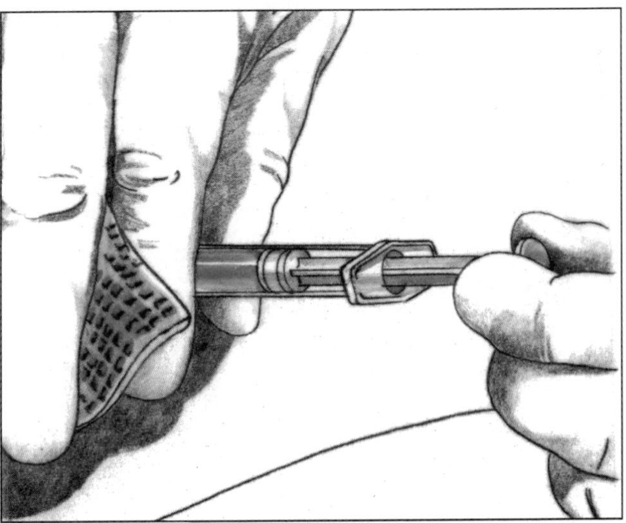

4. When the injection is completed, place the second alcohol swab over the insertion site and apply gentle downward pressure while quickly withdrawing the needle. Massage the site with the alcohol swab to help promote circulation to the area and decrease pain.

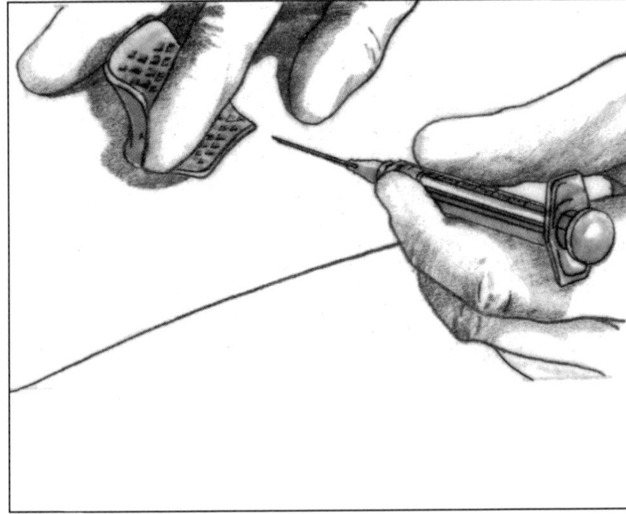

Injection sites and techniques *(continued)*

Intravenous injection sites and techniques

Common sites for I.V. injections include the superficial veins in the dorsum of the hand and in the forearm, because they offer the most choices. When trauma renders these sites impractical, the feet and legs offer acceptable injection sites.

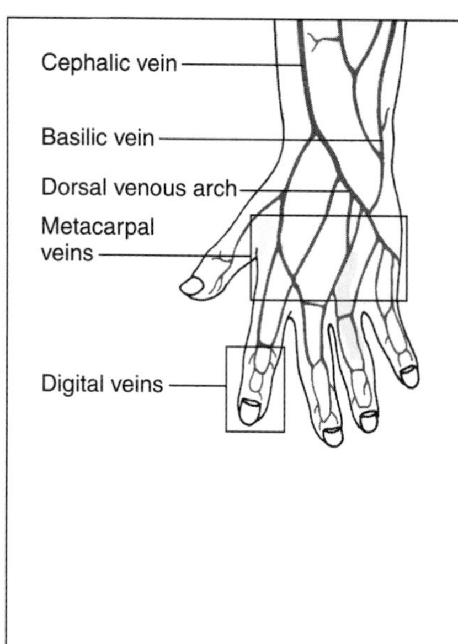

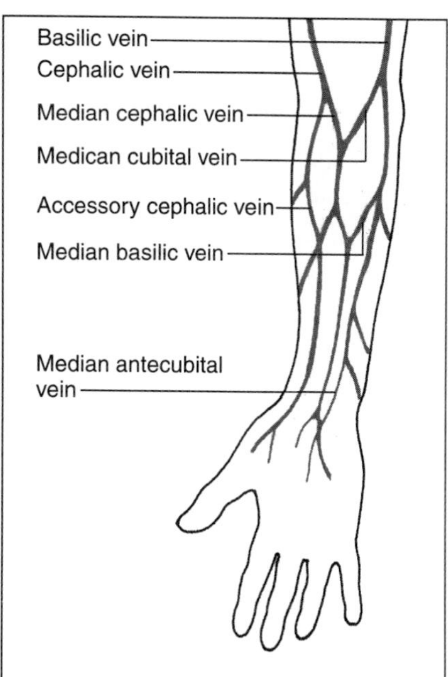

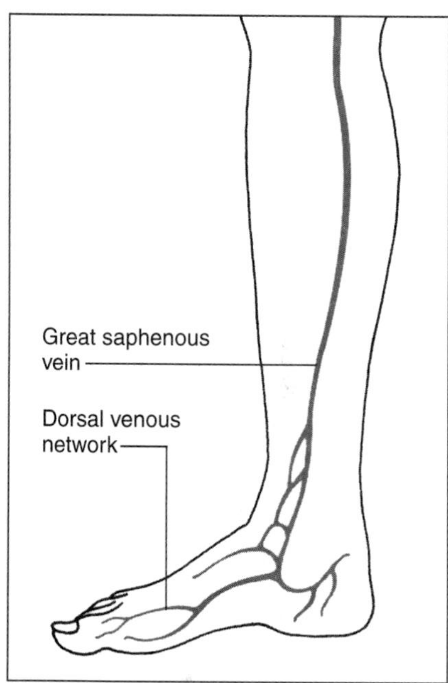

The I.V. injection technique varies with the type of administration prescribed: direct bolus, intermittent infusion, continuous infusion, or central venous catheter administration. The nurse should follow institutional policy and the general guidelines in this text when administering any type of I.V. injection.

medication is not available in another form and when the patient cannot tolerate the medication via other routes.

Sites used for I.V. administration include the veins on the hand and wrist, the forearm veins that traverse the antecubital fossa, the veins in the scalp and the umbilical vessels (for infants), the subclavian and internal and external jugular veins (for long-term administration or for medications that require rapid blood dilution), and the superficial veins of the leg and foot when other sites cannot be used.

The equipment used for an I.V. injection depends on several factors. The vein chosen for the injection or infusion in part determines the type of needle used. For a one-time bolus of a medication, the nurse may use an antecubital vein because of the vein's accessibility and large size. For a bolus type of injection at an antecubital site, the nurse may use a syringe with a needle. For continuous or intermittent infusions lasting a few days, the nurse would select a vein of the hand, wrist, forearm, scalp, or umbilicus. For such an infusion, the nurse would use a cannula. For a single-dose infusion, the nurse would use a scalp vein needle (also called a butterfly because of the winglike tabs used to hold the needle during insertion). If the solution is irritating, a smaller-gauge needle is recommended to create greater dilution by the blood flow.

Special catheters, called central venous (CV) catheters, are used for infusions that require rapid blood dilution and infusions or injections administered frequently over a prolonged time. They must be inserted into a large vein, such as the subclavian vein. Temporary venous access catheters, such as triple-lumen catheters, may be inserted for emergency access, blood sampling, or short-term therapy with antibiotics, blood or blood products, or agents used for chemotherapy or total parenteral nutrition.

For long-term venous access, the physician may insert a catheter, such as a Hickman, Broviac, or Groshong catheter; these catheters have from one to three lumens. A vascular access port may also be used for long-term access. A certified RN may insert a peripherally inserted central catheter (PICC) line, commonly used in long-term and home care.

After determining the appropriate site and needle, the nurse performs a venipuncture. When the venipuncture has been completed, the nurse documents the date and time of the insertion, the type and gauge of needle inserted, and the initials of the person inserting the I.V. on the tape that se-

Vascular access port

The illustration below provides a cutaway view of drug injection through a vascular access port (VAP). The inset shows the entire VAP device.

Implantable VAP

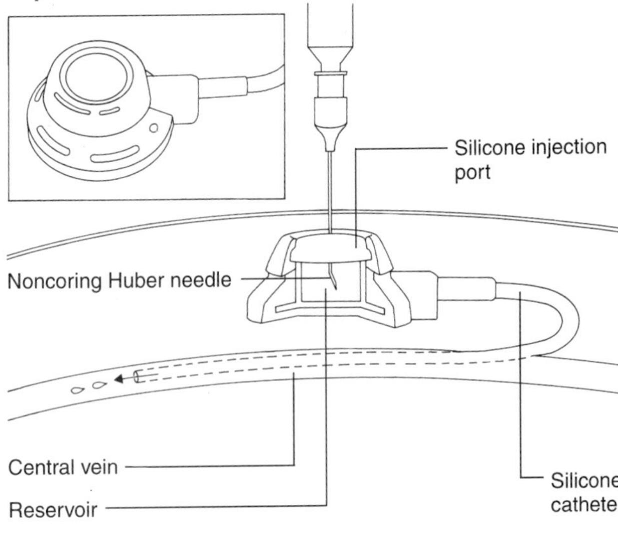

cures the gauze pad. Once a venipuncture has been performed, I.V. administration of medication can begin.

Direct bolus. To administer medication by direct bolus, the nurse will need two syringes and 20G or smaller needles filled with 1 ml of 0.9% sodium chloride (normal saline) solution, a syringe and needle with the prescribed medication, a syringe and needle with 1 ml of heparin flush solution (if required by facility policy), and three iodophor or alcohol swabs to clean all ports and vials prior to puncturing them with a needle.

To administer the bolus, the nurse should identify the patient and explain the medication and procedure. Clean the intermittent infusion port with a swab or remove the cap from the needleless system. Puncture the port with the syringe containing the normal saline solution. Gently aspirate for a blood return to ensure correct placement. Inject the saline.

Use the syringe containing the medication and slowly inject the medication through the line over the recommended time interval. Withdraw the syringe, and clean the port. Inject the saline from the second syringe to rinse all medication from the port and needle. Then inject the saline solution. Swab the port, and inject the heparin flush solution (if required). Remove the needle and syringe.

Intermittent infusion. To administer medication using the intermittent infusion method, the nurse will need alcohol or iodophor swabs, a syringe and needle with 1 ml of heparin flush solution (if required), two syringes and needles with 2 ml of normal saline solution, I.V. administration tubing, a 20G or smaller needle or needleless system, the I.V. container of medication, and an I.V. pole.

To administer the infusion, the nurse should identify the patient and explain the procedure. Remove the tubing from the container and the protective cover from the medication bottle or bag. Close the roller clamp, which regulates fluid flow through the tubing. Remove the cap from the I.V. tubing spike, and insert it into the outlet port of the medication bag or bottle. Invert the bag or bottle and hang it from the I.V. pole.

Fill the drip chamber, and then remove the protective cap on the end of the tubing and replace it with a 20G needle or needleless system. Remove the needle cap or needleless system cap, and slowly open the roller clamp, allowing the fluid to clear the tubing of air. Close the roller clamp when the liquid reaches the tip of the needle or tubing, and replace the cap or system cap. Swab the intermittent infusion port, and insert a saline syringe needle. Aspirate to verify blood return. Inject the saline. Remove the syringe and needle.

Swab the port. Attach the tubing and needle to the port. Secure the connection with tape for the duration of the infusion. Open the roller clamp slightly, and infuse the medication over the recommended time interval. When the infusion is completed, remove the infusion set, clean the port, and inject the saline solution. Clean the port again, and inject the heparin flush solution (if required).

Central venous catheter administration. The procedures for injecting or infusing medication resemble those used for intermittent infusion or direct bolus. A heparin flush, usually 3 ml, is used after the final saline flush.

Continuous infusion. The procedure for administering a continuous I.V. infusion is similar to that used for the intermittent infusion, except for a longer duration of infusion. The tubing is usually used for 24 to 72 hours; however, the medication bottle or bag may need to be replaced during that period. To do so, the nurse clamps the tubing, inserts the sterile spike into the new bottle or bag of medication, unclamps the tubing, and continues the infusion.

Continuous I.V. medication administration often is facilitated by using an infusion pump. The nurse sets the electric or battery-powered infusion pump to deliver a constant amount of solution per minute or hour. To determine the pump settings, the nurse considers the total amount of fluid to be given and the interval over which it must be infused. Each of the different infusion pumps available comes with its own set of operating instructions. The nurse must follow the manufacturer's guidelines to ensure adequate pump functioning.

PICC line use. A peripherally inserted central catheter (PICC) line, easier to insert than other central access devices, provides safe, reliable access for administering drugs and taking blood samples. The device may remain in place up to 140 days, making it cost-effective. It is available with a single or double lumen and in lengths that range from 16" to 24" (40 to 60 cm).

Infusions commonly given through a PICC line include total parenteral nutrition, chemotherapy, antibiotics, narcotics, analgesics, and blood products. PICC therapy works best when introduced early in treatment. The patient receiving PICC therapy must have a peripheral vein large enough to accept the introducer needle and catheter.

A specially-trained nurse or physician inserts a PICC into the basilic, median antecubital basilic, cubital, or cephalic vein. Then the catheter is threaded into the superior vena cava or subclavian vein or a noncentral site, such as the axillary vein.

Before and after drug administration, the nurse should flush the PICC line with 3 ml of 0.9% normal saline. A heparin flush may also be used. The nurse also should perform sterile dressing changes according to the institution's protocol for home or hospital care. If a patient or caregiver will care for the PICC and administer drugs through it at home, the nurse should teach the appropriate techniques.

Use of a vascular access port. A vascular access port (VAP) is an implanted device, inserted under local anesthesia in a patient who needs intermittent I.V. therapy for 3 months or more. VAPs reduce the risk of infection because they are not exposed to the external environment. To access a VAP, the nurse inserts a non-coring needle through subcutaneous tissue and into the port. Then the nurse secures the VAP access needle for the drug administration or I.V. infusion. (See *Vascular access port.*)

Other routes of drug administration

Other routes are used for medication administration, including the **intrathecal, epidural, intra-articular, dermal,** ophthalmic, otic, nasal and sinus, respiratory, urethral, and **vaginal routes.**

INTRATHECAL ADMINISTRATION

During intrathecal administration, an access device implanted beneath the scalp delivers medication to the brain. The access device, which consists of a dome-shaped reservoir and a ventricular catheter, is implanted surgically below the scalp on the top portion of the head. The catheter is threaded into a lateral ventricle.

Then a bolus of medication is injected into the pliable reservoir. When the filled reservoir is compressed, medication is ejected through the catheter into the brain. Intrathecal reservoir injections usually are not administered by nurses.

Intrathecal administration is used for patients requiring frequent chemotherapy treatments for lymphoma, leukemia, or meningeal metastases. The intrathecal device delivers chemotherapeutic agents at regular intervals and also provides greater patient mobility and freedom from repeated lumbar punctures. It also is used to administer antibiotics to patients with central nervous system infections.

EPIDURAL ADMINISTRATION

Using the epidural route requires that a catheter be placed into the spinal column via a lumbar puncture. Drugs are injected or infused through the catheter into the epidural space. From there, they diffuse slowly through the dura mater into the intrathecal space, which contains cerebrospinal fluid (CSF). CSF carries the drug directly into the spinal cord, bypassing the blood-brain barrier.

The epidural route may be used to: administer anesthetics and narcotic analgesics, such as morphine; to treat acute pain postoperatively; to treat chronic pain in terminal illness; administer a single injection of a corticosteroid to reduce back pain caused by inflammation or a bulging disk; or administer a series of injections to treat a condition, such as acute herpes zoster.

The procedure for injecting or infusing medication by the epidural route resembles that used for the I.V. route. However, the epidural route may require much lower doses of medication than the I.V. route. Therefore, patients typically are more alert and have fewer adverse reactions during long-term therapy. Also, the medication's effects last longer. Postoperative patients become ambulatory sooner, which reduces their risk of pulmonary complications and shortens their hospitalization.

INTRA-ARTICULAR ADMINISTRATION

Intra-articular injections seldom are given because of their high risk of infection. Furthermore, intra-articular injections may reduce the chances of success of future joint replacement surgery. Occasionally, patients with severe joint inflammation receive an intra-articular injection of corticosteroids, but these injections usually are not repeated. When giving an intra-articular injection, the physician uses a long needle to deposit the medication directly into the joint and observes strict aseptic technique.

DERMAL ADMINISTRATION

The dermal route also is known as the dermatomucosal route and, more commonly, the topical route. Dermal medications usually are used for their local rather than systemic effects. One of several exceptions, nitroglycerin is given by the dermal route for its systemic rather than local effect.

Medication forms given by the dermal route include creams, lotions, ointments, powders, and patches. The medication is absorbed through the epidermal layer into the dermis. The extent of absorption depends on the vascularity

Inserting a vaginal medication

The procedure is similar for administering all forms of vaginal medication, such as creams, suppositories, ointments, and gels. However, the nurse should follow the manufacturer's instructions for administering the prescribed medication.

Before inserting a vaginal medication, the nurse identifies the patient according to standard procedure and states the drug's name and action or use. To administer the medication, the nurse will need these supplies: the prescribed medication, applicator, gloves, water-soluble lubricant, tissues, bedsaver pad, several cotton balls, perineal pads, drape, and soap and water. The nurse should provide for the patient's privacy and explain the procedure to her. The nurse should ask the patient to void and then should use the following procedure.

1. Help the patient lie down with her knees flexed and legs spread apart. Place a bedsaver pad under her to protect the bed linen, and a drape over her legs, leaving only her perineum exposed. Put on gloves.
2. Using one cotton ball per stroke, clean the perineum with soap and water. Then spread the labia and clean this area.
3. Insert the medication into the applicator, and lubricate the applicator tip.
4. Spread the labia with one hand, and insert the applicator into the vagina with the other. Advance the applicator about 2" (5 cm), while angling it toward the sacrum. Release the labia and depress the plunger to expel the medication from the applicator.

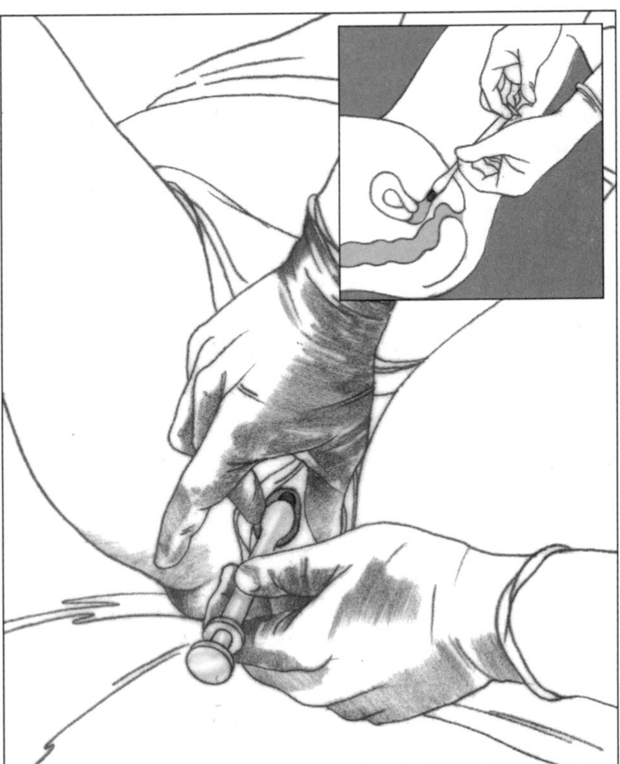

5. Remove the applicator and wipe any excess lubricant from the perineum. Instruct the patient to remain supine for about 30 minutes to retain the medication.
6. Give the patient tissues to wipe away any medication that may drain when she stands. Instruct her to wear a perineal pad to prevent drainage stains on her clothes.

of and circulation in the region. To apply a cream, lotion, or ointment, the nurse begins at the midline and uses long, even strokes outward and downward, in the direction of hair growth. This application pattern reduces the risk of follicle irritation and skin inflammation. After applying a cream, lotion, or ointment, the nurse usually should rub the medication into the patient's skin; powders should not be rubbed into the skin.

Patches contain a measured dose of medication that is delivered over an extended time. Medications in patch form include nitroglycerin, scopolamine, clonidine, and estrogen. The nurse should apply the patch over clean, dry skin. Removal of excessive hair will ensure proper absorption. The drug is released through a thin membrane or from a gel base in the patch.

OPHTHALMIC ADMINISTRATION

Liquid and ointment medications are administered topically into the eye. The nurse usually instills liquid medications by the **drop** method, described later in this chapter.

OTIC ADMINISTRATION

Liquid medications are administered topically into the ear. The nurse instills liquid medications by the drop method, described later in this chapter.

NASAL AND SINUS ADMINISTRATION

The nurse administers liquid and powdered forms of medications into the patient's nose and sinuses by instillation or by an atomizer or nasal aerosol device. Vasoconstrictors represent one kind of drug commonly administered by this route.

The nasal aerosol device seldom is used. The technique for its use resembles that for the atomizer and drop instillation methods. The package insert provides specific information regarding the administration technique for this device.

RESPIRATORY ADMINISTRATION

Almost all drugs given by the respiratory route produce a systemic effect because of the rich blood supply in the lungs. The drug forms administered by this route include gas, such as oxygen; liquid, such as isoproterenol; and powder, such as cromolyn sodium.

Nebulization is a commonly used method for administering drugs by the respiratory route. The two major kinds of nebulizers are the ultrasonic nebulizer and the metered-dose aerosol or turbo inhaler. The ultrasonic nebulizer uses a small volume of medication (usually under 1 ml) combined with about 3 ml of normal saline solution. Air forced through the nebulizer delivers the medication in a fine mist, which the patient inhales by breathing deeply through a mouthpiece attached to the nebulizer.

Administering drugs by a metered-dose aerosol or turbo inhaler requires a nebulizer that is prefilled by the manufacturer with several doses of the drug. Each patient receives an individual nebulizer filled with the appropriate medication and dosage. The nebulizer may be used with a spacer, which suspends the medication for a few seconds before the patient inhales.

Powder is administered with a turbo inhaler. The nurse places a capsule of powdered drug inside the inhaler, and the patient inhales deeply through the mouth. As a result, the contents of the capsule are delivered in a fine powdered form to the lungs.

URETHRAL ADMINISTRATION

Physicians and nurses use urethral administration for local antibiotic or antifungal therapy. After identifying the patient according to standard procedure and stating the drug's name and action or use, the nurse instills the liquid medication into the urethra through a small-diameter urinary catheter using sterile technique. The catheter then is removed or clamped so the medication can reach and bathe the bladder walls. How long the catheter remains clamped determines the duration of medication retention in the bladder. Occasionally, an intracath (the type used for I.V. administration), with the needle removed, is inserted into the urethra for the instillation of liquid medication. Severe cases of epididymitis may be treated in this manner.

Urethral administration may be repeated several times a day for about a week or only performed once. For repeated treatment, the nurse probably will use a special urinary catheter with an extra lumen for medication instillation. The volume of medication can range from a few milliliters to almost a liter.

VAGINAL ADMINISTRATION

Vaginal administration is used for topical antibiotic or antifungal medications, in liquid, suppository, cream, ointment, tablet, or gel form. When administering drugs in liquid form, the nurse performs what commonly is called a douche or vaginal irrigation. The procedure resembles that used for a rectal retention enema except for the use of a special vaginal catheter. (See the "Rectal" section for a description of the retention enema procedure.) When the nurse inserts the catheter tip into the vagina, the patient should be on a bedpan or toilet because no sphincter controls the vagina and the fluid will flow immediately out of the vaginal vault.

Other forms of vaginal medication are administered with the patient lying supine in bed. (See *Inserting a vaginal medication.*)

Pediatric administration techniques

Administering drugs safely to a child requires special attention to the five rights because any medication error can have a much greater impact on a child than on an adult. For each route of administration, the nurse must modify adult administration techniques for a pediatric patient. No matter which route is used, the nurse should try to elicit the child's cooperation to make medication administration as easy as possible. If the child is unable to cooperate, the nurse should enlist help to hold the child still during administration. (See *Administering pediatric medications,* page 80.)

ORAL ADMINISTRATION

Although absorption from the GI tract is less predictable than by other routes, oral administration frequently is prescribed because it is the least traumatic for the child. However, oral administration to a child can challenge a nurse's skills. Although a child willingly may swallow a medication at first, the child may begin to spit, drool, or choke after realizing that the medication tastes unpleasant. When this happens, the nurse must try to give the medication with as little distress as possible to the child. To do this, a nurse might hold a child in a bottle-feeding position, placing the child's inner arm behind the nurse's back, supporting the head in the crook of the nurse's elbow, and holding the child's free hand with the hand of the supporting arm. This position immobilizes the child's head in the crook of the nurse's arm and prevents the child from spilling the medication with either hand.

If an infant or small child must be restrained for medication administration, the nurse should use a syringe without a needle to administer small, controlled doses. To minimize the risk of choking or aspirating, the nurse should hold the child's head upright or to the side.

Then the nurse should slide the syringe into the child's mouth about halfway back between the gums and cheeks and squirt in a small amount of medication. This administration technique offers several advantages. Placement of the medication deep in the side of the mouth makes it difficult for the child to lose the medication by spitting or drooling. Although medication administration takes longer because the drug is given in small amounts, this technique reduces the risk of choking, coughing, and vomiting because it does not stimulate the gag reflex.

The nurse never should place medication in an infant's formula because it can lead to several problems. For example, the infant may not take the feeding if the medication alters its taste. If this happens, the nurse will not be able to determine how much medication the child actually took, and the child will not receive the drug's therapeutic effects or the formula's nutrition. Administration with formula can also alter the absorption of some medications. For example,

Administering pediatric medications

To administer pediatric medications effectively, the nurse must understand how children of different ages think about and react to drugs and know how to intervene appropriately.

AGE-GROUP	PATIENT CHARACTERISTICS AND REACTIONS TO MEDICATION	NURSING INTERVENTIONS
Infant	• In a very young infant, lack of experience eliminates fear; the infant may take medication willingly. • Between ages 5 and 8 months, the infant begins to observe visual cues and anticipate unpleasant events. • By age 10 months, the infant will try to get away from anticipated unpleasantness and may spit, drool, or choke to avoid taking medication.	• Hold the infant still when giving an oral medication. • Make the medication palatable; if appropriate, mix it with syrup or applesauce. • Administer mediation in a syringe placed in the side of the mouth or from a spoon placed far back on the tongue. • Allow the infant to suck medication from a nipple. • Give medication slowly to prevent choking or spitting. • Ask the parent or a coworker to hold the infant still during a painful administration. • Cuddle, rock, and speak soothingly to the infant after a painful procedure.
Toddler	• A toddler has limited ability to express anger in words but will protest loudly. • A toddler may try to escape from the nurse or physician. • A toddler has a limited understanding of explanations and a poor concept of time. • The child may not be able to cooperate and may squirm because of a lack of self-control.	• Explain the procedure very simply just before performing it. • Mention that the child has no options about taking the medication. • Tell the child that you realize the procedure is unpleasant. Warn the child before a painful procedure. • Let the toddler exercise some control over the situation by allowing a choice of a spoon, straw, cup, or syringe to take an oral medication. • Try to improve the medication's taste by mixing it with a small amount of syrup or food, if appropriate. • Use the child's rituals to administer medication whenever possible. • Hold the child still, if necessary. Praise any attempts the child makes to hold still. • Encourage the child to express feelings, and offer reassurance that the child is not being punished. • Allow the parents to comfort the child after the procedure.
Preschooler	• A child in this age-group has a limited ability to understand a detailed explanation. • A preschooler will attempt to cooperate. • After an I.M. injection, a preschooler may think that body fluids will leak out of the injection site.	• Express faith in the child's ability to cooperate even with an unpleasant procedure. • Provide options, whenever possible, to give the child a sense of control over the situation. • Explain the procedure simply. • Warn the child before a painful procedure. • Praise the child for all attempts to cooperate. • Encourage the child to express feelings. • Offer the child an adhesive bandage after an I.M. injection. • Allow the parents or caregiver to comfort the child after the procedure. • Use therapeutic play before and after the procedure. Listen carefully to the child's play. Clear up any misconceptions, and provide further explanations as needed.
School-age child	• The older the school-age child, the greater the ability to exercise restraint and to cooperate.	• Explain the procedure in detail. • Allow the child to make choices, whenever possible. • Warn the child in advance when a painful procedure is scheduled. • Reassure the child that no one likes the procedure. • Praise the child for cooperating. • Listen to the child's concerns and feelings.
Adolescent	• An adolescent's reaction to medication is similar to an adult's. The ability to cooperate is highly developed.	• Include the adolescent in discussions and decisions about the procedure. • Allow the adolescent to make choices and to exercise as much control as possible. • Give support and encouragement, but do not treat the adolescent like a child.

I.M. injection sites for pediatric patients

The nurse can use several landmarks to identify I.M. injection sites for pediatric patients. The vastus lateralis and rectus femoris muscles are the recommended sites for an infant or a toddler. The dorsogluteal and ventrogluteal sites can be used only after the toddler has been walking for about 1 year.

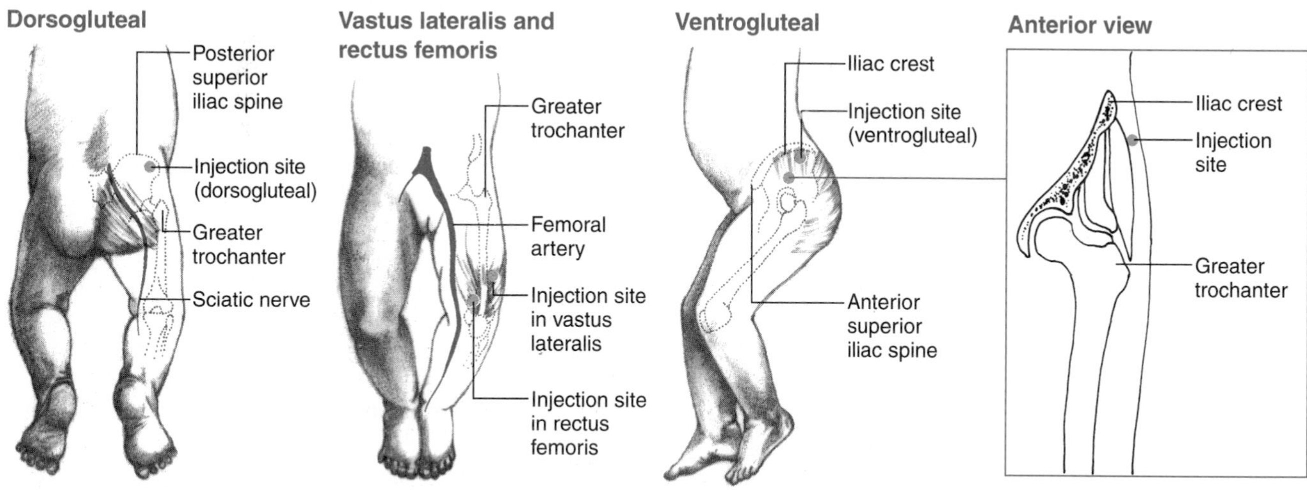

Osmolite can inhibit the absorption of phenytoin suspension.

INTRAMUSCULAR ADMINISTRATION

For an I.M. injection, the nurse should use the smallest gauge needle appropriate for the medication. This usually is a needle that is 25G to 22G. The needle length should not exceed 1" (2.5 cm), except for an adult-size adolescent, who may require a 1½" (3.8-cm) needle.

The recommended injection sites vary with age. The vastus lateralis and rectus femoris muscles are the recommended sites for an infant or toddler. For a child who has been walking for about 1 year, the nurse can give an I.M. injection in the ventrogluteal or dorsogluteal area. Walking develops these muscles, thus reducing the risk of sciatic nerve damage during an I.M. injection. (See *I.M. injection sites for pediatric patients.*) For an older child, the nurse may use an adult I.M. injection site, such as the deltoid, gluteus maximus, ventrogluteal, vastus lateralis, or rectus femoris muscle. The nurse uses the same I.M. injection technique for a child as for an adult. If necessary, the nurse may ask the child's parent or another nurse to hold the child still during the injection.

SUBCUTANEOUS ADMINISTRATION

Subcutaneous administration is the same in a child as in an adult. Injection sites include the abdomen or the middle third of the upper outer arm or thigh. The needle should be 27G to 23G and ⅜" to ⅝" (1 to 1.5 cm) long. The nurse must remember to provide an age-appropriate explanation.

INTRADERMAL ADMINISTRATION

To administer a drug intradermally, the nurse should insert the needle, bevel up, at a 10- to 15-degree angle just beneath the skin layer. Then the nurse should inject the medication slowly and watch for a bleb to appear. To remove the needle, the nurse should withdraw it quickly, while maintaining the proper injection angle. If appropriate, the nurse may draw a circle around the injection. The area should not be massaged.

INTRAVENOUS ADMINISTRATION

Pediatric I.V. administration poses several challenges for the nurse. For example, the nurse must assist with or perform the I.V. insertion, which can be traumatic for the child and parents. The nurse also must monitor the I.V. frequently to maintain its patency.

The nurse should explain the procedure to the parents of a neonate or an infant, to prepare them for the necessity of the I.V. and the possibility that the infant's head will be shaved if the I.V. catheter is inserted in the scalp. The nurse also should tell the parents that the procedure may take some time so that they do not expect to see the infant again in a few minutes. For a toddler, the nurse should explain the procedure briefly just before taking the child to the treatment room, because the toddler's concept of time is not fully developed. A toddler probably will not be able to cooperate, so the nurse should plan to restrain the child carefully to ensure safe insertion of the I.V. catheter. For a preschooler, who has a better concept of time, the nurse may explain the procedure a short time before performing it. A preschooler needs to know that crying is permitted and that he or she is expected to hold still. Although a young school-age child should be able to hold still without help, the nurse should help by holding the child's hand or taking other comfort measures. Generally, an older school-age child or an adolescent can hold still for this procedure.

The nurse should insert the I.V. catheter as for an adult. After inserting the catheter, tape the I.V. so that the insertion site is visible for frequent monitoring. If the extremity will be immobilized, secure the I.V. so that the site can be observed hourly to detect complications and so that circulation in the fingers can be assessed. If the child complains of pain at the I.V. site or if an infant or young child becomes unusually irritable, check closely for signs of infiltration or phlebitis, such as redness or swelling.

Just as adults do, children may also need CV catheters. The catheters are inserted by a specially trained nurse or physician. Parents need to understand the purpose of the catheter and how to use and care for it, if it will remain in place when the child is discharged. Age-appropriate teaching about the catheter should also be done for the child prior to discharge. The nurse should monitor the patient closely for signs and symptoms of complications related to the catheter or to the administration of I.V. medications.

Infants, small children, and children with compromised cardiopulmonary status are particularly vulnerable to fluid overload with I.V. medication administration. To prevent this problem, a volume control set and an infusion pump or syringe should be used. No more than 2 hours' worth of I.V. fluid at a time should be placed in the volume control set, to limit the amount of fluid infused.

Other factors can influence the amount and rapidity of medication administration. In tubing with a narrow lumen, the medication will reach the child faster than in tubing with a wide lumen because of increased pressure in the narrow tubing. If a child has a delicate fluid balance, an infusion (auto) syringe can deliver small amounts of fluid. With this technique, a syringe containing medication is secured in the cradle of an autoinfusion mechanism. The nurse can set the correct rate on the syringe to infuse the medication automatically.

Careful monitoring of intake and output can help prevent fluid overload and ensure that the child gets the amount of fluid ordered. Careful observation of the infusion will detect clot formation in the catheter, which is especially likely with a slow I.V. rate or a narrow catheter lumen. Frequent assessment of the flow rate — particularly with gravity infusion — is important because position changes, crying, and restraints can impede the flow of fluids.

With all I.V. medications, the nurse must flush the volume control set and tubing before and after administration. Some medications are not compatible, and if they are mixed they may form a precipitate in the I.V. administration set.

The nurse should check with the pharmacist if a question arises about medication compatibility. If a precipitate forms, the nurse must stop the infusion immediately and change all of the tubing.

TOPICAL ADMINISTRATION

In a neonate, infant, or small child, thin epidermis and large body-surface area allow for increased drug absorption of topical medications and explain why a young pediatric patient is more likely to develop a toxic, systemic drug reaction than an older patient. Topical corticosteroids can produce particularly severe reactions. To decrease the risk of toxic effects, the nurse should wash a cleansing solution off an infant's skin, unless otherwise instructed, and apply a topical medication as thinly as possible and to as small a body-surface area as possible. When removing a topical medication from a jar, the nurse should use a tongue depressor to avoid contaminating the medication with the hand used to apply the medication.

RECTAL ADMINISTRATION

Drug absorption from the rectum may be unpredictable. The presence of stool in the rectum can delay, decrease, or block drug absorption. Nevertheless, medications often are administered rectally when oral administration is contraindicated or when they are designed for rectal administration. Children who are neutropenic or thrombocytopenic, however, should not receive rectal medications because of the increased risk of infection and bleeding caused by tissue trauma.

Before administering the rectal medication, the nurse should explain the procedure and the importance of retaining the suppository rather than expelling it. To administer the medication, the nurse uses a gloved hand to insert the unwrapped, lubricated suppository past the rectal sphincters. Then the nurse should hold the buttocks together so the child cannot expel the medication.

Some suppositories are scored and can be halved easily and accurately, if necessary. If an unscored suppository must be halved, the nurse should split it lengthwise to ensure even distribution of its medication.

ADMINISTRATION OF EYE-, EAR-, AND NOSE DROPS

To administer eyedrops, the nurse may need to have a coworker restrain an infant or toddler. For a pediatric patient, the nurse places the hand that holds the dropper on the child's forehead so that it will move as the child's head moves and decrease the risk of injury. With the other hand, the nurse can pull down the lower lid to expose the conjunctival sac. If the child is old enough to cooperate, the nurse should ask the child to look up and then instill the drops in the lower conjunctival sac. If the child will not cooperate, the nurse can place the eyedrops at the inner canthus while the child's eyes are closed. As the child's eyes open, the drops will be dispersed. After instillation, the nurse should encourage the child to blink or close the eyelids and rotate the eyes to distribute the medication.

Before administration, the nurse should warm eardrops almost to body temperature to prevent pain or vertigo when the drops come in contact with the child's tympanic membrane. The nurse should assist the child into a supine position with the head turned to the side and the affected ear up. For a child under age 3, the nurse will have to pull the pinna down and back to straighten the external auditory canal. For a child over age 3, the nurse should pull the pinna up and back. Then the nurse can administer the drops and massage the area in front of the tragus to promote their entry into the ear. If only one ear is affected, the child should lie on the unaffected side for several minutes after administration. If both ears are affected, the nurse should place a cotton ball in each external canal to prevent the medication from escaping.

To prevent nose drops from entering the throat rather than the nasal passages, the nurse should administer them to a child whose head is suspended over the edge of a pillow or bed or to an infant who is being held in the football position (tucked against the nurse's side with the infant on its back, and its feet against the nurse's waist). The nurse should keep the child in this position for 1 minute after medication administration to allow the drops to come in contact with as much of the nasal passages as possible.

CHAPTER SUMMARY

Chapter 5 presented the different drug forms and routes of administration, including detailed descriptions of techniques used for the different routes. Here are the chapter highlights.

Drugs are packaged in the unit-dose format (one dose in a labeled container) and bulk style (multiple doses in a labeled container).

The major drug forms include solids, liquids, suppositories, and inhalants. The form of a drug affects the way the patient uses the drug.

Solids include tablets, capsules, enteric-coated tablets, and wax matrix tablets. Solid drug forms are given orally and by the sublingual and buccal routes. Enteric-coated and wax matrix tablets should not be crushed because doing so alters the drug action and may irritate the esophageal and gastric mucosa. Buccal and sublingual medications are absorbed into the bloodstream without going through the GI tract.

Liquids include syrups, suspensions, tinctures, and elixirs. Liquids usually are administered orally or parenterally via injection.

Suppositories, administered rectally and vaginally, carry medications in a solid base that melts at body temperature.

Inhalants are powdered or liquid forms of a drug administered via the respiratory route using an ultrasonic nebulizer, metered-dose aerosol or turbo inhaler, or vaporizer.

Most medications are administered by the GI tract, which provides a fairly safe, but relatively slow-acting, site for drug absorption. Oral, sublingual, buccal, and rectal preparations are given using the GI tract.

The technique for administering an enema depends on whether the drug requires retention.

Parenteral liquids are packaged in vials, ampules, and self-contained or prefilled syringes. Parenteral medications in powdered form must be reconstituted before administration.

Parenteral medications commonly are administered by the intradermal, S.C., I.M., and I.V. routes. Rotating injection sites improves absorption and minimizes patient discomfort. The nurse must match the type of syringe and appropriate needle size with the correct parenteral administration route. Alcohol most commonly is used to clean the skin before administration of parenteral medications.

I.V. medications may be administered as a bolus, intermittent infusion, or continuous infusion. An infusion pump may be used to deliver continuous I.V. medication. A PICC line or VAP may also be used for intermittent I.V. medications.

Other administration routes include intrathecal, epidural, intra-articular, dermal, ophthalmic, otic, nasal and sinus, respiratory, urethral, and vaginal.

Intrathecal administration delivers medication to the brain through an access device implanted under the scalp.

Epidural administration delivers medication to the spinal cord through a catheter.

Intra-articular administration deposits medication directly into the joint.

Medications administered by the dermal route include creams, lotions, ointments, powders, and patches.

Ophthalmic medications are administered topically into the eyes; otic medications, into the ears.

Liquid and powdered forms of medications may be administered to the patient's nose and sinuses by instillation, atomizer, or nasal aerosol device.

Drug forms administered by the respiratory route include gas, such as oxygen; liquid, such as isoproterenol; and powder, such as cromolyn sodium.

Urethral administration commonly is used for local antibiotic and antifungal therapy and involves instillation of liquid medication through a catheter.

Vaginal administration is used for topical antibiotic or antifungal medications in liquid, suppository, cream, ointment, tablet, or gel form.

Although pediatric and adult routes of medication administration are the same, pediatric sites and techniques of administration vary with the patient's age. The nurse must be familiar with the drug to be administered as well as the appropriate administration techniques for the child's age.

Questions to consider

See Appendix 1 for answers.

1. To treat hypertension for Ron Musolf, age 57, the physician prescribes an oral medication that comes in capsule form. Where do capsules dissolve?
   (a) In the mouth
   (b) In the stomach
   (c) In the intestine
   (d) In the rectum

2. John Campanella, age 39, has angina pectoris. His physician orders nitroglycerin $^1/_{150}$ gr sublingual p.r.n. for chest pain. What should the nurse teach Mr. Campanella about taking this medication?
   (a) Place the tablet under the tongue.
   (b) Place the tablet between the cheek and gum.
   (c) Chew the tablet thoroughly before swallowing.
   (d) Swallow the tablet with at least 3 oz of water.

3. The nurse must administer a retention enema to Helen Adams, age 92. After administering the drug, the nurse should instruct Mrs. Adams to retain the enema for how long?
   (a) At least 40 minutes
   (b) At least 30 minutes
   (c) At least 20 minutes
   (d) At least 10 minutes

4. Terry Smith, age 30, contracts syphilis. Her physician prescribes 2.4 million U of penicillin G benzathine (Bicillin L-A) I.M. When should the nurse use the Z-track technique for I.M. injections?
   (a) When the drug is extremely potent
   (b) When the patient is uncooperative
   (c) When a large dose is being administered
   (d) When the drug is extremely irritating to tissue

5. For Herman Cullen, age 55, the nurse must administer epoetin alfa (Epogen) subcutaneously. What is the maximum amount of fluid that may be given by the subcutaneous route?
   (a) 3 ml
   (b) 2 ml
   (c) 1 ml
   (d) 0.5 ml

6. Darcy Bennet, age 16, has just received a diagnosis of diabetes. When teaching her about insulin injections, the nurse should be sure to include which of the following points?
   (a) Site rotation promotes proper insulin absorption.
   (b) Site rotation causes hard nodules in subcutaneous tissue.
   (c) Adolescent diabetics don't need to rotate injection sites.
   (d) Random site rotation is effective and easy to do.

7. Lisa Karl brings her son Sam, age 2, to the pediatrician because Sam has an earache. After determining that Sam has otitis externa in the right ear, the nurse practitioner prescribes neomycin sulfate, 3 drops into the external auditory canal q.i.d. for 10 days. When administering eardrops to a toddler, how should the nurse straighten the ear canal?
   (a) Pull the tragus up and back.
   (b) Pull the pinna down and back.
   (c) Pull the pinna up and forward.
   (d) Pull the tragus down and forward.

UNIT

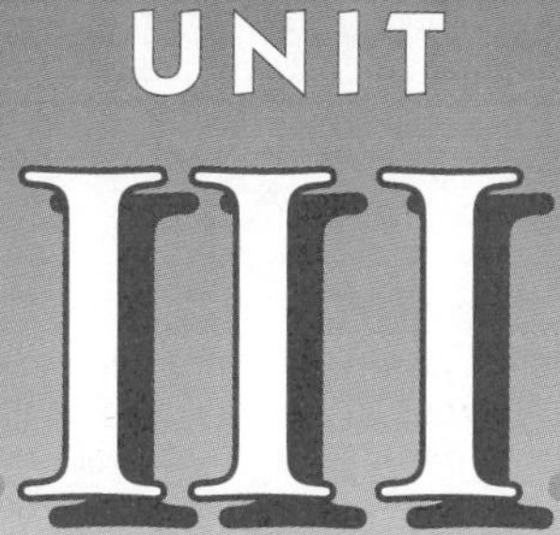

Drugs affecting the autonomic nervous system

Many drugs influence one component of the nervous system: the efferent, or motor, limb of the peripheral nervous system. The nurse must remember the interrelationship of all components of the nervous system when planning and monitoring drug therapy. The nurse can achieve clinical objectives for many **autonomic nervous system** disorders by applying an understanding of the system, how it communicates, and how it adapts to alterations in its environment.

The nervous system, which controls and coordinates functions throughout the body, has two major divisions: the central nervous system (CNS) containing the brain and spinal cord and the peripheral nervous system containing afferent, or sensory, neurons (carrying information to the CNS) and efferent, or motor, neurons (carrying information from the CNS). The peripheral nervous system, which mediates between the CNS and the external and internal environments, is subdivided into the somatic nervous system and the autonomic nervous system.

The drugs discussed in unit 3 affect information transmittal by the motor neurons of the somatic and the autonomic divisions of the peripheral nervous system. To apply the nursing process when caring for a patient receiving such drug therapy, the nurse needs a working knowledge of this system.

Anatomy and physiology

Different neurons of the autonomic nervous system innervate smooth and cardiac muscles, glands, and other viscera. Unlike the somatic nervous system, the autonomic nervous system is subdivided into the **sympathetic nervous system (adrenergic)** and the **parasympathetic nervous system (cholinergic).**

The sympathetic and parasympathetic nervous systems have two **neurons** (rather than one, as in the somatic nervous system) carrying information to the target sites. The cell bodies of the first neurons, like those of the somatic nervous system, originate in the CNS. The neurons of the sympathetic nervous system originate in the thoracic and lumbar regions of the spinal cord, and those of the parasympathetic nervous system originate in the brain stem or the sacral region of the spinal cord. The two systems are referred to, respectively, as the thoracolumbar and craniosacral divisions.

Axons from these first neurons leave the CNS and travel to **ganglia** where they **synapse** with a second neuron that travels to the target site. Because of the intervening ganglia, the axons of the first neurons are called preganglionic fibers; those of the second neurons, postganglionic fibers.

The preganglionic fibers of the sympathetic nervous system are short, terminating in ganglia that lie adjacent to the spinal cord (paravertebral chain) or a short distance from the cord (such as the celiac ganglion). The preganglionic fiber that innervates the adrenal medulla is an exception. It goes directly from the spinal cord to special cells in the adrenal medulla without synapsing. The adrenal medulla is analogous to a sympathetic postganglionic neuron (its secretory cells originate in nervous tissue) and releases norepinephrine and epinephrine directly into the circulation. Postganglionic fibers travel some distance to reach their target sites. (See *Sympathetic division activity,* page 86.)

In contrast, most preganglionic fibers of the parasympathetic nervous system are long and travel to ganglia located close to or in the walls of their target sites. The postganglionic fibers of the parasympathetic nervous system are short. This dissimilarity in the distribution pattern of preganglionic and postganglionic fibers facilitates the contrasting effects of the two systems. The characteristics of the sympathetic nervous system permit a more generalized, widespread effect; those of the parasympathetic nervous system permit a more discrete, localized effect. (See *Parasympathetic division activity,* page 87.)

Usually, both systems send information to the same target sites. Exceptions include the adrenal medulla, sweat glands, spleen, and hair follicles, which are innervated by the sympathetic nervous system only. Because the physiologic functions of the two systems usually are opposite, dual innervation balances physiologic effects. Drug therapy

Sympathetic division activity

The sympathetic branch of the autonomic nervous system has two neurons that carry information to effector organs. Neurons originate from the thoracolumbar region within the central nervous system. Preganglionic and postganglionic fibers transmit nerve impulses. Preganglionic fibers are short, terminating in ganglia that lie adjacent to the spinal cord or a short distance from it. The preganglionic fiber that directly innervates the adrenal medulla without synapsing at a ganglion causes release of norepinephrine and epinephrine directly into the circulation. Postganglionic fibers are long and travel some distance through effector cells to reach effector organs. This transmittal is carried out by chemicals (neurotransmitters). Major neurotransmitters are norepinephrine, epinephrine and, to a lesser extent, dopamine and acetylcholine (ACh).

Major physiologic effects are alpha and beta adrenergic: vasoconstriction; vasodilation; increased heart rate, force of contraction, and conduction velocity; bronchial smooth muscle relaxation; gastrointestinal (GI) tract smooth muscle relaxation; GI sphincter contraction; urinary system smooth muscle relaxation; sphincter contraction; pupillary dilation and ciliary muscle relaxation; sweat gland secretion increase; pancreatic secretion decrease; and thick salivary secretions.

Drugs that influence these functions include adrenergic agonists and antagonists and ganglionic blocking agents.

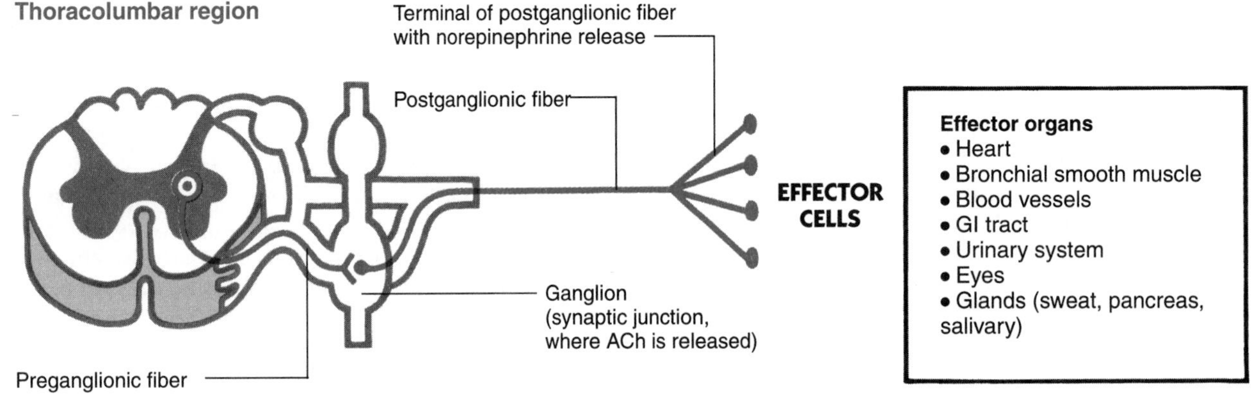

sometimes disrupts this critical balance, as when the parasympathetic nervous system is blocked and the activity of the sympathetic nervous system is unopposed. Knowing the physiologic effects of each system allows the nurse to predict what may happen when a particular drug is used therapeutically.

Stimulation of the somatic nervous system can be viewed as initiating a single activity, skeletal muscle contraction; however, the physiologic effects of the subdivisions of the autonomic nervous system are much more complex. In general, however, the sympathetic nervous system can be viewed as an activity-response system, and the parasympathetic nervous system as a vegetative-homeostatic system.

Stimulation of the sympathetic nervous system increases heart and respiratory rate, metabolic rate, and fat and glycogen breakdown; produces pupillary dilation, smooth muscle vasoconstriction, and skeletal muscle vasodilation; and decreases gastrointestinal (GI) activity. These effects sometimes are called the "fight or flight" response because they prepare the individual to face or run from something threatening.

Conversely, stimulation of the parasympathetic nervous system produces heart and respiratory rate decrease, pupil constriction and enhanced accommodation, digestion and elimination increase, GI tone enhancement, and sphincter tone relaxation. These activities are considered energy conserving and homeostatic.

Neuron communication

The nervous system communicates via chemicals called neuroregulators, or **neurotransmitters,** that transmit neuron information between adjacent cells. In the motor limb of the peripheral nervous system, the major neurotransmitters are **acetylcholine,** norepinephrine, epinephrine and, to a lesser extent, dopamine.

Acetylcholine. This neurotransmitter is released from all preganglionic neurons of the autonomic nervous system, from all postganglionic neurons of the parasympathetic nervous system, from some postsynaptic neurons of the sympathetic nervous system, and at neuromuscular junctions within the somatic nervous system. Acetylcholine's duration of action is short; it is degraded rapidly by the enzyme acetylcholinesterase.

Norepinephrine and epinephrine. These chemicals are released from the adrenal medulla. Norepinephrine also is released from the postganglionic adrenergic fibers of the sympathetic nervous system. The epinephrine and norepinephrine released from the adrenal medulla have

Parasympathetic division activity

The parasympathetic branch of the autonomic nervous system has two neurons that carry information to the cells of effector organs. Neurons originate in the craniosacral region of the central nervous system. Preganglionic and postganglionic fibers transmit nerve impulses. Most preganglionic fibers are long and travel to ganglia located close to or in the walls of the effector organs. In contrast, the postganglionic fibers are short. The major neurotransmitter is acetylcholine (Ach).

The physiologic effects include vasodilation of salivary glands; decreased heart rate, force of contraction, and conduction velocity decrease; bronchial smooth muscle constriction; gastrointestinal (GI) tract tone and peristalsis increase with sphincter relaxation; urinary system sphincter relaxation and bladder tone increase; pupillary constriction; and increased pancreatic, salivary, and lacrimal secretions increase.

Drugs that influence these functions include cholinergic agonists and antagonists and ganglionic blocking agents.

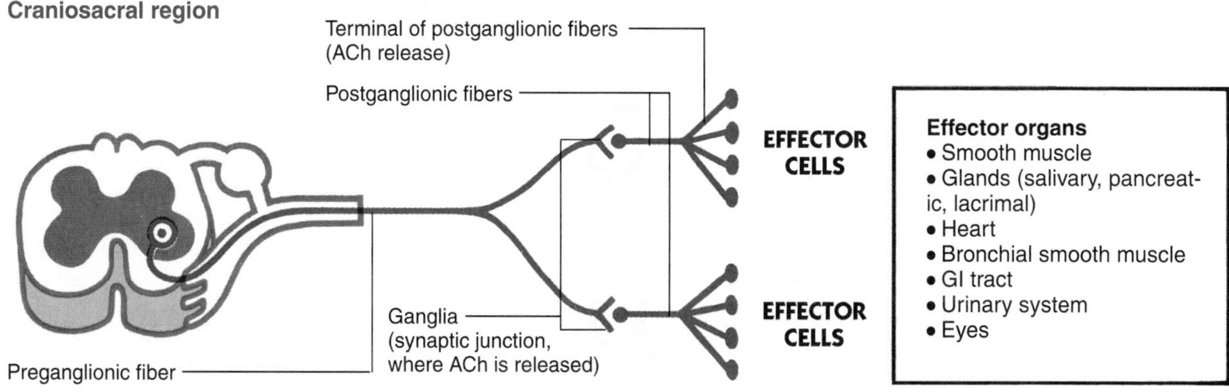

effects similar to direct adrenergic neuronal stimulation but can reach and stimulate target sites that do not receive direct innervation from adrenergic fibers.

The duration of action of norepinephrine released at the synapse is extremely short because it rapidly re-enters the neuron from which it was released (reuptake), diffuses from the area, or is degraded by the enzymes **monoamine oxidase** or **catechol-O-methyltransferase.** The duration of action of the epinephrine and norepinephrine released from the adrenal medulla, however, may last 10 times longer because removal from the circulation is less rapid than from neuronal synapses. This slower removal from the circulation emphasizes the potential difference between the effects of administered drugs and endogenous substances released within the body.

Dopamine. This neurotransmitter is a precursor to norepinephrine. It can interact with dopaminergic as well as alpha- and beta-adrenergic receptors and can stimulate the release of norepinephrine from adrenergic fibers.

DRUG EFFECTS

Effects sometimes are achieved through a drug's interaction with specific receptors on a target cell. Receptors are dynamic cellular components that can be altered by many conditions. Knowledge of receptor physiology has improved drug specificity and the understanding of how the body adapts to exogenous drugs or an altered internal environment. The mechanisms of action for drugs discussed in this unit depend on receptor types, presynaptic receptors, receptor regulation, and nonspecific drug effects.

Types of receptors

The major classes of receptors currently identified in the motor limb of the peripheral nervous system include **alpha-adrenergic receptors, beta-adrenergic receptors,** dopamine receptors, **muscarinic receptors,** and **nicotinic receptors.** Target tissues may have one or a combination of these receptors. A drug's effects are determined by the numbers of each receptor and the drug's specificity.

The **catecholamines** norepinephrine and epinephrine exert their effects by interacting with alpha- and beta-adrenergic receptors. Each has two subtypes: $alpha_1$ and $alpha_2$ and $beta_1$ and $beta_2$. Norepinephrine has a greater effect on $alpha_1$, $alpha_2$, and $beta_1$ receptors than on $beta_2$ receptors; epinephrine has an equal effect on alpha and beta receptors. Thus epinephrine can exert greater metabolic, vasodilatory, and bronchodilatory effects than norepinephrine can.

Over the past decade, alpha-adrenergic receptors that regulate sympathetic transmission to the cardiovascular system also have been identifed in the CNS. Therefore, drugs that act on receptors in the CNS can influence the peripheral nervous system. Dopamine can also interact with dopaminergic, alpha, and beta receptors, depending on its concentration.

Acetylcholine exerts its effect by interacting with nicotinic and muscarinic receptors. Nicotinic receptors are located in the autonomic ganglia (between pre- and postsynaptic fibers of the autonomic nervous system), in the motor end plates at the neuromuscular junction of the somatic nervous system, and in the CNS. The nicotinic receptors on skeletal muscle have different properties than those in the autonomic ganglia. Muscarinic receptors are found at the synapses of the postsynaptic fibers of the parasympathetic nervous system, on some postsynaptic fibers of the sympathetic nervous system, and in the CNS.

Presynaptic receptors

The amount of a neurotransmitter released from a neuron is modulated by neuroregulators and presynaptic receptors on the neuron. Presynaptic alpha-adrenergic receptors are $alpha_2$ receptors.

Presynaptic receptors have clinical importance. For example, an adrenergic blocking agent that nonselectively blocks $alpha_1$ and $alpha_2$ receptors will block the contraction of vascular smooth muscle ($alpha_1$) and the negative feedback to adrenergic fibers ($alpha_2$). The negative feedback block will release more norepinephrine that can stimulate the heart's beta-adrenergic receptors and cause tachycardia.

Receptor regulation

Altered environmental conditions can change receptor number or density (up or down regulation) or change the affinity of a receptor for an agonist or antagonist (uncoupling). Drug effects and withdrawal effects relate to receptor number or affinity. For instance, long-term administration of a beta agonist can decrease the density of beta receptors and reduce the drug's effect. In contrast, long-term administration of a beta antagonist, or blocker, can increase the density of receptors and the response to sudden withdrawal of a beta-blocking agent.

A number of clinical conditions, such as diabetes mellitus and hypothyroidism or hyperthyroidism, can affect receptor concentration or affinity. Thus the nurse must consider the patient's current clinical status when assessing drug therapy.

Nonspecificity

Drugs cannot be directed to a select body area or tissue site. Rather, they act on all receptors to which they have access and can bind. Because the CNS contains receptors for acetylcholine, norepinephrine, and epinephrine, drugs given to affect acetylcholine in the peripheral neurons can exert unwanted CNS effects if they cross the blood-brain barrier.

DRUG SELECTION AND USE

Drugs affect the neural transmission of information in several ways. For example, they may imitate a neurotransmitter's action, block its effect at a receptor site, or enhance or inhibit its synthesis, storage, release, or breakdown. Drugs also may alter the ability of postsynaptic target cells to recover from stimulation.

Drug selection is based on mechanism of action and clinical objectives. For example, if hypertension treatment is aimed at lowering norepinephrine levels to minimize vasoconstriction, a drug that inhibits norepinephrine's effects will be considered. Drug selection is based on specificity for a particular target tissue, efficacy, adverse effects and toxicity, and cost. The cost must be evaluated in dollars and effects on the patient's physical and psychological functioning (such as impotence from antihypertensive agents).

Drugs that influence the somatic or autonomic nervous systems can be categorized according to (1) location of their primary effect, (2) primary effect, such as facilitation or inhibition of sympathetic or parasympathetic effects, and (3) the receptor with which they interact. The drug categories discussed in this unit produce effects similar to acetylcholine, norepinephrine, or epinephrine, or inhibit the effects of those substances.

Drug categories that produce effects similar to acetylcholine include cholinergic agents, parasympathomimetic agents, cholinesterase inhibitors, muscarinic agents, and nicotinic agents. Drugs that inhibit the sympathetic nervous system also can permit acetylcholine's unopposed activity within the parasympathetic nervous system.

Drug categories that inhibit the effects of acetylcholine include cholinergic blocking agents, anticholinergic agents, **parasympatholytic** agents, **antimuscarinic** agents, ganglionic blocking agents, and neuromuscular blocking agents. Drugs that facilitate sympathetic nervous system activity also may antagonize acetylcholine's effects.

Drug categories that produce effects similar to norepinephrine and epinephrine include adrenergic agents (catecholamines or noncatecholamines that are alpha, beta, dopaminergic, or nonselective), **sympathomimetic** agents, and monoamine oxidase inhibitors. Drugs that inhibit the parasympathetic nervous system also may allow unopposed sympathetic nervous system activity.

Drug categories that inhibit the effects of norepinephrine and epinephrine include **sympatholytic** agents, adrenergic blocking agents, and ganglionic blocking agents, which block the sympathetic and parasympathetic nervous systems at the preganglionic level. Drugs that facilitate parasympathetic activity also indirectly may antagonize the effects of norepinephrine and epinephrine.

6 Cholinergic agents

OBJECTIVES

After reading and studying this chapter, the student should be able to:

1. discuss the three major clinical indications for the cholinergic agents.
2. compare the pharmacokinetics of the cholinergic agonists and anticholinesterase agents.
3. identify significant adverse effects of the cholinergic and anticholinesterase agents.
4. describe how to apply the nursing process when caring for a patient who is receiving a cholinergic or anticholinesterase agent.

INTRODUCTION

Cholinergic agents are drugs that directly or indirectly promote the function of the **neurotransmitter acetylcholine.** The cholinergics also are called **parasympathomimetics** because they produce effects that imitate parasympathetic nerve stimulation.

Cholinergic agents have three major clinical indications. They are used to reduce intraocular pressure in patients with glaucoma or during ocular surgery, to treat atony of the gastrointestinal (GI) tract or bladder, and to diagnose and treat myasthenia gravis. Some of the cholinergic agents are important antidotes to neuromuscular blocking agents, tricyclic antidepressants, and belladonna alkaloids.

Cholinergic agents achieve their effects in one of two ways: They mimic the action of acetylcholine or inhibit its destruction at cholinergic receptor sites.

Chapter 6 discusses the two main classes of drugs used as cholinergic agents: cholinergic agonists and **anticholinesterase** agents. (See *Selected major cholinergic agents,* page 90.) Cholinergic agents in this chapter include:

- ambenonium
- bethanechol chloride
- carbachol
- edrophonium chloride
- neostigmine
- physostigmine salicylate
- pilocarpine hydrochloride
- pyridostigmine.

Cholinergic agonists

Cholinergic agonists directly stimulate cholinergic receptors, thus mimicking the action of endogenous acetylcholine. They include synthetic acetylcholine; choline esters, such as bethanechol chloride and carbachol; and naturally occurring cholinomimetic alkaloids, such as pilocarpine hydrochloride.

Acetylcholine rarely is used clinically because it can act at **nicotinic** and **muscarinic receptor** sites, which can cause unpredictable effects, and because it is rapidly destroyed by acetylcholinesterase. Although the choline esters and cholinomimetic alkaloids resist breakdown by acetylcholinesterase, they too lack specificity of action. Clinically, they are used for their effects on the eye, the intestine, and the urinary bladder, but because of their widespread parasympathomimetic actions, cholinergic agonists have many adverse effects.

PHARMACOKINETICS

The action and metabolism of the cholinergic agonists vary widely, depending on their affinity for nicotinic or muscarinic receptors and on their susceptibility to inactivation by the enzyme acetylcholinesterase.

The cholinergic agonists rarely are administered by intramuscular (I.M.) or intravenous (I.V.) injection because they are subject to immediate breakdown by cholinesterases in the interstitial and intravascular spaces. In addition, cholinergic agonists administered I.M. and I.V. take effect rapidly and increase the likelihood of a cholinergic crisis.

Usually, the cholinergic agonists are administered intraocularly, orally, or subcutaneously (S.C.). With oral administration, adverse effects seem to be reduced when the drugs are given on an empty stomach. S.C. administration may result in a more rapid and effective response.

The most useful cholinergic agonists are parasympathomimetic agents, which bind primarily with muscarinic receptors and are less susceptible to cholinesterases. For example, bethanechol has an affinity for muscarinic receptors in the bladder and GI tract and is resistant to cholinesterases.

All cholinergic agonists are metabolized by cholinesterases at the muscarinic and nicotinic receptor sites, in the plasma, and in the liver. All drugs in this class are excreted by the kidneys.

Selected major cholinergic agents

This table summarizes the major cholinergic agents currently in clinical use.

DRUG	MAJOR INDICATIONS AND USUAL DOSAGES	CONTRAINDICATIONS AND PRECAUTIONS
Cholinergic agonists		
bethanechol chloride (Duvoid, Myotonachol, Urecholine)	*Urine retention secondary to hypotonic or atonic bladder* ADULT: 1q 10 to 50 mg P.O. t.i.d. or q.i.d. *Acute urine retention* ADULT: 5 mg S.C. t.i.d. or q.i.d. as required	• Bethanechol is contraindicated in a breast-feeding patient or one with known hypersensitivity to any component of the drug, hyperthyroidism, peptic ulcer disease, latent or active bronchial asthma, pronounced bradycardia or hypotension, vasomotor instability, coronary artery disease, epilepsy, parkinsonism, impaired strength or integrity of the GI or bladder wall, actual or potential GI or bladder obstruction, any condition in which increased muscular activity of the GI or urinary bladder may cause harm (as after recent urinary bladder surgery), spastic GI disturbances, acute inflammatory lesions of the GI tract, peritonitis, or marked vagotonia. • This drug requires cautious use in a pregnant patient. • Safety and efficacy in children have not been established.
Anticholinesterase agents		
edrophonium chloride (Enlon, Reversol, Tensilon)	*Differential diagnosis of cholinergic toxicity and myasthenic crisis* ADULT: 1 mg I.V. followed by an additional 1 mg if patient is not impaired further *Diagnosis of myasthenia gravis* ADULT: initially, 10 mg I.M. or 1 to 2 mg I.V., followed by 8 mg I.V. if no response occurs PEDIATRIC: in infants, 0.5 mg I.V.; in children weighing up to 75 lb (34 kg), 1 mg I.V. followed by titration up to 5 mg given in increments of 1 mg every 30 to 45 seconds as needed to elicit a response or alternately a one-time dose of 2 mg I.M.; in children weighing 75 lb or more, 2 mg I.V. followed by titration up to 10 mg given in increments of 1 mg every 30 to 45 seconds as needed to elicit a response or alternately a one-time dose of 5 mg I.M. *Neuromuscular blockade* ADULT: 10 mg I.V. given over 30 to 45 seconds, repeated to a maximum of 40 mg *Paroxysmal supraventricular tachycardia* ADULT: 5 to 10 mg slow I.V. push, repeated as necessary	• Edrophonium is contraindicated in a patient with known hypersensitivity to anticholinesterase agents or a mechanical intestinal or urinary obstruction. • This drug requires cautious administration in a pregnant or breast-feeding patient or in one with cardiac arrhythmias or bronchial asthma.
neostigmine (Prostigmin)	*Myasthenia gravis* ADULT: 15 mg P.O. every 3 to 4 hours or 0.5 to 2 mg I.V., I.M., or S.C. based on patient's response *Postoperative distention or urine retention* ADULT: 0.5 mg I.M. or S.C. every 4 to 6 hours *Neuromuscular blockade* ADULT: 0.5 to 2 mg I.V., repeated as necessary	• Neostigmine is contraindicated in a breast-feeding patient or one with known hypersensitivity to the drug, a history of hypersensitivity to bromides, or with peritonitis or mechanical obstruction of the intestinal or urinary tract. • This drug requires cautious use in a pregnant patient or one with epilepsy, bronchial asthma, bradycardia, recent coronary occlusion, vagotonia, hyperthyroidism, cardiac arrhythmias, or peptic ulcer. • Oral neostigmine requires cautious use in a patient receiving concurrent therapy with an anticholinergic drug. • Acute toxicity is treated with atropine. • Safety and efficacy in children have not been established.

Pharmacologic actions of cholinergic agents

Cholinergic agents produce different parasympathomimetric effects on various body systems. To provide quality patient care, the nurse should be aware of these differences.

DRUG	SITE OF ACTION							
	Bronchi	Cardio-vascular system	Central nervous system	Eye	Gastro-intestinal system	Myoneural junction	Salivary glands	Urinary bladder
Cholinergic agonists								
bethanechol	++	++	-	++	+++	-	+	+++
carbachol	+	+	-	+++	++	-	+	++
pilocarpine	++	+++	++	+++	++	-	+++	++
Anticholinesterase agents								
ambenonium	+	+	+	+	+	+++	+	+
edrophonium	+	+	-	+	+	++	+	+
neostigmine	+	+	+	+	++	+++	+	+++
physostigmine	+	+	+++	+	+	+++	+	+
pyridostigmine	+	+	+	+	+	+++	+	+

KEY: + minor effect ++ moderate effect +++ major effect - no effect

Route	Onset	Peak	Duration
I.V.	2-5 min	15 min	2-3 hr
I.M.	10-20 min	20-30 min	Up to 4 hr
S.C.	5-15 min	5-30 min	2 hr
P.O.	30 min	60-120 min	Variable
Intraocular	10-30 min	30 min	Variable

PHARMACODYNAMICS

Cholinergic agonists mimic the action of acetylcholine at the autonomic effector site. They bind with receptors on the cell membrane of target organs, changing the permeability of the cell membrane and permitting calcium and sodium to flow into the cells. This depolarizes the cell membrane, causing muscle stimulation. (See *Pharmacologic actions of cholinergic agents.*)

PHARMACOTHERAPEUTICS

Cholinergic agonists are used to treat atonic bladder conditions; to treat GI disorders, such as postoperative distention and GI atony; and to reduce intraocular pressure in the anterior chamber of the eye. The last indication is useful in patients with glaucoma and in those undergoing ocular surgery.

Drug interactions

The effect of the cholinergic agonists is intensified by the simultaneous presence of anticholinesterase agents, which inhibit the breakdown of acetylcholine at the receptor sites. The action of cholinergic agonists is limited by interaction with **antimuscarinic** drugs and **sympathomimetics.** Antimuscarinic drugs, such as atropine, block the action of the cholinergic agonists on the autonomic effector. Sympathomimetics produce a response opposite to that of the cholinergic agonists at muscarinic receptors. (See Drug Interactions: *Cholinergic agonists,* page 92.)

ADVERSE DRUG REACTIONS

Adverse drug reactions to the cholinergic agonists usually result from their nonspecific effects throughout the **parasympathetic nervous system.** The cholinergic agonists typically bind with receptors in the parasympathetic nervous system, creating undesirable parasympathomimetic effects outside the target organ. For example, the use of bethanechol to reduce urine retention also will increase GI motility, which may cause nausea, belching, vomiting, intestinal

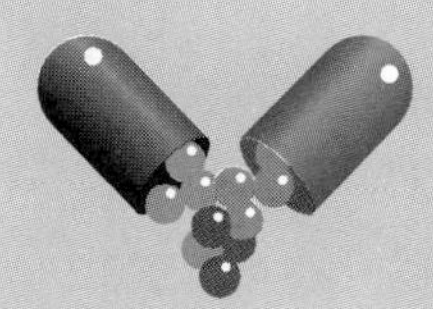

DRUG INTERACTIONS

Cholinergic agonists

Drug interactions involving the cholinergic agonists typically occur with drugs that also act at the autonomic effector cells.

DRUG	INTERACTING AGENTS	POSSIBLE EFFECTS	NURSING IMPLICATIONS
bethanechol, carbachol, pilocarpine	other cholinergic agents, particularly anticholinesterase agents (ambenonium, edrophonium, neostigmine, physostigmine, pyridostigmine)	Increased potential for cholinergic toxicity	• Observe the patient for signs of a toxic response, including generalized weakness, fasciculations, dysphagia, and respiratory weakness. • Observe the patient for signs of cardiovascular dysfunction, including bradycardia and hypotension.
	cholinergic blocking agents (atropine, belladonna, homatropine, methantheline, methscopolamine, propantheline, scopolamine)	Decreased effect of acetylcholine at the muscarinic receptors	• Have atropine on hand as an antidote. • Have respiratory support equipment available: suction, oxygen, and mechanical ventilator. • Have atropine available as the antidote for cholinergic agonists. • Monitor the patient for decreased response to the prescribed cholinergic agonist.
	quinidine	Decreased effects of cholinergic agonists	• Monitor cardiovascular status in a patient with paroxysmal supraventricular tachycardia.

cramps, and diarrhea. Effects of the drug on the eye may include blurred vision and decreased accommodation. With high doses, cardiovascular responses may include vasodilation, decreased cardiac rate, and decreased force of cardiac contraction, which may cause hypotension. Salivation or sweating may increase greatly. The drug's bronchoconstrictor effect may produce shortness of breath. Even the desired effect on the urinary bladder is problematic because urinary frequency may replace urine retention. Usually, the greater the dose, the greater the generalized parasympathomimetic effect.

Cholinergic overstimulation can result from patient hypersensitivity, drug overdose, or, rarely, subcutaneous administration. This overstimulation may cause circulatory collapse, resulting in hypotension, shock, and cardiac arrest.

NURSING PROCESS APPLICATION

The following information assists the nurse in caring for a patient who is receiving a cholinergic agonist. It includes an overview of assessment activities as well as examples of appropriate nursing diagnoses and related interventions (under "Planning and implementation"). It also highlights the importance of evaluation.

Assessment

Before drug therapy begins, review the patient's history for conditions that contraindicate or require cautious use of the prescribed cholinergic agonist. Also, review the patient's medication history to identify use of drugs that may interact with this drug. During therapy, assess the patient for adverse drug reactions and signs of drug interactions. Also, periodically assess the effectiveness of therapy. Finally, evaluate the patient's and family's knowledge about the prescribed cholinergic agonist.

Nursing diagnoses

- Risk for injury related to a preexisting condition that contraindicates or requires cautious use of a cholinergic agonist
- Risk for injury related to adverse drug reactions or drug interactions with the prescribed cholinergic agonist
- Altered health maintenance related to potential ineffectiveness of the cholinergic agonist
- Knowledge deficit related to the prescribed cholinergic agonist

Planning and implementation

- Do not administer a cholinergic agonist to a patient with a condition that contraindicates its use.
- Administer a cholinergic agonist cautiously to a patient at risk because of a preexisting condition.
- Monitor the patient for adverse reactions when administering a cholinergic agonist.

∗ *Keep respiratory support equipment readily available.*

∗ *Observe the patient for 30 minutes to 1 hour after S.C. administration of bethanechol; have atropine (0.6 mg) available in a syringe to use as an antidote.*

- Check vital signs and auscultate for breath sounds when administering a cholinergic agonist.
- Administer the cholinergic agonist when the patient's stomach is empty to minimize adverse reactions.

• Advise the physician if the patient has been taking another cholinergic agent or cholinergic blocking agent.
• Notify the physician if the patient displays decreased effectiveness of the prescribed cholinergic agonist.
• Monitor for urination in a patient who is receiving bethanechol for acute urine retention. Urination should occur within 1 hour. If not, notify the physician and expect to perform urinary catheterization.
• Teach the patient about the prescribed agent. (See Patient Teaching: *Cholinergic agonists.*)

Evaluation

For each nursing diagnosis, prepare an evaluation statement that describes the patient's or family's response to nursing interventions.

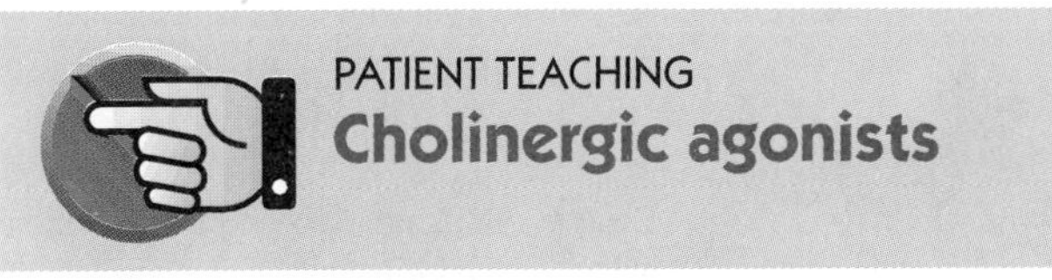

PATIENT TEACHING
Cholinergic agonists

- Teach the patient and family the name, dose, frequency, action, and adverse effects (such as headache, dizziness, and decreased night vision) of the prescribed cholinergic agonist.
- Instruct the patient to take the cholinergic agonist 1 hour before or 2 hours after meals to minimize adverse reactions.
- Show the patient how and where to apply pressure when instilling a cholinergic agonist in the eye.
- Advise the patient that vision may blur and accommodation may decrease.
- Teach the patient to notify the physician if adverse reactions occur.

Anticholinesterase agents

Anticholinesterase agents inhibit the enzyme acetylcholinesterase, thus slowing the destruction of acetylcholine. The subsequent buildup of acetylcholine produces continued stimulation of cholinergic receptors throughout the body. This action is short term in drugs that are used therapeutically, the so-called reversible anticholinesterase agents. The following reversible anticholinesterase agents are discussed here: ambenonium, edrophonium chloride, neostigmine, physostigmine salicylate, and pyridostigmine.

Other anticholinesterase agents, the organophosphates, have a long-term or irreversible action. Used primarily as toxic insecticides and pesticides, they also have been used as nerve gases in chemical warfare. Only two of them, echothiophate and isoflurophate, have therapeutic usefulness. They are used to treat glaucoma and esotropia.

PHARMACOKINETICS

Reversible and *irreversible* refer to the duration of the anticholinesterase agents' blocking effect. With reversible anticholinesterase agents, the blocking effect lasts for minutes to hours; with the irreversible anticholinesterase agents, the effects are sustained for days or weeks. The major differences between these agents are their pharmacokinetics and adverse effects.

Many anticholinesterase agents are absorbed readily from the GI tract, subcutaneous tissue, and mucous membranes. The exceptions are neostigmine and related quaternary ammonium compounds, which are absorbed poorly from the GI tract and are given in larger doses when administered orally. If absorption from the GI tract is enhanced, overdose may occur.

Only physostigmine readily penetrates the blood-brain barrier. Most anticholinesterase agents are metabolized in the body by the plasma esterases and excreted in the urine.

Oral neostigmine has a half-life of 40 to 60 minutes and an onset of action of 45-75 minutes; injectable neostigmine has a half-life of 50 to 90 minutes.

Route	Onset	Peak	Duration
P.O.	20-75 min	1-2 hr	2-12 hr
I.M.	2-20 min	20-30 min	5 min-4 hr
I.V.	30 sec-8 min	5-30 min	5 min-5 hr

PHARMACODYNAMICS

The anticholinesterase agents, like the cholinergic agonists, increase the effect of acetylcholine at receptor sites in the central nervous system (CNS), at autonomic **ganglia,** at autonomic effector cells on the viscera, and at the **motor end plate.** Depending on the site and the drug's dose and duration of action, they can have stimulant and depressant effects on the cholinergic receptors.

PHARMACOTHERAPEUTICS

Anticholinesterase agents are important therapeutically because of their effects on the eye, the GI tract, and the skeletal **neuromuscular junction.** Their ability to reduce intraocular pressure makes them useful adjuncts to ocular surgery and glaucoma treatment. They stimulate tone and peristalsis in the GI tract in patients with gastroparesis. Probably their most important use is to promote muscle contraction in patients with myasthenia gravis. (Neostigmine and edrophonium also are used to diagnose myasthenia gravis.) Anticholinesterase agents also are antidotes to the competitive neuromuscular blocking agents, tricyclic antidepressants, belladonna alkaloids, and narcotics. They also are used to increase bladder tone.

Drug interactions

Interacting drugs usually alter the actions of the anticholinesterase agents at the nicotinic or muscarinic receptor sites. Cholinergic agonists and other acetylcholinesterase inhibitors act at both sites. Therefore, combinations of the drugs must be used with caution to avoid precipitating a

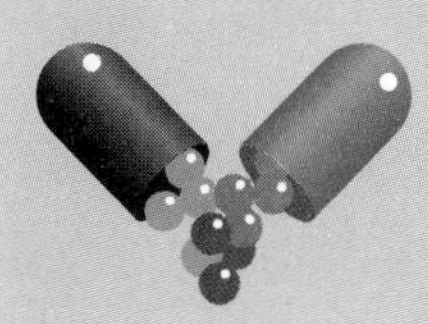

DRUG INTERACTIONS
Anticholinesterase agents

Drug interactions involving the anticholinesterase agents usually occur at nicotinic or muscarinic receptor sites.

DRUG	INTERACTING AGENTS	POSSIBLE EFFECTS	NURSING IMPLICATIONS
ambenonium, edrophonium, neostigmine, physostigmine, pyridostigmine	other cholinergic agents, particularly cholinergic agonists (bethanechol, carbachol, pilocarpine)	Increased effect of acetylcholine at the neuromuscular junction	• Observe the patient for signs of a toxic response, including generalized weakness, fasciculations, dysphagia, abdominal cramps, diarrhea, excessive salivation, perspiration with chills, and respiratory weakness. • Observe the patient for signs of cardiovascular dysfunction, including bradycardia and hypotension. • Have I.V. atropine on hand as an antidote. • Have respiratory support equipment on hand: suction, oxygen, and mechanical ventilator.
	cholinergic blocking agents (atropine, belladonna, homatropine, methantheline, methscopolamine, propantheline, scopolamine), magnesium, corticosteroids, aminoglycosides, anesthetics, antiarrhythmic agents	Decreased effect of anticholinesterase agents, masking early signs of cholinergic crisis	• Monitor for signs and symptoms of cholinergic overdose.
	nondepolarizing neuromuscular blocking agents (atracurium, metocurine, pancuronium, tubocurarine, vecuronium)	Decreased effect of acetylcholine at the neuromuscular junction	• Monitor the patient for decreased therapeutic response to the anticholinesterase agent.
	ester anesthetics	Increased risk of toxicity of anticholinesterase agents	• Monitor the patient for a decreased therapeutic response to nondepolarizing neuromuscular blocker.

toxic response. Drugs with neuromuscular blocking action antagonize the effect of the anticholinesterase agents at the nicotinic receptors in the skeletal muscle. These include selected antibiotics and anesthetics as well as neuromuscular blocking agents. Antimuscarinic agents such as atropine interfere with the anticholinesterase agents in the central and peripheral nervous systems. Therefore, they may be used as antidotes. Ganglionic blocking agents antagonize the effect of these drugs at the nicotinic receptor sites only. (See Drug Interactions: *Anticholinesterase agents.*)

ADVERSE DRUG REACTIONS

Adverse reactions to the anticholinesterase agents almost invariably result from the increased action of acetylcholine at parasympathetic, motor, and CNS receptors. These reactions are difficult to control, particularly at high doses.

Parasympathomimetic effects are common. In the eye, they include blurred vision, decreased accommodation, and miosis; in the skin, increased sweating; in the GI system, increased salivation, belching, nausea, vomiting, intestinal cramps, and diarrhea. The bronchoconstrictor effect may occur as shortness of breath, wheezing, or tightness in the chest. Vasodilation, decreased cardiac rate, and decreased cardiac contraction can result in hypotension, although this effect is offset partially by decreased acetylcholine metabolism at the preganglionic receptor sites in the **sympathetic nervous system.** At the motor end plate, hyperpolarization of the skeletal muscles reduces effective contractions. Adverse reactions in the CNS include irritability, anxiety or fear, and in some cases, seizures.

Reaction to the anticholinesterase agents is difficult to predict in a patient with myasthenia gravis. The therapeutic dose varies from day to day, and increased muscle weakness may result from underdosage, resistance to the drug, or overdosage. Differentiating between a toxic response and myasthenic crisis may be difficult. A physician who uses edrophonium to distinguish between the two must have respiratory support equipment (a suction machine, oxygen, and a mechanical ventilator) and emergency drugs, such as atropine, available to counteract cholinergic crisis.

NURSING PROCESS APPLICATION

The following information assists the nurse in caring for a patient who is receiving an anticholinesterase agent. It includes an overview of assessment activities as well as examples of appropriate nursing diagnoses and related interventions (under "Planning and implementation"). It also highlights the importance of evaluation.

Assessment

Before drug therapy begins, review the patient's history for conditions that contraindicate or require cautious use of the prescribed anticholinesterase agent. Also, review the patient's medication history to identify use of drugs that may interact with these agents. During therapy, assess the patient for adverse drug reactions and signs of drug interactions. Also, periodically assess the effectiveness of therapy. Finally, evaluate the patient's and family's knowledge about the prescribed anticholinesterase agent.

Nursing diagnoses

• Risk for injury related to a preexisting condition that contraindicates or requires cautious use of an anticholinesterase agent
• Risk for injury related to adverse drug reactions or drug interactions
• Anxiety related to the adverse CNS effects of the anticholinesterase agent
• Knowledge deficit related to the prescribed anticholinesterase agent

Planning and implementation

• Do not administer an anticholinesterase agent to a patient with a condition that contraindicates its use.
• Administer an anticholinesterase agent cautiously to a patient at risk because of a preexisting condition.
*** *Have respiratory support equipment available. Keep suction equipment, oxygen, and a mechanical ventilator on hand if edrophonium is used.***
• Observe the patient periodically for adverse reactions and drug interactions.
• Monitor vital signs and auscultate for breath sounds at least once every 4 hours.
• Monitor the patient closely for signs of a toxic response, such as generalized weakness, fasciculations, dysphagia, and respiratory weakness.
*** *Keep atropine (0.6 mg) readily available in a syringe as an antidote.***
*** *Take seizure precautions.***
• Notify the physician if adverse reactions or drug interactions occur.
• Monitor the patient's emotional state periodically.
• Maintain a calm environment.
• Encourage the patient to verbalize feelings of anxiety.
• Notify the physician if anxiety occurs. Also reassure the patient and family that anxiety is an adverse reaction to the anticholinesterase agent. (See Patient Teaching: *Anticholinesterase agents.*)
• Monitor and record changes in muscle strength daily when administering an anticholinesterase agent.

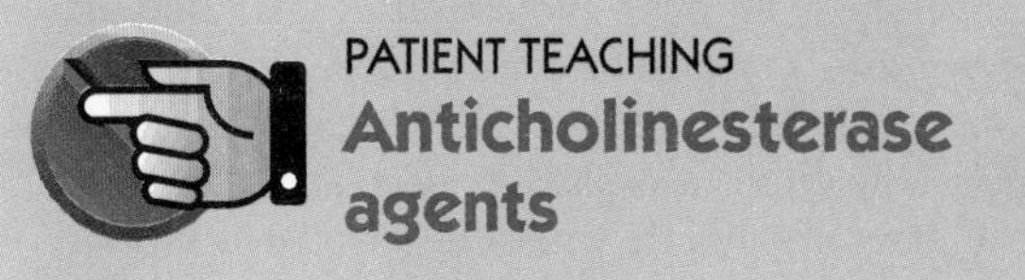

PATIENT TEACHING
Anticholinesterase agents

➤ Teach the patient and family the name, dose, frequency, action, and adverse effects of the prescribed anticholinesterase agent.
➤ Help the patient develop a system for keeping track of each dose and its effect.
➤ Describe ways to manage common adverse reactions. For example, tell the patient to take the drug with food or milk if nausea occurs after oral administration.
➤ Show the patient how to assess and record changes in muscle strength and help the patient practice this assessment.
➤ Advise the patient to report adverse reactions to the physician.

Evaluation

For each nursing diagnosis, prepare an evaluation statement that describes the patient's or family's response to nursing interventions.

CHAPTER SUMMARY

Chapter 6 presented cholinergic agonists and anticholinesterase agents and explained their actions on the parasympathetic nervous system. Here are the chapter highlights.

Cholinergic agents directly or indirectly mimic the effects of acetylcholine in the body. Because these effects usually are similar to the effects of the parasympathetic nervous system, the cholinergic agents also are called parasympathomimetic drugs.

Cholinergic agonists replicate the action of acetylcholine at the autonomic effector site. They bind with receptors on the cell membrane of target organs, changing cell membrane permeability and permitting calcium and sodium to flow into the cells. This depolarizes the cell membrane, causing muscle stimulation. Therapeutically, they are used for their actions on the eye, the GI tract, and the urinary bladder.

The anticholinesterase agents facilitate the action of acetylcholine by inhibiting its destruction by the acetylcholinesterase enzyme at the autonomic effector sites and at the neuromuscular junction. Their primary therapeutic use is to diagnose and treat myasthenia gravis and to counteract neuromuscular blocking agents. Occasionally, they are used to treat glaucoma, to treat hypotonia of the GI tract or urinary bladder, and in ocular surgery.

The adverse effects of the cholinergic agents result primarily from their nonspecific effects on the parasympathetic nervous system; those of the anticholinesterase agents almost invariably result from the increased action of acetylcholine at parasympathetic, motor, and CNS receptors.

Nursing care for a patient receiving a cholinergic agent should include managing and teaching about adverse drug reactions. For a patient who takes an anticholinesterase agent for long-term treatment of myasthenia gravis, the nurse should supply detailed instructions.

Questions to consider

See Appendix 1 for answers.

1. Alice Jensen, age 42, comes to the emergency department because she has not been able to void for the past 16 hours. Her history reveals multiple sclerosis of 2 years' duration. The physician orders bethanechol (Duvoid), 10 mg S.C., to relieve acute urine retention. During bethanechol therapy, the nurse should assess Mrs. Jensen for which of the following common adverse reactions?
   - (a) Dry mouth, flushed face, and constipation
   - (b) Fasciculations, dysphagia, and respiratory distress
   - (c) Nausea, vomiting, diarrhea, and intestinal cramps
   - (d) Rash, shortness of breath, and nasal congestion

2. After administering bethanechol to Richard Woods, age 57, the nurse monitors for signs of cholinergic overstimulation. Because this adverse reaction may occur in some patients, the nurse should keep which of the following drugs readily available as an antidote to bethanechol?
   - (a) atropine
   - (b) ambenonium
   - (c) epinephrine
   - (d) neostigmine

3. Nina Aarons, age 30, takes neostigmine 15 mg P.O. every 4 hours to treat myasthenia gravis. What is the onset of action of oral neostigmine?
   - (a) 5 to 15 minutes
   - (b) 20 to 30 minutes
   - (c) 45 to 75 minutes
   - (d) 90 to 120 minutes

4. When teaching Nathan Wells, age 64, about neostigmine therapy, the nurse should tell him to note and report which of the following adverse reactions?
   - (a) Wheezing
   - (b) Increased heart rate
   - (c) Hypertension
   - (d) CNS depression

5. After 6 months of neostigmine therapy, Elizabeth Varshaw, age 44, is hospitalized for myasthenic crisis. Before Ms. Varshaw is discharged, the nurse should remind her to monitor and record which parameter daily to assess the effectiveness of neostigmine therapy?
   - (a) Pulse rate
   - (b) Temperature
   - (c) Bowel movement
   - (d) Muscle strength

7 Cholinergic blocking agents

OBJECTIVES

After reading and studying this chapter, the student should be able to:

1. discuss the actions of the cholinergic blocking agents.
2. describe the pharmacokinetics of the cholinergic blocking agents.
3. list the major clinical indications for the cholinergic blocking agents.
4. describe the major adverse reactions to these drugs.
5. describe how to apply the nursing process when caring for a patient who is receiving a cholinergic blocking agent.

INTRODUCTION

Cholinergic blocking agents interrupt parasympathetic nerve impulses in the central and **autonomic nervous systems.** Their primary clinical indications include spastic conditions of the gastrointestinal (GI) and urinary tracts, cardiac arrhythmias, motion sickness, and parkinsonism. They also are used as preanesthesia medications and as relaxants for the GI tract during diagnostic procedures and for the eye and pupil during ophthalmologic surgery. They serve as antidotes to cholinergic agents and certain organophosphate pesticides.

Cholinergic blocking agents constitute two classes: ganglionic blocking agents and **antimuscarinic** drugs. Although ganglionic blockers block the transmission of **adrenergic** and cholinergic stimuli, their clinical use has been limited to their adrenergic effects. The drugs that comprise this class of blocking agents have recently been taken off the market.

The antimuscarinic drugs, of which atropine sulfate is the prototype, exert their blockade effect at postganglionic cholinergic nerve endings at the **muscarinic receptor** sites. They are the focus of this chapter. (See *Selected major cholinergic blocking agents,* page 98.)

Drugs covered in this chapter include:

- atropine sulfate
- belladonna
- clidinium bromide
- dicyclomine hydrochloride
- glycopyrrolate
- hyoscyamine sulfate
- oxybutynine chloride
- propantheline bromide
- scopolamine hydrobromide.

Cholinergic blockers

The cholinergic blockers block the action of **acetylcholine** at muscarinic receptors in the **parasympathetic nervous system.** The major drugs in this class are the belladonna alkaloids (atropine sulfate, belladonna, homatropine hydrobromide, hyoscyamine sulfate, and scopolamine hydrobromide), their synthetic derivatives (the quaternary ammonium agents clidinium bromide, glycopyrrolate, and propantheline bromide), and the tertiary amines (benztropine mesylate, dicyclomine hydrochloride, ethopropazine hydrochloride, oxybutynin chloride, and trihexyphenidyl hydrochloride). Because benztropine, ethopropazine, and trihexyphenidyl are almost exclusively treatments for parkinsonism, they are discussed fully in another chapter.

PHARMACOKINETICS

The belladonna alkaloids are absorbed from the GI tract, the mucous membranes, the skin, and the eyes. The quaternary ammonium derivatives and tertiary amines are absorbed primarily through the GI tract, although much less readily than the alkaloids.

The belladonna alkaloids are distributed more widely than the quaternary ammonium derivatives or dicyclomine. The alkaloids readily cross the blood-brain barrier; the other drugs in this class do not.

The belladonna alkaloids have low to moderate binding with serum proteins, are metabolized in the liver, and are excreted by the kidneys as unchanged drug and metabolites. The metabolism of the quaternary ammonium derivatives is more complicated. Hydrolysis occurs in the GI tract and the liver; excretion is in feces and urine. Dicyclomine's metabolism is unknown, but it is excreted approximately 50% in urine and 50% in feces.

Selected major cholinergic blocking agents

This table summarizes the major cholinergic blockers currently in clinical use.

DRUG	MAJOR INDICATIONS AND USUAL DOSAGES	CONTRAINDICATIONS AND PRECAUTIONS
atropine sulfate (Atropine Sulfate Injection)	*Reversal of arrhythmias, bradycardia, and sinus arrest* ADULT: 0.4 to 1 mg I.V. every 2 hours, as needed, up to a maximum of 2 mg PEDIATRIC: 0.02 mg/kg I.V., up to a maximum of 1 mg *Preanesthesia medication* ADULT: 0.2 to 0.6 mg I.M. 30 to 60 minutes before surgery PEDIATRIC: Dose given I.M. or S.C. Infants $\leq$ 5 kg, give 0.04 mg/kg; infants > 5 kg, give 0.03 mg/kg, repeat every 4 to 6 hours; in children give 0.01 mg/kg to a maximum dose of 0.4 mg repeated every 4 to 6 hours as needed *Adjunct to drugs used to reverse neuromuscular blockade* ADULT: 0.6 to 1.2 mg I.V. before or concurrently with 2 to 2.5 mg of neostigmine in a separate syringe	• Atropine is contraindicated in a breast-feeding patient or one with hypersensitivity, narrow-angle glaucoma, obstructive uropathy, severe ulcerative colitis, obstructive disease of the GI tract, cardiospasm, paralytic ileus, intestinal atony, myasthenia gravis (unless the drug is used to reduce adverse muscarinic effects of an anticholinesterase), tachycardia caused by cardiac insufficiency or thyrotoxicosis, or acute hemorrhage and unstable cardiovascular status. • This drug requires cautious use in a pregnant, pediatric, or geriatric patient or in one with autonomic neuropathy, GI infection, diarrhea, mild to moderate ulcerative colitis, partial obstructive uropathy, fever, hyperthyroidism, hepatic or renal disease, gastric ulcer, hypertension, tachyarrhythmias, heart failure, coronary artery disease, chronic pulmonary disease (in a debilitated patient), esophageal reflux, or hiatal hernia associated with reflux esophagitis.
dicyclomine hydrochloride (Antispas, Bentyl, Di-Spaz)	*Irritable bowel syndrome* ADULT: 20 mg P.O. q.i.d., up to a maximum of 160 mg/day, or 20 mg I.M. daily in four divided doses	• Dicyclomine is contraindicated in infants under age 6 months, breast-feeding patients, or patients with hypersensitivity, glaucoma, obstructive uropathy, severe ulcerative colitis, obstructive disease of the GI tract, myasthenia gravis, reflux esophagitis, or acute hemorrhage and unstable cardiovascular status. • This drug requires cautious use in a pregnant patient or one with autonomic neuropathy, hepatic or renal failure, mild to moderate ulcerative colitis, hyperthyroidism, hypertension, coronary heart disease, heart failure, tachyarrhythmia, hiatal hernia, or prostatic hypertrophy. • Safety and efficacy in children have not been established.
propantheline bromide (Pro-Banthine)	*Peptic ulcer (adjunctive therapy)* ADULT: 15 mg P.O. q.i.d. 30 minutes before meals and at bedtime	• Propantheline is contraindicated in a patient with glaucoma, obstructive disease of the GI tract, obstructive uropathy, intestinal atony (in a geriatric or debilitated patient), severe ulcerative colitis, ulcerative colitis complicated by toxic megacolon, myasthenia gravis, or acute hemorrhage and unstable cardiovascular status. • This drug requires cautious use in a pregnant, breast-feeding, or geriatric patient or in one with autonomic neuropathy, hepatic or renal disease, hyperthyroidism, coronary heart disease, heart failure, tachyarrhythmias, hypertension, hiatal hernia associated with reflux esophagitis, or mild to moderate ulcerative colitis. • Safety and efficacy in children have not been established.
scopolamine hydrobromide (Transderm Scōp)	*Motion sickness* ADULT: 0.5 mg transdermal patch 1 hour before the effect is desired *Preanesthesia medication* ADULT: 0.3 to 0.6 mg I.M., I.V., or S.C. 30 to 60 minutes before surgery	• Scopolamine is contraindicated in a child or any patient with hypersensitivity, narrow-angle glaucoma, partial or complete obstruction of the GI tract, paralytic ileus, obstructive uropathy, thyrotoxicosis, or tachycardia caused by cardiac insufficiency. • This drug requires cautious use in a pregnant, breast-feeding, or geriatric patient or in one with metabolic, hepatic, or renal dysfunction.

How atropine speeds the heart rate

When acetylcholine is released, the vagus nerve stimulates the sinoatrial (SA) and atrioventricular (AV) nodes, which inhibits electrical conduction. This slows the heart rate. The cholinergic blocker atropine competes with acetylcholine for binding with cholinergic receptors on SA and AV nodal cells. By blocking the effects of acetylcholine, atropine speeds the heart rate.

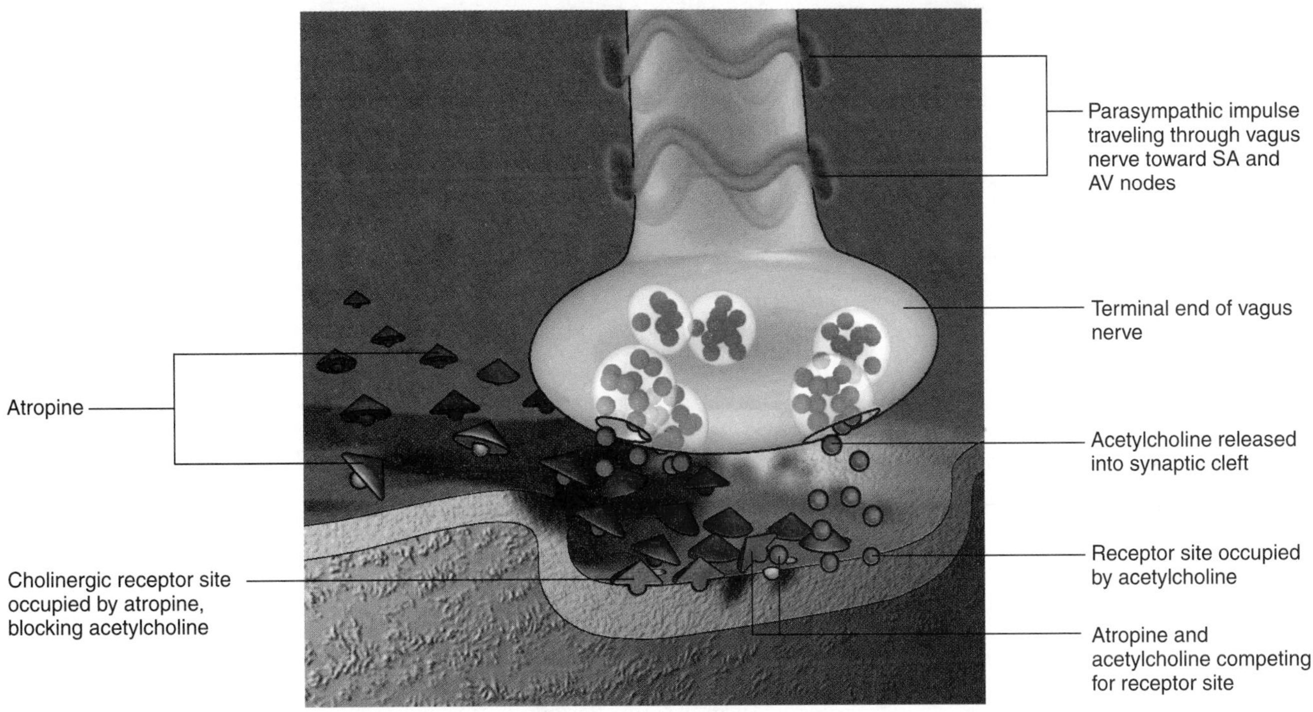

Route	Onset	Peak	Duration
P.O.	30-120 min	60-120 min	Up to 6 hr
I.V.	1 min	2-4 min	Variable
I.M.	30 min	15-20 min	Up to 4 hr
S.C.	30 min	Variable	Variable

PHARMACODYNAMICS

The action of the cholinergic blockers is stimulating or depressing, depending on the target organ. In the brain, they seem to do both — low drug levels stimulate, and high levels depress. Drug effects are also determined by the condition being treated. Parkinsonism, for example, is characterized by a dopamine deficiency that intensifies the stimulating effects of acetylcholine. Antimuscarinic agents depress this effect. In other cases, the effects of these drugs on the central nervous system (CNS) seem to be stimulatory.

PHARMACOTHERAPEUTICS

All the cholinergic blockers are used to treat spastic conditions of the GI and urinary tracts because they relax muscles and decrease GI secretions. The quaternary ammonium compounds, such as propantheline, are the drugs of choice for these conditions because they cause fewer adverse reactions than the belladonna alkaloids. However, the alkaloids are used with morphine to treat biliary colic. Parenteral doses of cholinergic blocking agents are used before such diagnostic procedures as endoscopy or sigmoidoscopy to relax the GI smooth muscle.

As preanesthesia medications, cholinergic blockers such as atropine reduce salivation and gastric secretions and depress the respiratory system. They also block cardiac vagal inhibition during anesthesia.

The belladonna alkaloids have several therapeutic CNS effects. Scopolamine, given with morphine or meperidine, reduces excitement and produces amnesia in the preanesthesia patient. It is also used in treating motion sickness. Although other drugs are more effective for other dyskinesias, the cholinergic blockers play an important role in treating extrapyramidal symptoms from drugs and in treating parkinsonism.

The belladonna alkaloids also have important therapeutic effects on the heart. Parenteral atropine is the drug of choice to treat sinus bradycardia. (See *How atropine speeds the heart rate.*) It is particularly useful when arrhythmia results from anesthetics, choline esters, or succinylcholine.

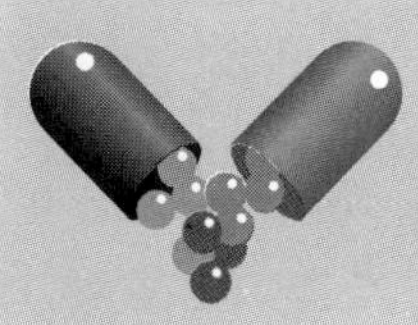

DRUG INTERACTIONS

Cholinergic blockers

The nurse must be aware of the many commonly administered medications that interact with cholinergic blockers.

DRUG	INTERACTING AGENTS	POSSIBLE EFFECTS	NURSING IMPLICATIONS
atropine, belladonna, clidinium, dicyclomine, glycopyrrolate, hyoscyamine, oxybutynin, propantheline, scopolamine	disopyramide, tricyclic and tetracyclic antidepressants, antidyskinetics (including amantadine), antiemetics and antivertigo agents (including buclizine, cyclizine, meclizine, and diphenhydramine), antipsychotics (including haloperidol, phenothiazines, and thioxanthenes), cyclobenzaprine, orphenadrine	Enhanced anticholinergic effect	• Monitor the patient for signs of adverse reactions to cholinergic blockers. • Monitor for constipation, which may become severe or result in paralytic ileus.
	cholinergic agonists (bethanechol), anticholinesterase agents (neostigmine, pyridostigmine)	Decreased antimuscarinic effect, antagonism of cholinergic effect	• Monitor the patient for therapeutic effects of the cholinergic blocking agents. • Monitor the patient for therapeutic effects of cholinergic agonists.
	digoxin	Increased serum concentration levels of digoxin	• Monitor the patient's apical pulse frequently. • Observe the patient for signs of digitalis toxicity, such as GI, cardiac, and neurologic effects.
	opiate-like analgesics	Decreased GI motility	• Monitor the patient for constipation, which may become severe or result in paralytic ileus. • Monitor the patient's bowel sounds frequently.
	nitroglycerin	Delayed sublingual absorption of nitroglycerin	• Offer the patient sips of water before administering nitroglycerin.

Cholinergic blockers also are used as cycloplegics to paralyze the ciliary muscles of the eye, altering the shape of the lens, and as mydriatics to dilate the pupils. They make it easier to measure refractive errors during an ophthalmic examination or to perform ophthalmologic surgery. Occasionally, they are used as adjuncts to antibiotics in treating eye infections.

The belladonna alkaloids, particularly atropine and hyoscyamine, are effective antidotes to cholinergic and anticholinesterase agents. Atropine is the drug of choice to treat poisoning from organophosphate pesticides. Atropine and hyoscyamine also counteract the effects of the neuromuscular blocking agents by competing for the same receptor sites.

Drug interactions

Because cholinergic blockers decrease gastric motility and delay gastric emptying, they may increase the absorption of other medications. Additionally, the delayed gastric emptying keeps the drugs in prolonged contact with the GI mucosa, which can increase their adverse effects. (See Drug Interactions: *Cholinergic blockers.*)

ADVERSE DRUG REACTIONS

The widespread action of the cholinergic blockers commonly produces therapeutic benefits that are accompanied by undesirable effects. The use of drugs that interact with cholinergic blockers further increases the possibility of adverse reactions.

Adverse reactions are a function of the affinity of the muscarinic receptors for specific drugs and of the drug dosage. Dosage is particularly crucial: the difference between a therapeutic and a toxic dosage is small with the cholinergic blockers. Also, some people are much more susceptible than others to the effects of these drugs. These include infants, geriatric patients, fair-skinned children with Down syndrome, and children with spastic paralysis or brain damage.

Adverse reactions increase in severity as the dosage increases. Small doses are accompanied by decreased salivation, bronchial secretions, and sweating — reducing the patient's ability to cope with heat. As the dosage increases, the pupils dilate, visual accommodation decreases, and heart rate increases. Still larger doses inhibit urination and intestinal motility, followed by a decrease in gastric secretions and motility.

With drug overdose, all these effects are exaggerated. CNS excitation is prominent at toxic levels. The patient becomes restless, irritable, and disoriented, even hallucinatory or delirious. If the process is not reversed, the excitatory phase is followed by CNS depression, unconsciousness, medullary paralysis, and death.

Cholinergic blockers may precipitate problems in patients with some underlying diseases. The drugs sometimes cause a dangerous rise in intraocular pressure in those with unrecognized narrow-angle glaucoma.

In a patient with coronary artery disease, tachycardia secondary to the administration of cholinergic blockers can lead to circulatory failure. This may be compounded by the atrial and ventricular arrhythmias that sometimes occur with the cholinergic blockers.

In a patient with benign prostatic hypertrophy, cholinergic blockers may cause urine retention. The agents therefore should be used cautiously in geriatric male patients.

Heatstroke is another potential complication with these drugs because they inhibit such heat-regulating mechanisms as sweating. It produces extreme elevation in body temperature, dehydration, flushing, and mental changes. Heatstroke occurs more commonly with strenuous activity and high environmental temperatures. (See Geriatric Considerations: *Heatstroke and cholinergic blockers.*)

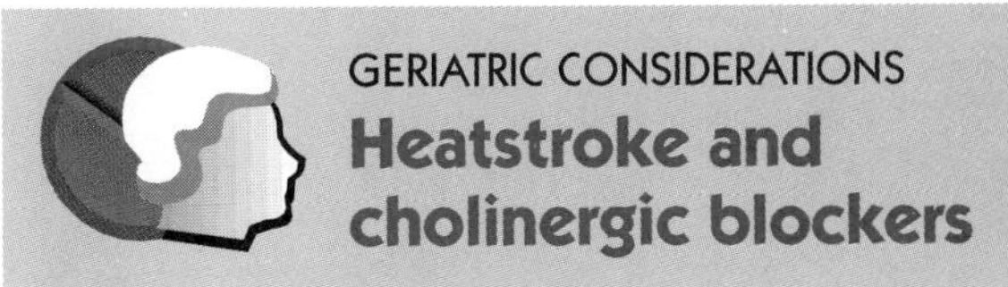

GERIATRIC CONSIDERATIONS

Heatstroke and cholinergic blockers

For a geriatric patient who takes a cholinergic blocker and lives in a warm climate or an area with hot summers, discuss heatstroke. Cholinergic blockers increase the risk of heatstroke, especially in geriatric patients. The risk is even greater in geriatric patients with cardiovascular disease. Instruct the patient to remain indoors during hot weather, use an air conditioner or fan, and drink plenty of cool liquids.

NURSING PROCESS APPLICATION

The following information assists the nurse in caring for a patient who is receiving a cholinergic blocking agent. It includes an overview of assessment activities as well as examples of appropriate nursing diagnoses and related interventions (under "Planning and implementation"). It also highlights the importance of evaluation.

Assessment

Before drug therapy begins, review the patient's history for conditions that contraindicate or require cautious use of the prescribed cholinergic blocker. Also review the patient's medication history to identify use of drugs that may interact with it. During therapy, assess the patient for adverse drug reactions, such as heatstroke, and drug interactions. Also, periodically assess the effectiveness of drug therapy. Finally, evaluate the patient's and family's knowledge about the prescribed cholinergic blocker.

Nursing diagnoses

- Risk for injury related to a preexisting condition that contraindicates or requires cautious use of a cholinergic blocker
- Risk for injury related to adverse drug reactions or drug interactions
- Risk for altered body temperature related to risk of heatstroke caused by the cholinergic blocker
- Knowledge deficit related to the prescribed cholinergic blocker

Planning and implementation

- Do not administer a cholinergic blocker to a patient with a condition that contraindicates its use.
- Administer a cholinergic blocker cautiously to a patient at risk because of a preexisting condition.

* ***Monitor the patient regularly for adverse reactions and drug interactions. Frequently monitor an infant, a geriatric patient, a fair-skinned child with Down syndrome, or a child with spastic paralysis or brain damage because such a patient is at increased risk for developing adverse reactions to a cholinergic blocker. Keep in mind that adverse reactions increase in severity as the dosage increases.***

- Administer a cholinergic blocker 30 minutes before meals and at bedtime when used to reduce GI motility.
- Notify the physician if adverse drug reactions occur.
- Monitor the patient for signs of heatstroke, such as dehydration, flushing, and altered level of consciousness. Heatstroke induced by a cholinergic blocker is more common during strenuous activity, in hot weather, and in geriatric patients with cardiovascular disease.
- Keep the patient's room temperature cool.
- Encourage the patient to drink additional fluids (if not contraindicated) when engaging in a strenuous activity or when the weather is hot. (See Patient Teaching: *Cholinergic blockers,* page 102.)
- Be prepared to perform emergency interventions if heatstroke occurs.
- Monitor the patient for signs and symptoms of urine retention, such as urinary frequency with voiding of small amounts.
- Notify the physician if urine retention occurs.

Evaluation

For each nursing diagnosis, prepare an evaluation statement that describes the patient's or family's response to nursing interventions.

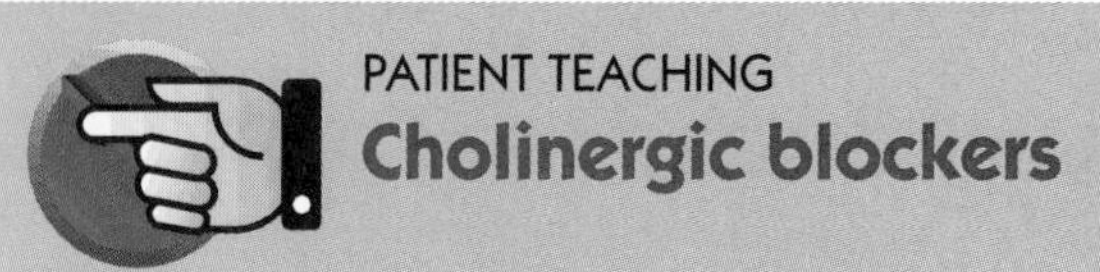

PATIENT TEACHING

Cholinergic blockers

- Teach the patient and family the name, dose, frequency, action, and adverse reactions of the prescribed cholinergic blocker.
- Teach the patient to avoid drug toxicity by taking only the amount of medicine ordered. Advise the patient who misses a dose to take it as soon as possible. If it is almost time for the next dose, the patient should wait until then and take a single dose only. Stress that the patient should not double the dose without consulting the physician.
- Teach the patient to reduce the risk of heatstroke by moving slowly and staying in the shade in hot weather, avoiding strenuous exercise, and using fans or air conditioners.
- Advise the patient to limit milk and bedtime snacks because they increase gastric secretions.
- Teach the patient to consume a high-fiber diet and plenty of fluids to help prevent constipation. If needed, suggest the use of an over-the-counter stool softener.
- Teach the patient how to stroke the abdomen or use Credé's maneuver (bladder massage) if voiding becomes difficult.
- Recommend that the patient wear dark glasses and avoid driving if drug therapy produces mydriasis and cycloplegia.
- Teach the patient about the need for scrupulous oral hygiene to decrease the likelihood of caries and periodontal disease caused by decreased salivation.
- Recommend sugarless gum, hard sugarless candies, or ice to reduce dry mouth.

CHAPTER SUMMARY

Chapter 7 focused on the antimuscarinic cholinergic blockers. Here are the chapter highlights.

Cholinergic blockers interrupt parasympathetic nerve impulses in the central and autonomic nervous systems by competing with the neurotransmitter acetylcholine at muscarinic receptor sites. These drugs include the belladonna alkaloids, their quaternary ammonium derivatives, and the tertiary amines.

Clinical indications for cholinergic blockers include cardiac arrhythmias, motion sickness, parkinsonism, spastic conditions of the GI and urinary tracts, poisoning by organophosphate pesticides, and toxicity from cholinergic agents or neuromuscular blockers. They also are used to decrease salivary and respiratory secretions during anesthesia, relax the GI tract during diagnostic procedures, and relax eye muscles and dilate the pupil during ophthalmologic examinations and surgery.

Because of the drugs' lack of selectivity, even therapeutic doses of the cholinergic blockers may cause multiple adverse reactions, usually extensions of the anticholinergic actions. Adverse reactions increase in severity as the dosage increases. The margin of safety between therapeutic and toxic doses is extremely small.

The nurse should teach the patient about the prescribed cholinergic blocker, including its adverse effects and how to prevent, recognize, and obtain treatment for toxicity.

Questions to consider

See Appendix 1 for answers.

1. Richard Ahearn, age 64, is scheduled for a hip replacement. The physician prescribes preoperative sedation with midazolam hydrochloride 2 mg I.V. and the cholinergic blocker atropine 0.4 mg I.M. What is the purpose of atropine as a preanesthetic agent?
   (a) To reduce hyperreflexia during surgery
   (b) To minimize the risk of postoperative ileus
   (c) To prevent respiratory depression during surgery
   (d) To reduce excess salivation and gastric secretions

2. Because Linda Russo, age 56, is about to begin therapy with dicyclomine hydrochloride, the nurse checks her medication history carefully. Which of the following agents may enhance the anticholinergic effects of this cholinergic blocker?
   (a) digoxin
   (b) nitroglycerin
   (c) haloperidol
   (d) neostigmine

3. Connie Baker, age 32, has irritable bowel syndrome for which her physician prescribes propantheline bromide (Pro-Banthine) 15 mg P.O. q.i.d. When should Ms. Baker take this medication?
   (a) On an empty stomach between meals and at bedtime
   (b) 30 minutes before meals and at bedtime
   (c) 30 minutes after meals and at bedtime
   (d) With meals and a snack at bedtime

4. Steven Legg, age 43, becomes constipated during propanthelene therapy. He asks the nurse what he should do about this problem. What should the nurse recommend?
   (a) Stop taking the drug and notify the physician.
   (b) Increase his fluid and fiber intake.
   (c) Increase his milk intake.
   (d) Avoid eating fruits.

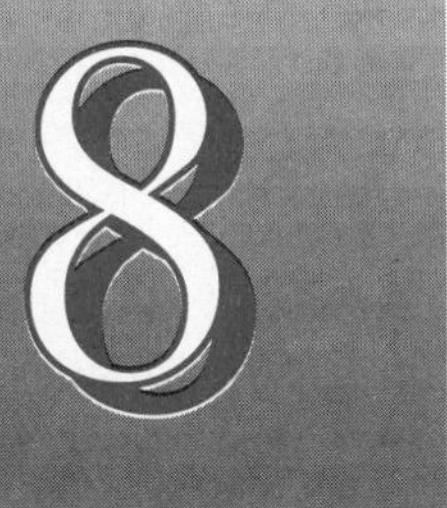

Adrenergic agents

OBJECTIVES

After reading and studying this chapter, the student should be able to:

1. differentiate between catecholamines and noncatecholamines.
2. compare the methods of action of adrenergic agents: direct, indirect, or dual.
3. differentiate among the effects of alpha-, $beta_1$-, and $beta_2$-receptor stimulation.
4. describe clinical situations that require catecholamine use.
5. describe clinical situations in which the noncatecholamines are useful.
6. discuss the adverse effects of catecholamines and noncatecholamines.
7. describe how to apply the nursing process when caring for a patient who is receiving a catecholamine or noncatecholamine.

INTRODUCTION

Adrenergic agents, which also are called **sympathomimetics,** include a large number of endogenous substances and synthetic drugs that have a wide range of therapeutic uses. Classifying adrenergic agents is thus difficult. The classification system used in this chapter divides adrenergic agents into two groups: **catecholamines** (including endogenous and synthetic agents) and noncatecholamines.

Adrenergic agents may be divided further by their method of action. They may be direct-acting (acting directly on the sympathetically innervated organ or tissue), indirect-acting (triggering the release of a **neurotransmitter,** usually norepinephrine), or dual-acting (combining direct and indirect actions).

Therapeutic use of an adrenergic agent depends on its receptor activity. (See *Adrenergic receptor sites,* page 104.) Most adrenergic agents stimulate **alpha-adrenergic** or **beta-adrenergic receptors** to produce their pharmacologic effects, thus mimicking the action of norepinephrine or epinephrine. Other adrenergic agents, called dopaminergic agents, act primarily on receptors in the **sympathetic nervous system** (SNS) stimulated by dopamine. (See *Selected major adrenergic agents,* pages 105 and 106.)

Drugs in this chapter include:

- albuterol
- amphetamine sulfate
- bitolterol mesylate
- dextroamphetamine sulfate
- dobutamine hydrochloride
- dopamine hydrochloride
- ephedrine sulfate
- epinephrine, epinephrine bitartrate, epinephrine hydrochloride
- isoetharine hydrochloride, isoetharine mesylate
- isoproterenol hydrochloride, isoproterenol sulfate
- mazindol
- mephentermine sulfate
- metaproterenol sulfate
- metaraminol sulfate
- methoxamine hydrochloride
- methylphenidate hydrochloride
- norepinephrine (levarterenol)
- phenylephrine hydrochloride
- phenylpropanolamine hydrochloride
- pirbuterol acetate
- ritodrine hydrochloride
- terbutaline sulfate.

Catecholamines

Catecholamines include dobutamine hydrochloride, dopamine hydrochloride, epinephrine, epinephrine bitartrate, epinephrine hydrochloride, isoproterenol hydrochloride, isoproterenol sulfate, and norepinephrine (levarterenol). These drugs may be endogenous or synthetic. Because of their common basic chemical structure, catecholamines share certain properties.

PHARMACOKINETICS

Catecholamines are destroyed by digestive enzymes — **monoamine oxidase (MAO)** and **catechol-O-methyltransferase (COMT)** — but are absorbed rapidly from mucous membranes. When given sublingually, a catecholamine must be absorbed completely to prevent its rapid metabolism by swallowed saliva.

Subcutaneous (S.C.) absorption is slowed by local vasoconstriction secondary to the drug's administration.

Intramuscular absorption is more rapid because this route results in less local vasoconstriction. These drugs are distributed widely in the body.

Adrenergic receptor sites

This chart lists receptor types and locations and the effects of adrenergic or dopaminergic drugs on receptors

RECEPTOR TYPE	LOCATION	EFFECT
Adrenergic agents		
$alpha_1$	Arterioles	Constriction
	Urinary bladder sphincters	Contraction
	Eye (radial) and skin (pilomotor) muscles	Contraction
	Liver	Glyconeogenesis Glycogenolysis
$alpha_2$	Pancreas	Decreased insulin secretion
	Skeletal blood vessels	Constriction
$beta_1$	Heart	Increased rate, conduction, and contractility
	Adipose tissue	Lipolysis
	Kidneys	Renin release
$beta_2$	Bronchi, GI, and urinary bladder smooth muscles	Relaxation
	Skeletal blood vessels	Dilation
	Uterus	Relaxation
	Liver	Glyconeogenesis Glycogenolysis
Dopaminergic agents		
dopaminergic	Coronary arteries, renal blood vessels, and mesenteric or visceral blood vessels	Dilation

Metabolism with inactivation of the drugs occurs in the gastrointestinal (GI) tract, lungs, kidneys, plasma, and other tissues, but most occurs in the liver.

Metabolites and some unchanged drug are excreted primarily in the urine; a small amount of isoproterenol is excreted in the feces, and some epinephrine is excreted in breast milk.

Route	Onset	Peak	Duration
I.V.	1-10 min	Unknown	1-20 min
I.M.	10-15 min	Unknown	30-120 min
S.C.	Variable	Unknown	50-60 min
S.L.	15-30 min	Unknown	60-120 min
Inhalation	2-5 min	Unknown	30-120 min

PHARMACODYNAMICS

When catecholamines combine with alpha or beta receptors, chemical or electrical events occur that produce excitatory or inhibitory effects. In most cases, alpha-receptor activation generates an excitatory response (except for intestinal relaxation). Beta-receptor activation is mostly inhibitory (except in the myocardial cells, where norepinephrine elicits excitatory effects).

The clinical effects of catecholamines depend on the dosage and the route of administration. In the cardiovascular system, these effects also may depend on the vascular bed. The positive **inotropic** action (marked increase in strength of contraction) results from the influx of calcium into cardiac fibers, producing more complete emptying of the ventricles and increasing cardiac workload and oxygen consumption. Also, the positive inotropic action may occur with catecholamines as well as a positive chronotropic effect from the increased rate of membrane depolarization in the pacemaker cells of the sinus node. This produces a more rapid attainment of the action potential threshold, so the pacemaker cells fire more often. Reflex bradycardia may occur from increased vasoconstriction and blood pressure. Catecholamines may precipitate spontaneous firing in the Purkinje fibers, producing pacemaker activity and possibly producing premature ventricular contractions and fibrillation. Epinephrine is likelier than norepinephrine to produce this spontaneous firing.

PHARMACOTHERAPEUTICS

The particular receptor activity that exists alone or predominates if more than one receptor type is activated determines how the drug is used therapeutically. Of the catecholamines, norepinephrine has the most nearly pure alpha activity. Drugs with only beta-related therapeutic uses include dobutamine and isoproterenol; epinephrine stimulates alpha and beta receptors. Dopamine primarily exhibits dopaminergic activity.

The therapeutic uses of catecholamines are related not only to their systemic effects, but also to their local effects. These drugs are not effective if given orally.

The alpha stimulators can be used systemically to relieve hypotension. Hypotension may be caused by numerous conditions, including sympathectomy, pheochromocytomectomy, spinal anesthesia, myocardial infarction, transfusion reaction, septicemia, drug reactions, or shock. As a rule, the pressor effects are used for conditions related to loss of vasomotor tone or loss of adequate circulating blood volume.

Selected major adrenergic agents

This table summarizes the major adrenergic agents currently in clinical use.

DRUG	MAJOR INDICATIONS AND USUAL DOSAGES	CONTRAINDICATIONS AND PRECAUTIONS
Catecholamines		
dobutamine hydrochloride (Dobutrex)	*Acute heart failure, cardiopulmonary bypass surgery* ADULT: 2.5 to 20 mcg/kg/minute I.V. infusion of a 250 mcg/ml, 500 mcg/ml, or 1,000 mcg/ml solution in D_5W or normal saline solution; increased up to 40 mcg/kg/minute, if required	• Dobutamine is contraindicated in a patient with known hypersensitivity to the drug or idiopathic hypertrophic subaortic stenosis. • This drug requires cautious use in a pregnant patient or one with acute myocardial infarction. • Safety and efficacy in children have not been established.
dopamine hydrochloride (Intropin)	*Shock, decreased renal function* ADULT: initially, 1 to 5 mcg/kg/minute I.V. infusion, diluted as recommended; may increase every 10 to 30 minutes, as needed, by 5- to 10-mcg/kg/minute increments to 20 to 50 mcg/kg/minute in a critically ill patient	• Dopamine is contraindicated in a patient with pheochromocytoma, uncorrected tachyarrhythmias, or ventricular fibrillation. • This drug requires cautious use in a pregnant patient or one who inhales cyclopropane or halogenated hydrocarbon anesthetics or has a history of occlusive vascular disease. • Safety and efficacy in children have not been established.
epinephrine hydrochloride and epinephrine bitartrate (Parenteral: Adrenalin, Sus-Phrine, Epi-pen. Inhalation: AsthmaHaler, Medihaler-Epi), epinephrine (Inhalation: Bronkaid Mist, Primatene Mist)	*Cardiac arrest* ADULT: 1 to 10 ml of a 1:10,000 solution I.V. repeated at 5-minute intervals; 10 ml of 1:10,000 solution via endotracheal tube *Bronchospasm, hypersensitivity reactions, anaphylaxis* ADULT: 0.1 to 0.5 ml of a 1:1,000 solution S.C. or I.M., or 0.1 to 0.3 ml of 1:200 solution S.C.; one inhalation of a 1:100 solution, repeat once after at least 1 minute, if needed PEDIATRIC: 0.01 mg/kg or 0.3 mg/m^2 of a 1:1000 injection S.C. *Hemostasis* ADULT: 1:50,000 or 1:1,000 applied topically *Local anesthetic adjunct* ADULT: 1:200,000 to 1:20,000 mixed with local anesthetic *Spinal anesthetic* ADULT: 0.2 to 0.4 ml 1:1,000 added to anesthetic solution and administered intraspinally	• Epinephrine is contraindicated in a patient with narrow-angle glaucoma, shock, cardiac dilation, coronary insufficiency, organic brain syndrome, or cerebral arteriosclerosis. It also is contraindicated during general anesthesia with halogenated hydrocarbons or cyclopropane, local anesthesia of the fingers and toes, and labor. • This drug requires cautious use in a pregnant or geriatric patient or one with a cardiovascular disease, hypertension, diabetes, hyperthyroidism, psychoneurotic disorder, thyrotoxicosis, or bronchial asthma or emphysema accompanied by degenerative heart disease.
isoproterenol hydrochloride (Oral: Isuprel. Inhalation: Vapo-Iso), isoproterenol sulfate (Inhalation: Medihaler-Iso)	*Bronchospasm during anesthesia* ADULT: 0.01 to 0.02 mg I.V. of 1:50,000 solution in normal saline or D_5W *Shock* ADULT: 0.25 to 2.5 ml/minute (0.5 to 5 mcg/minute) I.V. of a 1:500,000 solution in D_5W *Cardiac arrest* ADULT: I.V. injection of 1 to 3 ml (0.0 to 0.06 mg) or 1:50,000 dilution, or I.V. infusion of 1.25 ml/minute (5 mcg/minute) of 1:250,000 solution or 1 ml (0.2 mg) undiluted I.M. or S.C.; for intracardiac administration, 0.1 ml (0.02 mg) of 1:5,000 solution *Heart block* ADULT: initially, 10 to 20 mg sublingually, with range of 5 to 50 mg, or initially 5 mg rectally, with 5 to 15 mg for maintenance *Bronchospasm* ADULT: 10 to 20 mg t.i.d. or q.i.d. sublingually or rectally up to 60 mg/day; or one to two inhalations four to six times a day	• Isoproterenol is contraindicated in a patient with tachyarrhythmia, tachycardia or heart block caused by digitalis intoxication, ventricular arrhythmias that require inotropic therapy, or angina pectoris. • This drug requires cautious use in a pregnant or breast-feeding patient or one with coronary artery disease, coronary insufficiency, diabetes, hyperthyroidism, or unusual sensitivity to sympathomimetic amines. • Appropriate dosages have not been established for children.

(continued)

Selected major adrenergic agents *(continued)*

DRUG	MAJOR INDICATIONS AND USUAL DOSAGES	CONTRAINDICATIONS AND PRECAUTIONS
Catecholamines *(continued)*		
norepinephrine, formerly levarterenol (Levophed)	*Acute hypotension, shock, cardiac arrest, myocardial infarction, anaphylaxis* ADULT: initially, 2 to 3 ml/minute I.V. of a 4-mg norepinephrine:1,000 ml D_5W solution (4 mg/1,000 ml); for maintenance, 0.5 to 1 ml/minute I.V.	• Norepinephrine is contraindicated in a patient with profound hypoxia, hypercarbia, concomitant use of cyclopropane or a halothane anesthetic, hypotension caused by blood volume deficit, or mesenteric or peripheral vascular thrombosis (except when administered as a lifesaving procedure). • This drug requires cautious use in a pregnant or breast-feeding patient or one who is receiving guanethidine, bretylium, a monoamine oxidase inhibitor, or a tricyclic antidepressant. • Safety and efficacy in children have not been established.
Noncatecholamines		
albuterol (Proventil, Ventolin)	*Bronchospasm* ADULT: one to two inhalations every 4 to 6 hours or 2 to 4 mg P.O. t.i.d. or q.i.d., up to a total daily dosage of 32 mg PEDIATRIC: for ages 6 to 12, 2 mg P.O. q.i.d.	• Albuterol is contraindicated in a patient with known hypersensitivity to the drug's components. • This drug requires cautious use in a pregnant or breast-feeding patient or one with a cardiovascular disorder, convulsive disorder, hyperthyroidism, diabetes mellitus, or unusual sensitivity to sympathomimetic amines. • Safety and efficacy in children under age 6 have not been established for regular tablets, inhalation aerosol, inhalation solution, and syrup.
metaproterenol sulfate (Alupent, Metaprel)	*Asthma, bronchitis, emphysema* ADULT: 20 mg P.O. t.i.d. or q.i.d.; 10 inhalations of 5% solution by hand-held nebulizer; 2 to 3 sprays by aerosol nebulizer every 3 to 4 hours up to 12 per day; or 2 inhalations from a metered-dose inhaler t.i.d. PEDIATRIC: for ages 6 to 9, or less than 60 lb (27 kg), 10 mg P.O. t.i.d. or q.i.d.	• Metaproterenol is contraindicated in a patient with known hypersensitivity to the drug or arrhythmias associated with tachycardia. • This drug requires cautious use in a pregnant or breast-feeding patient or one with a cardiovascular disorder, hyperthyroidism, diabetes mellitus, convulsive disorder, or unusual sensitivity to sympathomimetic amines. • Metaproterenol is not recommended for use in children under age 6.
ritodrine hydrochloride (Yutopar)	*Preterm labor* ADULT: initially, 0.5 mg/minute I.V. infusion, increased by 0.05 mg/minute every 10 minutes up to 0.35 mg/minute; continued for 12 hours after labor has ceased	• Ritodrine is contraindicated in a pregnant patient (before 20 weeks) or one with known hypersensitivity to the drug, a condition in which pregnancy continuation would be hazardous, eclampsia or severe preeclampsia, intrauterine fetal death, chorioamnionitis, maternal cardiac disease, pulmonary hypertension, maternal hyperthyroidism, uncontrolled maternal diabetes mellitus, or any maternal condition that would be adversely affected by a betamimetic drug.
terbutaline sulfate (Brethaire, Brethine, Bricanyl)	*Bronchial asthma, bronchitis, and emphysema* ADULT: 2.5 to 5 mg P.O. t.i.d.; 0.25 mg S.C., repeated in 15 to 30 minutes, if needed; two inhalations separated by 1 minute no more than every 6 hours PEDIATRIC: over age 12, 2.5 mg P.O. t.i.d. or q.i.d.	• Terbutaline requires cautious use in a breast-feeding patient or one with preterm labor (follow manufacturer's directions), cardiovascular disorder, hyperthyroidism, diabetes, history of seizures, or known hypersensitivity or unusual sensitivity to any of the drug's components or to sympathomimetic amines. • Safety and efficacy in children under age 12 have not been established.

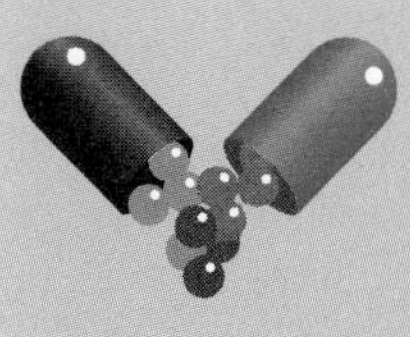

DRUG INTERACTIONS

Catecholamines

Drug interactions involving catecholamines can be among the most serious, causing hypotension, hypertension, cardiac arrhythmias, seizures, and hyperglycemia in diabetic patients. If catecholamines must be administered with other drugs, the patient must be monitored frequently. Note that all interactions may not occur between all catecholamines and the drugs listed.

DRUG	INTERACTING AGENTS	POSSIBLE EFFECTS	NURSING IMPLICATIONS
dobutamine, dopamine, epinephrine, isoproterenol, norepinephrine	alpha blockers (phentolamine)	Hypotension	• Administer with caution. • Monitor the patient's blood pressure.
	insulin, oral hypoglycemic agents	Hyperglycemia	• Monitor the patient's blood glucose level.
	beta blockers (propranolol)	Hypertension; bronchial constriction or asthma	• Monitor the patient's blood pressure.
	sympathomimetics	Additive effects (hypertension, cardiac arrhythmias); enhanced adverse effects	• Alternate drugs as prescribed, or monitor closely. • Monitor the patient's pulse rate and blood pressure.
	tricyclic antidepressants	Increased pressor effect	• Monitor the patient's blood pressure.

$Beta_1$-active drugs are used to treat bradycardia, heart block (as seen in Adams-Stokes disease and carotid sinus syndrome), and insufficient cardiac output. They also may be used to terminate paroxysmal atrial or nodal tachycardia. Because they are believed to make the heart more responsive to defibrillation, they are used in cases of ventricular fibrillation, asystole, or cardiac arrest.

Catecholamines that exert $beta_2$ activity are used to treat acute and chronic bronchial asthma, emphysema, bronchitis, and acute hypersensitivity reactions to drugs.

The dopaminergic stimulator, dopamine, is used in low doses to promote renal perfusion becuase it dilates the renal blood vessels.

The effects of drugs that are exogenously administered differ somewhat from the natural effects of endogenous catecholamines. Thus the patient's response also will differ somewhat from the normal physiologic response to endogenous catecholamines. The effects of catecholamines administered exogenously will be of short duration, which may limit their therapeutic usefulness.

Drug interactions

Knowledge of the interactions between catecholamines and other agents is essential because of the potential for additive effects, which might lead to a hypertensive crisis or cardiac arrhythmias. (See Drug Interactions: *Catecholamines.*)

ADVERSE DRUG REACTIONS

Because of the widespread actions of the catecholamines, adverse reactions affect the central nervous system (CNS), cardiovascular system, GI tract, skeletal and smooth muscles, and all other body systems. Although the reactions vary from drug to drug, the nurse must be aware of their possibility and must monitor and assess patients carefully when they are receiving catecholamine therapy.

Many CNS manifestations may be noted, including restlessness, nervousness, anxiety, fear, dizziness, vertigo, headache (throbbing to severe), and insomnia. Adverse cardiovascular reactions include pallor or flushing, palpitations, cardiac arrhythmias, tachycardia or slow and forceful heartbeat, hypotension or hypertension, cerebrovascular accident, and angina. Skeletal muscle adverse reactions may include weakness or mild tremors. The most common GI adverse reactions include nausea, vomiting (which may be severe), and diarrhea. Catecholamines can induce hyperglycemia, which may require insulin dosage adjustments in diabetic patients. They also may cause vasoconstriction, which can lead to hypertensive crisis.

With extravasation of intravenous (I.V.) catecholamines, necrosis can occur from local vasoconstriction. Tissue sloughing may follow. Injury to the area can be minimized by injecting phentolamine, an alpha-adrenergic anatagonist.

NURSING PROCESS APPLICATION

The following information assists the nurse in caring for a patient who is receiving a catecholamine. It includes an overview of assessment activities as well as examples of appropriate nursing diagnoses and related interventions (under "Planning and implementation"). It also highlights the importance of evaluation.

Proper preparation and administration of catecholamines

The nurse should remember these important points before administering any catecholamines.

Preparation

- Do not expose solutions to heat, light, or air; they may deteriorate rapidly.
- Do not use any solution that is yellow or amber-colored or that contains a precipitate.
- In patients dependent on catecholamines for blood pressure support, keep an additional bag of solution available.
- Use a syringe with calibrations small enough to ensure accurate dosage measurement.
- Always have an antidotal drug (phentolamine) on hand when administering I.V. dopamine or norepinephrine to manage extravasation.

Administration

- Always aspirate with the syringe before S.C. or I.M. injection to avoid systemic effects.
- For I.V. infusion, use a large vein (preferably a central line) when possible and rotate peripheral I.V. insertion sites to minimize the risk of necrosis from infiltration.
- Never administer catecholamines for hypotension through the proximal port of a pulmonary artery catheter being used for cardiac output measurement; the patient inadvertently might receive a bolus of the drug.
- Use an infusion control device to ensure accurate drug delivery and prevent overdose.
- With I.V. administration, gradually titrate the dose upward and monitor blood pressure and pulse rate every 3 to 5 minutes until they stabilize, then every 15 minutes.
- With all catecholamines, gradually decrease the infusion rate when weaning off the drug. Continue monitoring vital signs every 15 minutes to ensure circulatory stability.
- With I.V. administration, observe for cyanosis or pallor (signs of shock or excessive peripheral vasoconstriction).
- During drug infusion, continually monitor electrocardiogram, blood pressure, cardiac rate, cardiac rhythm and, when possible, cardiac output and pulmonary wedge pressure.
- Monitor for bradycardia; the rate of the infusion of alpha stimulants should be decreased as prescribed to return the heart rate to normal; atropine, isoproterenol, dopamine, or dobutamine may be ordered if necessary.
- With I.V. drugs, decrease or discontinue the drug as prescribed if the heart rate exceeds 120 beats/minute.
- Note that duration of I.V. drug action is brief, and the effects terminate shortly after discontinuation of I.V. infusion.
- Massage S.C. and I.M. injection sites to hasten absorption.
- Always dilute dopamine, dobutamine, isoproterenol, and norepinephrine as prescribed before I.V. administration.
- Do not give I.V. infusion of vasoconstrictors into leg veins, especially in geriatric patients, because of the possibility of occlusive vascular disease.
- With inhalant drugs, allow 1 to 5 minutes between inhalations to prevent systemic effects.
- Monitor urine output frequently to assess for renal perfusion and urine retention.
- To prevent systemic effects with inhalation drugs, use the minimum number of inhalations to relieve the symptoms.
- If I.V. dopamine or norepinephrine extravasates, stop the infusion immediately and infiltrate with 10 to 15 ml of normal saline solution containing 5 to 10 mg phentolamine as prescribed.
- Do not infuse concurrently in I.V. lines being used to administer blood products or heparin because of incompatibility.

Assessment

Before drug therapy begins, review the patient's history for conditions that contraindicate or require cautious use of the prescribed catecholamine. Also review the patient's medication history to identify use of drugs that may interact with it. During therapy, assess the patient for adverse drug reactions and signs of drug interactions. Also, periodically assess the effectiveness of therapy. Finally, evaluate the patient's and family's knowledge about the prescribed catecholamine.

Nursing diagnoses

- Risk for injury related to a preexisting condition that contraindicates or requires cautious use of a catecholamine
- Risk for injury related to adverse drug reactions or drug interactions
- Knowledge deficit related to the prescribed catecholamine

Planning and implementation

- Do not administer a catecholamine to a patient with a condition that contraindicates its use.
- Administer a catecholamine cautiously to a patient at risk because of a preexisting condition.

**** Have oxygen and emergency respiratory equipment readily available.***

- Correct hypovolemia, as prescribed, before catecholamine therapy begins.
- Check the prescription closely, particularly noting the solution concentration, dosage, and rate.
- Do not administer isoproterenol and inhaled epinephrine concurrently; space 4 hours apart.
- Monitor the patient for adverse reactions and drug interactions.
- Obtain blood glucose levels, as needed, for the diabetic patient.

**** Monitor the patient's respiratory rate when administering isoproterenol to detect rebound bronchospasm.***

- Prepare and administer the catecholamine carefully. (See *Proper preparation and administration of catecholamines.*)
- Notify the physician if adverse reactions or drug interactions occur.
- Teach the patient about the prescribed agent. (See Patient Teaching: *Catecholamines.*)

Evaluation

For each nursing diagnosis, prepare an evaluation statement that describes the patient's or family's response to nursing interventions.

Noncatecholamines

Noncatecholamine adrenergic drugs have a wide variety of therapeutic uses. This wide use is related to the many physiologic effects of these drugs, including local or systemic vasoconstriction (mephentermine sulfate, metaraminol bitartrate, methoxamine hydrochloride, phenylephrine hydrochloride), nasal and ophthalmic decongestion and bronchodilation (albuterol, ephedrine sulfate, isoetharine hydrochloride, isoetharine mesylate, metaproterenol sulfate, terbutaline sulfate), and smooth muscle relaxation (ritodrine hydrochloride, terbutaline sulfate). In this chapter, drugs are discussed in relation to their direct- or dual-acting mechanism of action and their adrenergic receptor activity (alpha, $beta_1$, or $beta_2$).

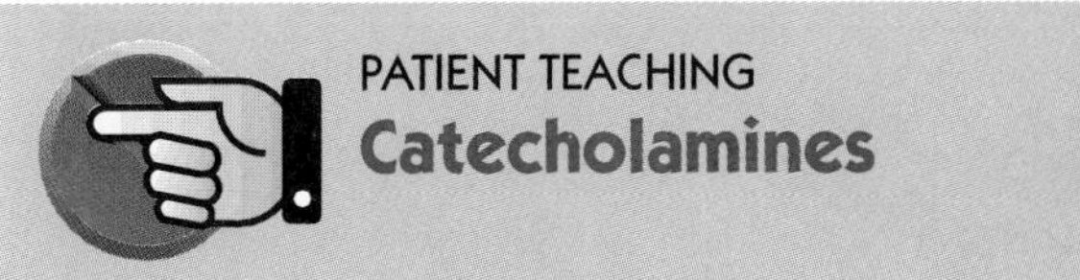

PATIENT TEACHING

Catecholamines

- Teach the patient and family the name, dose, frequency, action, and adverse effects of the prescribed catecholamine.
- Teach the family and patient how to take a pulse rate.
- Show the patient and family how to use inhalant devices correctly. Emphasize using the lowest number of inhalations possible.
- Teach the patient using an inhaler to rinse the mouth with water after administration to prevent dry mouth.
- Advise the patient using an intranasal drug that rebound congestion and hyperemia commonly occur with too frequent use of epinephrine.
- Advise the patient using an intranasal drug that it will sting, but that the discomfort will be temporary.
- Teach the diabetic patient to notify the physician if glucose test results change or if signs and symptoms of hyperglycemia occur.
- Tell the patient to notify the physician if adverse reactions occur.

PHARMACOKINETICS

Absorption of the noncatecholamines depends on the route of administration. Drugs administered by inhalation, such as albuterol, are absorbed gradually from the bronchi, causing lower systemic drug levels after the patient inhales recommended doses. Oral drugs are absorbed well from the GI tract and are distributed widely in the body fluids and tissues. Some drugs cross the blood-brain barrier (for example, ephedrine) and may be found in high concentrations in the brain and cerebrospinal fluid.

Metabolism and inactivation of the noncatecholamines occur primarily in the liver, where large concentrations of MAO are found, but also occur in the lungs, GI tract, and other tissues.

These drugs and their metabolites are excreted primarily in the urine. Some, such as inhaled albuterol, are excreted within 24 hours; others, such as oral albuterol, within 3 days. Of minor clinical importance, acidic urine increases excretion of many noncatecholamines; alkaline urine slows excretion.

Route	Onset	Peak	Duration
P.O.	10-120 min	1-8 hr	Variable
I.V.	1-60 min	30-60 min	Variable
I.M.	5-60 min	30-60 min	Variable
S.C.	5-60 min	30-60 min	Variable
Topical	5-60 min	30-60 min	Variable
Inhalation	1-30 min	5-15 min	Variable

PHARMACODYNAMICS

Noncatecholamines may be direct-acting, indirect-acting, or dual-acting (unlike catecholamines, which are primarily direct-acting). Direct-acting noncatecholamines achieve their effects by occupying receptor sites on organs and structures innervated by the CNS. Drugs that exhibit primarily alpha activity include methoxamine and phenylephrine; those that selectively exert $beta_2$ activity include albuterol, isoetharine, metaproterenol, ritodrine, and terbutaline.

Indirect-acting noncatecholamines exert their effects by stimulating norepinephrine release from its storage sites. Dual-acting noncatecholamines combine both actions; they include ephedrine, mephentermine, and metaraminol.

PHARMACOTHERAPEUTICS

Because noncatecholamines stimulate the SNS and produce varied physiologic effects, they are used widely. Many differences exist among the drugs, however, making general statements difficult. The various drugs are more or less effective depending on the route of administration, the dose, and the desired therapeutic effect and patient tolerance.

Drug interactions

Many drugs are known to interact with the noncatecholamines. Because interactions vary from drug to drug, the nurse should be aware of potentially serious interactions. (See Drug Interactions: *Noncatecholamines,* page 110.)

ADVERSE DRUG REACTIONS

Adverse reactions to noncatecholamines primarily affect the CNS, cardiovascular system, GI and genitourinary tracts, skeletal and smooth muscles, and all other body systems. The adverse effects of any noncatecholamine depend on its

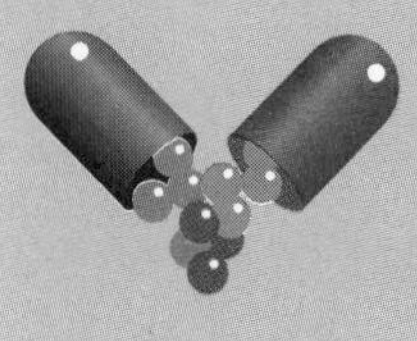

DRUG INTERACTIONS

Noncatecholamines

Noncatecholamines can produce significant reactions, including hypotension, hypertension, cardiac arrhythmias, seizures, and hyperglycemia in diabetic patients. If noncatecholamines must be administered with other drugs, the patient must be monitored frequently. Note that all interactions may not occur between all noncatecholamines and the drugs listed.

DRUG	INTERACTING AGENTS	POSSIBLE EFFECTS	NURSING IMPLICATIONS
albuterol, ephedrine, isoetharine, mephentermine, metaproterenol, metaraminol, methoxamine, phenylephrine, ritodrine, terbutaline	anesthetics (general), cyclopropane, and halogenated hydrocarbons	Arrhythmias from increased cardiac irritability; increased hypotension if used with agents having predominant $beta_2$ activity (ritodrine, terbutaline)	• Avoid administration, or administer with extreme caution, to patients scheduled for surgery if general anesthesia is to be used. • Monitor the patient's blood pressure.
	monoamine oxidase inhibitors	Severe hypertension from potentiation	• Avoid concurrent administration. • Monitor the patient's blood pressure.
	oxytocics	Reversal of oxytocic effects (terbutaline and ritodrine); hypertensive crisis; cerebrovascular accident	• Avoid concurrent use; maintain blood pressure under 130/80 mm Hg.
	tricyclic antidepressants	Increased pressor effects; hypertension; arrhythmias	• If administered concurrently, reduce adrenergic dosage as prescribed. • Monitor the patient's pulse rate and blood pressure.
	urine alkalinizers (acetazolamide, sodium bicarbonate)	Decreased excretion; prolonged action	• Monitor the patient for increased adverse reactions.

receptor activity. Other considerations include the intended therapeutic effect of the drug and whether the drug crosses the blood-brain barrier. For example, if ephedrine given for its bronchodilation effects interferes with sleep, the insomnia is considered an adverse reaction; however, if the drug is given to treat narcolepsy, the insomnia is the desired therapeutic effect. Although adverse reactions vary from drug to drug, the nurse must be aware of their potential and must monitor the patient appropriately.

In the CNS, adverse reactions to the noncatecholamines include headache, restlessness, nervousness, anxiety or euphoria, irritability, trembling, drowsiness or insomnia, lethargy, dizziness, light-headedness, incoherence, and seizures. Possible adverse cardiovascular reactions include hypertension or hypotension, palpitations, bradycardia or tachycardia, arrhythmias, cardiac arrest, cerebral hemorrhage, tingling or coldness in the extremities, pallor or flushing, anginal pain, and alterations in maternal and fetal heart rates and blood pressures. Geriatric patients are particularly susceptible to CNS reactions, such as confusion and anxiety, and to cardiovascular reactions, such as increased systolic blood pressure, coldness in the extremities, and anginal pain.

Skeletal muscle reactions may include weakness, mild tremors, or muscle cramps. Other possible adverse reactions include sweating, urinary urgency or incontinence, pilomotor stimulation, stinging and burning of the nasal mucosa or eyes, blurred vision, sneezing, dryness of the oropharynx, nausea, vomiting, unusual taste, erythema, and transient elevations in blood glucose level and increased insulin requirements in diabetic patients.

Prolonged use of certain noncatecholamines, such as metaraminol, may result in shock because continued vasoconstriction prevents volume expansion. Hypotension can occur after discontinuation of these drugs because of depletion of the intrinsic catecholamines in the storage granules of the nerve endings.

Although rare, overdose of nasal decongestants can cause marked somnolence, sedation, hypotension, bradycardia, and even coma. Methoxamine and other drugs can cause severe headache and sustained, severe hypertension. In rare instances, ephedrine and other agents may cause respiratory depression.

Confusion, delirium, hallucinations, or tremors may follow large doses of ephedrine. This drug also may produce paradoxical bronchospasm or aggravate ketoacidosis. Parotid gland enlargement is a rare result of metaproterenol administration. Care must be exercised with I.V. ritodrine and terbutaline because hypokalemia, lactic acidosis, chest pain, arrhythmias, dyspnea, bloating, chills, or anaphylactic shock may occur.

NURSING PROCESS APPLICATION

The following information assists the nurse in caring for a patient who is receiving a noncatecholamine. It includes an overview of assessment activities as well as examples of appropriate nursing diagnoses and related interventions (under "Planning and implementation"). It also highlights the importance of evaluation.

Assessment

Before drug therapy begins, review the patient's history for conditions that contraindicate or require cautious use of the prescribed noncatecholamine. Also review the patient's medication history to identify use of drugs that may interact with it. During therapy, assess the patient for adverse drug reactions and drug interactions. Also, periodically assess the effectiveness of drug therapy. Finally, evaluate the patient's and family's knowledge about the prescribed noncatecholamine.

Nursing diagnoses

• Risk for injury related to a preexisting condition that contraindicates or requires cautious use of a noncatecholamine
• Risk for injury related to adverse drug reactions or drug interactions
• Knowledge deficit related to the prescribed noncatecholamine

Planning and implementation

• Do not administer a noncatecholamine to a patient with a condition that contraindicates its use.
• Administer a noncatecholamine cautiously to a patient at risk because of a preexisting condition.
• Monitor vital signs, mental status, and muscle strength at least every 4 hours.
• Obtain electrolyte levels in all patients who are beginning therapy; obtain blood pH, $Paco_2$, and bicarbonate levels in patients who are receiving prolonged drug therapy, as prescribed.
• Monitor the serum potassium level to detect hypokalemia in a patient receiving prolonged infusion of ritodrine or terbutaline.
• Obtain the diabetic patient's serum glucose level, as prescribed, and observe for signs of hyperglycemia.
***** ***Monitor the patient for 12 hours after terbutaline is discontinued; cardiovascular symptoms may recur.***
• Monitor the patient for drug interactions.
• Administer an oral noncatecholamine with food to reduce GI symptoms unless otherwise indicated.
• Administer S.C. terbutaline in the lateral deltoid area.
***** ***Place the patient in a left lateral recumbent position to prevent hypotension during I.V. infusion of ritodrine or terbutaline.***
• Infuse I.V. ritodrine or terbutaline into a large vein to avoid extravasation. If extravasation occurs, inject the area within 12 hours with 10 to 15 ml of normal saline solution containing phentolamine (Regitine), as prescribed.

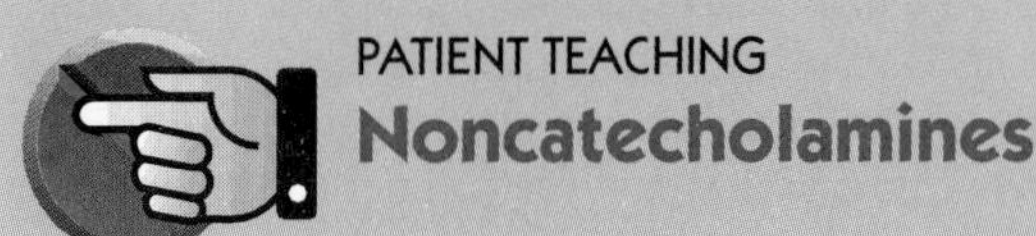

PATIENT TEACHING
Noncatecholamines

➤ Teach the patient and family the name, dose, frequency, action, and adverse effects of the prescribed noncatecholamine.
➤ Instruct the patient to initiate inhalation therapy before meals to improve lung ventilation and to reduce fatigue caused by eating.
➤ Teach the patient self-assessment techniques to determine the need for administration or repeat administration of the drug. For example, instruct the patient to assess for dyspnea, wheezing, and chest discomfort.
➤ Teach the patient the proper inhalation technique.
➤ Teach the patient to blow the nose gently, with both nostrils open to clear nasal passages before administering a nasal medication.
➤ Instruct the patient to avoid contact between the inhaled drug and the eyes.
➤ Advise the patient to rinse the mouth after inhalation to minimize dryness and irritation.
➤ Teach the patient to use no other aerosol bronchodilator during terbutaline inhalation therapy.
➤ Advise the patient of the prescribed interval between albuterol inhalations, which may vary from 1 to 10 minutes.
➤ Teach the patient to take the drug only as prescribed because of possible adverse reactions.
➤ Instruct the patient to protect these drugs from light, excessive heat or cold, and moisture and not to use discolored drugs.
➤ Teach the patient to notify the physician if symptoms are not relieved or if adverse reactions occur.

***** ***Discontinue ephedrine and notify the physician if wheezing or bronchospasm occurs after therapy.***
• Be aware that a patient may greatly exceed the prescribed dose because of tolerance and dependence.
• Notify the physician if adverse reactions or drug interactions occur.
• Teach the patient about the prescribed agent. (See Patient Teaching: *Noncatecholamines.*)

Evaluation

For each nursing diagnosis, prepare an evaluation statement that describes the patient's and family's response to nursing interventions.

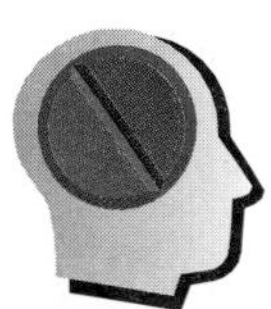

CRITICAL THINKING: To enhance your critical thinking about adrenergic agents, consider the following situation and its analysis.
Situation: Ralph Sawyer, age 61, has emphysema and is recovering from hernia repair. He awakens in the middle of the night, with wheezing and postoperative pain. Mr. Sawyer rates his pain as a 7 on a 1-to-10 scale. His respirations are 20, and his oxygen saturation is 91%. His medication orders include metaproterenol sulfate (Alupent) 2 to 3 inhalations q 3 to 4 hours, as need-

ed; oxygen 2 L via nasal cannula; morphine sulfate 2.5 mg I.V. q 4 hours, as needed for pain; and Tylenol with codeine No. 3 1 tab P.O. q 6 hours for pain. He received morphine 2.5 mg I.V. 6 hours earlier. Now he will not use the Alupent inhaler because of his postoperative pain. What should the nurse do?

Analysis: The nurse could administer a dose of morphine because this small dose will reduce pain quickly without suppressing respirations. (Tylenol with codeine, an oral drug, would take longer to work.) After 5 to 10 minutes, when the morphine has taken effect, the nurse may again urge Mr. Sawyer to use the Alupent inhaler. With pain relief, he may be more cooperative and able to deep breathe, cough, and use the incentive spirometer. Alupent should open his airway, decrease wheezing, and improve his oxygenation. The nurse also should monitor this patient's respiratory status closely.

Other adrenergic agents

This section contains information about cerebral stimulating agents, such as CNS stimulants and appetite suppressants. These drugs share many noncatecholamine characteristics.

A Schedule II drug, amphetamine sulfate may be used to treat narcolepsy, attention deficit hyperactivity disorder (ADHD), or exogenous obesity.

Bitolterol mesylate (Tornalate) is a long-acting bronchodilator similar to albuterol. It is used primarily to treat bronchial asthma.

A Schedule II drug, dextroamphetamine sulfate (Dexedrine, Spancap) is used to treat narcolepsy, exogenous obesity, and ADHD. Its CNS-stimulating effect is about twice that of amphetamine, and it sometimes is given with amphetamine in the combination product Biphetamine.

A Schedule IV drug, mazindol (Mazanor, Sanorex) is used only as a short-term adjunct in treating exogenous obesity.

A Schedule II drug, methylphenidate hydrochloride (Ritalin) is used to treat narcolepsy in adults and ADHD in children.

Pirbuterol acetate (Maxair) is indicated for the prevention and reversal of bronchospasm in patients with reversible bronchospasm, including asthma. It may be used with or without concurrent theophylline or steroid therapy.

Phenylpropanolamine hydrochloride (Acutrim, Dexatrim, Prolamine) directly stimulates alpha and beta receptors. It is used primarily in nasal decongestant products and sold over the counter in appetite-suppressing products as well as many cold and influenza preparations.

CHAPTER SUMMARY

Chapter 8 covered catecholamine and noncatecholamine adrenergic drugs. Here are the chapter highlights.

Adrenergic drugs produce biological responses similar to those produced by the SNS. The therapeutic use of these drugs depends on their receptor activity. Alpha activation produces primarily vasoconstrictive and smooth muscle contraction effects; $beta_1$ activation produces primarily cardiac stimulant effects; and $beta_2$ activation produces primarily smooth muscle relaxation as well as bronchodilatory and vasodilatory effects. Adverse reactions to adrenergic agents can involve all body systems.

Catecholamines may be endogenous or synthetic, but all catecholamines are ineffective when administered orally. Alpha-active drugs are used primarily to relieve hypotension. Beta-active drugs are used primarily to treat respiratory disorders and acute hypersensitivity reactions to drugs and for cardiac stimulation.

Noncatecholamines are active orally and generally have a longer duration of action than catecholamines. Noncatecholamines exert effects on sympathetic receptor sites through direct, indirect, or dual action. They primarily produce bronchodilation, vasopression, smooth muscle relaxation, and cardiac stimulation.

Other drugs that share noncatecholamine characteristics include cerebral stimulating agents, such as CNS stimulants and appetite suppressants.

When caring for a client who is receiving an adrenergic agent, the nurse should apply the nursing process. Care typically includes monitoring the patient for therapeutic and adverse effects based on the drug's indications, preparing and administering the drugs properly, and teaching the patient how to self-administer the drugs correctly.

Question to consider

See Appendix 1 for answers.

1. Dwayne Eberle, age 43, is undergoing excretory urography to determine the cause of acute pain in his left flank. Four minutes after the radiographic dye is injected, he develops shortness of breath and chest pain. One minute later, he begins to wheeze, and his eyes, lips, and tongue begin to swell. The radiologist administers epinephrine 0.5 ml of 1:1,000 solution S.C. Like the other catecholamines, epinephrine is not administered orally. Why not?
   (a) Catecholamines are destroyed by digestive enzymes.
   (b) Absorption after oral administration is delayed and unpredictable.
   (c) Normal intestinal flora block their absorption from the GI tract.
   (d) Catecholamines produce toxic effects when administered orally.

2. After back surgery, Jake Heller, age 62, develops oliguria. In addition to fluid replacement and diuretic therapy, he is to receive dopamine at 3 mcg/kg/min. Why?
   (a) It promotes renal perfusion.
   (b) It increases blood pressure.
   (c) It helps replace fluids.
   (d) It acts as a diuretic.

3. During surgery, Allen Winkler's blood pressure drops to 80/60 mm Hg. To maintain his blood pressure, the physician prescribes a dopamine drip 1 to 5 mcg/kg/minute. While receiving dopamine, Mr. Winkler complains of a headache. What may this symptom indicate?
   (a) Catecholamine toxicity
   (b) Catecholamine hypersensitivity
   (c) Inadequate catecholamine dosage
   (d) Adverse reaction to the catecholamine

4. When administering dobutamine, what does the nurse need to know?
   (a) Sedation is a major adverse effect.
   (b) The drug is used to treat hypertension.
   (c) The drug is given S.C. or I.M. only.
   (d) Tachycardia is major adverse effect.

5. JoEllen Marzani, age 24, takes the noncatecholamine albuterol (Ventolin) 2 mg q.i.d., for asthma. Which of the following statements best describes how catecholamines differ from noncatecholamines?
   (a) Catecholamines cross the blood-brain barrier; noncatecholamines do not.
   (b) Catecholamines are not effective when given orally; most noncatecholamines are.
   (c) Catecholamines stimulate alpha receptors; noncatecholamines stimulate beta receptors.
   (d) Catecholamines do not affect the heart; noncatecholamines affect the heart in many ways.

6. What makes albuterol effective in treating asthma?
   (a) It is a direct-acting $alpha_1$-selective agent.
   (b) It is a direct-acting $beta_2$-selective agent.
   (c) It is an indirect-acting $alpha_1$-selective agent.
   (d) It is an indirect-acting $beta_1$-selective agent.

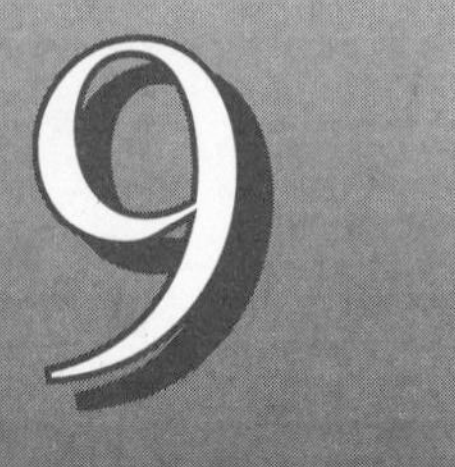

Adrenergic blocking agents

OBJECTIVES

After reading and studying this chapter, the student should be able to:
1. distinguish among alpha-adrenergic and beta-adrenergic blocking agents.
2. identify the major drugs in each class of adrenergic blocking agent.
3. describe the major physiologic effects and mechanisms of action of each class of adrenergic blocking agent.
4. discuss therapeutic uses for each class of adrenergic blocking agent.
5. identify the major drug interactions and adverse reactions for each class of adrenergic blocking agent.
6. describe how to apply the nursing process when caring for a patient who is receiving an adrenergic blocking agent.

INTRODUCTION

Adrenergic blocking agents, or **sympatholytics,** are used therapeutically to disrupt **sympathetic nervous system** (SNS) function. These agents may block impulse transmission (and thus SNS stimulation) at adrenergic **neurons** or adrenergic receptor sites. This action at these sites may be exerted by interrupting the action of **sympathomimetic** (adrenergic) agents, by reducing available norepinephrine, or by preventing the action of **cholinergic** agents.

Adrenergic blocking agents are classified according to their site of action as, respectively, alpha blockers, beta blockers, or autonomic ganglionic blockers. (Drugs in this class have recently been taken off the market). (See *Selected major adrenergic blocking agents.*)

Drugs covered in this chapter include:
- acebutolol
- atenolol
- betaxolol hydrochloride
- carteolol
- ergoloid mesylates
- ergotamine tartrate
- esmolol hydrochloride
- labetalol hydrochloride
- metoprolol tartrate
- nadolol
- phenoxybenzamine hydrochloride
- pindolol
- prazosin hydrochloride
- propranolol hydrochloride
- timolol maleate.

Alpha-adrenergic blockers

Alpha-adrenergic blocking agents interrupt the actions of sympathomimetic agents at **alpha-adrenergic receptors,** relaxing vascular smooth muscle, increasing peripheral vasodilation, and decreasing blood pressure. Drugs in this class include ergoloid mesylates, ergotamine tartrate, phenoxybenzamine hydrochloride, phentolamine mesylate, and prazosin hydrochloride. Ergotamine tartrate is a mixed alpha agonist and antagonist; at high doses, it acts as an alpha-adrenergic blocker.

PHARMACOKINETICS

The action of alpha-adrenergic blocking agents in the body is not well understood. Most of these agents are absorbed erratically when administered orally and more rapidly and completely when administered sublingually. The various alpha-adrenergic blocking agents vary considerably in their onset of action, peak concentration levels, and duration of action.

Route	Onset	Peak	Duration
P.O.	15-90 min	2-4 hr	7-24 hr
S.L.	Variable	Unknown	Unknown

PHARMACODYNAMICS

Alpha-adrenergic blockers exert two main pharmacologic actions: They interfere with or block the synthesis, storage, release, and reuptake of norepinephrine by neurons; and they competitively or noncompetitively antagonize epinephrine, norepinephrine, or sympathomimetic agents at alpha-receptor sites.

Alpha-receptor sites are categorized as $alpha_1$ or $alpha_2$. Pharmacologic classification does not recognize the specificity of alpha-receptor activity; the category of alpha-adrenergic blockers includes drugs that block the stimulation of $alpha_1$ receptors and that also may or may not block $alpha_2$ stimulation.

Alpha-adrenergic blockers occupy alpha-receptor sites on the vascular smooth muscle. (See *How alpha-adrenergic blockers affect peripheral blood vessels,* page 117.) This action prevents the excitatory response to sympathetic stimulation or sympathomimetic agents. In most patients, this action

Selected major adrenergic blocking agents

This table summarizes the major adrenergic blocking agents currently in clinical use.

DRUG	MAJOR INDICATIONS AND USUAL DOSAGES	CONTRAINDICATIONS AND PRECAUTIONS
Alpha-adrenergic blockers		
ergotamine tartrate (Ergomar, Ergostat)	*Vascular headaches* ADULT: 2 mg P.O. or sublingually at onset of attack, then 2 mg every 30 minutes until resolution occurs, with maximum dosage of 6 mg per attack or 10 mg per week	• Ergotamine is contraindicated in a pregnant patient or one with known hypersensitivity, peripheral vascular disease, coronary heart disease, hypertension, impaired hepatic or renal function, severe pruritus, or sepsis. • This drug requires cautious use in a breast-feeding patient. • Safety and efficacy in children have not been established.
phentolamine mesylate (Regitine)	*Hypertension associated with pheochromocytoma* ADULT: 5 mg I.M. or I.V. before surgery, 5 mg I.V., if needed, during surgery PEDIATRIC: 1 mg I.M. or I.V. 1 to 2 hours before surgery and repeated if needed; 1 mg I.V., if needed during surgery *Necrosis prevention* ADULT: 5 to 10 mg in 10 ml normal saline solution injected into the area of extravasation, within 12 hours of the extravasation	• Phentolamine is contraindicated in a breast-feeding patient or one with known hypersensitivity to the drug or related compounds, myocardial infarction (MI), history of MI, coronary insufficiency, angina, or other signs of coronary artery disease. • This drug requires cautious use in a pregnant patient or one with peptic or gastric ulcers.
Beta-adrenergic blockers		
atenolol (Tenormin)	*Hypertension or prophylactic management of stable angina pectoris* ADULT: initially, 50 mg P.O. once a day; increased to 100 mg once a day, if necessary, after 1 to 2 weeks; reduced to 50 mg on alternate days for patients with renal failure *Acute MI* ADULT: 5 mg I.V. over 5 minutes, followed by 5 mg I.V. 10 minutes later, then 50 mg P.O. 10 minutes later, followed by 50 mg P.O. 12 hours later, then 100 mg P.O. daily or 50 mg P.O. b.i.d. for 6 to 9 days	• Atenolol is contraindicated in a patient with sinus bradycardia, heart block greater than first degree, hypotension, shock, or overt cardiac failure. • This drug requires cautious use in a pregnant or breast-feeding patient or one with heart failure controlled by a digitalis glycoside or diuretics, bronchospastic disease, diabetes, hypoglycemia, hyperthyroidism, or impaired renal function. • Safety and efficacy in children have not been established.
metoprolol tartrate (Lopressor)	*Hypertension or prophylactic management of stable angina pectoris* ADULT: initially, 100 mg/day P.O. in single or divided doses, increased weekly as needed (usual range is 100 to 450 mg/day for hypertension or 100 to 400 mg/day for angina) *Acute MI* ADULT: 5 mg I.V., 2 minutes apart, for three doses; then 50 mg P.O. every 6 hours for 48 hours, then 100 mg P.O. every 12 hours	• Metoprolol is contraindicated in a patient with sinus bradycardia, heart block greater than first degree, cardiogenic shock, or overt cardiac failure. • This drug requires cautious use in a pregnant or breast-feeding patient or one with heart failure controlled by a digitalis glycoside or diuretics, bronchospastic disease, diabetes, hypoglycemia, hyperthyroidism, or impaired hepatic function. • Safety and efficacy in children have not been established.
nadolol (Corgard)	*Hypertension* ADULT: initially, 40 mg/day P.O., increased gradually in 40- to 80-mg doses to a maximum of 640 mg/day as needed *Angina* ADULT: initially, 40 mg P.O. once a day, increased every 3 to 7 days as needed (usual range is 80 to 240 mg once a day)	• Nadolol is contraindicated in a breast-feeding patient or one with bronchial asthma, sinus bradycardia and greater than first-degree block, cardiogenic shock, or overt cardiac failure. • This drug requires cautious use in a pregnant patient or one with a history of cardiac failure, nonallergic bronchospasm, diabetes, hypoglycemia, hyperthyroidism, or impaired renal function. • Safety and efficacy in children have not been established.

(continued)

Selected major adrenergic blocking agents *(continued)*

DRUG	MAJOR INDICATIONS AND USUAL DOSAGES	CONTRAINDICATIONS AND PRECAUTIONS
Beta-adrenergic blockers *(continued)*		
propranolol hydrochloride (Inderal)	*Hypertension* ADULT: initially, 40 mg P.O. b.i.d., increased as needed to a maximum of 640 mg/day PEDIATRIC: 1 mg/kg/day given in two equally divided doses and adjusted as needed *Essential tremor* ADULT: initially, 40 mg P.O. b.i.d., increased as needed to a maximum of 320 mg/day *Pheochromocytoma* ADULT: 60 mg P.O. daily in divided doses for 3 days before surgery *Angina* ADULT: initially, 10 to 20 mg P.O. t.i.d. or q.i.d., increased every 3 to 7 days as needed to a maximum of 320 mg/day *Arrhythmias* ADULT: 10 to 30 mg P.O. t.i.d. or q.i.d.; in emergencies, 1 to 3 mg I.V. push (1 mg/ minute) repeated in 2 to 3 minutes, as needed PEDIATRIC: 1.5 to 2 mg/kg P.O. daily and adjusted as needed; maximum dosage of 16 mg/kg/day given in four divided doses *Hypertrophic subaortic stenosis* ADULT: 20 to 40 mg P.O. t.i.d. or q.i.d., or 80 to 160 mg of sustained-release capsules once a day *Acute MI* ADULT: 180 to 240 mg P.O. daily in three or four divided doses to a maximum of 240 mg/ day *Migraine headache (prophylaxis)* ADULT: 80 mg P.O. daily in divided doses, increased as needed	• Propranolol is contraindicated in a patient with cardiogenic shock, sinus bradycardia and greater than first-degree block, malignant hypertension, Raynaud's disease, bronchial asthma, or heart failure (unless the failure is caused by a tachyarrhythmia that can be treated with the drug). • This drug requires a cautious use in a pregnant or breast-feeding patient or one with a history of cardiac failure, nonallergic bronchospasm, diabetes, hypoglycemia, hyperthyroidism, or impaired hepatic or renal function. • I.V. administration of Inderal is not recommended in children.

produces vasodilation, which increases local blood flow to the skin and other organs. The decreased peripheral vascular resistance decreases blood pressure.

The degree of therapeutic effect depends on the sympathetic tone before drug administration. Only a small change in blood pressure is produced with the patient in a supine position; however, orthostatic hypotension develops when the patient shifts to a standing position because the ability of the SNS to prevent peripheral blood pooling is blocked.

PHARMACOTHERAPEUTICS

Therapeutic use of alpha-adrenergic blockers is based on their smooth muscle relaxation and vasodilation and the resultant increased local blood flow to skin and other organs and decreased blood pressure from decreased peripheral vascular resistance. Conditions in which these effects prove beneficial include hypertension, peripheral vascular disorders, and pheochromocytoma.

Certain peripheral vascular disorders — mainly those with a vasospastic component causing poor local blood flow, such as Raynaud's disease (intermittent pallor, cyanosis, or redness of fingers), acrocyanosis (symmetrical mottled cyanosis of the hands and feet), and aftereffects of frostbite — respond well to alpha-adrenergic therapy.

Drug interactions

Many agents interact synergistically with alpha-adrenergic blocking agents and can potentiate or cause mutually additive effects, often with serious sequelae. The most serious include severe hypotension or vascular collapse. (See Drug Interactions: *Alpha-adrenergic blockers,* page 118.)

ADVERSE DRUG REACTIONS

Adverse reactions caused by blockade of alpha receptors are related primarily to the vasodilation effect of the drugs. However, because of the varied mechanisms of action of the

How alpha-adrenergic blockers affect peripheral blood vessels

By occupying alpha-receptor sites, the alpha-adrenergic blockers cause vessel muscle-wall relaxation, vasodilation, and reduced peripheral vascular resistance. These effects can cause orthostatic hypotension when the patient changes position from supine to standing because of altered blood flow redistribution.

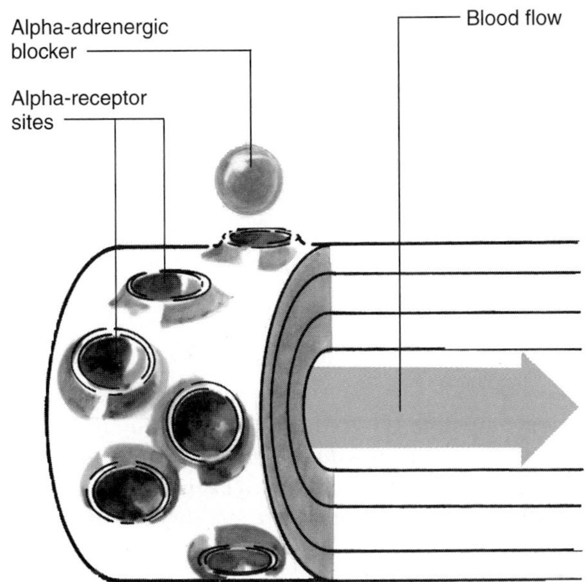

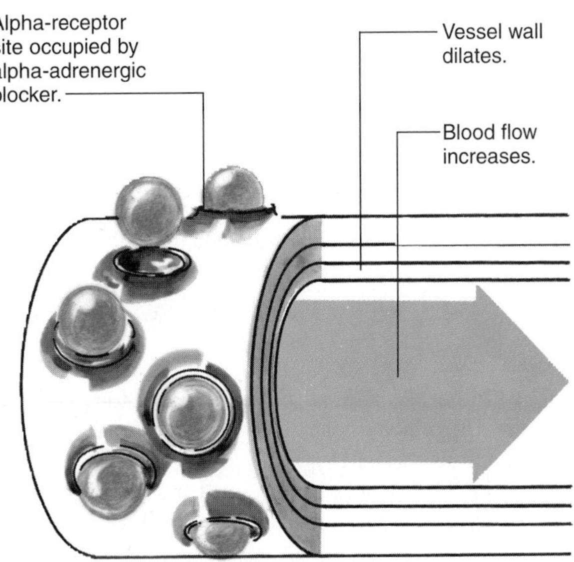

alpha-adrenergic blocking agents, many adverse reactions are possible with these drugs.

Reactions may include such cardiovascular manifestations as orthostatic hypotension or severe hypertensive episodes, bradycardia or tachycardia, edema, dyspnea, lightheadedness, flushing, arrhythmias, angina, myocardial infarction (MI), cerebrovascular spasm, or a shocklike state. With long-acting noncompetitive alpha-adrenergic blockers, such as phenoxybenzamine, the beta-adrenergic receptors are left unopposed, possibly leading to an exaggerated hypotensive response and tachycardia.

Central nervous system (CNS) manifestations may include paresthesia, tingling of extremities, muscle weakness, fatigue, nervousness, depression, insomnia, drowsiness, lethargy, sedation, vertigo, syncope, confusion, headache, or CNS stimulation.

The nurse also may note eye, ear, nose, and throat manifestations, such as nasal stuffiness, blurred vision, increased nasopharyngeal secretions, epistaxis, miosis (pinpoint pupil), conjunctival infection, reddened sclera, ptosis (drooping of the eyelids), tinnitus, or dry mouth.

Gastrointestinal (GI) manifestations are common and may consist of sublingual irritation, nausea, vomiting, heartburn, diarrhea, abdominal pain, or exacerbation of peptic ulcer.

Genitourinary reactions may include urinary frequency, impotence, incontinence, or priapism.

Hematologic manifestations are rare; however, granulocytopenia, leukopenia, thrombocytopenia, and pancytopenia have been reported with some agents.

Various dermatologic manifestations may occur, including rash, allergic dermatitis, pruritus, alopecia, or lichen planus. Other adverse reactions reported are allergic phenomena, including shock, diaphoresis, and arthralgia. Increased serum uric acid and blood urea nitrogen levels also may occur.

NURSING PROCESS APPLICATION

The following information assists the nurse in caring for a patient who is receiving an alpha-adrenergic blocker. It includes an overview of assessment activities as well as examples of appropriate nursing diagnoses and related interventions (under "Planning and implementation"). It also highlights the importance of evaluation.

Assessment

Before drug therapy begins, review the patient's history for conditions that contraindicate or require cautious use of the prescribed alpha-adrenergic blocker. Also review the patient's medication history to identify use of drugs that may

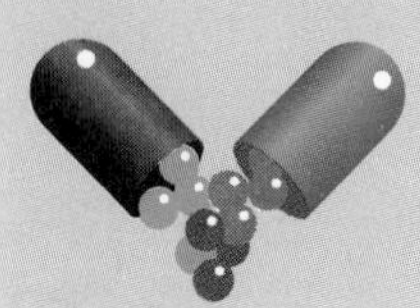

DRUG INTERACTIONS

Alpha-adrenergic blockers

Drug interactions involving alpha-adrenergic blocking agents primarily affect the cardiovascular system and may include profound hypotension or vascular collapse, hypertension, and cardiac arrhythmias.

DRUG	INTERACTING AGENTS	POSSIBLE EFFECTS	NURSING IMPLICATIONS
ergoloid mesylates, ergotamine	caffeine, macrolides	Increased ergotamine effect	• Monitor the patient for an increased therapeutic effect.
	dopamine	Increased pressor effects	• Monitor the patient's blood pressure frequently.
	nitroglycerin	Hypotension caused by excessive vasodilation	• Monitor the patient's blood pressure frequently.
	sympathomimetics, including many over-the-counter medications	Enhanced cardiac stimulation; hypotension with rebound hypertension	• Monitor the patient's blood pressure and heart rate frequently.

interact with this agent. During therapy, assess the patient for adverse drug reactions, such as impotence, and signs of drug interactions. Also, periodically assess the effectiveness of therapy. Finally, evaluate the patient's and family's knowledge about the prescribed alpha-adrenergic blocker.

Nursing diagnoses

- Risk for injury related to a preexisting condition that contraindicates or requires cautious use of an alpha-adrenergic blocker
- Risk for injury related to adverse drug reactions or drug interactions
- Sexual dysfunction related to impotence caused by the alpha-adrenergic blocker
- Knowledge deficit related to the prescribed alpha-adrenergic blocker

Planning and implementation

- Do not administer an alpha-adrenergic blocker to a patient with a condition that contraindicates its use.
- Administer an alpha-adrenergic blocker cautiously to a patient at risk because of a preexisting condition.
- Monitor the patient for adverse reactions and signs of drug interactions.
- Measure the patient's vital signs frequently, noting a change in blood pressure from the supine to standing position. Auscultate breath sounds frequently during therapy with an alpha-adrenergic blocker.
- Take safety measures if the patient develops light-headedness, weakness, or changes in mental status. For example, raise the side rails and assist with ambulation, as appropriate.

*** *Notify the physician immediately if the patient develops chest pain. Obtain an electrocardiogram and treat the patient as prescribed.***

*** *Place the patient in the Trendelenburg position if a shocklike state occurs (and if not contraindicated). Also, notify the physician immediately and begin emergency interventions according to health care facility guidelines.***

- Administer oral drugs with food or milk to reduce GI distress.
- Notify the physician if the patient displays adverse reactions or drug interactions.
- Encourage the patient to report impotence; notify the physician if it occurs. (See Patient Teaching: *Alpha-adrenergic blockers.*)
- Offer to arrange for sexual counseling for the patient and partner if the alpha-adrenergic agent cannot be replaced with another agent that does not cause impotence.

Evaluation

For each nursing diagnosis, prepare an evaluation statement that describes the patient's or family's response to nursing interventions.

Beta-adrenergic blockers

Beta-adrenergic blocking agents, the most widely used adrenergic blockers, prevent SNS stimulation by inhibiting the action of **catecholamines** and other sympathomimetic agents at **beta-adrenergic receptors.**

Many beta-adrenergic blocking agents (including carteolol, labetalol hydrochloride, nadolol, propranolol hydrochloride, and timolol maleate) are nonselective in their blocking action, affecting $beta_1$-receptor sites (located mainly in the heart) and $beta_2$-receptor sites (located in bronchi, blood vessels, and the uterus). The beta-adrenergic blocking agents acebutolol, atenolol, betaxolol hydrochloride, esmolol hydrochloride, and metoprolol tartrate are se-

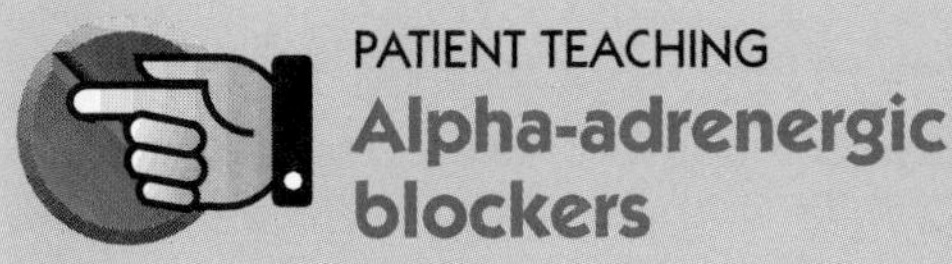

PATIENT TEACHING
Alpha-adrenergic blockers

- Teach the patient and family the name, dose, frequency, action, and adverse effects of the prescribed alpha-adrenergic blocker.
- Teach the patient to minimize orthostatic hypotension by rising slowly from a supine position and by dangling the feet for a few minutes before standing.
- Instruct the patient to assume a head-low position or to lie down if light-headedness, faintness, or weakness occurs.
- Advise the patient not to exceed the prescribed dosage. Explain that adverse reactions can result from higher dosages.
- Teach the patient to avoid alcohol consumption. Explain that alcohol used with alpha-adrenergic blocking agents may cause hypotension.
- Instruct the patient to avoid over-the-counter cough, cold, allergy, or weight-loss medications that contain alcohol or caffeine unless they have been approved by the physician.
- Advise the patient to store medications in a light-resistant, airtight container.
- Instruct the patient to notify the physician if adverse reactions occur.

lective: they primarily affect $beta_1$-receptor sites. Some beta-adrenergic blockers also exhibit a pharmacologic property known as intrinsic sympathetic activity (ISA). Drugs that exhibit ISA, such as pindolol and acebutolol, sometimes are classified as partial agonists.

PHARMACOKINETICS

Beta-adrenergic blockers usually are absorbed rapidly and well from the GI tract and are protein-bound to some extent. Food does not inhibit their absorption and may enhance absorption of some agents. Some beta-adrenergic blockers are absorbed more completely than others.

Beta-adrenergic blockers are distributed widely in body tissues, with the highest concentrations found in the heart, liver, lungs, and saliva.

With the exception of nadolol and atenolol, beta-adrenergic blockers are metabolized to some extent in the liver. Excretion is primarily in the urine, as metabolites or in unchanged form, with some excretion also occurring in feces and bile, and some secretion in breast milk.

The onset of action of beta-adrenergic blockers is primarily dose- and drug-dependent; peak concentration levels are route-dependent.

Route	Onset	Peak	Duration
P.O.	15-30 min	1-2 hr	4-24 hr
I.V.	1-5 min	20 min	5 min-8 hr

PHARMACODYNAMICS

Beta-adrenergic blocking agents produce a competitive blocking action not only at adrenergic nerve endings but also in the adrenal medulla; that accounts for their widespread effects. Some researchers speculate that certain beta-adrenergic blockers, such as metoprolol and propranolol, produce CNS activity, with effects exerted at the vasomotor center in the brain stem to reduce tonic sympathetic nerve impulse transmission. These agents can reduce or block myocardial stimulation, vasodilation, bronchodilation, glycogenolysis (production of glucose from glycogen), and lipolysis (fat hydrolysis). The effects of this blockade include increased peripheral vascular resistance, decreased systemic blood pressure, decreased contractile force, decreased myocardial oxygen consumption, slowed atrioventricular (AV) conduction, and decreased cardiac output. Pulmonary manifestations include increased bronchial smooth muscle tone; metabolic manifestations include inhibition of the sympathetic response to hypoglycemia. CNS manifestations include weakness, lethargy, and fatigue. Other manifestations include decreased plasma renin activity (particularly in patients with high levels before beta-adrenergic blocker therapy) and decreased production of aqueous humor in the eye, not accompanied by miosis or hyperemia (increased blood).

Some physiologic manifestations of the various beta-adrenergic blocking agents are related to the drugs' classification as selective or nonselective. Selective beta-adrenergic blockers, which preferentially block $beta_1$-receptor sites, produce effects primarily related to prevention of cardiac excitation. Nonselective beta-adrenergic blockers, which block $beta_1$- and $beta_2$-receptor sites, prevent not only cardiac excitement but also bronchiolar dilation. For instance, nonselective beta-adrenergic blockers can cause bronchospasm in patients with chronic obstructive lung disorders, but this adverse effect largely is eliminated with the use of selective drugs, which have minimal $beta_2$ activity at certain doses.

PHARMACOTHERAPEUTICS

Beta-adrenergic blockers are used to treat many conditions and are under investigation for use in many more. As mentioned earlier, their clinical usefulness is based largely (but not exclusively) on their cardiovascular effects. (See *Major effects of beta-adrenergic blockers,* page 120.) Cardiovascular indications for beta-adrenergic blockers include hypertension, angina pectoris, prevention of reinfarction after MI, supraventricular arrhythmias, and hypertrophic cardiomyopathy. Other uses include the treatment of migraine headaches, anxiety, wide-angle glaucoma, pheochromocytoma, and the cardiovascular symptoms associated with thyrotoxicosis.

Drug interactions

Many agents can interact synergistically with beta-adrenergic blocking agents to cause potentially dangerous effects,

Major effects of beta-adrenergic blockers

By blocking the action of endogenous catecholamines and other sympathomimetic agents at beta-receptor sites, beta-adrenergic blockers counteract the stimulating effects of these agents. The illustration below shows the effects of beta-adrenergic blockers on the pulmonary and cardiovascular systems.

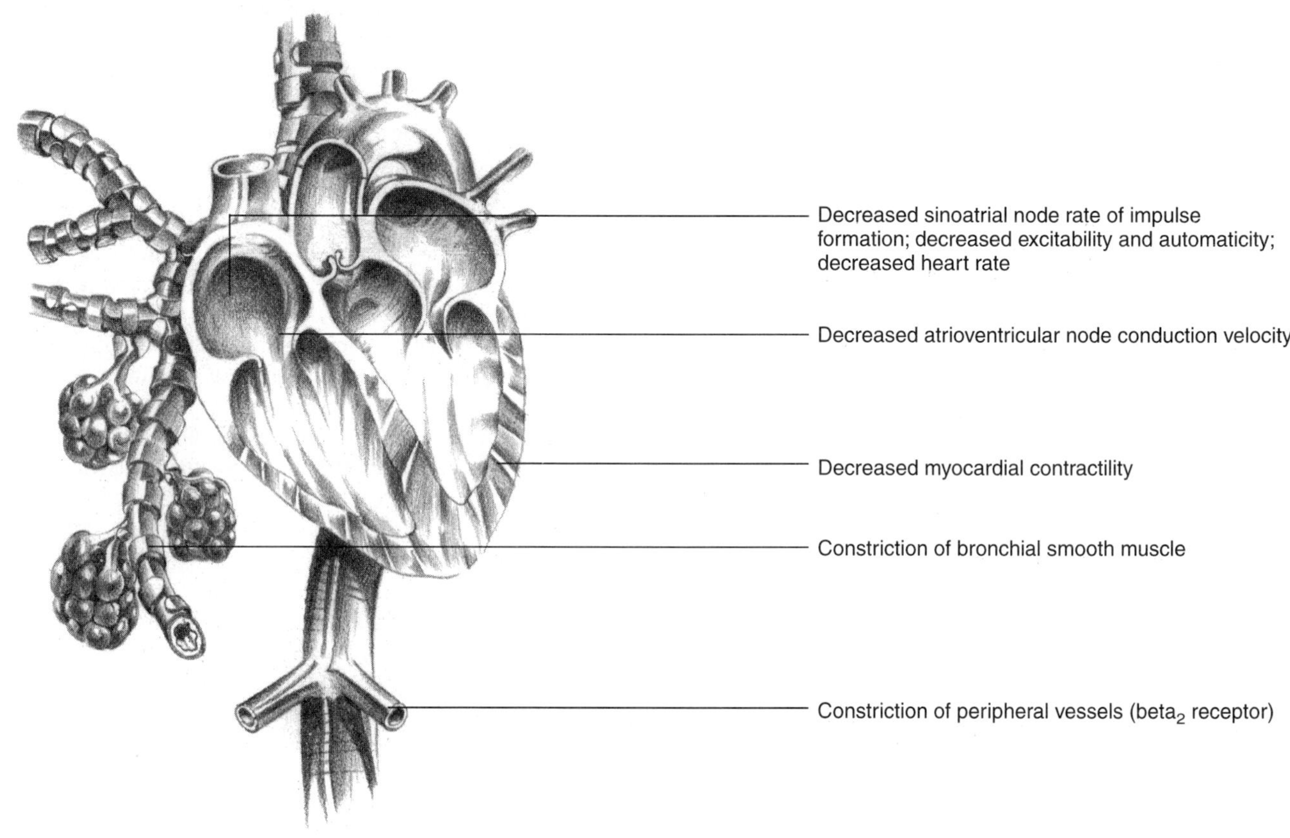

by potentiating or creating additive effects of one or both drugs or by inhibiting the desired effects of the drugs. Some of the most serious potential effects include cardiac depression, arrhythmias, respiratory depression, severe bronchospasm, and severe hypotension that could lead to vascular collapse. (See Drug Interactions: *Beta-adrenergic blockers.*)

ADVERSE DRUG REACTIONS

Generally, beta-adrenergic blockers cause few adverse reactions. Most that do occur are drug- or dose-dependent. Adverse reactions occur most often from intravenous (I.V.) rather than oral administration and in geriatric patients and those with impaired renal or hepatic function.

Beta-adrenergic blocker toxicity is marked primarily by arrhythmias, orthostatic hypotension, CNS disturbances, and GI or respiratory distress. Cardiovascular reactions include hypotension, bradycardia, peripheral vascular insufficiency (Raynaud's disease), AV block, and heart failure. Geriatric patients are especially likely to experience peripheral vascular insufficiency and heart failure.

The most common respiratory reaction is bronchospasm. Although selective agents are less likely than nonselective agents to cause bronchospasm, caution is nevertheless advisable when administering all beta-adrenergic blockers, particularly to patients with bronchial asthma, bronchitis, or emphysema. GI manifestations commonly include diarrhea, nausea, vomiting, constipation, abdominal discomfort, anorexia, and flatulence.

CNS effects may include dizziness, insomnia, fatigue, weakness, lethargy, disorientation, memory loss, visual disturbances, sedation, hallucinations, or behavioral changes. Geriatric patients, in particular, are at increased risk for CNS effects, such as cognitive impairment and depression.

Hematologic adverse reactions, also rare, include decreased platelet agglutination, granulocytopenia, and thrombocytopenic purpura. Other reported adverse reactions include headache, impotence or decreased libido, nasal stuffiness, diaphoresis, tinnitus, and dry mouth, eyes, and skin.

Adverse reactions indicating an allergic response include rash, fever with sore throat, laryngospasm, and possibly respiratory distress. Although most patients tolerate beta-

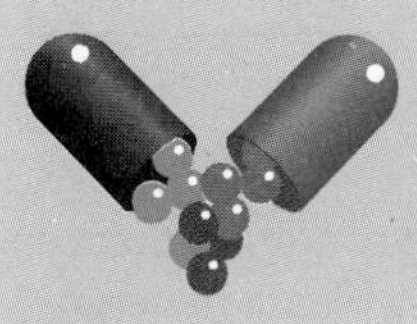

DRUG INTERACTIONS

Beta-adrenergic blockers

Drug interactions involving beta-adrenergic blockers primarily affect the cardiovascular and respiratory systems.

DRUG	INTERACTING AGENTS	POSSIBLE EFFECTS	NURSING IMPLICATIONS
acebutolol, atenolol, labetalol, metoprolol, nadolol, pindolol, propranolol, timolol	antacids, calcium salts, cholestyramine, penicillin	Delayed drug absorption from GI tract	• Administer several hours apart. • Monitor the patient for a decreased therapeutic effect.
	lidocaine	Increased plasma levels of lidocaine (potential toxicity); additive cardiac depressant effects	• Monitor the patient for signs of lidocaine toxicity, such as confusion, restlessness, and tremors.
	insulin and oral hypoglycemic agents	Hypoglycemia or hyperglycemia; masking of tachycardia as a sign of hypoglycemia (diaphoresis and agitation still present)	• Administer these drugs cautiously. • Monitor the diabetic patient's blood glucose levels frequently.
	anti-inflammatories (indomethacin, salicylates)	Decreased hypotensive effects of beta-adrenergic blockers	• Monitor the patient for altered beta-adrenergic blocker effects.
	barbiturates	Increased rate of metabolism of beta-adrenergic blockers that are metabolized extensively	• Monitor the patient for altered response to beta-adrenergic blockers that are metabolized by the liver (propranolol, metoprolol).
	cardiac glycosides	Additive bradycardia and depression of atrioventricular conduction	• Monitor the patient's blood pressure and heart rate frequently.
	calcium channel blockers (primarily verapamil)	Increased pharmacologic and toxicologic effects of both agents	• Monitor the patient for adverse reactions.
	sympathomimetics (albuterol, dobutamine, dopamine, epinephrine, isoproterenol, metaproterenol, ritodrine, terbutaline)	Hypertension and reflex bradycardia from unopposed alpha effects (vasoconstriction) and increased vagal tone	• Monitor the patient's blood pressure and heart rate frequently.
	cimetidine	Reduced metabolism of beta-adrenergic blockers; enhanced ability of beta-adrenergic blockers to reduce pulse rate	• Monitor the patient for altered response to the beta-adrenergic blocker.
	rifampin	Inhibited therapeutic response to metoprolol and propranolol	• Monitor the patient for altered response to the beta-adrenergic blocker.
	theophyllines	Impaired bronchodilating effects of theophyllines by nonselective beta-adrenergic blockers	• Monitor the patient's therapeutic response.
	clonidine	Unopposed alpha effects when clonidine is discontinued, leading to a life-threatening increase in blood pressure	• Monitor the patient's blood pressure closely.
labetalol	halothane anesthetics	Increased hypotension	• Monitor the patient's blood pressure closely.

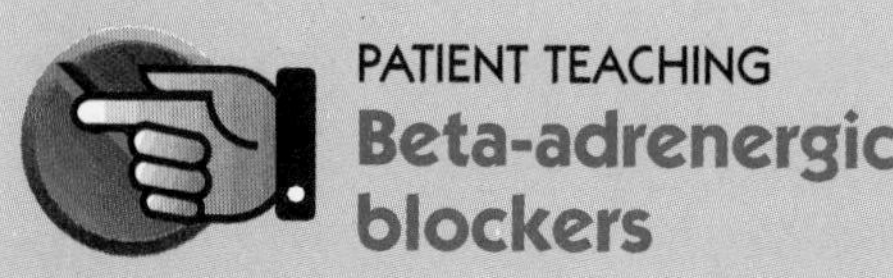

PATIENT TEACHING
Beta-adrenergic blockers

- ➤ Teach the patient and family the name, dose, frequency, action, and adverse effects of the prescribed beta-adrenergic blocker.
- ➤ Advise the patient not to stop taking the drug abruptly or alter the prescribed dosage, unless ordered. Explain that abrupt withdrawal can cause myocardial infarction, arrhythmias, or other serious complications.
- ➤ Teach the patient to measure the pulse rate and report slowing or irregularity to the physician.
- ➤ Teach the patient to minimize the effects of orthostatic hypotension by changing position slowly, especially supine to upright, and by dangling the legs over the bedside for a few minutes before standing.
- ➤ Instruct the patient to sit or lie down immediately if dizziness or faintness occurs.
- ➤ Advise the patient not to drive or operate machinery until after adjusting to the drug's central nervous system effects.
- ➤ Advise the patient receiving metoprolol that the drug may take up to 1 week to produce optimal effects; if the drug produces insomnia, the patient should avoid late-evening doses.
- ➤ Teach the patient with impaired renal function to report a weight gain of 3 to 4 lb (1.4 to 1.8 kg) per day, cough, orthopnea, fatigue, tachycardia, dyspnea on exertion, edema, or anxiety.
- ➤ Teach the patient to store the beta-adrenergic blocker at room temperature and to protect it from moisture, light, and air.
- ➤ Tell the patient and family to notify the physician of any adverse drug reactions.

adrenergic blockers fairly well, patients with various preexisting chronic conditions are at special risk for adverse reactions to beta-adrenergic blocker therapy.

NURSING PROCESS APPLICATION

The following information assists the nurse in caring for a patient who is receiving a beta-adrenergic blocker. It includes an overview of assessment activities as well as examples of appropriate nursing diagnoses and related interventions (under "Planning and implementation"). It also highlights the importance of evaluation.

Assessment

Before drug therapy begins, review the patient's history for conditions that contraindicate or require cautious use of the prescribed beta-adrenergic blocker. Also review the patient's medication history to identify use of drugs that may interact with the agent. During therapy, assess the patient for adverse drug reactions and signs of drug interactions. Also, periodically assess the effectiveness of therapy. Finally, evaluate the patient's and family's knowledge about the prescribed beta-adrenergic blocker.

Nursing diagnoses

- Risk for injury related to a preexisting condition that contraindicates or requires cautious use of a beta-adrenergic blocker
- Risk for injury related to adverse drug reactions or drug interactions
- Altered cardiopulmonary tissue perfusion related to drug interaction between the beta-adrenergic blocker and another prescribed drug
- Knowledge deficit related to the prescribed beta-adrenergic blocker

Planning and implementation

- Do not administer a beta-adrenergic blocker to a patient with a condition that contraindicates its use.
- Administer a beta-adrenergic blocker cautiously to a patient at risk because of a preexisting condition.
- Monitor the patient periodically for adverse reactions to the beta-adrenergic blocker. Be aware that adverse reactions most commonly occur from I.V. rather than oral administration and in geriatric patients and those with impaired renal or hepatic function.
- Obtain blood glucose levels frequently for the diabetic patient because beta-adrenergic blockers can potentiate hypoglycemia and mask its signs and symptoms.
- ***Keep the following emergency drugs on hand when administering an I.V. beta-adrenergic blocker: atropine for possible bradycardia, epinephrine (or another vasopressor) for possible hypotension, and isoproterenol and aminophylline for possible bronchospasm.***
- Administer oral beta-adrenergic blockers before meals or at bedtime to facilitate absorption. Avoid late-evening doses if insomnia occurs.
- Check the patient's apical pulse rate before drug administration (especially if the patient is taking digitalis). Withhold the drug if the patient has a pulse rate below 60 or exhibits adverse reactions to the beta-adrenergic blocker.
- ***Notify the physician immediately if the patient experiences cardiac or respiratory depression, arrhythmias, severe bronchospasm, or severe hypotension. Institute emergency care according to the health care facility's guidelines.***
- Administer antacids several hours before or after the oral beta-adrenergic blocker.
- Teach the patient about the prescribed agent. (See Patient Teaching: *Beta-adrenergic blockers.*)

Evaluation

For each nursing diagnosis, prepare an evaluation statement that describes the patient's or family's response to nursing interventions.

CHAPTER SUMMARY

Chapter 9 discussed adrenergic blockers as they are used therapeutically to disrupt sympathetic nervous system function. Here are the chapter highlights.

Adrenergic blocking agents, also called sympatholytics, are used therapeutically to block sympathetic nervous system function. This drug class includes alpha-adrenergic blockers, beta-adrenergic blockers, and autonomic ganglionic blockers. (The latter have recently been taken off the market.)

Alpha-adrenergic blockers block alpha-adrenergic receptors, decreasing blood pressure by relaxing the smooth muscles surrounding the arterioles. As a result, these drugs are used to treat certain types of hypertension. Their pharmacokinetics are not well understood. Most of these agents are absorbed erratically when administered orally and more rapidly and completely when administered sublingually or by inhalation. Adverse reactions to alpha-adrenergic blockers primarily are related to their vasodilation effect and mainly involve the cardiovascular system.

Selective beta-adrenergic blockers preferentially block $beta_1$-receptor sites; nonselective beta-adrenergic blockers block $beta_1$- and $beta_2$-receptor sites. Both types prevent cardiac excitation. They are used extensively to treat hypertension, cardiac arrhythmias, and angina pectoris. They also are used to treat hyperthyroidism and related disorders of sympathetic nervous system overstimulation. Beta-adrenergic blockers are absorbed rapidly and well, distributed widely in the body, and excreted primarily in the urine.

When caring for a patient who receives an adrenergic blocking agent, the nurse should apply the nursing process, providing care that includes monitoring for adverse reactions, screening for drug interactions, and providing patient teaching.

Questions to consider

See Appendix 1 for answers.

1. When Susan Mesnick, age 22, experiences a migraine headache, she takes ergotamine tartrate (Ergostat) as prescribed, 2 mg P.O. at the onset of an attack. If the headache continues, how long should she wait before taking another dose?
   (a) 10 minutes
   (b) 30 minutes
   (c) 1 hour
   (d) 2 hours

2. Before administering atenolol to Andrew Ames, age 49, the nurse reviews his medical history. Which of the following conditions would contraindicate atenolol therapy for Mr. Ames?
   (a) Diabetes mellitus
   (b) Hyperthyroidism
   (c) Impaired hepatic function
   (d) Sinus bradycardia

3. Which of the following classes of drugs is used to treat essential hypertension, Raynaud's disease, and pheochromocytoma?
   (a) Beta-adrenergic blockers
   (b) Cholinergic blockers
   (c) Alpha-adrenergic blockers
   (d) CNS stimulants

4. Amanda Pechin, age 55, develops hypertension. Her physician prescribes the beta-adrenergic blocker atenolol (Tenormin) 50 mg P.O. once a day. How do beta-adrenergic blockers produce their therapeutic effects?
   (a) They act as competitive adrenergic antagonists at beta-receptor sites.
   (b) They chemically inactivate neurotransmitters at receptor sites.
   (c) They stimulate metabolism of neurotransmitters.
   (d) They inhibit neurotransmitter production.

5. Which of the following drugs is most likely to induce bronchospasm in a patient with a history of asthma?
   (a) Phenoxybenzamine
   (b) Propranolol
   (c) Ergotamine
   (d) Prazosin

6. Jamie Van Der Pelt, age 36, takes ergotamine 2 mg sublingually at the onset of a vascular headache. Ergotamine belongs to which of the following groups of adrenergic blocking agents?
   (a) Alpha-adrenergic blockers
   (b) Beta-adrenergic blockers
   (c) Autonomic ganglionic blockers
   (d) Selective adrenergic blockers

7. If a patient's vascular headache is not relieved by a dose of ergotamine, how soon after the initial dose can the patient repeat it?
   (a) 5 minutes
   (b) 10 minutes
   (c) 15 minutes
   (d) 30 minutes

10 Neuromuscular blocking agents

OBJECTIVES

After reading and studying this chapter, the student should be able to:

1. list the major clinical indications for the neuromuscular blocking agents.
2. describe the pharmacokinetics of the neuromuscular blockers.
3. differentiate between the actions of nondepolarizing and depolarizing neuromuscular blockers.
4. explain the additive effects that result when drugs interact with the neuromuscular blockers.
5. identify the antidotes to the neuromuscular blockers.
6. describe how to apply the nursing process when caring for a patient who is receiving a neuromuscular blocker.

INTRODUCTION

Neuromuscular blocking agents are drugs that act to relax the skeletal muscles by disrupting the transmission of nerve impulses at the **motor end plate.** (See *Motor end plate.*) Because the drugs do not cross the blood-brain barrier, the patient remains conscious and aware of pain.

Neuromuscular blockers have three major clinical indications: to relax skeletal muscles during surgery, to reduce the intensity of muscle spasms in drug or electrically induced convulsions, or to manage patients who are fighting mechanical ventilation. Chapter 10 discusses the two main classes of natural and synthetic drugs used as neuromuscular blockers: nondepolarizing and depolarizing blocking agents. (See *Selected major neuromuscular blocking agents,* page 126.)

Drugs in this chapter include:

- atracurium besylate
- cisatracurium
- doxacurium
- metacurine iodide
- mivacurium
- pancuronium bromide
- rocuronium
- succinylcholine
- tubocurarine chloride
- vecuronium bromide.

Nondepolarizing blocking agents

The nondepolarizing blocking agents, also called competitive or stabilizing agents, are derived curare alkaloids and their synthetic analogues. They include atracurium besylate, cisatracurium, doxacurium, metocurine iodide, mivacurium, pancuronium bromide, pipecuronium bromide, rocuronium, tubocurarine chloride, and vecuronium bromide. These agents produce intermediate to prolonged muscle relaxation, such as that required for intubation and ventilation during surgery.

PHARMACOKINETICS

Because nondepolarizing blockers are absorbed poorly from the gastrointestinal (GI) tract, they are administered parenterally. The intravenous (I.V.) route is preferred because the action is more predictable. The drugs, which are distributed rapidly throughout the body, act on the motor end plates and, to a lesser degree, on the autonomic **ganglia.** A variable but large proportion of the nondepolarizing agents is excreted unchanged in the urine. Some of the newer drugs, such as atracurium, pancuronium, pipecuronium, and vecuronium, are metabolized partially in the liver.

The duration of action of metocurine and tubocurarine is related directly to the total dosage and the depth of anesthesia produced by the accompanying anesthetic agent. Repeated doses of metocurine and tubocurarine result in a cumulative effect.

Route	Onset	Peak	Duration
I.V.	2 min	3-6 min	Variable

PHARMACODYNAMICS

The nondepolarizing blockers compete with **acetylcholine** at the **cholinergic** receptor sites of the skeletal muscle membrane. This blocks acetycholine's **neurotransmitter** action, preventing the muscle membrane from depolarizing. The effect can be counteracted clinically by **anticholinesterase** drugs, such as neostigmine or pyridostigmine, which inhibit

Motor end plate

The motor nerve axon divides to form branching terminals called motor end plates. These are enfolded in muscle fibers but are separated from the fibers by the synaptic cleft.

A stimulus to the nerve causes the release of acetylcholine into the synaptic cleft. There, acetylcholine occupies receptor sites on the muscle cell membrane, depolarizing the membrane and causing muscle contraction. Neuromuscular blocking agents act at the motor end plate by competing with acetylcholine for the receptor sites or by blocking depolarization.

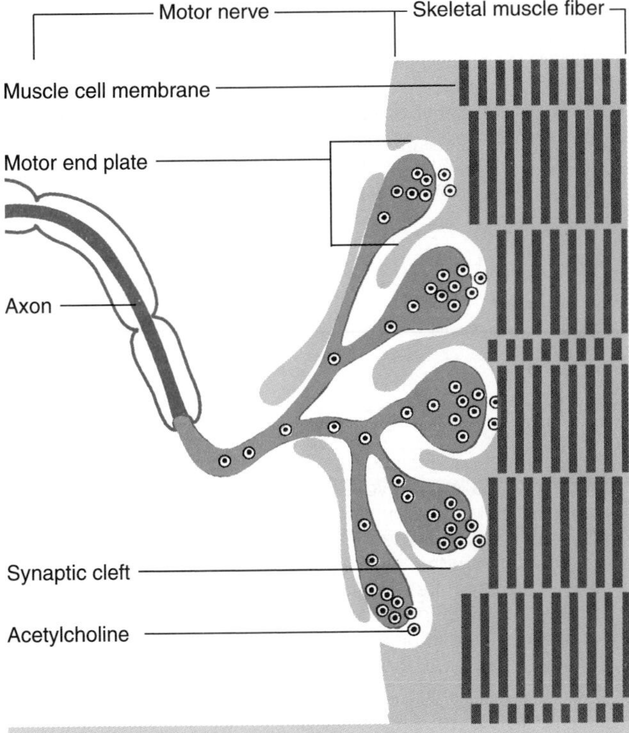

the action of acetylcholinesterase, the enzyme that destroys acetylcholine.

The initial muscle weakness produced by the drugs quickly changes to a flaccid paralysis that affects the muscles in a specific sequence. The first muscles to exhibit flaccid paralysis are those innervated by the motor portions of the cranial nerves and small, rapidly moving muscles in the eyes, face, and neck. Next, the limb, abdomen, and trunk muscles become flaccid. Finally, the intercostal muscles and diaphragm are paralyzed. Recovery from the paralysis usually occurs in the reverse order.

Because these drugs do not cross the blood-brain barrier, no alterations in consciousness or pain perception occur. Patients are aware of what is happening to them and may experience extreme anxiety and pain, but they cannot communicate their feelings.

PHARMACOTHERAPEUTICS

Nondepolarizing blockers are used for intermediate or prolonged muscle relaxation. They facilitate endotracheal intubation and are used during surgery to decrease the amount of anesthetic required and to facilitate manipulations. They also are used to paralyze patients who need ventilatory support but who fight the endotracheal tube and ventilator. Some nondepolarizing blockers also prevent muscle injury during electroconvulsive therapy (ECT) by reducing the intensity of muscle spasms.

Drug interactions

Most drugs that interact with the nondepolarizing blockers have an additive effect. For example, some antibiotics and anesthetics potentiate the neuromuscular blockade. Drugs that alter the serum levels of calcium, magnesium, or potassium also alter the effects of the nondepolarizing blockers. The anticholinesterases (neostigmine, pyridostigmine, and edrophonium) are antagonistic to nondepolarizing blockers and are used as antidotes to them. (See Drug Interactions: *Nondepolarizing blocking agents*, page 127.)

ADVERSE DRUG REACTIONS

Nondepolarizing blockers most commonly produce adverse reactions when given to patients who are debilitated, have fluid and electrolyte imbalances, or have respiratory, hepatic, neuromuscular, or renal disorders.

The prolonged pharmacologic effects of these drugs are responsible for most adverse reactions. The most serious adverse reaction is apnea. Ganglionic blockade and histamine release may cause a cardiovascular reaction, usually hypotension. Histamine release also may produce skin reactions, bronchospasm, and excessive bronchial and salivary secretions. Antidotes used to restore breathing may accentuate the hypotension and bronchospasms. Allergic reactions to nondepolarizing blockers are rare.

Pancuronium selectively blocks the vagus nerve and may result in tachycardia, cardiac arrhythmias, and hypertension.

NURSING PROCESS APPLICATION

The following information assists the nurse in caring for a patient who is receiving a nondepolarizing blocking agent. It includes an overview of assessment activities as well as examples of appropriate nursing diagnoses and related interventions (under "Planning and implementation"). It also highlights the importance of evaluation.

Assessment

Before drug therapy begins, review the patient's history for conditions that contraindicate or require cautious use of the prescribed nondepolarizing blocker. Also review the patient's medication history to identify use of drugs that may interact with it. During therapy, assess the patient for ad-

Selected major neuromuscular blocking agents

This table summarizes the major neuromuscular blocking agents currently in clinical use.

DRUG	MAJOR INDICATIONS AND USUAL DOSAGES	CONTRAINDICATIONS AND PRECAUTIONS
Nondepolarizing blocking agents		
pancuronium bromide (Pavulon)	*Facilitation of intubation and mechanical ventilation* ADULT: 0.06 to 0.1 mg/kg of body weight I.V. bolus PEDIATRIC: for children over age 1 month, 0.06 to 0.1 mg/kg of body weight I.V.; for neonates 1 month or younger, highly individualized dosage *Adjunct to anesthesia* ADULT: 0.04 to 0.1 mg/kg of body weight I.V., followed by 0.01 to 0.02 mg/kg administered every 25 to 60 minutes PEDIATRIC: for children over age 1 month, 0.04 to 0.1 mg/kg of body weight I.V., followed 0.01 mg/kg administered every 25 to 60 minutes, as needed; for neonates age 1 or younger, highly individualized dosage	• Pancuronium is contraindicated in a patient with hypersensitivity to it or to bromides, preexisting tachycardia, or any condition in which even a minor heart rate increase is undesirable. • This drug requires cautious use in a pregnant, geriatric, or debilitated patient or in one with myasthenia gravis; hepatic, renal, or pulmonary impairment; respiratory depression; lung cancer; dehydration; thyroid disorder; collagen disease; porphyria; familial periodic paralysis; electrolyte disturbances, especially hyperkalemia; digitalis glycoside therapy; or fractures or muscle spasms.
Depolarizing blocking agents		
succinylcholine (Anectine, Quelicin, Sucostrin)	*Facilitation of intubation or orthopedic manipulation; prevention of trauma during electroconvulsive therapy* ADULT: for short procedures or treatments, 0.3 to 1.1 mg/kg I.V.; for longer procedures or treatments, continuous I.V. infusion of 0.1% to 0.2% solution at a rate of 0.5 to 10 mg/minute for up to 1 hour; then 0.04 to 0.07 mg/kg as needed PEDIATRIC: 1 to 2 mg/kg initially; maintenance dosage is highly individualized, but must not exceed 150 mg total	• Succinylcholine is contraindicated in a patient with a family history of malignant hyperthermia, hypersensitivity to the drug, acute narrow-angle glaucoma, penetrating eye injury, myopathy with elevated creatinine phosphokinase, or genetic plasma pseudocholinesterase. • This drug requires cautious use in a pregnant patient or one with a renal, pulmonary, or neuromuscular disorder; fluid or electrolyte imbalance; increased intraocular pressure; or low serum pseudocholinesterase levels.

verse drug reactions, such as apnea and bronchospasm, and signs of drug interactions. Periodically assess the effectiveness of therapy. Finally, evaluate the patient's and family's knowledge about the prescribed nondepolarizing blocker.

Nursing diagnoses

• Risk for injury related to a preexisting condition that contraindicates or requires cautious use of a nondepolarizing blocker
• Risk for injury related to adverse drug reactions or drug interactions
• Ineffective breathing pattern related to respiratory muscle paralysis
• Knowledge deficit related to the nondepolarizing blocker

Planning and implementation

• Do not administer a nondepolarizing blocker to a patient with a condition that contraindicates its use.
• Administer a nondepolarizing blocker cautiously to a patient at risk because of a preexisting condition.
• Keep antidotes to the nondepolarizing blocker readily available.
*** *Keep endotracheal equipment, oxygen, and suction equipment available for respiratory support.***
• Monitor the patient for signs of adverse reactions to the nondepolarizing blocker. Keep in mind that a patient who is debilitated or has a fluid or electrolyte imbalance or a respiratory, hepatic, or neuromuscular disorder has increased susceptibility to adverse drug reactions. Also monitor for drug interactions.
• Notify the physician if adverse reactions or drug interactions occur.

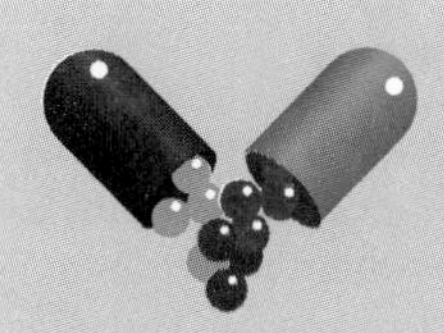

DRUG INTERACTIONS

Nondepolarizing blocking agents

Most interacting drugs enhance the blocking action of the neuromuscular blocking agents and require that the patient be observed closely to prevent fatal complications.

DRUG	INTERACTING AGENTS	POSSIBLE EFFECTS	NURSING IMPLICATIONS
atracurium, cisatracurium, doxacurium, metocurine, mivacurium, pancuronium, pipecuronium, rocuronium, tubocurarine, vecuronium	inhalation anesthetics, aminoglycosides, clindamycin, polymyxin, verapamil, quinine derivatives, ketamine, lithium, nitrates, pipercillin, thiazide diuretics, magnesium salts	Increased neuromuscular blockade	• Anticipate possible prolonged apnea. • Keep equipment available to provide mechanical ventilation. • Monitor the patient's heart rate and rhythm and blood pressure for signs of cardiovascular collapse. • Be prepared to replace fluid and electrolytes, as necessary. • Monitor patient for adverse drug reactions and consult the physician regarding a dosage decrease. • Keep the antidotes neostigmine and pyridostigmine available.
	corticosteroids, hydantoins, rantidine, theophylline	Decreased neuromuscular blockade	• Monitor patient closely. Dosage adjustments may be necessary.

***** ***Monitor respirations frequently until the patient is fully recovered from neuromuscular blockade, as evidenced by tests of muscle strength (peripheral nerve stimulator, hand grip, head lift, and ability to cough).***
- Keep the nondepolarizing blocker refrigerated to maintain potency.

***** ***Check mechanical ventilator settings and functions frequently to ensure that it is operating properly. Never turn off the ventilator alarm.***
- Turn the patient every 2 hours and provide chest physiotherapy, as prescribed.
- Suction the patient, as needed, because the nondepolarizing blocker suppresses the cough reflex and may increase respiratory secretions.
- Reassure the patient that breathing will return to normal after the nondepolarizing blocker is discontinued. (See Patient Teaching: *Nondepolarizing blocking agents,* page 128.)
- Notify the physician of any changes in the patient's respiratory status during administration of a nondepolarizing blocker.

Evaluation

For each nursing diagnosis, prepare an evaluation statement that describes the patient's or family's response to nursing interventions.

Depolarizing blocking agents

Succinylcholine is the only therapeutic depolarizing blocking agent. Although it is similar to the nondepolarizing blockers in its therapeutic effect, its mechanism of action differs.

PHARMACOKINETICS

Because succinylcholine is absorbed poorly from the GI tract, the preferred administration route is I.V., but the intramuscular route may be used if necessary. Succinylcholine is hydrolyzed in the liver and plasma by pseudocholinesterase, and a resulting metabolite, succinylmonocholine, produces a nondepolarizing blocking action. Succinylcholine is excreted via the kidneys; approximately 10% is excreted unchanged.

Route	Onset	Peak	Duration
I.V.	30 sec	1 min	4-10 min
I.M.	2-3 min	Unknown	10-30 min

PHARMACODYNAMICS

Succinylcholine produces a biphasic effect. In phase I blockade, it acts like acetylcholine and depolarizes the postsynaptic membrane of the muscle. However, succinylcholine is not inactivated by cholinesterase, so the depolarization persists. This results in brief periods of repetitive excitation — manifested by muscle fasciculations (uncoordinated contractions of muscle fibers) — followed by muscle paralysis and flaccidity. Phase II blockade normally is not seen except with a high drug concentration or repeated doses. In this phase, the muscle gradually repolarizes toward normal, although the drug persists in the synaptic cleft. It remains unresponsive to nerve stimulation, causing prolonged blockade. This action may result from desensitization of acetylcholine receptors and other factors.

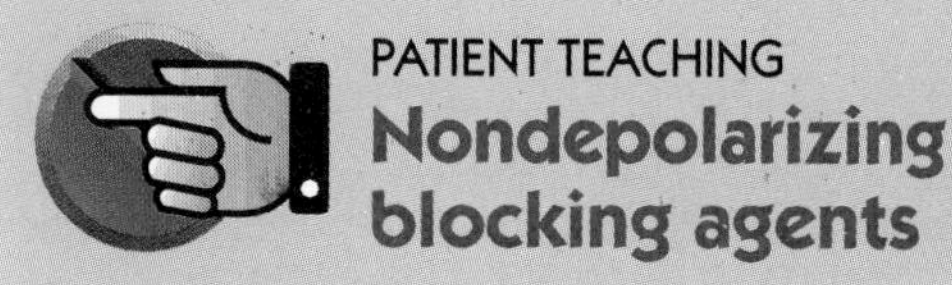

PATIENT TEACHING

Nondepolarizing blocking agents

- Teach the patient and family the name, dose, frequency, action, and adverse effects of the prescribed nondepolarizing blocking agent.
- Encourage the patient and family to ask questions about the nondepolarizing blocker before administration, if possible.
- Inform the patient and family fully of all procedures in advance. Provide reassurance that the nurse will monitor the patient continually during administration of the nondepolarizing blocker.

PHARMACOTHERAPEUTICS

Succinylcholine is the drug of choice for short-term muscle relaxation, such as during intubation and ECT.

Drug interactions

The action of succinylcholine is potentiated by a number of anesthetics and antibiotics. However, succinylcholine does not interact with most drugs that alter serum electrolyte levels. In contrast to their interaction with nondepolarizing blockers, anticholinesterases increase succinylcholine blockade.

ADVERSE DRUG REACTIONS

The primary adverse drug reactions to succinylcholine are the same as those to the nondepolarizing blockers: prolonged apnea and cardiovascular alterations.

Patients commonly experience muscle pain from the fasciculations that occur in phase I. These also may cause myoglobinemia and myoglobinuria, especially in children. The concomitant rise in the serum potassium level can be dangerous to patients with renal or neuromuscular disorders. The transient elevation of intraocular pressure that occurs during phase I may be harmful to patients with previously elevated intraocular pressure.

Neuromuscular blockade may be potentiated by certain genetic predispositions, such as a low pseudocholinesterase level and the tendency to develop malignant hyperthermia. A low pseudocholinesterase level also is present in liver disorders because pseudocholinesterase is synthesized in the liver. To determine the patient's sensitivity to succinylcholine, an initial test dose of 10 mg may be administered.

Phase II blockade may occur with repeated doses of succinylcholine.

NURSING PROCESS APPLICATION

The following information illustrates general application of the nursing process for a patient who is receiving succinylcholine. It includes an overview of assessment activities as well as examples of appropriate nursing diagnoses and related interventions (under "Planning and implementation"). It also highlights the importance of evaluation.

Assessment

Before drug therapy begins, review the patient's history for conditions that contraindicate or require cautious use of succinylcholine. Also review the patient's medication history to identify use of drugs that may interact with it. During therapy, assess the patient for adverse drug reactions — especially apnea — and signs of drug interactions. Also, periodically assess the effectiveness of therapy. Finally, evaluate the patient's and family's knowledge about succinylcholine.

Nursing diagnoses

- Risk for injury related to a preexisting condition that contraindicates or requires cautious use of succinylcholine
- Risk for injury related to adverse drug reactions or drug interactions
- Ineffective breathing pattern related to succinylcholine's effect on respiratory muscles
- Knowledge deficit related to succinylcholine

Planning and implementation

- Do not administer succinylcholine to a patient with a condition that contraindicates its use.
- Administer succinylcholine cautiously to a patient at risk because of a preexisting condition.
- Monitor the patient periodically for adverse reactions. Keep in mind that genetic factors, such as a low pseudocholinesterase level and a tendency to develop malignant hyperthermia, may potentiate neuromuscular blockade. Also monitor for drug interactions.

* ***Notify the physician immediately if adverse reactions or drug interactions occur. Be prepared to give emergency care according to facility guidelines.***

- Maintain a patent airway for the patient.

* ***Keep endotracheal equipment, oxygen, suction equipment, and a mechanical ventilator available for respiratory support.***

- Check the patient's respiratory rate and pattern every 5 to 10 minutes during infusion.

* ***Monitor the patient closely until recovery from neuromuscular blockade is complete. Signs of complete recovery include a renewed ability to cough and a return to previous levels of muscle strength on hand-grip and head-lift tests.***

- Notify the physician of any change in the patient's respiratory status.
- Teach the patient about succinylcholine. (See Patient Teaching: *Depolarizing blocking agents.*)

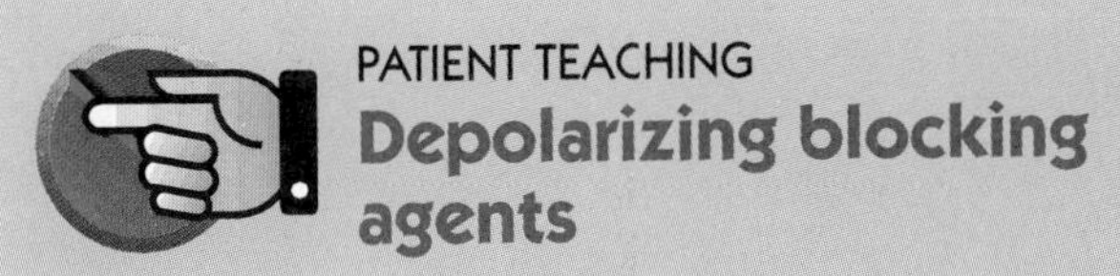

PATIENT TEACHING
Depolarizing blocking agents

- Teach the patient and family the name, dose, frequency, action, and adverse effects of succinylcholine.
- Encourage the patient and family to ask questions about succinylcholine before administration, if possible.
- Inform the patient and family fully of all procedures in advance. Provide reassurance that the nurse will monitor the patient continually during succinylcholine administration.

Evaluation

For each nursing diagnosis, prepare an evaluation statement that describes the patient's or family's response to nursing interventions.

CHAPTER SUMMARY

Chapter 10 discussed nondepolarizing and depolarizing neuromuscular blocking agents, which are used to relax the skeletal muscles by disrupting the transmission of nerve impulses. Here are the chapter highlights.

Neuromuscular blockers have three major uses: to relax skeletal muscles during surgery, to reduce the intensity of muscle spasms in drug-induced or electrically induced convulsions, or to manage patients who are fighting mechanical ventilation. They fall into two classes: nondepolarizing and depolarizing blocking agents.

Nondepolarizing blockers are used when intermediate or prolonged duration of action is required. They compete with acetylcholine at the cholinergic receptor sites of the skeletal muscle membrane, blocking the depolarization required for muscle contraction. This class is composed of curare alkaloids and their synthetic derivatives.

Succinylcholine is the only therapeutic depolarizing blocker. It acts like acetylcholine and results in depolarization of the postsynaptic membrane. However, unlike acetylcholine, succinylcholine is not inactivated by cholinesterase. Therefore, the depolarization lasts longer. With continued drug use, succinylcholine changes to a nondepolarizing blocking action. It is the drug of choice for short-term muscle relaxation.

The nurse must monitor the vital functions of any patient receiving these drugs. Maintenance of respiratory function is the top priority. However, because these drugs also alter cardiovascular function and fluid and electrolyte balance, careful monitoring is required.

Questions to consider

See Appendix 1 for answers.

1. After extensive surgery, Sarah Kiley, age 31, is admitted to the intensive care unit, where she soon develops acute respiratory distress syndrome. When placed on a mechanical ventilator, she fights it, which interferes with its effectiveness. To help maintain adequate ventilation, the physician orders the nondepolarizing blocker pancuronium (Pavulon) 0.1 mg/kg of body weight. How does pancuronium exert its therapeutic effect?
   (a) It stimulates muscarinic receptors at effector organs.
   (b) It inhibits the action of cholinesterase at the motor end plate.
   (c) It enhances the muscle's ability to respond to the neurotransmitter.
   (d) It competes with acetylcholine at cholinergic receptor sites in the skeletal muscle.

2. After receiving pancuronium, Lawrence Bingham, age 56, experiences paralysis. The nurse can expect paralysis to occur in which of the following sequences?
   (a) Diaphragm, eyes, and legs
   (b) Face, arms, and diaphragm
   (c) Diaphragm, arms, and legs
   (d) Neck, diaphragm, and legs

3. Jack Quigley, age 38, is receiving ECT as a part of therapy for a manic depressive disorder. Before ECT, Mr. Quigley receives succinylcholine. Why is succinylcholine administered before ECT?
   (a) To provide short-term muscle relaxation
   (b) To increase muscle contractions
   (c) To sedate the patient
   (d) To relieve pain

4. Which of the following is a common adverse reaction to nondepolarizing and depolarizing blocking agents?
   (a) Renal failure
   (b) Prolonged apnea
   (c) Bone fractures
   (d) Liver failure

5. After succinylcholine administration and ECT, the nurse assesses Barbara Cole, age 24, for muscle pain, a common adverse reaction to succinylcholine. What is the most likely cause of this reaction?
   (a) Adverse effects of ECT
   (b) Succinylcholine toxicity
   (c) Action of succinylcholine in phase I
   (d) Action of succinylcholine in phase II

UNIT IV

Drugs to treat neurologic and neuromuscular system disorders

This unit discusses pharmacologic agents used to treat neurologic and neuromuscular system disorders, such as musculoskeletal spasms, **Parkinson's disease,** and seizure disorders. The agents discussed include skeletal muscle relaxing, antiparkinsonian, and anticonvulsant agents. Although their pharmacokinetics, pharmacodynamics, and pharmacotherapeutics vary greatly, they all affect the neurologic or neuromuscular system.

To help the nurse understand the actions and uses of these agents, this introduction provides an overview of the anatomy and physiology of the nervous system.

Anatomy and physiology of the nervous system

The nervous system is composed of the central and peripheral divisions. The central nervous system (CNS) consists of the brain and spinal cord. (See *Structures of the central nervous system.*)

The peripheral nervous system is composed of the cranial and spinal nerves, which carry sensory messages from organs and tissues to the brain and motor instructions from the brain to target organs.

The 12 pairs of cranial nerves provide primarily for the sensory and motor needs of the head but also of the neck, chest, and abdomen. Cranial nerves I and II originate in the frontal lobe; III through XII originate in the brain stem.

The 31 pairs of spinal nerves originate in the spinal cord. These paired nerves include 8 cervical, 12 thoracic, 5 lumbar, 5 sacral, and 1 coccygeal. Cervical 3 to thoracic 2 supply the upper extremities; thoracic 9 through 12 supply the lower extremities.

Physiology of the nervous system

The nervous system governs all movement, sensation, thought, and emotion. Two types of cells constitute the nervous system: neuroglial cells and neurons. Neuroglial cells perform specialized support functions, such as supplying nutrients to the neurons, assisting in the production of cerebrospinal fluid, and providing electrical insulation for the **axons** of the CNS neurons.

The neuron consists of a cell body and two types of appendages—a long one (an axon) and one or more shorter ones (**dendrites**). Cell bodies form the gray matter in the brain, brain stem, and spinal cord. The axon transmits impulses from the cell body to other neurons, whereas dendrites receive impulses from nearby cells and conduct them toward the cell body.

Neurons perform one of three roles in transmitting impulses: reception of sensory stimuli, transmission of motor responses, or integration of activities and coordination of communication between body parts. Sensory neurons carry stimuli from the peripheral sensory organs, such as the skin, to the spinal cord and brain. Motor neurons carry impulses from the brain and spinal cord to tissues and organs. **Interneurons** relay impulses within the CNS.

All human functions rely on the electrical and chemical transmission of impulses from neuron to neuron. This transmission occurs across a **synapse,** or the contact point between two neurons. Neurotransmission is facilitated by **neurotransmitters,** such as acetylcholine and **dopamine.**

Structures of the central nervous system

The brain, brain stem, and spinal cord function synergistically to control movement, sensation, thought, and emotion. Major structures and their functions are shown below.

The brain is composed of the cerebrum, diencephalon, cerebellum, and brain stem. Two structurally matched hemispheres make up the cerebrum, the largest portion of the brain. Each hemisphere contains four lobes—frontal, parietal, temporal, and occipital. The surface of the cerebrum (cortex) is composed of gray matter made of neuron cell bodies, axon terminals, and dendrites. The interior of the cerebrum is composed of white matter made of basal ganglia. The corpus callosum facilitates communication between corresponding areas in the two hemispheres.

The diencephalon, located anterior to the brain stem, includes the hypothalamus and thalamus. The cerebellum lies at the base of the brain below the occipital lobes of the cerebrum.

The brain stem, composed of the midbrain, pons, and medulla oblongata, relays all messages between the upper and lower levels of the nervous system; cranial nerves III through XII originate there.

The spinal cord serves as a communication pathway between the brain and the peripheral nervous system, and its gray matter functions as a reflex center for spinal reflexes. It joins the brain stem at the level of the foramen magnum and terminates near the second lumbar vertebra. The spinal cord comprises a central H-shaped mass of gray matter divided into dorsal (or posterior) and ventral (or anterior) horns. Cell bodies in the dorsal horn relay sensory (afferent) impulses, and those in the ventral horn relay motor (efferent) impulses. White matter surrounding these horns consists of myelinated axons of sensory and motor nerves grouped in ascending and descending tracts.

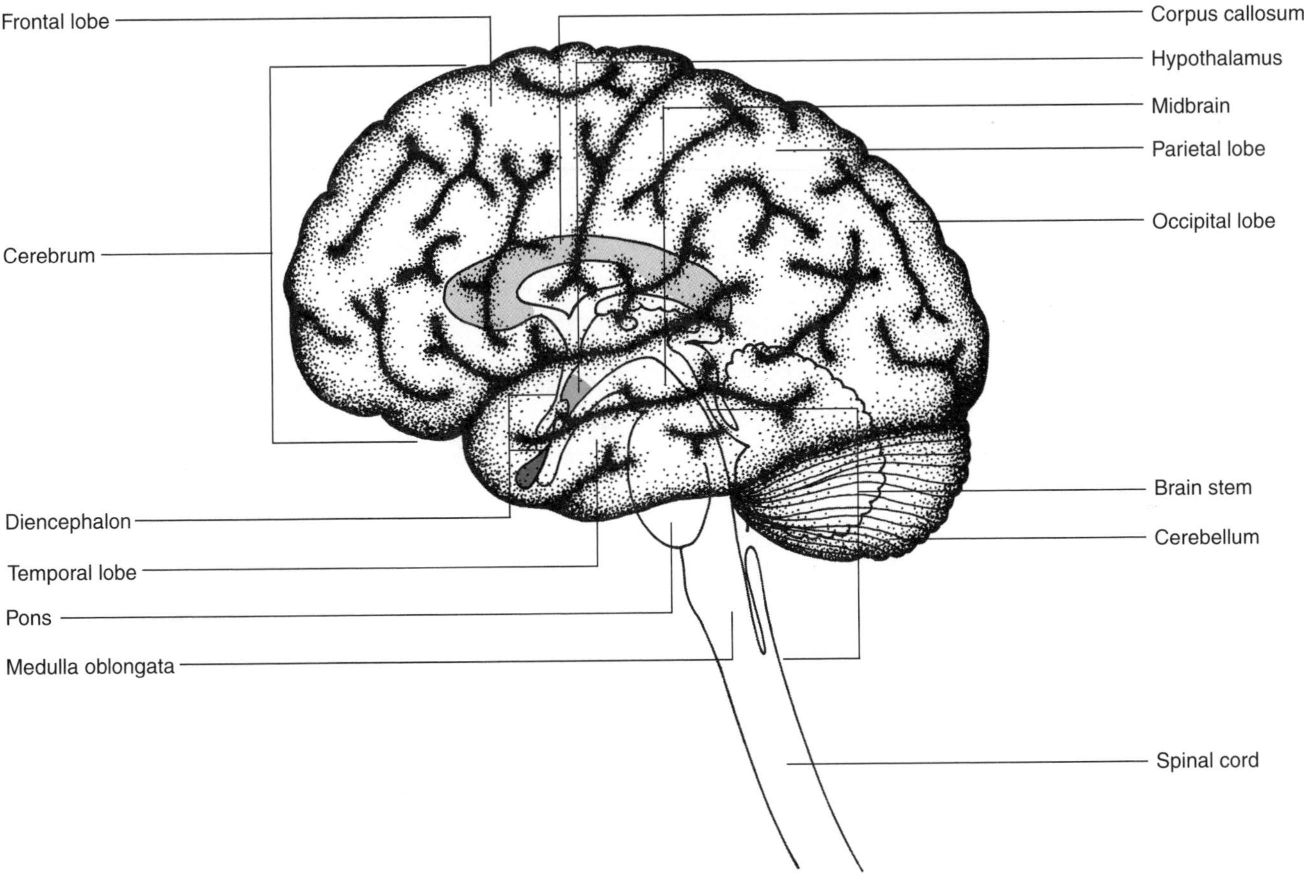

Skeletal muscle relaxing agents

OBJECTIVES

After reading and studying this chapter, the student should be able to:

1. define spasm and spasticity.
2. differentiate the skeletal muscle relaxants that act centrally from those that act peripherally.
3. describe the mechanisms of action of the centrally and peripherally acting skeletal muscle relaxants.
4. list the therapeutic uses for the various groups of skeletal muscle relaxants.
5. describe the adverse reactions that occur when these agents are given with central nervous system (CNS) depressants.
6. describe how to apply the nursing process when caring for a patient who is receiving a skeletal muscle relaxant.

INTRODUCTION

Skeletal muscle **relaxants** relieve musculoskeletal pain or **spasm** and severe musculoskeletal **spasticity.** They are used to treat acute, painful musculoskeletal conditions and the muscle spasticity associated with multiple sclerosis (MS), cerebral palsy, cerebrovascular accident (CVA), and spinal cord injuries. Chapter 11 discusses the two main classes of skeletal muscle relaxants — centrally acting and peripherally acting — and baclofen and diazepam, two other drugs used to manage musculoskeletal disorders.

The drugs covered in this chapter include:

- baclofen
- carisoprodol
- chlorphenesin carbamate
- cyclobenzaprine hydrochloride
- dantrolene sodium
- diazepam
- metaxalone
- methocarbamol
- orphenadrine citrate.

Acute spasms and spasticity

Severe cold, lack of blood flow to a muscle, or overexertion can elicit pain or other sensory impulses that are transmitted by the posterior sensory nerve fibers to the spinal cord and the higher levels of the CNS. These sensory impulses may cause a reflex (involuntary) muscle contraction, or spasm from trauma, epilepsy, hypocalcemia, or muscular disorders. The muscle contraction further stimulates the sensory receptors to a more intense contraction, establishing a cycle. Centrally acting muscle relaxants are believed to break this cycle by acting as CNS depressants.

Spasticity is a motor disorder characterized by an increase in muscle tone from hyperexcitability of the anterior motor neurons. This hyperexcitability may arise from a lack of inhibition or from excess stimulation produced by signals transmitted from the brain through the interneurons in the spinal cord to the anterior motor neurons. Spasticity is associated with various clinical conditions, called upper motor neuron disorders, including MS, cerebral palsy, CVA (stroke), and spinal cord injuries. The skeletal muscle relaxants vary in their efficacy; they apparently reduce spasticity by reducing hyperexcitability. (See *Selected major skeletal muscle relaxing agents.*)

Centrally acting skeletal muscle relaxants

Such conditions as trauma, inflammation, anxiety, and pain can be associated with acute muscle spasms. The following drugs may relieve such spasms: carisoprodol, chlorphenesin carbamate, chlorzoxazone, cyclobenzaprine hydrochloride, metaxalone, methocarbamol, and orphenadrine citrate. However, they are ineffective in treating spasticity associated with chronic neurologic disease. Lack of controlled clinical trials makes assessing these agents difficult.

PHARMACOKINETICS

Currently, the pharmacokinetic properties of the centrally acting skeletal muscle relaxants are not well defined. In general, these drugs are absorbed from the gastrointestinal (GI) tract, widely distributed in the body, metabolized in the liver, and excreted by the kidneys. (See *Pharmacokinetics of centrally acting skeletal muscle relaxants,* page 134.)

Route	Onset	Peak	Duration
P.O.	30 min-1 hr	1-8 hr	3-24 hr
I.M.	5 min	30 min	Unknown
I.V.	Immediate	Immediate	Unknown

Selected major skeletal muscle relaxing agents

This table summarizes the major skeletal muscle relaxants currently in clinical use. Diazepam is discussed in chapter 42, Antianxiety Agents.

DRUG	MAJOR INDICATIONS AND USUAL DOSAGES	CONTRAINDICATIONS AND PRECAUTIONS
Centrally acting agents		
carisoprodol (Soma)	*Acute muscle spasms* ADULT: 350 mg P.O. t.i.d. and h.s.	• Carisoprodol is contraindicated in a patient with acute intermittent porphyria or known hypersensitivity to the drug, to metabisulfite in Soma. • This drug requires cautious use in a pregnant or breast-feeding patient or one with impaired hepatic or renal function. • Safety and efficacy in children under age 12 have not been established.
cyclobenzaprine (Flexeril)	*Musculoskeletal conditions* ADULT: 10 mg P.O. t.i.d. to a maximum of 60 mg/day for no longer than 2 to 3 weeks	• Cyclobenzaprine is contraindicated in a patient with known hypersensitivity to the drug, arrhythmias, heart block or conduction disturbances, heart failure, or hyperthyroidism; during the acute recovery phase of a myocardial infarction; or within 14 days of monoamine oxidase inhibitor therapy.
Peripherally acting agents		
dantrolene sodium (Dantrium)	*Spasticity* ADULT: 25 mg P.O. daily, increased to 25 mg b.i.d., t.i.d., or q.i.d., and then by increments of 25 mg to a maximum of 100 mg q.i.d. PEDIATRIC: 0.5 mg/kg b.i.d., increased to t.i.d. or q.i.d. and then by increments of 0.5 mg/kg up to 3 mg/kg b.i.d. to q.i.d to a maximum of 100 mg q.i.d. *Prevention of malignant hyperthermic crisis* ADULT: 4 to 8 mg/kg of body weight P.O. daily in four divided doses for 1 to 2 days before surgery with the last dose 3 to 4 hours before surgery; or 2.5 mg/kg I.V. 1 hour before surgery infused over 1 hour *Treatment of malignant hyperthermic crisis* ADULT and PEDIATRIC: 1 mg/kg of body weight by rapid I.V. infusion repeated up to a maximum cumulative dose of 10 mg/kg	• Dantrolene is contraindicated in a pregnant or breast-feeding patient or one with hepatic disease. • This drug requires cautious use in a female patient, any patient over age 35, or a patient with impaired pulmonary function, severely impaired cardiac function, or previous history of liver disease. • The patient should take potective measures against exposure to sunlight because photosensitization may occur. • Because of high pH of the I.V. formulation, take measures to prevent extravasation into surrounding tissues. • Safety and efficacy in children under age 5 have not been established.
Other agents		
baclofen (Lioresal)	*Spasticity* ADULT: initially, 5 mg P.O. t.i.d. increased by 15 mg at 3-day intervals up to a maximum of 80 mg P.O. daily. Intrathecal use: Test dose of 50 to 100 mcg/ml administered in 25-mcg increments at intervals of at least 24 hours, beginning with a 50-mcg dose; the initial intrathecal dose is twice the test dose that produced a positive response. Daily dose can be increased by increments of 10% to 30%	• Baclofen is contraindicated in a patient with known hypersensitivity to the drug. • This drug requires cautious use in a breast-feeding or geriatric patient or one with a cerebrovascular accident or other brain disorder. • Safety and efficacy in children under age 12 have not been established.

Pharmacokinetics of centrally acting skeletal muscle relaxants

As this chart shows, the onset of action of the centrally acting skeletal muscle relaxants administered orally varies from 30 minutes to 1 hour. Cyclobenzaprine has the longest duration of action at 12 to 14 hours.

DRUG	ONSET OF ACTION	TIME TO PEAK CONCENTRATION	DURATION OF ACTION
carisoprodol	30 minutes	4 hours	4 to 6 hours
chlorphenesin	Not known	1 to 3 hours	4 to 6 hours
chlorzoxazone	1 hour	1 to 2 hours	3 to 4 hours
cyclobenzaprine	1 hour	4 to 8 hours	12 to 24 hours
metaxalone	1 hour	2 hours	4 to 6 hours
methocarbamol	30 minutes	1 to 2 hours	Not known
orphenadrine	1 hour	2 hours	4 to 6 hours

PHARMACODYNAMICS

The skeletal muscle relaxant effects of the centrally acting agents are minimal and may be related to their sedative effects. The drugs do not relax skeletal muscle directly or depress neuronal conduction, neuromuscular transmission, or muscle excitability. The precise mechanism of action of these drugs is unknown. However, they are known to be CNS depressants.

PHARMACOTHERAPEUTICS

The centrally acting skeletal muscle relaxants are used as adjuncts to rest and physical therapy in treating acute, painful musculoskeletal conditions. Their beneficial effects probably derive from their sedative properties, and they do not appear to be as effective as diazepam for treating musculoskeletal pain. They are ineffective in treating skeletal muscle hyperactivity secondary to such chronic neurologic disorders as cerebral palsy.

Drug interactions

The centrally acting skeletal muscle relaxants interact with few drugs, but all interact with other CNS depressants (including alcohol), causing additive depression of the CNS. Cyclobenzaprine interacts with **monoamine oxidase (MAO) inhibitors:** 14 days must elapse between the last dose of an MAO inhibitor and the first dose of cyclobenzaprine. Cyclobenzaprine may decrease the effects of the antihypertensive agents guanethidine and clonidine. Orphenadrine and cyclobenzaprine sometimes enhance the effects of cholinergic blocking agents. Methocarbamol may antagonize the cholinergic effects of the anticholinesterase agents used to treat myasthenia gravis. (See Drug Interactions: *Centrally acting skeletal muscle relaxants.*)

The centrally acting skeletal muscle relaxants also interfere with some laboratory tests. Metaxalone may produce false-positive results for urine glucose with the copper reduction method. (It does not interfere with the glucose oxidase method.) Methocarbamol may cause false-positive results for urine 5-hydroxyindoleacetic acid and for urine vanillylmandelic acid.

ADVERSE DRUG REACTIONS

The most common adverse reactions to the centrally acting skeletal muscle relaxants are extensions of their therapeutic effects on the CNS.

Drowsiness and dizziness are the most common adverse reactions to drugs in this class. Occasionally, nausea, vomiting, diarrhea, constipation, heartburn, abdominal distress, or **ataxia** occurs. Areflexia, flaccid paralysis, respiratory depression, and hypotension are seen occasionally after oral administration of any of these drugs except methocarbamol. With parenteral administration, reactions may include syncope, hypotension, flushing, blurred vision, asthenia, lethargy, vertigo, lack of coordination, and bradycardia.

Because orphenadrine has an anticholinergic effect, adverse reactions may include dry mouth, urine retention, urinary hesitancy, blurred vision, and tachycardia. Orphenadrine overdose may cause seizures, shock, respiratory arrest, coma, or death. At high doses, cyclobenzaprine, which is structurally similar to the tricyclic antidepressants, shares their toxic potential; reactions include tachycardia and orthostatic hypotension. Physical and psychological dependence is a possibility after long-term use of these agents; abrupt cessation of the drug may cause severe withdrawal symptoms.

Rarely, parenteral orphenadrine causes an anaphylactic reaction. Chlorphenesin contains tartrazine dye, which may

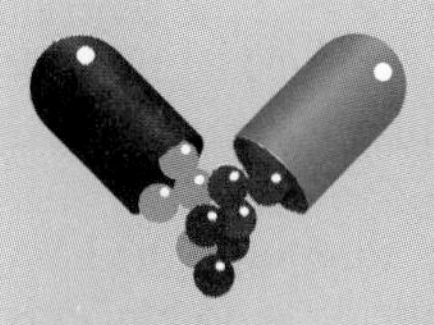

DRUG INTERACTIONS

Centrally acting skeletal muscle relaxants

Drug interactions involving centrally acting skeletal muscle relaxants are infrequent and most commonly result from simultaneous administration of central nervous system (CNS) depressants including alcohol.

DRUG	INTERACTING AGENTS	POSSIBLE EFFECTS	NURSING IMPLICATIONS
carisoprodol, chlorphenesin, chlorzoxazone, cyclobenzaprine, metaxalone, methocarbamol, orphenadrine	CNS depressants (alcohol, narcotics, barbiturates, anticonvulsants, tricyclic antidepressants, antianxiety agents)	Increased sedative and other CNS effects, including motor skill impairment and respiratory depression	• Monitor the patient for changes in level of consciousness. • Monitor the patient for signs of respiratory depression. • Advise the patient of possible additive effects, especially with alcohol.
cyclobenzaprine	monoamine oxidase (MAO) inhibitors	Hyperpyrexia, excitation, and seizures	• Expect 14 days to elapse between the administration of the last does of an MAO inhibitor and the first dose of cyclobenzaprine. • Monitor the patient's CNS status and body temperature frequently.
	cholinergic blockers	Increased anticholinergic effects, including confusion and hallucinations	• Monitor the patient for signs and symptoms of an adverse reaction; be prepared to administer a reduced dosage of the cholinergic blocker as prescribed.
orphenadrine	cholinergic blockers	Increased anticholinergic effects, including confusion and hallucinations	• Monitor the patient for signs and symptoms of an adverse reaction; be prepared to administer a reduced dosage of the cholinergic blocker as prescribed.
	phenothiazines	Decreased effects of phenothiazines	• Monitor the patient for a decreased effect of the phenothiazine (for example, psychotic behavior).
	propoxyphene	Additive CNS effects	• Monitor the patient for signs and symptoms of mental confusion, anxiety, and tremors. • Reduced dosage of one or both agents is recommended.

cause an allergic reaction. Methocarbamol injectable contains polyethylene glycol that may increase preexisting acidosis and urea retention in patients with renal impairment.

NURSING PROCESS APPLICATION

The following information assists the nurse in caring for a patient who is receiving a centrally acting skeletal muscle relaxant. It includes an overview of assessment activities as well as examples of appropriate nursing diagnoses and related interventions (under "Planning and implementation"). It also highlights the importance of evaluation.

Assessment

Before drug therapy begins, review the patient's history for conditions that contraindicate or require cautious use of the prescribed centrally acting skeletal muscle relaxant. Also review the patient's medication history to identify use of drugs that may interact with it. During therapy, assess the patient for adverse drug reactions and signs of drug interactions. Also, periodically assess the effectiveness of therapy with the centrally acting skeletal muscle relaxant. Because the drug may be addictive, assess the patient for signs of physical or psychological dependence. Finally, evaluate the patient's and family's knowledge about the prescribed drug.

Nursing diagnoses

- Risk for injury related to a preexisting condition that contraindicates or requires cautious use of a centrally acting skeletal muscle relaxant
- Risk for injury related to adverse drug reactions or drug interactions
- Impaired adjustment related to physical and psychological dependence on the centrally acting skeletal muscle relaxant
- Knowledge deficit related to the prescribed centrally acting skeletal muscle relaxant

Planning and implementation

- Do not administer a centrally acting skeletal muscle relaxant to a patient with a condition that contraindicates its use. (See Patient Teaching: *Centrally acting skeletal muscle relaxants*, page 136.)

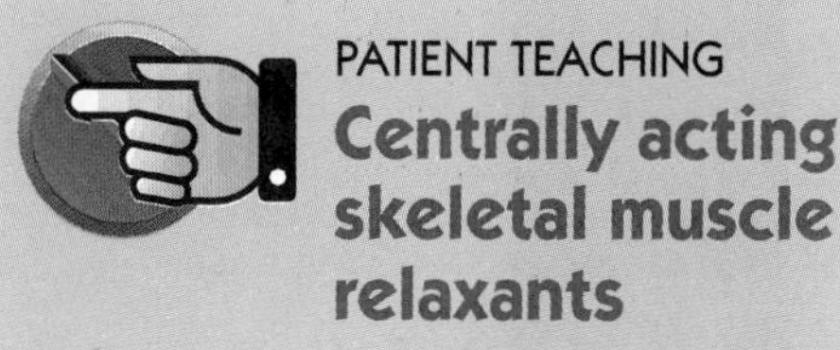

PATIENT TEACHING

Centrally acting skeletal muscle relaxants

- Teach the patient and family the name, dose, frequency, action, and adverse effects of the prescribed centrally acting skeletal muscle relaxant.
- Inform the patient that a centrally acting skeletal muscle relaxant may impair mental alertness or physical coordination, increasing the risk of operating machinery or driving a motor vehicle.
- Instruct the patient to take an oral centrally acting agent with meals or milk to prevent gastrointestinal distress.
- Advise the patient taking orphenadrine to relieve dry mouth with sugarless candy or gum and cool beverages, if permitted. Also, advise the patient to contact the physician if urine retention occurs.
- Inform the patient that chlorzoxazone may harmlessly discolor urine orange or purple-red; methocarbamol, green, black, or brown.
- Teach the diabetic patient that metaxalone may cause false-positive results for urine glucose with the copper reduction method.
- Teach the patient to notify the physician if adverse reactions occur.

• Administer a centrally acting skeletal muscle relaxant cautiously to a patient at risk because of a preexisting condition.
• Monitor the patient periodically for adverse reactions during therapy with a centrally acting skeletal muscle relaxant.
• Avoid abrupt discontinuation of a centrally acting skeletal muscle relaxant.
• Give parenteral orphenadrine over 5 minutes with the patient in the supine position; keep the patient supine for 5 to 10 more minutes. Then help the patient to a sitting position and supervise ambulation.
• Monitor the I.V. site in a patient who receives parenteral methocarbamol. Watch for extravasation because thrombophlebitis, sloughing, and pain may result.
• Administer I.V. methocarbamol slowly at a maximum rate of 3 ml/minute. Inject I.M. methocarbamol deeply and slowly, only in the upper outer quadrant of the buttocks, with a maximum of 5 ml in each buttock.
• Keep epinephrine, antihistamines, and corticosteroids on hand during methocarbamol therapy to correct syncope that does not resolve with supportive therapy.
• Avoid administering methocarbamol subcutaneously.
Monitor respiratory status for a patient receiving a CNS depressant along with a centrally acting skeletal muscle relaxant. Keep emergency equipment available.
• Notify the physician if the centrally acting skeletal muscle relaxant does not relieve pain or muscle spasm.
• Verify the patient's need for continued use of the centrally acting skeletal muscle relaxant.
• Reduce the dosage gradually for a centrally acting skeletal muscle relaxant, as prescribed.
• Provide a referral for psychological evaluation if the patient refuses to reduce drug use when the drug no longer is needed.

Evaluation

For each nursing diagnosis, prepare an evaluation statement that describes the patient's or family's response to nursing interventions.

Peripherally acting skeletal muscle relaxants

Dantrolene sodium is a peripherally acting skeletal muscle relaxant. Similar to the centrally acting agents in its therapeutic effect, dantrolene differs in its mechanism of action. Because its major effect is on the muscle, dantrolene has a lower incidence of adverse CNS effects, but high therapeutic doses are hepatotoxic. Clinically, dantrolene seems most effective for spasticity of cerebral origin. Because it produces muscle weakness, dantrolene is of questionable benefit in patients with borderline strength.

PHARMACOKINETICS

Dantrolene is absorbed poorly from the GI tract. It is highly plasma protein–bound, metabolized by the liver, and excreted in the urine. Although the peak concentration level of a single dose of dantrolene occurs about 5 hours after it is ingested, the drug's therapeutic benefit may not be evident for a week or more. Dosage increases should not exceed two per week. Dantrolene's elimination half-life in healthy adults is about 9 hours. Because dantrolene undergoes significant hepatic metabolism, however, its half-life may be prolonged in patients with impaired liver function.

Route	Onset	Peak	Duration
P.O.	Unknown	5 hr	Unknown
I.V.	Unknown	Unknown	Unknown

PHARMACODYNAMICS

Dantrolene is chemically and pharmacologically unrelated to the other skeletal muscle relaxants. It may act by inhibiting calcium release from the sarcoplasmic reticulum in muscle cells. The sarcoplasmic reticulum stores calcium until the muscle is activated electrically by an action potential; then it releases calcium, which triggers muscle contraction.

Although dantrolene appears to affect the CNS as well, any central effect remains unproven. CNS effects, such as drowsiness, possibly result indirectly from decreased skeletal muscle activity. At therapeutic concentrations, dantrolene has little effect on cardiac or intestinal smooth muscle.

PHARMACOTHERAPEUTICS

Dantrolene helps manage all types of spasticity, regardless of lesion location, but is most effective when the lesion is cerebral. Patients with MS, cerebral palsy, spinal cord injury, or CVA may benefit from dantrolene. It is particularly useful for reducing spasticity in patients whose nursing care is impeded by severe muscle contractions. It also benefits patients whose rehabilitation program has been slowed by spasticity. If these patients have reversible spasticity, its relief should speed restoration of residual function. The patients' gait or ability to stand or sit also may improve. (See Patient Teaching: *Peripherally acting skeletal muscle relaxants.*)

Dantrolene also is used to treat and prevent malignant hyperthermic crisis.

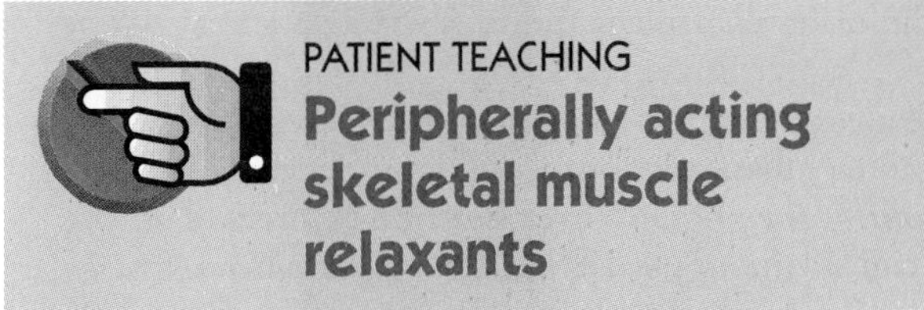

PATIENT TEACHING

Peripherally acting skeletal muscle relaxants

- Teach the patient and family about dantrolene, including its name, dose, frequency, action, and adverse effects.
- Teach the patient about dantrolene's possible effects, such as weakness, drowsiness, and dizziness. Reassure the patient that these effects usually subside in a few days.
- Instruct the patient to take dantrolene with meals or milk to prevent gastric irritation.
- Advise the patient to expect frequent blood testing of liver function.
- Teach the patient and family to notify the physician if adverse reactions occur.

Drug interactions

CNS depressants combined with dantrolene increase CNS depression, which may lead to sedation, motor skill impairment, and respiratory depression. No other interactions are reported.

ADVERSE DRUG REACTIONS

Dose-related adverse reactions to dantrolene usually are transient, lasting up to 4 days after therapy begins. The most common is muscle weakness, rarely severe enough to cause slurring of speech, drooling, and enuresis. Other common reactions include drowsiness, dizziness, lightheadedness, diarrhea, nausea, malaise, and fatigue. If weakness or diarrhea is severe, the dosage may be decreased or the drug discontinued. Other adverse GI reactions that may respond to a dosage decrease include anorexia, vomiting, gastric irritation, abdominal cramps, constipation, difficulty swallowing, and GI bleeding. Constipation sometimes is severe enough to resemble bowel obstruction.

Neurologic adverse reactions include visual and speech disturbances, headache, taste alteration, depression, confusion, hallucinations, nervousness, insomnia, and seizures.

Urogenital reactions include urinary frequency, incontinence, nocturia, difficult urination, urine retention, hematuria, crystalluria, and difficult erection.

Cardiovascular reactions include tachycardia, erratic blood pressure, phlebitis, and pleural effusion with pericarditis.

Fatal and nonfatal hepatitis from dantrolene appear to be idiosyncratic reactions. In most cases, nausea, anorexia, vomiting, and abdominal discomfort precede hepatitis, which occurs most commonly in patients receiving more than 300 mg daily for longer than 2 months. The risk of dantrolene hepatotoxicity is greatest in women over age 35 who simultaneously take estrogens and in patients with baseline liver function test abnormalities. The abnormal liver function test results induced by dantrolene may return to normal when the drug is discontinued.

Other reactions include acneiform rash, erratic blood pressure, pruritus, urticaria, excessive tearing, chills and fever, and a feeling of suffocation.

NURSING PROCESS APPLICATION

The following information assists the nurse in caring for a patient who is receiving dantrolene. It includes an overview of assessment activities as well as examples of appropriate nursing diagnoses and related interventions (under "Planning and implementation"). It also highlights the importance of evaluation.

Assessment

Before drug therapy begins, review the patient's history for conditions that contraindicate or require cautious use of dantrolene. Also review the patient's medication history to identify use of drugs that may interact with it. During therapy, assess the patient for adverse drug reactions and signs of drug interactions. Also, periodically assess the effectiveness of dantrolene therapy. Finally, evaluate the patient's and family's knowledge about the drug.

Nursing diagnoses

- Risk for injury related to a preexisting condition that contraindicates or requires cautious use of dantrolene
- Risk for injury related to adverse drug reactions or drug interactions
- Impaired physical mobility related to ineffectiveness of dantrolene
- Knowledge deficit related to dantrolene

Planning and implementation

- Do not administer dantrolene to a patient with a condition that contraindicates its use.

- Administer dantrolene cautiously to a patient at risk because of a preexisting condition.
- Frequently monitor any patient with severe cardiac or pulmonary disease who receives dantrolene.

*** *Monitor the patient's liver function before and during dantrolene therapy with the alanine aminotransferase (ALT; formerly SGPT), aspartate aminotransferase (AST; formerly SGOT), alkaline phosphatase, and total bilirubin tests, as prescribed.***

- Observe closely for adverse drug reactions.
- Empty dantrolene capsules into fruit juice or another liquid immediately before administration to a patient who has difficulty swallowing.
- Reconstitute dantrolene with 60 ml of sterile, not bacteriostatic, water for I.V. administration.
- Notify the physician if adverse reactions occur.
- Monitor for sedation, motor skill impairment, and respiratory depression in a patient receiving dantrolene and a CNS depressant.

*** *Keep emergency equipment nearby to treat respiratory depression.***

- Monitor the patient's level of spasticity during therapy.
- Notify the physician if physical mobility does not improve while the patient is taking dantrolene.

Evaluation

For each nursing diagnosis, prepare an evaluation statement that describes the patient's or family's response to nursing interventions.

Other skeletal muscle relaxants

Two other drugs, diazepam and baclofen, are used as skeletal muscle relaxants, although diazepam is primarily an antianxiety agent. (See *Diazepam as a skeletal muscle relaxant.*) This section discusses baclofen only.

PHARMACOKINETICS

Baclofen is absorbed rapidly from the GI tract. It is distributed widely (with only small amounts crossing the blood-brain barrier), undergoes minimal liver metabolism, and is excreted primarily unchanged in the urine.

The beneficial effects of baclofen may or may not occur immediately — the onset of therapeutic effect ranges from hours to weeks. The elimination half-life of baclofen is 2.5 to 4 hours. Abrupt withdrawal of the drug may precipitate hallucinations, seizures, and acute exacerbations of spasticity.

Route	Onset	Peak	Duration
P.O.	Hours-weeks	2-3 hr	8 hr
Intrathecal	0.5-1 hr	4 hr	4-8 hr

Diazepam as a skeletal muscle relaxant

Diazepam (Valium) is a benzodiazepine with antispastic effects besides its antianxiety, hypnotic, and anticonvulsant ones. Useful in various chronic disorders in which spasticity is a component, diazepam is one of the most effective agents available for treating acute muscle spasms. It seems to work by enhancing the inhibitory effect on muscle contraction of the neurotransmitter gamma-aminobutyric acid.

In treating spasticity, diazepam is useful alone or with other drugs, especially in patients with spinal cord lesions and occasionally in patients with cerebral palsy. It is useful in patients who have painful continuous muscle spasms and are not too susceptible to the drug's sedative effect; its tranquilizing properties may be helpful in anxious patients. However, diazepam's use is limited by its central nervous system effects and the tolerance that develops with prolonged use.

Diazepam therapy is initiated with 2 mg P.O. b.i.d.; the dosage is increased slowly every few days until adverse reactions develop or until it reaches 10 mg t.i.d or q.i.d. Children may be given initial doses of 2.5 mg t.i.d. or q.i.d., increased as needed and as tolerated. A slow upward titration will minimize the sedation associated with diazepam. In the geriatric patient, the initial dosage should not exceed 2 mg daily.

PHARMACODYNAMICS

The exact mechanism of action of baclofen has not been established. Baclofen is an analogue of the neurotransmitter gamma-aminobutyric acid and probably acts in the spinal cord.

Baclofen seems to depress neuron activity, decreasing the degree and frequency of muscle spasms and reducing muscle tone. Its overall effect reduces the frequency and severity of painful flexor or extensor muscle spasms. Baclofen also reduces protracted muscle spasms of the lower extremities in patients with spinal spasticity.

Because baclofen produces less sedation than diazepam and less peripheral muscle weakness than dantrolene, it is the drug of choice to treat spasticity.

PHARMACOTHERAPEUTICS

Baclofen's principal clinical indication is for the paraplegic or quadriplegic patient with spinal cord lesions, most commonly caused by MS or trauma. For these patients, baclofen significantly reduces the number and severity of painful flexor spasms. Aside from these benefits, however, baclofen does not improve stiff gait, increase manual dexterity, or improve residual muscle function.

Drug interactions

Few drug interactions are reported with baclofen; the most significant is an increase in CNS depression when baclofen is administered with other CNS depressants, including alcohol. Other drug interactions include prolonged analgesia when fentanyl and baclofen are administered concomitantly, aggravation of **hyperkinesia** when lithium carbonate and baclofen are administered concomitantly, and increased muscle relaxation when tricyclic antidepressants and baclofen are administered concomitantly.

ADVERSE DRUG REACTIONS

The most common adverse reaction to baclofen is transient drowsiness. Other, less frequent adverse reactions include nausea, fatigue, vertigo, **hypotonia,** muscle weakness, depression, and headache. These can be avoided by a slow titration of the dose.

Geriatric patients or patients with CVA and brain disorders may experience psychiatric disturbances, such as hallucinations, euphoria, depression, confusion, and anxiety. Dosage increases should be made even more slowly in these patients.

Other rare neuropsychiatric disturbances include insomnia, muscle pain, paresthesia, tinnitus, slurred speech, **tremor, rigidity,** ataxia, seizures, blurred vision, strabismus, nystagmus, diplopia, and dysarthria. Abrupt discontinuation of baclofen may precipitate seizures. Baclofen rarely causes adverse genitourinary reactions. Cardiovascular reactions include hypotension and, rarely, dyspnea, chest pain, and syncope. Adverse GI reactions include nausea, vomiting, constipation and, rarely, dry mouth, anorexia, taste disorders, and diarrhea.

Rash, allergic skin disorders, and pruritus have occurred with baclofen, as have ankle edema, weight gain, and excessive diaphoresis.

NURSING PROCESS APPLICATION

The following information assists the nurse in caring for a patient who is receiving baclofen. It includes an overview of assessment activities as well as examples of appropriate nursing diagnoses and related interventions (under "Planning and implementation"). It also highlights the importance of evaluation.

Assessment

Before drug therapy begins, review the patient's history for conditions that contraindicate or require cautious use of baclofen. Also review the patient's medication history to identify use of drugs that may interact with it. During therapy, assess the patient for adverse drug reactions and signs of drug interactions. Also, periodically assess the effectiveness of baclofen therapy. Finally, evaluate the patient's and family's knowledge about the drug.

Nursing diagnoses

- Risk for injury related to a preexisting condition that contraindicates or requires cautious use of baclofen
- Risk for injury related to adverse drug reactions or drug interactions

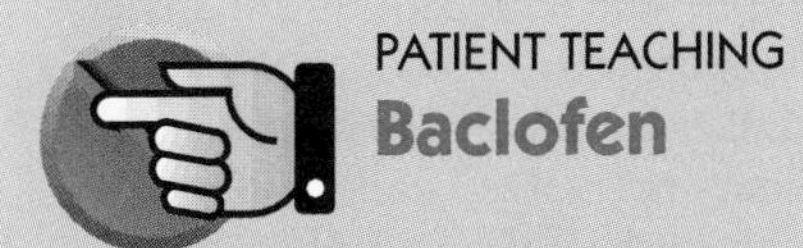

PATIENT TEACHING
Baclofen

- Teach the patient and family the name, dose, frequency, action, and adverse effects of baclofen.
- Inform the patient that baclofen may impair mental alertness or physical coordination, increasing the risks associated with operating machinery or driving a motor vehicle.
- Advise the patient to avoid alcohol while taking baclofen.
- Instruct the patient to take baclofen with meals or milk to prevent GI distress.

- Activity intolerance related to possible ineffectiveness of baclofen
- Knowledge deficit related to baclofen

Planning and implementation

- Do not administer baclofen to a patient with a condition that contraindicates its use.
- Administer baclofen cautiously to a patient at risk because of a preexisting condition.
- Monitor the patient periodically for adverse reactions.

* ***Monitor for impaired renal function by documenting the patient's fluid intake and output and body weight daily. Impaired renal function may require dosage reduction because baclofen is excreted primarily in the urine.*** (See Patient Teaching: *Baclofen.*)

- Do not discontinue baclofen abruptly.
- Notify the physician if adverse reactions occur.
- Monitor the number and severity of painful flexor spasms.
- Assess the patient's degree of bowel and bladder control.
- Notify the physician if baclofen does not improve the patient's spasticity or bowel and bladder control.

Evaluation

For each nursing diagnosis, prepare an evaluation statement that describes the patient's or family's response to nursing interventions.

CHAPTER SUMMARY

Chapter 11 investigated the skeletal muscle relaxants, which act to relieve musculoskeletal pain or spasm and severe musculoskeletal spasticity. Here are the chapter highlights.

Some skeletal muscle relaxants have minimal skeletal muscle relaxing effects, and their actions may be related to their CNS depressant effects; these are centrally acting drugs. Others act on the skeletal muscle itself; these are peripherally acting drugs. Two other drugs — baclofen, which may act on the spinal cord, and diazepam, an antianxiety agent — have valuable antispastic effects.

The centrally acting skeletal muscle relaxants include carisoprodol, chlorphenesin, chlorzoxazone, cyclobenzaprine, metaxalone, methocarbamol, and orphenadrine.

Patients with MS, cerebral palsy, spinal cord injury, or CVA may benefit from the peripherally acting agent dantrolene, although it has hepatotoxic potential.

Baclofen's principal indication is for the paraplegic or quadriplegic patient with spinal cord lesions, most commonly caused by MS or trauma.

Questions to consider

See Appendix 1 for answers.

1. Mary Ellis, age 45, develops low back strain. Her physician prescribes methocarbamol (Robaxin) 1.5 g P.O. q.i.d. What is this drug's mechanism of action?
   (a) It may inhibit calcium release from the sarcoplasmic reticulum in muscle cells.
   (b) It enhances the inhibitory effect on muscle contraction of the neurotransmitter gamma-aminobutyric acid.
   (c) It acts directly on the skeletal muscle.
   (d) Its precise action is unknown.

2. Ken Walker, age 50, has cerebral palsy and takes dantrolene (Dantrium) 50 mg P.O. t.i.d. to control his spasticity. What is the most common dose-related adverse reaction associated with this drug?
   (a) Muscle weakness
   (b) Hypotension
   (c) Hepatitis
   (d) Seizures

3. Jim Davis, age 30, develops muscle spasms in his lower back after an automobile accident. His physician prescribes diazepam (Valium). This drug is not indicated for prolonged use because it may cause which of the following problems?
   (a) Hepatotoxicity
   (b) Constipation
   (c) Hypotension
   (d) Tolerance

4. Which of the following explanations best explains why dantrolene is often given to patients with skeletal muscle spasm?
   (a) It acts by depressing the central nervous system.
   (b) It acts by directly acting on skeletal muscle.
   (c) It acts by causing vasodilation.
   (d) It acts on the spinal cord.

5. Which of the following is not true about baclofen?
   (a) It should not be abruptly discontinued.
   (b) It is used to decrease muscle spasm.
   (c) Hypertension is a common adverse effect.
   (d) It should be taken with meals.

12 Antiparkinsonian agents

OBJECTIVES

After reading and studying this chapter, the student should be able to:
1. identify the four cardinal features that characterize Parkinson's disease.
2. identify the major adverse effects of the antiparkinsonian agents.
3. compare the uses of anticholinergic and dopaminergic agents in treating parkinsonism.
4. describe how to apply the nursing process when caring for a patient who is receiving an antiparkinsonian agent.

INTRODUCTION

Drug therapy is an important part of the treatment for **Parkinson's disease,** also known as paralysis agitans. Parkinson's disease is a progressive, idiopathic neurologic disorder caused by depletion, degeneration, or destruction of **dopamine** in the neurons of the brain's basal ganglia. With Parkinson's disease, there is disruption of transmission in the striatum of the extrapyramidal system due to an imbalance of the two neurotransmitters, dopamine (an inhibitory transmitter) and **acetylcholine** (an excitatory transmitter). When the dopaminergic neurons that produce dopamine are damaged, the acetylcholine or cholinergic neurons are not inhibited by the dopamine. Excessive excitation causes the movement disorders of Parkinson's disease. Pharmacologic intervention is aimed at promoting the secretion of dopamine and inhibiting the cholinergic effects. Parkinsonism is an involuntary movement disorder characterized by four cardinal features: **tremor** at rest, **akinesia** (complete or partial loss of muscle movement), **rigidity** (increased muscle tone), and disturbances of posture and equilibrium. Parkinsonism also can result from drugs, encephalitis, neurotoxins, trauma, arteriosclerosis, or other neurologic disorders and environmental factors.

This chapter includes synthetic anticholinergic and **dopaminergic** agents used to treat parkinsonism. (See *Selected major antiparkinsonian agents,* page 142.)

The drugs that will be covered in this chapter include:
- amantadine hydrochloride
- benztropine mesylate
- biperiden hydrochloride
- biperiden lactate
- bromocriptine meslyate
- carbidopa-levadopa
- diphenhydramine hydrochloride
- ethopropazine
- levodopa
- orphenadrine citrate
- pergolide mesylate
- procyclidine hydrochloride
- selegiline hydrochloride
- trihexyphenidyl hydrochloride

Anticholinergic agents

Anticholinergics are sometimes called parasympatholytics because they antagonize functions controlled primarily by the parasympathetic nervous system. Anticholinergics used to treat parkinsonism are classified in three chemical categories: synthetic tertiary amines, phenothiazine derivatives, and antihistamines. The synthetic tertiary amines constitute the largest group, including benztropine mesylate, biperiden hydrochloride, biperiden lactate, procyclidine hydrochloride, and trihexyphenidyl hydrochloride. Ethopropazine (a phenothiazine derivative) and diphenhydramine hydrochloride and orphenadrine citrate (antihistamines) constitute the remainder of these anticholinergics.

PHARMACOKINETICS

In general, the anticholinergics are well absorbed from the gastrointestinal (GI) tract and cross the blood-brain barrier to their action site in the brain. Most of them undergo hepatic metabolism and renal excretion.

After oral administration, nearly complete absorption occurs readily in the GI tract. Food does not significantly reduce absorption of anticholinergics. The exact distribution of most of these agents is undetermined. The liver metabolizes most anticholinergics at least partially. Anticholinergics are usually excreted in urine as metabolites and unchanged drug.

Benztropine is a long-acting drug with a duration of action up to 24 hours in some patients. For most anticholinergics, half-life is undetermined. Some anticholinergics may also be given I.M. or I.V.

Selected major antiparkinsonian agents

This table summarizes the major antiparkinsonian agents currently in clinical use.

DRUG	MAJOR INDICATIONS AND USUAL DOSAGES	CONTRAINDICATIONS AND PRECAUTIONS
Anticholinergic agents		
benztropine mesylate (Cogentin)	*Initial or adjunct treatment of all forms of parkinsonism* ADULT: 0.5 to 1 mg P.O. daily as a single dose h.s., increased by 0.5 mg every few days, until most effective dosage is reached; maintenance dosage, 1 to 2 mg P.O., I.V., or I.M. daily	• Benztropine is contraindicated in a patient with known hypersensitivity to the drug, angle-closure glaucoma, obstructive uropathy, tachycardia secondary to cardiac insufficiency or thyrotoxicosis, acute hemorrhage causing unstable cardiovascular status, severe ulcerative colitis, toxic megacolon that complicates ulcerative colitis, obstructive gastrointestinal (GI) disease, myasthenia gravis, or tardive dyskinesia. • This drug requires cautious use in a pregnant patient or one with autonomic neuropathy, diarrhea, mild to moderate ulcerative colitis, known or suspected GI infections, fever or exposure to elevated environmental temperatures, hyperthyroidism, hepatic or renal disease, gastric ulcers, esophageal reflux, hiatal hernia associated with reflux esophagitis, hypertension, tachyarrhythmias, heart failure or coronary artery disease (CAD), or chronic pulmonary disease with debilitation. • Benztropine is contraindicated in children under age 3 and should be used with caution in older children because of the drug's adverse anticholinergic effects.
trihexyphenidyl hydrochloride (Artane)	*Initial or adjunct treatment of all forms of parkinsonism* ADULT: 3 to 15 mg P.O. t.i.d.	• Trihexyphenidyl is contraindicated in a breast-feeding patient or one with known hypersensitivity to the drug, angle-closure glaucoma, obstructive uropathy, tachycardia secondary to cardiac insufficiency or thyrotoxicosis, acute hemorrhage that causes unstable cardiovascular status, severe ulcerative colitis, toxic megacolon that complicates ulcerative colitis, obstructive GI disease, or myasthenia gravis. • This drug requires cautious use in a pregnant patient or one with autonomic neuropathy, diarrhea, mild to moderate ulcerative colitis, known or suspected GI infections, fever or exposure to elevated environmental temperatures, hyperthyroidism, hepatic or renal disease, gastric ulcers, esophageal reflux, hiatal hernia associated with reflux esophagitis, hypertension, tachyarrhythmias, heart failure, CAD, or chronic pulmonary disease with debilitation. • Safety and efficacy in children have not been established.
diphenhydramine hydrochloride (Benadryl)	*All forms of parkinsonism* ADULT: initially, 25 mg P.O. t.i.d., increased gradually to 25 to 50 mg P.O. t.i.d. or q.i.d. at 4- to 6-hour intervals, based on the patient's response and tolerance; 10 to 100 mg I.M. or I.V.	• Diphenhydramine is contraindicated in a neonate or premature infant, a breast-feeding patient, or a patient with known hypersensitivity to the drug or to any structurally similar antihistamine. • This drug requires cautious use in a pregnant patient or one with angle-closure glaucoma, stenosing peptic ulcer, pyloric or duodenal obstruction, symptomatic prostatic hypertrophy, or bladder-neck obstruction.
Dopaminergic agents		
levodopa (Dopar, Larodopa)	*Parkinsonism, especially with moderate to severe symptoms* ADULT: 3 to 6 g P.O. daily in three or more divided doses	• Levodopa is contraindicated in a breast-feeding patient or one with known hypersensitivity to the drug, angle-closure glaucoma, suspicious undiagnosed skin lesions, a history of melanoma, or a need for monoamine oxidase (MAO) inhibitors. • This drug requires cautious use in a pregnant patient or one with severe cardiovascular or pulmonary disease; bronchial asthma; renal, hepatic, or endocrine disease; psychiatric disorder; history of myocardial infarction (MI) with residual atrial, nodal, or ventricular arrhythmias; or history of active peptic ulcer disease. • Safety and efficacy in children under age 12 have not been established.

Selected major antiparkinsonian agents *(continued)*

DRUG	MAJOR INDICATIONS AND USUAL DOSAGES	CONTRAINDICATIONS AND PRECAUTIONS
Dopaminergic agents *(continued)*		
carbidopa-levodopa (Sinemet Sinemet CR)	*Parkinsonism, especially with moderate to severe symptoms* ADULT: 75/300 to 200/2,000 mg P.O. daily in divided doses	• Carbidopa-levodopa is contraindicated in a breast-feeding patient or one with known hypersensitivity to these drugs, angle-closure glaucoma, suspicious undiagnosed skin lesions, history of melanoma, or need for MAO inhibitors. • This drug requires cautious use in a pregnant patient or one with severe cardiovascular or pulmonary disease; bronchial asthma; renal, hepatic, or endocrine disease; psychiatric disorder; history of MI with residual atrial, nodal, or ventricular arrhythmias; or history of active peptic ulcer disease. • Safety and efficacy in children under age 18 have not been established.
pergolide mesylate (Permax)	*Adjunct treatment with carbidopa-levodopa for Parkinson's disease* ADULT: initially, 0.05 mg P.O. daily for 2 days, increased by 0.1 to 0.15 mg daily every third day for 12 days, then increased by 0.25 mg daily every third day until a therapeutic dosage is reached	• Pergolide is contraindicated in a breast-feeding patient or one with known hypersensitivity to this drug or other ergot derivatives. • This drug requires cautious use in a pregnant patient or one prone to cardiac arrhythmias. • Safety and efficacy in children have not been established.
selegiline hydrochloride (Eldepryl)	*Adjunct treatment with levodopa or carbidopa-levodopa for Parkinson's disease* ADULT: 5 to 10 mg P.O. daily	• Selegiline is contraindicated in a patient with known hypersensitivity to the drug or one who is taking meperidine, fluoxetine, or a tricyclic antidepressant. • This drug requires cautious use in a pregnant or breast-feeding patient. • Use of selegiline in children has not been evaluated.

Route	Onset	Peak	Duration
P.O.	1 hr	1-4 hr	6-24 hr
I.M.	15 min	1-4 hr	6-24 hr
I.V.	Immediate	1-4 hr	6-24 hr

PHARMACODYNAMICS

In the brain, anticholinergics counteract the cholinergic activity believed to be present in Parkinson's disease. Because dopamine helps control motor activity, a lack of it will cause problems in coordinating smooth motor movements. At the same time, a relative excess of acetylcholine activity develops, producing an excitatory effect on the central nervous system (CNS), which may cause the parkinsonian tremor. The mechanism of action of the anticholinergics is not known.

PHARMACOTHERAPEUTICS

Anticholinergics are used to treat all forms of parkinsonism, but they are used most commonly in the early stages of Parkinson's disease when symptoms are mild and do not have a major impact on the patient's lifestyle. These agents effectively control sialorrhea (excessive flow of saliva) and are about 20% effective in reducing the incidence and severity of akinesia and rigidity. Anticholinergics may be used alone or with amantadine in the early stages of Parkinson's disease. They may be given with levodopa during the later stages to relieve symptoms further. Trihexyphenidyl is the most widely used drug of the group.

Most anticholinergics maintain their effectiveness with long-term administration and rarely require dosage adjustment after the proper dosage is reached. Abrupt withdrawal of anticholinergics can produce confusion, exhaustion, and exacerbation of parkinsonian symptoms.

Drug interactions

A few drugs, such as amantadine, levodopa, and the antipsychotics, produce clinically significant interactions when used with anticholinergics. (See Drug Interactions: *Anticholinergics*, page 144.)

ADVERSE DRUG REACTIONS

Most of the adverse effects of the anticholinergics are an extension of their pharmacologic effects. Mild, dose-related adverse reactions are seen in 30% to 50% of patients.

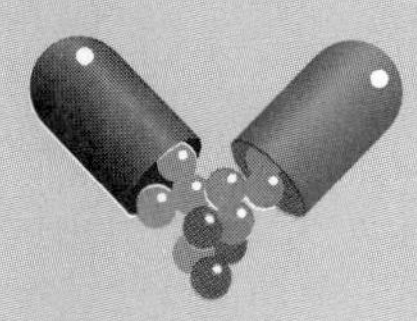

DRUG INTERACTIONS

Anticholinergcs

The most common interactions occur between anticholinergic agents and drugs that have anticholinergic properties. Other interactions involving antipsychotic drugs may produce serious problems.

DRUG	INTERACTING AGENTS	POSSIBLE EFFECTS	NURSING IMPLICATIONS
benztropine, biperiden, diphenhydramine, ethopropazine, orphenadrine procyclidine, trihexyphenidyl	amantadine	Increased anticholenergic adverse effects	• Monitor the patient for changes in mental status and other adverse reactions, such as urine retention, dry mouth, blurred vision, and constipation. • Expect to reduce the dose of either agent, as prescribed, if intolerable anticholinergic adverse reactions occur.
	levodopa	Decreased levodopa absorption, which could lead to worsening Parkinsonian signs and symptoms	• Monitor the patient for increased rigidity, bradykinesia, and tremor. Instruct the patient to report these problems to the physician. • Expect to increase the levodopa dosage, as prescribed.
	antipsychotics (phenothiazines, thiothixene, haloperidol, loxapine)	Decreased effectiveness of anticholinergics; decreased effectiveness of antipsychotics; increased incidence of anticholinergic adverse reactions	• Avoid concomitant use of anticholinergics and antipsychotics. • Observe the patient for an increase in parkinsonian signs or deterioration in mental status. Instruct the patient and family to report these problems to the physician. • Monitor the patient for increased anticholinergic adverse reactions.
	over-the-counter cough or cold preparations, diet aids, or analeptics (agents used to stay awake)	Increased anticholinergic effects	• Advise the patient not to take these drugs without consulting the physician because they may contain ingredients that have anticholinergic properties.
	alcohol	Increased depression of the central nervous system	• Teach the patient that alcohol may increase the drowsiness produced by the anticholinergic agent.

Typically, reactions decrease as treatment continues, but they may limit the dosage that the patient can tolerate. One way to review the various dose-related adverse reactions is to start at the head of the body and move down. (See *Dose-related adverse reactions to anticholinergics.*)

Anticholinergics also can produce various patient-sensitivity-related adverse reactions, including urticaria and allergic rashes that may lead to exfoliation. Diphenhydramine also can produce a photosensitivity reaction (abnormal reaction of the skin to sunlight), causing burning and redness with minimal exposure.

Rare adverse effects include blood dyscrasias. Prolonged therapy with some antihistamines may precipitate angle-closure glaucoma. High dosages of an anticholinergic can cause psychiatric disturbances that differ from the confusion usually associated with anticholinergic therapy.

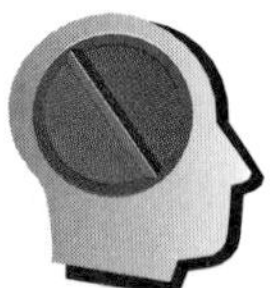

CRITICAL THINKING: To enhance your critical thinking about antiparkinsonian agents, consider the following situation and analysis.

Situation: Ms. Patel is a 69-year-old female with recently diagnosed Parkinson's disease. She is brought to the emergency room by her daughter with a 12-hour history of blurred vision and deteriorating mental status. The patient has been taking benztropine (Cogentin) 2 mg P.O. at bedtime following her diagnosis of Parkinson's disease 1 year ago. Her daughter states that Ms. Patel has been self-medicating a recent cold (onset, 5 days) with an over-the-counter antihistamine-decongestant. She has also been taking an over-the-counter sleeping pill since the onset of her cold symptoms to help her rest. On examination, the patient's pupils are dilated and weakly reactive to light. She is oriented to person only. How might you explain her signs and symptoms?

Analysis: The patient is experiencing significant anticholinergic toxicity secondary to overmedication. The cough-cold

Dose-related adverse reactions to anticholinergics

Common dose-related adverse reactions to anticholinergic agents are listed below. Use this illustration as a head-to-toe guide when assessing a patient.

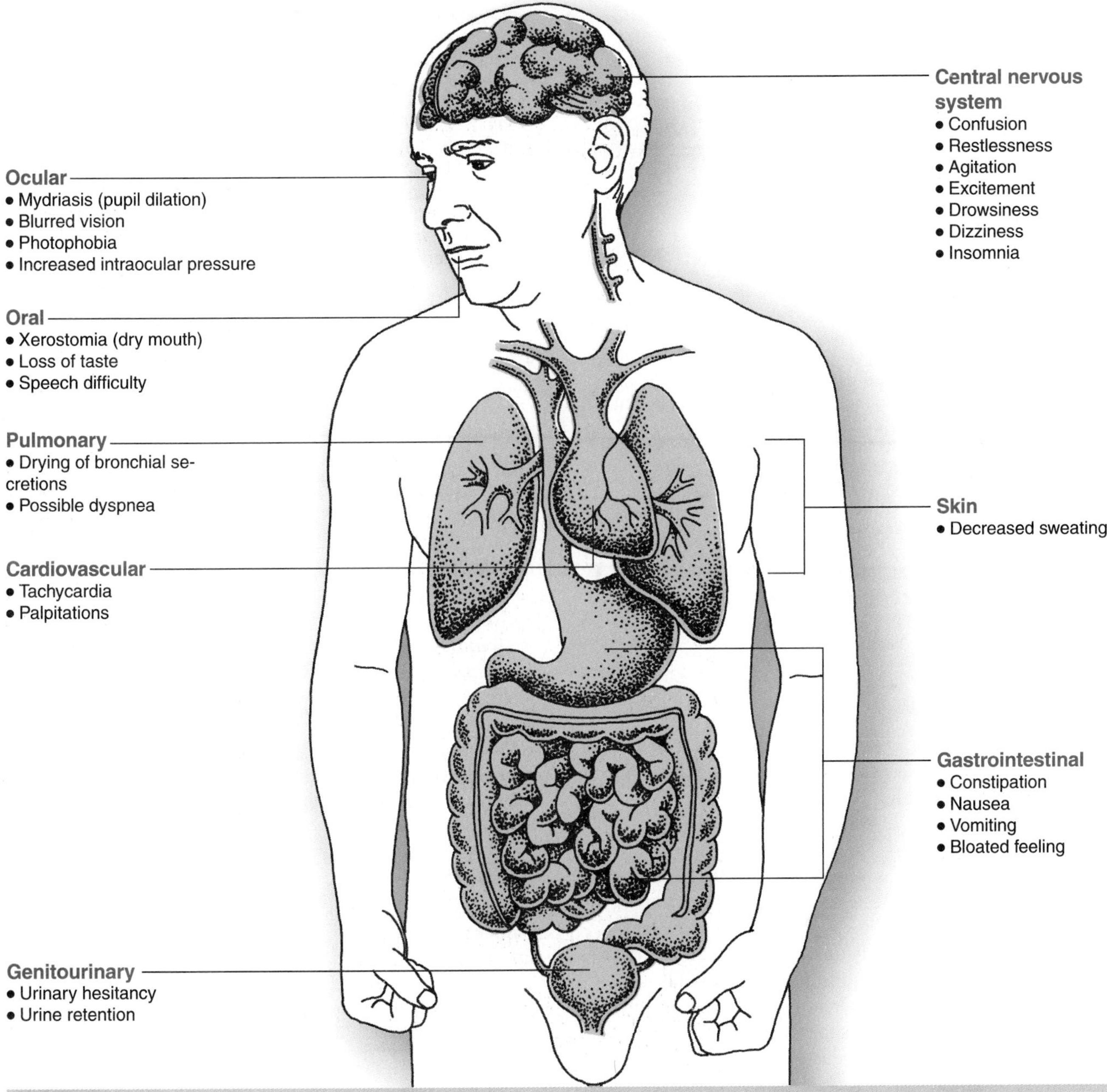

preparation and the sleeping pill (most likely an antihistamine) will have additive anticholinergic effects with her anticholinergic agent, benztropine. A patient who is taking an anticholinergic agent should be instructed not to take over-the-counter cough-cold preparations, diet aids, or analeptics (agents used to stay awake) because of potential interactions with the prescribed anticholinergic agent.

NURSING PROCESS APPLICATION

The following information assists the nurse in caring for a patient who is receiving an anticholinergic. It includes an overview of assessment activities as well as examples of appropriate nursing diagnoses and related interventions (un-

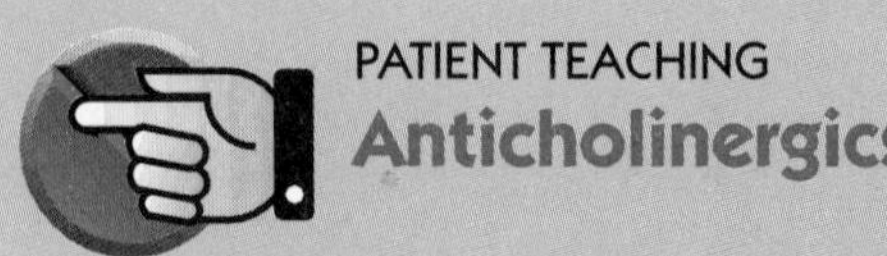

PATIENT TEACHING

Anticholinergics

- Teach the patient and family the name, dose, frequency, action, and adverse effects of the prescribed anticholinergic agent.
- Encourage the patient and family to ask questions about the prescribed anticholinergic agent.
- Teach the patient to relieve xerostomia by drinking cold beverages, sucking on sugarless hard candy, or using a nonprescription saliva substitute. Encourage proper oral hygiene.
- Instruct the patient to use caution when performing tasks that require alertness because of the risk from adverse reactions, such as drowsiness or blurred vision.
- Advise the patient to avoid prolonged exposure to high temperatures because an anticholinergic agent increases the risk of heat stroke by reducing sweating.
- Teach the patient not to discontinue long-term anticholinergic therapy before consulting the physician.
- Instruct the patient not to take over-the-counter cough or cold preparations, diet aids, or analeptics (agents used to stay awake) without consulting the physician because of potential interactions with the prescribed anticholinergic agent.
- Teach the patient that alcohol may increase the drowsiness produced by the anticholinergic agent.
- Advise the patient and family to inform the physician of improving or worsening of parkinsonian signs and symptoms.
- Advise the patient to notify the physician of adverse drug reactions.
- Instruct family members to inform the physician of any signs of confusion or mental changes in the patient, especially in an elderly patient.
- Give the patient written instructions about the prescribed anticholinergic agent.

der "Planning and implementation"). It also highlights the importance of evaluation.

Assessment

Before drug therapy begins, review the patient's history for conditions that contraindicate or require cautious use of the prescribed anticholinergic agent. Also review the patient's medication history to identify use of drugs that may interact with it. During therapy, assess the patient for adverse drug reactions, such as urine retention, and signs of drug interactions. Periodically assess the effectiveness of anticholinergic therapy. Finally, evaluate the patient's and family's knowledge about the prescribed drug.

Nursing diagnoses

- Risk for injury related to a preexisting condition that contraindicates or requires cautious use of an anticholinergic agent
- Risk for injury related to adverse drug reactions or drug interactions
- Urinary retention related to use of an anticholinergic agent

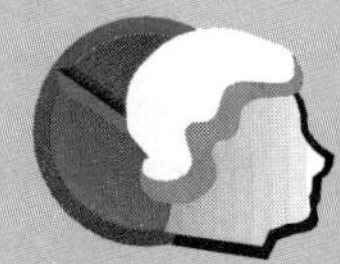

GERIATRIC CONSIDERATIONS

Anticholinergics

Although therapeutically necessary, anticholinergic agents can cause serious adverse effects in a geriatric patient. For example, xerostomia may decrease the patient's desire to eat and increase the risk of oral infections, thus impacting overall nutrient intake. Mydriasis decreases the ability to accommodate and increases the risks for falls. Decreased gastrointestinal motility and constipation may lead to fecal impaction. Tachycardia associated with anticholinergic use may worsen an existing cardiac condition. Hyperthermia may occur secondary to poor thermoregulation. Finally, the effects of anticholinergic agents on the central nervous system may worsen confusion, impaired concentration, and dementia.

- Knowledge deficit related to the prescribed anticholinergic agent

Planning and implementation

- Do not administer an anticholinergic agent to a patient with a condition that contraindicates its use. (See Patient Teaching: *Anticholinergics.*)
- Administer an anticholinergic agent cautiously to a patient at risk because of a preexisting condition. (See Geriatric Considerations: *Anticholinergics*).
- Monitor the patient's vital signs and respiratory status.

* ***Administer an anticholinergic agent during or shortly after meals to prevent adverse GI reactions.***

- Notify the physician if the patient experiences adverse reactions.

* ***Record fluid intake and output during anticholinergic therapy. Observe for decreased urine output.***

- Notify the physician if the patient experiences urine retention.

Evaluation

For each nursing diagnosis, prepare an evaluation statement that describes the patient's or family's response to nursing interventions.

Dopaminergic agents

Dopaminergics include six chemically unrelated drugs: levodopa, the metabolic precursor to dopamine; carbidopa-levodopa, a combination drug composed of the substance carbidopa along with levodopa; amantadine hydrochloride, an antiviral agent; bromocriptine mesylate, a semisynthetic ergot alkaloid; pergolide mesylate, a dopamine agonist; and selegiline, a type B **monoamine oxidase (MAO) inhibitor.**

PHARMACOKINETICS

Like anticholinergics, dopaminergics are absorbed from the GI tract into the bloodstream and are delivered to their action site in the brain. They are metabolized extensively in various areas of the body and eliminated by the liver, kidneys, or both.

Levodopa absorption is slowed and reduced when the drug is ingested with food. The body absorbs most of a levodopa, carbidopa-levodopa, or amantadine dose from the GI tract after oral administration, but it absorbs only about 28% of a bromocriptine dose. The body may absorb a significant amount of pergolide, although its absorption percentage is not fully known. It absorbs about 73% of an oral dose of selegiline.

Levodopa is widely distributed into most body tissues, including the GI tract, liver, pancreas, kidneys, salivary glands, and skin. Carbidopa-levodopa also is widely distributed. Amantadine is distributed in saliva, nasal secretions, and breast milk. Bromocriptine is 90% to 96% bound to serum albumin. Pergolide is approximately 90% protein-bound. The distribution of selegiline is unknown.

Large amounts of levodopa are metabolized in the lumen of the stomach and during the first pass through the liver. It is metabolized extensively to various compounds that are excreted by the kidneys. Carbidopa is not metabolized extensively. The kidneys excrete approximately one-third of it as unchanged drug within 24 hours. The pharmacokinetic processes of amantadine and bromocriptine are not understood completely. Amantadine is excreted mostly unchanged by the kidneys. Almost all of a bromocriptine dose is metabolized hepatically to pharmacologically inactive compounds and primarily eliminated in the feces; only 2.5% to 5.5% is excreted in the urine. After pergolide is metabolized, it is excreted by the kidneys. Selegiline is metabolized to amphetamine, methamphetamine, and N-desmethylselegin (the major metabolite), which are eliminated in the urine.

The onset of action, peak concentration levels, and duration of action of levodopa — with or without carbidopa — vary widely in patients. Administration of levodopa with food may delay its onset. Levodopa produces a short-term improvement that subsides 5 hours after a dose and a long-term improvement with prolonged therapy. The half-life of carbidopa-levodopa is approximately 2 hours, or about double that of levodopa alone. Amantadine's peak concentration is reached approximately 1 to 4 hours after administration. Its half-life varies greatly but averages 24 hours. Bromocriptine's onset varies somewhat; improvement in parkinsonian signs may occur 30 to 90 minutes after a single dose. Peak concentration occurs in approximately 2 hours, and the duration of action is 3 to 5 hours. Bromocriptine has a half-life of 6 hours.

Pergolide's onset ranges from 15 to 20 minutes. It reaches peak concentration in 1 to 3 hours. Its duration of action and half-life are unknown. After oral administration, selegiline attains peak concentration in 2 hours. Its onset, duration, and half-life have not been identified.

Route	Onset	Peak	Duration
P.O.	15-90 min	1-4 hr	3-5 hr

PHARMACODYNAMICS

The dopaminergics act in the brain by increasing the dopamine concentration or by enhancing neurotransmission of dopamine, thereby improving motor function.

Levodopa is pharmacologically inactive until it crosses the blood-brain barrier and is converted to dopamine by enzymes in the brain. After this conversion, levodopa acts primarily by increasing dopamine concentrations in the basal ganglia. Carbidopa enhances levodopa's effectiveness. Amantadine's mechanism of action is less clear. It may increase the amount of dopamine in the brain by increasing dopamine release or by blocking dopamine reuptake from presynaptic neurons. Bromocriptine stimulates dopamine receptors in the brain, producing effects that are similar to dopamine's. Pergolide directly stimulates postsynaptic dopamine receptors in the CNS. Selegiline may increase dopaminergic activity by inhibiting type B MAO activity or by other mechanisms.

PHARMACOTHERAPEUTICS

Usually, dopaminergics are used to treat patients with severe parkinsonism or those who do not respond to anticholinergics alone. Levodopa, a dopaminergic agent, is the most effective drug used to treat Parkinson's disease.

Carbidopa given with levodopa is preferred because it reduces the levodopa dosage, decreasing adverse GI and cardiovascular effects. In a patient switching from levodopa alone to carbidopa-levodopa, levodopa must be discontinued at least 8 hours before initiating combination therapy.

Some dopaminergics, such as amantadine and bromocriptine, must be withdrawn gradually to avoid precipitating parkinsonian crisis and possible life-threatening complications.

Drug interactions

The most serious interactions between the dopaminergics and other drugs occur when levodopa is combined with a type A MAO inhibitor, which can cause hypertensive crisis, or with meperidine, which can lead to death. Selegiline has the potential to produce a similar interaction. Other interactions between dopaminergics and other drugs usually decrease the effectiveness of the dopaminergics. (See Drug Interactions: *Dopaminergics,* page 148.)

In some patients, levodopa may produce a significant interaction with foods. Dietary amino acids can decrease levodopa's effectiveness by competing with it for absorption from the intestine and slowing its transport to the brain. Therefore, if a patient's response deteriorates regularly after

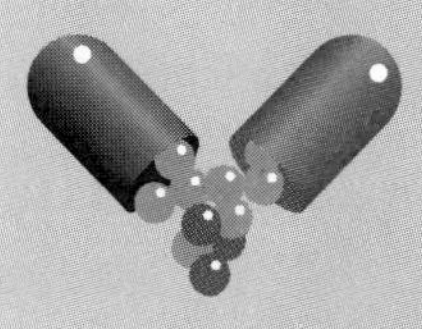

DRUG INTERACTIONS

Dopaminergics

Among the dopaminergics, levodopa causes most of the significant interactions with other drugs and with foods. Levodopa and monoamine oxidase (MAO) inhibitors can produce a hypertensive crisis when given concomitantly. Selegiline and meperidine may cause a fatal reaction. Less serious drug interactions can also occur with other dopaminergics, producing additive toxicities or decreasing the effectiveness of the dopaminergic agent.

DRUG	INTERACTING DRUGS	POSSIBLE EFFECTS	NURSING IMPLICATIONS
levodopa	pyridoxine (vitamin B_6)	Decreased effectiveness of levodopa by increasing peripheral conversion of levodopa to dopamine by vitamin B_6	• Instruct the patient taking levodopa without carbidopa to avoid vitamin B_6 supplements or multiple vitamins containing vitamin B_6. • Expect that this drug interaction may not occur in a patient taking carbidopa-levodopa.
	type A MAO inhibitors and furazolidone	Hypertensive crisis; increased toxic effects of levodopa	• Monitor the patient for hypertension if this combination is given. • Document and inform the physician if the patient starting levodopa has taken an MAO inhibitor in the past 2 weeks.
	phenytoin	Decreased effectiveness of levodopa	• Observe the patient for increased parkinsonian signs, such as bradykinesia, rigidity, and tremor. • Tell the patient to report any worsening of parkinsonian symptoms to the physician.
	benzodiazepines	Inhibited effectiveness of levodopa	• Avoid concomitant administration of these drugs, if possible. • Observe the patient for increased parkinsonian signs, such as bradykinesia, rigidity, and tremor, if this combination is given.
	papaverine	Decreased effectiveness of levodopa	• Avoid concomitant administration, if possible.
levodopa, pergolide	antipsychotics (phenothiazines, thiothixene, haloperidol, loxapine)	Decreased effectiveness of levodopa and pergolide	• Avoid concomitant use of antipsychotics. If an antipsychotic medication is required, thioridazine usually is preferred. • Observe the patient for increased parkinsonian signs, such as bradykinesia, rigidity, and tremor, if this combination is given.
	reserpine	Decreased therapeutic response to levodopa by depleting dopamine stores in the brain	• Avoid administering reserpine to a patient receiving levodopa. • Observe the patient for increased parkinsonian signs, such as bradykinesia, rigidity, and tremor, if this combination is given.
levodopa, amantadine	anticholinergics	Increased anticholinergic effects with amantadine, including adverse effects on mental function; decreased levodopa absorption, possibly leading to worsening of parkinsonian signs and symptoms or exacerbation of abnormal involuntary movements	• Monitor the patient taking amantadine for changes in mental status and other adverse reactions, such as urine retention, dry mouth, blurred vision, and constipation. • Expect to reduce the dosage of either agent, as prescribed, if intolerable anticholinergic adverse reactions occur. • Monitor the patient taking levodopa for increased rigidity, bradykinesia, and tremor and for exacerbation of abnormal involuntary movements.
selegiline	meperidine	Fatal reactions	• Avoid concomitant administration.

meals, the patient may need to reduce protein intake and avoid taking levodopa with meals to minimize this interaction.

ADVERSE DRUG REACTIONS

Among the dopaminergics, amantadine produces the fewest adverse reactions. Adverse reactions to bromocriptine, pergolide, and levodopa are mainly dose-related and can occur peripherally or in the CNS. With daily recommended dosages, selegiline produces few adverse reactions.

Adverse reactions to levodopa or carbidopa-levodopa usually are dose-related and reversible. Carbidopa decreases levodopa's peripheral effects but not its CNS effects. Levodopa commonly produces adverse GI reactions, such as nausea, vomiting, and anorexia. It also can cause orthostatic (postural) hypotension as well as other, less common adverse cardiovascular reactions, such as palpitations, tachycardia, arrhythmias, flushing, and hypertension. Additional adverse reactions include dark-colored urine and sweat, urinary frequency or urine retention, CNS disturbances (irritability, confusion, and hallucinations), and visual difficulties.

After withdrawal of levodopa, some patients experience **hyperpyrexia** (extreme elevation of body temperature) and neuroleptic malignant syndrome (characterized by hyperthermia, akinesia, altered consciousness, muscular rigidity, and profuse sweating). Both of these reactions can be fatal. Hematologic effects — such as leukopenia, granulocytopenia, thrombocytopenia, hemolytic anemia, and decreased hemoglobin and hematocrit levels — may also occur. When used alone, levodopa can cause transient elevations of liver enzymes, bilirubin, and blood urea nitrogen (BUN). When combined with carbidopa, levodopa may produce lower BUN, serum creatinine, and uric acid laboratory test values.

The most distressing problem with levodopa is the drug's loss of effectiveness after 3 to 5 years. The problem takes one of two forms: the on-off phenomenon, characterized by sharp fluctuations between mobility and immobility, or the end-of-dose deterioration (also known as the wearing-off effect), a progressive decrease in the duration of beneficial effects from each levodopa dose. The use of smaller, more frequent doses of levodopa and adjunctive therapy (e.g., selegiline and pergolide) can reduce both problems.

Amantadine produces relatively few adverse reactions at usual dosages. However, long-term therapy may produce livedo reticularis (diffuse, mottled reddening of the skin usually confined to the lower extremities), which commonly is accompanied by mild ankle edema. Other relatively common adverse reactions include urine retention, orthostatic hypotension, anorexia, nausea, and constipation. Adverse CNS reactions may include inability to concentrate, confusion, light-headedness, anxiety, insomnia, irritability, dizziness, and hallucinations. Rare reactions include rash, leukopenia, eczematoid dermatitis, seizures, oculogyric episodes, and lingual and facial dyskinesias.

Besides cost, adverse reactions are the most important factor limiting the use of bromocriptine. Adverse reactions are more common at the start of therapy and when dosage exceeds 20 mg/day. Adverse GI reactions, such as nausea, occur commonly. Other common initial adverse reactions include orthostatic hypotension, vomiting, acute anxiety, dizziness, and sedation. Erythromelalgia also may occur. Bromocriptine can cause adverse reactions in the cardiovascular system by producing persistent orthostatic hypotension (which may result in syncope), edema in the ankles and feet, palpitations, ventricular tachycardia, bradycardia, and exacerbation of angina. Confusion, hallucinations, delusions, nightmares, and erythromelalgia are notable especially during long-term or high-dosage (100 mg or more daily) bromocriptine therapy, but they usually are reversible. The presence of adverse CNS reactions usually limits the dosage and is the main reason for discontinuation of bromocriptine therapy.

Bromocriptine therapy has been associated with pleuropulmonary reactions, such as pulmonary infiltrates, pleural effusions, and thickening of the pleura. Bladder dysfunction with incontinence, urinary frequency, and urine retention have also been reported. Signs and symptoms of ergotism, including numbness and tingling of the extremities, cold feet, and muscle cramps in the legs and feet, also may occur.

The most common adverse reactions to pergolide include confusion, dyskinesia, hallucinations, nausea, and constipation. Hypertension is less common. Other adverse reactions may include abdominal pain, dizziness, drowsiness, flulike symptoms, orthostatic hypotension, lower back pain, rhinitis, and weakness; they may require medical attention if they continue or are bothersome. Rarely, pergolide has been associated with cerebrovascular hemorrhage, myocardial infarction, chills, diarrhea, xerostomia, facial edema, appetite loss, and vomiting.

Selegiline usually does not cause serious adverse reactions. However, it may produce nausea, dry mouth, dizziness, light-headedness, fainting, confusion, and hallucinations. Additional adverse reactions include vivid dreams, dyskinesia, headache, generalized achiness, anxiety, tension, diarrhea, insomnia, lethargy, leg pain, low back pain, palpitations, urine retention, and weight loss.

NURSING PROCESS APPLICATION

The following information assists the nurse in caring for a patient who is receiving a dopaminergic agent. It includes an overview of assessment activities as well as examples of appropriate nursing diagnoses and related interventions (under "Planning and implementation"). It also highlights the importance of evaluation.

Assessment

Before drug therapy begins, review the patient's history for conditions that contraindicate or require cautious use of the prescribed dopaminergic agent. Also review the patient's

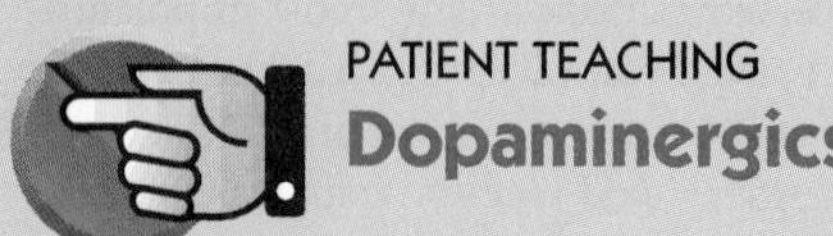

PATIENT TEACHING

Dopaminergics

- Teach the patient and family the name, dose, frequency, action, and adverse effects of the prescribed dopaminergic agent.
- Advise the patient not to exceed the prescribed daily dosage because serious adverse reactions could result.
- Explain the importance of frequent blood pressure measurements, and teach the patient to recognize the symptoms of hypotension (such as dizziness and light-headedness) as well as hypertension (such as headache and vision changes).
- Instruct the family on how to maintain a safe environment to prevent patient injury during periods of confusion.
- Inform the patient that levodopa may cause harmless discoloration of urine and sweat.
- Teach the patient who is taking levodopa about the on-off phenomenon.
- Instruct the female patient to notify her physician if she becomes pregnant or is breast-feeding during dopaminergic therapy.
- Inform the patient that the levodopa-carbidopa dosage may be decreased after adjunct therapy begins with another dopaminergic agent.
- Instruct the patient who is beginning levodopa therapy that the drug may take several weeks or months to reach its maximum effectiveness.
- Teach the patient not to discontinue long-term levodopa, amantadine, or bromocriptine therapy before consulting the physician.
- Teach the diabetic patient how to monitor glucose levels using a blood glucose test.
- Instruct the patient to notify the physician if adverse reactions occur.
- Instruct family members to inform the physician if the patient experiences confusion or mental changes.
- Give the patient written instructions about the prescribed dopaminergic agent.

medication history to identify use of drugs that may interact with it. During therapy, assess the patient for adverse drug reactions and signs of drug interactions. If the patient is receiving levodopa, assess the diet for consumption of foods that may interact with it. Also, periodically assess the effectiveness of dopaminergic therapy. Evaluate the patient's and family's knowledge about the prescribed drug.

Nursing diagnoses

- Risk for injury related to a preexisting condition that contraindicates or requires cautious use of a dopaminergic agent
- Risk for injury related to adverse drug reactions or drug or food interactions
- Impaired physical mobility related to ineffectiveness of a dopaminergic agent, particularly levodopa
- Knowledge deficit related to the prescribed dopaminergic agent

Planning and implementation

- Do not administer a dopaminergic agent to a patient with a condition that contraindicates its use.
- Administer a dopaminergic agent cautiously to a patient at risk because of a preexisting condition.

* ***Monitor the patient's blood pressure for orthostatic hypotension or, if the patient is taking an MAO inhibitor, hypertension.***

- Be aware that levodopa or carbidopa-levodopa may produce false-positive or false-negative results with urine glucose test strips (Tes-Tape, Diastix). (See Patient Teaching: *Dopaminergics.*)

* ***Avoid administering levodopa with meals to prevent a drug-food interaction that may result in a decreased rate and extent of drug absorption.***

- Give the second daily dose of amantadine earlier in the evening if the patient experiences insomnia.
- Monitor the patient's degree of physical mobility.
- Report decreased mobility to the physician.

Evaluation

For each nursing diagnosis, prepare an evaluation statement that describes the patient's or family's response to nursing interventions.

CHAPTER SUMMARY

Chapter 12 concentrated on drugs for Parkinson's disease. Here are the chapter highlights.

Two major drug classes, the anticholinergics and the dopaminergics, are used to treat parkinsonism, which may result from idiopathic Parkinson's disease or other causes.

Anticholinergics may be used alone or with amantadine in the early stages of Parkinson's disease and with levodopa in the more advanced stages.

Most adverse reactions to anticholinergics are an extension of their pharmacologic effects. Typically, they decrease as treatment continues, but may limit the dosage that the patient can take.

Levodopa, a dopaminergic agent, is the most effective drug used to treat Parkinson's disease. Levodopa therapy usually begins during advanced stages, either alone or with other drugs. Carbidopa given with levodopa is preferred because it reduces the levodopa dosage, decreasing GI and cardiovascular adverse effects.

Levodopa presents two major therapeutic problems after 3 to 5 years of treatment: sharp fluctuations between mobility and immobility in the patient and a progressive decrease in beneficial effects. Although smaller, more frequent doses help, both problems become increasingly difficult to manage as the disease progresses.

Amantadine may be used by itself in the early stages of Parkinson's disease or with other drugs in the advanced stages. Patients taking amantadine commonly develop a tolerance to it shortly after therapy begins. Tolerance does not develop, however, when the drug is used with levodopa or bromocriptine.

Bromocriptine, another dopaminergic agent, serves primarily as an adjunct to levodopa in advanced stages of Parkinson's disease. Bromocriptine's major drawbacks are its high cost and its adverse effects.

When given with carbidopa-levodopa, pergolide and selegiline may decrease the levodopa dosage, improve the duration of response, and decrease on-off fluctuations.

Questions to consider

See Appendix 1 for answers.

1. Roy Somers, age 72, takes amantadine 100 mg b.i.d. to treat early-stage Parkinson's disease. Which of the following adverse reactions might he experience with long-term use of this drug?
   (a) Livedo reticularis
   (b) Liver cirrhosis
   (c) Atrial arrhythmias
   (d) Pleural effusions

2. Jean Jones has been prescribed trihexyphenidyl for her Parkinson's disease. Which of the following adverse reactions may be dose-related?
   (a) Excessive salivation
   (b) Dryness of mouth
   (c) Bradycardia
   (d) Diarrhea

3. Sarah Jackson, age 65, has just received a diagnosis of Parkinson's disease. The physician initially prescribes procyclidine 2.5 mg P.O. b.i.d. after meals. Before administering this drug to Ms. Jackson, the nurse assesses her history. Which of the following history findings contraindicates procyclidine use?
   (a) Nystagmus
   (b) Angle-closure glaucoma
   (c) Cataracts
   (d) Blurred vision

4. The nurse warns Ms. Jackson not to use any over-the-counter cough or cold preparations without first consulting the physician. Why is this warning necessary for a patient on procyclidine therapy?
   (a) Procyclidine can decrease the effectiveness of over-the-counter cough or cold preparations.
   (b) Procyclidine interferes with the metabolism of over-the-counter cough or cold preparations.
   (c) Over-the-counter cough or cold preparations can delay the absorption of procyclidine.
   (d) Over-the-counter cough or cold preparations can increase the anticholinergic effects of procyclidine.

5. Which of the following symptoms does *not* characterize the progressive neurologic disorder known as Parkinson's disease?
   (a) Tremor at rest
   (b) Akinesia
   (c) Flaccidity
   (d) Disturbance in posture and equilibrium

6. How do dopaminergic agents work?
   (a) In the periphery by increasing the dopamine concentration or by enhancing neurotransmission of dopamine
   (b) In the brain by counteracting the cholinergic activity that may be present in Parkinson's disease
   (c) In the brain by increasing the dopamine concentration or by enhancing neurotransmission of dopamine
   (d) In the periphery by counteracting the cholinergic activity that may be present in Parkinson's disease

7. Which of the following antiparkinsonian agents is associated with the on-off phenomenon and end-of-dose deterioration?
   (a) amantadine
   (b) benztropine
   (c) selegiline
   (d) carbidopa-levodopa

13 Anticonvulsant agents

OBJECTIVES

After reading and studying this chapter, the student should be able to:

1. describe the mechanisms of action of and the types of seizures treated by hydantoins, barbiturates, iminostilbenes, benzodiazepines, succinimides, and valproic acid.
2. discuss the important adverse reactions associated with each of the six major classes of anticonvulsants.
3. identify the contraindications and precautions for each agent in the six major classes of anticonvulsants.
4. describe how to apply the nursing process when caring for patients who are receiving drugs from each class of anticonvulsants.

INTRODUCTION

Anticonvulsants are prescribed for long-term management of chronic **epilepsy** (recurrent seizures) and for short-term management of acute isolated seizures not caused by epilepsy. The short-term use of anticonvulsants also provides prophylaxis after trauma or a craniotomy. Selected anticonvulsants are indicated in the emergency treatment of **status epilepticus,** which is characterized by a series of rapidly repeating seizures without intervening periods of consciousness.

Seizures can be classified in various ways, but health care professionals usually use the international classification of epileptic seizures as the standard system. (See *International classification of epileptic seizures.*)

The accurate diagnosis of a seizure requires a reliable patient history, careful patient observations, and an electroencephalogram. It also may require a computerized tomography scan or magnetic resonance imaging. The pharmacologic therapy used to treat seizures varies, depending on the type of seizure. The goal of anticonvulsant therapy is to control or prevent seizures. For many patients, anticonvulsant therapy is lifelong. Some patients, however, may have their drug therapy tapered off and eventually discontinued if they do not experience any seizures for a year.

Anticonvulsants fall into six major classes: hydantoins, barbiturates, iminostilbenes, benzodiazepines, succinimides, and valproic acid. (See *Selected major anticonvulsant agents,* pages 154 and 155.)

The drugs that will be covered in this chapter include:

- carbamazepine
- clonazepam
- clorazepate dipotassium
- diazepam
- divalproex sodium
- ethosuximide
- ethotoin
- fosphenytoin
- mephenytoin
- mephobarbital
- methsuximide
- phenobarbital
- phensuximide
- phenytoin
- phenytoin sodium
- primidone
- valproate sodium.

Hydantoins

Phenytoin and phenytoin sodium, the most commonly prescribed anticonvulsant agents, belong to the hydantoin class of drugs. Fosphenytoin is a prodrug of phenytoin. Mephenytoin and ethotoin are also hydantoin anticonvulsants.

PHARMACOKINETICS

Hydantoin anticonvulsants usually are absorbed slowly, rapidly distributed, and extensively protein-bound. These drugs usually are metabolized by hepatic microsomal enzymes and excreted as metabolites in the urine.

Phenytoin is absorbed slowly after oral administration and absorbed poorly after I.M. administration. It is distributed rapidly to all tissues and bound extensively (90%) to plasma proteins, primarily albumin. Phenytoin is metabolized in the liver. Inactive metabolites of phenytoin are excreted in bile and then reabsorbed from the gastrointestinal (GI) tract. Eventually, however, they are excreted in the urine.

Mephenytoin is absorbed rapidly after oral administration. The drug then exhibits moderate protein binding (60%) in the plasma. Metabolism of mephenytoin by the liver results in 5,5-ethylphenylhydantoin, an active metabolite believed to possess the therapeutic and toxic effects attributed to mephenytoin. Excretion occurs via the urine.

Ethotoin is metabolized by the hepatic microsomal enzyme system. Extensively protein-bound, ethotoin is excreted in the urine, primarily as metabolites.

Fosphenytoin is indicated for short-term intravenous (I.V.) or intramuscular (I.M.) administration. Fosphenytoin has a water-soluble formula that eliminates propylene gly-

International classification of epileptic seizures

Anticonvulsant therapy depends primarily on the accurate diagnosis of the seizure type. The following two classifications conform with the international classification scheme and reflect the current practice related to seizure types and their clinical characteristics. A third category of epileptic seizures remains unclassified because of inadequate or incomplete data. Earlier terminology appears in parentheses.

SEIZURE CLASSIFICATION	CLINICAL CHARACTERISTICS
Partial seizures — focal or local seizures	
Simple partial seizures (focal; jacksonian) • Sensory • Motor • Autonomic • Psychic	Most common in older children and adults. Consciousness not impaired; an aura is a simple partial seizure.
Complex partial seizures (psychomotor epilepsy) or **temporal lobe seizures**	Most common in older children and adults; brief impairment of consciousness; characterized by loss of contact with reality, automatisms (automatic behaviors, such as chewing and lip smacking), and confusion that may last 1 to 2 minutes after seizure subsides.
Partial seizures evolving to secondarily generalized seizures	Partial seizures may spread, or "march," and ultimately involve all other parts of the brain with subsequent loss of consciousness. A tonic-clonic seizure follows.
Generalized seizures — convulsive or nonconvulsive	
Absence seizures (petit mal) • Typical	Onset between ages 4 and 8; abrupt loss of consciousness, amnesia, or unawareness characterized by staring and a 3-cycle/second spike and waveform on electroencephalogram; attack lasts 10 to 30 seconds; may occur as frequently as 50 to 100 times/day. No postictal or confused state follows the attack.
• Atypical	Slower onset and cessation of attacks than is usually seen with absence seizures.
Myoclonic seizures	Occur in older children and adults; myoclonic, lightning jerks (flexor or extensor) without loss of consciousness; last from seconds to minutes or longer and may occur daily.
Clonic seizures	Rhythmic clonic contraction and relaxation of muscles, loss of consciousness, and marked autonomic signs and symptoms.
Tonic seizures	Abrupt increase in muscle tone (contraction), loss of consciousness, and marked autonomic signs and symptoms.
Tonic-clonic seizures (grand mal)	Can occur at any age. May be preceded by an aura or an outcry. Contraction of all skeletal muscle masses occurs in rhythmic, alternating clonic and tonic patterns, followed by depression of all central functions, a state called the postictal period. Urinary and fecal incontinence may occur. Usually lasts 2 to 5 minutes but may last much longer. The frequency of attacks varies.
Atonic seizures	Seen in older children and adults. Consciousness usually lost, accompanied by loss of postural tone or akinesia. Lasts a few seconds to minutes and may occur daily.

Adapted from the Commission on Classification and Terminology of the International League Against Epilepsy. "Proposal for Classification of Epilepsies and Epileptic Syndromes," *Epilepsia* 26:268-278, 1985. Used with the permission of Raven Press, Ltd., New York.

col and can be infused three times faster than I.V. phenytoin. Fosphenytoin is well tolerated when administered I.M.

When administered orally, phenytoin demonstrates a variable onset of action, from 30 minutes to 2 hours. When phenytoin is administered I.V., the onset occurs within 3 to 5 minutes. The peak plasma concentration level for prompt-acting phenytoin preparations occurs in 1.5 to 3 hours, although the sustained-release preparation produces peak serum concentrations in 4 to 12 hours. The duration of action for phenytoin depends on the time the drug remains in the therapeutic range.

Mephenytoin exhibits a rapid onset of action, achieving peak serum concentration in 2 to 4 hours. The duration of action of mephenytoin and its major metabolite, 5,5-ethyl-

Selected major anticonvulsant agents

This table summarizes the major anticonvulsants currently in clinical use.

DRUG	MAJOR INDICATIONS AND USUAL DOSAGES	CONTRAINDICATIONS AND PRECAUTIONS
Hydantoins		
phenytoin and phenytoin sodium (Dilantin)	*Complex partial seizures, tonic-clonic seizures* ADULT: 300 to 400 mg P.O. daily in three divided doses if a prompt-acting preparation is used; sustained-release preparations are administered as single doses, usually at bedtime PEDIATRIC: 5 mg/kg/day administered in two to three equally divided doses *Status epilepticus* ADULT: 10 to 15 mg/kg I.V. at a rate not exceeding 50 mg/minute followed by a maintenance dose of 100 mg P.O. or I.V. every 6 to 8 hours PEDIATRIC: 15 to 20 mg/kg I.V. at a rate not exceeding 1 to 3 mg/kg/minute	• Phenytoin is contraindicated in a breast-feeding patient or one with known hypersensitivity to the drug or other hydantoins, sinus bradycardia, sinoatrial block, second- or third-degree atrioventricular block, or Adams-Stokes syndrome. • This drug requires cautious use in a pregnant patient or a woman of childbearing age.
Barbiturates		
phenobarbital, phenobarbital sodium (Luminal, Solfoton)	*Partial seizures, tonic-clonic seizures* ADULT: 100 to 300 mg P.O. daily in divided doses PEDIATRIC: 3 to 5 mg/kg P.O. daily in two equal doses *Status epilepticus* ADULT: 15 to 20 mg/kg I.V. over 10 to 15 minutes	• Phenobarbital is contraindicated in a patient with known hypersensitivity to barbiturates, a history of manifest or latent porphyria, marked impairment of liver function, or respiratory disease in which dyspnea or obstruction is evident. • This drug requires cautious use in a pregnant, breast-feeding, geriatric, debilitated, or pediatric patient or one with acute or chronic pain, mental depression, suicidal tendencies, a history of drug abuse, hepatic dysfunction, or borderline hypoadrenal function.
Iminostilbenes		
carbamazepine (Tegretol)	*Partial seizures; tonic-clonic seizures* ADULT: initially, 200 mg P.O. b.i.d.; gradually increased in small increments up to 400 mg P.O. t.i.d. until desired response is obtained; maintenance dosage, 1,200 mg P.O. daily in adults and children over age 15 PEDIATRIC: for children ages 6 to 12, 20 to 30 mg/kg, beginning with 100 mg P.O. b.i.d.; increased by 100 mg P.O. daily using at least a t.i.d. regimen; for children over age 12, 200 mg P.O. b.i.d.; maintenance dosage for children under age 12, 400 to 800 mg P.O. daily in three divided doses; for children ages 12 to 15, 800 to 1,200 mg P.O. daily	• Carbamazepine is contraindicated in a breast-feeding patient, one with known hypersensitivity to the drug or tricyclic compounds or a history of previous bone marrow depression, or one who currently takes monoamine oxidase inhibitors. • This drug requires cautious use in a pregnant patient or one with a mixed seizure disorder that includes atypical absence seizures. • Safety and efficacy in children under age 6 have not been established.
Benzodiazepines		
clonazepam (Klonopin)	*Absence seizures; atypical absence, atonic, and myoclonic seizures* ADULT: 1.5 mg P.O. daily in three divided doses; dosage is highly individualized PEDIATRIC: for children up to age 10 or weighing up to 30 kg, 0.01 to 0.03 mg/kg P.O. daily in three divided doses; maintenance dosage, 0.1 to 0.2 mg/kg P.O. daily in three divided doses	• Clonazepam is contraindicated in a breast-feeding patient or one with known hypersensitivity to benzodiazepines, significant liver disease, or acute angle-closure glaucoma. • This drug requires cautious use in a pregnant patient or one with impaired renal function or a chronic respiratory disorder. • Clonazepam should be administered to a child only if the potential benefit justifies the risk; possible adverse effects on physical or mental development could become apparent only after many years.

Selected major anticonvulsant agents *(continued)*

DRUG	MAJOR INDICATIONS AND USUAL DOSAGES	CONTRAINDICATIONS AND PRECAUTIONS
Succinimides		
ethosuximide (Zarontin)	*Absence seizures* ADULT: 250 mg P.O. b.i.d., with maintenance dosage of 20 to 40 mg/kg P.O. daily; dosage is highly individualized PEDIATRIC: initially, for children over age 6, 250 mg P.O. b.i.d.; for children ages 3 to 6, 250 mg P.O. daily; maintenance dosage, 20 mg/kg, with a maximum dosage of 1 g for children up to age 6	• Ethosuximide is contraindicated in a patient with known hypersensitivity to succinimides. • This drug requires cautious use in a pregnant or breast-feeding patient or one with known liver or renal disease or mixed types of epilepsy.
Valproic acid		
valproate sodium (Depakene), divalproex sodium (Depakote, Depacon)	*Absence seizures; myoclonic and tonic-clonic seizures* ADULT: 15 mg/kg P.O. daily up to a maximum dosage of 60 mg/kg P.O. daily; dosage is highly individualized and should be divided if it exceeds 250 mg daily.	• Valproic acid is contraindicated in a patient with known hypersensitivity to the drug or with hepatic disease or significant dysfunction. • This drug requires cautious use in a pregnant or breast-feeding patient.

phenylhydantoin, is longer than that of phenytoin: 24 to 48 hours. Half-lives of 32 to 144 hours have been reported with mephenytoin.

Ethotoin demonstrates a rapid onset of action, achieving peak serum concentrations in 2 to 4 hours. Ethotoin half-life ranges from 3 to 9 hours.

Route	Onset	Peak	Duration
P.O.	Variable	45 min-12 hr	4-48 hr
I.M.	Variable	30 min	Unknown
I.V.	3-5 min	Post-infusion	Unknown

PHARMACODYNAMICS

In most cases, the hydantoin anticonvulsants can stabilize nerve cells against hyperexcitability. Phenytoin's primary site of action appears to be the motor cortex, where the drug inhibits the spread of seizure activity. The pharmacodynamics of mephenytoin and ethotoin are thought to mimic those of phenytoin. Phenytoin also exhibits antiarrhythmic properties similar to those of quinidine or procainamide. In addition, phenytoin exerts a membrane-stabilizing effect on the pancreas and may inhibit effective insulin release.

PHARMACOTHERAPEUTICS

Because of its clinical efficacy and relatively low toxicity, phenytoin is the most commonly prescribed anticonvulsant. Phenytoin represents one of the drugs of choice to treat complex partial (also called psychomotor or temporal lobe) and tonic-clonic seizures. Physicians sometimes prescribe mephenytoin and ethotoin as adjunct therapy for partial and tonic-clonic seizures in patients who are refractory to, or intolerant of, other anticonvulsants.

Drug interactions

Hydantoins interact with a number of other drugs. As a result, the activities of phenytoin, the other drug, or both are altered. (See Drug Interactions: *Hydantoins*, page 156.)

ADVERSE DRUG REACTIONS

The adverse effects of hydantoin anticonvulsants involve the central nervous, cardiovascular, GI, and hematopoietic systems, as well as cosmetic effects. The adverse reactions presented here relate directly to phenytoin. Ethotoin produces similar reactions; mephenytoin may produce more serious blood dyscrasias, including aplastic anemia.

In the central nervous system (CNS), adverse reactions to hydantoins include drowsiness, ataxia, irritability, headache, restlessness, nystagmus, dizziness, vertigo, and dysarthria. Adverse CNS reactions to phenytoin reflect the drug's blood concentration. For example, nystagmus and diplopia occur at 25 to 30 mcg/ml; ataxia, lethargy, and asterixis, at 30 to 40 mcg/ml; and decreased consciousness and coma, at 40 to 50 mcg/ml. Phenytoin also may cause toxic amblyopia and mental dullness.

The major adverse GI reactions include nausea, vomiting, epigastric pain, and anorexia. The adverse cardiovascular reactions are depressed atrial and ventricular conduction and, in toxic states, ventricular fibrillation. With I.V. administration, the adverse cardiovascular reactions include bradycardia, hypotension, and potential cardiac arrest. The

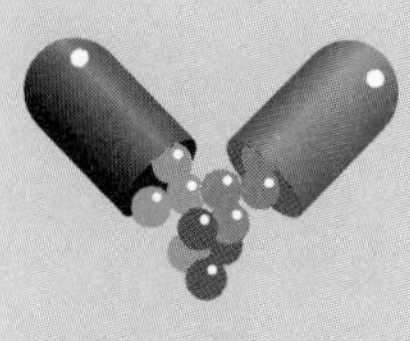

DRUG INTERACTIONS

Hydantoins

The following drug interactions may occur with the use of phenytoin or any other hydantoin anticonvulsant. Because phenytoin interacts with many drugs, this chart has been limited to interactions that have major to moderate clinical significance. Drug interactions of lesser clinical significance, involving such drugs as acetaminophen and dopamine, are not included.

DRUG	INTERACTING AGENTS	POSSIBLE EFFECTS	NURSING IMPLICATIONS
phenytoin, fosphenytoin, mephenytoin, ethotoin	allopurinol, cimetidine, disulfiram, fluconazole, isoniazid, omeprazole, sulfonamides	Increased toxic adverse effects of phenytoin	• Monitor serum phenytoin concentration; phenytoin dosage may need to be decreased. • Advise the patient to report adverse reactions. • Carefully monitor complete blood count (CBC), platelet and reticulocyte counts, and liver function tests.
	oral anticoagulants	Increased serum phenytoin concentrations when phenytoin therapy begins; transient increase in anticoagulant effect followed by a decrease in anticoagulant effect when oral anticoagulant therapy begins	• Monitor serum phenytoin concentration; phenytoin dosage may need to be decreased. • Advise the patient to report adverse reactions. • Carefully monitor CBC, platelet and reticulocyte counts, and liver function tests.
	phenobarbital	Decreased phenytoin concentration; occasionally, increased phenytoin concentration	• Monitor for anticoagulant effects. • Monitor phenytoin and phenobarbital serum concentrations. • Monitor CBC, platelet and reticulocyte counts, and liver function tests. • Advise the patient to report changes in adverse reactions or seizure frequency.
	diazoxide	Decreased efficacy of phenytoin	• Monitor serum phenytoin concentration.
	levodopa	Decreased efficacy of levodopa	• Observe for increased signs or symptoms of Parkinson's disease. • Advise the patient to report any change in parkinsonian signs or symptoms. • Expect to increase the levodopa dosage.
	chloramphenicol	Increased toxic adverse effects of phenytoin; decreased efficacy of chloramphenicol	• Monitor serum phenytoin concentration; advise the patient to report adverse reactions. Phenytoin dose may need to be reduced. • Monitor CBC, platelet and reticulocyte counts, and liver function tests. • Monitor serum chloramphenicol concentration. • Expect to increase the chloramphenicol dosage.
	amiodarone	Twofold to threefold increase in phenytoin concentration; decreased amiodarone efficacy	• Monitor serum phenytoin concentration. • Observe the patient for signs of phenytoin toxicity. • Expect to decrease the phenytoin dosage. • Expect to increase the amiodarone dosage. • Advise the patient to see the physician frequently for monitoring of cardiac status. • Alert the patient to report signs or symptoms of arrhythmias, such as palpitations and irregular pulse.
	corticosteroids	Decreased efficacy of corticosteroids	• Expect to increase the corticosteroid dosage. • Monitor the patient's blood pressure and weight. • Monitor serum electrolyte levels.

Hydantoins *(continued)*

DRUG	INTERACTING AGENTS	POSSIBLE EFFECTS	NURSING IMPLICATIONS
fosphenytoin, phenytoin, mephenytoin, ethotoin *(continued)*	doxycycline	Decreased efficacy of doxycycline	• Monitor the patient frequently because of decreased effect. • Expect to increase the doxycycline dosage.
	methadone	Decreased efficacy of methadone	• Expect to increase the methadone dosage. • Alert the patient to watch for signs of withdrawal.
	metyrapone	Decreased efficacy of metyrapone	• Monitor the patient frequently. • Expect to increase the metyrapone dosage.
	quinidine, mexiletine	Decreased efficacy of these drugs	• Expect to increase the dosage of these drugs. • Advise the patient to see the physician frequently for monitoring of cardiac status. • Alert the patient to report signs or symptoms of arrhythmias, such as palpitations and irregular pulse.
	theophylline	Decreased efficacy of phenytoin; decreased efficacy of theophylline	• Expect to increase the phenytoin and theophylline dosages. • Monitor serum concentrations of both drugs. • Advise the patient to report increased shortness of breath to the physician. • Monitor CBC, platelet and reticulocyte counts, and liver function tests.
	thyroid hormone	Increased metabolism of thyroid hormone	• Monitor the patient frequently because of increased thyroid hormone metabolism. • Expect to increase the thyroid hormone dosage.
	oral contraceptives	Decreased efficacy of contraceptives	• Expect the patient to need an alternative contraceptive method.
	valproic acid	Transient decrease in phenytoin concentrations; increased phenytoin concentrations; decrease in valproic acid levels	• Monitor phenytoin and valproic acid concentrations. • Be alert for breakthrough seizures, which may occur with use of valproic acid-phenytoin combination.
	cyclosporine	Decreased cyclosporine concentrations	• Monitor cyclosporine concentration.
	digitoxin	Decreased digitoxin effect	• Monitor the patient frequently. • Monitor digitoxin level. • Expect to increase the digitoxin dosage.
	carbamazepine	Decreased phenytoin and carbamazepine levels	• Monitor phenytoin and carbamazepine levels. • Monitor seizure frequency.
	rifampin	Decreased phenytoin effects	• Monitor phenytoin level. • Monitor seizure frequency.
	antacids, sucralfate	Decreased absorption of phenytoin	• Monitor phenytoin level.
	charcoal-broiled meats	May decrease phenytoin level	• Monitor phenytoin level. • Inform the patient of this interaction.

primary adverse reaction of the hematopoietic system is a folic acid deficiency that can cause macrocytic anemia.

Cosmetic toxicity includes gingival hyperplasia, hirsutism, and facial skin coarsening. Other adverse reactions include hyperglycemia, glycosuria, and osteomalacia. Toxic doses of phenytoin paradoxically may induce seizures.

Hypersensitivity reactions to hydantoins typically are manifested as pruritus, fever, arthralgia, and a measleslike rash; exfoliative, purpuric, or bullous dermatitis; Stevens-

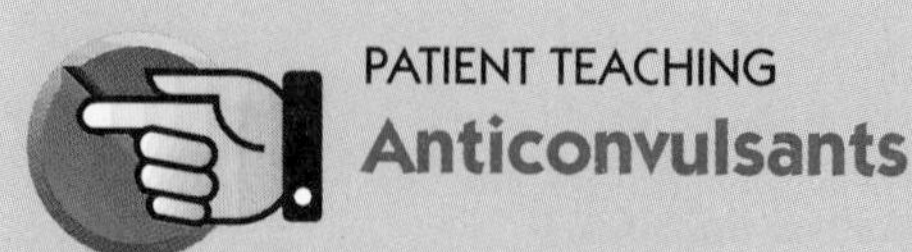

PATIENT TEACHING
Anticonvulsants

Regardless of the anticonvulsant prescribed, the following patient-teaching tips apply.

- Instruct the patient not to alter the prescribed drug regimen.
- Instruct the patient to notify the physician if seizure control deteriorates.
- Alert the patient that abrupt discontinuation of the prescribed drug can precipitate seizures or status epilepticus.
- Remind the patient to check all prescription refills to ensure that the drug preparation is the same as the previous preparation.
- Advise the patient to avoid hazardous activities until the dosage and adverse effects become stabilized.
- Teach the patient's family how to care for the patient during a seizure.
- Advise the patient not to medicate with over-the-counter drugs.
- Advise the patient to refrain from ingesting alcohol because of its possible interactive effects with some anticonvulsants.
- Emphasize the importance of frequent follow-up care for the patient, and provide information about voluntary community organizations that provide information and support.

Johnson syndrome; lymphadenopathy; acute renal failure; hepatitis; and liver necrosis. Several adverse reactions also relate to the hematopoietic system, including thrombocytopenia, leukopenia, leukocytosis, agranulocytosis, pancytopenia, eosinophilia, macrocytosis, and various anemias.

NURSING PROCESS APPLICATION

The following information assists the nurse in caring for a patient who is receiving a hydantoin. It includes an overview of assessment activities as well as examples of appropriate nursing diagnoses and related interventions (under "Planning and implementation"). It also highlights the importance of evaluation.

Assessment

Before drug therapy begins, review the patient's history for conditions that contraindicate or require cautious use of the prescribed hydantoin. Also review the patient's medication history to identify use of drugs that may interact with it. During therapy, assess the patient for adverse drug reactions and signs of drug interactions. If the patient develops adverse cosmetic reactions, assess for perceived changes in body image. Periodically assess the effectiveness of hydantoin therapy. Finally, evaluate the patient's and family's knowledge about the prescribed drug.

Nursing diagnoses

• Risk for injury related to a preexisting condition that contraindicates or requires cautious use of a hydantoin
• Risk for injury related to adverse drug reactions and drug interactions
• Body image disturbance related to cosmetic toxicity from hydantoin use
• Knowledge deficit related to the prescribed hydantoin

Planning and implementation

• Do not administer a hydantoin to a patient with a condition that contraindicates its use.
• Administer a hydantoin cautiously to a patient at risk because of a preexisting condition.
• Monitor the patient's serum phenytoin concentration because many adverse reactions are dose-related.
• Keep oxygen, suction, and resuscitation equipment available when administering phenytoin I.V.
• Monitor the patient regularly for signs of adverse reactions to the prescribed hydantoin.
Administer I.V. phenytoin at a rate not to exceed 50 mg/minute (or 50 mg/3 minutes in a geriatric patient with heart disease) because of its cardiotoxicity. Also monitor the patient's blood pressure, pulse, and respirations every 5 minutes during administration and every 15 minutes thereafter until the patient becomes stable. If blood pressure decreases during drug administration, reduce the infusion rate.
Administer I.V. fosphenytoin at a rate not to exceed 150 phenytoin equivalents per minute.
• Minimize vein irritation by infusing normal saline solution after I.V. phenytoin administration, as prescribed.
Do not mix I.V. phenytoin with any other drug to avoid phenytoin precipitation.
• Avoid I.M. injections (except for fosphenytoin) because phenytoin precipitates in muscle tissue, which decreases drug bioavailability.
• Administer an oral hydantoin with meals to minimize GI distress.
• Shake suspension preparations vigorously before pouring to ensure uniform distribution and exact measurement of the drug.
• Advise the patient not to discontinue the drug abruptly.
• Encourage the patient to express feelings about body image if cosmetic adverse reactions occur. (See Patient Teaching: *Anticonvulsants*, and Patient Teaching: *Hydantoins*, page 160.)
• Explore ways to mask undesired cosmetic changes, such as by using makeup and hair removal preparations for the female patient.
• Consult with the physician about switching to a different anticonvulsant agent if the patient is disturbed greatly by cosmetic adverse reactions.

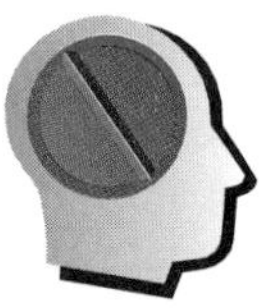

CRITICAL THINKING. To enhance your critical thinking about anticonvulsant agents, consider the following situation and analysis.
Situation: Your neighbor Mary, age 35, has been taking phenytoin 300 mg at bedtime for the past 5 years following seizures after a motor vehicle accident in which she suffered a head injury. She has been seizure-free for 4 years. She tells you that she is going to

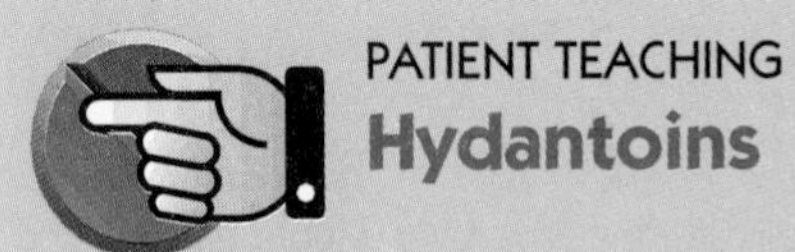

PATIENT TEACHING
Hydantoins

- ➤ Teach the patient and family the name, dose, frequency, action, and adverse effects of the prescribed hydantoin agent.
- ➤ Recommend that the female patient taking an oral contraceptive and a hydantoin use an additional or different contraceptive method. Discuss the advantages and disadvantages of various contraceptive methods, if requested.
- ➤ Encourage the patient with gingival hyperplasia to brush the teeth meticulously and floss daily.
- ➤ Remind the patient to notify the dentist about hydantoin therapy.
- ➤ Inform the patient that phenytoin may cause harmless pink, red, or red-brown discoloration of urine.
- ➤ Advise the patient to report adverse drug reactions to the physician.
- ➤ Advise the diabetic patient to monitor blood glucose levels because the hydantoin may increase them.

stop taking the phenytoin because she doesn't need it anymore. What is your response?
Analysis: Anticonvulsant medications should never be discontinued abruptly. Mary should make an appointment with her physician and discuss a possible tapering schedule if feasible. You may want to warn Mary that if she should stop her medication abruptly, it would lower her seizure threshold, resulting in a generalized seizure.

Evaluation

For each nursing diagnosis, prepare an evaluation statement that describes the patient's or family's response to nursing interventions.

Barbiturates

The long-acting barbiturate phenobarbital is also one of the most widely employed anticonvulsants. Phenobarbital is used in long-term treatment of epilepsy and is prescribed selectively for acute treatment of status epilepticus. Mephobarbital, also a long-acting barbiturate, is used less commonly as an anticonvulsant. Primidone, which is closely related chemically to the barbiturates, is also used in the chronic treatment of epilepsy.

PHARMACOKINETICS

The barbiturate anticonvulsants are metabolized in the liver. Metabolites and unchanged drug are excreted in the urine.

Phenobarbital is absorbed slowly but well from the GI tract. Peak plasma concentration levels occur 8 to 12 hours after a single dose. The drug is 20% to 45% bound to serum proteins and to a similar extent to other tissues, including the brain. About 75% of a phenobarbital dose is metabolized by hepatic microsomal enzymes, and 25% is excreted unchanged in the urine.

Almost 50% of a mephobarbital dose is absorbed from the GI tract and well distributed in body tissues. The drug is bound to tissue and plasma proteins. Mephobarbital undergoes extensive metabolism by hepatic microsomal enzymes. Only 1% to 2% is excreted unchanged in the urine.

Approximately 60% to 80% of a primidone dose is absorbed from the GI tract and distributed evenly among body tissues. The drug is protein-bound to a small extent in the plasma. Primidone is metabolized by hepatic microsomal enzymes to two active metabolites, phenobarbital and phenylethylmalonamide (PEMA). From 15% to 25% of primidone is excreted unchanged in the urine, 15% to 25% is metabolized to phenobarbital, and 50% to 70% is excreted in the urine as PEMA. Primidone also is excreted in breast milk.

Phenobarbital provides an onset of action within 30 minutes after oral administration. Peak anticonvulsant effect occurs in 8 to 12 hours. The onset after I.V. administration occurs within 5 minutes, with peak anticonvulsant effect within 30 minutes. Phenobarbital has an extremely long half-life of 50 to 170 hours. Mephobarbital demonstrates a rapid onset, with peak anticonvulsant effect in 6 to 8 hours. The half-life of mephobarbital is 11 to 67 hours. Primidone displays a rapid onset, with peak anticonvulsant effect in 4 hours. The half-life of primidone varies from 10 to 21 hours.

Route	Onset	Peak	Duration
P.O.	30 min-1 hr	4-12 hr	10-16 hr
I.V.	5 min	30 min	10-12 hr

PHARMACODYNAMICS

The barbiturates exhibit anticonvulsant action at subhypnotic dosages. For this reason, the barbiturates usually do not produce addiction when used to treat epilepsy. (See Drug Interactions: *Barbiturates,* page 160.)

PHARMACOTHERAPEUTICS

The barbiturate anticonvulsants are effective in treating partial, tonic-clonic, and febrile seizures when used alone or with other anticonvulsants. I.V. phenobarbital also is used to treat status epilepticus. The major disadvantage of using phenobarbital for status epilepticus is delayed onset of action. Barbiturate anticonvulsants are ineffective in treating absence seizures.

Mephobarbital offers no advantage over phenobarbital; it is used when the patient cannot tolerate the adverse effects of phenobarbital. Primidone is used primarily with other anticonvulsants. Some clinicians, however, consider it the drug of choice for complex partial seizures.

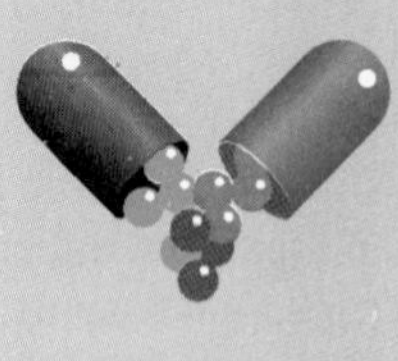

DRUG INTERACTIONS

Barbiturates

Most of the clinically significant interactions involving barbiturates occur with phenobarbital. Mephobarbital and primidone interact with the same drugs as phenobarbital. Because primidone is converted to phenobarbital in the body, concurrent administration of primidone and phenobarbital may result in an elevated serum phenobarbital concentration.

DRUG	INTERACTING AGENTS	POSSIBLE EFFECTS	NURSING IMPLICATIONS
phenobarbital, mephobarbital, primidone	hydantoins	Increased, decreased, or no change in phenytoin level; may increase phenobarbital level	• Monitor serum concentrations; phenobarbital dosage may need to be decreased. • Advise the patient to report adverse reactions. • Alert the patient not to drive or operate heavy machinery until the effect of the drug combination on the patient is known. • Advise the patient to avoid alcohol consumption.
	beta blockers (metoprolol, propranolol)	Decreased effectiveness of beta blockers	• Monitor desired effect in the patient (antianginal, antihypertensive, and antiarrhythmic); beta blocker dosage may need to be increased. • Instruct the patient to report changes in desired effect in drug therapy. • Advise the patient to report periodically for blood pressure and pulse checks.
	chloramphenicol	Decreased effectiveness of chloramphenicol; inhibited phenobarbital metabolism	• Monitor desired effect in the patient (anti-infective); chloramphenicol dosage may need to be increased. • Monitor serum chloramphenicol and phenobarbital concentrations.
	corticosteroids	Decreased effectiveness of corticosteroids	• Expect to increase the corticosteroid dosage. • Monitor the patient's weight and blood pressure. • Monitor serum electrolyte levels.
	doxycycline	Decreased effectiveness of doxycycline	• Expect to increase the doxycycline dosage or to substitute tetracycline.
	oral anticoagulants	Decreased effectiveness of oral anticoagulants	• Monitor prothrombin level; anticoagulant dosage may need to be increased. • Advise the patient to be alert for signs and symptoms of thrombus formation, such as pain, tenderness, and edema in the calf.
	oral contraceptives	Decreased effectiveness of oral contraceptives	• Alert the patient that contraceptive effect may be impaired; breakthrough bleeding may occur. • Suggest alternative or additional contraceptive methods.
	quinidine	Decreased effectiveness of quinidine	• Expect to increase the quinidine dosage. • Advise the patient to see the physician frequently for monitoring of cardiac status. • Alert the patient to report any signs and symptoms of arrhythmias, such as palpitations and irregular pulse. • Monitor quinidine level.
	methoxyflurane	Metabolism of methoxyflurane to nephrotoxic metabolites	• Avoid concurrent administration of phenobarbital and methoxyflurane.
	phenothiazines	Decreased effectiveness of phenothiazine	• Expect to increase the phenothiazine dosage. • Monitor the patient's behavior frequently. • Advise the patient and family members to report changes in behavior promptly to the physician.

Barbiturates *(continued)*

DRUG	INTERACTING AGENTS	POSSIBLE EFFECTS	NURSING IMPLICATIONS
phenobarbital, mephobarbital, primidone *(continued)*	tricyclic antidepressants	Decreased effectiveness of tricyclic antidepressant; increased adverse effects of tricyclic antidepressant (lowered seizure threshold)	• Expect to increase the tricyclic antidepressant dosage. • Monitor adverse effects of the tricyclic antidepressant, such as respiratory depression. • Advise the patient to report change in therapeutic effect, such as lack of mood elevation.
	central nervous system depressants (antianxiety agents, sedative-hypnotics, most narcotic analgesics, alcohol)	Increased sedative toxicity	• Assess frequently for changes in level of consciousness and respirations. • Supervise ambulation; raise side rails, especially with geriatric patients. • Alert the patient not to drive or use heavy machinery until the effects of the drug combination in the patient is known. • Advise the patient not to drink alcohol while taking these medications.
	valproic acid	Inhibited metabolism of phenobarbital	• Monitor for excessive phenobarbital effect, such as drowsiness. • Expect to decrease the phenobarbital dosage.
	metronidazole	Increased metronidazole metabolism	• Expect to increase the metronidazole dosage.
	digitoxin	Decreased digitoxin effectiveness	• Monitor the patient for signs of digitoxin's effectiveness; monitor digitoxin level. • Expect to increase the digitoxin dosage.
	theophylline	Decreased serum theophylline concentration	• Monitor theophylline concentration, as prescribed. • Expect to increase the theophylline dosage.
	cyclosporine	Decreased plasma cyclosporine concentration	• Monitor cyclosporine concentration regularly. • Expect to increase the cyclosporine dosage.
	rifampin	Decreased effectiveness of barbiturate	• Monitor phenobarbital level.
	carbamazepine	Decreased carbamazepine level	• Monitor carbamazepine level. • Monitor seizure frequency.
	felodipine, verapamil	May decrease plasma level of felodipine and verapamil	• Monitor desired effect (antihypertensive or antianginal) in the patient.

Drug interactions

Phenobarbital interacts with many drugs, usually altering their metabolic rate. For example, such drugs as the hydantoins and chloramphenicol inhibit phenobarbital metabolism, increasing the drug's toxic effects. Mephobarbital and primidone interact with the same drugs and in the same way as phenobarbital because both drugs are metabolized to phenobarbital.

ADVERSE DRUG REACTIONS

The toxicity of the barbiturate anticonvulsants results primarily in adverse reactions in the CNS. Significant GI reactions, blood dyscrasias, and emotional or psychiatric reactions also occur.

The most common dose-related CNS effects of phenobarbital include drowsiness, lethargy, and dizziness; nystagmus; confusion; and ataxia with large doses.

The adverse GI reactions include nausea and vomiting. These adverse reactions are most common when primidone therapy begins, which explains why the primidone dosage is increased gradually.

Folate deficiencies and osteomalacia secondary to the induced metabolism of vitamin D also may occur. When administered I.V., phenobarbital can cause laryngospasm, respiratory depression, and hypotension secondary to de-

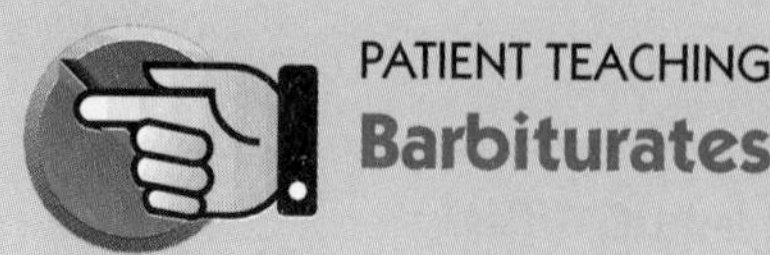

PATIENT TEACHING
Barbiturates

- Teach the patient and family the name, dose, frequency, action, and adverse effects of the prescribed barbiturate.
- Reassure the patient that the prescribed barbiturate is not addictive when used in subhypnotic doses for seizures.
- Advise the patient to keep the prescribed barbiturate in a secure place to prevent others, including children, from taking the drug.
- Inform the male patient that impotence may occur.
- Inform the patient that a barbiturate can impair mental alertness, which may require avoidance of activities that require alertness.
- Instruct the patient to report adverse reactions to the physician.
- Advise the patient to refrain from ingesting alcohol.

creased cardiac output. Signs of overdose include respiratory depression, pupillary constriction, oliguria, hypothermia, circulatory collapse, and pulmonary edema.

Mephobarbital produces adverse reactions similar to phenobarbital. Primidone evokes the same CNS and GI adverse reactions as phenobarbital. Primidone also has been implicated in the development of acute psychoses in patients with complex partial seizures. It also may cause alopecia, impotence, and osteomalacia.

Rare hematologic adverse effects of the barbiturates include agranulocytosis, thrombocytopenia, leukopenia, eosinophilia, decreased serum folate levels, and megaloblastic anemia. All three barbiturate anticonvulsants can produce a hypersensitivity rash. These drugs also may produce a morbilliform rash, lupus erythematosus–like syndrome, and lymphadenopathy. Paradoxical excitement in elderly patients and children and hyperkinetic behavior in children may occur.

NURSING PROCESS APPLICATION

The following information assists the nurse in caring for a patient who is receiving a barbiturate anticonvulsant. It includes an overview of assessment activities as well as examples of appropriate nursing diagnoses and related interventions (under "Planning and implementation"). It also highlights the importance of evaluation.

Assessment

Before drug therapy begins, review the patient's history for conditions that contraindicate or require cautious use of the prescribed barbiturate anticonvulsant. Also review the patient's medication history to identify use of drugs that may interact with it. During therapy, assess the patient for adverse drug reactions and signs of drug interactions. Particularly note the patient's physical mobility during barbiturate therapy and compare it to baseline levels. Also, periodically assess the effectiveness of therapy. Finally, evaluate the patient's and family's knowledge about the prescribed drug.

Nursing diagnoses

- Risk for injury related to a preexisting condition that contraindicates or requires cautious use of a barbiturate
- Risk for injury related to adverse drug reactions or drug interactions
- Impaired physical mobility related to the sedative effects of a barbiturate
- Knowledge deficit related to the prescribed barbiturate

Planning and implementation

- Do not administer a barbiturate to a patient with a condition that contraindicates its use. (See Patient Teaching: *Barbiturates.*)
- Administer a barbiturate cautiously to a patient at risk because of a preexisting condition.
- Keep resuscitative drugs and equipment nearby when administering an I.V. barbiturate.

*** *Do not exceed a rate of 60 mg/minute when giving an I.V. barbiturate.***

- Do not use a cloudy solution when giving an I.V. barbiturate. Administer a reconstituted solution within 30 minutes of preparation.

*** *Monitor vital signs frequently — especially respirations and blood pressure — when administering an I.V. barbiturate.***

- Monitor the patient's physical mobility during barbiturate therapy.
- Notify the physician if the barbiturate's sedative effects interfere with the patient's physical mobility.

Evaluation

For each nursing diagnosis, prepare an evaluation statement that describes the patient's or family's response to nursing interventions.

Iminostilbenes

Carbamazepine, an iminostilbene derivative, acts as an effective anticonvulsant for partial and generalized tonic-clonic seizures and mixed seizure types. Carbamazepine also produces sedative, anticholinergic, antidepressant, muscle-relaxant, antiarrhythmic, antidiuretic, and neuromuscular transmission–inhibiting actions. Also, carbamazepine is the only anticonvulsant compound that has a chemical structure similar to the tricyclic antidepressant drugs, such as imipramine. This similarity helps explain the drug's effects on behavior and emotions.

PHARMACOKINETICS

Carbamazepine is absorbed slowly and erratically from the GI tract. The drug is distributed rapidly to all tissues, and

75% to 90% is bound to plasma proteins. Metabolism occurs in the liver, and carbamazepine is excreted in the urine. A small amount crosses the placenta, and some is secreted in breast milk. The half-life also varies greatly.

Route	Onset	Peak	Duration
P.O.	Unknown	1.5-12 hr	Unknown

PHARMACODYNAMICS

Carbamazepine exerts an anticonvulsant effect similar to that of phenytoin. The drug's anticonvulsant action may occur because of its ability to inhibit the spread of seizure activity or neuromuscular transmission in general.

PHARMACOTHERAPEUTICS

Carbamazepine is used to treat generalized tonic-clonic seizures as well as simple and complex partial seizures in adults and children. The efficacy of carbamazepine makes it a drug of choice for treating these seizures. The drug also relieves pain when used to treat trigeminal neuralgia (tic douloureux).

Drug interactions

Carbamazepine possesses enzyme-inducing properties and generally decreases the steady-state levels of other drugs. Some anticonvulsant drugs, however, decrease the steady-state levels of carbamazepine. (See Drug Interactions: *Iminostilbenes,* page 164.)

ADVERSE DRUG REACTIONS

Most adverse reactions produced by carbamazepine are tolerable and relatively minor, if the drug therapy begins slowly at a low dosage and advances gradually to tolerance. Occasionally, however, serious hematologic toxicity occurs. Furthermore, because carbamazepine is related structurally to the tricyclic antidepressants, it can cause similar toxicities.

Dose-related adverse reactions include drowsiness, diplopia, ataxia, vertigo, nystagmus, headaches, tremor, and dry mouth. Because carbamazepine is related to the tricyclic antidepressants, it can produce many of the same adverse reactions, including heart failure, hypertension or hypotension, syncope, arrhythmias, and myocardial infarction. Carbamazepine's action as a mild anticholinergic may result in urine retention, constipation, and increased intraocular pressure. With long-term use, the drug also can cause syndrome of inappropriate antidiuretic hormone secretion and water intoxication.

Urticaria and Stevens-Johnson syndrome have been reported with carbamazepine use. The occasional but significant hematologic reactions include aplastic anemia (rare), agranulocytosis, thrombocytopenia, and leukopenia. Rare instances of cholestatic and hepatocellular jaundice also have been noted. Rare psychiatric reactions have been noted, including activation of latent psychosis, mental depression with agitation, and talkativeness.

NURSING PROCESS APPLICATION

The following information assists the nurse in caring for a patient who is receiving the iminostilbene carbamazepine. It includes an overview of assessment activities as well as examples of appropriate nursing diagnoses and related interventions (under "Planning and implementation"). It also highlights the importance of evaluation.

Assessment

Before drug therapy begins, review the patient's history for conditions that contraindicate or require cautious use of carbamazepine. Also review the patient's medication history to identify use of drugs that may interact with it. During therapy, assess the patient for adverse drug reactions and signs of drug interactions. In a patient who is receiving long-term therapy, assess for signs of fluid overload. Also, periodically assess the effectiveness of carbamazepine therapy. Finally, evaluate the patient's and family's knowledge about the prescribed drug.

Nursing diagnoses

- Risk for injury related to a preexisting condition that contraindicates or requires cautious use of carbamazepine
- Risk for injury related to adverse drug reactions and drug interactions
- Fluid volume excess related to water intoxication with long-term use of carbamazepine
- Knowledge deficit related to carbamazepine

Planning and implementation

- Do not administer carbamazepine to a patient with a condition that contraindicates its use.
- Administer carbamazepine cautiously to a patient at risk because of a preexisting condition.
- Monitor the patient for adverse drug reactions.
- Take bleeding and infection precautions, if the patient develops thrombocytopenia or leukopenia.
- Take safety precautions if the patient exhibits drowsiness, diplopia, ataxia, vertigo, or syncope.
- Notify the physician if the patient develops any adverse reactions to carbamazepine.

✱ ***Assess the patient for signs of fluid retention, such as crackles, dependent edema, and weight gain.***

- Document fluid intake and output and note changes in vital signs, such as increased blood pressure, pulse, and respirations, at least daily.
- Limit the patient's fluid and salt intake. (See Patient Teaching: *Iminostilbenes,* page 165.)
- Notify the physician if the patient develops signs of fluid excess, such as shortness of breath.

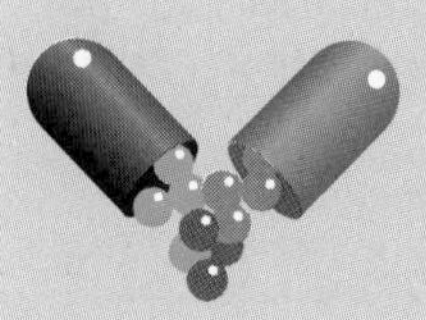

DRUG INTERACTIONS
Iminostilbenes

The following chart lists the drug interactions between carbamazepine, an iminostilbene derivative, and other drugs.

DRUG	INTERACTING AGENTS	POSSIBLE EFFECTS	NURSING IMPLICATIONS
carbamazepine	erythromycin, isoniazid, propoxyphene, troleandomycin, cimetidine, danazol, diltiazem, verapamil	Increased toxic adverse reactions to carbamazepine	• Monitor serum carbamazepine concentrations carefully; decreased carbamazepine dosage may be needed. • Monitor complete blood count and platelet and reticulocyte counts; hematopoietic toxicity warrants immediate withdrawal. • Advise the patient and family to notify the physician immediatley if the following signs or symptoms occur: fever, sore throat or mouth, malaise, unusual fatigue, or tendency to bruise or bleed. • Monitor the pulse and cardiac function frequently in a patient with heart disease because toxic doses may precipitate cardiac arrhythmias. • Advise the patient to avoid hazardous tasks that require mental alertness and physical coordination, such as operating a motor vehicle or using heavy machinery, because dizziness, drowsiness, and ataxia may occur.
	doxycycline	Decreased therapeutic effect of doxycycline	• Expect to increase the doxycycline dosage.
	theophylline	Increased or decreased therapeutic effect of theophylline	• Expect to increase the theophylline dosage.
	warfarin	Decreased carbamazepine level; decreased therapeutic effect of warfarin	• Monitor prothrombin time frequently. • Expect to increase warfarin dosage. • Observe for signs of thrombus formation, such as Homans' sign, tenderness, or edema.
	lithium	Neurotoxicity	• Assess for changes in level of consciousness. • Instruct the patient to report dizziness, headache, fatigue, or slurred speech immediately. • Advise the patient not to operate a motor vehicle or heavy machinery until the drug combination effects on the patient are known.
	oral contraceptives	Decreased efficacy of contraceptives	• Advise the patient to use an alternative contraceptive method during carbamazepine therapy.
	antihistamines, nonsedating	Increased carbamazepine level	• Monitor carbamazepine level.
	barbiturates	Decreased carbamazepine level; increased phenobarbital level	• Monitor carbamazepine and phenobarbital levels.
	felbamate	Decreased felbamate and carbamazepine levels	• Monitor carbamazepine and felbamate levels. • Monitor seizure frequency.
	phenytoin	Decreased carbamazepine level; variable effects on phenytoin	• Monitor phenytoin and carbamazepine levels. • Monitor for increased seizure frequency. • Monitor for adverse effects of phenytoin.
	valproic acid	Increased carbamazepine level; decreased valproic acid level	• Monitor carbamazepine and valproic acid levels.
	selective serotonin reuptake inhibitors	Increased carbamazepine level	• Monitor carbamazepine level.

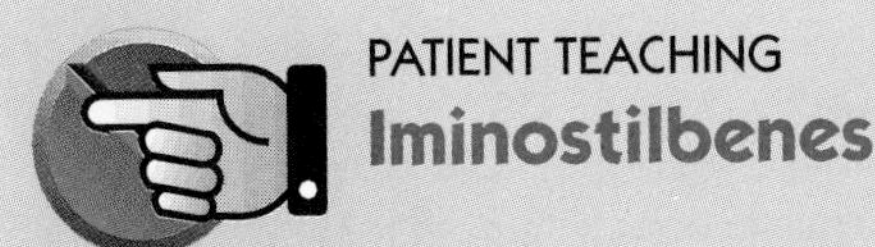

PATIENT TEACHING
Iminostilbenes

- Teach the patient and family about carbamazepine's name, dose, frequency, action, and adverse effects.
- Advise the patient to take carbamazepine with meals to decrease gastrointestinal distress and enhance absorption.
- Recommend that the female patient who uses an oral contraceptive use an additional or different contraceptive method. Discuss the advantages and disadvantages of various contraceptive methods, if requested.
- Instruct the patient and family to notify the physician immediately if the patient displays early signs of hematologic problems, such as fever, sore throat, malaise, unusual fatigue, or a tendency to bruise or bleed.

Evaluation

For each nursing diagnosis, prepare an evaluation statement that describes the patient's or family's response to nursing interventions.

Benzodiazepines

The three drugs from the benzodiazepine class that provide anticonvulsant effects are diazepam (parenteral), clonazepam, and clorazepate dipotassium. Only clonazepam is recommended for long-term treatment of epilepsy; diazepam is restricted to acute treatment of status epilepticus. Clorazepate is prescribed as an adjunct in treating partial seizures.

PHARMACOKINETICS

The benzodiazepines may be given orally or parenterally and are metabolized in the liver to multiple metabolites, which subsequently are excreted in the urine. They are absorbed rapidly and almost completely from the GI tract, but are distributed at different rates. Protein-binding of benzodiazepines ranges from 85% to 90%. Based on the rate of excretion or elimination, benzodiazepines are classified as long-acting, intermediate-acting, or short-acting. The metabolites of the benzodiazepines eventually are excreted in urine. The benzodiazepines are distributed readily across the placenta and are excreted in breast milk.

Route	Onset	Peak	Duration
P.O.	Unknown	1 to 2 hr	Unknown
I.V.	1-5 min	Immediate	15 min-1 hr

PHARMACODYNAMICS

The benzodiazepines provide anticonvulsant, antianxiety, sedative-hypnotic, and muscle-relaxant effects. Their mechanism of action is poorly understood.

PHARMACOTHERAPEUTICS

Clonazepam is used to treat absence (petit mal), atypical absence (Lennox-Gastaut syndrome), atonic, and myoclonic seizures. Diazepam is not recommended for long-term treatment because of the high serum concentrations required to control seizures and its addictive potential. Intravenously, it is used routinely as the initial control for status epilepticus. Because it is distributed so rapidly, diazepam provides only short-term effects of less than 1 hour. Consequently, a long-acting anticonvulsant, such as phenytoin or phenobarbital, also must be given during diazepam therapy. Clorazepate is used with other drugs to treat partial seizures. The therapeutic serum concentrations for the benzodiazepines have not been well established.

Drug interactions

Drug interactions between benzodiazepines and other CNS depressant drugs can occur. (See Drug Interactions: *Benzodiazepines*, page 166.)

ADVERSE DRUG REACTIONS

The dose-related adverse reactions to the benzodiazepines are primarily neurologic and include drowsiness, confusion, ataxia, weakness, dizziness, nystagmus, vertigo, syncope, dysarthria, headache, tremor, and a glassy-eyed appearance. These dose-related reactions diminish as therapy continues. Cardiorespiratory depression may occur with high doses and with I.V. diazepam. Geriatric patients are particularly susceptible to confusion, ataxia, and paradoxical excitement.

Idiosyncratic reactions to the benzodiazepines include a rash and acute hypersensitivity reactions. Hepatomegaly, leukopenia, thrombocytopenia, and eosinophilia have been reported rarely.

NURSING PROCESS APPLICATION

The following information assists the nurse in caring for a patient who is receiving a benzodiazepine. It includes an overview of assessment activities as well as examples of appropriate nursing diagnoses and related interventions (under "Planning and implementation"). It also highlights the importance of evaluation.

Assessment

Before drug therapy begins, review the patient's history for conditions that contraindicate or require cautious use of the prescribed benzodiazepine. Also review the patient's medication history to identify use of drugs that may interact

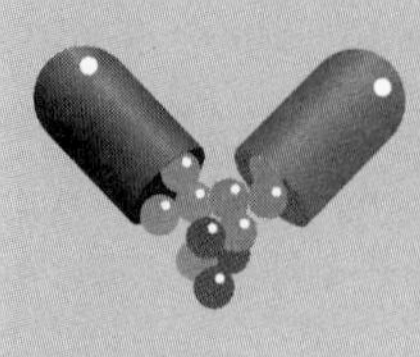

DRUG INTERACTIONS

Benzodiazepines

Drug interactions involving the benzodiazepines discussed in this chapter occur infrequently. However, when interactions occur, they usually involve concurrent use of other central nervous system (CNS) depressant drugs, including alcohol. The additive effects of CNS drugs with benzodiazepines can be lethal.

DRUG	INTERACTING AGENTS	POSSIBLE EFFECTS	NURSING IMPLICATIONS
clonazepam, clorazepate, diazepam	CNS depressants	Enhanced sedative and other CNS depressant effects. Effects may be supra-additive, causing motor skill impairment and respiratory depression. Lethal effect is possible, especially with high doses. Combination with anticonvulsant drugs can cause changes in seizures, especially in frequency or severity.	• Monitor for changes in level of consciousness and muscle coordination. • Monitor for signs of respiratory depression. • Advise the patient about possible additive effects of other CNS depressant drugs. • Warn the patient that alcohol increases the effect of the drug and can cause serious CNS depression. • Supervise ambulation; raise side rails, especially with geriatric patients. • Advise the patient against operating a motor vehicle or heavy machinery because of possibly impaired motor skills. • Observe for changes in frequency and severity of seizures when these drugs are used with anticonvulsant drugs.
	cimetidine	Excessive sedation and increasing CNS depression	• Monitor for signs of increasing CNS depressant effects; notify the physician if changes are noted. • Advise the patient against operating a motor vehicle or heavy machinery because increased sedation is possible. • Supervise ambulation; raise side rails, especially with geriatric patients.
	oral contraceptives	Decreased oxidative metabolism of these benzodiazepines	• Monitor for signs of excessive sedation. • Expect to decrease the benzodiazepine dosage.

with it. During therapy, assess the patient for adverse drug reactions and signs of drug interactions. Also, periodically assess the effectiveness of benzodiazepine therapy. Finally, evaluate the patient's and family's knowledge about the prescribed drug.

Nursing diagnoses

• Risk for injury related to a preexisting condition that contraindicates or requires cautious use of a benzodiazepine
• Risk for injury related to adverse drug reactions or drug interactions
• Knowledge deficit related to the prescribed benzodiazepine

Planning and implementation

• Do not administer a benzodiazepine to a patient with a condition that contraindicates its use. (See Patient Teaching: *Benzodiazepines.*)
• Administer a benzodiazepine cautiously to a patient at risk because of a preexisting condition.
• Monitor the patient for adverse drug reactions.
• Monitor vital signs during I.V. administration of diazepam, and keep resuscitation equipment readily available.
**** Administer I.V. diazepam no faster than 5 mg/minute in adults and over at least 3 minutes in children. Avoid starting an I.V. line in small veins. Use care to prevent extravasation.***
**** Do not mix I.V. diazepam with other drugs in the same syringe. Give direct I.V. push only. Do not give the drug as an infusion.***
• Store an oral benzodiazepine in a light-resistant container at room temperature, unless otherwise specified by the manufacturer.
• Notify the physician if the patient develops adverse reactions to the prescribed benzodiazepine.

Evaluation

For each nursing diagnosis, prepare an evaluation statement that describes the patient's or family's response to nursing interventions.

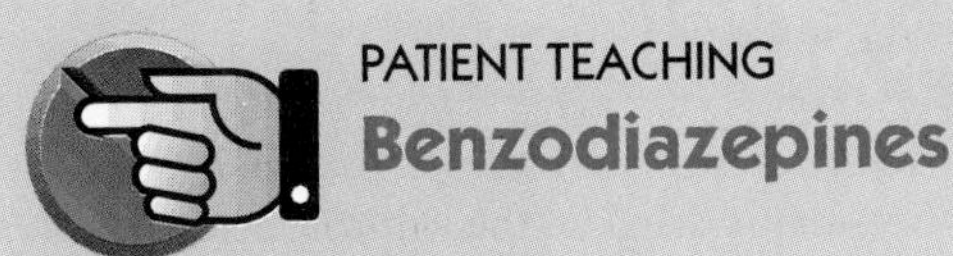

PATIENT TEACHING
Benzodiazepines

- Teach the patient and family the name, dose, frequency, action, and adverse effects of the prescribed benzodiazepine.
- Instruct the patient to contact the physician if adverse reactions occur.
- Instruct the patient to notify the physician if seizure control deteriorates.
- Instruct the patient to take the benzodiazepine exactly as prescribed to prevent drug dependence. Teach the patient and family to recognize and report to the physician signs of drug dependence, such as nervousness, insomnia, or diarrhea.

Succinimides

Three drugs from the succinimide class are used to treat absence (petit mal) seizures: ethosuximide, methsuximide, and phensuximide.

PHARMACOKINETICS

The succinimides are absorbed well from the GI tract and distributed widely throughout body tissues. Plasma protein-binding of the drugs is negligible. The succinimides are metabolized in the liver by microsomal enzymes. Almost 50% of ethosuximide is metabolized to a primary metabolite. This metabolite, as well as those of the other succinimides, is excreted as a glucuronoside in the urine. Approximately 20% of ethosuximide is excreted unchanged in the urine.

The onset of action for the succinimides is rapid. Peak serum concentration levels are reached at the following rates: methsuximide, 2 hours; phensuximide, 1 to 4 hours; ethosuximide, about 4 hours. The half-life is 4 to 12 hours for phensuximide, 23 to 57 hours for methsuximide and its active metabolite, and 60 hours for ethosuximide.

Route	Onset	Peak	Duration
P.O.	Rapid	1-4 hr	Unknown

PHARMACODYNAMICS

The succinimides reduce the frequency of absence seizures in children and adults, apparently by depressing nerve transmission in the motor cortex and increasing the seizure threshold for stimulus.

PHARMACOTHERAPEUTICS

Ethosuximide is the drug of choice for treating absence seizures. Methsuximide is prescribed less frequently because of the high incidence of toxicity associated with it. Methsuximide is indicated, however, for absence seizures and with other anticonvulsants to treat complex partial seizures. Phensuximide rarely is used because it is less effective. If used alone for mixed types of seizures, succinimides may increase the frequency of tonic-clonic seizures. However, methsuximide is least likely to precipitate tonic-clonic seizures.

Drug interactions

The succinimides may inhibit the metabolism of hydantoin anticonvulsants. Carbamazepine may decrease the concentration of a succinimide by induction.

ADVERSE DRUG REACTIONS

The succinimides produce GI, neurologic, hematologic, and genitourinary adverse reactions. In the GI tract, adverse reactions include nausea, vomiting, weight loss, abdominal pain, constipation, and diarrhea. The neurologic complaints include ataxia, dizziness, drowsiness, headache, euphoria, restlessness, irritability, lethargy, and confusion. Psychosis and suicidal ideation have occurred, but rarely. The hematologic adverse reactions include eosinophilia, leukopenia, thrombocytopenia, agranulocytosis, and aplastic anemia. The genitourinary adverse reactions include urinary frequency, hematuria, and albuminuria.

Methsuximide also can produce renal and hepatic damage. Other toxic reactions include increased libido, hirsutism, alopecia, and gum hypertrophy. The following hypersensitivity reactions to succinimides can occur: Stevens-Johnson syndrome, pruritic skin eruptions, exfoliative dermatitis, and systemic lupus erythematosus.

NURSING PROCESS APPLICATION

The following information assists the nurse in caring for a patient who is receiving a succinimide. It includes an overview of assessment activities as well as examples of appropriate nursing diagnoses and related interventions (under "Planning and implementation"). It also highlights the importance of evaluation.

Assessment

Before drug therapy begins, review the patient's history for conditions that contraindicate or require cautious use of the prescribed succinimide. Also review the patient's medication history to identify use of drugs that may interact with it. During therapy, assess the patient for adverse drug reactions, such as CNS changes, and signs of drug interactions. Also, periodically assess the effectiveness of succinimide therapy. Finally, evaluate the patient's and family's knowledge about the prescribed drug.

Nursing diagnoses

- Risk for injury related to a preexisting condition that contraindicates the use of a succinimide

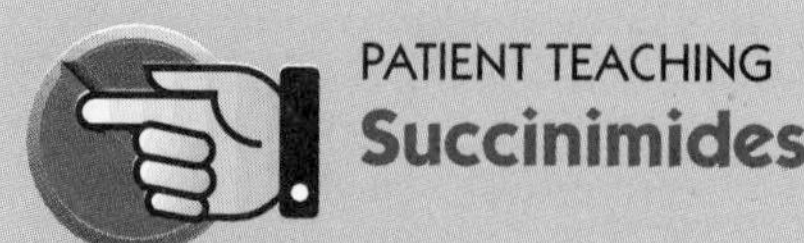

PATIENT TEACHING
Succinimides

- Teach the patient and family the name, dose, frequency, action, and adverse effects of the prescribed succinimide.
- Instruct the patient with gastrointestinal distress to take the prescribed succinimide with meals.
- Inform the patient that phensuximide may cause harmless pink, red, or red-brown discoloration of urine.
- Instruct the patient to contact the physician if adverse reactions occur.

• Risk for injury related to a preexisting condition that requires cautious use of a succinimide
• Risk for injury related to adverse drug reactions or drug interactions
• Altered thought processes related to the adverse CNS effects of a succinimide
• Knowledge deficit related to the prescribed succinimide

Planning and implementation

• Do not administer a succinimide to a patient with a condition that contraindicates its use. (See Patient Teaching: *Succinimides.*)
• Administer a succinimide cautiously to a patient at risk because of a preexisting condition.
• Observe the patient for adverse drug reactions.
• Monitor the patient for signs of toxicity when adjusting the dosage or when adding or eliminating any other medication.
*** *Administer a succinimide with meals if adverse GI reactions occur.***
• Store a succinimide away from heat. Shake all suspensions well before administration.
• Monitor the serum drug concentration.
• Report evidence of adverse drug reactions to the physician.
• Monitor the patient for signs of efficacy when adjusting the dosage or when adding or eliminating any other medication.
• Monitor seizure activity.
• Monitor the patient's mental status frequently.
*** *Take safety precautions if mental status alters. For example, keep the side rails up at all times, keep the bed in a low position, and supervise ambulation.***
• Reorient the confused patient, as needed.
• Notify the physician if the patient displays mental status changes.

Evaluation

For each nursing diagnosis, prepare an evaluation statement that describes the patient's or family's response to nursing interventions.

Valproic acid

Valproic acid is unrelated structurally to the other anticonvulsants. The two major drugs in the valproic acid class are valproate sodium and divalproex sodium.

PHARMACOKINETICS

Valproate sodium is converted rapidly to valproic acid in the stomach. Divalproex is a prodrug (precursor) of valproic acid and dissociates (separates into molecular fragments) to valproic acid in the GI tract. Valproic acid is absorbed well when administered as valproate or divalproex. Once absorbed, it is strongly protein-bound and is metabolized in the liver. Metabolites and unchanged drug are excreted in urine. Valproic acid readily crosses the placental barrier and also appears in breast milk.

The peak serum concentration level of valproate sodium occurs in 1 to 4 hours. Serum concentration of divalproex sodium peaks in 3 to 5 hours. The time needed to reach peak concentration is longer if the patient has a full stomach or receives enteric-coated tablets. In patients not taking other drugs, the half-life is 13 to 16 hours. For patients taking other anticonvulsants, the half-life drops to 6 to 10 hours, probably as a result of hepatic enzyme induction.

Route	Onset	Peak	Duration
P.O.	20-30 min	1-5 hr	Unknown

PHARMACODYNAMICS

The mechanism of action for valproic acid remains unknown.

PHARMACOTHERAPEUTICS

Valproic acid is prescribed for long-term treatment of absence, myoclonic, and tonic-clonic seizures. It also is administered rectally for status epilepticus refractory to other anticonvulsants. Valproic acid must be used cautiously in a young child or a patient receiving multiple anticonvulsants because of possible fatal hepatotoxicity. This risk limits the use of valproic acid as a drug of choice for seizure disorders.

Drug interactions

The most clinically significant drug interactions associated with valproic acid are inhibition of platelet aggregation, which may cause prolonged bleeding times in patients who also are receiving anticoagulants, and inhibition of the hepatic metabolism of phenobarbital. Valproic acid also can produce a false-positive result on urine ketone tests.

ADVERSE DRUG REACTIONS

Most adverse reactions associated with valproic acid are tolerable and dose related; however, rare fatal hepatotoxicity has occurred. The drug is not prescribed routinely because of the possibility of hepatotoxicity.

The dose-related adverse reactions affect the GI tract and CNS. The adverse GI reactions include nausea, vomiting, appetite changes, diarrhea, and constipation. Divalproex produces fewer adverse GI reactions than valproate. The adverse CNS reactions include sedation, drowsiness, dizziness, ataxia, headache, decreased alertness, and muscle weakness.

Adverse hematologic reactions include inhibited platelet aggregation and prolonged bleeding time. Rare adverse psychiatric reactions include depression, hallucinations, and behavioral disorders in children.

The rare, fatal hepatotoxicity that has been reported usually is preceded by nonspecific symptoms, such as loss of seizure control, malaise, jaundice, weakness, lethargy, facial edema, anorexia, and vomiting. The reaction may develop at any time from 3 days to 6 months after initiation of therapy. At the greatest risk are children and patients who receive other anticonvulsants along with valproic acid.

A drug rash may occur, as may hyperammonemia with normal liver function. The use of valproic acid also may produce blood dyscrasias, such as anemia, leukopenia, and thrombocytopenia.

NURSING PROCESS APPLICATION

The following information assists the nurse in caring for a patient who is receiving valproic acid. It includes an overview of assessment activities as well as examples of appropriate nursing diagnoses and related interventions (under "Planning and implementation"). It also highlights the importance of evaluation.

Assessment

Before drug therapy begins, review the patient's history for conditions that contraindicate or require cautious use of valproic acid. Also review the patient's medication history to identify use of drugs that may interact with it. During therapy, assess the patient for adverse drug reactions and signs of drug interactions. Also, periodically assess the effectiveness of valproic acid therapy. Finally, evaluate the patient's and family's knowledge about the drug.

Nursing diagnoses

- Risk for injury related to a preexisting condition that contraindicates or requires cautious use of valproic acid
- Risk for injury related to adverse drug reactions or drug interactions
- Altered health maintenance related to ineffectiveness of valproic acid
- Knowledge deficit related to valproic acid

Planning and implementation

- Do not administer valproic acid to a patient with a condition that contraindicates its use.

Administer valproic acid cautiously to a pregnant or breast-feeding patient.

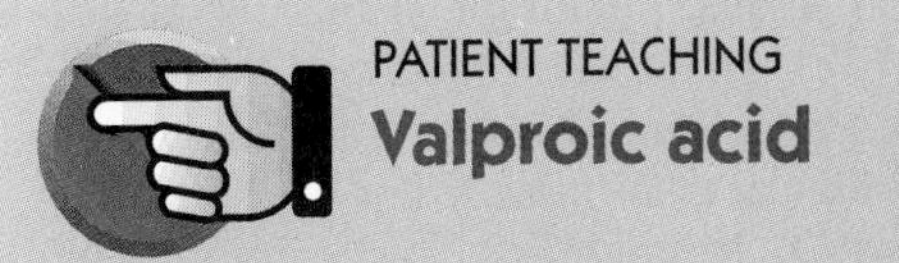

PATIENT TEACHING
Valproic acid

- Teach the patient and family the name, dose, frequency, action, and adverse effects of valproic acid.
- Instruct the patient to swallow each capsule whole because the free drug can irritate the gastrointestinal mucosa.
- Alert the diabetic patient that the drug may produce a false-positive result on a urine ketone test.
- Teach the patient to recognize the signs and symptoms of hepatotoxicity and to contact the physician immediately if any occur.
- Remind the patient to report immediately signs of bleeding so that platelet function can be assessed.
- Instruct the patient to inform the physician of valproic acid therapy before surgery, including dental surgery.

- Monitor the patient for adverse reactions.
- Take safety measures, if decreased mental alertness occurs. For example, keep the bed side rails up at all times, maintain the bed in a low position, and supervise all patient activity.

Administer valproic acid with meals to decrease adverse GI reactions. Keep the flavorful red syrup out of the reach of children. (See Patient Teaching: *Valproic acid.*)

- Notify the physician if adverse drug reactions occur.
- Monitor the serum concentration of valproic acid regularly.
- Monitor seizure activity.
- Notify the physician of any change in seizure activity and serum drug concentrations.

Evaluation

For each nursing diagnosis, prepare an evaluation statement that describes the patient's or family's response to nursing interventions.

Other anticonvulsants

This section contains information about other drugs used less frequently to treat seizure disorders.

Acetazolamide is used primarily as a diuretic, but also possesses anticonvulsant properties. Acetazolamide sometimes is used as adjunct or intermittent therapy in absence, partial, and generalized tonic-clonic seizures. Its mechanism of action remains unknown. Hypokalemia and metabolic acidosis represent potentially serious effects associated with the use of acetazolamide.

Since the introduction of the succinimides, trimethadione and paramethadione are used only occasionally as sole or adjunct treatment for refractory absence seizures. Both drugs are metabolized to an active metabolite that has a prolonged half-life of 10 days to 2 weeks. Trimethadione and paramethadione cause significant GI and CNS toxicity and are less effective than the succinimides.

Magnesium sulfate prevents or controls seizures by blocking neuromuscular transmission. It is used primarily as an anticonvulsant in preeclampsia or eclampsia and hypomagnesemic seizures.

Felbamate is a drug recently reintroduced for seizure control. Felbamate is recommended for use only in those patients who do not respond to alternative treatments. It is not a first line drug. The drug is well absorbed orally. It is a pregnancy C category and is detected in breast milk. The main adverse reaction is an associated increased incidence of aplastic anemia with use of felbamate.

CHAPTER SUMMARY

Chapter 13 centered on anticonvulsant drugs. Here are the highlights of the chapter.

Anticonvulsants are prescribed for long-term treatment of epilepsy and for short-term control of acute isolated seizures not caused by epilepsy.

The major classes of drugs used to treat patients with seizure disorders include hydantoins, barbiturates, iminostilbenes, benzodiazepines, succinimides, and valproic acid.

The drugs of choice for complex partial seizures are phenytoin and carbamazepine, and possibly primidone. Phenobarbital is one of the most widely used anticonvulsants in long-term treatment of epilepsy. It also may be used for acute treatment of status epilepticus. Ethosuximide is the drug of choice for absence seizures.

Anticonvulsants commonly interact with other drugs, sometimes producing drug toxicity. To help prevent drug interactions, the nurse should maintain an up-to-date drug history.

Some anticonvulsants are an increased risk factor when administered to women of childbearing age or to pregnant or lactating women. Teratogenic effects have occurred in patients using anticonvulsants.

The nurse should monitor serum concentrations of anticonvulsants frequently. Additional laboratory studies are recommended depending on the potential for toxicity.

Questions to consider

See Appendix 1 for answers.

1. Mary Anderson, age 15, has a tonic-clonic seizure disorder and takes phenytoin 300 mg P.O. h.s. daily. Which of the following terms best describes the absorption rate of oral phenytoin?
   (a) Rapid
   (b) Slow
   (c) Erratic
   (d) Poor

2. Harry Phillips, age 36, has had partial seizures for 10 years and takes phenobarbital 60 mg P.O. daily. Where is phenobarbital primarily metabolized?
   (a) Stomach
   (b) Liver
   (c) Kidneys
   (d) Brain

3. Sarah Frank, age 12, has a history of tonic-clonic seizures and takes carbamazepine 100 mg P.O. b.i.d. This iminostilbene derivative is structurally related to which of the following drugs?
   (a) Tricyclic antidepressants
   (b) Phenothiazines
   (c) Benzodiazepines
   (d) Barbiturates

4. A patient develops status epilepticus and is brought to the emergency department. Which of the following drugs is preferred for status epilepticus?
   (a) clorazepate dipotassium
   (b) phenytoin
   (c) diazepam
   (d) mephobarbital

5. Joseph Cirano, age 9, takes ethosuximide 250 mg P.O. b.i.d. This anticonvulsant is the drug of choice for which of the following types of seizures?
   (a) Partial
   (b) Tonic-clonic
   (c) Atonic
   (d) Absence

6. Amy Henderson, age 11, develops myoclonic seizures. The physician could prescribe valproate sodium, but this drug is not administered routinely. Which of the following major adverse reactions limits the use of valproate?
   (a) Hepatotoxicity
   (b) CNS sedation
   (c) Respiratory depression
   (d) Muscle weakness

7. Which of the following medications can be given I.M. for the short term if a patient is unable to take his oral anticonvulsant medicine?
   (a) phenytoin
   (b) fosphenytoin
   (c) valproic acid
   (d) phenobarbital

8. Which of the following administration principles is important to remember when administering phenytoin I.V.?
   (a) It is best given by I.V. push.
   (b) It can be mixed with other medications or additives.
   (c) It should be diluted in normal saline and not mixed with other medications.
   (d) It should never be given I.V.

UNIT

V

Drugs to prevent and treat pain

A basic protective mechanism, pain is a symptom of an underlying physiologic or psychological problem. Pain usually indicates that something is wrong and that health care is desirable.

Because pain is subjective, only the patient can describe it. Pain is whatever sensation the patient perceives it to be; one person's pain perceptions may vary widely from another's. Emotional states and ethnic, cultural, and religious factors all contribute to the patient's pain perception.

Pain detection and transmission

Pain sensation begins in the **nociceptors,** which are part of an afferent neuron. Nociceptors are free nerve endings located primarily in the skin, periosteum, joint surfaces, and arterial walls. They may be activated by mechanical, chemical, or thermal stimuli. They also are activated by chemical mediators that are released or synthesized in response to tissue damage. Regardless of the etiology, even if only minor tissue damage occurs, the chemical mediators are synthesized and stimulate the nociceptors.

Prostaglandins, histamine, bradykinin, and serotonin are chemical mediators that sensitize the nociceptors.

Once the pain process is initiated, the impulse is communicated from the peripheral terminals of the nociceptors to the spinal cord. (See *Pain pathways,* page 172.)

Somatostatin, cholecystokinin, and substance P have been identified as possible neurotransmitters in the afferent neurons. Analgesics may act to block the effects of any of those neurotransmitters. Two types of nociceptors exist: the myelinated A-delta fibers and the smaller, unmyelinated, more numerous C fibers. The faster-conducting A-delta fibers signal sharp, well-localized pain; the slower-conducting C fibers signal dull, poorly localized pain.

All nociceptors terminate in the dorsal horn of the spinal cord. The dorsal horn is the control center for incoming information from the afferent neurons, for local modulation (pain impulse regulation), and for descending influences from higher centers in the central nervous system (CNS), such as emotion, attention, and memory.

Pain theory

The Melzack-Wall gate-control theory, the most widely accepted pain theory, states that neural mechanisms in the dorsal horn act as a regulator between the peripheral fibers and the higher processing centers in the CNS. The dorsal horn receives pain- and non-pain-related signals from the various peripheral nerves; pain messages depend on the total information. This process, or gating effect, modulates, or regulates, afferent input before an impulse is sent to the CNS and pain is perceived. Therefore, pain perception may be inhibited by the simultaneous activation of sensory neurons carrying nonpain information.

Mechanisms of inflammation

Pain may occur alone or with **inflammation.** Both are reactions to tissue irritation. Inflammation is an immune-mediated process characterized by redness, heat, swelling, loss of function, and pain at the site. Some of the chemical mediators of pain, including prostaglandins, bradykinin, and histamine, also mediate the inflammatory response.

Temperature regulation

The hypothalamus regulates body temperature by balancing heat production and loss. **Pyrogens,** secreted by toxic bacteria or released from protein breakdown, can cause the hypothalamic thermostat to rise. This in turn increases body temperature. Pyrogens may also increase body temperature by causing production of prostaglandin E_1 in the hypothalamus. Some of the drugs used to control pain inhibit prostaglandins and produce an antipyretic effect.

Pain pathways

When stimulated, the A-delta fiber and C fiber nociceptors transmit an afferent impulse through the dorsal root ganglia to the dorsal horn. Peripheral nerves also transmit information to the dorsal horn. The dorsal horn then controls this information and may transmit an impulse via the spinothalamic tract to the cerebral cortex. Descending pathways carry inhibitory information from the brain to the dorsal horn to be used by the peripheral nervous system.

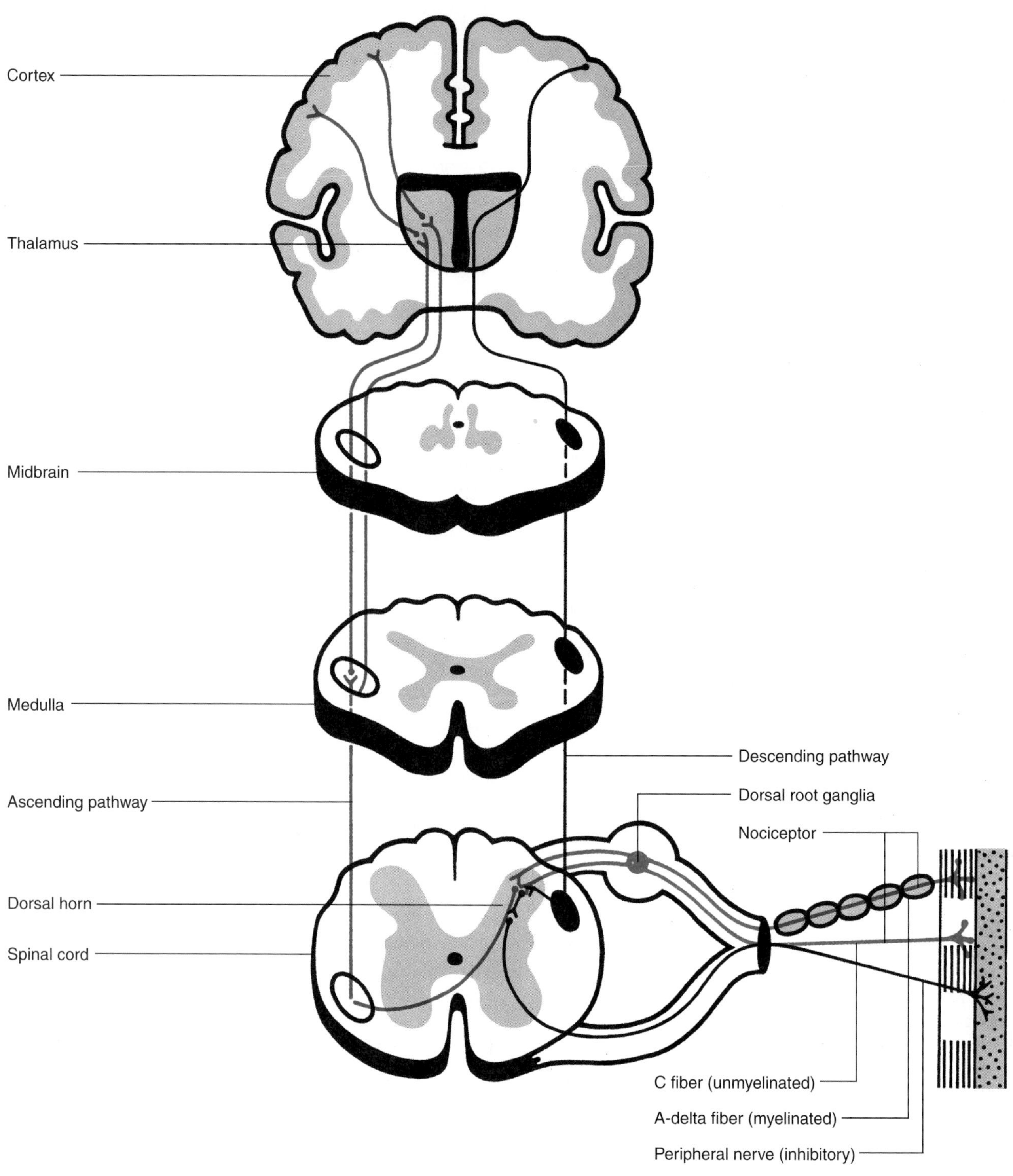

14 Nonnarcotic analgesic, antipyretic, and nonsteroidal anti-inflammatory agents

OBJECTIVES

After reading and studying this chapter, the student should be able to:

1. describe the pharmacodynamics of salicylates, acetaminophen, and nonsteroidal anti-inflammatory drugs (NSAIDs).
2. compare the therapeutic uses of salicylates, acetaminophen, and NSAIDs.
3. contrast the drug interactions associated with salicylates, acetaminophen, and NSAIDs.
4. compare the adverse drug reactions to salicylates, acetaminophen, and NSAIDs.
5. describe how to apply the nursing process when caring for a patient who is receiving a salicylate, acetaminophen, or an NSAID.

INTRODUCTION

The drugs discussed in this chapter form a heterogenous collection that produce analgesic, antipyretic, and anti-inflammatory effects. Among these drugs, salicylates — especially aspirin — are the most widely used. This chapter discusses the salicylates, the para-aminophenol derivative acetaminophen, NSAIDs, and the urinary tract analgesic phenazopyridine hydrochloride. (See *Selected major nonnarcotic analgesic, antipyretic, and nonsteroidal anti-inflammatory drugs,* pages 174 to 176.)

The drugs covered in this chapter include:

- acetominophen
- aspirin
- choline magnesium-trisalicylate
- choline salicylate
- diclofenac
- diflunisal
- etodolac
- fenoprofen calcium
- flurbiprofen
- ibuprofen
- indomethacin
- ketoprofen
- ketorolac tromethamine
- meclofenamate
- mefenamic acid
- nabumetone
- naproxen
- naproxen sodium
- piroxicam
- phenylbutazone
- salsalate
- sodium salicylate
- sulindac
- tolmetin sodium.

Salicylates

These agents possess analgesic, antipyretic, and anti-inflammatory properties. They usually cost less than other analgesics and most are readily available without a prescription. In fact, many over-the-counter (OTC) medications for pain, colds, and influenza contain salicylates along with other agents. This section discusses the following salicylates: aspirin, choline magnesium trisalicylate, choline salicylate, diflunisal, salsalate, and sodium salicylate. Despite the recent development of new products, however, aspirin remains the cornerstone of anti-inflammatory drug therapy.

PHARMACOKINETICS

After oral administration, salicylate absorption occurs partly in the stomach but mainly in the upper part of the small intestine through passive diffusion. Although absorption usually occurs within 30 minutes, the rate depends on the dosage form, the gastric and intestinal pH, the presence of food or antacids in the stomach, and the gastric-emptying time. The pure and buffered forms of aspirin are absorbed readily, but sustained-release and enteric-coated salicylate preparations or food or antacids in the stomach delay absorption. Salicylates may also be given rectally.

Salicylates are distributed widely throughout the body tissues and fluids, including breast milk. They cross the placenta easily. The liver metabolizes salicylates extensively into several metabolites. Therapeutic salicylate concentrations range from 30 to 300 mcg/ml. Blood levels that exceed this amount may be toxic. The kidneys excrete the salicylate metabolites and some unchanged drug.

Route	Onset	Peak	Duration
P.O.	30-60 min	1-3 hr	3-6 hr
P.R.	1-2 hr	4-5 hr	7 or more hr

PHARMACODYNAMICS

The salicylates produce **analgesia** primarily by inhibiting **prostaglandin** synthesis; reduce fever through hypothalamic stimulation leading to vasodilation and increased diaphoresis; and reduce **inflammation** through a poorly understood process that may involve their ability to inhibit

(Text continues on page 176.)

Selected major nonnarcotic analgesic, antipyretic, and nonsteroidal anti-inflammatory drugs

This table summarizes the major analgesic, antipyretic, and nonsteroidal anti-inflammatory drugs (NSAIDs) currently in clinical use.

DRUG	MAJOR INDICATIONS AND USUAL DOSAGES	CONTRAINDICATIONS AND PRECAUTIONS
Salicylates		
aspirin (A.S.A., Bayer Timed-Release, Empirin)	*Mild to moderate pain, fever* ADULT: 325 to 650 mg P.O. every 3 to 4 hours as needed PEDIATRIC: 10 to 15 mg/kg/dose P.O. every 4 hours up to 60 to 80 mg/kg/day *Dysmenorrhea* ADULT: 650 mg P.O. every 4 to 6 hours, beginning 1 or 2 days before the onset of menses and continuing until the 2nd or 3rd day of menses *Acute rheumatic fever* ADULT: initially, 5 to 8 g/day P.O. PEDIATRIC: 100 mg/kg/day P.O. for 2 weeks, then decreased to 75 mg/kg/day for 4 to 6 weeks *Rheumatoid arthritis* ADULT: 3.2 to 6 g P.O. daily in divided doses *Juvenile rheumatoid arthritis* PEDIATRIC: 60 to 110 mg/kg/day in divided doses P.O. every 6 to 8 hours *Myocardial infarction prophylaxis* ADULT: 300 to 325 mg/day P.O. *Transient ischemic attacks* ADULT: 325 mg P.O. q.i.d. or 650 mg P.O. b.i.d.	• Aspirin in contraindicated in a pediatric patient with varicella or influenza due to the possibility of Reye's syndrome (unless directed by a physician), a patient during the last 3 months of pregnancy, and one with a bleeding disorder, known hypersensitivity to the drug, or aspirin-induced acute asthmatic attacks, urticaria, or rhinitis. • This drug requires cautious use in a breast-feeding or pregnant patient during the first 6 months of pregnancy, one receiving anticoagulant therapy, or one with impaired renal function, hypoprothrombinemia, vitamin K deficiency, thrombocytopenia, thrombotic thrombocytopenic purpura, severe hepatic impairment, or gastrointestinal (GI) lesions. Highly buffered aspirin solutions require cautious use in a patient with congestive heart failure or other conditions in which a high sodium intake would be harmful.
diflunisal (Dolobid)	*Mild to moderate musculoskeletal pain* ADULT: 500 to 1,000 mg P.O. initially, followed by 250 to 500 mg every 8 to 12 hours; not to exceed 1,500 mg/day *Osteoarthritis* ADULT: 500 to 1,000 mg P.O. daily in two divided doses	• Diflunisal is contraindicated in a pediatric patient with varicella or influenza (unless directed by a physician), a patient during the last 3 months of pregnancy, a breast-feeding patient, or one with known hypersensitivity to the drug or diflunisal-induced acute asthmatic attacks, urticaria, or rhinitis. • This drug requires cautious use in a pregnant patient during the first 6 months of pregnancy; one receiving anticoagulant therapy; one with a history of bleeding disorders, peptic ulceration, or GI bleeding; or one with renal dysfunction, compromised cardiac function, hypertension, or other conditions that predispose to fluid retention. • Safety and efficacy in children have not been established.
Para-aminophenol derivatives		
acetaminophen (Datril, Panadol, Tylenol)	*Headache, mild to moderate pain, fever* ADULT: 325 to 650 mg P.O. or rectally every 4 to 6 hours as needed, not to exceed 4 g/day PEDIATRIC: 5 to 10 mg/kg P.O. every 4 to 6 hours, not to exceed five doses in 24 hours *Osteoarthritis* ADULT: 325 to 650 mg P.O. or rectally every 3 to 4 hours as needed, not to exceed 4 g/day	• Acetaminophen is contraindicated in a patient with known hypersensitivity to the drug. Repeated administration is contraindicated in a patient with anemia or cardiac, pulmonary, renal, or hepatic disease. • This drug requires cautious use in a patient with anemia.
Nonsteroidal anti-inflammatory drugs		
diclofenac (Voltaren)	*Ankylosing spondylitis* ADULT: 100 to 125 mg P.O. daily in 25-mg doses q.i.d. with an additional 25 mg at bedtime as needed	• Diclofenac is contraindicated in a breast-feeding or pregnant patient during the last 3 months of pregnancy or one with known hypersensitivity to the drug, hepatic porphyria, or a history of diclofenac-, aspirin-, or other NSAID-induced asthma, urticaria, or other allergic reactions.

Selected major nonnarcotic analgesic, antipyretic, and nonsteroidal anti-inflammatory drugs *(continued)*

DRUG	MAJOR INDICATIONS AND USUAL DOSAGES	CONTRAINDICATIONS AND PRECAUTIONS
Nonsteroidal anti-inflammatory drugs *(continued)*		
diclofenac (Voltaren) *(continued)*	*Osteoarthritis* ADULT: 100 to 150 mg P.O. daily in two or three divided doses *Rheumatoid arthritis* ADULT: 150 to 200 mg P.O. daily in two to four divided doses	• This drug requires cautious use in a pregnant patient during the first 6 months of pregnancy or one with significant renal impairment or a history of cardiac decompensation, hypertension, or other conditions that predispose to fluid retention. • Dosage recommendations and indications for use in children have not been established.
ibuprofen (Advil, Motrin, Nuprin)	*Mild to moderate pain* ADULT: 200 to 400 mg P.O. every 4 to 6 hours, not to exceed 3.2 g/day PEDIATRIC: for children age 6 months or older, 20 to 40 mg/kg P.O. daily in three or four divided doses *Dysmenorrhea* ADULT: 400 mg P.O. every 4 hours as needed, given as soon as pain begins *Arthritis* ADULT: 400 to 800 mg P.O. t.i.d. or q.i.d. PEDIATRIC: for rheumatoid arthritis, 20 to 70 mg/kg/day P.O. in three or four divided doses *Fever* ADULT: 400 mg P.O. every 4 to 6 hours as needed PEDIATRIC: 5 mg/kg if baseline temperature is 102.5° F or less or 10 mg/kg if baseline temperature is above 102.5° F (39° C); not to exceed 40 mg/kg/day	• Ibuprofen is contraindicated in a pregnant or breast-feeding patient or one with known hypersensitivity to the drug or a history of aspirin- or NSAID-induced bronchospasm, angioedema, nasal polyps, urticaria, severe rhinitis, or shock. • This drug requires cautious use in a patient with peptic ulcer disease, GI perforation or bleeding, bleeding abnormalities, impaired renal function, hypertension, or compromised cardiac function. • Safety and efficacy in children under age 6 months have not been established.
indomethacin (Indocin)	*Rheumatoid arthritis, osteoarthritis, ankylosing spondylitis* ADULT: 25 to 50 mg P.O. t.i.d., increased to a maximum of 200 mg/day *Acute gouty arthritis* ADULT: 50 mg P.O. t.i.d. *Bursitis and tendinitis* ADULT: 75 to 150 mg P.O. daily in three or four divided doses	• Indomethacin is contraindicated in a pregnant or breast-feeding patient or one with known hypersensitivity to the drug, active GI lesions or a history of recurrent GI lesions (unless high risk is warranted and the patient is closely monitored), or aspirin- or NSAID-induced acute asthmatic attacks, urticaria, or rhinitis. Indomethacin suppositories are contraindicated in a patient with a history of proctitis or recent rectal bleeding. • This drug requires cautious use in a patient with depression or other psychiatric disturbances; epilepsy; infections; parkinsonism; or renal impairment, coagulation defects, cardiac dysfunction, hypertension, or other conditions that predispose to fluid retention. • Safety and efficacy in children have not been established.
naproxen (Naprosyn, Aleve)	*Osteoarthritis, rheumatoid arthritis, ankylosing spondylitis* ADULT: 250 to 500 mg P.O. in morning and evening, increased to a maximum of 1,500 mg/day, if needed *Tendinitis, bursitis, dysmenorrhea, mild to moderate pain* ADULT: 250 to 500 mg P.O. in morning and evening, increased to a maximum of 1,500 mg/day if needed *Juvenile arthritis* PEDIATRIC: 10 mg/kg P.O. daily in two divided doses	• Naproxen is contraindicated in a breast-feeding or pregnant patient during the last 3 months of pregnancy or one with known hypersensitivity to the drug, a history of aspirin- or NSAID-induced asthma, rhinitis, or nasal polyps. • This drug requires cautious use in a geriatric patient, a patient during the first 6 months of pregnancy, or one with impaired renal function, chronic alcoholic liver disease, anemia, fluid retention, hypertension, heart failure, liver dysfunction, or diuretic therapy. • Safety and efficacy in children under age 2 have not been established.

(continued)

Selected major nonnarcotic analgesic, antipyretic, and nonsteroidal anti-inflammatory drugs *(continued)*

DRUG	MAJOR INDICATIONS AND USUAL DOSAGES	CONTRAINDICATIONS AND PRECAUTIONS
Nonsteroidal anti-inflammatory drugs *(continued)*		
tolmetin sodium (Tolectin)	*Osteoarthritis, rheumatoid arthritis* ADULT: 400 mg P.O. t.i.d. initially, including a dose upon arising and at bedtime, increased as needed to a maximum of 1,800 mg/day in four divided doses *Juvenile rheumatoid arthritis* PEDIATRIC: for children age 2 and over, initially 20 mg/kg/day in three or four divided doses; then 15 to 30 mg/kg/day	• Tolmetin is contraindicated in a breast-feeding patient or one with known hypersensitivity to the drug or other NSAIDs or aspirin- or NSAID-induced acute asthmatic attacks, urticaria, or rhinitis. • This drug requires cautious use in a pregnant or geriatric patient or one with liver dysfunction, diuretic therapy, or heart failure, impaired renal function, bleeding disorder, compromised cardiac function, hypertension, or other conditions that predispose to fluid retention. • Safety and efficacy in children under age 2 have not been established.

prostaglandin synthesis and release during inflammation. The salicylate aspirin inhibits platelet aggregation through irreversible pathways by interfering with thromboxane A_2 production, which is necessary for platelet clumping.

PHARMACOTHERAPEUTICS

Salicylates are used primarily to relieve pain and reduce fever. However, they cannot effectively relieve visceral pain or severe pain from trauma.

Salicylates have little or no effect on normal body temperature but cause a marked fall if body temperature is elevated. This is especially true of aspirin. Salicylates are often the drugs of choice for relief of fever associated with common colds or influenza because they can relieve headache and muscle ache as well.

Salicylates suppress inflammation, probably by inhibiting prostaglandin synthesis. Used to reduce inflammation in rheumatic fever and rheumatoid arthritis, they can provide considerable relief in 24 hours. No matter what the clinical indication, the main guideline of salicylate therapy is to use the lowest dose that provides relief.

Drug interactions

Because salicylates are highly protein bound, they may interact with many other protein-bound drugs by displacing them from their binding sites. This increases the serum concentration of unbound active drug, thereby increasing the pharmacologic effects of the displaced drug. Salicylates also may potentiate the effects of other drugs. Rarely, they can cause false-positive reactions in diabetic patients using the copper reduction test (Clinitest) for urine glucose and false-negative reactions to the glucose oxidase test (Tes-Tape). (See Drug Interactions: *Salicylates.*)

ADVERSE DRUG REACTIONS

The most common adverse reactions to salicylates involve the gastrointestinal (GI) system. Other reactions may include respiratory alkalosis and metabolic acidosis, hearing problems, salicylate toxicity, and hypersensitivity reactions.

Gastric distress, nausea, and vomiting commonly result from the central action of the salicylates on the emetic center of the medulla and their local action on the gastric mucosa secretions that protect the stomach from gastric acid. Although sodium bicarbonate may help prevent GI irritation, it also promotes salicylate excretion by the kidneys.

Large or toxic salicylate doses can cause respiratory alkalosis and increase the rate and depth of respiration. If the respiratory problem is not corrected, metabolic acidosis can occur as the body attempts to compensate for the respiratory alkalosis.

Prolonged use of salicylates sometimes causes bilateral hearing loss of 30 to 40 decibels that usually resolves within 2 weeks after therapy is discontinued. Tinnitus may occur with dosage levels used to treat arthritis, requiring a small dosage reduction. A geriatric patient or a patient with impaired hearing, who may not notice the ringing sound until it is severe, should be monitored closely.

Mild salicylate toxicity, or **salicylism,** characteristically causes nausea, vomiting, diarrhea, thirst, diaphoresis, tinnitus, confusion, dizziness, impaired vision, and hyperventilation. When these signs and symptoms appear with doses used to treat rheumatic conditions, a reduction of 325 mg/day usually reduces them to a tolerable level. Indications of severe toxicity include metabolic acidosis and related acid-base imbalances, hemorrhagic tendencies, hypoglycemia, restlessness, incoherent speech, apprehension, delirium, hallucinations, and seizures.

In a child with a varicella infection or flulike symptoms, salicylates may lead to Reye's syndrome, a potentially fatal

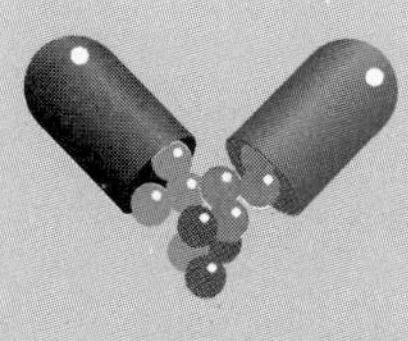

DRUG INTERACTIONS

Salicylates

Drug interactions involving salicylates are common and sometimes severe. They typically occur with concurrent use of other highly protein-bound or ulcerogenic agents. Because salicylates are so widely used, the nurse must obtain a thorough drug history and be alert for possible drug interactions.

DRUG	INTERACTING AGENTS	POSSIBLE EFFECTS	NURSING IMPLICATIONS
aspirin, choline magnesium trisalicylate, choline salicylate, diflunisal, salsalate, sodium salicylate	alcohol	Increased ulcerogenic effect, leading to gastrointestinal (GI) bleeding	• Monitor the patient for signs of GI bleeding, such as epigastric pain, abdominal pain or cramps, or black or tarry stools.
	oral anticoagulants and heparin	Increased anticoagulant effect, increasing risk of bleeding	• Monitor the patient for signs of increased anticoagulant effect, such as gingival bleeding, black or tarry stools, blood in the urine, petechiae, and bruises.
	corticosteroids	Decreased plasma salicylate concentrations and increased ulcerogenic effect	• Assess the patient for the salicylate's effectiveness. If it does not provide relief, obtain a prescription for a different analgesic. • Monitor the patient for epigastric pain, especially 1 to 2 hours after meals. Also assess for other signs of GI bleeding, such as abdominal pain or cramps or black or tarry stools.
	methotrexate	Increased methotrexate effect and toxicity, causing pancytopenia	• Question any prescription for salicylates for a patient receiving methotrexate. Avoid concurrent use, if possible. • Monitor the patient for signs of methotrexate toxicity, such as diarrhea and stomatitis. • Monitor the patient for signs of severe bone marrow depression, such as fatigue, pallor, and fever.
	probenecid, sulfinpyrazone	Decreased uricosuric effect, even with small doses of salicylates	• Instruct the patient not to take aspirin or other over-the-counter drugs containing salicylates unless directed by the physician.
	antacids	Alkaline urine, leading to reduced renal tubular reabsorption and increased renal excretion of salicylates	• Observe the patient for signs and symptoms of reduced salicylate response, such as increased pain and inflammation. • Expect serum salicylate concentrations to decrease, requiring a dosage adjustment.
	oral hypoglycemics (sulfonylureas) and exogenous insulin	Increased hypoglycemic effect	• Monitor the patient for signs and symptoms of hypoglycemia, such as fatigue, tremors, hunger, drowsiness, headache, diaphoresis, anxiety, numb mouth, or incoherent speech.
	zidovudine	Inhibited zidovudine metabolism, possibly causing toxicity	• Avoid concurrent use of these drugs.
	alkalinizing agents	Increased salicylate excretion, if salicylate dosage exceeds 50 mg/kg/day	• Monitor the patient for decreased salicylate effectiveness.
	spironolactone	Reduced spironolactone diuretic effects	• Monitor the patient's fluid intake and output. • Monitor the patient's serum potassium level.
	acetazolamide	Acetazolamide intoxication	• Monitor the patient for signs and symptoms of central nervous system toxicity, such as lethargy, confusion, or anorexia.

(continued)

Salicylates *(continued)*

DRUG	INTERACTING AGENTS	POSSIBLE EFFECTS	NURSING IMPLICATIONS
aspirin, choline magnesium trisalicylate, choline salicylate, diflunisal, salsalate, sodium salicylate *(continued)*	nizatidine	Increased serum salicylate levels	• Monitor for signs of salicylate toxicity
	angiotensin converting enzyme inhibitors, beta blockers	Decreased antihypertensive effectiveness	• Monitor blood pressure and teach the patient about salicylate use and antihypertensive medications.
	nonsteroidal anti-inflammatory drugs (NSAIDs)	Decreased serum concentration of NSAID and increased incidence of GI effects	• Instruct the patient not to take salicylates and NSAIDs together.
	valproic acid, phenytoin	Displaced from protein binding sites and increased effect of valproic acid	• Monitor serum valproic acid and phenytoin levels.

disorder that causes encephalopathy and fatty infiltration of the internal organs. Although a direct causal relationship has not been established, the U.S. Food and Drug Administration discourages the use of salicylates in children and teenagers who have varicella or influenza infections.

Common hypersensitivity reactions to salicylates include rash and, in asthmatics with nasal polyps, bronchospasm and asthma. Anaphylaxis rarely occurs.

NURSING PROCESS APPLICATION

The following information assists the nurse in caring for a patient who is receiving a salicylate. It includes an overview of assessment activities as well as examples of appropriate nursing diagnoses and related interventions (under "Planning and implementation"). It also highlights the importance of evaluation.

Assessment

Before drug therapy begins, review the patient's history for conditions that contraindicate or require cautious use of the prescribed salicylate. Also review the patient's medication history to identify use of drugs that may interact with it. During therapy, assess the patient for adverse drug reactions and signs of drug interactions. Also, periodically assess the effectiveness of therapy. Finally, evaluate the patient's and family's knowledge about the prescribed salicylate.

Nursing diagnoses

- Risk for injury related to a preexisting condition that contraindicates or requires cautious use of a salicylate
- Risk for injury related to adverse drug reactions or drug interactions
- Pain related to salicylate ineffectiveness
- Knowledge deficit related to the salicylate

Planning and implementation

- Do not administer a salicylate to a patient with a condition that contraindicates its use. Keep in mind that an asthmatic patient with nasal polyps is particularly vulnerable to acute asthmatic attack and bronchospasm, usually 15 to 30 minutes after salicylate ingestion. (See Patient Teaching: *Salicylates.*)
- Do not administer aspirin to a patient in the third trimester of pregnancy. If she ingests aspirin or an aspirin-containing product up to 2 weeks before delivery, observe the neonate for bleeding.
- Do not administer diflunisal for antipyretic therapy.
- Administer a salicylate cautiously to a patient at risk because of a preexisting condition.
- Question any prescription of sodium salicylate for a patient with hypertension or on a sodium-restricted diet. Advise such a patient not to use effervescent aspirin products, which have a high sodium content.
- Observe the patient frequently for adverse reactions to the salicylate.
- Check the diflunisal dose carefully before administration. Small dosage changes may cause large changes in the blood concentration, leading to toxicity.
- Administer the salicylate with at least 8 oz (240 ml) of liquid, unless contraindicated.
- Do not check the diabetic patient's urine for glucose with the copper reduction test (Clinitest) or glucose oxidase test (Tes-Tape). These tests may provide incorrect results during salicylate use.
- Expect to discontinue aspirin 1 week before major surgery to reduce the risk of bleeding.

✱ ***Observe for early signs and symptoms of salicylate toxicity. Expect to reduce the salicylate dosage.***

- Notify the physician of other adverse reactions or evidence of salicylate toxicity.

***** ***Encourage the patient to report hearing changes because bilateral hearing loss of 30 to 40 decibels can occur with prolonged use of a salicylate.***

• Monitor the patient for pain relief during salicylate therapy. If pain relief does not occur, obtain a prescription for a different analgesic. Be aware that concomitant use of certain drugs, such as corticosteroids and antacids, may decrease the analgesic effect of salicylates.

Evaluation

For each nursing diagnosis, prepare an evaluation statement that describes the patient's or family's response to nursing interventions.

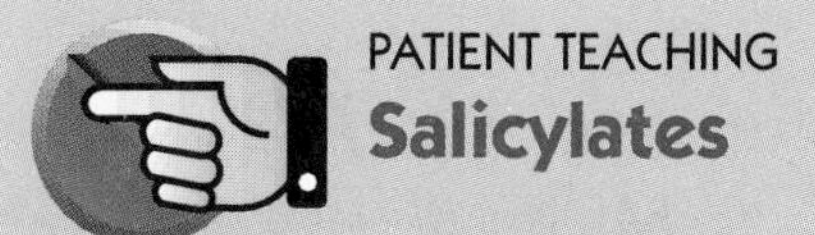

PATIENT TEACHING

Salicylates

- Teach the patient and family the name, dose, frequency, action, and adverse effects of the prescribed salicylate.
- Discourage the use of salicylates — even "children's aspirin" — in a patient under age 18.
- Advise an aspirin-sensitive patient to read labels carefully on over-the-counter (OTC) drugs because many contain aspirin or another salicylate.
- Teach the patient to recognize such signs as gingival bleeding, prolonged bleeding from a cut, black or tarry stools, dark urine (which may indicate blood in the urine), petechiae, and bruises. Advise the patient to report these signs to the physician immediately.
- Inform the patient to keep the salicylate in a cool, dry place because exposure to heat and moisture will weaken its potency.
- Advise the patient to discard tablets with a vinegar–like odor — a sign of salicylate deterioration.
- Inform the patient that buffered aspirin contains too little antacid to reduce gastric irritation. Suggest that the patient take plain aspirin with food, milk, or 1 to 2 teaspoons of antacid to prevent gastrointestinal distress more effectively at less expense. (If aspirin is taken with an antacid, the patient may require an increased aspirin dosage.)
- Advise the patient taking sodium salicylate tablets not to crush or chew them or take them within 1 hour of ingesting milk or antacids, which may disrupt the enteric coating.
- Advise the patient taking diflunisal tablets not to crush or chew them. Expect to administer a decreased diflunisal dosage to a patient with renal failure.
- Encourage the patient to use the salicylate as prescribed. Because many salicylates have been available for years and can be purchased OTC, some patients question their therapeutic effectiveness.
- Inform the patient that concurrent use of alcohol and a salicylate increases the risk of bleeding.
- Tell the diabetic patient who must test urine for glucose to use products other than Clinitest or Tes-Tape and to be alert for signs of hypoglycemia.
- Caution the pregnant patient not to take salicylates during the last trimester.
- Advise the asthmatic patient with nasal polyps to avoid using salicylates when self-medicating for minor aches and pains because these drugs may induce an acute asthma attack.
- Instruct the patient to notify the physician of adverse reactions to the salicylate.

Para-aminophenol derivatives

Although this subclass contains two substances — phenacetin and acetaminophen — only acetaminophen is available in the United States. Phenacetin was removed from all preparations in the United States because it was associated with anemia, acidosis, kidney damage, and methemoglobinemia. Acetaminophen, an analgesic and antipyretic, appears in many products to relieve pain, colds, and influenza. It has no anti-inflammatory properties. Physicians frequently choose acetaminophen over a salicylate for a patient with a history of GI bleeding, ulcers, or salicylate hypersensitivity.

PHARMACOKINETICS

Acetaminophen is absorbed rapidly and completely from the GI tract and is absorbed well from the rectal mucosa. It is distributed widely in body fluids and readily crosses the placenta. After acetaminophen undergoes metabolism by hepatic enzymes, it is excreted by the kidneys and, in small amounts, in breast milk. Acetaminophen's plasma protein binding is about 25%, and its half-life ranges from 1 to 3 hours.

Route	Onset	Peak	Duration
P.O., P.R.	Variable	1-3 hr	3-4 hr

PHARMACODYNAMICS

Acetaminophen offers significant analgesic and antipyretic actions, but unlike salicylates, does not act on inflammation or platelet function.

Although acetaminophen's mechanism of analgesic action is not understood fully, the drug may act centrally by inhibiting prostaglandin synthesis and peripherally in some unknown way. The drug's antipyretic effect results from its direct action on the heat-regulating center in the hypothalamus.

PHARMACOTHERAPEUTICS

Acetaminophen offers an alternative to patients who cannot tolerate aspirin and who do not need an analgesic with anti-inflammatory properties. An OTC drug, acetaminophen reduces fever and relieves headache, muscle ache, and pain in general but cannot relieve intense or visceral pain. It is the drug of choice to treat fever and flulike symptoms in children. Recently, the American Arthritis Association has indicated that acetaminophen is an effective pain reliever for some types of arthritis.

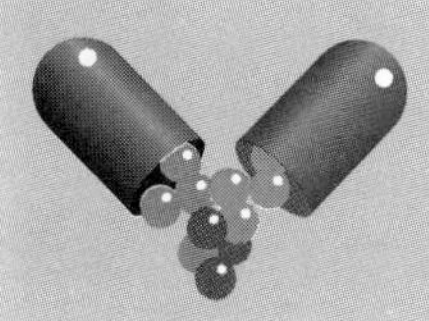

DRUG INTERACTIONS

Para-aminophenol derivatives

When acetaminophen is given with certain drugs, its absorption may decrease. This interaction requires that the nurse time the doses properly. Other interactions require different nursing interventions.

DRUG	INTERACTING AGENTS	POSSIBLE EFFECTS	NURSING IMPLICATIONS
acetaminophen	alcohol (chronic use), phenytoin, barbiturates, carbamazepine, isoniazid	Increased risk of hepatotoxicity	• Inform a patient with known or suspected chronic alcoholism of the increased risk of liver damage. Because acetaminophen is available over-the-counter, patient teaching is the only way to prevent this problem.
	charcoal	Reduced gastrointestinal absorption of acetaminophen	• Administer the charcoal and acetaminophen doses several hours apart unless charcoal is being administered for acetaminophen overdose.
	oral contraceptives	Decreased half-life of acetaminophen	• Inform the patient of medication interaction because the therapeutic effects of acetaminophen may be reduced.
	lamotrigine	Decreased therapeutic effects of lamotrigine	• Monitor for increased seizure activity.
	loop diuretics	Decreased effect of loop diuretics	• Monitor the patient for effects of increased fluid retention.
	zidovudine	Decreased effect of zivdovudine	• Monitor for progression of the signs and symptoms of human immunodeficiency virus infection and bone marrow suppression.

Drug interactions

Few significant interactions occur between acetaminophen and other drugs. (See Drug Interactions: *Para-aminophenol derivatives.*)

Acetaminophen may increase slightly the effects of oral anticoagulants. Antacids, anticholinergics, and narcotics may reduce acetaminophen's absorption by slowing intestinal motility; however, these interactions are not clinically significant.

ADVERSE DRUG REACTIONS

Most patients tolerate acetaminophen well. Unlike the salicylates, acetaminophen rarely causes gastric irritation or hemorrhagic tendencies.

Similar to an overdose, chronic use of high doses of acetaminophen can cause hypoglycemia, methemoglobinemia, leukopenia, kidney damage, renal failure, hepatotoxicity leading to coagulation defects, cyanosis, and vascular collapse.

Hypersensitivity reactions to acetaminophen usually take the form of rashes but rarely may include fever and angioedema. Such reactions are much less common with acetaminophen than with aspirin.

NURSING PROCESS APPLICATION

The following information assists the nurse in caring for a patient who is receiving acetaminophen. It includes an overview of assessment activities as well as examples of appropriate nursing diagnoses and related interventions (under "Planning and implementation"). It also highlights the importance of evaluation.

Assessment

Before drug therapy begins, review the patient's history for conditions that contraindicate or require cautious use of acetaminophen. Also review the patient's medication history to identify use of drugs that may interact with it. During therapy, assess the patient for adverse drug reactions and signs of drug interactions. Also, periodically assess the effectiveness of therapy. Finally, evaluate the patient's and family's knowledge about acetaminophen.

Nursing diagnoses

- Risk for injury related to a preexisting condition that contraindicates or requires cautious use of acetaminophen
- Risk for injury related to adverse drug reactions and drug interactions

• Pain related to ineffectiveness of acetaminophen
• Knowledge deficit related to acetaminophen

Planning and implementation

• Do not administer acetaminophen to a patient with a condition that contraindicates its use.
• Administer acetaminophen cautiously to a patient at risk because of a preexisting condition.
• Obtain a baseline liver function test before beginning acetaminophen therapy and monitor liver function test results periodically during therapy, as prescribed.
• Monitor the patient for adverse reactions, and notify the physician as needed.
*** *Withhold acetaminophen and notify the physician if the patient develops a rash, unexplained fever, or angioedema.***
• Monitor the patient for pain relief. If pain does not subside, obtain a prescription for a different analgesic. (See Patient Teaching: *Para-aminophenol derivatives.*)

Evaluation

For each nursing diagnosis, prepare an evaluation statement that describes the patient's or family's response to nursing interventions.

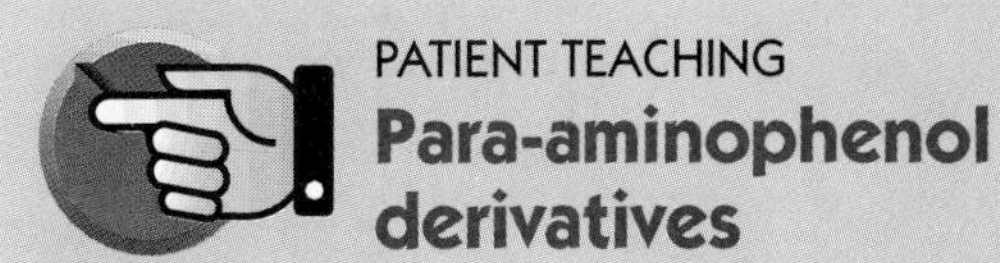

PATIENT TEACHING
Para-aminophenol derivatives

➤ Teach the patient and family the name, dose, frequency, action, and adverse effects of acetaminophen.
➤ Inform the patient that high doses or unsupervised long-term use of this drug can cause liver damage and that excessive alcohol ingestion may increase this risk.
➤ Teach the patient that acetaminophen is safe and effective only when used as directed on the label. Because this drug is readily available over-the-counter (OTC) and is advertised widely, many patients assume that it is nontoxic. This assumption can lead to accidental overdose when a patient attempts to relieve severe or persistent fever or pain.
➤ Advise the asthmatic or hypersensitive patient to read all drug labels carefully. Acetaminophen is an ingredient in many OTC drugs with brand names that do not signal its presence.
➤ Explain that if fever or pain lasts more than 3 days, the patient should obtain medical advice.
➤ Teach the patient to store the drug in a light-resistant container, because transfer to a clear glass or plastic container eventually may affect the drug's potency.
➤ Advise the diabetic patient on long-term, high-dose acetaminophen therapy to monitor blood glucose levels at least daily for hypoglycemia.
➤ Instruct the patient to notify the physician if adverse reactions occur.

Nonsteroidal anti-inflammatory drugs

With chemical structures that differ from those of corticosteroids, NSAIDs have anti-inflammatory, analgesic, and antipyretic properties, although they are seldom prescribed for fever. Their anti-inflammatory action equals that of aspirin.

The NSAIDs are derived from many different chemical sources. Fenoprofen calcium, flurbiprofen, ibuprofen, ketoprofen, meclofenamate, naproxen, naproxen sodium, and nabumetone are propionic acid derivatives (fenamates). Mefenamic acid is an anthranilic acid derivative. Phenylbutazone is a pyrazolone derivative. Piroxicam is an oxicam derivative. Indomethacin, ketorolac tromethamine, and etodolac are indoleacetic acid derivatives. Tolmetin sodium is a pyrrole acetic acid derivative. Sulindac is an indene derivative. Diclofenac is a phenylacetic acid derivative.

PHARMACOKINETICS

All NSAIDs are absorbed in the GI tract. NSAIDs are mostly metabolized in the liver and excreted primarily by the kidneys. NSAIDs may be given orally or parenterally.

Route	Onset	Peak	Duration
P.O.	30 min-4 hr	1-4 hr	4-72 hr
I.M.	10-30 min	30-60 min	4-8 hr
I.V.	1-3 min	1-3 min	4-8 hr

Note: It may take 1 to 4 weeks for peak antirheumatic effects to be obtained.

PHARMACODYNAMICS

Researchers believe that NSAIDs inhibit prostaglandin synthesis, retard polymorphonuclear leukocyte motility, and affect the release and activity of lysosomal enzymes. Their ability to decrease prostaglandin concentrations in peripheral tissues may account for their anti-inflammatory effects. Fenamates may act in another way because studies have shown that they compete with prostaglandins at receptor-binding sites. (See Drug Interactions: *Nonsteroidal anti-inflammatory drugs,* page 182.)

PHARMACOTHERAPEUTICS

NSAIDs are used primarily to decrease inflammation and secondarily to relieve pain. Although the NSAIDs share similar indications and mechanisms of action, individual responses vary greatly: A patient may respond poorly to one drug and very well to another. Therefore, the choice of an NSAID must be made empirically. Usually, a patient receives an NSAID for a trial period of 2 to 4 weeks. If this NSAID does not produce a therapeutic response, it usually is discontinued and replaced with a second drug for another trial period. This procedure may be repeated until relief is obtained.

Indications for NSAIDs include ankylosing spondylitis; moderate to severe rheumatoid arthritis; osteoarthritis in the hip, shoulder, or other large joints; osteoarthritis accompanied by inflammation; and acute gouty arthritis.

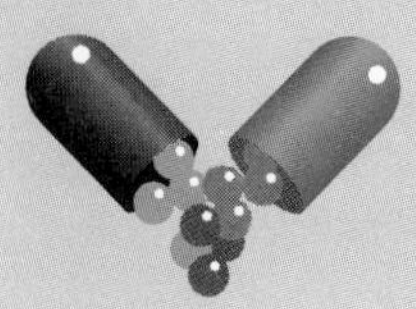

DRUG INTERACTIONS

Nonsteroidal anti-inflammatory drugs

Drug interactions with the nonsteroidal anti-inflammatory drugs (NSAIDs) are common and can be severe. They typically require dosage adjustment, drug discontinuation, or drug substitution.

DRUG	INTERACTING AGENTS	POSSIBLE EFFECTS	NURSING IMPLICATIONS
diclofenac, etodolac, fenoprofen, flurbiprofen, ibuprofen, indomethacin, ketorolac, ketoprofen, meclofenamate, mefenamic acid, naproxen, naproxen sodium, nabumetone, phenylbutazone, piroxicam, sulindac, tolmetin	corticosteroids	Increased ulcerogenic effect	• Monitor the patient for epigastric and abdominal pain, abdominal cramps — especially 1 to 2 hours after eating — and signs of GI bleeding, such as bloody or tarry stools.
	loop diuretics	Decreased antihypertensive and diuretic effects	• Monitor the patient's blood pressure and fluid intake and output to detect decreased effects. • Anticipate substitution of a different NSAID, such as sulindac, for indomethacin.
	oral anticoagulants	Increased anticoagulant effect	• Monitor the patient for gingival bleeding, black or tarry stools, blood in the urine, petechiae, bruises, or prolonged bleeding from a cut. • Monitor the patient's prothrombin time and partial thromboplastin time, and adjust the anticoagulant dosage as prescribed.
	lithium	Increased lithium concentration (except with sulindac)	• Monitor the patient's lithium concentration.
	beta-adrenergic blockers	Inhibited synthesis of renal prostaglandins, possibly causing hypertension	• Monitor the patient's blood pressure frequently.
	methotrexate	Increased methotrexate toxicity (bone marrow depression, nephrotoxicity, stomatitis)	• Avoid concurrent use. If this is unavoidable, monitor for increased adverse reactions to methotrexate, such as fatigue, bone marrow suppression, and stomatitis.
	zidovudine	Inhibited zidovudine metabolism, which may lead to toxicity	• Avoid concomitant use of these agents.
	cyclosporin	Nephrotoxicity of both agents may be increased	• Monitor blood urea nitrogen and serum creatinine level.
	phenytoin	Phenytoin levels increased resulting in an increased pharmacologic effect	• Monitor serum phenytoin level.
	probenecid	Increased concentrations and toxicity of NSAIDs	• Monitor for signs and symptoms of NSAID toxicity. • Teach the patient about concomitant use of NSAIDs and salicylates.
	salicylates	Increased incidence of gastrointestinal (GI) effects	• Avoid concurrent use.
indomethacin	sympathomimetics	Hypertension	• Monitor the patient's blood pressure when concurrent use is unavoidable.
	digoxin	Increased serum digoxin level	• Monitor serum digoxin level and observe for signs of digitalis toxicity.
	dipyridamole	Fluid retention	• Monitor for effects of fluid retention.

Nonsteroidal anti-inflammatory drugs *(continued)*

DRUG	INTERACTING AGENTS	POSSIBLE EFFECTS	NURSING IMPLICATIONS
indomethacin *(continued)*	captopril	Decreased antihypertensive effect	• Monitor the patient's blood pressure.
indomethacin & naproxen	thiazide diuretics	Decreased antihypertensive and diuretic effects	• Monitor the patient's blood pressure and watch for signs of fluid retention.
ibuprofen	digoxin	Increased serum digoxin levels	• Monitor serum digoxin level and watch for signs of digitalis toxicity.
ketorolac	food in general	Reduces rate, but not extent, of drug absorption	• Inform the patient that although drug should be taken with food, delayed effects may occur.
etodolac	food in general	Reduces peak concentration by about 50% and delays peak concentration by 1.4 to 3.8 hours	• Teach the patient about food interactions.
flurbiprofen	food in general	Alters rate, but not extent, of drug absorption	• Teach the patient about food interactions.
ketoprofen	food in general	Slows absorption rate; delays and reduces peak concentrations	• Teach the patient about food interactions.
ketorolac	salicylates	Increased plasma concentrations of unbound ketorolac	• Avoid concurrent use.

Some NSAIDs have been approved for OTC use with recommended dosage at half the usual prescribed dose. Patients may be taking one or more of these OTC preparations, and some patients take more than the recommended dose. If an NSAID is prescribed for a patient, make sure that OTC NSAIDs are not being used concurrently.

Drug interactions

A wide variety of drugs can interact with NSAIDs, especially with indomethacin, mefenamic acid, phenylbutazone, piroxicam, and sulindac. Because they are highly protein bound, NSAIDs are likely to interact with other protein-bound drugs, such as oral anticoagulants. They also may interfere with antihypertensive drugs, such as beta-adrenergic blockers and thiazides, decreasing their antihypertensive effects. This interaction is not documented fully, however, and may not occur with all NSAIDs.

ADVERSE DRUG REACTIONS

All NSAIDs produce similar adverse reactions that rarely require discontinuation of therapy. In general, the NSAIDs are better tolerated than salicylates or corticosteroids.

GI tract disturbances are the most common adverse reactions to NSAIDs. Other reactions affect the central nervous system (CNS), the renal system, and the eyes. Adverse CNS and renal reactions are particularly common in geriatric patients. (See *Adverse reactions to nonsteroidal anti-inflammatory drugs,* page 184.)

Phenylbutazone has an unusually high incidence of adverse reactions, commonly causing nausea, vomiting, abdominal discomfort, dyspepsia, diarrhea, and rashes. Other reactions include gastric ulceration and hemorrhage, vertigo, insomnia, and the combination of sodium and water retention, increased plasma volume, and decreased urine volume — which may lead to peripheral edema, acute pulmonary edema, and cardiac symptoms. Phenylbutazone sometimes causes thrombocytopenia, aplastic anemia, granulocytopenia, and other blood dyscrasias. At highest risk for adverse reactions are elderly patients, especially women, and patients receiving high doses or long-term therapy. Adverse reactions limit phenylbutazone's use to short-term therapy: 1 week or less for a patient over age 60.

NSAIDs can cause hypersensitivity reactions, evidenced by rashes, urticaria, angioedema, hypotension, dyspnea, and an asthmalike syndrome. With phenylbutazone, hypersensitivity reactions include pruritus, fever, arthralgia, polyarthritis, Stevens-Johnson syndrome, and anaphylaxis. With piroxicam, rashes and photosensitivity occur more commonly than with the other NSAIDs. With any NSAID, ther-

Adverse reactions to nonsteroidal anti-inflammatory drugs

NSAIDs can produce numerous adverse reactions in the central nervous system, gastrointestinal system (most common site), renal system, and the eyes and skin.

CENTRAL NERVOUS SYSTEM

- Drowsiness
- Headache
- Dizziness
- Confusion
- Tinnitus
- Vertigo
- Depression

GASTROINTESTINAL SYSTEM

- Abdominal pain
- Bleeding
- Anemia
- Diarrhea
- Nausea
- Ulcerations
- Perforation
- Hepatotoxicity

RENAL SYSTEM

- Cystitis
- Hematuria
- Kidney necrosis
- Nephrotic syndrome (rare)

EYES

- Blurred vision
- Decreased acuity
- Corneal deposits

SKIN

- Rash

apy should be discontinued at the first sign of a hypersensitivity reaction.

NURSING PROCESS APPLICATION

The following information assists the nurse in caring for a patient who is receiving an NSAID. It includes an overview of assessment activities as well as examples of appropriate nursing diagnoses and related interventions (under "Planning and implementation"). It also highlights the importance of evaluation.

Assessment

Before drug therapy begins, review the patient's history for conditions that contraindicate or require cautious use of the prescribed NSAID. (See Cultural Considerations: *Nonsteroidal anti-inflammatory drugs.*) Also review the patient's medication history to identify use of drugs that may interact with it. During therapy, assess the patient for adverse drug reactions, such as water retention, and signs of drug interactions. Also, periodically assess the effectiveness of therapy. Finally, evaluate the patient's and family's knowledge about the prescribed NSAID.

Nursing diagnoses

- Risk for injury related to a preexisting condition that contraindicates or requires cautious use of an NSAID
- Risk for injury related to adverse drug reactions or drug interactions
- Fluid volume excess related to sodium and water retention caused by an NSAID
- Knowledge deficit related to the prescribed NSAID

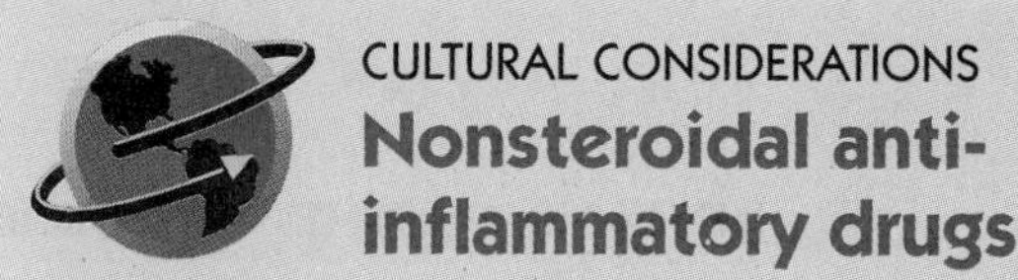

CULTURAL CONSIDERATIONS
Nonsteroidal anti-inflammatory drugs

Because black males have a high risk of hypertensive disease, it is important for the nurse to educate them regarding nonsteroidal anti-inflammatory drug (NSAID) and antihypertensive drug interactions. NSAIDs decrease the effects of some antihypertensive agents due to the sodium retention properties of nonsteroidals. NSAIDs also compete with some diuretic agents at their sites of action within the renal tubules.

Planning and implementation

- Do not administer an NSAID to a patient with a condition that contraindicates its use. Keep in mind that a patient with aspirin hypersensitivity also may be hypersensitive to NSAIDs. (See Patient Teaching: *Nonsteroidal anti-inflammatory drugs.*)
- Administer an NSAID cautiously to a patient at risk because of a preexisting condition.
- Observe the patient for adverse reactions to the NSAID.
- Discontinue NSAID therapy and notify the physician at the first sign of a hypersensitivity reaction to the drug.
- Monitor the patient's vision. If an alteration or problem develops, expect to discontinue the NSAID until an ophthalmic examination rules out drug therapy as the cause.

* ***Administer the prescribed NSAID with food or milk to decrease GI irritation, unless directed otherwise.***

- Monitor the patient with a history of peptic ulcer for ulcer reactivation and gastric bleeding during NSAID therapy.

* ***Monitor the patient for signs of GI irritation, such as nausea, vomiting, abdominal pain, or black, tarry stools. Notify the physician immediately if the patient displays signs of GI irritation.***

- Monitor the patient for signs of infection. Keep in mind that indomethacin may mask some signs.
- Notify the physician of adverse reactions to the prescribed NSAID.
- Evaluate the degree of pain relief during NSAID therapy. Note that 2 to 4 weeks may elapse before the prescribed NSAID provides relief.
- Expect to administer a different NSAID if pain is not relieved within 4 weeks of NSAID therapy.
- Expect to administer a larger dose of naproxen in the evening to a patient who awakens with morning pain.
- Monitor the patient's vital signs at least every 8 hours. Note a significant increase in blood pressure, which may indicate increased plasma volume.

• Weigh the patient daily and report sudden, unexplained weight gain. Be aware that fluid retention and edema may occur during NSAID therapy.
• Monitor the patient regularly for signs of fluid retention, such as ankle edema, crackles, and shortness of breath.
• Limit the patient's sodium and fluid intake, unless prescribed by the physician.
• Document the patient's intake and output daily to detect a fluid imbalance.
* ***Alert the physician if the patient displays signs of fluid retention.***

Evaluation

For each nursing diagnosis, prepare an evaluation statement that describes the patient's or family's response to nursing interventions.

Phenazopyridine hydrochloride

Phenazopyridine hydrochloride (Pyridium), an azo dye, produces a local analgesic effect on the urinary tract, usually within 24 to 48 hours after therapy begins. It relieves the pain, burning, urgency, and frequency that occur with urinary tract infections.

The usual dosage ranges from 100 to 200 mg P.O. t.i.d. after meals for 2 days only. After oral administration, phenazopyridine is 35% metabolized in the liver, with the remainder excreted unchanged in the urine. The drug colors the urine orange or red, which permanently may stain fabrics it contacts. A yellow tinge to the skin or sclera may indicate drug accumulation and the need to discontinue phenazopyridine therapy. Because this drug can alter the results of some urine glucose tests, such as Tes-Tape and Clinistix, the nurse should use Clinitest for a more accurate urine glucose determination.

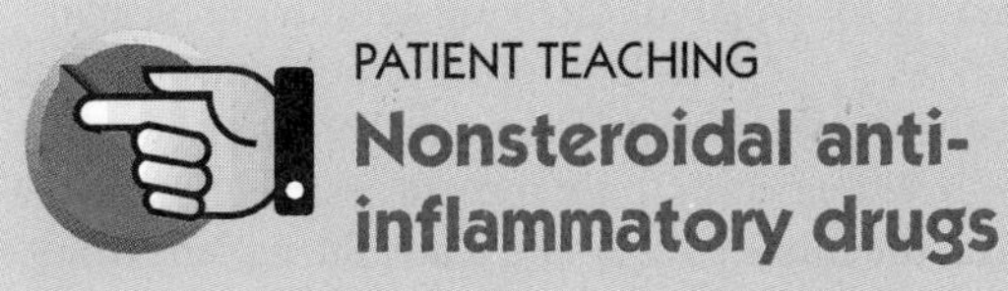

PATIENT TEACHING

Nonsteroidal anti-inflammatory drugs

- Teach the patient and family the name, dose, frequency, action, and adverse effects of the prescribed nonsteroidal anti-inflammatory drug (NSAID).
- Stress the importance of returning for periodic blood tests as prescribed.
- Advise the patient receiving indomethacin to avoid driving or operating machinery until the drug's effects are evaluated because drowsiness and dizziness commonly occur at the beginning of therapy.
- Advise the patient that some NSAIDs, such as naproxen, ibuprofen, and fenoprofen, may take several weeks to produce the maximum therapeutic effect.
- Instruct the patient to take the prescribed NSAID with milk or food to decrease gastric irritation, unless directed otherwise.
- Advise the patient with aspirin hypersensitivity to avoid ibuprofen.
- Instruct the patient who self-medicates with an NSAID to discontinue the drug and consult a physician if pain lasts longer than 72 hours.
- Advise the patient to avoid alcohol, aspirin, and other drugs that may cause gastrointestinal irritation and bleeding.
- Instruct the patient taking an oral anticoagulant along with the prescribed NSAID to be alert for bleeding tendencies, such as easy bruising, nosebleeds, and black, tarry stools. Also advise the patient to institute bleeding precautions, such as using an electric razor when shaving and avoiding forceful nose blowing and bumps and trauma to the skin.
- Teach the diabetic patient taking an oral hypoglycemic and phenylbutazone to monitor blood glucose levels frequently and watch for signs of hypoglycemia, such as tremors, lightheadedness, and diaphoresis.
- Instruct the patient taking indomethacin to avoid nonamphetamine anorexigenic agents to prevent hypertension.
- Advise the patient taking ketorolac not to take a salicylate concurrently.
- Teach the patient to avoid high-sodium foods and to limit fluid, unless directed by the physician, because fluid retention can occur.
- Instruct the patient to notify the physician if adverse reactions occur.

CHAPTER SUMMARY

Chapter 14 covered nonnarcotic analgesic, antipyretic, and NSAIDs. Here are the highlights of the chapter.

The three subclasses of nonnarcotic analgesics include salicylates, para-aminophenol derivatives, and NSAIDs.

Aspirin, a salicylate and the most widely used analgesic, is available alone or with other ingredients in OTC remedies for pain, colds, and influenza. Salicylates produce analgesia by inhibiting prostaglandin synthesis. They also can act as antipyretics. The anti-inflammatory action of salicylates is understood poorly. Salicylates are used to treat headache, neuralgia, myalgia, dysmenorrhea, and arthritis. The major adverse reactions involve the GI system.

Acetaminophen is currently the only para-aminophenol derivative used in the United States. Its effects are antipyretic and analgesic but not anti-inflammatory. A common ingredient in many OTC analgesics, acetaminophen causes few adverse reactions when taken in recommended doses.

The NSAID category includes many drugs that may act by inhibiting prostaglandin synthesis, retarding polymorphonuclear leukocyte motility, and affecting the release and activity of lysosomal enzymes. These drugs are used primarily to relieve the symptoms of arthritis and related conditions as well as mild to moderate pain in such conditions as dysmenorrhea. They commonly cause adverse reactions in the GI system.

The only urinary tract analgesic, phenazopyridine, acts locally. It is used to relieve the pain, burning, and urinary urgency and frequency associated with urinary tract infections.

When caring for a patient receiving a nonnarcotic analgesic, antipyretic, or NSAID, the nurse should monitor the patient frequently for adverse reactions. Because many of these drugs are used commonly and are available without a prescription, the nurse also should teach the patient about the drug and its effects.

Questions to consider

See Appendix 1 for answers.

1. Edward Smith, age 28, takes 3.6 g of aspirin daily for rheumatoid arthritis. He is likely to experience which of the following common adverse reactions to aspirin?
   (a) Increased rate and depth of respirations
   (b) Nausea, vomiting, and GI distress
   (c) Dizziness and vision changes
   (d) Tinnitus and hearing loss

2. During a follow-up visit, Mr. Smith tells the nurse his 6-year-old son has influenza and asks if he should give his son aspirin to make him more comfortable. The nurse tells Mr. Smith that aspirin should not be used to treat flulike symptoms in children. Why not?
   (a) Salicylates are too irritating to a child's GI mucosa.
   (b) Salicylates may lead to excessive bleeding.
   (c) Salicylates are not effective in children.
   (d) Salicylates may cause Reye's syndrome.

3. Gloria Anderson, age 48, seeks medical attention because of frequent, severe headaches. Her medication history reveals that she has been taking 3 to 4 g of acetaminophen daily for pain relief. Long-term use of high doses of acetaminophen can increase Ms. Anderson's risk for which of the following adverse reactions?
   (a) Hepatotoxicity
   (b) Hypertension
   (c) Peptic ulcer
   (d) Hemorrhage

4. Melvin Quigley, age 57, has osteoarthritis. His physician prescribes the NSAID diclofenac 100 mg P.O. daily in two divided doses. The nurse teaches Mr. Quigley about potential adverse reactions to this drug. Which of the following adverse reactions most commonly occurs with NSAID use?
   (a) Dyspnea
   (b) Pruritus
   (c) Hypotension
   (d) GI disturbances

5. The nurse should include which of the following instructions when teaching Mr. Quigley about NSAID therapy?
   (a) Drink plenty of fluids.
   (b) Take the drug with aspirin.
   (c) Avoid high-sodium foods.
   (d) Take the drug on an empty stomach.

15 Narcotic agonist and antagonist agents

OBJECTIVES

After reading and studying this chapter, the student should be able to:

1. discuss how narcotic agonists act to relieve pain.
2. distinguish between narcotic agonists and narcotic antagonists.
3. discuss the clinical indications for the various narcotic agents.
4. identify the common adverse reactions to narcotic drugs.
5. describe the pain-relieving action of mixed narcotic agonist-antagonists.
6. describe the action of naloxone hydrochloride and its use in treating narcotic overdose.
7. describe how to apply the nursing process when caring for a patient who is receiving a narcotic agonist, mixed narcotic agonist-antagonist, or narcotic antagonist.

INTRODUCTION

Narcotic agonists (analgesics), which include opium derivatives and synthetic drugs with similar pharmacologic properties, can relieve or decrease pain without causing loss of consciousness. Some narcotic agonists also possess antitussive and antidiarrheal actions.

Narcotic agonists provide **analgesia,** relieving pain by attaching to opiate receptor sites. Narcotic antagonists block the effects of narcotic agonists, including pain relief and adverse drug reactions, most notably respiratory depression. Some narcotic analgesics, called mixed narcotic agonist-antagonists, display agonist and antagonist properties: The agonist component relieves pain; the antagonist component decreases the risk of toxicity and drug dependence. These mixed narcotic agonist-antagonists are less likely than pure agonists to result in respiratory depression and drug abuse. (See *Selected major narcotic agonist and antagonist agents,* pages 188 and 189.)

The drugs that will be covered in this chapter include:

- buprenorphine hydrochloride
- butorphanol tartrate
- codeine
- dezocine
- fentanyl citrate
- hydrocodone bitrate and acetaminophen
- hydrocodone and phenyltoloxamine
- hydromorphone hydrochloride
- hydrocodone and phenyltoloxamine
- levorphanol tartrate
- meperidine hydrochloride
- methadone hydrochloride
- morphine sulfate
- nalbuphine hydrochloride
- naloxone hydrochloride
- naltrexone hydrochloride
- oxycodone hydrochloride
- pentazocine hydrochloride
- propoxyphene hydrochloride
- propoxyphene napsylate.

Narcotic agonists

The term *narcotic* refers to any analgesic derived from active opium poppy alkaloids as well as to compounds chemically similar to the alkaloids. Because the Harrison Narcotic Act of 1914 established a legal definition of narcotics based on their habit-forming nature, however, the term *narcotic* commonly is used inaccurately to refer to any drug that can produce dependence or is restricted by the Controlled Substance Act of 1970.

This chapter presents the following narcotic agonists: codeine, fentanyl citrate, hydrocodone bitartrate and acetaminophen, hydrocodone and phenyltoloxamine, hydromorphone hydrochloride, levorphanol tartrate, meperidine hydrochloride, methadone hydrochloride, morphine sulfate (including morphine sulfate sustained-release tablets and intensified oral solution), oxycodone hydrochloride (alone or with acetaminophen or aspirin), oxymorphone hydrochloride, propoxyphene hydrochloride, and propoxyphene napsylate.

Morphine sulfate serves as a standard against which the effectiveness and adverse reactions of other narcotic drugs as well as nonnarcotic analgesics are measured.

PHARMACOKINETICS

The narcotic agonists are administered by the oral, intravenous (I.V.), subcutaneous (S.C.), intramuscular (I.M.),

Selected major narcotic agonist and antagonist agents

This table summarizes the major narcotic agonist and antagonist agents currently in clinical use.

DRUG	MAJOR INDICATIONS AND USUAL DOSAGES	CONTRAINDICATIONS AND PRECAUTIONS
Narcotic agonists		
meperidine hydrochloride (Demerol)	*Moderate to severe pain* ADULT: 50 to 150 mg parenterally or P.O. every 2 to 3 hours, as needed PEDIATRIC: 0.75 mg/kg S.C., I.V.or I.M. up to the adult dose every 2 to 3 hours, as needed *Preoperative analgesia* ADULT: 50 to 100 mg I.M. or S.C. 30 to 90 minutes before surgery PEDIATRIC: 1.2 to 2 mg/kg S.C. or I.M. up to the adult dose, 30 to 90 minutes before surgery *Obstetric analgesia* ADULT: 50 to 100 mg I.M. or S.C., possibly repeated at 1- to 3-hour intervals	• Meperidine hydrochloride is contraindicated in a patient with known hypersensitivity or one who is receiving a monoamine oxidase (MAO) inhibitor. • This drug requires cautious use in a pregnant, breast-feeding, geriatric, or debilitated patient or one with head injury, increased intracranial pressure, asthma or other respiratory condition, susceptibility to hypotension (as from surgery or volume depletion), hypothyroidism, Addison's disease, prostatic hypertrophy, urethral stricture, severe hepatic or renal impairment, supraventricular tachycardia, or therapy with another central nervous system (CNS) depressant, a phenothiazine, or certain anesthetics.
morphine sulfate (Duramorph)	*Severe pain* ADULT: initially, 10 mg/70 kg of body weight parenterally or an equianalgesic dose orally (a 60-mg oral dose is equianalgesic to a 10-mg parenteral dose)	• Morphine sulfate is contraindicated in a patient with known hypersensitivity to the drug. I.V. administration is contraindicated in a patient with acute bronchial asthma or upper airway obstruction. • This drug requires cautious use in a pregnant, breast-feeding, geriatric, or debilitated patient or one with increased intracranial or intraocular pressure, head injury, decreased respiratory reserve, acute asthmatic attack, severe obesity, kyphoscoliosis, seizures, hepatic or renal dysfunction; reduced blood volume, or impaired myocardial function. • Safety and efficacy in children have not been established.
morphine sulfate sustained-release tablets (MS Contin, Roxanol SR)	*Prolonged relief of chronic, severe pain* ADULT: dosage titrated to the patient's individual needs, beginning with a starting dose of 30 mg P.O. every 8 to 12 hours when the narcotic need is not known	• Morphine sulfate sustained-release tablets are contraindicated in a patient with known hypersensitivity to the drug, severe CNS depression, bronchial asthma, heart failure secondary to chronic lung disease, cardiac arrhythmias, increased intracranial or cerebrospinal pressure, head injury, brain tumor, acute alcoholism, delirium tremens, convulsive disorder, or a suspected disorder that may require abdominal surgery. It is also contraindicated after biliary tract surgery, surgical anastomosis, or during or up to 14 days after MAO inhibitor therapy. • This drug requires cautious use in a pregnant, breast-feeding, geriatric, or debilitated patient; one who is receiving another narcotic analgesic, a general anesthetic, or phenothiazine; or one with asthma or other respiratory conditions, severe hepatic or renal impairment, hypothyroidism, Addison's disease, prostatic hypertrophy, urethral stricture, or reduced blood volume. • Safety and efficacy in children have not been established.
morphine sulfate intensified oral solution (Roxanol)	*Severe acute pain, severe chronic pain* ADULT: initially, 10 to 30 mg P.O. every 3 to 4 hours, then titrated to the patient's needs	• Morphine sulfate intensified oral solution is contraindicated under the same conditions as morphine sulfate sustained-release tablets.
propoxyphene hydrochloride (Darvon)	*Mild pain* ADULT: 65 mg P.O. every 4 hours, as needed, not to exceed 390 mg/day	• Propoxyphene hydrochloride is contraindicated in a patient with known hypersensitivity to the drug or one who is suicidal or addiction-prone.

Selected major narcotic agonist and antagonist agents *(continued)*

DRUG	MAJOR INDICATIONS AND USUAL DOSAGES	CONTRAINDICATIONS AND PRECAUTIONS
Narcotic agonists *(continued)*		
propoxyphene hydrochloride (Darvon) *(continued)*		• Propoxyphene requires cautious use in a pregnant or breast-feeding patient, one with hepatic or renal impairment, or one who uses other CNS depressants or alcohol. • Safety and efficacy in children have not been established.
Mixed narcotic agonist-antagonists		
butorphanol tartrate (Stadol)	*Moderate to severe pain, obstetric analgesia during labor, preoperative medication* ADULT: 2 mg I.M. every 3 to 4 hours, with a dosage range of 1 to 4 mg; or 1 mg I.V. every 3 to 4 hours, with a dosage range of 0.5 to 2 mg	• Butorphanol is contraindicated in a breast-feeding patient or one with narcotic addiction or known hypersensitivity to the drug. • This drug requires cautious use in a pregnant patient or one with emotional instability, a history of drug addiction, head injury, increased intracranial pressure, acute myocardial infarction, ventricular dysfunction, coronary insufficiency, respiratory depression, severely limited respiratory reserve, bronchial asthma, obstructive respiratory conditions, cyanosis, renal or hepatic impairment, biliary surgery, or hypertension. • Safety and efficacy in children under age 18 have not been established.
nalbuphine hydrochloride (Nubain)	*Moderate to severe pain, obstetric analgesia, preoperative medication* ADULT: 10 mg/70 kg of body weight I.V., I.M., or S.C. every 3 to 6 hours, as needed; not to exceed 160 mg/day	• Nalbuphine is contraindicated in a patient with known hypersensitivity to the drug. • This drug requires cautious use in a pregnant patient or one with head injury, increased intracranial pressure, emotional instability, a history of narcotic abuse, impaired respirations, renal or hepatic dysfunction, or nausea and vomiting in the presence of myocardial infarction. It also requires cautious use in a patient who has had biliary tract surgery or who uses another CNS depressant. • Safety and efficacy in children under age 18 have not been established.
Narcotic antagonists		
naloxone hydrochloride (Narcan)	*Reversal of respiratory depression caused by narcotic overdose, diagnosis of narcotic overdose* ADULT: initially, 0.4 to 2 mg I.V., I.M., or S.C., repeated every 2 to 3 minutes as needed, depending on the degree of counteraction achieved *Opiate-induced asphyxia neonatorum* PEDIATRIC: initially, 0.01 mg/kg I.V. via the umbilical vein; if no response, 0.1 mg/kg I.V. (or I.M., S.C., or by endotracheal tube if an I.V. route is unavailable).	• Naloxone hydrochloride is contraindicated in a patient with known hypersensitivity to the drug. • This drug requires cautious use in a pregnant or breast-feeding patient, a neonate of a mother who is known or suspected to be physically dependent on opioids, or a patient who has cardiac disease or uses cardiotoxic drugs.

epidural, intrathecal, sublingual, rectal, and transdermal routes. Oral doses are absorbed readily from the gastrointestinal (GI) tract. I.V. administration produces the most rapid (almost immediate) and reliable analgesic effects. The S.C. and I.M. routes may result in delayed absorption and peak concentration of the drug, especially in patients with impaired tissue perfusion. Intravenous morphine reaches peak concentration in 20 to 40 minutes.

Narcotic agonists are distributed widely throughout body tissues, displaying relatively low plasma protein-binding capacity (30% to 35%). The drugs are metabolized extensively in the liver. For example, meperidine is metabolized to normeperidine, a toxic metabolite with a longer half-life than meperidine. Metabolites are excreted by the kidneys. A minor amount, 7% to 10% of the dose, is excreted in feces via the biliary tract. Narcotic agonist half-life varies, depending on the drug administered and the route of administration.

Route	Onset	Peak	Duration
P.O.	15-90 min	1- 2.5 hr	2-12 hr
I.M.	7-30 min	20 min-2 hr	1-6 hr
S.C.	10-90 min	30-90 min	2-6 hr
I.V.	1-20 min	3-4 min	0.5-8 hr
Intrathecal	15-60 min	Unknown	Up to 24 hr
Epidural	15-60 min	15-60 min	Up to 24 hr
Rectal	15-60 min	20 to 60 min	4-6 hr
Sublingual	Variable	20-15 min	Variable
Transdermal	12-24 hr	1-3 days	Variable

PHARMACODYNAMICS

Narcotic agonists act primarily at opiate receptor sites, binding to the receptors centrally and peripherally and activating the endogenous pain relief system. (See *Narcotic sites of action.*) This receptor-site binding produces the therapeutic effects of analgesia and cough suppression along with narcotic adverse reactions, including respiratory depression and constipation. (See *How opiates control pain.*)

Narcotic agonists, especially morphine, affect the smooth muscle of the GI and genitourinary tracts, causing bladder and ureter contraction and decreased intestinal peristalsis. These drugs also cause blood vessel dilation, especially in the face, head, and neck. In addition, they depress the cough center in the brain, thereby producing antitussive effects and causing constriction of the bronchial musculature. Any of these effects can become adverse reactions.

Narcotic sites of action

Narcotics act at many different body sites, producing effects that usually are therapeutic but that occasionally may be adverse. Major effects are highlighted in this illustration.

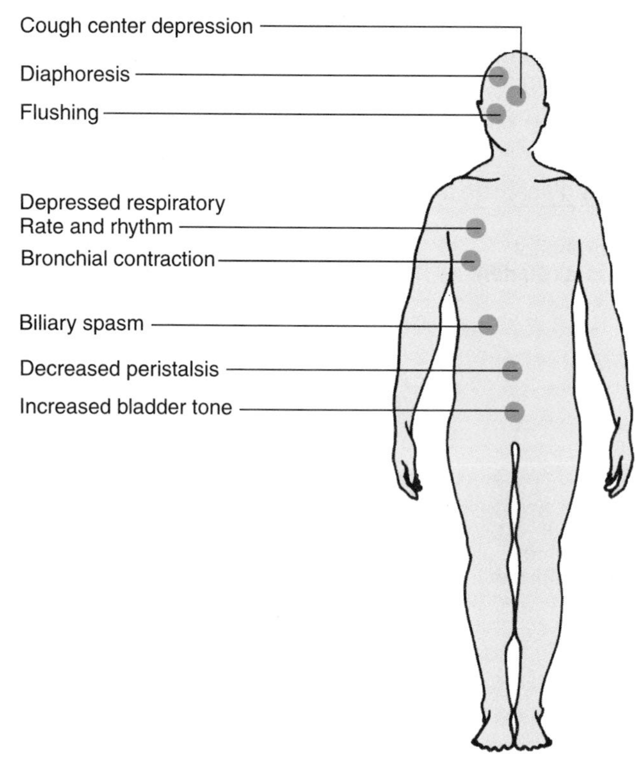

PHARMACOTHERAPEUTICS

Narcotic agonists are used to relieve severe pain in acute, chronic, and terminal illnesses and to reduce preanesthesia patient anxiety. They also have antidiarrheal and antitussive effects. Morphine reduces the dyspnea of pulmonary edema and left ventricular failure.

An **equianalgesic dose** of a narcotic drug is a dose that produces the same level of analgesia as an agent and dose selected as a standard, usually 10 mg of morphine I.M. Occasionally, a patient must be changed from one narcotic drug to another (for example, when the postoperative patient is allowed to take drugs orally). When this is necessary, referring to the equianalgesic dose decreases the risk of toxicity and inadequate pain relief.

Drug interactions

The use of narcotic agonists with any other drugs known to decrease respiration, including alcohol, sedatives, hypnotics, and anesthetics, increases the patient's risk of severe respiratory depression. Concomitant therapy with tricyclic antidepressants, phenothiazines, or anticholinergics may cause severe constipation and urine retention.

ADVERSE DRUG REACTIONS

Narcotic agonists produce numerous adverse reactions that affect most body systems. Central nervous system (CNS) reactions, the most common, usually affect the respiratory and GI tracts.

One of the most common adverse reactions to the opium derivatives is decreased rate and depth of respiration that worsens as the dosage is increased. This may cause periodic, irregular breathing or precipitate asthmatic attacks in susceptible patients. The cough-suppressant effect of narcotic agonists usually is considered therapeutic; however, as these adverse reactions indicate, it sometimes may be undesirable.

Dilation of peripheral arteries and veins from narcotic agonists leads to flushing and orthostatic hypotension; the patient may feel drowsy or light-headed, and the extremities may feel warm and heavy. (Little change in blood pressure or pulse rate occurs when the patient is recumbent.)

How opiates control pain

Opiates such as meperidine inhibit pain transmission by mimicking the body's natural pain-control mechanisms, as shown.

In the dorsal horn of the spinal cord, peripheral pain neurons meet central nervous system (CNS) neurons. At the synapse, the pain neuron releases substance P (a pain neurotransmitter). This agent helps transfer pain impulses to the CNS neurons that carry the impulses to the brain.

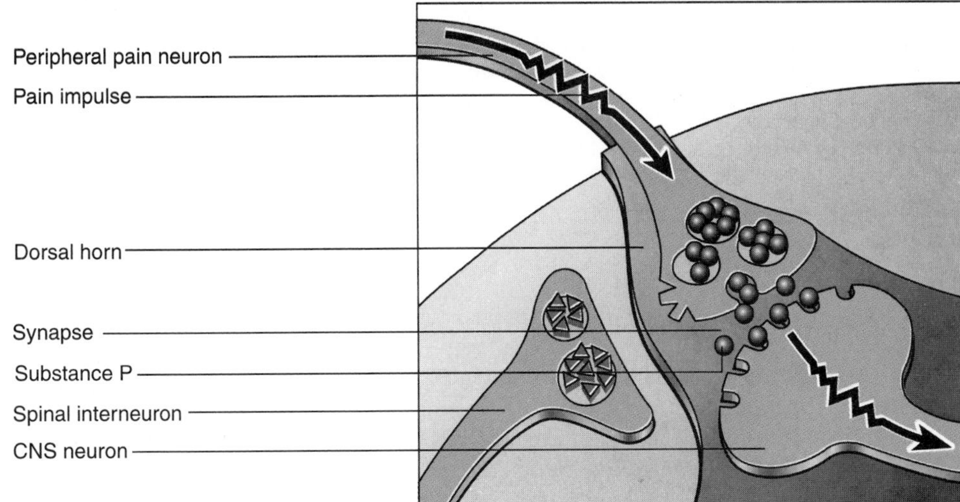

In theory, the spinal interneurons respond to stimulation from the descending neurons of the CNS by releasing endogenous opiates. These opiates bind to the peripheral pain neuron to inhibit substance P's release and to retard the transmission of pain impulses.

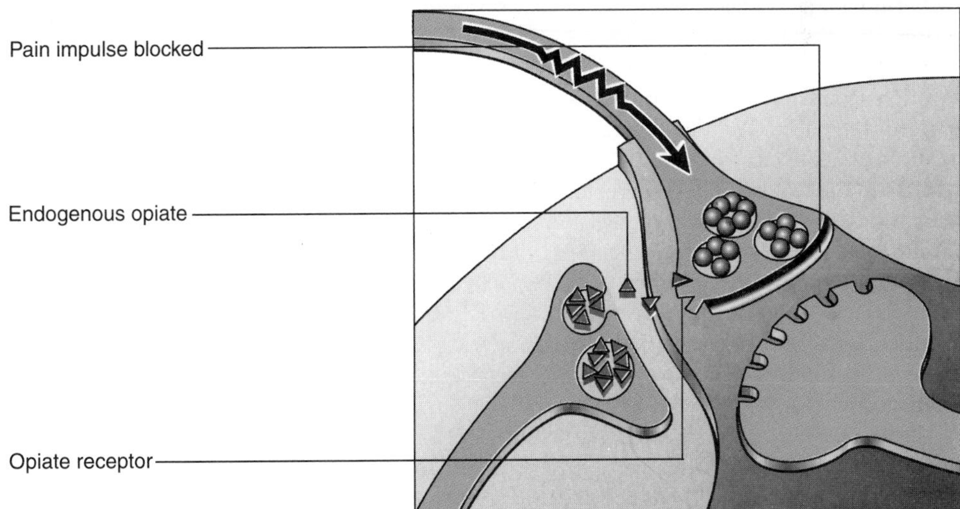

Synthetic opiates supplement this pain-blocking effect by binding with free opiate receptors to inhibit the release of substance P. Opiates also alter consciousness of pain, but how this mechanism works remains unknown.

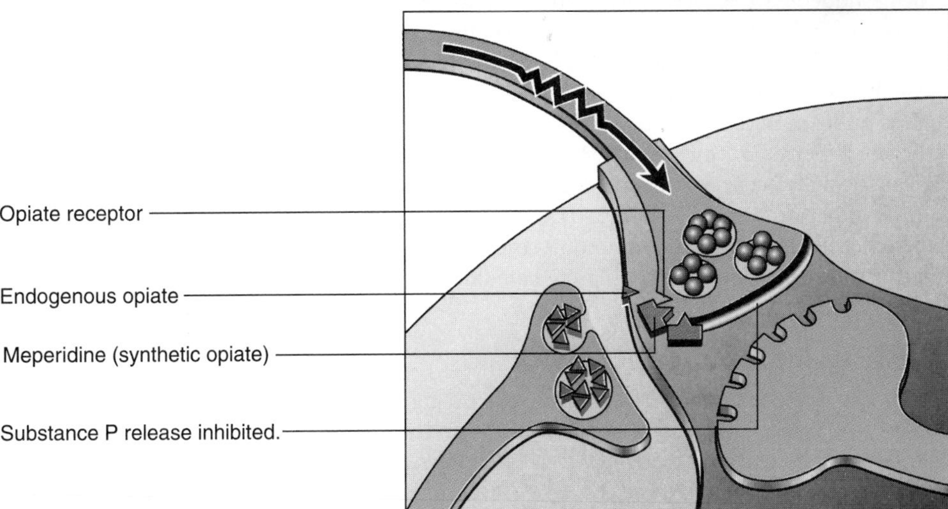

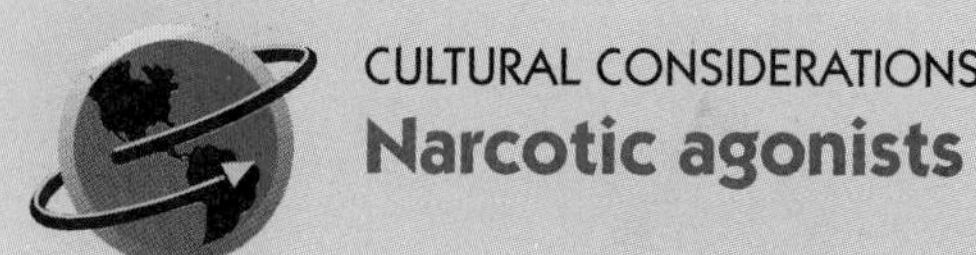

CULTURAL CONSIDERATIONS
Narcotic agonists

Sickle cell disease occurs predominantly in the black population. Sickle cell crisis is a painful exacerbation of the disease that requires prompt medical attention and timely pain medicine administration. I.V. opiates are the drugs of choice to treat the pain of these patients, and morphine is the preferred agent. If a patient is discharged with pain relief or decrease, oral opiate analgesics should be given for home use.

Increased respirations may result from a medullary effect of the drug.

Adverse GI reactions include nausea, vomiting, biliary colic, and constipation. Nausea and vomiting are more likely to occur in ambulatory patients; however, this reaction differs with specific narcotic agonists, even in the same patient. Biliary colic is most likely to occur with morphine; meperidine is least likely to produce or exacerbate this condition. Narcotic agonists may cause constipation through sedation that reduces response to the defecation impulse, through significant reduction in peristalsis, and through increased water absorption from intestinal contents.

Some patients receiving these drugs, especially males with prostatic hypertrophy, experience urine retention. Narcotic agonists also may prolong labor and produce respiratory depression in the neonate. (See Cultural Considerations: *Narcotic agonists.*)

All narcotic agonists may cause pupil constriction (miosis) that persists throughout long-term therapy. Meperidine frequently produces tremors, palpitations, tachycardia, and delirium.

Health care professionals should always be alert for the development of patient tolerance to the effects of narcotic drugs. When a patient who has become tolerant to a narcotic drug suddenly stops receiving it, withdrawal symptoms may occur, including increased sensory perceptions (especially those of pain and touch), tactile hallucinations, increased GI secretions, nasopharyngeal secretions, diarrhea, dilated pupils, and photophobia.

Severe hypersensitivity reactions to narcotic agonists are rare and usually occur as urticaria or a rash; even I.V. administration rarely causes anaphylaxis. Some patients may experience itching or wheal formation at the injection site, but this is usually a local, histamine-mediated response.

NURSING PROCESS APPLICATION

The following information assists the nurse in caring for a patient who is receiving a narcotic agonist. It includes an overview of assessment activities as well as examples of appropriate nursing diagnoses and related interventions (under "Planning and implementation"). It also highlights the importance of evaluation.

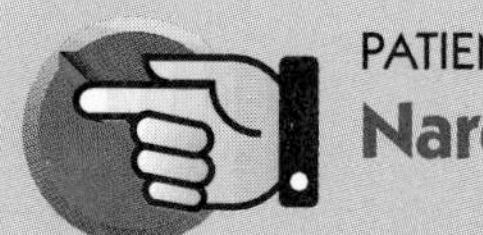

PATIENT TEACHING
Narcotic agonists

- Teach the patient and family the name, dose, frequency, action, and adverse effects of the prescribed narcotic agonist.
- Instruct the patient not to smoke or walk immediately after receiving a narcotic agonist because of its sedative effects. Also caution the patient against operating a motor vehicle or performing any other activity that requires alertness.
- Advise the patient to avoid alcohol or other central nervous system depressants, which may cause excessive sedation and respiratory depression.
- Instruct the patient to lie down if drowsiness, nausea, or light-headedness occurs.
- Teach the patient ways to prevent constipation, such as increasing fluid and fiber intake.
- Advise the patient to note any change in voiding patterns because urine retention may occur.
- Caution the patient to take the narcotic agonist exactly as prescribed because misuse can lead to dependence.
- Teach the patient pain management techniques, such as guided imagery, distraction, and meditation, to minimize the need for prolonged use or large doses of the narcotic agonist.
- Instruct the patient to take the prescribed narcotic agonist before the pain becomes severe for greatest effectiveness.
- Instruct the patient taking morphine sulfate sustained-release tablets not to crush or break them because this will negate the sustained-release effect.
- Advise the patient and family to notify the physician if adverse reactions occur.
- Provide written instructions about the prescribed narcotic agonist.

Assessment

Before drug therapy begins, review the patient's history for conditions that contraindicate or require cautious use of the prescribed narcotic agonist. Also review the patient's medication history to identify use of drugs that may interact with it. During therapy, assess the patient for adverse drug reactions or signs of drug interactions. Also, periodically assess the effectiveness of therapy. Finally, evaluate the patient's and family's knowledge about the prescribed narcotic agonist. (See Patient Teaching: *Narcotic agonists.*)

Nursing diagnoses

- Risk for injury related to a preexisting condition that contraindicates or requires cautious use of a narcotic agonist
- Risk for injury related to adverse drug reactions or drug interactions
- Impaired adjustment related to dependence on a narcotic agonist
- Knowledge deficit related to the prescribed narcotic agonist

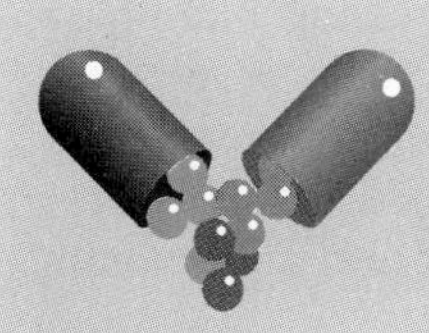

DRUG INTERACTIONS
Narcotic agonists

Drug interactions involving the narcotic agonists commonly lead to increased (and possibly lethal) respiratory and central nervous system (CNS) depression.

DRUG	INTERACTING AGENTS	POSSIBLE EFFECTS	NURSING IMPLICATIONS
codeine, fentanyl, hydromorphone, levorphanol, meperidine, methadone, morphine, oxycodone, oxymorphone, propoxyphene, sufentanil	alcohol, general anesthetics, tranquilizers, sedatives, hypnotics, anti-depressants	Increased CNS depression, especially respiratory depression	• Advise the patient to avoid concomitant alcohol ingestion. Teach the patient to read labels on all over-the-counter cough syrups and cold remedies for possible alcohol content. • Monitor the patient's respirations every 30 minutes for 2 hours if alcohol ingestion occurs, and report change to the physician.
	barbiturates	Additive CNS effects; increased sedation	• Administer doses at least 2 hours apart, as prescribed, to avoid extreme patient drowsiness or deep sleep. • Monitor the patient for signs of respiratory depression every 20 to 30 minutes for 2 hours after concomitant administration.
	cimetidine	Inhibited narcotic metabolism, leading to increased respiratory and CNS depression	• Monitor the patient for increased sedation. • Monitor the patient's respiratory rate every 20 to 30 minutes for 2 hours after concomitant administration.
meperidine	monoamine oxidase (MAO) inhibitors	Increased effects of meperidine; rigidity, hypotension, excitation	• Avoid administering meperidine to a patient within 10 days after administration of a MAO inhibitor.
methadone	hydantoins	Analgesic effects of meperidine may be decreased, while the toxic effects may be increased	• Monitor for analgesic effectiveness and opiate toxicity.
	hydantoins, rifampin	Increased methadone metabolism	• Monitor the patient for signs of withdrawal. • Expect to increase the methadone dosage.
propoxyphene	warfarin	Effects of warfarin may be potentiated	• Monitor PT and observe for increased bleeding tendencies.
	carbamazepine	Effects of carbamazepine may be increased	• Monitor for carbamazepine toxicity.

Planning and implementation

• Do not administer a narcotic agonist to a patient with a condition that contraindicates its use. (See Drug Interactions: *Narcotic agonists.*)
• Administer a narcotic agonist cautiously to a patient at risk because of a preexisting condition.
• Observe the patient periodically for adverse reactions to the prescribed narcotic agonist.
• Obtain the patient's baseline blood pressure, pulse, and respirations before administering the initial dose of a narcotic agonist. Continue to monitor these vital signs throughout narcotic agonist therapy.
∗ ***Note the patient's respiratory rate, depth, and rhythm before administering each narcotic agonist dose. Withhold the dose and consult the physician if the patient's respiratory rate is 8 to 10 breaths/minute or less. Keep in mind that an infant or a patient with compromised respiratory function may be particularly sensitive to the respiratory effects of a narcotic agonist.***
• Notify the physician of adverse reactions to the narcotic agonist.
• Observe for signs of patient tolerance to the effects of the narcotic agonist, such as inadequate pain relief and requests for increased drug administration.
• Do not discontinue the narcotic agonist suddenly in a drug-dependent patient. This may cause withdrawal symptoms, such as increased sensory perceptions, tactile halluci-

nations, increased GI or nasopharyngeal secretions, diarrhea, dilated pupils, and photophobia.
• Encourage the patient to seek help in combating drug dependence.
• Assess the patient's pain before and after each dose of narcotic agonist. Keep in mind that narcotic agonists are most effective when administered before pain becomes severe.
• Do not crush or break morphine sulfate sustained-release tablets; this will negate the sustained-release effect.
• Discuss with the physician the addition of a nonnarcotic analgesic agent to improve pain control, if needed.

Evaluation

For each nursing diagnosis, prepare an evaluation statement that describes the patient's or family's response to nursing interventions.

Mixed narcotic agonist-antagonists

The mixed narcotic agonist-antagonists — buprenorphine hydrochloride, butorphanol tartrate, dezocine, nalbuphine hydrochloride, and pentazocine hydrochloride (combined with pentazocine lactate, naloxone hydrochloride, aspirin, or acetaminophen) — originally appeared to have less abuse potential than the pure narcotic agonists. However, butorphanol and pentazocine have reportedly caused dependence.

PHARMACOKINETICS

The mixed narcotic agonist-antagonists can be administered orally or by the S.C., I.M., or I.V. route, but pentazocine is the only drug in this category available in oral form. Absorption occurs rapidly from parenteral sites. These drugs are distributed to most body tissues and also cross the placenta. They are metabolized in the liver and excreted primarily by the kidneys, although more than 10% of a butorphanol dose and a small amount of dezocine and pentazocine doses are excreted in the feces.

Route	Onset	Peak	Duration
P.O.	15-30 min	60-180 min	3 hr
I.M.	10-20 min	15-60 min	3-6 hr
I.V.	2-15 min	30-60 min	3-6 hr
S.C.	15-20 min	15-60 min	3-6 hr

PHARMACODYNAMICS

The exact mechanism of action of the mixed narcotic agonist-antagonists has not been established. Buprenorphine seems to dissociate slowly from binding sites and therefore has a longer duration of action than the other drugs in this class. The site of action of butorphanol may be opiate receptors in the limbic system. Like pentazocine, butorphanol also acts on pulmonary circulation, increasing pulmonary artery and pulmonary capillary wedge pressures and pulmonary vascular resistance. Both drugs also increase systemic arterial pressure and the overall cardiac workload. Dezocine reportedly increases cardiac index, stroke volume, and pulmonary vascular resistance.

PHARMACOTHERAPEUTICS

Mixed narcotic agonist-antagonists are prescribed primarily for the relief of moderate to severe pain, for obstetric analgesia in selected cases, and for preoperative medication to reduce anxiety and pain perception.

Mixed narcotic agonist-antagonists sometimes are preferred because the risk of drug dependence is lower with them than with the narcotic agonists. Mixed narcotic agonist-antagonists also are less likely to cause respiratory depression.

Drug interactions

Patients who have become dependent on narcotic agonists almost always will experience withdrawal symptoms if they are given mixed narcotic agonist-antagonists. The exception is nalbuphine, which can be administered just before, together with, or just after an injection of a narcotic agonist without antagonizing it. Patients with a known or suspected history of narcotic abuse should not receive any of the mixed narcotic agonist-antagonists. Supportive measures should be readily available in the event that one of these drugs is administered inadvertently to a narcotic-dependent patient.

Increased CNS depression and an additive decrease in respiratory rate and depth may result if mixed narcotic agonist-antagonists are administered to patients taking or using other CNS depressants, such as barbiturates or alcohol. If concomitant administration is necessary, the dosage of one of the drugs should be reduced.

ADVERSE DRUG REACTIONS

Adverse reactions to the mixed narcotic agonist-antagonists are less common than reactions to narcotic agonists and usually affect the CNS and the GI tract.

The most common adverse reactions to these drugs include nausea, vomiting, light-headedness, sedation, and euphoria. Dysphoria, visual hallucinations, confusion, and disorientation also may occur (especially in geriatric patients). These effects limit the long-term use of these agents in patients with severe pain. Respiration may be depressed with initial doses but does not worsen with increased dosage. Insomnia and disturbed dreams may occur, especially with pentazocine and nalbuphine, and anticholinergic effects (dry mouth, blurred vision, constipation, and urine retention) are common. The patient may experience blood pressure changes, primarily hypertension, especially with nalbuphine. The mixed narcotic agonist-antagonists also can cause hypersensitivity reactions.

NURSING PROCESS APPLICATION

The following information assists the nurse in caring for a patient who is receiving a mixed narcotic agonist-antagonist. It includes an overview of assessment activities as well as examples of appropriate nursing diagnoses and related interventions (under "Planning and implementation"). It also highlights the importance of evaluation.

Assessment

Before drug therapy begins, review the patient's history for conditions that contraindicate or require cautious use of the prescribed mixed narcotic agonist-antagonist. Also review the patient's medication history to identify use of drugs that may interact with it. During therapy, assess the patient for adverse drug reactions and signs of drug interactions. Also, periodically assess the effectiveness of therapy. Finally, evaluate the patient's and family's knowledge about the prescribed mixed narcotic agonist-antagonist.

Nursing diagnoses

- Risk for injury related to a preexisting condition that contraindicates or requires cautious use of a mixed narcotic agonist-antagonist
- Risk for injury related to adverse drug reactions or drug interactions
- Pain related to ineffectiveness of the prescribed mixed narcotic agonist-antagonist
- Knowledge deficit related to the prescribed mixed narcotic agonist-antagonist

Planning and implementation

- Do not administer a mixed narcotic agonist-antagonist to a patient with a condition that contraindicates its use. (See Patient Teaching: *Mixed narcotic agonist-antagonists.*)
- Administer a mixed narcotic agonist-antagonist cautiously to a patient at risk because of a preexisting condition.
- Monitor the patient for adverse reactions throughout drug therapy.

* ***Monitor respiratory status during therapy. Have emergency equipment readily available.***

* ***Do not administer a mixed narcotic agonist-antagonist to a narcotic-dependent patient; it may precipitate withdrawal symptoms.***

- Take safety precautions and provide psychological support if a mixed narcotic agonist-antagonist is administered inadvertently to a narcotic-dependent patient. Observe the patient frequently and take necessary safety precautions if the patient develops mental status changes. For example, keep the bed rails up and place the bed in the low position.

* ***Do not mix pentazocine in the same syringe as a barbiturate.***

- Question any prescription for S.C. pentazocine because it may cause severe tissue damage when administered by S.C. injection. If the patient must receive the drug S.C., record, inspect, and rotate injection sites.

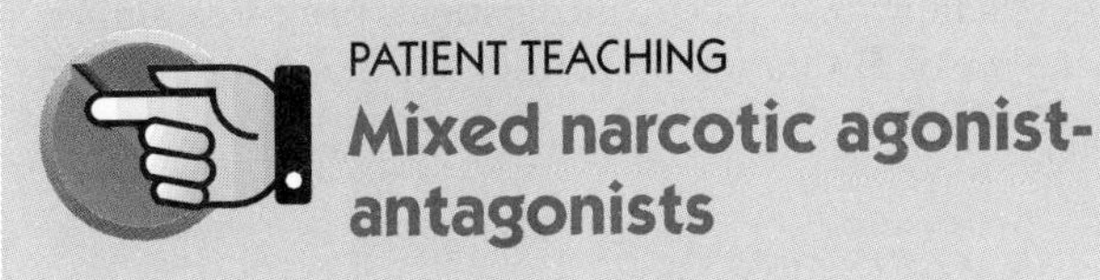

PATIENT TEACHING

Mixed narcotic agonist-antagonists

- Teach the patient and family the name, dose, frequency, action, and adverse effects of the prescribed mixed narcotic agonist-antagonist.
- Advise the patient to avoid activities that require alertness until response to the drug has been determined.
- Inform the narcotic-dependent patient that administration of a mixed narcotic agonist-antagonist may precipitate withdrawal symptoms; encourage honesty in reporting all drug use.
- Advise the patient not to take alcohol or any over-the-counter medication containing alcohol without consulting the physician because of the increased risk of central nervous system and respiratory depression.
- Instruct the patient to drink 2 to 3 qt (2 to 3 L) of fluid daily and increase dietary fiber to prevent constipation.
- Alert the patient and family that dysphoria, blurred vision, visual hallucinations, confusion, and disorientation may occur. Instruct the family to handle these adverse reactions by taking safety measures, such as constant supervision, until the effects of the drug wear off.
- Instruct the patient to relieve dry mouth by drinking cold beverages, sucking on hard candy, or using a nonprescription saliva substitute. Also encourage frequent oral hygiene.
- Instruct the patient and family to notify the physician if adverse reactions occur or if pain is not relieved.

- Provide emergency care if an overdose occurs; use mechanical ventilation, as prescribed. Keep in mind that naloxone can reverse the effects of pentazocine and nalbuphine, but will not reverse totally the effects of buprenorphine.
- Notify the physician if adverse drug reactions occur.
- Rate the patient's pain before and after each dose of a mixed narcotic agonist-antagonist agent; determine and record the onset, duration, location, intensity, and quality of the pain as well as the degree of pain relief obtained after drug administration.
- Notify the physician if the prescribed mixed narcotic agonist-antagonist does not relieve the patient's pain.

Evaluation

For each nursing diagnosis, prepare an evaluation statement that describes the patient's or family's response to nursing interventions.

Narcotic antagonists

The pure narcotic antagonists naloxone hydrochloride and naltrexone hydrochloride have an affinity for opiate receptors but do not stimulate them. Instead, these drugs attach to the receptors and prevent narcotic drugs, **enkephalins,** and **endorphins** from producing their effects. Naloxone is used to treat narcotic overdose. Naltrexone is used as an adjunct therapy to keep detoxified patients drug-free, similar to the use of disulfiram (Antabuse) to prevent resumption of alcohol abuse.

PHARMACOKINETICS

Naloxone is administered I.M., S.C., or I.V.; naltrexone is administered orally in tablet or liquid form. Both drugs are metabolized by the liver and excreted by the kidneys.

Naloxone has an immediate onset of action, but its duration of action depends on the dose and administration route. For example, I.M. administration produces a more prolonged effect than I.V. administration. The nurse must monitor the patient carefully because the effects of the narcotic overdose in many cases last longer than the effects of the antagonist, and repeated doses may be necessary. Onset of naltrexone occurs in 20 to 30 minutes; peak concentration occurs in 1 hour. The plasma half-life of naloxone is 60 to 90 minutes. The half-life of naltrexone is 13 hours.

Route	Onset	Peak	Duration
P.O.	20-30 min	1 hr	Up to 24 hr
I.M.	2-5 min	Unknown	1-4 hr
I.V.	2 min	Unknown	1-4 hr
S.C.	2-5 min	Unknown	1-4 hr

PHARMACODYNAMICS

Narcotic antagonists block the effects of narcotics by occupying the opiate receptor sites, displacing any narcotic molecules already present, and blocking further narcotic binding at these sites. This is known as **competitive inhibition.**

PHARMACOTHERAPEUTICS

Naloxone is the drug of choice for managing a narcotic overdose because it reverses the respiratory depression and sedation and helps stabilize the patient's vital signs within seconds after administration. Naloxone administration also reverses the analgesic effects of narcotic drugs, so a patient who was given a narcotic drug for pain relief may complain of pain or even experience withdrawal symptoms. The severity of these symptoms depends on the narcotic used and the amount.

If repeated injections of naloxone are needed but the patient does not improve after receiving three doses or 10 mg, supportive methods such as mechanical ventilation should be instituted as prescribed; lingering depressant effects may be from nonnarcotic drugs or a mixed overdose. (See *Adverse reactions of naltrexone.*)

Naltrexone is used only as an adjunct to psychotherapy or counseling for patients who have been detoxified from narcotic drugs and wish to remain so. Before naltrexone treatment is initiated, a naloxone challenge test may be given after the patient has been without narcotics for 7 to 10 days. In this test, the patient receives naloxone I.V. or S.C. and is observed for withdrawal symptoms. If withdrawal symptoms occur, the patient is at risk and should not begin naltrexone therapy.

Adverse reactions of naltrexone

Adverse reactions to naltrexone can take many forms, as this chart demonstrates. (Hepatotoxicity may occur occasionally.)

Cardiopulmonary
- Edema
- Hypertension
- Palpitations
- Phlebitis
- Shortness of breath

Central nervous system
- Anxiety
- Depression
- Disorientation
- Dizziness
- Headache
- Nervousness

Eye, ear, nose, and throat
- Blurred vision
- Cough
- Epistaxis
- Fatigue, insomnia
- Nasal congestion
- Tinnitus

Gastrointestinal
- Anorexia
- Diarrhea or constipation
- Nausea
- Thirst
- Vomiting

Genitourinary
- Changes in libido
- Delayed ejaculation
- Urinary frequency

Skin
- Acne
- Alopecia
- Itching
- Rash

Drug interactions

Naloxone produces no significant drug interactions. Naltrexone will cause withdrawal symptoms if given to a patient receiving a narcotic agonist or to a narcotic addict.

ADVERSE DRUG REACTIONS

Naloxone may cause nausea, vomiting, and, occasionally, hypertension and tachycardia. An unconscious patient returned to consciousness abruptly after naloxone administration may hyperventilate and experience tremors.

Naltrexone produces numerous adverse reactions affecting various body systems. The variety and number of adverse reactions to this drug have delayed its full acceptance in maintaining narcotic abstinence. Patients should be monitored frequently, even if they receive the drug on an outpatient basis.

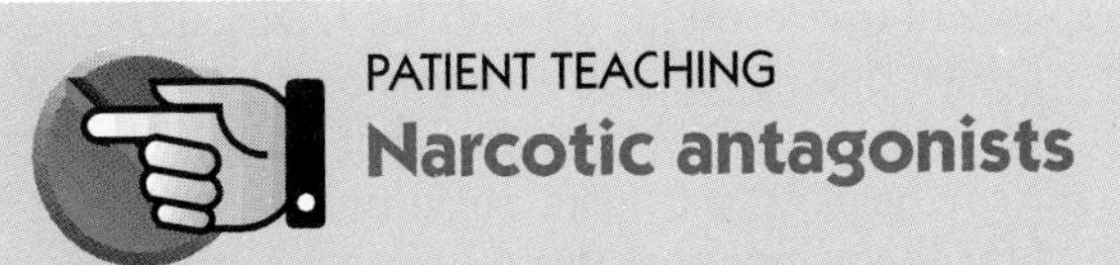

PATIENT TEACHING
Narcotic antagonists

- Teach the family about the use and purpose of naloxone to treat narcotic overdose in the patient.
- Inform the family that naloxone cannot reverse the effects of all drugs and that other emergency care may be required, such as mechanical ventilation.
- Advise the family that an unconscious patient returned to consciousness abruptly after naloxone administration may hyperventilate and experience tremors.
- Encourage the family to ask questions about naloxone use.
- Teach the patient and family the name, dose, frequency, action, and adverse effects of naltrexone.
- Inform the patient that naltrexone blocks the action of narcotics and may precipitate narcotic withdrawal. Advise the patient to be honest with the physician about narcotic use.
- Instruct the patient about the naloxone challenge test.
- Teach the patient how to manage a nosebleed, which may occur during naltrexone therapy.
- Advise the patient to change positions slowly and not to engage in activities that require concentration if naltrexone produces dizziness, blurred vision, or mental status changes.
- Instruct the patient to eat small, frequent meals if naltrexone produces anorexia. Also advise the patient to consume 2 to 3 qt (2 to 3 L) of fluid a day and adequate fiber to prevent naltrexone-induced constipation.
- Inform the patient about naltrexone's genitourinary effects, such as change in libido and delayed ejaculation.
- Instruct the patient to notify the physician if adverse reactions to naltrexone occur.

NURSING PROCESS APPLICATION

The following information assists the nurse in caring for a patient who is receiving a narcotic antagonist. It includes an overview of assessment activities as well as examples of appropriate nursing diagnoses and related interventions (under "Planning and implementation"). It also highlights the importance of evaluation.

Assessment

Before drug therapy begins, review the patient's history for conditions that contraindicate or require cautious use of the prescribed narcotic antagonist. Also review the patient's medication history to identify use of drugs that may interact with it. During therapy, assess the patient for adverse drug reactions, such as sexual dysfunction, and signs of drug interactions. Also, periodically assess the effectiveness of therapy. Finally, evaluate the patient's and family's knowledge about the prescribed narcotic antagonist.

Nursing diagnoses

- Risk for injury related to a preexisting condition that contraindicates or requires cautious use of the prescribed narcotic antagonist
- Risk for injury related to adverse drug reactions or drug interactions
- Sexual dysfunction related to the genitourinary effects of naltrexone
- Knowledge deficit related to the prescribed narcotic antagonist

Planning and implementation

- Do not administer a narcotic antagonist to a patient with a condition that contraindicates its use.
- Do not administer naltrexone until a negative naloxone challenge test is obtained. Also, do not administer naltrexone to a patient who is receiving narcotic drugs, is addicted to narcotic drugs, or is in the acute phase of narcotic withdrawal because acute withdrawal may occur or worsen.
- Administer a narcotic antagonist cautiously to a patient at risk because of a preexisting condition.
- Observe the patient for adverse reactions throughout narcotic antagonist therapy.

✱ ***Be prepared to administer another dose of naloxone, as prescribed, if respiratory depression occurs.*** Keep in mind that a narcotic's duration of action may exceed naloxone's duration, and that naloxone does not reverse respiratory depression produced by diazepam.

- Encourage the patient taking naltrexone to report signs and symptoms of sexual dysfunction, such as changes in libido and delayed ejaculation. Reassure the patient that these effects will disappear when naltrexone is discontinued. (See Patient Teaching: *Narcotic antagonists.*)

Evaluation

For each nursing diagnosis, prepare an evaluation statement that describes the patient's or family's response to nursing interventions.

CHAPTER SUMMARY

Chapter 15 explored narcotic agonists, mixed narcotic agonist-antagonists, and narcotic antagonists. Here are the chapter highlights.

Narcotic agonists modify the sensation of pain by inhibiting the transmission of pain impulses in sensory pathways in the spinal cord, reducing cortical responses to painful stimuli, and altering behavioral responses to pain. Narcotic agonists include the opium derivatives and the synthetic narcotics used to relieve pain. Oral, rectal, parenteral, and transdermal forms are available.

Morphine is considered the narcotic standard; all narcotic drugs are compared with it. Adverse reactions to narcotic agonists include respiratory depression, orthostatic hypotension, and constipation. Tolerance as well as psychological and physical dependence may occur with long-term narcotic use.

Mixed narcotic agonist-antagonists produce analgesic effects similar to those of morphine. They have few or no antitussive effects. The respiratory depression caused by mixed narcotic agonist-antagonists does not worsen with higher doses.

The narcotic antagonists naloxone and naltrexone work by competitive inhibition at the opiate receptor sites, displacing narcotic molecules and preventing them from exerting their effects. Naloxone is used to treat narcotic overdose. Naltrexone is used as an adjunct treatment with detoxified addicts who are highly motivated to remain drug-free.

Questions to consider

See Appendix 1 for answers.

1. Ann Marie Giovanni, age 26, experiences severe pain from metastatic bone cancer. For her pain, the physician initially prescribes the narcotic agonist morphine sulfate intensified oral solution 10 mg P.O. every 4 hours. Which of the following is a common adverse reaction to a narcotic agonist?
   (a) Decreased repiratory rate
   (b) Urine retention
   (c) Blurred vision
   (d) Diarrhea

2. A friend brings Tony Campbell, age 21, to the emergency department with pain in the right lower abdominal quadrant. After performing an emergency appendectomy on Mr. Campbell, the physician prescribes dezocine 10 mg I.M. for postoperative pain. Before administering dezocine, the nurse asks Mr. Campbell about narcotic use. Administering a mixed narcotic agonist-antagonist to a patient dependent on narcotic agonists may cause which of the following reactions?
   (a) Hypersensitivity reaction
   (b) Withdrawal symptoms
   (c) Urinary incontinence
   (d) Hepatotoxicity

3. What is the difference between a narcotic agonist and a mixed narcotic agonist-antagonist?
   (a) A mixed narcotic agonist-antagonist is less likely to cause respiratory depression.
   (b) A mixed narcotic agonist-antagonist is more likely to cause drug dependence.
   (c) More of a mixed narcotic agonist-antagonist is needed to relieve pain.
   (d) Less of a mixed narcotic agonist-antagonist is needed to relieve pain.

4. Despondent over breaking up with her boyfriend, Jennifer Brown, age 16, takes an overdose of oxycodone hydrochloride and acetaminophen. When her parents bring her to the emergency department, she is unresponsive. Which of the following drugs is commonly prescribed to treat a narcotic overdose?
   (a) butorphanol
   (b) pentazocine
   (c) naltrexone
   (d) naloxone

5. Which of the following adverse reactions can occur if an unconscious patient is returned to consciousness abruptly after the administration of a narcotic antagonist?
   (a) Seizures
   (b) Vomiting
   (c) Hyperventilation
   (d) Hypertensive crisis

16 Anesthetic agents

OBJECTIVES

After reading and studying this chapter, the student should be able to:

1. differentiate between inhalation and injection general anesthetic agents.
2. differentiate between local and topical anesthetic agents.
3. discuss the pharmacokinetics of general, local, and topical anesthetic agents.
4. describe the drug interactions and adverse effects associated with inhalation and injection general anesthetics.
5. describe the drug interactions and adverse effects associated with local and topical anesthetics.
6. describe how to apply the nursing process when caring for a patient who is receiving an anesthetic agent.

INTRODUCTION

Anesthetic agents can be divided into three main groups: general, local, and topical anesthetic agents. General anesthetic agents can be subdivided into two main types: inhalation and injection anesthetics.

General anesthetics depress the central nervous system (CNS) to produce loss of consciousness, loss of responsiveness to sensory stimulation including pain, and muscle relaxation. General **anesthesia** may result from one or a combination of drugs.

These drugs are volatile liquids or gases vaporized in oxygen and administered by inhalation or nonvolatile solutions administered by injection.

The practice of general anesthesia includes more than proper administration of anesthetic agents. Monitoring and maintaining vital signs, fluids, electrolytes, acid-base balance, body temperature, and positioning, and assuring the patient's well-being from before surgery through recovery are vital components of anesthesia practice.

The choice of a particular general anesthetic agent for a patient involves several considerations, including the patient's physiologic state and medical history, the type of surgical procedure, and the anticipated postoperative course.

Local and topical anesthetics are used to interrupt pain impulse transmission from peripheral nerves by causing a temporary loss of sensation in a limited area of the body. Local anesthetics must be injected to produce anesthesia, whereas topical anesthetics are applied directly to the skin or mucous membranes. Some local anesthetics can be used topically.

The drugs covered in this chapter include:

- benzocaine
- benzyl alcohol
- butamben picrate
- bupivacaine hydrochloride
- chloroprocaine hydrochloride
- clove oil
- cocaine hydrochloride
- desflurane
- dibucaine hydrochloride
- dyclonine hydrochloride
- enflurane
- etidocaine hydrochloride
- etomidate
- ethyl chloride
- halothane
- isoflurane
- ketamine hydrochloride
- lidocaine
- lidocaine hydrochloride
- menthol
- mepivacaine hydrochloride
- nitrous oxide
- pramoxime hydrochloride
- prilocaine hydrochloride
- procaine hydrochloride
- propofol
- ropivacaine hydrochloride
- sevoflurane
- tetracaine
- tetracaine hydrochloride.

Inhalation anesthetics

Commonly used inhalation anesthetics include desflurane, sevoflurane, enflurane, halothane, isoflurane, and nitrous oxide.

PHARMACOKINETICS

The absorption and elimination rates of an anesthetic are governed by its solubility in blood. Inhalation anesthetics enter the blood from the lungs and are distributed to other tissues. Distribution is most rapid to organs with high blood flow: the brain, liver, kidneys, and heart. The inhalation anesthetics are eliminated primarily by the lungs, but also by the liver in the case of enflurane, halothane, and sevoflurane. Metabolites are excreted in the urine.

Onset of action and peak concentration levels of the inhalation anesthetics vary greatly, depending on therapeutic

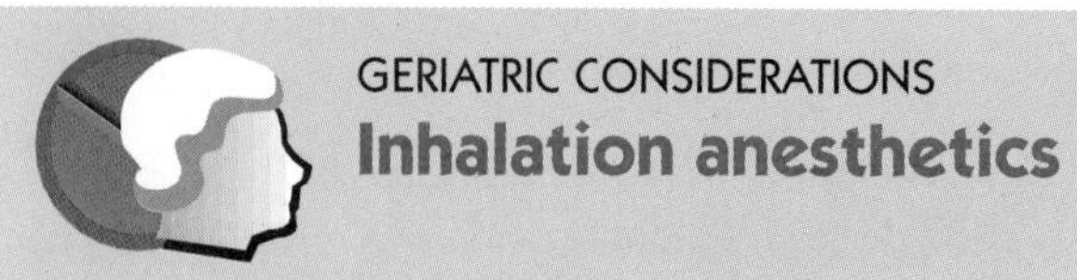

GERIATRIC CONSIDERATIONS
Inhalation anesthetics

Inhalation anesthetics must be used carefully in the geriatric population. An elderly patient may present with multiple coexisting conditions that have had an effect on his overall health. A debilitated surgical patient is predisposed to an exaggerated response to the drugs, and even smaller-than-normal drug doses may result in hypotension, prolonged respiratory depression, and longer recovery. In addition, confusion, agitation, and memory loss may accompany a prolonged recovery from an anesthetic agent and may be mistaken for signs of dementia.

and patient factors. Therapeutic variables include the anesthetic concentration and the presence of other CNS-depressant drugs in the blood. Patient variables include age, pregnancy, respiratory and circulatory status, hypotension, and hypothermia.

The duration of action for each inhalation anesthetic is determined by the rate at which it leaves the brain.

Route	Onset	Peak	Duration
Inhalation	Dose-dependent	Dose-dependent	Dose-dependent

PHARMACODYNAMICS

Inhalation anesthetics are general depressants of the CNS, although they affect other organ systems.

PHARMACOTHERAPEUTICS

Inhalation anesthetics are used for surgery because they offer more precise and rapid control of depth of anesthesia than injection anesthetics. These anesthetics, which are liquids at room temperature, require a vaporizer and special delivery system for safe use. They may be administered only by skilled practitioners.

Of the inhalation anesthetics available, desflurane and isoflurane are the most commonly used, usually with nitrous oxide. Which anesthetic is used depends on a careful evaluation of the patient's physical condition, medical history, and medication profile; the type of surgical procedure; and an assessment of anticipated postoperative needs. (See Geriatric Considerations: *Inhalation anesthetics.*)

Inhalation anesthetics are administered as gases, so dosages are not expressed in weight, as with other drugs. Because the amount of anesthetic in the lungs is known to be proportional to the amount in the brain at equilibrium, the quantity of anesthetic agent needed can be determined by a measurement called the minimum alveolar concentration (MAC). MAC is the alveolar anesthetic concentration at which 50% of patients do not move during a surgical incision.

Inhalation anesthetics are contraindicated in a patient with known hypersensitivy to the drug, a hepatic disorder, or malignant hyperthermia. They require cautious use in a pregnant or breast-feeding patient.

Drug interactions

The most important drug interactions involving inhalation anesthetics are with other CNS, cardiac, or respiratory depressant drugs. The potent anesthetics greatly enhance the depressant effects of normally safe concentrations of these drugs. (See Drug Interactions: *Inhalation anesthetics.*)

ADVERSE DRUG REACTIONS

The most common adverse reaction associated with inhalation anesthetics is an exaggerated patient response to a normal dose. The postoperative reactions are much the same as those seen with other CNS depressant drugs: cardiopulmonary depression, confusion, sedation, nausea, vomiting, ataxia, and hypothermia.

Malignant hyperthermia, characterized by a sudden and often lethal increase in body temperature, is a serious and unexpected reaction to inhalation anesthetic agents. It occurs in genetically susceptible patients only and may result from a failure in calcium uptake by muscle cells. The skeletal muscle relaxant dantrolene is used to treat this condition.

In approximately 1 in 35,000 cases, liver necrosis develops several days after halothane use. Although it is not infective in origin, the necrosis resembles hepatitis clinically, so it is called halothane hepatitis. Symptoms include rash, fever, jaundice, nausea, vomiting, eosinophilia, and alterations in liver function. This often fatal syndrome occurs most commonly with multiple exposures to the drug. An immunologic or chemical response to a toxic metabolite may explain this phenomenon. Treatment is symptomatic.

NURSING PROCESS APPLICATION

The following information assists the nurse in caring for a patient receiving an inhalation anesthetic. It includes an overview of assessment activities as well as examples of appropriate nursing diagnoses and related interventions (under "Planning and implementation"). It also highlights the importance of evaluation.

Assessment

Before drug therapy begins, review the patient's history for conditions that contraindicate or require cautious use of the prescribed inhalation anesthetic. .

Also review the patient's medication history to identify use of drugs that may interact with it. During therapy, assess the patient for adverse drug reactions, such as body temperature changes, and signs of drug interactions. Periodically assess the effectiveness of therapy. Finally, eval-

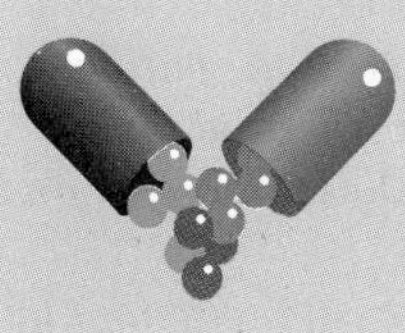

DRUG INTERACTIONS

Inhalation anesthetics

The most significant drug interactions involving inhalation anesthetics are caused by other central nervous system (CNS) depressants. Not every drug listed reacts adversely with each interacting agent.

DRUG	INTERACTING AGENTS	POSSIBLE EFFECTS	NURSING IMPLICATIONS
desflurane, enflurane, halothane, isoflurane, nitrous oxide, sevoflurane	labetalol	Increased hypotensive effects	• Monitor the patient's blood pressure frequently.
	CNS depressants	Increased CNS and respiratory depression and hypotension	• Monitor the patient's rate and rhythm of respirations, level of consciousness, and blood pressure.
	xanthines (caffeine, theophylline)	Increased risk of arrhythmias	• Monitor the patient's pulse rate and characteristics, blood pressure, and respirations.
enflurane, halothane, isoflurane	neuromuscular blocking agents	Increased neuromuscular blockade	• Monitor the patient's respirations. • Monitor the patient's ability to move limbs as anesthesia diminishes.
	catecholamines (dopamine, epinephrine, norepinephrine), doxapram, ephedrine, metaraminol, methoxamine; other sympathomimetics	Increased risk of arrhythmias	• Monitor the patient's pulse rate and characteristics and blood pressure.
	ketamine	Increased risk of hypotension, decreased cardiac output, decreased pulse rate	• Monitor the patient's blood pressure and level of consciousness. • Provide supportive therapy, such as drugs, fluids, and volume expanders, as prescribed.
	ritodrine	Increased risk of hypotension and arrhythmias	• Monitor the patient's vital signs frequently.
	succinylcholine	Increased risk of malignant hyperthermia and neuromuscular blockade; with repeated use, increased risk of bradycardia, arrhythmias, sinus arrest, and apnea	• Monitor the patient's temperature and other vital signs frequently. • Monitor the patient's airway and ability to move limbs.
enflurane	isoniazid	Increased release of nephrotoxic fluorine from enflurane	• Monitor the patient's urine output and blood urea nitrogen (BUN) and serum creatinine levels.
	aminoglycosides	Increased risk of nephrotoxicity	• Monitor the patient's urine output and BUN and serum creatinine levels.
desflurane	midazolam	Decreased anesthetic requirements	• Monitor the amount of medication administered.
	fentanyl	Decreased anesthetic requirements	• Monitor the amount of medication administered.
	succinycholine, atracurium, pancuronium	Increased neuromuscular blockade	• Monitor the patient's respirations and his ability to move limbs as anesthesia diminishes.
sevoflurane	benzodiazepines, opioids, nitrous oxide	Decreased anesthetic requirements	• Same as for desflurane.
	pancuronium, vecuronium, atracurium	Increased neuromuscular blockade	• Monitor the patient's respirations and his ability to move limbs as anesthesia diminishes.

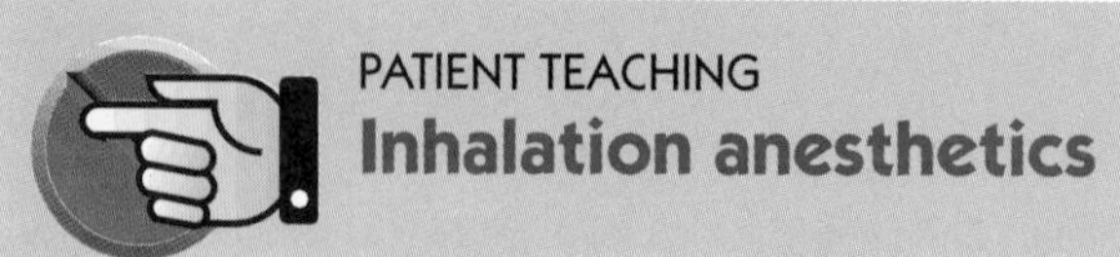

PATIENT TEACHING
Inhalation anesthetics

- Teach the patient and family the name, action, and adverse effects of the inhalation anesthetic to be used.
- Advise the patient not to eat for at least 8 hours before surgery to prevent aspiration of stomach contents into the lungs during anesthesia.
- Inform the patient that psychomotor functions may be impaired for 24 hours or more after inhalation anesthesia.
- Advise the patient not to drink alcohol or use any other central nervous system depressants for at least 24 hours after anesthesia.
- Instruct the patient to report adverse reactions or unusual symptoms to the physician immediately.

uate the patient's and family's knowledge about the prescribed inhalation anesthetic.

Nursing diagnoses

- Risk for injury related to a preexisting condition that contraindicates or requires cautious use of an inhalation anesthetic
- Risk for injury related to adverse drug reactions or drug interactions
- Risk for altered body temperature related to potential development of hypothermia or malignant hyperthermia during inhalation anesthetic administration
- Knowledge deficit related to the inhalation anesthetic

Planning and implementation

- Know that an inhalation anesthetic must not be administered to a patient with a condition that contraindicates its use. (See Patient Teaching: *Inhalation anesthetics*.)
- Know that an inhalation anesthetic must be administered cautiously to a patient at risk because of a preexisting condition.
- Observe the patient for adverse reactions to the inhalation anesthetic throughout administration and recovery.
- Monitor the patient's vital signs frequently to detect potential problems. Assess the adequacy, rate, and depth of the patient's respirations. Maintain a patent airway. Assess the patient's level of consciousness, arousal, and orientation.
- Provide symptomatic care for a patient with adverse reactions, such as cardiovascular and respiratory depression, prolonged sedation, and nausea and vomiting; these reactions usually are reversible. Inform the anesthesiologist of severe adverse reactions.
- Keep atropine available to reverse bradycardia, if it occurs.
- Monitor the patient's temperature frequently. Be aware that hypothermia is a common effect of inhalation anesthesia and that shivering is normal during recovery. If the patient is shivering, administer oxygen, as prescribed, to compensate for the increased oxygen demand.
- Keep the patient warm if hypothermia occurs.

* ***Notify the anesthesiologist immediately if the patient's temperature increases suddenly. This may signal malignant hyperthermia, a sudden, potentially lethal reaction to the inhalation anesthetic.***

* ***Keep dantrolene readily available to treat malignant hyperthermia.***

Evaluation

For each nursing diagnosis, prepare an evaluation statement that describes the patient's or family's response to nursing interventions.

Injection anesthetics

Injection anesthetics usually are used in situations requiring a short duration of anesthesia, such as outpatient surgery. They also are used to promote rapid induction of anesthesia or to supplement inhalation anesthetics.

Three agents in this class — etomidate, propofol, and ketamine hydrochloride — are used solely as injected general anesthetics. The rest are drawn from other chemical categories, such as barbiturates (methohexital sodium, thiamylal sodium, and thiopental sodium) and benzodiazepines (diazepam, lorazepam, and midazolam hydrochloride), and are used secondarily as anesthetics. In addition, various opiates and opiate-like drugs may be used as injected general anesthetics, such as alfentanil hydrochloride, fentanyl citrate, meperidine hydrochloride, morphine sulfate, and sufentanil citrate.

PHARMACOKINETICS

All injection anesthetics bypass the mechanisms that reduce bioavailability, distributing rapidly into the CNS. Effects of the injection anesthetics appear quickly, beginning 15 seconds to a few minutes after administration. Intramuscular (I.M.) injection of the opiates may delay absorption and decrease peak effect when compared to intravenous (I.V.) administration. The barbiturates depend on hepatic transformation for elimination, as do the benzodiazepine and opiate agents and the hypnotic etomidate.

All injection anesthetics have a rapid onset of action and are short-acting, except for diazepam, which is long-acting. Etomidate, the opiates, propofol, and the barbiturates begin to act within 60 seconds; the benzodiazepines act within 1 to 15 minutes. The opiates reach peak concentration levels in 3 to 20 minutes. Rapid redistribution of barbiturates, propofol, etomidate, and ketamine from the brain to other tissues ends anesthetic action; therefore, their duration of action is much shorter than would be anticipated from their half-lives.

Route	Onset	Peak	Duration
I.V.	Variable	Few min	Variable
I.M.	3-4 min	Unknown	12-25 min

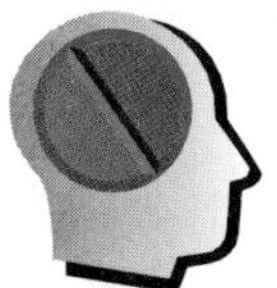

CRITICAL THINKING To enhance your critical thinking about anesthetic agents, consider the following situation and analysis.
Situation: Inez Turner is admitted for removal of a ganglion cyst on her hand. She receives a general anesthetic with sodium pentathol. She awakens in about 30 minutes and is discharged home in 2 hours. Sodium pentathol has a half-life of about 12 hours. What characteristic of injection anesthetics is responsible for her rapid awakening and discharge?
Analysis: The recovery from injection anesthetics is due to the rapid redistribution of the drug from the CNS to nonnervous peripheral sites. Therefore, metabolism and rapid elimination does not account for recovery. The half-life of injection anesthetics is much less important than for usual pharmacologic agents.

PHARMACODYNAMICS

Barbiturates seem to enhance responses to the CNS neurotransmitter gamma-aminobutyric acid (GABA) and to depress the excitability of CNS neurons. The benzodiazepines also stimulate responses to GABA, thus inhibiting the brain's response to stimulation of the reticular activating system, the area of the brain stem that controls alertness. Etomidate, too, may have GABA-like effects, including direct inhibition of the RAS. The opiates occupy sites on specialized receptors scattered throughout the CNS and modify the release of neurotransmitters from sensory nerves entering the CNS. Ketamine appears to interact with N-methyl-D-aspartate receptors, which may account for its inhibitory anesthetic action.

PHARMACOTHERAPEUTICS

The short duration of action of these agents is an advantage in shorter surgical procedures — including outpatient surgery. However, only skilled practitioners may administer these agents for anesthesia.

The subcategories of injection anesthetics have various pharmacologic characteristics. The barbiturates are used alone in surgery that is not expected to be painful and as adjuncts to other agents in more extensive procedures. The benzodiazepines produce sedation and amnesia, but not **analgesia.** Etomidate is used to induce anesthesia and to supplement low-potency inhalation anesthetics such as nitrous oxide. The opiates provide analgesia and supplement other anesthetic agents.

Etomidate, propofol, and ketamine are contraindicated in a patient with known hypersensitivity to them. Avoid ketamine in a patient with significant hypertension, severe cardiac decompensation, any condition in which a significant blood pressure increase would endanger the patient, or a history of cerebrovascular accident or during surgery of the pharynx, larynx, or bronchial tree (unless used with muscle relaxants).

Ketamine should be administered cautiously to a pregnant or breast-feeding patient or one with chronic alcoholism, alcohol intoxication, or elevated cerebrospinal fluid (CSF) pressure.

Drug interactions

Injection anesthetics interact with many other drugs. As with the inhalation anesthetics, most of these interactions require the nurse to monitor the patient's vital signs, airway, and level of consciousness. (See Drug Interactions: *Injection anesthetics*, page 204.) The opiates, barbiturates, and benzodiazepines and their interactions are discussed elsewhere in this text.

ADVERSE DRUG REACTIONS

Adverse reactions to the injection anesthetics frequently are extensions of their therapeutic effects.

Adverse CNS reactions are most common after ketamine anesthesia; they include prolonged recovery, unpleasant dreams, irrational behavior, excitement, disorientation, delirium, and hallucinations. The barbiturates and propofol cause respiratory depression. Thiopental, etomidate, and propofol can produce airway reflex hyperactivity with hiccoughs, coughing, and muscle twitching and jerking. Thiopental also depresses cardiac function and causes peripheral vasodilation; ketamine increases heart rate, cardiac output, and blood pressure in patients who are not severely ill. The opiates sometimes cause changes in heart rate, including arrhythmias. The rare circulatory failure and respiratory arrest seen with the benzodiazepines appear to be associated with too-rapid drug administration or concomitant **narcotic** administration. Phlebitis has been reported with diazepam administration.

Muscle rigidity and spasms follow administration of ketamine and the opiates; the reaction seems to be directly proportional to the infusion rate. Fentanyl and ketamine may cause seizures.

Etomidate, ketamine, and propofol can cause nausea and vomiting. Ketamine also may produce excess salivation, tearing, shivering, and increased CSF and intraocular pressure. In a patient under stress, etomidate may cause reduced cortisol levels. The only other major adverse reaction to etomidate is pain on administration, which can be avoided by rapid administration into a large vein or with use of a preoperative analgesic.

Rash and hypersensitivity reactions are uncommon with etomidate, the opiates, and the barbiturates; anaphylaxis has been reported with the barbiturates only. Extravasation of the barbiturates may cause neuritis and vasospasm.

NURSING PROCESS APPLICATION

The following information assists the nurse in caring for a patient receiving an injection anesthetic. It includes an overview of assessment activities as well as examples of appropriate nursing diagnoses and related interventions (un-

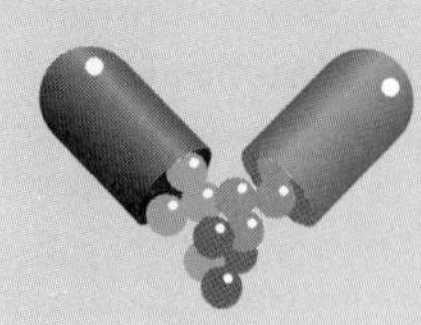

DRUG INTERACTIONS

Injection anesthetics

Because drug interactions involving the injection can cause increased central nervous system (CNS) depression and hypotension, the nurse must assess the patient's vital signs and level of consciousness frequently.

DRUG	INTERACTING AGENTS	POSSIBLE EFFECTS	NURSING IMPLICATIONS
etomidate	verapamil	Enhanced anesthetic effect of etomidate with respiratory depression and apnea	• Monitor the patient's vital signs, level of consciousness, and ability to move limbs.
ketamine	halothane	Increased risk of hypotension, decreased cardiac output	• Monitor the patient's vital signs closely.
	nondepolarizing muscle relaxants	Increased neuromuscular effects resulting in prolonged respiratory depression	• Observe the patient to assure adequate anesthetic effects.
	thiopental	Hypnotic effect of thiopental may be antagonized	• Monitor the patient's cardiopulmonary status.
	barbiturates/narcotics	Recovery time may be prolonged	• Monitor the patient's condition closely.
	theophylline	Seizures may occur	• Monitor the patient for seizures.
	thyroid hormones	Hypertension and tachycardia may occur	• Monitor the patient's blood pressure and heart rate.
propofol	opiates, inhalation anesthetics, hypnotics, sedatives	Increased effects of propofol	• Expect the propofol dosage to be reduced. • Monitor the patient's blood pressure and cardiac output.

der "Planning and implementation"). It also highlights the importance of evaluation.

Assessment

Before drug therapy begins, review the patient's history for conditions that contraindicate or require cautious use of the prescribed injection anesthetic. Also review the patient's medication history to identify use of drugs that may interact with it. During therapy, assess the patient for adverse drug reactions and signs of drug interactions. Also, periodically assess the effectiveness of therapy. Finally, evaluate the patient's and family's knowledge about the prescribed injection anesthetic.

Nursing diagnoses

- Risk for injury related to a preexisting condition that contraindicates or requires cautious use of an injection anesthetic
- Risk for injury related to adverse drug reactions or drug interactions
- Pain related to administration of an injection anesthetic
- Knowledge deficit related to the prescribed injection anesthetic

Planning and implementation

- Know that an injection anesthetic must not be administered to a patient with a condition that contraindicates its use. (See Patient Teaching: *Injection anesthetics.*)
- Know that an injection anesthetic must be administered cautiously to a patient at risk because of a preexisting condition.
- Monitor the patient for adverse reactions throughout injection anesthetic administration and recovery.

∗ ***Keep resuscitation equipment and emergency drugs readily available.***

- Be aware that barbiturates and ketamine should not be mixed in the same syringe; they are chemically incompatible.
- Expect to see methohexital used with dextrose 5% in water (D_5W) or normal saline solution because it is incompatible with lactated Ringer's solution or acid drug solutions, such as atropine.
- Know that ampules of propofol must be shaken well before use to distribute the emulsion evenly.
- Expect propofol to be prepared using sterile technique because it is dissolved in an I.V. fat emulsion, which gives it a high potential for bacterial infection.

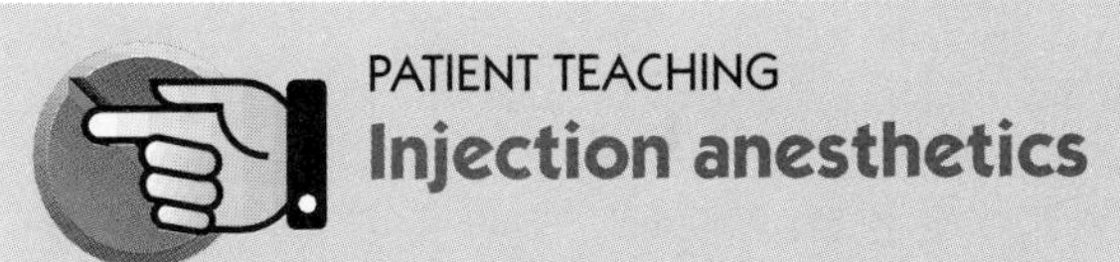

PATIENT TEACHING
Injection anesthetics

- Teach the patient and family the name, action, and adverse effects of the injection anesthetic to be used.
- Advise the patient not to eat for at least 8 hours before surgery.
- Instruct the patient not to drink alcohol or use any other central nervous system depressants for at least 24 hours after receiving an injection anesthetic.
- Stress the importance of notifying the nurse or physician of unusual symptoms up to 24 hours after receiving an injection anesthetic.

- Notify the physician immediately if adverse reactions occur.

*** *Know that a benzodiazepine should not be administered too rapidly or concurrently with a narcotic agent; respiratory arrest can result.***

- Watch for muscle rigidity and spasms after administration of ketamine or an opiate; these signs are directly proportional to the infusion rate.
- Expect to see etomidate administered rapidly into a large vein or with a preoperative analgesic to prevent pain during administration.
- Monitor the patient's I.V. site closely; barbiturate extravasation may cause neuritis and vasospasm, resulting in pain.
- Notify the physician if pain occurs with injection anesthetic administration.

Evaluation

For each nursing diagnosis, prepare an evaluation statement that describes the patient's or family's response to nursing interventions.

Local anesthetics

Many clinical situations require local anesthetics to prevent or relieve pain. These agents also offer a safe alternative to general anesthesia for geriatric or debilitated patients. Local anesthetics may be amide agents (ones with nitrogen in the molecular chain) or ester agents (ones with oxygen in the molecular chain). Amide anesthetics include bupivacaine hydrochloride, ropivacaine hydrochloride, etidocaine hydrochloride, lidocaine hydrochloride, mepivacaine hydrochloride, and prilocaine hydrochloride. Ester anesthetics include chloroprocaine hydrochloride, procaine hydrochloride, and tetracaine hydrochloride.

The physician can administer local anesthetics in various places to block different groups of nerves. Local anesthetics can be used for local effects as well as central, peripheral, I.V., regional, retrobulbar, or transtracheal **nerve blocks.** (See *Blocking the pain pathway,* page 206.)

Local infiltration involves injecting a local anesthetic into an area that has been injured or that will undergo surgery. One particularly useful type of local infiltration is the **field block,** which uses several injections to produce a wall of anesthetic around a lesion or an incision.

A *central nerve block* can be given in the spinal, perineal, epidural, caudal, or lumbar area to produce anesthesia in the CNS. A **spinal** (or subarachnoid) **block** requires penetrating the second layer of the spinal cord (the arachnoid membrane at the base of the spine) and injecting a local anesthetic into the CSF. In a *saddle block,* the anesthetic is administered near the lower end of the spinal column, where it is confined to the perineal or saddle area. An **epidural block** places the local anesthetic next to the outermost covering of the spinal cord, the dura mater. A *caudal block,* a special type of epidural block, is administered near the sacrum. A *lumbar block* is a type of epidural block administered low in the spinal column, near the lumbar vertebrae.

A **peripheral nerve block** places a local anesthetic next to nerve fibers in the peripheral nervous system. Paracervical and pudendal blocks are types of peripheral nerve blocks used in obstetric procedures. A **sympathetic block** is a peripheral nerve block of sympathetic nerve trunks that is used to relieve pain resulting from injury to the arms or legs and injury or disease of the internal organs. An *intercostal block* is a type of peripheral nerve block produced by injection of an anesthetic near the intercostal nerves.

An *I.V. regional nerve block* is reserved for specific surgical procedures, such as hand or foot surgery. To prepare the patient for this type of anesthesia, the physician applies a tourniquet to the proximal end of the patient's arm or leg and then applies a pressure bandage to force blood away from the area to be anesthetized. A local anesthetic solution is infused into the limb to provide **regional anesthesia** during the procedure.

A *retrobulbar nerve block* involves injecting a local anesthetic into nerves behind the eyeball in preparation for ocular surgery.

A *transtracheal nerve block* eliminates reflex activity that occurs from contact with mucous membranes during upper airway surgery. It requires inserting a needle through the cricoid cartilage into the larynx so that an anesthetic solution can be sprayed on the laryngeal mucosa.

PHARMACOKINETICS

Absorption of local anesthetics varies widely, yet distribution occurs throughout the body. Esters and amides undergo different types of metabolism, but both yield metabolites that are excreted in the urine.

The onset of action varies with the drug used, administration site, and technique. For example, a local lidocaine injection can cause anesthesia in 30 seconds, whereas a local chloroprocaine hydrochloride injection may require 10 minutes to take effect. Although lidocaine works quickly as

Blocking the pain pathway

Nerve endings transmit pain signals through the peripheral and central nervous systems to the brain. Administering a central nerve block can block the signal transmission and relieve pain. The illustration below shows two key points where an anesthetic may be administered to produce a central nerve block.

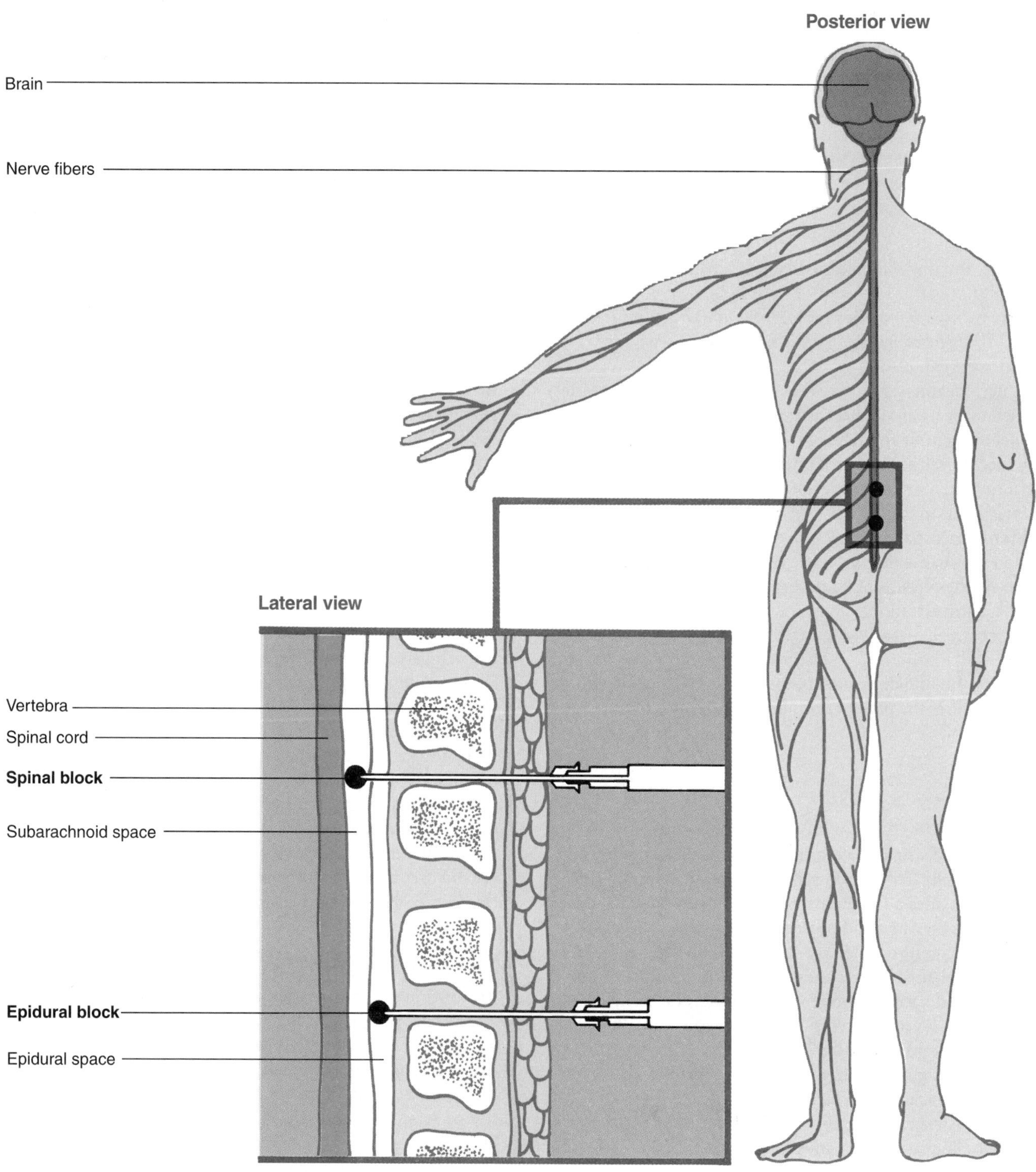

a local injection, it requires at least 5 minutes to produce anesthesia with epidural administration.

Route	Onset	Peak	Duration
Local Infiltration	30 sec-15 min	30-45 min	2-4 hr
Spinal	5-15 min	Unknown	0.5-5 hr
Epidural	5-30 min	30-45 min	0.5-5 hr
Peripheral	3-5 min	30-45 min	9 hr
Topical	1 min	5 min	30 min

PHARMACODYNAMICS

Local anesthetics block nerve impulses at the point of contact in all kinds of nerves. They apparently accumulate and cause the nerve cell membrane to expand. As the membrane expands, the cell loses its ability to depolarize, which is necessary for impulse transmission. Small nerves and nerves without myelin sheaths exhibit anesthetic effects before large, myelinated nerves.

PHARMACOTHERAPEUTICS

Clinical indications for local anesthetics include preventing and relieving pain from a medical procedure, disease, or injury. Local anesthetics are used for severe pain that topical anesthetics or analgesics cannot relieve. Also, they usually are preferred to general anesthetics for surgery in a geriatric or debilitated patient or a patient with a disorder that affects respiratory function, such as chronic obstructive pulmonary disease or myasthenia gravis.

For some procedures, a local anesthetic is combined with a vasoconstrictor, primarily epinephrine, to produce local vasoconstriction that controls local bleeding and reduces anesthetic absorption. Reduced absorption prolongs the anesthetic's action at the site and limits its distribution and CNS effects. However, the use of epinephrine with a local anesthetic is contraindicated in a patient with cardiovascular disease and in a geriatric patient because systemic absorption of this vasoconstrictor can cause tachycardia, palpitations, and chest pain. Epinephrine also should be avoided when anesthetizing an area with small vessels, such as the fingers, toes, nose, and ears, because ischemia and necrosis could result.

In other procedures, an anesthetic that contains a preservative (e.g., mepivacaine multidose container) may be used. However, this type of anesthetic would not be used for subarachnoid or epidural anesthesia because it can cause chronic **inflammation** of the arachnoid membrane.

For all local anesthetics, the dosage varies greatly, depending on the procedure to be performed, the depth and duration of anesthesia required, the degree of muscle relaxation needed, tissue vascularity, and the patient's physical condition. Therefore, only skilled practitioners may administer these agents.

Local anesthetics are contraindicated in a patient with known hypersensitivity to the drug or the group of local anesthetics (amide type or ester type), myasthenia gravis, severe shock, or impaired cardiac conduction. These anesthetics require cautious use in a severely debilitated patient or one with liver or cardiac disease, hyperthyroidism, or other endocrine disease.

Drug interactions

Local anesthetics produce few significant interactions with other drugs. Severe interactions can occur, however, when anesthetics with vasoconstrictors are given concurrently with certain other drugs. (See Drug Interactions: *Local anesthetics*, page 208.) No interactions between local anesthetics and food occur.

ADVERSE DRUG REACTIONS

Adverse reactions to local anesthetics usually result from three main causes: overdose, hypersensitivity, and improper injection technique.

High plasma concentrations of local anesthetics can cause CNS and cardiovascular reactions. Dose-related CNS reactions to stimulation include anxiety, apprehension, restlessness, nervousness, disorientation, confusion, dizziness, blurred vision, tremors, twitching, shivering, and seizures. CNS depression follows, with drowsiness, unconsciousness, and respiratory arrest. The stimulatory phase may not occur, however, if the patient has received lidocaine or another amide anesthetic. Other CNS reactions may include nausea, vomiting, chills, miosis, and tinnitus. Cardiovascular reactions usually are dose-related and typically occur with high plasma concentrations of local anesthetics. These effects may include myocardial depression, bradycardia, cardiac arrhythmias, hypotension, cardiovascular collapse, and cardiac arrest.

Local anesthetic solutions that contain vasoconstrictors such as epinephrine also can produce CNS and cardiovascular reactions, including anxiety, dizziness, headache, restlessness, tremors, palpitations, tachycardia, anginal pain, and hypertension. Extreme reactions include pulmonary edema and ventricular fibrillation. Norepinephrine may be less likely to cause cardiac arrhythmias, but it may cause reflex bradycardia. A burning sensation at the injection site also occurs commonly with these drugs. In rare cases, this reaction may be severe, producing pain, skin discoloration, tissue irritation, swelling, neuritis, **neurolysis,** and tissue necrosis and sloughing.

Ester anesthetics and preservatives in amide anesthetics can cause hypersensitivity reactions, with dermatologic symptoms, edema, status asthmaticus, or anaphylaxis. A patient who is hypersensitive to an ester anesthetic probably will not be sensitive to an amide agent, although the patient may be sensitive to other ester anesthetics. A local anesthetic solution with a preservative such as paraben, phenol, or bisulfite may produce chronic inflammation of the arach-

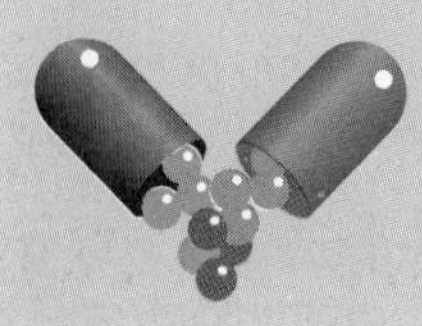

DRUG INTERACTIONS

Local anesthetics

Anesthetics with vasoconstrictors can interact with other drugs to produce serious adverse reactions. The nursing implications for these and other local anesthetics are detailed below.

DRUG	INTERACTING AGENTS	POSSIBLE EFFECTS	NURSING IMPLICATIONS
bupivacaine, chloroprocaine, etidocaine, lidocaine, mepivacaine, prilocaine, procaine, ropivacaine, tetracaine	central nervous system (CNS) depressants	Increased CNS depression	• Monitor the patient's vital signs and level of consciousness.
anesthetics with vasoconstrictors	anesthetics	Arrhythmias	• If concurrent use is unavoidable, monitor the electrocardiogram continuously while the patient is receiving an inhalation anesthetic.
	tricyclic antidepressants, monoamine oxidase inhibitors, ergot oxytocics	Severe hypotension	• Monitor the patient's blood pressure, and alert the physician to changes.
procaine, chloroprocaine, tetracaine	sulfonamides	Inhibits the action of sulfonamides	• Monitor for sulfonamide effectiveness.

noid membrane if it is used for subarachnoid or epidural anesthesia.

Local anesthetics may produce methemoglobinemia (the presence in the blood of oxidized hemoglobin that cannot combine irreversibly with oxygen). Although this reaction is rare, it occurs most commonly with prilocaine. Cyanosis may be the only symptom, but if it is severe, oxygen and methylene blue may be needed.

Because local anesthetics rapidly cross the placenta, they may produce adverse reactions in the fetus, such as bradycardia and acidosis.

NURSING PROCESS APPLICATION

The following information assists the nurse in caring for a patient receiving a local anesthetic. It includes an overview of assessment activities as well as examples of appropriate nursing diagnoses and related interventions (under "Planning and implementation"). It also highlights the importance of evaluation.

Assessment

Before drug therapy begins, review the patient's history for conditions that contraindicate or require cautious use of the prescribed local anesthetic. Also review the patient's medication history to identify use of drugs that may interact with it. During therapy, assess the patient for adverse drug reactions and signs of drug interactions. If the patient receives a local anesthetic with a vasoconstrictor, assess for anginal pain or discomfort at the injection site. Also, periodically assess the effectiveness of therapy. Finally, evaluate the patient's and family's knowledge about the prescribed local anesthetic.

Nursing diagnoses

- Risk for injury related to a preexisting condition that contraindicates or requires cautious use of a local anesthetic
- Risk for injury related to adverse drug reactions or drug interactions
- Pain related to use of a local anesthetic with a vasoconstrictor
- Knowledge deficit related to the prescribed local anesthetic

Planning and implementation

- Do not administer a local anesthetic to a patient with a condition that contraindicates its use.
- Administer a local anesthetic cautiously to a patient at risk because of a preexisting condition.
- Observe the patient for adverse reactions to the local anesthetic. Keep in mind that the higher the dose of a local anesthetic, the higher the incidence of adverse reactions.
- Keep emergency drugs and resuscitation equipment on hand when the patient must receive a parenteral local anesthetic.
- Position the patient as directed for a subarachnoid block to prevent CSF leakage and headache and to ensure proper anesthetic distribution. Afterward, ensure that the patient

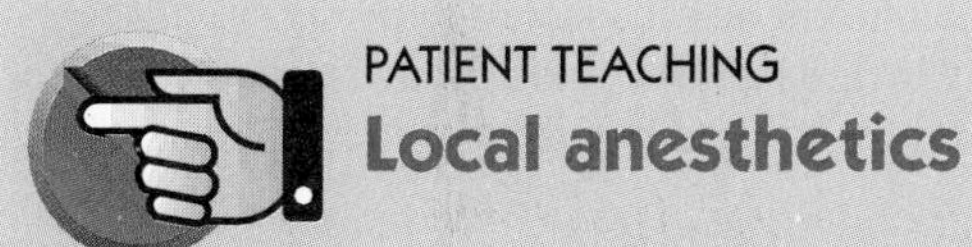

PATIENT TEACHING
Local anesthetics

- Teach the patient and family the name, action, and adverse effects of the prescribed local anesthetic.
- Stress the importance of remaining supine after receiving a spinal anesthetic.
- Teach the patient to protect numb areas until sensation returns.
- Instruct the patient to alert the nurse or physician immediately if adverse reactions occur.

stays flat in bed with the bed rails up for the time indicated by the physician.

*** *Do not administer a local anesthetic with a vasoconstrictor if a halogenated inhalation anesthetic may be used later.***

• Expect to see a test dose given before the full dose is administered for an epidural block with a local anesthetic agent.

• Expect that anesthesia for an obstetric procedure will not be injected during a contraction or when the patient is bearing down, because excess absorption could result.

• Help prevent maternal hypotension by elevating the patient's legs and positioning her on her left side after peripheral or epidural anesthesia.

• Observe the extremity that has undergone regional anesthesia. Check its peripheral pulse, color, and temperature, and compare it to the unaffected extremity.

*** *Ensure that the gag reflex has returned before feeding a patient whose throat has been anesthetized.***

• Discard partially used vials of local anesthetics that do not contain preservatives.

• Notify the physician if adverse reactions occur.

• Monitor the patient with angina for anginal pain when administering a local anesthetic that contains a vasoconstrictor. Ensure that the patient's nitroglycerin is nearby. (See Patient Teaching: *Local anesthetics.*)

• Alert the physician to the occurrence, frequency, and severity of anginal attacks. Be prepared to take emergency measures if anginal pain is not relieved.

• Reassure the patient that a burning sensation at the injection site is normal with use of a local anesthetic that contains a vasoconstrictor.

Evaluation

For each nursing diagnosis, prepare an evaluation statement that describes the patient's or family's response to nursing interventions.

Topical anesthetics

Applied directly to the skin or mucous membranes, topical anesthetics include benzocaine, benzyl alcohol, butacaine sulfate, butamben picrate, clove oil, cocaine hydrochloride, dibucaine hydrochloride, dyclonine hydrochloride, ethyl chloride, lidocaine, menthol, pramoxine hydrochloride, and tetracaine. Some injectable local anesthetics, such as lidocaine and tetracaine, also are effective topically. All these agents may be used to prevent or relieve minor pain.

Some of these agents also are used in combination products for **topical anesthesia.** Tetracaine also is used as a topical ophthalmic anesthetic. Benzocaine is used with other agents in several otic preparations.

PHARMACOKINETICS

Topical application of these anesthetics does not produce significant systemic absorption, except for mucosal application of cocaine. However, systemic absorption may occur with frequent or high-dose application to the eye or large areas of burned or injured skin. Tetracaine and other esters are metabolized extensively in the blood and to a lesser extent in the liver. Dibucaine, lidocaine, and other amides are metabolized primarily in the liver. Both types of topical anesthetics are excreted in the urine.

Route	Onset	Peak	Duration
Topical	Rapid	1-15 min	30-240 min

PHARMACODYNAMICS

Benzocaine, butacaine, butamben, cocaine, dyclonine, and pramoxine produce topical anesthesia by blocking nerve impulse transmission. They accumulate in the nerve cell membrane, causing it to expand and lose its ability to depolarize, thus blocking impulse transmission.

The aromatic compounds, such as benzyl alcohol and clove oil, appear to stimulate the nerve endings. Clove oil may stimulate the nerve endings by counterirritation that interferes with pain perception.

Ethyl chloride superficially freezes the tissue, stimulating the cold sensation receptors and blocking the nerve endings in the frozen area. Dibucaine, lidocaine, and tetracaine may block impulse transmission across the nerve cell membranes. Menthol selectively stimulates the sensory nerve endings for cold, causing a cool sensation and some local analgesic effects.

PHARMACOTHERAPEUTICS

Topical anesthetics relieve or prevent pain — especially minor burn pain — as well as itching and irritation. They also are used to anesthetize an area before an injection is given and to numb mucosal surfaces before a tube, such as an in-

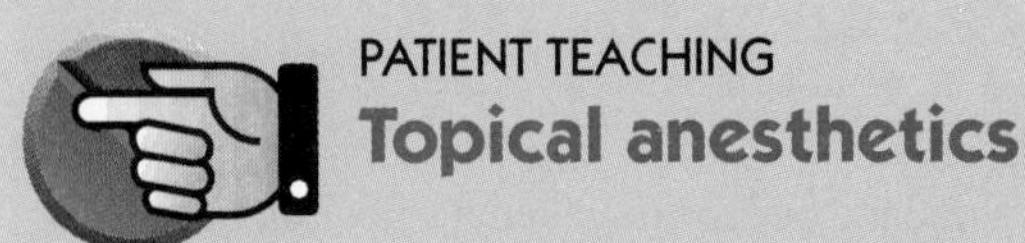

PATIENT TEACHING
Topical anesthetics

- Teach the patient and family the name, action, frequency, and adverse effects of the prescribed topical anesthetic.
- Show the patient and family how to apply a topical anesthetic if prescribed for home use. Instruct them to use it only as directed.
- Discourage prolonged use of a topical anesthetic without medical supervision.
- Advise the patient to keep dibucaine out of the reach of children to prevent ingestion and accidental poisoning.
- Advise the patient whose oropharyngeal mucosa has been anesthetized to delay eating until sensation returns.
- Instruct the patient to alert the nurse or physician if adverse reactions occur.

dwelling urinary catheter, is inserted. In a spray or solution, a topical anesthetic also is used to alleviate sore throat or mouth pain. (See Patient Teaching: *Topical anesthetics.*)

Topical anesthetics are contraindicated in a patient with known hypersensitivity to the drug, its group (ester type or amide type), or other ingredients that it contains, such as para-aminobenzoic acid (PABA). In addition, dibucaine should not be used in large quantities, especially over denuded or blistered areas.

Because of the possibility of rapid systemic absorption, dyclonine requires cautious use in areas with traumatized mucosa or localized sepsis. Butacaine and cocaine should be administered with caution to a patient with cardiovascular disease or hyperthyroidism. Butacaine also requires cautious use in a patient with open lesions; lidocaine, in a geriatric patient or one with large areas of broken skin or mucous membranes.

Drug interactions

Few interactions with other drugs occur with topical anesthetics because they are not absorbed well systemically. When used topically, lidocaine can interact with beta-adrenergic blockers and cimetidine, increasing the risk of lidocaine toxicity. When these medications must be given concurrently, the nurse must monitor the patient for signs of toxicity, such as confusion, restlessness, and tremors.

No interactions between the topical anesthetics and food have been described.

ADVERSE DRUG REACTIONS

Adverse reactions to topical anesthetics vary with the chemical class. Agents that are used as local anesthetics may produce CNS and cardiovascular reactions. Benzyl alcohol can cause topical reactions, such as skin irritation. Refrigerants such as ethyl chloride may produce frostbite in the application area.

Any topical anesthetic can cause a hypersensitivity reaction that may include a rash, pruritus, urticaria, swelling of the mouth and throat, and breathing difficulty.

NURSING PROCESS APPLICATION

The following information assists the nurse in caring for a patient receiving a topical anesthetic. It includes an overview of assessment activities as well as examples of appropriate nursing diagnoses and related interventions (under "Planning and implementation"). It also highlights the importance of evaluation.

Assessment

Before drug therapy begins, review the patient's history for conditions that contraindicate or require cautious use of the prescribed local anesthetic. Also review the patient's medication history to identify use of drugs that may interact with it. During therapy, assess the patient for adverse drug reactions and signs of drug interactions. Also, periodically assess the effectiveness of therapy. Finally, evaluate the patient's and family's knowledge about the prescribed local anesthetic.

Nursing diagnoses

- Risk for injury related to a preexisting condition that contraindicates or requires cautious use of the prescribed topical anesthetic
- Risk for injury related to adverse drug reactions or drug interactions
- Knowledge deficit related to the prescribed topical anesthetic

Planning and implementation

- Do not administer a topical anesthetic to a patient with a condition that contraindicates its use.
- Administer a topical anesthetic cautiously to a patient at risk because of a preexisting condition.
- Observe the patient regularly for adverse reactions to the topical anesthetic.
- Monitor for signs of localized frostbite in a patient receiving a refrigerant, such as ethyl chloride, and for skin irritation and other topical reactions in a patient receiving benzyl alcohol.

∗ ***Do not apply a refrigerant to broken skin or mucous membranes.***

∗ ***Use the lowest dose necessary for relief of symptoms.***

- Clean and dry the area thoroughly before applying an anesthetic rectally.
- Avoid contact with eyes.
- Discontinue use if a rash develops.
- Notify the physician if adverse reactions occur.

Evaluation

For each nursing diagnosis, prepare an evaluation statement that describes the patient's or family's response to nursing interventions.

CHAPTER SUMMARY

Chapter 16 described the types of anesthesia and presented the general, local, and topical anesthetics. Here are the chapter highlights.

General anesthetic agents may be subdivided into inhalation general anesthetic agents and injection general anesthetic agents.

General anesthesia may be induced with one or combined agents. These drugs are volatile liquids or gases vaporized in oxygen and administered by inhalation or nonvolatile solutions administered by injection.

Desflunane, enflurane, halothane, isoflurane, sevoflurane, and nitrous oxide are the inhalation general anesthetics in current use. Three agents — etomidate, ketamine, and propofol — are used solely as injection general anesthetics. Drugs from other categories, such as barbiturates and benzodiazepines, are used secondarily as injection general anesthetics. Many drugs interact with general anesthetics; thus, caution is needed when medicating a patient after anesthesia.

Local anesthetics produce their effect in a limited body area, but they are distributed throughout the body. When injected near nerves, these anesthetics can produce nerve block anesthesia for pain relief or surgery.

When applied to the skin or mucous membranes, topical anesthetics can relieve minor irritation or prevent discomfort during diagnostic testing or other procedures. In special formulations, they may also be used in the eyes and ears.

Hypersensitivity reactions may occur with local and topical anesthetic agents, especially with ester anesthetics.

Although an anesthesiologist or nurse anesthetist typically administers general anesthetics, the nurse uses the nursing process to provide patient care. For all general anesthetics, the nurse must monitor the patient's vital signs, maintain airway patency, and observe the return to consciousness. Nursing care for a patient receiving a local or topical anesthetic agent includes screening for potential drug interactions, monitoring for adverse drug reactions, and patient teaching.

Questions to consider

See Appendix 1 for answers.

1. During a hysterectomy, Arlene Richardson, age 42, received halothane and nitrous oxide. After the operation, the nurse monitors her for adverse reactions. What is the most common adverse reaction to inhalation anesthetics?
   (a) Exaggerated response to a normal dose
   (b) Hypersensitivity reaction
   (c) Nausea and vomiting
   (d) Respiratory distress

2. James Baskin, age 19, is about to receive ketamine, an injection general anesthetic, to repair a broken toe. During ketamine administration, the nurse should assess carefully for which of the following adverse reactions?
   (a) Increased respiratory rate
   (b) High blood pressure
   (c) Low blood pressure
   (d) Severe bradycardia

3. After sustaining multiple traumatic injuries in an automobile accident, Emma Gilman, age 41, must have a cutdown to provide access for I.V. administration of fluids and medications. Which of the following types of nerve block would the physician use to produce a wall of anesthesia around the incision?
   (a) Field block
   (b) Central nerve block
   (c) I.V. regional block
   (d) Peripheral nerve block

4. Harry Saunders, age 26, develops a sunburn after prolonged sun exposure on his first day of vacation. His wife applies the topical anesthetic benzocaine to relieve the pain. How does benzocaine relieve sunburn pain?
   (a) It numbs the skin surface, decreasing the perception of pain.
   (b) It freezes the skin, which prevents nerve impulse transmission.
   (c) It causes vasoconstriction to the area, minimizing the sense of pain.
   (d) It blocks nerve impulse transmission by preventing nerve cell depolarization.

5. Mary Wargo, age 28, has been admitted for routine delivery. She undergoes a pudendal block for delivery and episiotomy. Which of the following types of nerve block is a pudendal block?
   (a) Field block
   (b) Peripheral nerve block
   (c) Central nerve block
   (d) I.V. regional block

6. Andy Baskin, age 8, is admitted for the removal of tonsils. He receives a general anesthetic with desflurane and nitrous oxide. The nurse should observe for which of the following common adverse effects?
   (a) Nausea and vomiting
   (b) Seizures
   (c) Cyanosis
   (d) Hypotension

7. Jose´ Lopez is brought to the hospital for repair of multiple lacerations sustained in an industrial accident. He receives a large dose of lidocaine to anesthetize the area of suture. Shortly after injection, he exhibits anxiety, restlessness, shivering, and tremors. Which of the following conditions should the nurse suspect?

(a) An allergic reaction
(b) A drug interaction
(c) Stress
(d) An overdose

8. Joyce Kelly, age 7, is admitted for myringotomy. In the recovery room, the nurse notices a sudden rise in her body temperature. Which of the following conditions should the nurse suspect?

(a) Infection
(b) Stress
(c) Malignant hyperthermia
(d) Allergic reaction

UNIT

VI

Drugs to improve cardiovascular function

The circulatory system includes the heart and blood vessels. In this system, arteries generally carry oxygen and nutrients to the cells, and veins carry away the unoxygenated blood and the waste products of cellular metabolism. Because this system represents a vital function, a dysfunction in the heart or kidneys can seriously affect an individual's health. Unit 6 discusses drugs used to treat cardiovascular disease.

CIRCULATION

Blood flow results from pressure differences in the circulatory system, which are caused by the force of the blood flow through the vessels and the force or resistance to that blood flow.

Blood pressure refers to the force exerted by the blood against the vessel walls. Arterial blood pressure is determined by cardiac output and peripheral resistance. Usually, an increase or decrease in cardiac output or peripheral resistance will increase or decrease blood pressure correspondingly. Similarly, increases or decreases in blood flow and tissue perfusion will accompany blood pressure changes. Cardiac output is a function of the heart rate and stroke volume.

Peripheral circulation refers to blood ejected from the left side of the heart. Pulmonary circulation refers to blood ejected from the right side.

In peripheral circulation, the heart pumps blood to all body tissues and organs except the lungs. Arteries and arterioles carry the blood away from the heart; capillaries allow the exchange of nutrients for cellular waste products; then the venules and veins return the blood to the right side of the heart.

In pulmonary circulation, the heart pumps blood to the lungs via the pulmonary arteries, and the pulmonary veins return the blood to the left side of the heart. Unlike peripheral circulation, pulmonary circulation uses the veins to carry oxygen-rich blood and the arteries to carry unoxygenated blood and waste products.

HEART

Cardiac function depends on conduction of electrical impulses throughout the myocardium. When recorded by an electrocardiogram, the electrical activity of the heart appears as deflection points designated by the letters P, Q, R, S, T, and U. This electrical activity results in contraction of the heart and ejection of blood.

Coronary arteries, which arise from the aorta and fill during diastole, supply blood to the myocardium; coronary veins carry away the waste products of metabolism. (See *Coronary circulation*, page 214.)

The kidneys dispose of these waste products and regulate the body's fluid and electrolyte balance. Blood enters the kidneys through the renal arteries and is filtered at the glomerulus. The filtrate enters the renal tubular system, where it is altered and concentrated or diluted. Then the concentrated or diluted urine leaves the kidneys through the renal pelvis and ureters to the bladder for excretion. Blood leaves the kidneys through the renal veins.

The kidneys also help regulate blood pressure through the renin-angiotensin system. They release the hormone renin in response to a decrease in renal blood flow or, more specifically, to a decrease in the glomerular filtration rate. Renin acts on angiotensinogen (a plasma protein) to form angiotensin I. Angiotensin I is converted to angiotensin II as it circulates through the lungs. Angiotensin II, a potent vasoconstrictor, increases peripheral resistance and sodium and water reabsorption, contributing to an increase in blood pressure.

Coronary circulation

Coronary arteries arise from the aorta and supply blood to the myocardium. The coronary veins carry blood from the myocardium through the coronary sinus. The illustration below shows the location of the major structures of the heart.

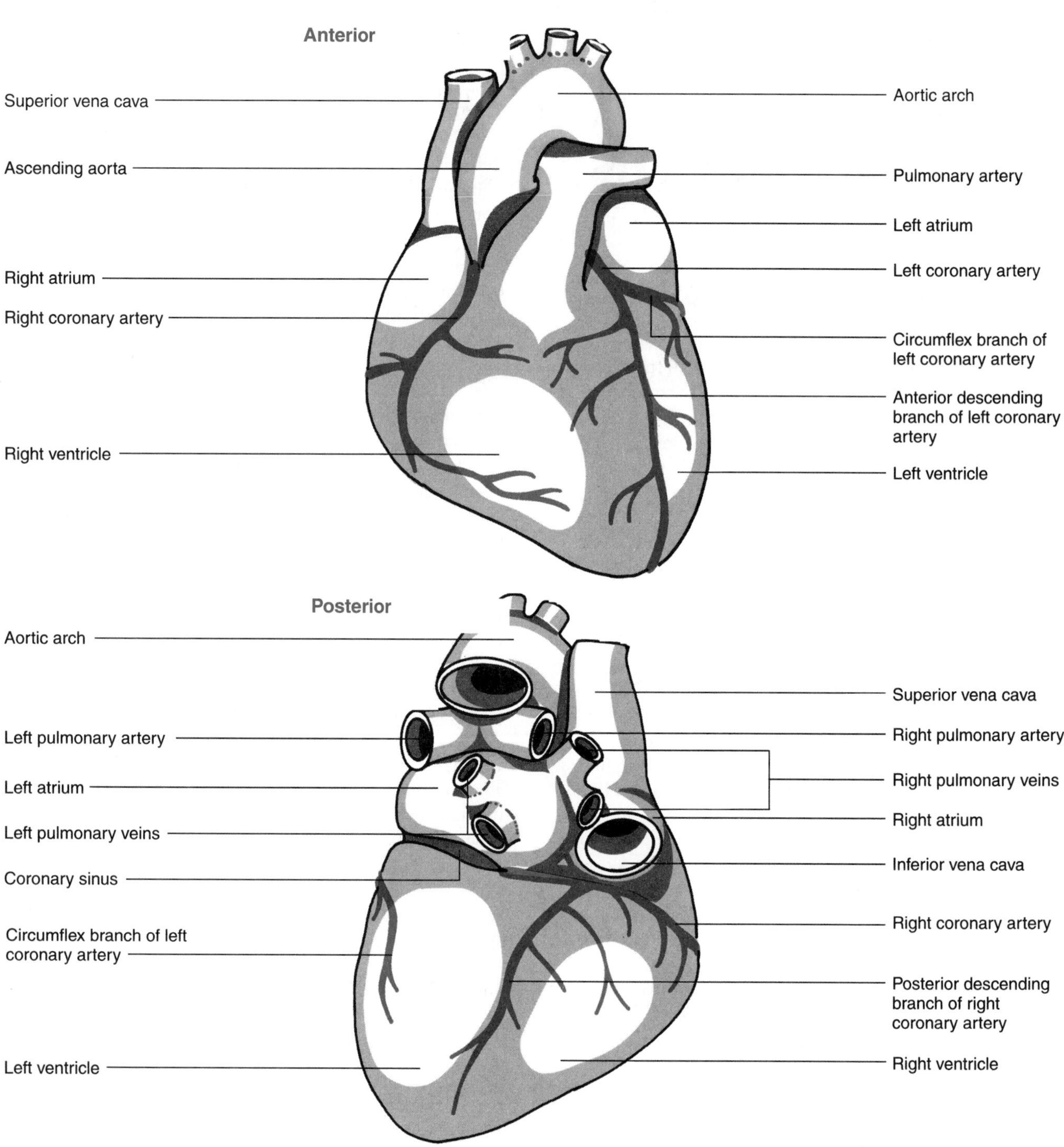

17 Cardiac glycoside agents and phosphodiesterase inhibitors

OBJECTIVES

After reading and studying this chapter, the student should be able to:

1. describe the clinical indications of the cardiac glycosides digoxin and digitoxin and the phosphodiesterase (PDE) inhibitors amrinone lactate and milrinone.
2. describe the actions of cardiac glycosides and PDE inhibitors in treating heart failure.
3. explain why digitalis toxicity commonly occurs, and describe its signs and symptoms.
4. describe how to apply the nursing process when caring for a patient receiving a cardiac glycoside or PDE inhibitor.

INTRODUCTION

Cardiac glycosides (digitalis compounds) and PDE inhibitors increase the force of cardiac contraction; that is, they exert a positive **inotropic** effect. For this reason, they also are called inotropic agents. Cardiac glycosides also slow the heart rate (a negative **chronotropic** effect) and slow electrical impulse conduction through the atrioventricular (AV) node (a negative **dromotropic** effect). These actions make cardiac glycosides and PDE inhibitors useful in treating heart failure and make cardiac glycosides useful in treating certain supraventricular **arrhythmias.**

Heart failure results from a decrease in **cardiac output.** It typically produces decreased myocardial contractility and increased **preload** and **afterload.** To try to maintain vital organ perfusion, the body uses compensatory mechanisms: It increases sympathetic tone and renin-angiotensin-aldosterone system activity and it causes ventricular dilation and hypertrophy (increased cardiac muscle size). Although these mechanisms help maintain adequate perfusion, they increase myocardial work. Eventually, the patient's condition worsens and drug treatment becomes necessary. When this occurs, the physician may prescribe cardiac glycosides or PDE inhibitors to improve myocardial contractility or diuretics or vasodilators to improve preload and afterload.

In supraventricular arrhythmias (such as atrial fibrillation or atrial flutter), cardiac glycosides are used to slow electrical impulse conduction through the AV node. By doing so, they slow the ventricular rate. Cardiac glycosides commonly are used with quinidine in these disorders. They are used to slow the ventricular response while quinidine converts the abnormal rhythm to a normal sinus rhythm. (See *Selected major cardiac glycoside agents and phosphodiesterase inhibitors,* page 216.)

Drugs covered in this chapter include:

- amrinone
- digitoxin
- digoxin
- milrinone.

Cardiac glycosides

Cardiac glycosides are a group of drugs derived from digitalis, a substance that occurs naturally in foxglove plants and certain toads. Also called digitalis compounds, these drugs are structurally similar. Digoxin and digitoxin are the two most frequently used cardiac glycosides.

PHARMACOKINETICS

The pharmacokinetic properties of digoxin and digitoxin differ significantly. The intestinal absorption of digoxin varies greatly, ranging from 60% to 80% in tablet form, from 70% to 85% in elixir form, and from 90% to 100% in capsule form. Digoxin is distributed widely throughout the body, is bound extensively to skeletal muscles, and does not penetrate body fat easily. About 20% to 30% of digoxin in the plasma binds to albumin.

A small percentage of digoxin is metabolized by the liver and by gastrointestinal (GI) flora. Several metabolites have been identified, some of which have pharmacologic activity. The remaining digoxin is eliminated by the kidneys as unchanged drug.

Oral digitoxin has an absorption rate of 90% to 100% and is distributed to most body tissues. About 90% of digitoxin in the blood is bound to plasma proteins, primarily albumin. Digitoxin is metabolized extensively in the liver to

Selected major cardiac glycoside agents and phosphodiesterase inhibitors

This table summarizes the major cardiac glycoside agents and phosphodiesterase (PDE) inhibitors currently in clinical use.

DRUG	MAJOR INDICATIONS AND USUAL DOSAGES	CONTRAINDICATIONS AND PRECAUTIONS
Cardiac glycosides		
digoxin (Lanoxin, Lanoxicaps)	*Heart failure, certain supraventricular arrhythmias* ADULT: 0.75 to 1.25 mg P.O. or 0.5 mg to 1 mg I.V. as a loading dose; 0.125 to 0.5 mg P.O. as a maintenance dosage PEDIATRIC: 10 to 60 mcg/kg P.O. or I.V. as a loading dose; 25% to 35% of the loading dose as a daily maintenance dosage, given in two divided doses	• Digoxin is contraindicated in a patient with ventricular fibrillation, digitalis toxicity, or known hypersensitivity. • This drug requires cautious use in a pregnant or breast-feeding patient or one who has hypertension and is receiving the drug I.V. or has atrial fibrillation or flutter and an anomalous conduction pathway disorder (such as Wolff-Parkinson-White syndrome). It also requires cautious use in a patient with idiopathic hypertrophic subaortic stenosis, renal failure, severe pulmonary disease, hypoxia, myxedema, acute myocardial infarction (MI), severe heart failure, acute myocarditis, other myocardial damage, chronic constrictive pericarditis, incomplete heart block, increased carotid sinus sensitivity, frequent premature ventricular contractions, or ventricular tachycardia.
digitoxin (Crystodigin)	*Heart failure, certain supraventricular arrhythmias* ADULT: for slow digitalization, a loading dose of 0.2 mg P.O. b.i.d. for 4 days, followed by a maintenance dosage of 0.05 to 0.3 mg P.O. daily; for rapid digitalization, a loading dose of 0.6 mg P.O. initially, followed by 0.4 mg and then 0.2 mg at 4- to 6-hour intervals, followed by a maintenance dosage of 0.05 to 0.3 mg P.O. daily with the most common maintenance dosage being 0.15 mg P.O. daily PEDIATRIC: 0.03 to 0.045 mg/kg P.O. as a loading dose, depending on the patient's age; 10% of the loading dose as a daily maintenance dosage	• Digitoxin is contraindicated in a patient with ventricular fibrillation, digitalis toxicity, or known hypersensitivity. • This drug requires cautious use in a pregnant or breast-feeding patient or one who has hypertension and is receiving the drug I.V. or has atrial fibrillation or flutter and an anomalous conduction pathway disorder (such as Wolff-Parkinson-White syndrome). It also requires cautious use in a patient with idiopathic hypertrophic subaortic stenosis, severe pulmonary disease, hypoxia, myxedema, acute MI, severe heart failure, acute myocarditis, other myocardial damage, chronic constrictive pericarditis, incomplete heart block, increased carotid sinus sensitivity, frequent premature ventricular contractions, or ventricular tachycardia.
PDE inhibitors		
amrinone lactate (Inocor)	*Heart failure* ADULT: 0.75 mg/kg I.V. over 2 to 3 minutes as a loading dose; 5 to 10 mcg/kg/minute by continuous I.V. infusion as a maintenance dosage	• Amrinone is contraindicated in a patient with acute MI, severe aortic or pulmonic valve disease, or known hypersensitivity to PDE inhibitors or disulfites. • This drug requires cautious use in a pregnant or breast-feeding patient.
milrinone (Primacor)	*Heart failure* ADULT: 50 mcg/kg I.V. over 10 minutes as a loading dose; 0.5 mcg/kg/minute I.V. (maintenance) dosage; total daily dosage of 0.77 mg/kg	• Milrinone is contraindicated in a patient with known hypersensitivity to the drug. • This drug requires cautious use in a pregnant or breast-feeding patient or one with renal impairment.

inactive metabolites. About 8% of the drug is converted to digoxin. The metabolites are eliminated by the kidneys.

The duration of action of cardiac glycosides varies with the patient's ability to eliminate the drug. The average duration for digoxin is 2 to 6 days with a half-life of 36 hours. For digitoxin, it is 2 to 3 weeks with a half-life of 5 to 7 days.

Route	Onset	Peak	Duration
P.O.	30 min-6 hr	2-12 hr	2 days-3 wk
I.V.	5-120 min	1-8 hr	2 days-3 wk

PHARMACODYNAMICS

Cardiac glycosides are used to treat heart failure because of their positive inotropic action, which may result from three mechanisms. First, they increase intracellular calcium availability to the contractile elements of the myocardium, leading to enhanced force of contraction. Cardiac glycosides also may enhance the movement of calcium into the myocardial cell and stimulate the release, or block the reuptake, of norepinephrine at the adrenergic nerve terminal.

Cardiac glycosides also have electrophysiologic properties that make them useful in managing specific supraventricular arrhythmias. They affect the autonomic nervous system by stimulating the parasympathetic division, which increases vagal tone. This vagal effect slows the heart rate, increases the refractory period, and slows conduction through the AV node and junctional tissue.

PHARMACOTHERAPEUTICS

Cardiac glycosides are prescribed to treat heart failure, atrial fibrillation and flutter, and paroxysmal atrial tachycardia. Supraventricular arrhythmias of the reentry type, such as paroxysmal supraventricular tachycardia, also may be treated with cardiac glycosides if the patient has a ventricular dysfunction that could worsen with the administration of other antiarrhythmic agents, such as verapamil or a beta blocker. Cardiac glycosides also may improve cardiac hemodynamics when used with diuretics or vasodilators in managing mild to moderate heart failure.

Because the cardiac glycosides have long half-lives, a loading dose must be given to a patient who requires immediate drug effects, as in supraventricular arrhythmia. (See *Dosage considerations for cardiac glycosides,* page 218.)

Drug interactions

Many drugs can interact with cardiac glycosides. Some drugs reduce their absorption, which can reduce their therapeutic effect; others enhance their absorption or pharmacologic effects, which can lead to toxicity. (See Drug Interactions: *Cardiac glycosides,* page 219.)

ADVERSE DRUG REACTIONS

Because cardiac glycosides have a narrow therapeutic index, they may produce digitalis toxicity. To prevent digitalis toxicity, the dosage should be individualized based on the patient's serum digitalis concentration. The therapeutic serum concentration of digoxin typically ranges from 0.5 to 2 ng/ml; of digitoxin, from 14 to 26 ng/ml. However, patients vary greatly in their response to cardiac glycosides.

The following conditions may predispose a patient to digitalis toxicity: hypokalemia, hypomagnesemia, hypothyroidism, hypoxemia, hypercalcemia, advanced myocardial disease, active myocardial ischemia, and altered autonomic (increased vagal) tone. Elevated sympathetic tone and hyperthyroidism may cause resistance to the drug's effect.

The signs and symptoms of digitalis toxicity fall primarily into three categories: GI, neurologic, and cardiac. (See *Signs and symptoms of digitalis toxicity,* page 220.) The GI and neurologic symptoms may precede or follow the potentially life-threatening cardiac symptoms.

A drug's half-life affects the duration of adverse reactions, such as digitalis toxicity. Because digoxin has a shorter half-life, most physicians prefer using it over digitoxin.

Less common and less severe adverse reactions to cardiac glycosides include gynecomastia and hypersensitivity reactions, such as rash, fever, and eosinophilia.

CRITICAL THINKING: To enhance your critical thinking about cardiac glycosides and PDE inhibitors, consider the following situation and its analysis.

Situation: Ramona Sweet, age 67, is being treated for end-stage heart failure. She continues to have dyspnea, despite digoxin 0.25 mg P.O. daily, furosemide 40 mg P.O. daily, and nitroglycerin paste 2" q.i.d. So the physician adds milrinone to her treatment regimen. Mrs. Sweet receives a loading dose of 50 mcg/kg I.V. over 10 minutes, and then begins a maintenance dosage of 0.25 mcg/kg/minute. Now her blood pressure has fallen to 88/66 mm Hg. What is the nurse's best course of action?

Analysis: The nurse should remove the nitroglycerin paste and call the physician. Because nitroglycerin is a vasodilator, it has added to the vasodilation caused by milrinone. This, in turn, has resulted in an excessive decrease in preload and therefore, cardiac output and blood pressure.

NURSING PROCESS APPLICATION

The following information assists the nurse in caring for a patient who is receiving a cardiac glycoside. It includes an overview of assessment activities as well as examples of appropriate nursing diagnoses and related interventions. It also highlights the importance of evaluation.

Assessment

Before drug therapy begins, review the patient's history for a preexisting condition that contraindicates or requires cautious use of a cardiac glycoside. Also review the patient's medication history to identify use of drugs that may interact with it. During therapy, assess the patient for adverse drug reactions and signs of drug interactions. Also, periodically assess the effectiveness of the prescribed cardiac glycoside. Finally, evaluate the patient's and family's knowledge about the prescribed drug.

Nursing diagnoses

- Risk for injury related to a preexisting condition that contraindicates or requires cautious use of a cardiac glycoside
- Risk for injury related to adverse drug reactions or drug interactions
- Decreased cardiac output related to the adverse effects of the prescribed cardiac glycoside

Dosage considerations for cardiac glycosides

Because the half-lives of digoxin (36 hours) and digitoxin (5 to 7 days) are relatively long, a loading (digitalizing) dose must be given to reach the therapeutic steady state concentration rapidly, followed by regular maintenance dosages. Specific dosage considerations vary, depending on the patient's age, the drug to be used, and whether the patient must receive a loading dose or a maintenance dosage.

ADULT DOSAGE CONSIDERATIONS

LOADING (DIGITALIZING) DOSE

- Expect to administer a digoxin loading dose that is 10 to 15 mcg/kg of the patient's ideal or lean body weight.
- Administer the drug I.V. or by mouth in divided doses.
- Give one-half of the loading dose initially, followed by one-quarter of the dose 3 to 6 hours later, and then the remainder of the dose if the patient does not respond 3 to 6 hours after the second dose.
- Expect to reduce the loading dose of digoxin if the patient has a condition that affects drug distribution to the receptor site, such as renal dysfunction or use of quinidine.
- Give the digitoxin loading dose as prescribed. The usual rapid loading dose is 0.6 mg initially, followed by 0.4 mg, then 0.2 mg every 4 to 6 hours.

MAINTENANCE DOSAGE

- Know that the maintenance dosage of a cardiac glycoside is determined by its half-life. The most common maintenance dosage of digoxin is 0.25 mg P.O. daily; of digitoxin, 0.15 mg P.O. daily.
- Expect to use a lower maintenance dosage of digoxin in a patient with renal dysfunction to avoid toxicity.
- Administer a lower maintenance dosage to a geriatric patient because of reduced renal function and increased drug sensitivity.
- Continue to monitor the patient after the maintenance dosage is discontinued because the cardiac glycoside's half-life determines the amount of time needed before the drug effect is diminished. In a patient with normal renal function, digoxin requires 6 to 8 days before the drug effect is eliminated completely; digitoxin, 3 to 5 weeks.

PEDIATRIC DOSAGE CONSIDERATIONS

DIGOXIN

- Know that an I.V. loading dose is 80% of an oral loading dose.
- Divide the loading dose and give half the total, followed by one-quarter after 4 hours and the remaining one-quarter after 8 hours.
- Be aware that loading dose and maintenance dosages for children are based on age and weight as shown in the chart below.

AGE	LOADING DOSE (ORAL)	DAILY MAINTENANCE DOSAGE
Under age 1 month (premature neonate)	20 to 30 mcg/kg	20% to 30% of loading dose
Under age 1 month (full-term neonate)	25 to 35 mcg/kg	25% to 35% of loading dose
Ages 1 to 24 months	35 to 60 mcg/kg	25% to 35% of loading dose
Ages 2 to 5 years	30 to 40 mcg/kg	25% to 35% of loading dose
Ages 5 to 10 years	20 to 35 mcg/kg	25% to 35% of loading dose
Over age 10 years	10 to 15 mcg/kg	25% to 35% of loading dose

DIGITOXIN

- Divide the loading dose into three or four portions, and give each portion at 6- to 8-hour intervals.
- Be aware that loading dose and maintenance dosages for children are based on age and weight as shown in the chart below.

AGE	LOADING DOSE (ORAL)	DAILY MAINTENANCE DOSAGE
Under age 1	45 mcg/kg	10% of loading dose
Ages 1 to 2 years	40 mcg/kg	10% of loading dose
Over age 2 years	30 mcg/kg or 750 mcg/m^2	10% of loading dose

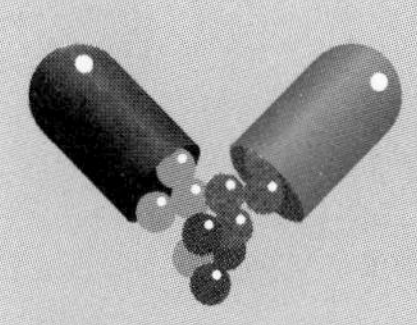

DRUG INTERACTIONS

Cardiac glycosides

Digoxin and digitoxin interact with several drugs. The interactions may result in decreased absorption (thereby reducing the therapeutic effect), digitalis toxicity, or arrhythmias.

DRUG	INTERACTING AGENTS	POSSIBLE EFFECTS	NURSING IMPLICATIONS
digoxin, digitoxin	rifampin, barbiturates, phenytoin (digitoxin only), cholestyramine resin, antacids, kaolin and pectin, sulfasalazine, neomycin, metoclopramide	Decreased therapeutic effect of digoxin and digitalis glycosides	• Monitor the patient for indications of effectiveness: decreased edema and jugular venous distention, weight loss, elimination of S_3 and basilar crackles (rales), increased urine output, improved oxygenation and pulse rate and rhythm, and increased well-being. • Increase the cardiac glycoside dosage, if prescribed.
	calcium preparations, quinidine, verapamil, anticholinergics, amiodarone, spironolactone, hydroxychloroquine, erythromycin, itraconazole, omeprazole	Digitalis toxicity	• Monitor the patient for signs and symptoms of digitalis toxicity: gastrointestinal, neurologic, and cardiac disturbances. • Monitor the patient's electrocardiogram (ECG) for arrhythmias or atrioventricular block.
	amphotericin B, potassium-wasting diuretics, steroids	Hypokalemia, digitalis toxicity	• Monitor the patient for signs and symptoms of hypokalemia: drowsiness, hypoperistalsis, depression, paresthesia, muscle weakness, anorexia, depressed reflexes, orthostatic hypotension, and polyuria. • Monitor the patient's serum digoxin or digitoxin level. • Monitor the patient's serum potassium level and administer a potassium supplement as prescribed; encourage the ingestion of dietary potassium.
	beta-adrenergic blockers	Excessive bradycardia and arrhythmias	• Monitor the patient's pulse rate frequently. • Monitor the patient's ECG as indicated. • Have resuscitation equipment available.
	succinylcholine, thyroid preparations	Arrhythmias	• Monitor the patient's pulse rate frequently. • Monitor the patient's ECG as indicated.

• Knowledge deficit related to the prescribed cardiac glycoside

Planning and implementation

• Do not administer a cardiac glycoside to a patient with a condition that contraindicates its use.

• Administer a cardiac glycoside cautiously to a patient at risk because of a preexisting condition.

∗ ***Assess the patient's baseline apical heart rate and rhythm before starting cardiac glycoside therapy; thereafter, take the apical rate before administering each dose. Withhold the drug and notify the physician if the pulse rate is below 60 beats/minute or the minimum specified by the physician.***

∗ ***Monitor the patient's serum digoxin or digitoxin levels as prescribed. To avoid a falsely elevated serum level, draw blood at least 8 hours after the last oral dose and preferably immediately before administering the daily maintenance dosage (about 24 hours after the last dose).***

• Expect to adjust the loading dose as prescribed for a pediatric or geriatric patient or one with renal failure, heart failure, or hypoalbuminemia, because these conditions affect the volume of drug distribution. The physician will prescribe a reduced dosage for a patient with renal dysfunction.

• Expect to administer a reduced dosage of digoxin capsules or elixir as prescribed because these drug forms have a higher bioavailability than tablets.

• Expect to decrease the digoxin dosage by half when quinidine is added to the patient's drug regimen because quinidine decreases digoxin's volume of distribution and elimination rate.

• Do not administer digoxin intramuscularly because it causes severe pain at the injection site and increases serum

Signs and symptoms of digitalis toxicity

Digitalis toxicity affects several body systems, most commonly the GI tract. The most common early symptoms are anorexia, nausea, vomiting, and diarrhea.

GASTROINTESTINAL

- Anorexia
- Nausea
- Vomiting
- Diarrhea
- Abdominal pain

NEUROLOGIC

- Headache
- Restlessness
- Irritability
- Depression
- Personality change
- Lassitude
- Confusion
- Disorientation
- Insomnia
- Psychosis
- Seizures
- Coma
- Blurred vision
- Blue-yellow color blindness
- Flickering lights
- White halos on dark objects
- Colored dots

CARDIAC

- Ventricular arrhythmias
- Sinoatrial arrest or block
- Accelerated junctional rhythms
- Atrial tachycardia with atrioventricular (AV) block
- Second-degree AV block (Wenckebach)
- Third-degree AV block (complete)

creatine phosphokinase levels, which complicates interpretation of enzyme elevation.

- Administer digoxin in two divided doses as prescribed for maintenance dosage in a pediatric patient to avoid a high peak serum concentration.
- Do not administer concurrently any drugs that reduce digoxin absorption, such as antacids or kaolin and pectin.
- As prescribed, administer the drug intravenously (I.V.) slowly (over 5 minutes), taking care to avoid extravasation, which can cause irritation, necrosis, and sloughing.
- Monitor the patient for adverse reactions, including signs and symptoms of digitalis toxicity, such as GI, neurologic, and cardiac dysfunction, even in a patient whose serum drug level falls within the therapeutic range. Be especially alert for these signs in a patient with hypokalemia, hypomagnesemia, hypothyroidism, hypoxemia, advanced myocardial disease, active myocardial ischemia, or altered autonomic tone; these conditions increase tissue sensitivity to digoxin or digitoxin.
- Withhold the prescribed cardiac glycoside, notify the physician, and obtain a serum drug level, as ordered, if digitalis toxicity is suspected.
- Notify the physician if arrhythmias occur during cardiac glycoside therapy. Withhold the prescribed cardiac glycoside and obtain a serum drug level, as ordered. Prepare for emergency treatment as prescribed. Also, notify the physician if the patient's condition does not improve or if adverse reactions or drug interactions occur.
- Teach the patient about the prescribed agent. (See Patient Teaching: *Cardiac glycosides.*)

PATIENT TEACHING
Cardiac glycosides

- ➤ Teach the patient and family the name, dose, frequency, action, and adverse effects of the prescribed cardiac glycoside.
- ➤ Stress the importance of taking the drug exactly as prescribed, even when the patient feels well. Instruct the patient not to take an extra dose if one dose is missed, but to notify the physician.
- ➤ Demonstrate how to take a pulse. Advise the patient to report a pulse rate below 60, a change in pulse regularity, or signs and symptoms of digitalis toxicity.
- ➤ Instruct the patient to recognize and report the following signs of heart failure: persistent cough; shortness of breath; weight gain of 1 to 2 lbs (0.45 to 0.90 kg) in 1 day or 5 lbs (2.25 kg) in a week; swelling of the ankles, legs, or hands; anorexia; nausea; and the sensation of abdominal fullness.
- ➤ Teach the patient treated for supraventricular arrhythmias to recognize and report signs of recurrence, such as a rapid heart rate (above 100 beats/minute), excessive fatigue, lightheadedness, or chest pain.
- ➤ Encourage the patient to eat high-potassium foods (orange juice, bananas, spinach, cantaloupe, watermelon, dates, raisins, soybeans, apples, prunes, beans, potatoes, molasses, squash) unless the patient is taking a potassium-sparing diuretic, an angiotensin-converting enzyme (ACE) inhibitor (such as captopril or enalapril), or a potassium supplement.
- ➤ Instruct the patient to store the drug in a tightly covered, light-resistant container and to consult the physician before taking any other drugs, including over-the-counter ones.
- ➤ Instruct the patient to consult with the pharmacist before each drug refill to ensure that the prescribed cardiac glycoside comes from the same manufacturer. Different formulations have different bioavailabilities.
- ➤ Refer a geriatric or debilitated patient who does not have adequate home supervision to a home health agency to ensure safe administration of the prescribed cardiac glycoside. Take periodic pill counts to evaluate compliance and detect accidental overdose.
- ➤ Reassure the patient that gastrointestinal distress should subside and vision should return to normal when the drug is eliminated from the body.
- ➤ Advise the patient to call the physician to discuss concerns about cardiac glycoside therapy. Give the patient written instructions about the drug for home use.

Evaluation

For each nursing diagnosis, prepare an evaluation statement that describes the patient's or family's response to nursing interventions.

Phosphodiesterase inhibitors

The PDE inhibitors are nonglycoside, noncatecholamine agents that are used for short-term management of heart failure. In addition to their positive inotropic effect, these drugs also dilate veins (which decreases preload) and arteries (which decreases afterload.) They produce minimal chronotropic effect. In the United States, two PDE inhibitors have been approved for use: amrinone lactate and milrinone.

PHARMACOKINETICS

Amrinone is administered intravenously, distributed rapidly, metabolized by the liver, and excreted by the kidneys. Amrinone is rapid-acting, increasing cardiac output within 5 minutes, but has a short duration of action. Amrinone's half-life is 3.6 hours in stable patients and 6 hours in patients with heart failure. The normal therapeutic plasma level of amrinone is 0.5 to 7 mcg/ml.

After I.V. administration, milrinone is distributed rapidly and excreted by the kidneys, primarily as unchanged drug. Milrinone acts rapidly, but has a short duration. Its half-life is 2 to 3 hours. The normal therapeutic plasma level of milrinone is approximately 200 ng/ml.

Route	Onset	Peak	Duration
I.V.	1-5 min	10 min	1-2 hr

PHARMACODYNAMICS

PDE inhibitors improve cardiac output by increasing contractility and decreasing peripheral vascular resistance (afterload) and venous return (preload). They do this by inhibiting cyclic adenosine monophosphate (cAMP) PDE activity in cardiac and vascular muscle tissue, causing a rise in intracellular cAMP levels.

PHARMACOTHERAPEUTICS

Amrinone and milrinone are indicated for the short-term management of heart failure in patients who have not responded adequately to treatment with cardiac glycosides, diuretics, or vasodilators. Prolonged use of these agents may increase morbidity and mortality.

Drug interactions

PDE inhibitors may interact with disopyramide, causing hypotension. Because these agents may enhance AV conduction in atrial fibrillation or atrial flutter and increase the ventricular response rate, they commonly are given with cardiac glycosides. PDE inhibitors reduce serum potassium levels; therefore, concurrent use with a potassium-wasting diuretic may lead to hypokalemia.

ADVERSE DRUG REACTIONS

Adverse reactions are uncommon and usually occur only in patients receiving prolonged therapy. PDE inhibitors can produce arrhythmias and should be withdrawn if arrhythmias occur. Other adverse reactions may include nausea, vomiting, headache, fever, chest pain, hypokalemia, thrombocytopenia, and a mild increase in heart rate. Amrinone also may increase liver enzyme levels and cause burning at the injection site. These effects, however, occur in only a small percentage of patients. Excessive vasodilation may lead to hypotension, which may require dosage reduction or drug discontinuation.

Patients on prolonged PDE inhibitor therapy have experienced hypersensitivity reactions. Signs and symptoms include pericarditis, pleurisy, and ascites.

NURSING PROCESS APPLICATION

The following information assists the nurse in caring for a patient who is receiving a PDE inhibitor. It includes an overview of assessment activities as well as examples of appropriate nursing diagnoses and related interventions. It also highlights the importance of evaluation.

Assessment

Before drug therapy begins, review the patient's history for conditions that contraindicate or require cautious use of a PDE inhibitor. Also review the patient's medication history to identify use of drugs that may interact with it. During therapy, assess the patient for adverse drug reactions and signs of drug interactions. Also, periodically assess the effectiveness of PDE-inhibitor therapy. Finally, evaluate the patient's and family's knowledge about the prescribed drug.

Nursing diagnoses

- Risk for injury related to a preexisting condition that contraindicates or requires cautious use of a PDE inhibitor
- Risk for injury related to adverse drug reactions or drug interactions
- Knowledge deficit related to the prescribed PDE inhibitor

Planning and implementation

- Do not administer a PDE inhibitor to a patient with a condition that contraindicates its use.
- Administer a PDE inhibitor cautiously to a patient at risk because of a preexisting condition.
- Monitor the patient regularly for adverse reactions and drug interactions during PDE-inhibitor therapy.
- Obtain baseline platelet counts and liver enzyme, electrolyte, blood urea nitrogen, and creatinine levels before starting PDE-inhibitor therapy. Monitor these values throughout therapy.

*** *Monitor the patient's heart rate, heart rhythm, and blood pressure frequently to detect arrhythmias or hypotension.***

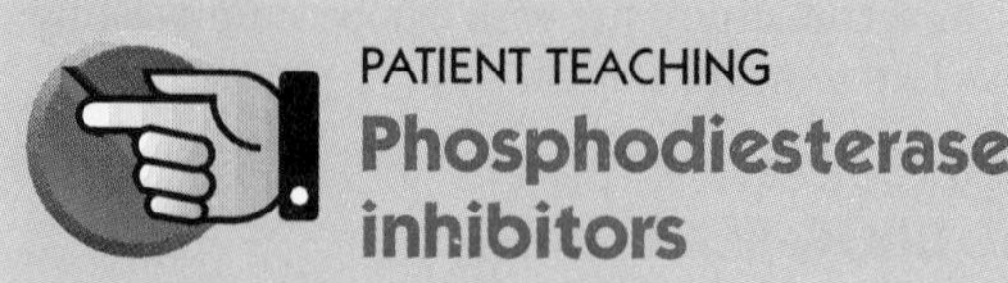

PATIENT TEACHING
Phosphodiesterase inhibitors

- Teach the patient and family the name, dose, frequency, action, and adverse effects of the prescribed phosphodiesterase inhibitor.
- Instruct the patient to report dyspnea, chest pain, palpitations, burning at the injection site, nausea, vomiting, abdominal pain, or anorexia.

Also monitor the patient's electrocardiogram to detect arrhythmias. If the patient develops hypotension or arrhythmias, expect to decrease the drug dosage or discontinue the drug, as prescribed.

- Dilute amrinone in normal saline solution before administration and use within 24 hours. Do not mix amrinone with dextrose 5% in water because this will result in an 11% to 13% decrease in activity after 24 hours.
- Administer I.V. infusions with an infusion pump. Amrinone produces burning but not tissue sloughing at the injection site; inject the drug using a central or peripheral line.
- Determine the effectiveness of PDE-inhibitor therapy by monitoring the patient for increased blood pressure; decreased pulmonary venous congestion, pulmonary artery pressure, and pulmonary capillary wedge pressure; decreased systemic venous congestion and central venous pressure; increased urine output; decreased weight, peripheral edema, and dyspnea; and elimination of S_3 and basilar crackles.
- Assess the patient for petechiae or ecchymosis. Note alterations in the patient's platelet count. A platelet count below 150,000/mm^3 usually requires dosage reduction; below 100,000/mm^3, usually requires drug discontinuation.
- Notify the physician if the patient's condition does not improve or if adverse reactions or drug interactions occur.
- Teach the patient about the prescribed agent. (See Patient Teaching: *Phosphodiesterase inhibitors.*)

Evaluation

For each nursing diagnosis, prepare an evaluation statement that describes the patient's or family's response to nursing interventions.

CHAPTER SUMMARY

Chapter 17 discussed the cardiac glycosides and PDE inhibitors. Here are the highlights of the chapter.

Cardiac glycosides are positive inotropic agents used to treat heart failure and supraventricular arrhythmias. Because these drugs have a narrow therapeutic range, they may cause digitalis toxicity.

When caring for a patient receiving a cardiac glycoside, the nurse uses the nursing process. Care focuses on teaching the patient how to monitor the pulse rate; recognize signs of digitalis toxicity, heart failure, and hypokalemia; and identify high-potassium foods.

PDE inhibitors are administered I.V. for short-term treatment of heart failure in patients who do not respond to digitalis compounds, diuretics, or vasodilators. Adverse reactions to these drugs are uncommon and usually occur only in patients receiving prolonged therapy.

For a patient receiving a PDE inhibitor, nursing care emphasizes close monitoring of cardiovascular status, regular assessment for such adverse reactions as hypotension and arrhythmias, and evaluation of the drug's effectiveness in treating heart failure.

Questions to consider

See Appendix 1 for answers.

1. Catherine Caldwell, age 71, is admitted to the critical care unit with atrial flutter and rapid ventricular response. Her physician prescribes a digoxin loading dose of 0.5 mg I.V., followed by a maintenance dosage of 0.125 mg P.O. daily. Why does Mrs. Caldwell need to receive a loading dose of digoxin?
   (a) A loading dose is required to treat ventricular fibrillation.
   (b) A loading dose provides an immediate drug effect.
   (c) A loading dose reduces the risk of digitalis toxicity.
   (d) A loading dose minimizes the risk of arrhythmias.

2. Alice Kuhl, age 62, must begin treatment with digitoxin (Crystodigin). The nurse plans to teach her to recognize signs and symptoms of digitalis toxicity. Which of the following are among the most common early signs and symptoms?
   (a) Headache and seizures
   (b) Nausea and diarrhea
   (c) Confusion and restlessness
   (d) Ventricular arrhythmias

3. James Barlow, age 65, is about to be discharged after being hospitalized for heart failure. Because Mr. Barlow will be taking a daily maintenance dosage of digoxin at home, the nurse should teach him about which of the following topics related to the effects of digoxin?
   (a) Pulse rate measurement
   (b) Blood pressure measurement
   (c) Use of potassium supplements
   (d) Dietary restrictions

4. Ralph Hendricks, age 73, is admitted to the coronary care unit for heart failure. The physician orders 0.5 mg of digoxin (Lanoxin) I.V. stat. Under which of the following circumstances might the physician prescribe amrinone (Inocor) for Mr. Hendricks?
(a) If his condition stabilizes and he needs long-term maintenance
(b) If he can return only infrequently for follow-up visits
(c) If his serum potassium level decreases significantly
(d) If he does not respond adequately to digoxin therapy

5. Rita Black, age 69, is receiving a maintenance dosage of amrinone (Inocor) 5 mcg/kg/minute I.V. for heart failure. The nurse should monitor Mrs. Black closely for which of the following adverse drug reactions?
(a) Renal failure
(b) Hypokalemia
(c) Hypertension
(d) Confusion

6. During the third week of amrinone therapy, Albert Weiss, age 75, develops petechiae on his chest, arms, back, and legs. He also has ecchymoses at each antecubital venipuncture site. What is the most likely cause of these findings?
(a) Traumatic venipuncture
(b) Thrombocytopenia caused by amrinone
(c) Fat embolus caused by subcutaneous tissue trauma
(d) Bacterial endocarditis caused by previous pulmonary artery catheter

18 Antiarrhythmic agents

OBJECTIVES

After reading and studying this chapter, the student should be able to:
1. describe the mechanism of action for each class of antiarrhythmics.
2. identify the clinical indications for treatment with each class of antiarrhythmics.
3. identify adverse effects of the agents in each class of antiarrhythmics.
4. describe how to apply the nursing process when caring for a patient receiving an antiarrhythmic.

INTRODUCTION

Arrhythmias (abnormal heart rhythms that can compromise cardiac function and cardiac output) have a high degree of morbidity and mortality. They may be classified as tachyarrhythmias, in which the heart rate is increased, or bradyarrhythmias, in which the heart rate is decreased.

Supraventricular arrhythmias originate in the atria, sinoatrial (SA) node, or atrioventricular (AV) node. They include supraventricular tachycardia, atrial flutter, and atrial fibrillation. Ventricular arrhythmias include sustained ventricular tachycardia, ventricular premature beats, and ventricular fibrillation. Supraventricular arrhythmias do not affect cardiac function and output as greatly as ventricular arrhythmias and are not as life-threatening.

Antiarrhythmic drugs are used to treat abnormal electrical activity of the heart. The drugs discussed in this chapter are used to treat, suppress, or prevent three major mechanisms of **arrhythmias:** increased **automaticity,** decreased **conductivity,** and **reentry.** They limit cardiac electrical activity to normal conduction pathways and decrease abnormally fast heart rates. Although mainly prescribed for adults, these drugs occasionally are prescribed for children.

Although ischemia is the most common cause of arrhythmias, other causes include congenital cardiac conditions, cardiac trauma or surgery, cardiomyopathy, electrolyte or acid-base imbalances, adverse drug reactions, emboli, invasive cardiac diagnostic procedures, cardiac valvular diseases, alcoholism, respiratory diseases, and viral infections.

An antiarrhythmic is used to treat an arrhythmia. However, the underlying condition must be treated to eliminate the need for continued antiarrhythmic therapy. Because most antiarrhythmic drugs also can cause new arrhythmias or worsen existing ones, the benefits need to be weighed against the risks of antiarrhythmic therapy.

Antiarrhythmics are categorized into four classes — I (which includes class IA, IB, and IC), II, III, and IV — and one agent that does not fall into any of these classes. (See *Selected major antiarrhythmic agents.*) Although the mechanisms of action of these drugs vary widely, a few drugs exhibit properties common to more than one class.

Drugs covered in this chapter include:

- acebutolol hydrochloride
- adenosine
- amiodarone hydrochloride
- bretylium tosylate
- diltiazem hydrochloride
- disopyramide phosphate
- esmolol hydrochloride
- flecainide acetate
- lidocaine hydrochloride
- mexiletine hydrochloride
- moricizine
- phenytoin
- procainamide hydrochloride
- propafenone hydrochloride
- propranolol hydrochloride
- quinidine sulfate or gluconate
- tocainide hydrochloride
- verapamil hydrochloride.

Class I antiarrhythmics

Moricizine is a class I antiarrhythmic agent with potent local anesthetic activity and myocardial membrane stabilizing effects.

PHARMACOKINETICS

After oral administration, approximately 38% of moricizine is absorbed. It undergoes extensive metabolism with less than 1% of a dose excreted unchanged in the urine. Plasma protein-binding is about 95%. The plasma half-life is about 3 hours.

Route	Onset	Peak	Duration
P.O.	< 2 hr	0.5-2 hr	10-24 hr

Selected major antiarrhythmic agents

This table summarizes the major antiarrhythmics currently in clinical use.

DRUG	MAJOR INDICATIONS AND USUAL DOSAGES	CONTRAINDICATIONS AND PRECAUTIONS
Class I antiarrhythmics		
moricizine hydrochloride (Ethmozine)	*Life-threatening ventricular arrhythmias such as sustained ventricular tachycardia* ADULT: 200 to 300 mg P.O. every 8 hours, individually titrated based on patient's response and tolerance	• Moricizine is contraindicated in a breast-feeding patient or one with preexisting second- or third-degree atrioventricular (AV) block or right bundle branch block when associated with left hemiblock (except if a pacemaker is in place), cardiogenic shock, or known hypersensitivity. • This drug requires cautious use in a pregnant patient or one with sick sinus syndrome, preexisting conduction abnormalities, hepatic disease, impaired renal function, or heart failure. • Safety and efficacy in children have not been established.
Class IA antiarrhythmics		
quinidine sulfate (Quinidex, Quinora); quinidine gluconate (Quinaglute); quinidine polygalacturonate (Cardioquin)	*Conversion of atrial fibrillation to normal sinus rhythm* ADULT: 300 to 400 mg of immediate-release quinidine sulfate P.O. every 6 hours, then 200 to 400 mg every 6 hours to maintain regular rhythm or 200 mg every 2 to 3 hours for 5 to 8 doses: increase daily until sinus rhythm is restored or toxic effects occur, up to a maximum of 4 g/day *Suppression of atrial or ventricular ectopic beats* ADULT: 200 to 300 mg of quinidine sulfate P.O. every 6 to 8 hours, 300 to 600 mg of sustained-release quinidine sulfate every 8 to 12 hours, or 324 to 660 mg of quinidine gluconate every 8 to 12 hours *Maintenance of regular rhythm* ADULT: 324 to 660 mg of sustained-release quinidine gluconate or 275 mg of quinidine polygalacturonate every 8 to 12 hours *Conversion of atrial fibrillation to normal sinus rhythm, suppression of atrial or ventricular ectopic beats, or maintenance of regular rhythm* PEDIATRIC: 30 mg/kg or 900 mg/m^2 P.O. daily, divided into five doses	• Quinidine is contraindicated in a patient with complete AV block, intraventricular conduction defects, ectopic impulses and rhythms due to escape mechanisms, cardiac glycoside–induced AV conduction disturbances, myasthenia gravis, or known hypersensitivity. • This drug requires cautious use in a pregnant or breast-feeding patient or one with incomplete nodal AV block, cardiac glycoside intoxication, heart failure, hypotension, asthma, muscle weakness, infection with fever, or hepatic or renal impairment.
Class IB antiarrhythmics		
lidocaine hydrochloride (Xylocaine)	*Suppression of ventricular ectopic beats; conversion of ventricular tachycardia; treatment of ventricular arrhythmias related to digitalis toxicity and other acute conditions; reduction in frequency and duration of abrupt, self-limiting ventricular tachycardia; or maintenance of sinus rhythm once ventricular fibrillation has been defibrillated electrically* ADULT: 50 to 100 mg I.V. bolus initially (at a rate of 25 to 50 mg/minute), followed by a second bolus of 50 to 100 mg in 5 minutes, then continuous I.V. infusion at 1 to 4 mg/minute, up to a maximum of 300 mg in 1 hour; or 300 mg (for 70-kg adult) or 4.3 mg/kg I.M., repeated in 60 to 90 minutes, if needed PEDIATRIC: 0.5 to 1 mg/kg I.V. bolus, which may be repeated but should not exceed 5 mg/kg; then a continuous infusion of 10 to 50 mcg/kg/minute	• Lidocaine is contraindicated in a patient with known hypersensitivity, Adams-Stokes disease, or severe degrees of sinoatrial, AV, or intraventricular heart block in the absence of a pacemaker. • This drug requires cautious use in a pregnant or breast-feeding patient or one with heart block, severe renal disease, liver disease, heart failure, marked hypoxia, severe respiratory depression, hypovolemia, shock, sinus bradycardia, or incomplete heart block.

(continued)

Selected major antiarrhythmic agents *(continued)*

DRUG	MAJOR INDICATIONS AND USUAL DOSAGES	CONTRAINDICATIONS AND PRECAUTIONS
Class IC antiarrhythmics		
flecainide acetate (Tambocor)	*Prevention or treatment of sustained ventricular tachycardia* ADULT: 100 to 200 mg P.O. every 12 hours, not to exceed 400 mg/day *Prevention of paroxysmal supraventricular tachycardia* ADULT: 50 mg P.O. every 12 hours, increased in 50-mg increments (given b.i.d.) every 4 days, up to a maximum of 300 mg daily, until the desired response occurs	• Flecainide is contraindicated in a breast-feeding patient or one with preexisting second- or third-degree AV block, bifascicular or trifascicular block, heart failure, left ventricular dysfunction, cardiogenic shock, or known hypersensitivity. • This drug requires cautious use in a pregnant patient or one with a history of heart failure or myocardial dysfunction, sick sinus syndrome (including tachycardia-bradycardia syndrome), a pacemaker in place, or renal or hepatic impairment. • Safety and efficacy in children have not been established.
Class II antiarrhythmics		
propranolol hydrochloride (Inderal, Inderal LA)	*Atrial or ventricular ectopy or sudden onset of self-limiting atrial or ventricular tachycardia* ADULT: 10 to 30 mg P.O. every 6 to 8 hours; 0.5 to 3 mg I.V. for life-threatening arrhythmias, followed by a second dose after 2 minutes if needed and additional I.V. doses at 4-hour intervals until oral therapy begins *Treatment of atrial or ventricular arrhythmias* PEDIATRIC: 2 to 4 mg/kg P.O., in two equally divided doses	• Propranolol is contraindicated in a patient with Raynaud's disease, malignant hypertension, bronchial asthma, sinus bradycardia and heart block greater than first degree, heart failure (unless failure is secondary to a tachyarrhythmia treatable with propranolol), cardiogenic shock, or myasthenia gravis. • This drug requires cautious use in a pregnant or breast-feeding patient or one with inadequate cardiac function, coronary artery disease, sinus node dysfunction, arrhythmias occurring during myocardial-depressant anesthesia, hyperthyroidism, diabetes mellitus, hypoglycemia, nonallergic bronchospastic disease, or renal or hepatic impairment. This drug also requires cautious use in a patient who is undergoing major surgery.
Class III antiarrhythmics		
amiodarone hydrochloride (Cordarone)	*Ventricular arrhythmias unresponsive to other antiarrhythmics* ADULT: 800 to 1,600 mg P.O. daily for 1 to 3 weeks or until a response occurs, reduced gradually to a maintenance dosage of 200 to 400 mg P.O. daily; or 15 mg/minute I.V. in D_5W for 10 minutes, followed by 1 mg/minute for 6 hours, then 0.5 mg/minute until arrhythmia is controlled or oral therapy begins	• Amiodarone is contraindicated in a breast-feeding patient or one with severe sinus node dysfunction resulting in marked sinus bradycardia, second- or third-degree AV block, bradycardia-induced syncope (except if a pacemaker is in place), or known hypersensitivity. • This drug requires cautious use in a pregnant patient or one with pulmonary disease or reduced pulmonary diffusion capacity. • Safety and efficacy in children have not been established.
Class IV antiarrhythmics		
verapamil hydrochloride (Calan, Isoptin)	*Paroxysmal supraventricular tachycardia* ADULT: 5 to 10 mg I.V. push over 2 minutes, followed by a second dose of 10 mg I.V. push after 15 to 30 minutes if the patient tolerates but does not respond to the first dose PEDIATRIC: in children under age 1, 0.75 to 2 mg I.V. push over 2 minutes; in children age 1 and older, 2 to 5 mg I.V. bolus over 2 minutes	• Verapamil is contraindicated in a breast-feeding patient or one with severe hypotension, cardiogenic shock, second- or third-degree AV block or sick sinus syndrome (except if a pacemaker is in place), or known hypersensitivity. • This drug requires cautious use in a pregnant patient or one with moderately severe to severe ventricular dysfunction or heart failure, hypertrophic car-

Selected major antiarrhythmic agents *(continued)*

DRUG	MAJOR INDICATIONS AND USUAL DOSAGES	CONTRAINDICATIONS AND PRECAUTIONS
Class IV antiarrhythmics *(continued)*		
verapamil hydrochloride (Calan, Isoptin) *(continued)*	*Prevention of recurrent paroxysmal supraventricular tachycardia* ADULT: 240 to 480 mg P.O. daily in 3 or 4 divided doses *Ventricular rate control in chronic atrial fibrillation or flutter* ADULT: 240 to 320 mg P.O. daily in three or four divided doses	diomyopathy, hepatic or renal impairment, Duchenne type (pseudohypertrophic) muscular dystrophy, or anesthesia induction for resection of a supratentorial tumor.
Other antiarrhythmics		
adenosine (Adenocard)	*Conversion of paroxysmal supraventricular tachycardia to normal sinus rhythm* ADULT: initially, 6 mg bolus given over 1 to 2 seconds directly into a vein or, if given through an I.V. line, as proximal as possible and followed by a rapid saline flush; if conversion does not occur within 1 to 2 minutes after the first dose, give 12 mg as a rapid I.V. bolus (the 12-mg dose may be repeated a second time if required)	• Adenosine is contraindicated in a patient with second- or third-degree AV block or sick sinus syndrome (except if a pacemaker is in place) or known hypersensitivity. • This drug requires cautious use in a pregnant patient or one with asthma. • Safety and efficacy in children have not been established.

PHARMACODYNAMICS

Moricizine decreases the fast inward current in cardiac tissue caused by the influx of sodium ions. This depresses the depolarization rate and decreases the action potential duration and effective refractory period. The drug has a local anesthetic activity and has a stabilizing effect on the myocardial membrane. It prolongs the PR interval and QRS complex, and decreases conduction velocity in the atria, ventricles, bundle of His, and Purkinje fibers.

PHARMACOTHERAPEUTICS

Moricizine is the newest class I antiarrhythmic agent currently in use. It is used to manage life-threatening ventricular arrhythmias such as sustained ventricular tachycardia.

Drug interactions

Administration of cimetidine may increase the moricizine plasma level. Therefore, a patient receiving cimetidine should begin moricizine therapy at a low dosage. Propranolol administration may increase the PR interval on an electrocardiogram (ECG), but the clinical significance of this interaction is unknown. During clinical trials, patients receiving moricizine showed increased theophylline clearance with decreased theophylline half-life.

ADVERSE DRUG REACTIONS

The appearance of new arrhythmias or the exacerbation of existing arrhythmias is the most serious adverse reaction reported. Other adverse reactions reported in more than 2% of patients in clinical trials include sustained ventricular tachycardia, hypoesthesia, abdominal pain, dyspepsia, vomiting, sweating, cardiac chest pain, heart failure, cardiac arrest, asthenia, nervousness, paresthesia, musculoskeletal pain, diarrhea, dry mouth, sleep disorders, and blurred vision. Those reported in more than 5% of patients include dizziness, nausea, headache, fatigue, palpitations, and dyspnea.

NURSING PROCESS APPLICATION

The following information assists the nurse in caring for a patient receiving the class I antiarrhythmic moricizine. It includes an overview of assessment activities as well as examples of appropriate nursing diagnoses and related interventions. It also highlights the importance of evaluation.

Assessment

Before drug therapy begins, review the patient's history for conditions that contraindicate or require cautious use of moricizine. Also review the patient's medication history to identify use of drugs that may interact with it. During therapy, assess the patient for adverse drug reactions and signs of drug interactions. Also, periodically assess the effective-

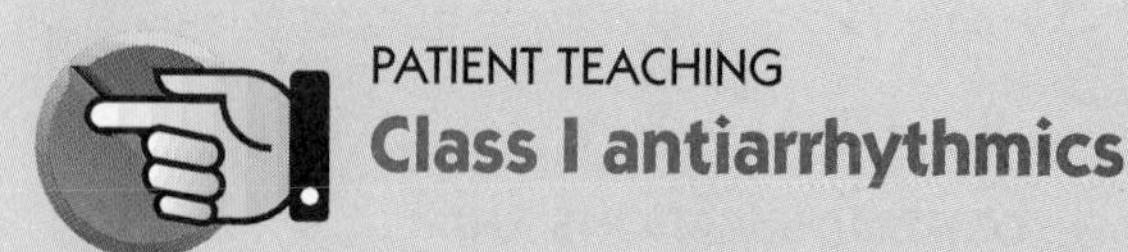

PATIENT TEACHING
Class I antiarrhythmics

- Teach the patient and family the name, dose, frequency, action, and adverse effects of moricizine.
- Inform the patient that moricizine may cause headache or abdominal, cardiac chest, or musculoskeletal pain. Advise the patient to immediately report such pain — especially cardiac chest pain — because prompt treatment is necessary.
- Instruct the patient to report signs and symptoms of heart failure, such as shortness of breath or sudden weight gain.
- Encourage the patient to limit sodium and fluid intake during moricizine therapy.
- Advise the patient that blurred vision is a dose-related adverse reaction and should subside when moricizine is discontinued.
- Instruct the patient to report any other adverse reactions.

ness of moricizine therapy. Finally, evaluate the patient's and family's knowledge about the prescribed drug.

Nursing diagnoses

- Risk for injury related to a preexisting condition that contraindicates or requires cautious use of moricizine
- Risk for injury related to adverse drug reactions or drug interactions
- Decreased cardiac output related to moricizine-induced development of new arrhythmias or exacerbation of existing arrhythmias
- Knowledge deficit related to moricizine

Planning and implementation

- Do not administer moricizine to a patient with a condition that contraindicates its use.
- Administer moricizine cautiously to a patient at risk because of a preexisting condition.
- Monitor the patient closely for adverse reactions during moricizine therapy. Check the patient's ECG for new arrhythmias or worsening of existing ones. Observe the patient for signs and symptoms of heart failure and decreased cardiac output, such as a weak pulse, hypotension, and dizziness. Also monitor for signs of drug interactions.

* ***Keep standard emergency equipment nearby when moricizine therapy begins because cardiac arrest can occur.***

- Notify the physician if the patient's condition does not improve or if arrhythmias, other adverse reactions, or drug interactions occur.
- Teach the patient about moricizine. (See Patient Teaching: *Class I antiarrhythmics.*)

Evaluation

For each nursing diagnosis, prepare an evaluation statement that describes the patient's or family's response to nursing interventions.

Class IA antiarrhythmics

Class IA antiarrhythmics include disopyramide phosphate, procainamide hydrochloride, and quinidine sulfate, gluconate, or polygalacturonate. These drugs are used to treat various atrial and ventricular arrhythmias.

PHARMACOKINETICS

When administered orally, class IA drugs undergo fairly rapid absorption and metabolism. Because of this, researchers have developed sustained-release forms of these drugs to help maintain therapeutic levels. In addition, food and extremes in gastric pH hasten or delay absorption of these drugs. Quinidine is absorbed almost completely, but its absorption rate depends on the salt with which it is combined: quinidine polygalacturonate and quinidine gluconate, although they are not sustained-release forms, are absorbed more slowly than quinidine sulfate. Procainamide and disopyramide are about 90% absorbed.

These three drugs are distributed through all body tissues except, in the case of quinidine, the brain. Disopyramide and quinidine also enter red blood cells. Plasma protein binding is 90% for quinidine, 20% for procainamide, and, depending on the concentration, 30% to 65% for disopyramide.

All class IA antiarrhythmics are metabolized in the liver and are excreted unchanged by the kidneys in the following amounts: 50% of disopyramide; 10% to 50% of quinidine, with the percentage decreasing as urine pH increases; and 40% to 70% of procainamide. A small percentage of disopyramide is excreted in the feces.

Disopyramide reaches a peak concentration level in 1 to 2 hours. Quinidine and oral procainamide capsules attain peak concentrations in 60 to 90 minutes. The sustained-release forms of these agents reach peak concentrations as follows: disopyramide in 5 hours, quinidine in 3 to 4 hours, and procainamide in 1½ to 2 hours. Procainamide given intramuscularly (I.M.) reaches peak concentrations in 15 to 60 minutes (one reason it is not used frequently).

Route	Onset	Peak	Duration
P.O.	0.5-3 hr	60-120 min	3 hr
P.O. (sustained release)	Later than P.O. above	1.5-5 hr	≥6 hr
I.M.	10-30 min	15-60 min	3-6 hr
I.V.	Immediate	Minutes	Unknown

The nurse must monitor the patient's serum concentration closely during therapy with a class IA antiarrhythmic to prevent toxicity. Normal therapeutic ranges are as follows: disopyramide, 2 to 6 mcg/ml; quinidine, 2 to 6 mcg/ml; and procainamide, 4 to 10 mcg/ml. N-acetyl procainamide (NAPA) levels resulting from procainamide metabolism usually range from 2 to 8 mcg/ml.

In healthy individuals, the half-life of disopyramide is from 5 to 12 hours; of quinidine, 6 to 8 hours; of procainamide, 3 hours; and of NAPA, about 7 hours in a patient with normal renal function.

PHARMACODYNAMICS

Class IA antiarrhythmics exert their effects by altering the myocardial cell membrane and interfering with autonomic nervous system control of pacemaker cells. All three drugs also block parasympathetic nervous system discharges to the SA and AV nodes, thereby increasing the conduction rate of the AV node. This anticholinergic (atropine-like) effect can produce dangerous increases in the ventricular heart rate if rapid atrial activity, as in atrial **fibrillation,** is present. In turn, the increased ventricular heart rate can offset the ability of the antiarrhythmics to convert atrial arrhythmias to a regular rhythm.

Disopyramide produces peripheral vasoconstriction, and procainamide and quinidine decrease **peripheral vascular resistance** (afterload). Disopyramide causes significant depression of myocardial contractility.

Procainamide and quinidine produce slight myocardial depression, widen the QRS complex, and prolong the QT interval. Quinidine's ventricular stimulation can be prevented by giving digoxin, a beta-blocker, or verapamil to decrease AV conduction.

PHARMACOTHERAPEUTICS

Based on their differing therapeutic and adverse effects, class IA antiarrhythmics are prescribed to treat various atrial and ventricular arrhythmias. The drugs (especially quinidine) are synergistic with digoxin. Because of decreased AV conduction time with digoxin therapy, quinidine can be added to a patient's drug regimen to convert atrial fibrillation to a regular rhythm. However, quinidine use has decreased because it increases cardiac mortality and because manufacturers have introduced other antiarrhythmic drugs. Procainimide is very effective with atrial and ventricular arrhythmias and is weakly anticholinergic.

Drug interactions

Class IA antiarrhythmics may exhibit additive or antagonistic effects with other antiarrhythmics as well as with anticholinergic drugs. (See Drug Interactions: *Class IA antiarrhythmics,* page 230.)

ADVERSE DRUG REACTIONS

Adverse reactions to class IA antiarrhythmics include anticholinergic effects, gastrointestinal (GI) changes, and reactions unique to quinidine's source, cinchona.

The anticholinergic effect of disopyramide commonly produces dry mouth, blurred vision, constipation, urinary hesitancy, and urine retention. The drug's negative inotropic effect combined with increased peripheral vasoconstriction sometimes results in heart failure, hypotension, chest pain, edema, and dyspnea.

The class IA antiarrhythmics, especially quinidine, may produce GI symptoms, such as diarrhea, cramping, nausea, vomiting, anorexia, and bitter taste.

Cinchonism, a reaction to the cinchona alkaloids, describes a set of quinidine-related reactions consisting of tinnitus, headache, vertigo, fever, light-headedness, and visual disturbances. Cinchonism may appear after the first dose or with quinidine toxicity. Quinidine-induced syncope also may occur, probably from transient ventricular tachycardia or ectopy.

Procainamide, especially the intravenous (I.V.) form, can produce hypotension. The drug's negative inotropic effect less commonly leads to heart failure. Because I.V. quinidine may lead to severe hypotension and cardiovascular collapse, the drug rarely is administered by this route.

All class IA antiarrhythmics can induce arrhythmias, especially conduction delays that may compound existing heart blocks. Apparent conduction through the AV node may be increased, precipitating a dangerously high ventricular rate. As the effective refractory period and the action potential duration increase, the ECG reflects a prolonged QT interval. This is a precursor to a special form of ventricular tachycardia known as torsades de pointes.

Up to 30% of patients using procainamide experience an adverse reaction that mimics systemic lupus erythematosus. Signs and symptoms include pain in small joints, pleuritic pain, dyspnea, fever, headache, pericardial effusion, blood dyscrasias, and positive serum antinuclear antibody titers. This reaction, called drug-induced systemic lupus, is not dose-dependent and resolves when procainamide is discontinued. Rarely, quinidine also causes lupus-like symptoms and hypersensitivity reactions manifested by fever, blood dyscrasias, skin eruptions, liver disorders, and anaphylaxis. All three of the class IA antiarrhythmics can precipitate heart failure and can produce confusion in geriatric patients.

NURSING PROCESS APPLICATION

The following information assists the nurse in caring for a patient who is receiving a class IA antiarrhythmic. It includes an overview of assessment activities as well as examples of appropriate nursing diagnoses and related interventions. It also highlights the importance of evaluation.

Assessment

Before drug therapy begins, review the patient's history for conditions that contraindicate or require cautious use of the prescribed class IA antiarrhythmic. Also review the patient's medication history to identify use of drugs that may interact with it. During therapy, assess the patient for adverse drug reactions and signs of drug interactions. Assess the patient receiving procainamide for drug-induced systemic lu-

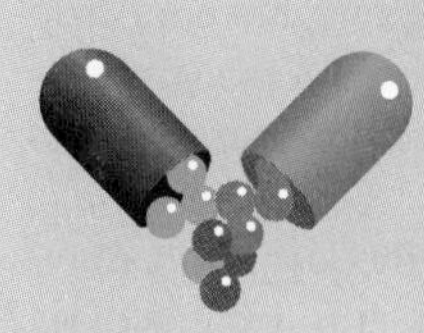

DRUG INTERACTIONS

Class IA antiarrhythmics

Class IA antiarrhythmics interact with several commonly administered drugs. To provide the best possible patient care, the nurse should be aware of these interactions and their implications.

DRUG	INTERACTING AGENTS	POSSIBLE EFFECTS	NURSING IMPLICATIONS
disopyramide	anticholinergics	Increased anticholinergic effects	• Observe the patient for adverse reactions, such as dry mouth, wheezing, urine retention, and orthostatic hypotension.
	verapamil	Myocardial depression	• Do not administer these drugs within 24 hours of each other. • Monitor for signs of heart failure or decreased peripheral perfusion, if concurrent administration is necessary.
procainamide	cimetidine, amiodarone	Increased serum procainamide levels	• Monitor for therapeutic levels of procainamide. • Assess the patient for signs and symptoms of procainamide overdose, such as tachycardia, confusion, drowsiness, nausea, and vomiting.
	quinidine	Increased plasma procainamide and N-acetyl procainamide (NAPA) levels	• Use caution during concomitant therapy.
quinidine	neuromuscular blockers	Increased skeletal muscle relaxation	• Observe the patient for hypoventilation when administering a class IA antiarrhythmic in the immediate postoperative period.
	oral anticoagulants	Hypoprothrombinemia	• Observe the patient for increased bruising, bleeding, or I.V. site oozing; monitor the patient's prothrombin time.
	digoxin	Increased serum digoxin level	• Monitor the patient's serum digoxin level. • Assess the patient for signs of digitalis toxicity: anorexia, nausea, vomiting, headache, malaise, visual disturbances, and changes in pulse rate or regularity.
	urine-alkalinizing agents, cimetidine, amiodarone	Increased serum quinidine levels	• Assess the patient for signs of quinidine toxicity, such as arrhythmias, hypotension, and syncope.
	procainamide	Increased plasma procainamide and NAPA levels	• Monitor therapeutic levels of procainamide.
quinidine, disopyramide	rifampin, phenytoin, phenobarbital	Increased metabolism of quinidine and disopyramide	• Monitor the patient's pulse rate and electrocardiogram for signs of decreased therapeutic effect. • Monitor the patient's quinidine and disopyramide levels.

pus erythematosus and the patient receiving quinidine for cinchonism. Also, periodically assess the effectiveness of class IA antiarrhythmic therapy. Finally, evaluate the patient's and family's knowledge about the prescribed drug. (See Patient Teaching: *Class IA antiarrhythmics.*)

Nursing diagnoses

- Risk for injury related to a preexisting condition that contraindicates or requires cautious use of a class IA antiarrhythmic
- Risk for injury related to adverse drug reactions or drug interactions
- Knowledge deficit related to the prescribed class IA antiarrhythmic

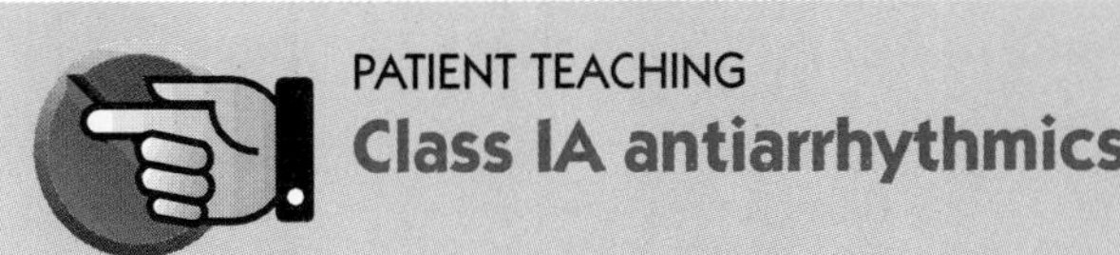

PATIENT TEACHING
Class IA antiarrhythmics

- Teach the patient and family the name, dose, frequency, action, and adverse effects of the prescribed class IA antiarrhythmic.
- Instruct the female patient to notify the physician if she is pregnant or plans to become pregnant.
- Instruct the patient to weigh self daily, at the same time every day and in similar clothes, to detect fluid retention. Advise the patient to notify the physician of sudden weight gain (2 pounds or more in one day), shortness of breath, or peripheral edema.
- Stress the importance of having drug concentration tests and electrocardiograms done regularly to detect abnormalities.
- Instruct the patient to take the prescribed class IA antiarrhythmic around-the-clock rather than just during the day to maintain therapeutic drug levels.
- Advise the family that a class IA agent may cause confusion in a geriatric patient. Instruct them to take safety measures, such as continual supervision, and to notify the physician if confusion occurs.
- Teach the patient how to manage the anticholinergic effects of class IA antiarrhythmics, such as dry mouth and constipation. Also advise the patient to report signs of urine retention, such as urinary frequency and a sensation of bladder fullness after voiding.
- Teach the patient to recognize and report to the physician any signs of drug-induced systemic lupus erythematosus before taking the next dose of procainamide.
- Teach the patient to recognize signs of infection and bleeding, especially with procainamide therapy.
- Teach the patient to recognize and report to the physician signs of cinchonism before taking the next dose of quinidine.
- Instruct the patient not to take the prescribed class IA antiarrhythmic with food, unless otherwise directed.
- Advise the patient receiving sustained-release tablets or capsules that the wax matrix may be excreted intact in the stool. Provide reassurance that this is normal and that all of the drug has been extracted in the intestines.
- Demonstrate how to take a pulse. Tell the patient to measure the pulse before taking the prescribed class IA antiarrhythmic. Advise the patient to notify the physician if the pulse is irregular or slow (below 60 beats/minute or the rate selected by the physician).
- Instruct the patient to notify the physician if adverse reactions occur.

Planning and implementation

- Do not administer a class IA antiarrhythmic to a patient with a condition that contraindicates it.
- Administer a class IA antiarrhythmic cautiously to a patient at risk because of a preexisting condition.
- Administer a digoxin loading dose, if prescribed, before the first dose of the prescribed class IA antiarrhythmic for a patient being treated for atrial tachycardia or fibrillation.
- Monitor the patient frequently for adverse reactions and drug interactions during class IA antiarrhythmic therapy.

* ***Assess for early signs of heart failure, such as hypotension, edema, and irregular heartbeat, by taking the patient's vital signs, auscultating for breath sounds regularly, recording the patient's fluid intake and output, and weighing the patient daily.***
* ***Monitor the patient's ECG for increased ventricular rate, a QT interval 50% greater than normal, and conduction disturbances.***

- Monitor electrolyte levels closely at the beginning of therapy and when administering diuretics with a class IA antiarrhythmic. Electrolyte abnormalities, especially hypokalemia, can predispose the patient to arrhythmias.
- Monitor the patient's serum drug concentration closely to detect early toxicity. Notify the physician if the concentration falls outside of the therapeutic range.
- Give around-the-clock doses (when appropriate and prescribed) rather than following a traditional t.i.d. or q.i.d. schedule to maintain therapeutic drug concentration.
- Observe for signs of drug-induced systemic lupus erythematosus during procainamide therapy.
- Monitor for signs of cinchonism during quinidine therapy.
- Do not administer a class IA antiarrhythmic with food unless prescribed because food may affect absorption.
- Expect to adjust the disopyramide dosage for a patient with renal impairment, the quinidine dosage for a patient with heart failure or liver dysfunction, and the procainamide dosage for a patient with renal or cardiac failure, as prescribed.
- Be aware that I.M. procainamide takes 15 to 60 minutes to reach peak concentration.
- Administer I.V. procainamide by using an infusion pump; monitor the patient's ECG and blood pressure frequently. When switching from the I.V. to the oral route, continue the infusion for 2 hours, or as prescribed, after the first oral dose.
- Notify the physician if the patient's condition does not improve or if adverse reactions or drug interactions occur.
- Teach the patient about the prescribed drug.

Evaluation

For each nursing diagnosis, prepare an evaluation statement that describes the patient's or family's response to nursing interventions.

Class IB antiarrhythmics

Class IB antiarrhythmics include lidocaine hydrochloride, mexiletine hydrochloride, and tocainide hydrochloride. Lidocaine is one of the most widely used antiarrhythmics in acute care. Mexiletine and tocainide were developed more recently. Although they have fewer clinical indications than class IA antiarrhythmics, class IB antiarrhythmics, especially lidocaine, are more effective for treating acute ventricular arrhythmias and cause fewer adverse reactions. Phenytoin,

Phenytoin for digitalis toxicity

Phenytoin sometimes is given I.V. to correct acute arrhythmias caused by digitalis toxicity. It is distributed throughout the body and is 95% protein-bound. The drug is metabolized in the liver by oxidation to an inactive metabolite, which then is excreted in the urine. Onset of action occurs within 5 minutes of intravenous (I.V.) administration. (Peak or therapeutic serum concentrations usually are not important when phenytoin is used to treat arrhythmias.) The duration of action is 4 to 6 hours, although the half-life of phenytoin usually is about 22 hours.

The mechanism of action of phenytoin in treating digitalis-induced arrhythmias resembles that of the class IB antiarrhythmics. The drug shortens the effective refractory period of the atrioventricular (AV) node and depresses the automaticity of ectopic myocardial cells. Phenytoin is used to shorten prolonged AV conduction time and to suppress premature ventricular beats.

The usual adult dosage is 100 mg I.V. push, repeated every 5 minutes until the arrhythmia disappears; if the total dosage reaches 1 gram without effect, another antiarrhythmic should be used.

Adverse reactions include pain at the infusion site, hypotension with cardiovascular collapse, a decreased level of consciousness, ventricular fibrillation, rash, and fever.

When administering phenytoin, the nurse should note the following considerations:
- Infuse the drug through a central line to avoid pain and phlebitis. If a peripheral site must be used, inject the drug into an I.V. line infusing normal saline solution.
- Do not dilute phenytoin; administer by I.V. push only at a rate of less than 50 mg/minute.
- Closely monitor the patient's heart rate and rhythm and blood pressure.
- Have standard emergency equipment nearby.

which resembles the class IB antiarrhythmics, also may be used to treat arrhythmias caused by digitalis toxicity. (See *Phenytoin for digitalis toxicity.*)

PHARMACOKINETICS

All class IB antiarrhythmics are absorbed well from the GI tract after oral administration; however, lidocaine is not available in oral form because most of an absorbed dose undergoes first-pass metabolism in the liver.

Lidocaine is distributed widely throughout the body, including the brain. Distribution data for mexiletine and tocainide are incomplete but may resemble that of lidocaine. Class IB antiarrhythmics are bound to plasma proteins in the following amounts: lidocaine, 65%; mexiletine, 55%; and tocainide, 15%.

Class IB antiarrhythmics are metabolized in the liver. Less than 10% of lidocaine, about 10% of mexiletine, and about 50% of tocainide are excreted unchanged in the urine. Mexiletine also is excreted in breast milk.

The half-life of lidocaine is 90 minutes; of mexiletine, 10 to 12 hours; and of tocainide, 11 to 15 hours.

Route	Onset	Peak	Duration
P.O.	0.5-2 hr	0.5-3 hr	Unknown
I.M.	Unknown	10 min	Unknown
I.V.	Immediate	1-2 min	5 min

PHARMACODYNAMICS

Class IB antiarrhythmics are used only to treat ventricular arrhythmias. These drugs slightly depress depolarization in myocardial cells. Class IB antiarrhythmics are cell membrane stabilizers, but do not affect the automaticity of the SA node or conductivity through the AV node.

As their major action, class IB antiarrhythmics decrease the action potential duration and, to a lesser extent, the effective refractory period. They especially affect the Purkinje fibers and myocardial cells in the ventricles. By shortening the effective refractory period, class IB antiarrhythmics eliminate unidirectional block, which can trigger a reentry arrhythmia. The drugs also decrease ventricular ectopy by blocking the slow influx of sodium during plateau (phase 2) and by decreasing the slope of phase 4 depolarization. (See *How lidocaine suppresses ventricular arrhythmias.*) Class IB antiarrhythmics neither block nor mimic autonomic control of the heart.

PHARMACOTHERAPEUTICS

Class IB antiarrhythmics are used to treat ventricular ectopic beats, ventricular tachycardia, and ventricular fibrillation. Because class IB antiarrhythmics usually do not produce serious adverse reactions, they are the drugs of choice in acute care.

Drug interactions

Class IB antiarrhythmics may exhibit additive or antagonistic effects when administered with other antiarrhythmics, such as phenytoin, propranolol, procainamide, and quinidine. Lidocaine toxicity may result from concurrent administration of propranolol or cimetidine. Phenytoin may reduce mexiletine concentrations, requiring a dosage increase; rifampin may reduce mexiletine or tocainide concentrations, requiring a dosage increase to maintain a therapeutic effect.

Narcotics decrease GI absorption of mexiletine. Theophylline plasma levels are increased when the drug is given with mexiletine. Plasma mexiletine levels are decreased during concomitant therapy with a hepatic enzyme inducer, such as rifampin or phenobarbital. Use of a beta-blocker or disopyramide with mexiletine may cause a negative inotropic effect.

ADVERSE DRUG REACTIONS

All class IB antiarrhythmics have a relatively high incidence of central nervous system (CNS) disturbances, especially drowsiness, confusion, light-headedness, paresthesia,

How lidocaine suppresses ventricular arrhythmias

Lidocaine works in injured or ischemic myocardial cells to retard sodium influx and restore cardiac rhythm. Normally, the ventricles contract in response to impulses from the sinoatrial (SA) node. But when tissue damage occurs in the ventricles, ischemic cells can create an ectopic pacemaker, which can trigger ventricular arrhythmias. How these arrythmias develop at the cellular level — and how lidocaine suppresses them — is shown in the illustrations below.

ISCHEMIC MYOCARDIAL CELL

Normal myocardial cells permit a limited amount of sodium ions to enter, which leads to controlled depolarization. Ischemic myocardial cells allow a rapid infusion of sodium ions. This causes the cells to depolarize much more quickly than normal and then begin firing spontaneously. The result: a ventricular arrhythmia.

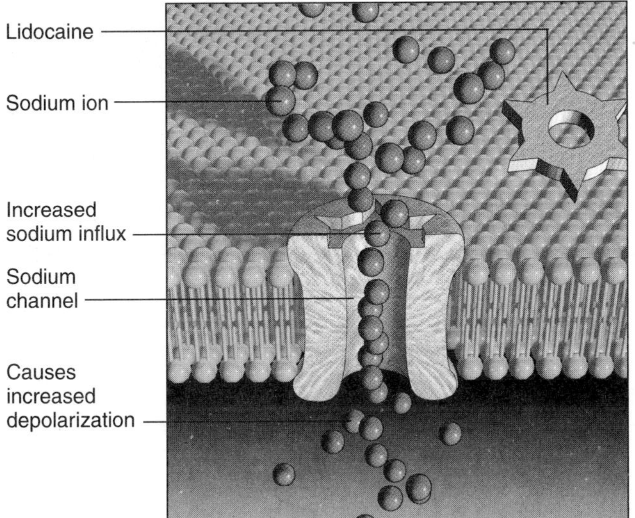

ISCHEMIC MYOCARDIAL CELL WITH LIDOCAINE

By slowing sodium's influx, lidocaine raises the cells' electrical stimulation threshold (EST). The increased EST prolongs depolarization in the ischemic cells and returns control to the SA node, the heart's main pacemaker.

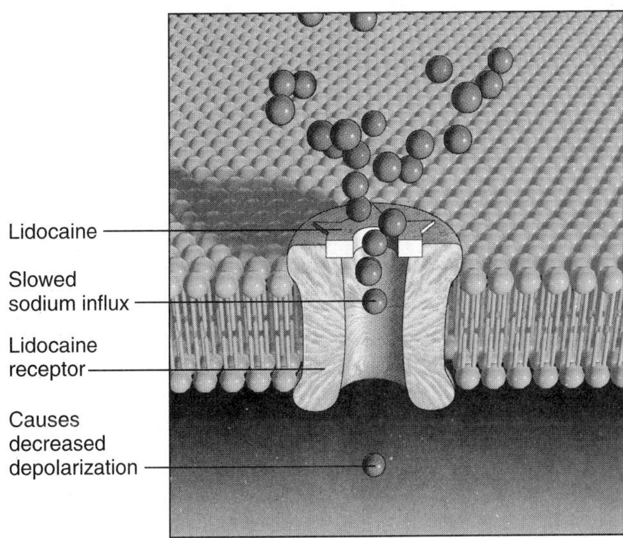

slurred speech, vision and hearing disturbances, tremor, seizures, and coma. Lowering the dosage or stopping the drug reverses these reactions. Hypotension and bradycardia sometimes occur.

Lidocaine toxicity can cause convulsions and respiratory arrest, requiring the use of resuscitation equipment. Up to 40% of patients taking mexiletine or tocainide experience upper GI distress, which usually is relieved by taking the drug with food or antacids. Adverse reactions to mexiletine occur in 70% of patients and commonly include hypotension, AV block, bradycardia, confusion, ataxia, and diplopia. Adverse reactions to tocainide occur in more than 50% of patients and commonly include GI distress and central nervous system (CNS) and cerebellar effects.

Tocainide can lead to two rare but serious reactions: blood dyscrasias and pulmonary fibrosis. These disappear when the drug is discontinued. Drug fever and hepatitis have occurred after tocainide therapy. Tocainide or mexiletine may produce allergic skin reactions. Generally, mexiletine poses less risk of causing an allergic reaction.

NURSING PROCESS APPLICATION

The following information assists the nurse in caring for a patient who is receiving a class IB antiarrhythmic. It includes an overview of assessment activities as well as examples of appropriate nursing diagnoses and related interventions. It also highlights the importance of evaluation.

Assessment

Before drug therapy begins, review the patient's history for conditions that contraindicate or require cautious use of the prescribed class IB antiarrhythmic. Also review the patient's medication history to identify use of drugs that may interact with it. During therapy, assess the patient for adverse drug reactions and signs of drug interactions. Also, periodically assess the effectiveness of class IB antiarrhythmic therapy. Finally, evaluate the patient's and family's knowledge about the prescribed drug. (See Patient Teaching: *Class IB antiarrhythmics*, page 234.)

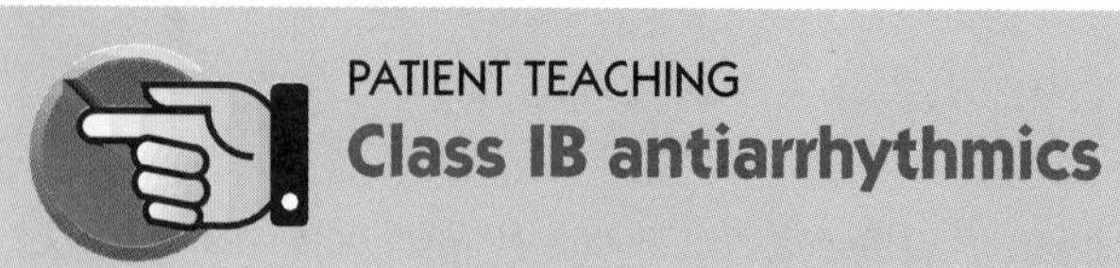

PATIENT TEACHING
Class IB antiarrhythmics

- Teach the patient and family the name, dose (if appropriate), frequency, action, and adverse effects of the prescribed class IB antiarrhythmic.
- Advise the patient not to perform activities that require alertness if adverse central nervous system reactions occur.
- Instruct the family that the class IB antiarrhythmic may cause confusion.
- Teach the patient and family to recognize and report to the physician signs of toxicity, such as change in level of consciousness, seizures, or vision or hearing disturbances. Reassure them that these reactions will disappear with dosage reduction or drug discontinuation.
- Instruct the patient to take mexiletine or tocainide with food or antacids.
- Instruct the patient to notify the physician if adverse reactions occur.

Nursing diagnoses

• Risk for injury related to a preexisting condition that contraindicates or requires cautious use of a class IB antiarrhythmic
• Risk for injury related to adverse drug reactions or drug interactions
• Sensory or perceptual alterations (auditory, tactile, and visual) related to the adverse CNS effects of the prescribed class IB antiarrhythmic
• Knowledge deficit related to the prescribed class IB antiarrhythmic

Planning and implementation

• Do not administer a class IB antiarrhythmic to a patient with a condition that contraindicates its use.
• Administer a class IB antiarrhythmic cautiously to a patient at risk because of a preexisting condition.
• Monitor the patient closely for CNS disturbances, sensory or perceptual alterations (such as vision or hearing disturbances or paresthesias) and other adverse reactions.
• Observe for signs of lidocaine toxicity, such as confusion and restlessness, when administering propranolol or cimetidine concurrently with the class IB antiarrhythmic.
• Monitor the patient's serum potassium level because hypokalemia exacerbates arrhythmias.
• Administer lidocaine I.M. in the deltoid muscle to enhance absorption. Keep in mind, however, that I.M. administration of lidocaine interferes with cardiac enzyme measurements used to help diagnose an acute myocardial infarction; the route should be changed to I.V. when possible.
• Use the 100-mg prefilled syringe of lidocaine for I.V. push. Use the 1- or 2-g prefilled syringe for mixing in 250 or 500 ml dextrose 5% in water.

***** *Do not use lidocaine solutions containing epinephrine when lidocaine is prescribed to treat arrhythmias; such solutions are for local anesthesia only.***
• Administer continuous I.V. infusions using an infusion pump, and monitor the patient's ECG constantly.
• Expect to reduce the dosage of the class IB antiarrhythmic, as prescribed, in a patient with heart failure, cardiogenic shock, liver disease, or severe renal or hepatic impairment. Expect to switch the patient from I.V. lidocaine to tocainide or mexiletine, as prescribed, if an oral anti-arrhythmic is needed.
• Administer mexiletine or tocainide with food or antacids to reduce GI distress.
• Notify the physician if the patient's condition does not improve or if adverse reactions or drug interactions occur.
• Reassure the patient that sensory and perceptual alterations should disappear with dosage reduction or drug discontinuation.

Evaluation

For each nursing diagnosis, prepare an evaluation statement that describes the patient's or family's response to nursing interventions.

Class IC antiarrhythmics

Flecainide acetate and propafenone hydrochloride are class IC antiarrhythmics used to treat certain types of severe, refractory ventricular arrhythmias.

PHARMACOKINETICS

After oral administration, class IC antiarrhythmics are absorbed well, distributed in varying degrees, probably metabolized by the liver, and excreted primarily by the kidneys, except for propafenone, which is excreted primarily in the feces.

The therapeutic plasma level of flecainide ranges from 0.2 to 1.0 mcg/ml. Its half-life ranges from 7 to 25 hours in healthy adults, with 13 to 16 hours as the average. The half-life may be increased in geriatric patients or those with premature ventricular contractions or severe renal impairment.

In patients who metabolize propafenone extensively, the half-life is 2 to 10 hours; in those who metabolize the drug poorly, the half-life ranges from 10 to 32 hours. Although the therapeutic concentration for propafenone is defined incompletely, it seems to range from 0.06 to 1.0 mcg/ml.

Route	Onset	Peak	Duration
P.O.	Unknown	3.5 hr	Unknown

PHARMACODYNAMICS

Class IC antiarrhythmics primarily block influx of sodium in the cell membrane fast channel during phase 0 of the ac-

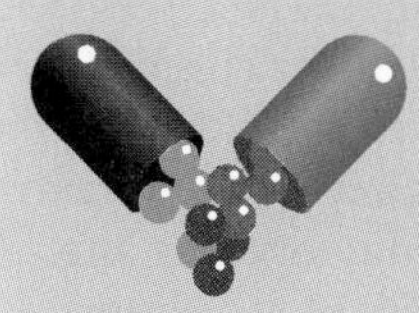

DRUG INTERACTIONS

Class IC antiarrhythmics

Class IC antiarrhythmics interact with several commonly administered drugs. To provide the best possible patient care, the nurse should be aware of these interactions and their implications.

DRUG	INTERACTING AGENTS	POSSIBLE EFFECTS	NURSING IMPLICATIONS
flecainide, propafenone	digoxin	Increased serum digoxin concentration	• Monitor the patient's serum digoxin concentration. • Assess the patient for signs of digitalis toxicity, such as central nervous system, cardiovascular, and gastrointestinal disturbances.
flecainide	alkalinizing agents, cimetidine, propranolol	Increased serum flecainide concentration	• Assess the patient for signs of flecainide toxicity, such as conduction disturbances, hypotension, and bradycardia.
	disopyramide, verapamil, diltiazem, beta-adrenergic blockers	Increased negative inotropic effects	• Assess the patient for signs of heart failure, such as shortness of breath and edema.
propafenone	warfarin	Increased prothrombin time	• Observe the patient for increased bruising, bleeding, or I.V. site oozing. • Monitor the patient's prothrombin time.
	metoprolol, propranolol	Increased serum concentrations and effects of metoprolol and propranolol	• Observe the patient for signs of increased beta-blocking effect, such as hypotension, bradycardia, intensified atrioventricular block, heart failure, and bronchoconstriction.
	quinidine	Inhibited propafenone metabolism	• Avoid concomitant administration.

tion potential, thereby decreasing depolarization. They inhibit the His-Purkinje conduction system, which widens the QRS complex. Flecainide produces a dose-related decrease in intracardiac conduction. It also increases endocardial pacing thresholds and exerts some negative inotropic effect.

Structurally similar to beta-adrenergic blocking agents, propafenone prolongs intracardiac conduction and produces minor effects on refractoriness (inability of the heart to be restimulated). It may suppress function in a diseased sinus node. Propafenone can alter pacing and sensing thresholds of artificial pacemakers.

PHARMACOTHERAPEUTICS

Like class IB antiarrhythmics, class IC drugs are used to treat life-threatening ventricular arrhythmias. Some arrhythmias respond better to class IC agents than to the class IB drugs. Flecainide and propafenone are used to treat supraventricular and ventricular arrhythmias. Flecainide also may be used to prevent paroxysmal supraventricular tachycardia (PSVT) in patients without structural heart disease.

Drug interactions

Class IC antiarrhythmics may exhibit additive effects with other antiarrhythmics. When used with digoxin, flecainide and propafenone can increase the serum digoxin concentration and predispose the patient to digitalis toxicity. When given with oral anticoagulants, propafenone can increase the patient's prothrombin time. Propafenone also can increase the negative inotropic effect of beta blockers or calcium antagonists. (See Drug Interactions: *Class IC antiarrhythmics.*)

ADVERSE DRUG REACTIONS

Class IC antiarrhythmics can produce serious adverse reactions, including the development of new arrhythmias, which limit the use of these drugs.

All class IC agents cause adverse CNS reactions, which may include dizziness, headache, paresthesia, fatigue, and blurred vision. They also may produce adverse GI reactions, such as nausea and vomiting and constipation or diarrhea. A metallic or bitter taste may result from propafenone use and, to a lesser extent, from flecainide use. The CNS and GI reactions may be dose-related in some patients and may abate with dosage reduction.

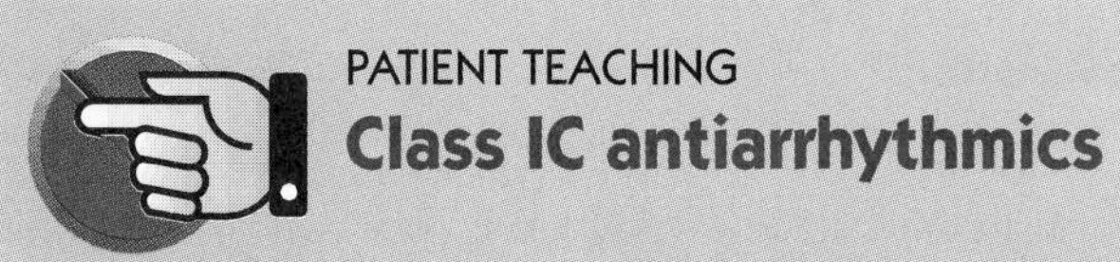

PATIENT TEACHING
Class IC antiarrhythmics

- Teach the patient and family the name, dose, frequency, action, and adverse effects of the prescribed class IC antiarrhythmic.
- Demonstrate how to take a pulse and tell the patient to do this before taking each dose of the prescribed class IC antiarrhythmic. Advise the patient to notify the physician if the pulse is irregular or lower than 60 beats/minute.
- Stress the importance of taking the drug exactly as prescribed. Instruct the patient to notify the physician if a dose is inadvertently forgotten.
- Teach the patient who is taking digoxin concurrently with flecainide or propafenone to watch for and report signs of digitalis toxicity.
- Instruct the patient taking propafenone and an oral anticoagulant to return regularly for prothrombin time testing to detect bleeding problems.
- Reassure the patient taking propafenone that adverse central nervous system (CNS) reactions, such as altered taste, may disappear if the dosage is reduced.
- Instruct the patient to avoid activities that require mental alertness if dizziness, blurred vision, or other CNS reactions occur.
- Instruct the patient to notify the physician and obtain a prescription for an antiemetic or antidiarrheal if nausea, vomiting, or diarrhea occurs. Suggest ways to relieve or prevent constipation, if necessary.
- Inform the patient that class IC antiarrhythmics can cause or worsen congestive heart failure. Review the signs and symptoms of this disorder, and advise the patient to notify the physician if fluid retention occurs. Instruct the patient to limit fluid and salt intake to minimize fluid retention.
- Instruct the patient to notify the physician if adverse reactions occur.

Adverse cardiovascular reactions to these agents include conduction abnormalities, exacerbation of heart failure, new arrhythmias, and hypotension. Paradoxically, class IC agents can aggravate existing arrhythmias.

Both class IC agents have some negative inotropic potential and can cause or worsen heart failure. This effect is most pronounced with flecainide.

Because propafenone possesses beta-blocking properties, it may cause bronchospasm, although only a few cases have been reported. Rarely, flecainide and propafenone have been associated with hematologic disturbances. More commonly, flecainide causes fever, rash, and allergic reactions.

NURSING PROCESS APPLICATION

The following information assists the nurse in caring for a patient who is receiving a class IC antiarrhythmic. It includes an overview of assessment activities as well as examples of appropriate nursing diagnoses and related interventions. It also highlights the importance of evaluation.

Assessment

Before drug therapy begins, review the patient's history for conditions that contraindicate or require cautious use of the prescribed class IC antiarrhythmic. Also review the patient's medication history to identify use of drugs that may interact with it. During therapy, assess the patient for adverse drug reactions and signs of drug interactions. Also, periodically assess the effectiveness of class IC antiarrhythmic therapy. Finally, evaluate the patient's and family's knowledge about the prescribed drug.

Nursing diagnoses

- Risk for injury related to a preexisting condition that contraindicates or requires cautious use of a class IC antiarrhythmic
- Risk for injury related to adverse drug reactions or drug interactions
- Fluid volume excess related to class IC antiarrhythmic-induced heart failure
- Knowledge deficit related to the prescribed class IC antiarrhythmic

Planning and implementation

- Do not administer a class IC antiarrhythmic to a patient with a condition that contraindicates its use.
- Administer a class IC antiarrhythmic cautiously to a patient at risk because of a preexisting condition.
- Monitor the patient closely for adverse reactions, especially CNS, cardiovascular, or GI disturbances. Reassure the patient that a dosage reduction may relieve adverse CNS reactions. (See Patient Teaching: *Class IC antiarrhythmics.*)
- Monitor the patient for drug interactions.

* ***Monitor the ECG continuously for a critical care patient when beginning or adjusting class IC antiarrhythmic therapy. Notify the physician if the original arrhythmia worsens, a new arrhythmia occurs, or the PR interval, QRS complex, or QT interval becomes excessively prolonged; the drug's arrhythmogenic effects may be misinterpreted as recurrence or spontaneous worsening of the original arrhythmia.***

- Monitor the patient's vital signs regularly, particularly noting an irregular heartbeat or hypotension.
- Monitor for additive effects in a patient who is receiving another antiarrhythmic agent.
- Observe the patient receiving digoxin with flecainide or propafenone for signs of digitalis toxicity.
- Make dosage adjustments several days apart, as prescribed, when administering a class IC antiarrhythmic. Expect to administer a lower dosage of flecainide, as prescribed, to a patient with renal or hepatic impairment.

* ***Monitor the patient closely for signs of heart failure, such as increasing shortness of breath, crackles, jugular venous distention, and peripheral edema.***

- Limit the patient's fluid and salt intake to decrease fluid retention, as prescribed.
- Record the patient's fluid intake and output to detect fluid retention.

• Notify the physician if the patient's condition does not improve or if adverse reactions or drug interactions occur.

Evaluation

For each nursing diagnosis, prepare an evaluation statement that describes the patient's or family's response to nursing interventions.

Class II antiarrhythmics

Class II antiarrhythmics are the beta-adrenergic blockers. Acebutolol hydrochloride, esmolol hydrochloride, and propranolol hydrochloride are antiarrhythmics approved by the Food and Drug Administration (FDA).

PHARMACOKINETICS

Acebutolol and propranolol are absorbed almost entirely from the GI tract after oral administration. Administered intravenously, esmolol is immediately available systemically.

Acebutolol, which has low lipid solubility, does not cross the blood-brain barrier. Distributed widely, propranolol has high lipid solubility and crosses readily. Esmolol is distributed rapidly throughout all body tissues. Acebutolol is 26% protein-bound in plasma; esmolol, about 55% protein-bound; and propranolol, 90% protein-bound.

Acebutolol and propranolol significantly bind to hepatic binding sites during first-pass metabolism, with propranolol being metabolized almost completely in the liver. Esmolol is hydrolyzed primarily in the cytosol of red blood cells and secondarily in highly perfused tissues.

About 35% of an acebutolol dose is excreted in the urine and 55% is excreted in the feces. Most of an esmolol dose is metabolized to an inactive metabolite, which is excreted in the urine. Only a small amount of unchanged drug is excreted in the urine (less than 2%) and possibly in the feces (less than 5%). Propranolol's metabolites are excreted in the urine.

The half-life of acebutolol is 6 to 12 hours; of esmolol, 5 to 23 minutes; of propranolol, 3.4 to 6 hours.

Route	Onset	Peak	Duration
P.O.	30 min	60-90 min	3-8 hr
P.O. (sustained release)	Unknown	Unknown	24 hr
I.V.	<5 min	Unknown	20-30 min

PHARMACODYNAMICS

Acebutolol, esmolol, and propranolol suppress arrhythmias by several different mechanisms of action. The drugs block receptor sites in the conduction system of the heart, thereby slowing automaticity of the SA node and the conductivity of the AV node and other cells. These effects probably convert unidirectional block to bidirectional block. The class II antiarrhythmics also exert a significant negative inotropic effect. By decreasing myocardial oxygen demand, this action also may decrease myocardial ischemia. As ischemia abates, myocardial cells lose their automaticity, and this effect suppresses atrial and ventricular ectopy.

PHARMACOTHERAPEUTICS

The class II drugs are not the drugs of choice to treat arrhythmias, in part because of their multiple effects and because of possible breakthrough ectopy. The use of these agents with other antiarrhythmics remains to be evaluated.

Drug interactions

Class II antiarrhythmics interact with phenothiazines and antihypertensive drugs, which potentiate hypotension. Interactions with anticholinergics and cimetidine alter the effects of class II antiarrhythmic drugs. (See Drug Interactions: *Class II antiarrhythmics*, page 238.)

ADVERSE DRUG REACTIONS

The most common adverse reactions to class II antiarrhythmics involve the cardiovascular system and usually occur when the drugs are first given. Because they inhibit sinus node stimulation, class II antiarrhythmics may produce bradycardia — a heart rate less than 60 beats/minute. Hypotension with peripheral vascular insufficiency also may occur, especially with esmolol. Syncope, angina, and shock may accompany these reactions. Occasionally, fluid retention and peripheral edema occur. Because class II antiarrhythmics reduce the force of myocardial contraction and increase preload, they may exacerbate or precipitate heart failure. Arrhythmias, especially AV block, also may occur.

Adverse CNS reactions include dizziness, confusion, fatigue, lassitude, and decreased libido. Typical GI reactions, such as nausea, vomiting, mild diarrhea, or constipation, usually are transient.

Acebutolol and propranolol block bronchial beta-receptors that otherwise dilate bronchioles; this action can lead to significant bronchoconstriction. Propranolol is more likely to cause this adverse reaction because it is a nonselective beta-adrenergic blocker. I.V. infusions of esmolol cause inflammation and induration at the injection site in about 80% of patients.

Other reactions to class II antiarrhythmics include rashes, blood dyscrasias, depression, and vivid dreams. These reactions, however, are rare.

NURSING PROCESS APPLICATION

The following information assists the nurse in caring for a patient who is receiving a class II antiarrhythmic. It includes an overview of assessment activities as well as examples of

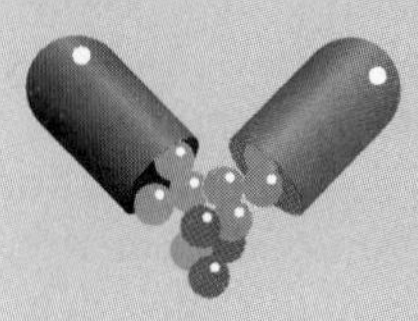

DRUG INTERACTIONS

Class II antiarrhythmics

Class II antiarrhythmics interact with several commonly administered drugs. To provide the best possible patient care, the nurse should be aware of these interactions and their implications.

DRUG	INTERACTING AGENTS	POSSIBLE EFFECTS	NURSING IMPLICATIONS
acebutolol, esmolol, propranolol	phenothiazines, antihypertensives	Increased hypotension	• Monitor the patient for dizziness and orthostatic hypotension.
	sympathomimetics (beta agonists)	Decreased sympathomimetic effect	• Monitor the patient for decreased therapeutic effect.
	anticholinergics	Potentiation of pressor effects, resulting in hypertension; reduced efficacy of the class II antiarrhythmics	• Monitor the patient's therapeutic response, heart rate and rhythm, and blood pressure.
	neuromuscular blockers	Enhanced skeletal muscle relaxation	• Monitor the patient for hypoventilation when administering class II antiarrhythmics in the immediate postoperative period.
	verapamil	Increased cardiac depression	• Monitor the patient for decreased heart rate.
	sulfonylureas	Reduced hypoglycemic effects	• Monitor the patient's glucose level and adjust the sulfonylurea dosage, as prescribed.
esmolol	digoxin	Increased serum digoxin concentration	• Monitor the patient's serum digoxin concentration. • Assess for signs of digitalis toxicity, such as cardiovascular, central nervous system, and GI disturbances.
	morphine	Increased blood esmolol concentration	• Monitor the patient for signs of esmolol toxicity, such as hypotension, bradycardia, and decreased level of consciousness.
propranolol	cimetidine	Decreased propranolol metabolism	• Observe the patient for adverse reactions even at low dosages of propranolol.

appropriate nursing diagnoses and related interventions. It also highlights the importance of evaluation.

Assessment

Before drug therapy begins, review the patient's history for conditions that contraindicate or require cautious use of the prescribed class II antiarrhythmic. Also review the patient's medication history to identify use of drugs that may interact with it. During therapy, assess the patient for adverse drug reactions and signs of drug interactions. Also, periodically assess the effectiveness of class II antiarrhythmic therapy. Finally, evaluate the patient's and family's knowledge about the prescribed drug. (See Patient Teaching: *Class II antiarrhythmics.*)

Nursing diagnoses

- Risk for injury related to a preexisting condition that contraindicates or requires cautious use of a class II antiarrhythmic
- Risk for injury related to adverse drug reactions or drug interactions
- Fluid volume excess related to fluid retention caused by the prescribed class II antiarrhythmic
- Knowledge deficit related to the prescribed class II antiarrhythmic

Planning and implementation

- Do not administer a class II antiarrhythmic to a patient with a condition that contraindicates its use.
- Administer a class II antiarrhythmic cautiously to a patient at risk because of a preexisting condition.

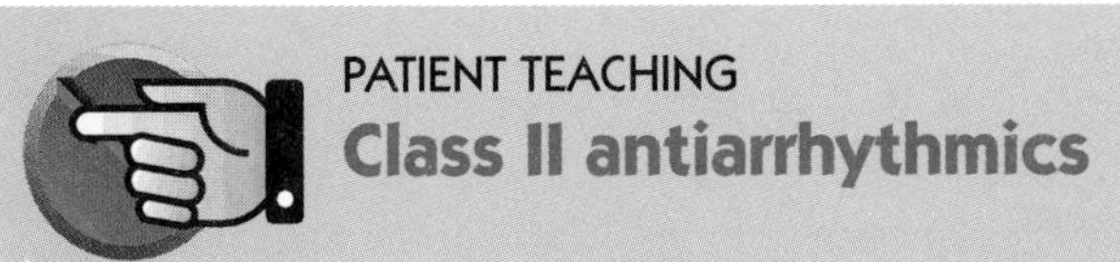

- Teach the patient and family the name, dose, frequency, action, and adverse effects of the prescribed class II antiarrhythmic.
- Demonstrate how to take a pulse. Tell the patient to check the pulse before each dose of the prescribed antiarrhythmic. If the pulse is slow (below 60 beats/minute or the rate selected by the physician), advise the patient to withhold the dose and notify the physician.
- Instruct the patient not to perform activities that require alertness if dizziness, fatigue, lassitude, or confusion occurs.
- Reassure the patient that libido, which may decrease during drug therapy, should return to normal when the drug is discontinued.
- Instruct the patient to notify the physician if nausea, vomiting, diarrhea, or constipation occurs. A prescription for an antiemetic, antidiarrheal, or laxative agent may be needed.
- Stress the importance of limiting fluid and salt intake to minimize fluid retention.
- Advise the patient to notify the physician if adverse reactions occur.

***** ***Monitor the patient closely for cardiovascular and other adverse reactions, especially when therapy first begins. Throughout therapy, monitor the patient closely for signs of fluid retention, such as peripheral edema, crackles, weight gain, shortness of breath, wheezing, or bronchospasm.***
- Monitor the patient's ECG to detect arrhythmias, especially AV block and bradycardia.
- Take the patient's vital signs, as prescribed. Particularly note decreased heart rate or blood pressure, especially during esmolol therapy.
- Withhold the dose and notify the physician if the pulse is less than 60 beats/minute or the systolic blood pressure is less than 90 mm Hg.
- Observe the esmolol infusion site for signs of inflammation and induration. Use an infusion pump when administering esmolol to control dosage titration. Carefully inspect the esmolol solution before administering. Discard the solution if it contains particles or is discolored. Monitor the heart rate and blood pressure continuously during esmolol infusion.
- Observe the patient receiving esmolol and digoxin concurrently for signs of digitalis toxicity.
- Notify the physician if the patient's condition does not improve or if adverse reactions (including fluid retention) or drug interactions occur.
- Teach the patient about the prescribed agents.

Evaluation

For each nursing diagnosis, prepare an evaluation statement that describes the patient's or family's response to nursing interventions.

Class III antiarrhythmics

The class III antiarrhythmics amiodarone hydrochloride and bretylium tosylate are used to treat ventricular arrhythmias.

PHARMACOKINETICS

After oral administration, amiodarone is absorbed slowly at widely varying rates. The drug is distributed extensively and accumulates in many sites, especially in highly vascular organs and adipose tissue. It is 96% protein-bound in plasma, mainly to albumin. Amiodarone probably is metabolized in the liver, and possibly in the intestinal lumen or GI mucosa, to at least one major metabolite with antiarrhythmic activity. The drug undergoes biliary excretion and is eliminated almost completely in feces.

Bretylium's erratic GI absorption mandates parenteral administration. Data about its distribution and protein binding are lacking. Bretylium is excreted unchanged by the kidneys over several days.

Amiodarone's onset of action may begin within 2 to 3 days in some patients, but usually does not occur until 1 to 3 weeks after therapy begins. After oral administration of amiodarone, the peak concentration level occurs within 3 to 7 hours. If a loading dose is not given, a steady-state concentration of amiodarone is not attained for at least 1 month and usually not for 5 months or longer. Effects of amiodarone may persist for weeks or even months after discontinuation. Amiodarone has an initial half-life of 2½ to 10 days and an average terminal half-life of 53 days.

In a patient with ventricular fibrillation, bretylium's onset begins within minutes of I.V. infusion. When the drug is given to suppress ventricular ectopy and ventricular tachycardia, however, the onset takes 20 minutes to 2 hours. Peak plasma concentration of bretylium occurs immediately after I.V. infusion and within 1 hour of I.M. administration. Bretylium's therapeutic serum level is 0.5 to 1.5 mcg/ml, its duration of action is 6 to 24 hours, and its half-life is 5 to 10 hours.

Route	Onset	Peak	Duration
P.O.	2 days-3 wk	3-7 hr	Weeks-months
I.M.	30 min	1 hr	6-24 hr
I.V.	Minutes-2 hr	Minutes-hours	6-24 hr

PHARMACODYNAMICS

The exact mechanism of action of class III antiarrhythmics that is most responsible for the antiarrhythmic effects remains uncertain. They may convert unidirectional block to bidirectional block, but they have little or no effect on depolarization. Amiodarone may decrease intracardiac conduction, as shown by increased PR and QT intervals; the QRS complex may be unchanged or increased. Bretylium does not prolong these intervals. However, bretylium exerts

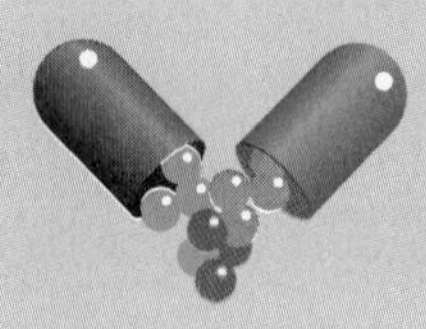

DRUG INTERACTIONS

Class III antiarrhythmics

Class III antiarrhythmics interact with several commonly administered drugs. To provide the best possible patient care, the nurse should be aware of these interactions and their implications.

DRUG	INTERACTING AGENTS	POSSIBLE EFFECTS	NURSING IMPLICATIONS
bretylium	sympathomimetics	Profound hypotension	• Monitor the patient for dizziness, orthostatic hypotension, and mental status changes.
bretylium, amiodarone	antihypertensives	Profound hypotension	• Monitor the patient for dizziness, orthostatic hypotension, and mental status changes.
amiodarone	warfarin	Increased hypoprothrombinemia	• Monitor the patient for increased bruising, bleeding, and I.V. site oozing; monitor prothrombin time.
	digoxin	Increased serum digoxin level	• Monitor the patient for signs of digitalis toxicity, such as anorexia, nausea, vomiting, diarrhea, visual disturbances, and arrhythmias.
	procainamide, quinidine, phenytoin	Increased serum antiarrhythmic concentration	• Monitor serum antiarrhythmic concentration; assess for increased antiarrhythmic effect.

a positive inotropic effect. Both drugs produce some peripheral and coronary vasodilation.

PHARMACOTHERAPEUTICS

In part because of their adverse effects, class III antiarrhythmics are not the drugs of choice for antiarrhythmic therapy. The drugs produce synergistic effects when combined with certain other antiarrhythmics.

Drug interactions

Significant interactions with other cardiovascular drugs, such as digoxin and antihypertensives vary. Interactions are more serious with amiodarone than with short-term bretylium therapy. Amiodarone increases quinidine, procainamide, and phenytoin levels and prolongs the prothrombin time — and may cause bleeding — in patients receiving coumadin. Bretylium cannot be given with epinephrine, norepinephrine, or other sympathomimetics. Bretylium may potentiate the effects of the drugs given to correct hypotension. (See Drug Interactions: *Class III antiarrhythmics.*)

ADVERSE DRUG REACTIONS

Adverse reactions to class III antiarrhythmics, especially amiodarone, vary widely and commonly lead to drug discontinuation.

Amiodarone may produce hypotension, nausea, and anorexia. It causes adverse CNS reactions in 20% to 40% of patients, including malaise, fatigue, tremor, involuntary movements, lack of coordination, abnormal gait, ataxia, dizziness, and paresthesia. Rarely, peripheral neuropathy and proximal myopathy occur.

Amiodarone causes several non-dose-related reactions. Pulmonary toxicity consisting of interstitial pneumonia and alveolitis occurs in 15% of patients and can be fatal; signs and symptoms include dyspnea, cough, and changes in X-ray findings. Corneal microdeposits occur in almost all patients, but only 10% experience visual disturbances. The deposits disappear with dosage reduction or drug discontinuation. Skin photosensitivity occurs, sometimes producing a blue-gray discoloration of exposed skin. The metabolic effects of amiodarone can produce hypothyroidism or hyperthyroidism.

Like most antiarrhythmics, amiodarone and bretylium can aggravate arrhythmias, especially bradycardia, and increase ventricular ectopic beats.

Upon initial bretylium administration, orthostatic and supine hypotension commonly occur, producing dizziness. Nausea and vomiting commonly accompany rapid I.V. administration.

NURSING PROCESS APPLICATION

The following information assists the nurse in caring for a patient who is receiving a class III antiarrhythmic. It includes an overview of assessment activities as well as examples of appropriate nursing diagnoses and related interventions. It also highlights the importance of evaluation.

Assessment

Before drug therapy begins, review the patient's history for conditions that contraindicate or require cautious use of the

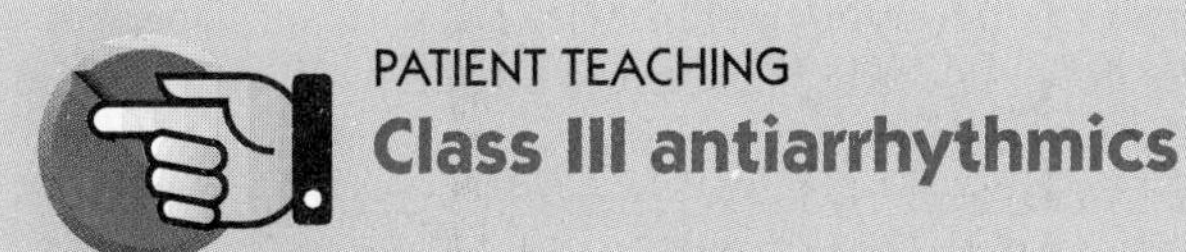

PATIENT TEACHING
Class III antiarrhythmics

- Teach the patient and family the name, dose, frequency, action, and adverse effects of the prescribed class III antiarrhythmic.
- Demonstrate how to take a pulse. Tell the patient to check the pulse before each dose of amiodarone and to notify the physician if the pulse falls below 60 beats/minute (or the rate selected by the physician) or becomes irregular.
- Instruct the patient receiving amiodarone to avoid activities that require alertness or coordination, if adverse central nervous system reactions occur.
- Advise the patient to consult with the physician about obtaining a prescription for an antiemetic if nausea or vomiting occurs.
- Inform the patient that the prescribed amiodarone dosage will be high for the first several weeks and then decreased gradually to a maintenance dosage.
- Instruct the patient taking amiodarone to notify the physician if signs of pulmonary toxicity occur, such as dyspnea or persistent cough.
- Teach the patient to recognize and report to the physician signs or symptoms of hypothyroidism or hyperthyroidism during amiodarone therapy.
- Teach the patient taking amiodarone to use protective clothing and sunscreen products or to avoid sunlight to protect against photosensitivity.
- Reassure the patient that corneal microdeposits produce visual disturbances in only 10% of all patients receiving amiodarone. However, tell the patient to notify the physician if visual changes occur.
- Advise the patient to notify the physician if adverse reactions occur.

prescribed class III antiarrhythmic. Also review the patient's medication history to identify use of drugs that may interact with it. During therapy, assess the patient for adverse drug reactions and signs of drug interactions. Also, periodically assess the effectiveness of class III antiarrhythmic therapy. Finally, evaluate the patient's and family's knowledge about the prescribed drug. (See Patient Teaching: *Class III antiarrhythmics.*)

Nursing diagnoses

• Risk for injury related to a preexisting condition that contraindicates or requires cautious use of a class III antiarrhythmic
• Risk for injury related to adverse drug reactions or drug interactions
• Ineffective breathing pattern related to amiodarone-induced pulmonary toxicity
• Knowledge deficit related to the prescribed class III antiarrhythmic

Planning and implementation

• Do not administer a class III antiarrhythmic to a patient with a condition that contraindicates its use.
• Administer a class III antiarrhythmic cautiously to a patient at risk because of a preexisting condition.
• Monitor the patient closely for adverse reactions and drug interactions during class III antiarrhythmic therapy.
*** *Monitor the patient's ECG. Be especially alert for bradycardia, increased ventricular ectopic beats, or, with amiodarone therapy, prolonged PR interval, QRS complex, and QT interval.***
*** *Monitor the patient receiving amiodarone closely for signs of pulmonary toxicity, such as dyspnea, cough, and changes in X-ray findings that show interstitial pneumonia or alveolitis. If the patient displays these signs, notify the physician and expect to discontinue amiodarone. Continue to monitor the patient for several months after amiodarone discontinuation; its effects may persist for weeks or months.***
• Take the patient's vital signs frequently, particularly noting a slow or irregular pulse or hypotension.
• Observe the patient receiving a class III antiarrhythmic and another antiarrhythmic for additive effects. Monitor the patient closely during concomitant therapy with a class III antiarrhythmic and another cardiovascular drug, such as digoxin or an antihypertensive.
• Notify the physician if the patient's condition does not improve or if adverse reactions or drug interactions occur.
• Place the patient with pulmonary toxicity in a position that enhances breathing.
• Prepare to treat pulmonary toxicity, as ordered; for example, by administering oxygen and antibiotics.
• Teach the patient about the prescribed agent.

Evaluation

For each nursing diagnosis, prepare an evaluation statement that describes the patient's or family's response to nursing interventions.

Class IV antiarrhythmics

Among the class IV antiarrhythmics, or calcium channel blockers, verapamil and diltiazem produce similar effects and are used to treat the same arrhythmias.

PHARMACOKINETICS

After oral administration, verapamil is about 90% absorbed, but its bioavailability is only 20% to 35% because of extensive first-pass metabolism. After oral or I.V. administration, the drug is 90% protein-bound. It is metabolized rapidly and almost completely in the liver to numerous metabolites, including the only active one — norverapamil. Verapamil metabolites are excreted primarily in the urine and to a lesser extent in the feces.

After oral administration, diltiazem is about 80% absorbed. However, only 40% of the drug reaches the systemic circulation because of extensive first-pass metabolism. The drug is metabolized rapidly and almost completely to one active and numerous inactive metabolites. About 24% of

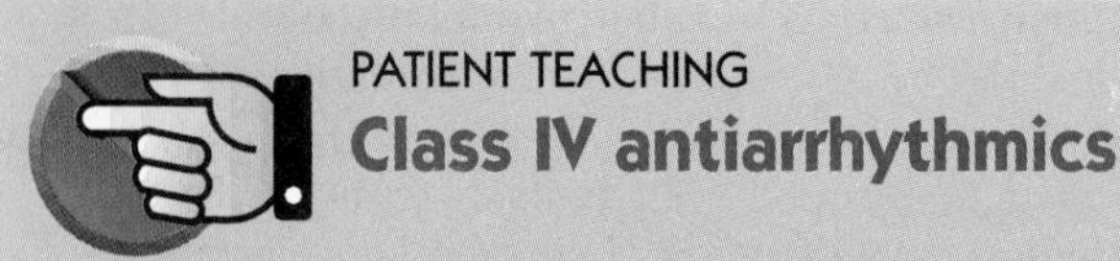

PATIENT TEACHING
Class IV antiarrhythmics

- Teach the patient and family the name, dose, frequency, action, and adverse effects of the prescribed class IV antiarrhythmic.
- Advise the patient to tell all personal physicians about class IV antiarrhythmic therapy to prevent drug interactions.
- Instruct the patient how to manage orthostatic hypotension.
- Caution the patient to avoid activities that require alertness if dizziness or weakness occurs.
- Teach the patient how to manage constipation, headache, and muscle cramps.
- Teach the patient to minimize fluid retention by limiting fluid and salt intake and to report to the physician signs of fluid retention, such as increasing shortness of breath or ankle swelling.
- Instruct the patient to notify the physician if adverse reactions occur.

the drug is excreted unchanged in urine; the remainder is eliminated as metabolites in the urine and feces.

Verapamil's half-life is 3 to 7 hours, but this may increase to 4.5 to 12 hours after long-term oral therapy, probably because of hepatic enzyme saturation. Diltiazem's half-life is 3.5 to 9 hours.

Route	Onset	Peak	Duration
P.O.	30 min	1-3 hr	<6 hr
P.O. (extended release)	Unknown	6-11 hr	Unknown
I.V.	5 min	10 min	Unknown

PHARMACODYNAMICS

Verapamil and diltiazem block the influx of calcium across the myocardial cell membrane. This blockade greatly increases the effective refractory period of the AV node and slows the conduction rate between the atria and the ventricles. Although these agents rarely affect normal sinus node function, they may reduce the resting heart rate and produce sinus arrest or sinus block in patients with SA node disease.

PHARMACOTHERAPEUTICS

Verapamil and diltiazem are used to treat supraventricular arrhythmias with rapid ventricular response rates.

Drug interactions

Verapamil and diltiazem interact with other antiarrhythmics, producing additive effects. (See Patient Teaching: *Class IV antiarrhythmics.*) Interactions with antihypertensives potentiate hypotension and heart failure; with digoxin, an increased serum digoxin level and digitalis toxicity may result. Concomitant use of verapamil and other highly protein-bound drugs, such as hydantoins, salicylates, sulfonamides, and sulfonylureas, can cause adverse reactions associated with verapamil or the other drugs. Verapamil and diltiazem competitively inhibit liver enzyme metabolism of other drugs. Conversely, drugs that inhibit (cimetidine) or stimulate (rifampin) liver enzymes may interact with these agents. For example, concomitant use of cimetidine may decrease the antiarrhythmic's metabolism; rifampin may increase it.

ADVERSE DRUG REACTIONS

Verapamil and diltiazem may cause alterations in the cardiovascular system. These drugs sometimes cause hypotension, particularly orthostatic hypotension. Hypotension usually is associated with I.V. verapamil, especially with rapid I.V. bolus administration or administration to patients with rapid, narrow, complex arrhythmias such as ventricular tachycardia. The class IV antiarrhythmics' effect on the SA and AV nodes causes arrhythmias, such as bradycardia, sinus block, and AV block. These drugs also depress myocardial contraction force, which may precipitate or exacerbate heart failure.

Vasodilation produced by these agents occasionally causes dizziness, headache, flushing, weakness, and persistent peripheral edema. Other dose-related reactions include constipation and other GI disturbances, leg fatigue, and muscle cramps.

Hypersensitivity reactions include worsening of angina, skin eruptions, photosensitivity, pruritus, nasal congestion, and mood changes.

NURSING PROCESS APPLICATION

The following information assists the nurse in caring for a patient who is receiving a class IV antiarrhythmic. It includes an overview of assessment activities as well as examples of appropriate nursing diagnoses and related interventions. It also highlights the importance of evaluation.

Assessment

Before drug therapy begins, review the patient's history for conditions that contraindicate or require cautious use of the prescribed class IV antiarrhythmic. Also review the patient's medication history to identify use of drugs that may interact with it. During therapy, assess the patient for adverse drug reactions and signs of drug interactions. Also, periodically assess the effectiveness of class IV antiarrhythmic therapy. Finally, evaluate the patient's and family's knowledge about the prescribed drug.

Nursing diagnoses

- Risk for injury related to a preexisting condition that contraindicates or requires cautious use of a class IV antiarrhythmic
- Risk for injury related to adverse drug reactions or drug interactions
- Fluid volume excess related to the adverse myocardial effects of the prescribed class IV antiarrhythmic
- Knowledge deficit related to the prescribed class IV antiarrhythmic

Planning and implementation

- Do not administer a class IV antiarrhythmic to a patient with a condition that contraindicates its use.
- Administer a class IV antiarrhythmic cautiously to a patient at risk because of a preexisting condition.
- Monitor the patient closely for adverse cardiovascular and other reactions and drug interactions.
- Monitor the patient's vital signs frequently. Take a resting apical pulse in a patient with SA node disease because class IV antiarrhythmics can reduce the resting heart rate in such a patient.

***Monitor the patient's ECG continuously while giving I.V. verapamil, being especially alert for SA or AV node effects, such as bradycardia, sinus block, and AV block.**

- Be alert for hypotension or heart failure in a patient receiving a class IV antiarrhythmic and an antihypertensive agent.
- Be alert for digitalis toxicity in a patient receiving a class IV antiarrhythmic and a digitalis compound.
- Notify the physician if the patient's condition does not improve or if adverse reactions or drug interactions occur.
- Monitor the patient closely for signs of fluid retention, such as increasing shortness of breath, crackles, jugular venous distention, or persistent peripheral edema.
- Limit the patient's salt and fluid intake to minimize fluid retention, as prescribed.
- Inform the physician immediately if the patient displays signs of fluid volume excess.
- Prepare to relieve fluid retention with the prescribed treatment such as diuretic administration.
- Teach the patient about the prescribed agent.

Evaluation

For each nursing diagnosis, prepare an evaluation statement that describes the patient's or family's response to nursing interventions.

Adenosine

Adenosine is an injectable antiarrhythmic agent indicated for acute treatment of PSVTs, including those associated with accessory bypass tracts, as in Wolff-Parkinson-White syndrome.

PHARMACOKINETICS

After I.V. administration, adenosine probably is distributed rapidly throughout the body and metabolized inside red blood cells as well as in vascular endothelial cells.

The half-life of adenosine is extremely short and may range from 0.6 to 10 seconds. An I.V. bolus of adenosine is removed completely from plasma in about 30 to 60 seconds. Most tachycardias terminate within 30 seconds after a bolus.

Route	Onset	Peak	Duration
I.V.	Immediate	30 sec	< 2 min

PHARMACODYNAMICS

Adenosine depresses pacemaker activity of the SA node and conductivity of the AV node. It produces negative chronotropic (bradycardia) and negative dromotropic (AV block) effects on the heart.

PHARMACOTHERAPEUTICS

Adenosine is available only as an I.V. preparation to treat arrhythmias. It is especially effective against reentry tachycardias that involve the AV node and is effective with more than 90% of PSVTs.

Drug interactions

When adenosine is administered concurrently with carbamazepine, the additive cardiovascular effects may increase the degree of heart block. Dipyridamole potentiates the effects of adenosine; therefore, smaller doses of adenosine may be necessary. Methylxanthines, such as caffeine and theophylline, antagonize the effects of adenosine; larger doses of adenosine may be necessary.

ADVERSE DRUG REACTIONS

Adverse reactions reported during clinical trials in more than 5% of patients include facial flushing, shortness of breath, dyspnea, and chest discomfort.

NURSING PROCESS APPLICATION

The following information assists the nurse in caring for a patient who is receiving adenosine. It includes an overview of assessment activities as well as examples of appropriate nursing diagnoses and related interventions. It also highlights the importance of evaluation.

Assessment

Before drug therapy begins, review the patient's history for conditions that contraindicate or require cautious use of adenosine. Also review the patient's medication history to

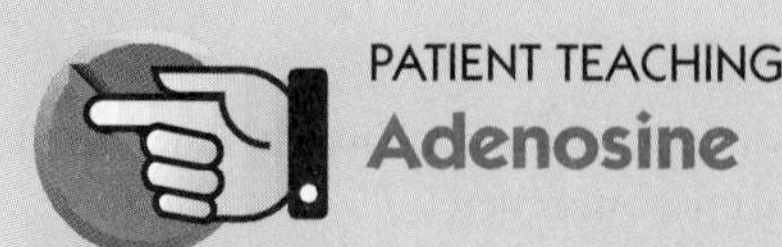

PATIENT TEACHING
Adenosine

- Teach the patient and family the name, dose, frequency, action, and adverse effects of adenosine.
- Advise the patient to tell the nurse if shortness of breath, dyspnea, or chest discomfort occurs.

identify use of drugs that may interact with it. During therapy, assess the patient for adverse drug reactions and signs of drug interactions. Also, periodically assess the effectiveness of adenosine therapy. Finally, evaluate the patient's and family's knowledge about the prescribed drug. (See Patient Teaching: *Adenosine.*)

Nursing diagnoses

- Risk for injury related to a preexisting condition that contraindicates or requires cautious use of adenosine
- Risk for injury related to adverse drug reactions or drug interactions
- Knowledge deficit related to adenosine

Planning and implementation

- Do not administer adenosine to a patient with a condition that contraindicates its use.
- Administer adenosine cautiously to a patient at risk because of a preexisting condition.
- Monitor the patient closely for adverse reactions and drug interactions during adenosine therapy.
- Administer adenosine as a rapid I.V. bolus only. If the drug must be given through an I.V. line, administer it as proximal as possible to the I.V. injection site and follow with a rapid saline flush.

* ***Monitor the patient's respiratory rate and pattern continuously to detect changes during adenosine administration.***
* ***Monitor the patient's ECG continuously during adenosine administration. Keep in mind that new rhythms may appear on the ECG during conversion to the normal sinus rhythm. These usually last for only a few seconds and do not require treatment. However, be prepared to treat heart block if it develops and persists. Be especially alert for heart block in a patient who also is receiving carbamazepine.***

- Expect to administer smaller doses of adenosine as prescribed if the patient also is receiving dipyridamole; higher doses as prescribed if the patient also is taking a methylxanthine.
- Inform the physician about the patient's cardiac status throughout adenosine therapy.
- Teach the patient about the prescribed agent.

Evaluation

For each nursing diagnosis, prepare an evaluation statement that describes the patient's or family's response to nursing interventions.

CHAPTER SUMMARY

Chapter 18 discussed antiarrhythmic agents. These drugs are used to treat abnormal electrical activity in the heart. Here are the highlights of the chapter.

Antiarrhythmics are divided into the following classes: Class I, Class IA, Class IB, Class IC, Class II, Class III, and Class IV.

Adenosine does not fall into any of these classes, but pharmacologically resembles the calcium channel blockers verapamil and diltiazem.

The different classes of antiarrhythmics have widely varying mechanisms of action but also share some pharmacologic properties. They possess different pharmacokinetics and pharmacodynamics and are used to treat different arrhythmias.

Administration of antiarrhythmics requires the nurse to monitor closely such data as heart rate and rhythm, blood pressure, plasma drug level (if appropriate), and interactions with other medications.

Questions to consider

See Appendix 1 for answers.

1. Ernest Parks, age 61, develops sustained ventricular tachycardia 3 days after experiencing an acute myocardial infarction. The physician prescribes moricizine hydrochloride (Ethmozine) 200 mg P.O. every 8 hours. While caring for Mr. Parks, the nurse monitors his response to moricizine and assesses him for adverse reactions. What is the most serious adverse reaction that can occur with this drug?
   (a) Arrhythmias
   (b) Hypoesthesia
   (c) Dyspnea
   (d) Seizures

2. Robert Gliboff, age 58, suffers a massive myocardial infarction and is admitted to the coronary care unit. Shortly after his admission, the nurse observes frequent premature ventricular beats on his ECG monitor. According to hospital protocol, she administers lidocaine (Xylocaine) 50 mg I.V. bolus. How soon should she administer a second bolus of the drug before initiating a continuous I.V. infusion of lidocaine?
   (a) 1 minute
   (b) 2 minutes
   (c) 5 minutes
   (d) 10 minutes

3. Loretta Danforth, age 75, is admitted to the coronary care unit with atrial fibrillation. The physician initially prescribes quinidine sulfate (Quinora) 300 mg P.O. every 6 hours. Sixteen hours later, the atrial fibrillation converts to normal sinus rhythm. To maintain this rhythm, the physician decreases the dosage of quinidine to 200 mg P.O. every 6 hours. The nurse monitors Ms. Danforth's serum quinidine concentration level closely for toxicity. What is the normal therapeutic range for quinidine?
   (a) 0.5 to 1 mcg/ml
   (b) 2 to 6 mcg/ml
   (c) 7 to 12 mcg/ml
   (d) 15 to 20 mcg/ml

4. Ruth Barnes, age 69, receives propranolol (Inderal) for ventricular tachycardia. During propranolol therapy, she is particularly susceptible to which of the following adverse drug reactions?
   (a) Tachycardia
   (b) Hypertension
   (c) Insomnia
   (d) Bronchoconstriction

5. James Wilson, age 66, has tachycardia that does not respond to propranolol. So the physician prescribes amiodarone (Cordarone). Before administering this class III antiarrhythmic, the nurse reviews Mr. Wilson's medication history. Which of the following drugs is most likely to interact with amiodarone?
   (a) digoxin
   (b) verapamil
   (c) morphine
   (d) theophylline

6. For Joan Morgan, age 57, the physician prescribes verapamil (Isoptin) to prevent the recurrence of supraventricular tachycardia. Which of the following statements best describes the action of verapamil?
   (a) It blocks sodium influx into myocardial cells.
   (b) It blocks calcium influx into myocardial cells.
   (c) It blocks potassium flow out of myocardial cells.
   (d) It blocks beta-receptor sites on myocardial cells.

19 Antianginal agents

OBJECTIVES

After reading and studying this chapter, the student should be able to:

1. identify the mechanisms of action and clinical indications for nitrates, beta-adrenergic blockers, and calcium channel blockers.
2. explain how routes of administration influence the onset of action and clinical uses of different nitrates.
3. list the most significant drug interactions and adverse reactions associated with various antianginal agents.
4. describe how to apply the nursing process when caring for a patient who is receiving an antianginal agent.

INTRODUCTION

To pump effectively, the heart needs its own blood supply, which the coronary arteries provide. These arteries originate from the aorta at the ostia situated above the cusps of the aortic valve (the sinus of Valsalva). From there, the arteries branch out to cover and penetrate all parts of the cardiac muscle, or myocardium. After delivering oxygen and nutrients throughout the myocardium, the blood moves through large coronary veins and returns to the right atrium via the coronary sinus. The myocardium cannot extract oxygen from blood inside the chambers of the heart; instead, it depends on blood from the coronary arteries for its supply of oxygen and nutrients.

Even when the body is at rest, the percentage of oxygen extracted from coronary arterial blood by the myocardium is high, approximately 80%. During exercise or other exertion, the amount of blood flowing through the coronary arteries must increase significantly to meet the increased myocardial demand for oxygen. This additional oxygen normally is provided by an increase in aortic blood pressure and by local factors that dilate the coronary arteries during a process called *autoregulation.*

When the myocardial oxygen demand exceeds the myocardial oxygen supply, areas become ischemic, causing chest pain. When the patient experiences symptoms from this myocardial ischemia, the condition is known as *angina* or *angina pectoris.*

Angina usually takes one of three main forms:

- Stable angina (also called predictable or chronic angina), in which pain occurs at a predictable level of physical or emotional stress, builds gradually, and reaches maximum intensity quickly.
- Unstable angina (also called preinfarction or crescendo angina, acute coronary insufficiency, or impending myocardial infarction [MI]), in which pain takes an unpredictable course and is more severe than in stable angina.
- Prinzmetal's angina (also called variant angina), in which pain usually occurs while the patient is at rest and resembles that of unstable angina. Occasionally, a patient may have stable and Prinzmetal's angina.

Although angina's cardinal symptom is chest pain, the drugs used to treat angina are not analgesics. The antianginal agents discussed in this chapter — nitrates, beta-adrenergic blockers, and calcium channel blockers — are used to treat angina by reducing myocardial oxygen demand, by increasing myocardial oxygen supply, or both. The nitrates and calcium channel blockers also treat angina by dilating the coronary arteries, which increases the myocardial oxygen supply. (See *How antianginal agents relieve angina.*)

Drugs covered in this chapter include:

- amlodipine besylate
- atenolol
- diltiazem hydrochloride
- erythrityl tetranitrate
- isosorbide dinitrate and mononitrate
- metoprolol tartrate
- nadolol
- nicardipine hydrochloride
- nifedipine
- nitroglycerin
- pentaerythritol tetranitrate
- propranolol hydrochloride
- verapamil hydrochloride.

Combination therapy with drugs from different classes of antianginal agents is indicated for symptoms that persist despite therapy with one or more drugs from a single class. Combining drugs from different classes provides antianginal effects from different mechanisms of action and reduces the risk of adverse reactions from high dosages of any one drug.

Combination therapy also is used to control different types of angina occurring in one patient. For example, a patient might take a beta-adrenergic blocker or a calcium channel blocker for long-term treatment of angina and supplement this therapy with rapid-acting nitrates for unusual,

How antianginal agents relieve angina

Angina occurs when the coronary arteries, the heart's primary source of oxygen, supply insufficient oxygen to the myocardium. This increases the heart's workload, increasing heart rate, preload (blood volume in ventricle at end of diastole), afterload (pressure in arteries leading from ventricle), and force of myocardial contractility. The antianginal agents (nitrates, beta-adrenergic blockers, and calcium channel blockers) relieve angina by *decreasing* one or more of these four factors. This diagram summarizes how antianginal agents affect the cardiovascular system.

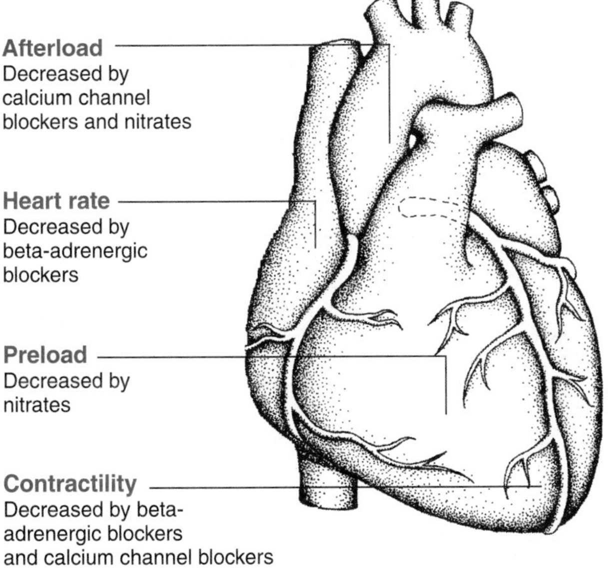

strenuous demands. Beta-adrenergic blockers prevent the reflex tachycardia sometimes reported with nitrates; nitrates, in turn, prevent the increased preload from beta-adrenergic blockers. Calcium channel blockers and beta-adrenergic blockers together more effectively treat Prinzmetal's angina that is unresponsive to beta-adrenergic blockers alone. (See *Selected major antianginal agents,* pages 248 and 249.)

Nitrates

Nitrates include erythrityl tetranitrate, isosorbide dinitrate, isosorbide mononitrate, nitroglycerin, and pentaerythritol tetranitrate. Used for many years to relieve angina, several of these drugs are available in multiple forms with several routes of administration. Nitrates act primarily as vasodilators, working directly on vascular smooth muscle to reduce the degree of vasoconstriction. They act primarily on venous but also on arterial smooth muscle.

PHARMACOKINETICS

Sublingual, buccal, and chewable tablets and lingual aerosols are absorbed almost completely through the richly vascularized oral mucosa. Nitrate capsules or tablets that are swallowed are absorbed through the gastrointestinal (GI) mucosa and are only about 50% to 60% absorbed. Transdermal nitrates are absorbed slowly and in varying amounts. The quantity of drug applied, the location and area of skin used for administration, and the amount of cutaneous circulation affect the percentage absorbed. Intravenous (I.V.) nitroglycerin, which does not require absorption, is delivered directly into the circulation.

Once in the body, nitrates are distributed widely; nitroglycerin is approximately 60% bound to plasma proteins. Nitrate metabolism occurs partly in the blood but mainly in the liver. Metabolite excretion occurs via the kidneys.

The rapidly acting nitrates absorbed in the mouth have the shortest duration of action: 20 to 30 minutes for sublingual nitroglycerin; up to 2 hours for sublingual erythrityl tetranitrate and isosorbide dinitrate. Oral forms of the nitrates produce antianginal effects for up to 6 hours for erythrityl tetranitrate, isosorbide dinitrate, isosorbide mononitrate, and nitroglycerin and for up to 5 hours for pentaerythritol tetranitrate.

The half-life of isosorbide dinitrate is 45 minutes; however, the half-life of one of its active metabolites is 2 to 5 hours, thus prolonging its duration of action. The duration of sustained-release oral forms of isosorbide dinitrate may persist for up to 12 hours. The half-life of isosorbide mononitrate is about 5 hours. For transdermal nitroglycerin, duration varies considerably. Nitroglycerin ointment exerts antianginal effects for 3 hours and hemodynamic effects for up to 6 hours. Longer-acting transdermal patches are replaced daily, although their actual duration may be somewhat less than 24 hours. With a plasma half-life of only 1 to 4 minutes, I.V. nitroglycerin is active for only a short time after discontinuation of the infusion.

Route	Onset	Peak	Duration
P.O.	20-60 min	1-2 hr	Up to 6 hr
Sublingual	1-3 min	1-3 min	20 min-2 hr
Transdermal	30-60 min	1-2 hr	<24 hr
I.V.	1-3 min	1-3 min	Unknown

PHARMACODYNAMICS

Nitrates act directly on vascular smooth muscle, producing relaxation and vessel dilation. These actions are independent of the autonomic nervous system's innervation of smooth muscle. Although veins have much less smooth muscle tissue than arteries have, nitrates dilate the veins considerably. Because the veins dilate, less blood is returned to the heart, decreasing the blood volume in the ventricles at the end of diastole, when the ventricles are full. (This blood volume in the ventricles and in the length of ventric-

Selected major antianginal agents

This table summarizes the major antianginal agents currently in clinical use.

DRUG	MAJOR INDICATIONS AND USUAL DOSAGES	CONTRAINDICATIONS AND PRECAUTIONS
Nitrates		
isosorbide dinitrate (Isordil, Sorbitrate)	*Relief of acute angina; prevention of angina attacks* ADULT: 2.5 to 10 mg sublingually or buccally or as a chewable tablet, repeated twice at 5- to 10-minute intervals if relief is not obtained; for angina prevention, the dosage may be repeated every 2 to 3 hours, but the initial dose of the chewable tablet should be no more than 5 mg *Long-term prevention of angina* ADULT: 10 to 20 mg P.O. t.i.d. or q.i.d. with the last daily dose taken no later than 7 p.m. to allow a 10- to 12-hour nitrate-free period; or 20 to 40 mg of sustained-release tablets or capsules every 6 to 12 hours, or 80 mg every 8 to 12 hours	• Isosorbide dinitrate is contraindicated in a patient with known hypersensitivity, increased intracranial pressure, severe anemia, or history of idiosyncratic reaction to the drug, other nitrates, or nitrites. Sustained-release preparations also are contraindicated in a patient with functional or organic GI hypermotility or malabsorption syndrome. • This drug requires cautious use in a pregnant or breast-feeding patient or one with acute myocardial infarction (MI), glaucoma, diuretic-induced fluid depletion, low systolic blood pressure, or hypertrophic cardiomyopathy. • Safety and efficacy in children have not been established.
isosorbide mononitrate (ISMO, IMDUR)	*Long-term prevention of chronic stable angina pectoris caused by coronary artery disease* ADULT: 20 mg P.O. b.i.d., with the first dose administered when the patient awakens and the second dose given 7 hours later; or 30 or 60 mg P.O. IMDUR once daily, increased over several days to 120 mg P.O. q.i.d., if needed	• Isosorbide mononitrate is contraindicated in a patient with severe anemia or known hypersensitivity to the drug, other nitrates, or nitrites. Sustained-release preparations also are contraindicated in a patient with functional or organic GI hypermotility or malabsorption syndrome. • This drug requires cautious use in a pregnant or breast-feeding patient or one with volume depletion, hypotension, acute MI, heart failure, increased intracranial pressure, or hypertrophic cardiomyopathy. • Safety and efficacy in children have not been established.
nitroglycerin (Nitro-Bid, Nitrostat, Nitro–Dur, Nitrogard)	*Relief of acute angina attack* ADULT: 0.15 to 0.6 mg sublingually repeated every 5 minutes up to three times, or 5 mcg /minute I.V., increased by 5 to 20 mcg every 3 to 5 minutes, up to a maximum of 400 mcg/minute, until pain is relieved *Prevention of expected angina attack* ADULT: 0.15 to 0.6 mg sublingually, repeated every 5 minutes up to three times *Long-term prevention of angina* ADULT: 1 to 3 mg of a sustained-release tablet between the upper gum and lip t.i.d. or q.i.d., or a sustained-release transdermal patch that releases 2.5 to 15 mg and is removed at bedtime to provide a 10- to 12-hour nitrate-free period	• Nitroglycerin is contraindicated in a patient with known hypersensitivity, severe anemia, or history of idiosyncratic reaction to organic nitrates. I.V. nitroglycerin also is contraindicated in a patient with hypotension, uncorrected hypovolemia, increased intracranial pressure, inadequate cerebral circulation, constrictive pericarditis, or pericardial tamponade. Sustained-release preparations also are contraindicated in a patient with functional or organic GI hypermotility or malabsorption syndrome. • This drug requires cautious use in a pregnant or breast-feeding patient or one with acute MI, glaucoma, diuretic-induced fluid depletion, or low systolic blood pressure. I.V. nitroglycerin also requires cautious use in a patient with severe hepatic or renal impairment. • Safety and efficacy in children have not been established.
Beta-adrenergic blockers		
propranolol hydrochloride (Inderal, Inderal LA)	*Long-term prevention of angina* ADULT: 10 to 20 mg P.O. b.i.d. to q.i.d.; if needed, the dosage may be increased over several days up to 320 mg divided into two to four daily doses; alternatively, 80 to 160 mg of the long-acting form once daily	• Propranolol is contraindicated in a patient with Raynaud's disease, malignant hypertension, bronchial asthma, sinus bradycardia and heart block greater than first-degree, heart failure (unless failure is secondary to a tachyarrhythmia treatable with propranolol), cardiogenic shock, or myasthenia gravis. • This drug requires cautious use in a pregnant or breast-feeding patient or one with inadequate cardiac function, coronary artery disease, sinus node dysfunction, hyperthyroidism, diabetes melli-

Selected major antianginal agents *(continued)*

DRUG	MAJOR INDICATIONS AND USUAL DOSAGES	CONTRAINDICATIONS AND PRECAUTIONS
Beta-adrenergic blockers *(continued)*		
propranolol hydrochloride (Inderal, Inderal LA) *(continued)*		tus, hypoglycemia, nonallergic bronchospastic disease, or renal or hepatic impairment. Propranolol also requires cautious use in a patient who is undergoing major surgery. • Safety and efficacy of sustained-release capsules, oral solutions, and injections in children have not been established.
Calcium channel blockers		
amlodipine besylate (Norvasc)	*Long-term prevention of chronic stable angina and Prinzmetal's angina* ADULT: 5 to 10 mg P.O. once daily	• Amlodipine is contraindicated in a breast-feeding patient or one with known hypersensitivity. • This drug requires cautious use in a pregnant patient or one with severe aortic stenosis, heart failure, or severe hepatic impairment. • Safety and efficacy in children have not been established.
diltiazem (Cardizem, Cardizem CD)	*Long-term prevention of chronic stable angina and angina caused by coronary artery spasm* ADULT: 30 mg P.O. q.i.d., increased every 1 to 2 days up to 360 mg daily in divided doses t.i.d. or q.i.d. if needed; or 120 to 180 mg of an extended-release preparation P.O. once daily, increased every 7 to 14 days to a maximum of 480 mg daily if needed	• Diltiazem is contraindicated in a breast-feeding patient or one with known hypersensitivity, sick sinus syndrome (unless a pacemaker is in place), second- or third-degree atrioventricular (AV) block (unless a pacemaker is in place), severe hypotension with a systolic pressure of less than 90 mm Hg, acute MI, or pulmonary congestion documented by X-ray. • This drug requires cautious use in a geriatric or pregnant patient or one with renal or hepatic impairment. • Safety and efficacy in children have not been established.
nifedipine (Adalat, Procardia)	*Long-term prevention of angina* ADULT: 10 mg P.O. t.i.d., gradually increased up to 40 mg P.O. q.i.d., if needed; or 30 to 60 mg of sustained-release tablets once daily, increased up to a maximum of 120 mg daily in the morning	• Nifedipine is contraindicated in a patient with known hypersensitivity. • This drug requires cautious use in a pregnant patient or one with heart failure, aortic stenosis, or severe GI narrowing. Liquid-filled, non-sustained release preparations should be used with caution.
verapamil (Calan, Calan SR)	*Long-term prevention of Prinzmetal's angina, chronic stable angina, and unstable angina* ADULT: 80 mg P.O. every 6 to 8 hours, increased weekly by 80-mg increments if needed, until angina is controlled, up to a maximum of 480 mg daily in divided doses t.i.d. or q.i.d.	• Verapamil is contraindicated in a breast-feeding patient or one with known hypersensitivity, cardiogenic shock, sick sinus syndrome (unless a pacemaker is in place), severe hypotension with a systolic pressure of less than 90 mm Hg), severe left ventricular dysfunction unless caused by a supraventricular tachycardia amenable to verapamil, or moderate to severe heart failure. • This drug requires cautious use in a pregnant patient or one with atrial fibrillation or flutter, an accessory bypass tract, ventricular tachycardia, moderate left ventricular dysfunction, AV conduction abnormalities, hypertrophic cardiomyopathy, hepatic or renal impairment, pseudohypertrophic muscular dystrophy, or supratentorial tumors. • Safety and efficacy in children have not been established.

ular fibers at the end of diastole is called **preload.**) By decreasing preload, nitrates reduce ventricular size and wall tension, which reduces the myocardial demand for oxygen needed to pump blood out of the ventricles.

Nitrates also dilate arteries by direct action on arterial smooth muscle, independent of autonomic nervous system innervation. In the arterial system, most resistance to ejection of blood from the left ventricle occurs in the arterioles. The more the arterioles constrict, the more they resist left ventricular ejection. The amount of resistance is called **afterload.** Nitrates decrease afterload by dilating the arterioles, thereby decreasing the energy required for the heart to pump blood and reducing myocardial oxygen demand.

Besides decreasing myocardial oxygen demand, nitrates promote coronary artery autoregulation to improve blood flow to ischemic areas of the myocardium and to decrease blood flow to unaffected areas. This combined effect may explain their antianginal action. Dilation of coronary arteries by nitrates explains their effectiveness in relieving Prinzmetal's angina, which is caused by arterial spasm. Overall, their ability to decrease oxygen demand usually is more important than their ability to increase oxygen supply.

PHARMACOTHERAPEUTICS

Nitrates are indicated for immediate relief of angina, prevention of angina when an attack can be expected, and long-term prevention of chronic angina. These drugs are synergistic with certain beta-adrenergic blockers and with calcium channel blockers.

The rapidly absorbed nitrates, such as nitroglycerin, are the drugs of choice for relief of acute angina because of their rapid onset of action, ease of administration, and low cost. Daily application of the inconspicuous, long-acting nitroglycerin transdermal patch is convenient and effective for preventing chronic angina, especially for the patient who may have difficulty complying with a regimen requiring frequent doses. Oral nitrates have the advantage of seldom producing serious adverse reactions. I.V. nitroglycerin is most effective for relieving severe, acute angina because of its rapid onset of action and short half-life.

Most of the controversy about nitrates concerns the best route of administration and the drug tolerance that develops with prolonged, continuous use, rather than which nitrate to administer. Of the five nitrates discussed in this chapter, the efficacy of nitroglycerin is the best established.

Drug interactions

Severe hypotension can result when nitrates interact with alcohol. Delayed sublingual absorption may occur when the patient's mouth is dry from using an anticholinergic agent. Marked symptomatic orthostatic hypotension has also been reported when calcium channel blockers and nitrates were used in combination therapy. A dosage adjustment for either class of drugs may be necessary.

ADVERSE DRUG REACTIONS

Most adverse reactions to nitrates are attributable to changes in the cardiovascular system. The reactions usually disappear when the dosage is reduced.

The decreased afterload produced by arteriolar dilation can cause hypotension that may be compounded by the reduced **cardiac output** after decreased preload. Hypotension is most noticeable when the patient assumes an upright position (**orthostatic hypotension**), because blood pressure is insufficient to perfuse the brain adequately. Besides a systolic blood pressure of less than 90 mm Hg, signs and symptoms of hypotension include syncope, dizziness, weakness, clammy skin, nausea, and vomiting. To compensate for the hypotension, the heart rate may increase to 150 beats/minute or more.

Although rare, complete collapse of the cardiovascular system can occur even with normal doses. Signs of complete cardiovascular collapse include thready or absent peripheral pulses, loss of blood pressure, loss of consciousness, and urinary and fecal incontinence.

Headache, the most common adverse reaction, probably is caused by blood vessel dilation in the meningeal layers between the brain and the cranium. The pain may be severe and persistent but usually disappears after several days of nitrate administration. Headache may be relieved by acetaminophen. For patients receiving transdermal patch therapy, the application site does not affect the incidence of headache.

Transdermal applications occasionally cause local skin irritation. A generalized rash after administration by any route is uncommon. If such a rash occurs, it is most likely a reaction to pentaerythritol tetranitrate. Many patients report a stinging sensation from the sublingual tablets, but the effect is not objectionable and even may indicate that the tablets are fresh. A few patients taking nitrates experience transient flushing of the face and neck.

Tolerance to nitrates may develop over time, especially with high-dose, long-term therapy. Patients appear to develop tolerance not just to the prescribed nitrate, but to the entire class. To minimize tolerance, nitrate therapy should be individualized, using the lowest effective dose and an intermittent dosage schedule.

I.V. nitroglycerin can produce alcohol intoxication when large doses are administered for long periods. This reaction results from the alcohol used to preserve nitroglycerin in ampules or vials from which I.V. infusions are prepared. The most prominent alcohol intoxication signs are an additive hypotensive effect and depression of myocardial contractility.

Other reactions may include blurred vision, dry mouth, increased peripheral edema, and methemoglobinemia, which occurs with large, continuous doses of nitrates.

NURSING PROCESS APPLICATION

The following information assists the nurse in caring for a patient who is receiving a nitrate. It includes an overview of assessment activities as well as examples of appropriate nursing diagnoses and related interventions. It also highlights the importance of evaluation.

Assessment

Before drug therapy begins, review the patient's history for conditions that contraindicate or require cautious use of the prescribed nitrate. Also review the patient's medication history to identify use of drugs that may interact with it. During therapy, assess the patient for adverse drug reactions and signs of drug interactions. Also, periodically assess the effectiveness of nitrate therapy. Finally, evaluate the patient's and family's knowledge about the prescribed drug. (See Patient Teaching: *Nitrates.*

Nursing diagnoses

- Risk for injury related to a preexisting condition that contraindicates or requires cautious use of a nitrate

• Risk for injury related to adverse drug reactions or drug interactions
• Pain related to nitrate-induced headache
• Knowledge deficit related to the prescribed nitrate

Planning and implementation

• Do not administer a nitrate to a patient with a condition that contraindicates its use.
• Do not administer erythrityl tetranitrate or isosorbide mononitrate to relieve acute angina.
• Administer a nitrate cautiously to a patient at risk because of a preexisting condition.
• Monitor the patient frequently for cardiovascular and other adverse reactions and drug interactions.
• Have the patient sit or lie down and take the pulse and blood pressure before administration of the first nitrate dose and again at the onset of action.
• Expect to repeat the isosorbide dinitrate dose two times at 5- to 10-minute intervals as prescribed if acute angina pain is not relieved, or to repeat the dose of sublingual or spray nitroglycerin up to three times.
• Do not administer more than 5 mg of chewable isosorbide dinitrate as an initial dose.
• Place nitroglycerin sustained-release tablets between the patient's upper gum and lips.
• Apply a subsequent dose of nitroglycerin ointment by removing the ointment remaining from the preceding dose and selecting a new administration site to avoid skin irritation. Remove a transdermal patch before electrical cardioversion.
• Prepare I.V. infusions of nitroglycerin cautiously. Mix the drug with dextrose 5% in water or normal saline solution in a glass bottle. Use administration tubing supplied by the manufacturer, if available, because nitroglycerin readily migrates into standard polyvinyl chloride tubing, greatly reducing the amount administered. (Some manufacturers add chemicals to the ampules to prevent such migration.)
*∗ **Monitor the blood pressure and pulse every 5 to 15 minutes while titrating the dosage and every hour thereafter for a patient receiving I.V. nitroglycerin. Use an infusion pump and calculate the dose in mcg/minute in addition to ml/hour, using the manufacturer's tables.***
• Begin infusing I.V. nitroglycerin as prescribed at 5 mcg/minute and increase it by 5 mcg every 3 to 5 minutes until pain is relieved in a patient with persistent angina accompanied by acute MI. When higher doses are reached, 10- to 20-mcg increases can be made until pain is relieved.
• Monitor the patient closely for signs of alcohol intoxication, such as hypotension or depressed myocardial contractility, during high-dosage, long-term, I.V. therapy with nitroglycerin.
*∗ **Have the patient sit up for a few minutes before standing to minimize the effects of orthostatic hypotension.***
• Take the patient's vital signs regularly and monitor closely for signs and symptoms of hypotension, such as a systolic blood pressure of less than 90 mm Hg, syncope, dizziness, weakness, clammy skin, nausea, vomiting, or tachycardia of at least 150 beats/minute.

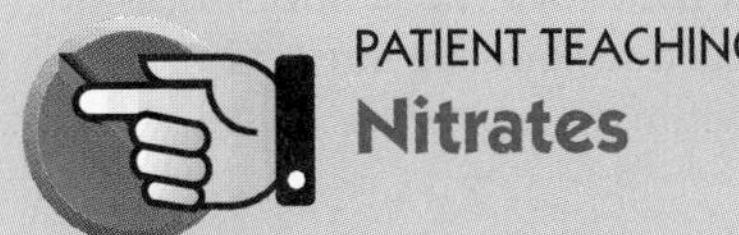

PATIENT TEACHING

Nitrates

➤ Teach the patient and family the name, dose, frequency, action, and adverse effects of the prescribed nitrate.
➤ Instruct the patient to store sublingual nitroglycerin tablets in the original container away from heat, including body heat. Advise the patient to discard the cotton filler after opening the container, because cotton may absorb some of the drug. Also instruct the patient to replace the tablets with fresh ones every 3 months and to discard any unused tablets.
➤ Instruct the patient to go to the nearest emergency department if angina is not relieved by three tablets taken 5 minutes apart while resting. Explain that the pain may indicate an acute myocardial infarction.
➤ Inform the patient using a lingual aerosol not to inhale the spray.
➤ Suggest that the patient use plastic wrap to cover a transdermal patch because nitroglycerin ointment may stain clothing.
➤ Instruct the patient using long-acting patches to change them at the same time every day; for example, right after showering.
➤ Encourage the patient to avoid drinking alcoholic beverages during nitrate therapy.
➤ Instruct the patient to take nitrate tablets or capsules half an hour before or 1 hour after meals, for better absorption.
➤ Teach the patient with dry mouth to take a few sips of water before taking sublingual or buccal tablets because a dry mouth can inhibit absorption.
➤ Instruct the patient not to stop taking nitrate medication without consulting the physician because vasospasm may follow abrupt discontinuation.
➤ Instruct the patient to take a sublingual dose, as prescribed, a few minutes before engaging in activities known or expected to induce angina.
➤ Inform the patient that the stinging sensation from sublingual nitroglycerin tablets is normal and indicates drug freshness.
➤ Advise the patient with local skin irritation to apply transdermal nitrate patches in a different location until the irritation disappears.
➤ Teach the patient to recognize and report signs and symptoms of hypotension. Also describe how to minimize the effects of orthostatic hypotension.
➤ Instruct the patient to relieve nitrate-induced headache with a mild analgesic, such as acetaminophen, as prescribed.
➤ Reassure the patient that, although headache pain may be severe and persistent, it usually disappears after several days of nitrate administration.
➤ Instruct the patient to notify the physician if adverse reactions occur or if the drug is ineffective.

• Position the hypotensive patient to promote venous return, such as in a supine or legs-elevated position, and recheck the blood pressure. If hypotension persists, remove the nitrate ointment or slow the I.V. infusion rate, notify the physician, and continue to monitor the patient's heart rate and blood pressure every 5 to 15 minutes.
• Monitor the patient for headache during nitrate therapy. Obtain a prescription for acetaminophen or another analgesic if the patient develops headache.

• Notify the physician if the patient's condition does not improve or if adverse reactions or drug interactions occur.

Evaluation

For each nursing diagnosis, prepare an evaluation statement that describes the patient's or family's response to nursing interventions.

Beta-adrenergic blockers

Also called beta-adrenergic antagonists, beta-adrenergic blockers are used for long-term prevention of angina. Atenolol, metoprolol tartrate, nadolol, and propranolol hydrochloride are the antianginal agents approved by the Food and Drug Administration.

PHARMACOKINETICS

Metoprolol and propranolol are absorbed almost entirely from the GI tract, whereas less than 50% of a dose of atenolol or nadolol is absorbed. These beta-adrenergic blockers are distributed widely. Each of the beta-adrenergic blockers is plasma protein-bound as follows: propranolol, 90%; nadolol, 30%; atenolol, 6% to 16%; and metoprolol, 12%.

Propranolol and metoprolol are hydroxylated in the liver. Atenolol and nadolol are not metabolized. Metabolites of metoprolol and propranolol are excreted in the urine. Atenolol and nadolol are excreted unchanged in the urine and feces.

Because beta-adrenergic blockers are not used for relief of acute angina, their onset of action is difficult to measure. Long-acting forms of these drugs take longer to appear in the plasma.

The peak concentration level of metoprolol occurs within 90 minutes and is increased when the drug is taken with food. Peak concentration of propranolol occurs within 6 hours for long-acting capsules; if the drug is taken with food, peak concentration is delayed but not reduced.

The half-life of atenolol is 6 to 9 hours; of nadolol, 10 to 24 hours. The duration of metoprolol is about 6 hours; its half-life varies from 3 to 7 hours. The duration of propranolol is 4 to 6 hours; long-acting capsules is up to 24 hours. Propranolol's half-life ranges from 3 to 6 hours.

Route	Onset	Peak	Duration
P.O.	10-30 min	1-6 hr	4-24 hr

PHARMACODYNAMICS

Beta-adrenergic blockers decrease blood pressure through one or more mechanisms. They also block beta-receptor sites in the myocardium and in the electrical conduction system of the heart. Subsequently, decreased heart rate and diminished force of myocardial contraction considerably reduce the oxygen requirements of the heart. The drugs also increase the patient's maximal exercise tolerance because they prevent the angina that commonly accompanies exertion.

PHARMACOTHERAPEUTICS

Beta-adrenergic blockers are indicated for long-term prevention of angina, not for immediate relief of an angina attack or prevention of an imminent one. The drugs act synergistically with other antianginal agents.

Drug interactions

Beta-adrenergic blockers may interact with many different types of drugs in a variety of ways. (See Drug Interactions: *Beta-adrenergic blockers.*)

ADVERSE DRUG REACTIONS

The most common adverse reactions to beta-adrenergic blockers involve the cardiovascular system and occur when the drug is administered initially. Because they inhibit sinus node stimulation, beta-adrenergic blockers can cause bradycardia and hypotension with peripheral vascular insufficiency. Angina, syncope, or shock may accompany these reactions. Fluid retention and peripheral edema also may occur.

Because of decreased force of myocardial contractility and increased preload, heart failure may be exacerbated or precipitated. Arrhythmias, especially **atrioventricular (AV) block,** also can occur.

Rapid discontinuation of a beta-adrenergic blocker may precipitate angina, hypertension, arrhythmias, or acute myocardial infarction.

Adverse central nervous system reactions include dizziness, fatigue, lethargy, confusion or depression (especially in geriatric patients), and decreased libido. They occur most commonly with propranolol therapy. GI reactions, such as nausea, vomiting, and diarrhea, usually are transient.

Significant bronchoconstriction is more likely to occur with nadolol and propranolol, which are nonselective beta-adrenergic blockers, but also can occur with high doses of atenolol and metoprolol.

Rarely, rashes, blood dyscrasias, depression, and vivid dreams occur.

NURSING PROCESS APPLICATION

The following information assists the nurse in caring for a patient who is receiving a beta-adrenergic blocker. It includes an overview of assessment activities as well as examples of appropriate nursing diagnoses and related interventions. It also highlights the importance of evaluation.

Assessment

Before drug therapy begins, review the patient's history for conditions that contraindicate or require cautious use of the

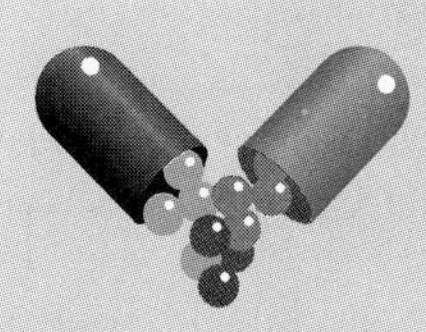

DRUG INTERACTIONS

Beta-adrenergic blockers

Drug interactions involving beta-adrenergic blockers primarily affect the cardiovascular and respiratory systems.

DRUG	INTERACTING DRUGS	POSSIBLE EFFECTS	NURSING IMPLICATIONS
atenolol, metoprolol, nadolol, propranolol	antacids	Delayed drug absorption from GI tract	• Administer drugs several hours apart. • Monitor the patient for a decreased therapeutic effect.
	lidocaine	Increased plasma levels of lidocaine (potential toxicity); increased cardiac depressant effects	• Monitor the patient for signs of lidocaine toxicity, such as confusion, restlessness, and tremors.
	insulin and oral hypoglycemic agents	Hypoglycemia or hyperglycemia; masking of tachycardia as a sign of hypoglycemia (diaphoresis and agitation still present)	• Administer these drugs cautiously. • Monitor the patient's blood glucose levels frequently.
	nonsteroidal anti-inflammatory drugs (indomethacin, salicylates)	Decreased hypotensive effects of beta-adrenergic blockers	• Monitor the patient for altered beta-adrenergic blocking effects.
	barbiturates	Stimulated metabolism of beta-adrenergic blockers that are metabolized extensively	• Monitor the patient for altered response to beta-adrenergic blockers that are metabolized by the liver (propranolol, metoprolol).
	cardiac glycosides	Increased bradycardia and depression of atrioventricular conduction	• Monitor the patient's blood pressure and heart rate frequently.
	calcium channel blockers	Increased pharmacologic and toxic effects of both agents	• Monitor the patient for adverse reactions.
	sympathomimetics (epinephrine, dobutamine, dopamine, isoproterenol, terbutaline, metaproterenol, albuterol, ritodrine)	Hypertension and reflex bradycardia from unopposed alpha effects (vasoconstriction) and increased vagal tone	• Monitor the patient's blood pressure and heart rate frequently.
	cimetidine	Reduced metabolism and enhanced ability of beta-adrenergic blockers to reduce pulse rate	• Monitor the patient for altered response to beta-adrenergic blockers.
	rifampin	Inhibited therapeutic response to metoprolol and propranolol	• Monitor the patient for altered response to beta-adrenergic blockers.
	theophyllines	Impaired bronchodilating effects of theophyllines	• Monitor the patient's therapeutic response.
	clonidine	Enhanced antihypertensive and bradycardic effects	• Monitor the patient's blood pressure closely.
	prazosin	Enhanced first-dose syncopal response to prazosin	• Monitor the patient's blood pressure closely. • Monitor the patient for dizziness and loss of consciousness.

prescribed beta-adrenergic blocker. Also review the patient's medication history to identify use of drugs that may interact with it. During therapy, assess the patient for adverse drug reactions and signs of drug interactions. Also, periodically assess the effectiveness of beta-adrenergic blocker therapy. Finally, evaluate the patient's and family's knowledge about the prescribed drug. (See Patient Teaching: *Beta-adrenergic blockers*, page 254.)

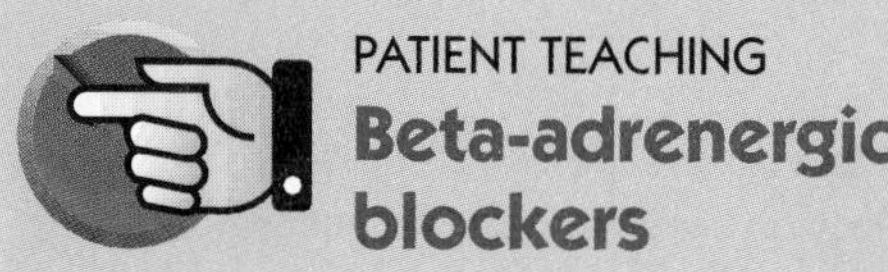

PATIENT TEACHING
Beta-adrenergic blockers

- ➤ Teach the patient and family the name, dose, frequency, action, and adverse effects of the prescribed beta-adrenergic blocker.
- ➤ Instruct the patient taking metoprolol or propranolol to take the drug at the same time each day — but not with meals. Inform the patient taking atenolol or nadolol that the drug can be taken at any time.
- ➤ Instruct the patient that a beta-adrenergic blocker should not be discontinued abruptly. The drug should be tapered off over several days, as prescribed, to prevent angina, hypertension, arrhythmias, or acute myocardial infarction.
- ➤ Inform the patient that central nervous system (CNS) effects may occur, especially during propranolol therapy. Advise the patient not to drive or operate heavy equipment if CNS effects occur.
- ➤ Reassure the patient that adverse GI effects are usually transient. If GI symptoms are severe or persistent, advise the patient to notify the physician, who may prescribe an antiemetic or antidiarrheal agent.
- ➤ Instruct the diabetic patient to test blood glucose levels regularly and to expect a change in the insulin or oral hypoglycemic dosage during beta-adrenergic blocker therapy.
- ➤ Instruct the patient to notify the physician if adverse reactions occur, especially increasing dyspnea, wheezing, or peripheral edema.

Nursing diagnoses

- Risk for injury related to a preexisting condition that contraindicates or requires cautious use of a beta-adrenergic blocker
- Risk for injury related to adverse drug reactions or drug interactions
- Fluid volume excess related to the adverse cardiovascular effects of the prescribed beta-adrenergic blocker
- Knowledge deficit related to the prescribed beta-adrenergic blocker

Planning and implementation

- Do not administer a beta-adrenergic blocker to a patient with a condition that contraindicates its use. Do not administer a beta-adrenergic blocker to relieve or prevent an angina attack.
- Administer a beta-adrenergic blocker cautiously to a patient at risk because of a preexisting condition.
- Monitor the patient closely for adverse reactions, especially for cardiovascular dysfunction during initial administration, and for drug interactions.

*** *Take the patient's vital signs regularly, particularly noting decreased blood pressure, heart rate, or irregular rhythm. Withhold the dose and notify the physician if the patient's apical pulse is less than 60 beats/minute or the systolic blood pressure is less than 90 mm Hg.***

- Monitor the diabetic patient's blood glucose level regularly. Expect to adjust the insulin or oral hypoglycemic dose, as needed.
- Do not administer metoprolol or propranolol with food because food delays their peak concentration effect.

*** *Auscultate the lungs frequently and assess the ease of breathing to detect bronchoconstriction. Notify the physician if bronchoconstriction occurs; prepare to administer bronchodilators and oxygen therapy.***

- Advise the patient not to stop taking propranolol suddenly; abrupt discontinuation may precipitate an acute MI or anginal symptoms.
- Assess for signs of fluid volume excess, such as crackles, increasing dyspnea, elevated blood pressure, peripheral edema, and jugular venous distention. Notify the physician if fluid volume excess occurs; prepare to reduce fluid overload with such measures as diuretic administration, as prescribed.
- Notify the physician if the patient's condition does not improve or if other adverse reactions or drug interactions occur.

Evaluation

For each nursing diagnosis, prepare an evaluation statement that describes the patient's or family's response to nursing interventions.

Calcium channel blockers

A class of drugs including amlodipine besylate, diltiazem hydrochloride, nicardipine hydrochloride, nifedipine, and verapamil hydrochloride, calcium channel blockers commonly are used to prevent angina unresponsive to drugs in either of the other antianginal classes.

PHARMACOKINETICS

When administered sublingually, nifedipine is absorbed quickly and almost completely. After oral administration, 64% to 90% of amlodipine, 80% of diltiazem, 90% of nifedipine and verapamil, and 100% of nicardipine is absorbed from the GI tract. Because of the first-pass effect, however, the bioavailability of these agents is much lower. The calcium channel blockers are highly bound to plasma proteins in the following amounts: diltiazem, 80%; nifedipine, nicardipine, amlodipine, and verapamil, over 90%.

All calcium channel blockers are metabolized rapidly and almost completely in the liver. The metabolites of all of these agents are excreted mostly in the urine and also in the feces. Only 2% to 10% of the drug is excreted unchanged in the urine.

The onset of action of oral diltiazem is 30 minutes; of nicardipine, 20 minutes; of nifedipine, 10 minutes; of verapamil, 30 to 60 minutes. The onset of action for amlodipine is unknown. The peak concentration level of oral diltiazem

How calcium channel blockers work

Calcium channel blockers prevent calcium transport across the cell membrane so the cardiac muscle and the smooth muscle of the coronary arteries will not contract as forcefully.

1. Under normal conditions, a protein complex prevents muscle contraction by keeping actin and myosin (the contractile proteins) apart. Actin and myosin must interact for a muscle to contract. When the muscle cell is stimulated, calcium ions enter the cell. This influx of calcium releases more calcium from the sarcoplasmic reticulum inside the muscle cell.

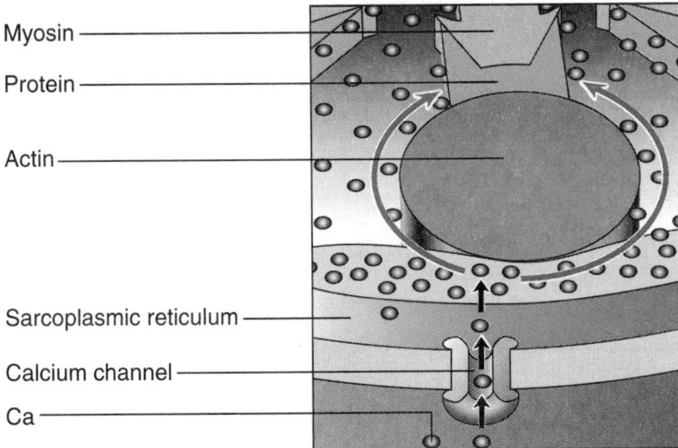

2. When enough calcium is released, it binds with the protein complex. Hence, the actin and myosin can interact and the muscle contracts.

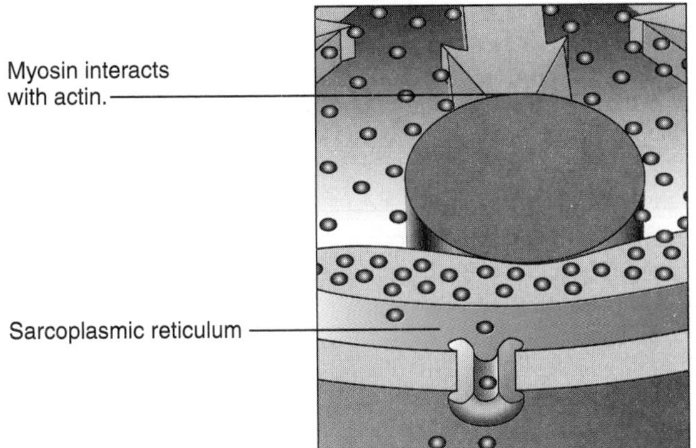

3. Calcium channel blockers prevent calcium from entering the cell, thereby preventing calcium release from the sarcoplasmic reticulum.

Although all the calcium channel blockers exert this effect on cardiac muscle, one compound may prove to be more effective for a specific heart condition than another. In general, however, calcium channel blockers can:

- reduce electrical excitation and mechanical contraction of the heart. (Arrhythmias, especially those of atrial origin, can be relieved and perhaps even prevented.)
- relieve excruciating anginal pain caused by spasms of the coronary arteries
- allow more rest for damaged tissue
- reduce peripheral arterial resistance and myocardial oxygen demand.

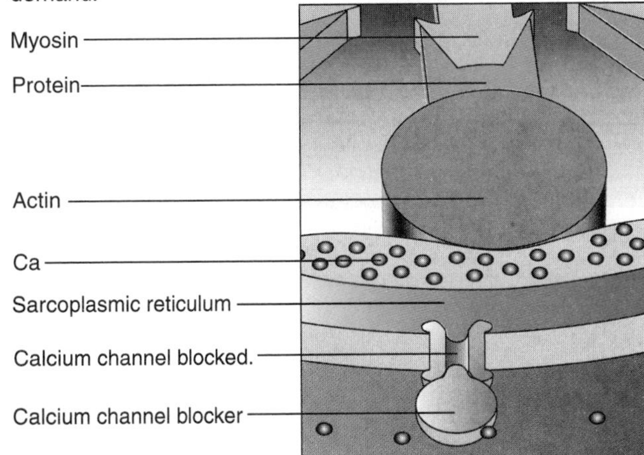

occurs within 2 to 3 hours; of nicardipine, in 0.5 to 2 hours; of nifedipine, within 30 minutes; of amlodipine, 6 to 12 hours; and of verapamil, 30 to 60 minutes after an oral dose.

In the absence of significant hepatic disease, the half-lives of the calcium channel blockers are as follows: diltiazem, 3.5 to 6 hours; nicardipine and nifedipine, 2 to 4 hours; verapamil, 3 to 7 hours. The elimination of amlodipine is biphasic; the terminal half-life of amlodipine is 30 to 50 hours.

Route	Onset	Peak	Duration
P.O.	10-60 min	0.5-12 hr	4-24 hr

PHARMACODYNAMICS

By preventing the influx of calcium ions into myocardial and vascular smooth muscle cells, calcium channel blockers inhibit the intracellular release of additional stores of calcium ions. (See *How calcium channel blockers work.*) These in-

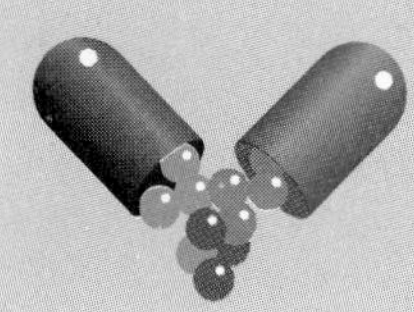

DRUG INTERACTIONS

Calcium channel blockers

Most drug interactions associated with calcium channel blockers result in adverse cardiovascular effects. The nurse must be aware of these interactions to monitor for these effects and to intervene appropriately.

DRUG	INTERACTING DRUGS	POSSIBLE EFFECTS	NURSING IMPLICATIONS
diltiazem, nicardipine, nifedipine, verapamil	cimetidine	Decreased hepatic clearance of the calcium channel blocker	• Monitor the patient for adverse reactions, which may occur more frequently. • Monitor the patient for orthostatic hypotension and for heart rate and rhythm changes.
	calcium salts, vitamin D	Reduced response to the calcium channel blocker	• Do not administer concurrently unless necessary; in that case, monitor the patient's therapeutic response and adjust the calcium channel blocker dosage, as prescribed.
	nondepolarizing blocking agents	Enhanced muscle relaxant action	• Monitor the patient's respiratory function closely.
diltiazem, verapamil micardipine	cyclosporine	Enhanced cyclosporine action	• Monitor the patient's renal function by recording the fluid intake and output and reviewing creatinine and blood urea nitrogen levels. • Monitor the patient's cyclosporine levels.
diltiazem, verapamil	digoxin	Increased serum digoxin concentration	• Monitor the patient for bradycardia, nausea, and vomiting. • Monitor the patient's serum digoxin level.
	carbamazepine	Enhanced carbamazepine action	• Monitor the patient's carbamazepine levels.
	beta-adrenergic blockers, diltiazem	Myocardial depression	• Do not administer these drugs within 24 hours of each other unless necessary; in that case, monitor the patient for signs of heart failure or decreased peripheral perfusion.

tracellular calcium ions otherwise would bind to the troponin-tropomyosin complex and allow actin and myosin to interact. The sliding of actin and myosin filaments past each other produces the contraction of a myocardial cell and, ultimately, of the whole ventricle. Thus, by inhibiting the release of intracellular calcium ions, calcium channel blockers decrease the force of myocardial contractility, thereby decreasing the oxygen demand.

Calcium channel blockers also prevent entry of calcium ions into arteriolar smooth muscle cells. This action decreases arteriolar constriction and thereby decreases systemic vascular resistance, or afterload. Decreasing afterload also decreases myocardial oxygen demand.

Myocardial oxygen demand also decreases when calcium channel blockers are used to slow the heart rate, regulated by the sinus node, and to decrease conduction velocity in the heart's conducting pathways, regulated by the AV node. This mechanism probably is significant only for patients with rapid heart rates.

Besides decreasing myocardial oxygen demand, calcium channel blockers increase the oxygen supply to the myocardium by dilating the coronary arteries. Because calcium channel blockers do not induce venous dilation appreciably, they have little effect on preload.

PHARMACOTHERAPEUTICS

Calcium channel blockers are indicated only for long-term prevention of angina. They are not used routinely to relieve acute attacks or to prevent expected ones. Calcium channel blockers are particularly effective in preventing Prinzmetal's angina, for which they are the drugs of choice. Nicardipine and nifedipine produce the greatest arteriolar dilation, followed by verapamil and then diltiazem. They act synergistically with other antianginal agents.

Drug interactions

Amlodipine has no known drug interactions. Other calcium channel blockers used as antianginal agents may interact with many different types of drugs in a variety of ways. (See Drug Interactions: *Calcium channel blockers.*)

ADVERSE DRUG REACTIONS

Undesirable alterations in the cardiovascular system are the most common and serious adverse reactions to calcium channel blockers. Because they decrease afterload and the force of ventricular contraction, calcium channel blockers sometimes cause an anticipated decrease in blood pressure, including orthostatic hypotension. Arrhythmias, such as bradycardia, sinus block, and AV block, result from inhibition of the sinus and AV nodes, especially by diltiazem and verapamil. The depressant action on myocardial contractility may account for the onset or worsening of heart failure.

Vasodilation can produce dizziness, headache, flushing, weakness, and persistent peripheral edema, especially with nicardipine, nifedipine, and amlodipine. Other possible adverse reactions include GI disturbances, such as nausea, vomiting, and diarrhea, as well as muscle fatigue and cramps.

Other reactions to calcium channel blockers may include worsening of angina and skin eruptions, photosensitivity, pruritus, nasal congestion, and mood changes.

NURSING PROCESS APPLICATION

The following information assists the nurse in caring for a patient who is receiving a calcium channel blocker. It includes an overview of assessment activities as well as examples of appropriate nursing diagnoses and related interventions. It also highlights the importance of evaluation.

Assessment

Before drug therapy begins, review the patient's history for conditions that contraindicate or require cautious use of the prescribed calcium channel blocker. Also review the patient's medication history to identify use of drugs that may interact with it. During therapy, assess the patient for adverse drug reactions and signs of drug interactions. Also, periodically assess the effectiveness of therapy with the prescribed calcium channel blocker. Finally, evaluate the patient's and family's knowledge about the prescribed drug.

Nursing diagnoses

- Risk for injury related to a preexisting condition that contraindicates or requires cautious use of a calcium channel blocker
- Risk for injury related to adverse drug reactions or drug interactions
- Pain related to the adverse central nervous system or muscular effects of the prescribed calcium channel blocker
- Knowledge deficit related to the prescribed calcium channel blocker

Planning and implementation

- Do not administer a calcium channel blocker to a patient with a condition that contraindicates its use.
- Administer a calcium channel blocker cautiously to a patient at risk because of a preexisting condition.

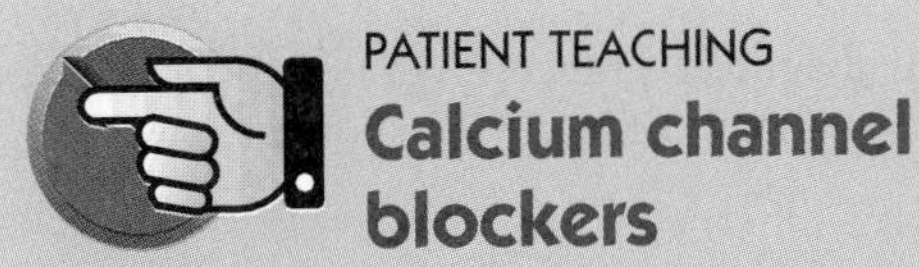

PATIENT TEACHING

Calcium channel blockers

- Teach the patient and family the name, dose, frequency, action, and adverse effects of the prescribed calcium channel blocker.
- Advise the female patient to tell the physician if she is pregnant or plans to become pregnant during calcium channel blocker therapy.
- Teach the patient to recognize and report to the physician the signs of fluid retention, such as peripheral edema and increasing shortness of breath.
- Demonstrate how to take a pulse, and tell the patient to take the pulse before each dose. Advise the patient to delay the dose and notify the physician if the pulse is less than 60 beats/minute.
- Emphasize that calcium channel blockers cannot relieve acute angina. If acute chest pain occurs, advise the patient to notify the physician immediately or go to the nearest emergency department.
- Teach the patient how to manage orthostatic hypotension.
- Advise the patient not to perform activities that require alertness if dizziness occurs.
- Instruct the patient to notify the physician if nausea, vomiting, or diarrhea occurs. If such gastrointestinal problems occur, advise the patient to request an appropriate medication.
- Instruct the patient to take diltiazem before meals.
- Instruct the patient to take a once-daily sustained-release tablet in the morning.
- Advise the patient with headaches or muscle cramps to take an analgesic, as prescribed.
- Instruct the patient to notify the physician if adverse reactions occur or if the drug is ineffective.

- Monitor the patient frequently for adverse reactions, especially cardiovascular alterations, and for drug interactions. ***Take the patient's vital signs regularly and monitor the electrocardiogram for arrhythmias, particularly when nicardipine or nifedipine is administered. Also monitor for fluid retention. Withhold the dose and notify the physician if the patient's heart rate is less than 60 beats/minute or if the systolic blood pressure is less than 90 mm Hg.***
- Expect to administer a calcium channel blocker as an antianginal agent when nitrates or beta-adrenergic blockers have been ineffective.
- Have the patient sit up for a few minutes before standing to minimize the effects of orthostatic hypotension. (See Patient Teaching: *Calcium channel blockers*.)
- Administer the once-daily dosage of a sustained-release tablet in the morning. Administer diltiazem before meals.
- Monitor the patient for headaches or muscle cramps. Ask the physician to prescribe an analgesic, if needed.
- Notify the physician if the patient's condition does not improve or if adverse reactions or drug interactions occur.

Evaluation

For each nursing diagnosis, prepare an evaluation statement that describes the patient's or family's response to nursing interventions.

CHAPTER SUMMARY

Chapter 19 discussed nitrates, beta-adrenergic blockers, and calcium channel blockers as they are used to prevent or relieve angina. Here are the highlights of the chapter.

Antianginal agents prevent or relieve myocardial ischemia by decreasing myocardial oxygen demand, increasing myocardial oxygen supply, or both.

Nitrates are used for the immediate relief of angina, prevention of an expected angina attack, and long-term prevention of chronic angina. Beta-adrenergic blockers and calcium channel blockers are used for long-term management of angina. Calcium channel blockers are especially useful in preventing Prinzmetal's angina.

Questions to consider

See Appendix 1 for answers.

1. Rosalie DaSilva, age 54, comes to the emergency department complaining of chest pain, which developed an hour ago while she was washing her car. The nurse administers nitroglycerin (Nitrostat) 0.4 mg sublingually stat, as prescribed. The nurse assesses Ms. DaSilva frequently for adverse reactions to nitroglycerin. Which of the following adverse reactions is most likely to occur?
   (a) GI distress
   (b) Headache
   (c) Diarrhea
   (d) Dizziness

2. After receiving sublingual nitroglycerin for chest pain in the emergency department, Abraham Goldman, age 63, is transferred to the coronary care unit. There, he must receive continuous I.V. nitroglycerin therapy. Which of the following steps should the nurse take to administer this antianginal agent?
   (a) Mix nitroglycerin with dextrose 5% in water and half-normal saline solution in a plastic infusion bag.
   (b) Infuse the nitroglycerin, using standard infusion tubing.
   (c) Begin infusing the nitroglycerin at 5 mcg/minute.
   (d) Increase the nitroglycerin at 20 mcg/minute after the first 3 minutes of infusion.

3. Linda Corman, age 59, is transferred to a medical-surgical unit after being treated with nitroglycerin for an angina attack. To prevent further chest pain, her physician prescribes the beta-adrenergic blocker propranolol 10 mg P.O. t.i.d. The nurse assesses Ms. Corman before administering each dose. Which of the following findings should prompt the nurse to withhold propranolol and notify the physician?
   (a) Complaints of chest pain
   (b) Pulse greater than 90 beats/minute
   (c) Systolic blood pressure less than 90 mm Hg
   (d) Diastolic blood pressure more than 80 mm Hg

4. Ben Majors, age 49, is about to be discharged with a prescription for the calcium channel blocker diltiazem (Cardizem), 30 mg P.O. before meals q.i.d. to take at home. Calcium channel blockers are the drugs of choice for which of the following types of angina?
   (a) Stable angina
   (b) Unstable angina
   (c) Preinfarction angina
   (d) Prinzmetal's angina

5. During a follow-up visit, the nurse is assessing Lawrence Tan, age 56, who has been taking oral diltiazem. The nurse is most likely to detect which of the following adverse reactions to diltiazem?
   (a) Heart failure
   (b) Hypertension
   (c) Tachycardia
   (d) Confusion

6. Four days after being discharged with a prescription for diltiazem, Anna Carter, age 63, calls the physician's office to report a stuffy nose and minor itching and extreme redness after sitting outside for a short time. Which of the following instructions should the nurse give this patient?
   (a) Stop taking the diltiazem and go to the emergency department immediately.
   (b) Continue taking the diltiazem and apply a lotion to reduce skin itching and redness.
   (c) Take an over-the-counter nasal decongestant and ignore the skin irritation.
   (d) Notify the physician, who may order palliative treatment.

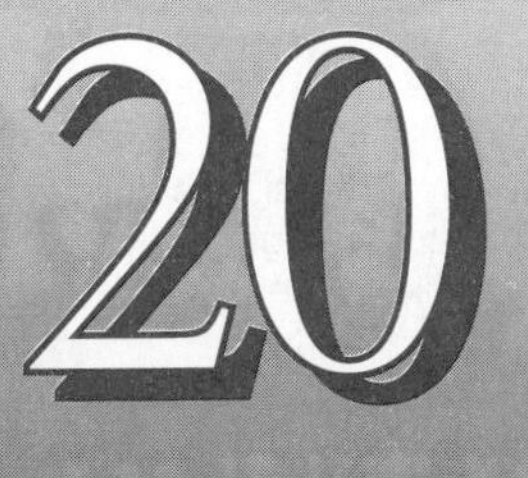

Antihypertensive agents

OBJECTIVES

After reading and studying this chapter, the student should be able to:

1. identify the four stages of hypertension.
2. explain the use of antihypertensive agents in the stepped-care approach to antihypertensive therapy.
3. list at least three examples of sympatholytics, vasodilators, and angiotensin-converting enzyme (ACE) inhibitors.
4. compare the actions of drugs in the three classes of antihypertensive agents.
5. identify the major adverse reactions that occur with each of the three major classes of antihypertensive agents.
6. describe how to apply the nursing process when caring for a patient who is receiving an antihypertensive agent.

INTRODUCTION

Antihypertensive agents, which act to reduce blood pressure, are used to treat **hypertension,** a disorder characterized by elevation in **systolic blood pressure, diastolic blood pressure,** or both.

Essential (primary) or secondary hypertension occurs when homeostatic mechanisms fail to regulate blood pressure. Essential hypertension affects about 95% of all hypertensive patients. Secondary hypertension affects about 5% of hypertensive patients and results from such underlying disorders as aortic regurgitation, renal artery stenosis, pheochromocytoma, and neurologic diseases. Treatment of the underlying disorder sometimes cures secondary hypertension.

Either form of hypertension can occur to varying degrees. According to the recent report issued by the Joint National Committee on Detection, Evaluation, and Treatment of High Blood Pressure (JNC) of the National Institutes of Health, the traditional terms *mild hypertension* and *moderate hypertension* have failed to convey the serious detrimental effects that high blood pressure has on the cardiovascular system. As a result, the JNC has devised a classification system based on impact of risk rather than severity. For example, high normal blood pressure now is considered a specific hypertensive category because it increases the patient's risk of developing definite hypertension and experiencing nonfatal and fatal cardiovascular events. This change, of course, simultaneously has created a new high normal blood pressure range that is lower than earlier guidelines have indicated.

The JNC's classification system describes four stages of hypertension. (See *Classification of blood pressure,* page 260). All stages of hypertension are associated with increased risk of cardiovascular and renal disease. The higher the blood pressure, the greater the risk. Stage 1 hypertension — previously termed *mild* — is the most common form of hypertension in the adult population. All stages of hypertension warrant effective long-term therapy.

The JNC also endorses the stepped-care approach in treating hypertension. In step one of this approach, the physician recommends nonpharmacologic therapies, if possible. In step two, the physician prescribes low doses of a beta-adrenergic blocker or a diuretic; these agents are the drugs of choice because of their proven ability to reduce the risk of morbidity and mortality when used to treat hypertension. If beta-adrenergic blockers or diuretics are contraindicated or unacceptable, or if other antihypertensive agents are indicated because certain diseases preexist or serious drug interactions may occur, ACE inhibitors, calcium channel blockers, and other antihypertensive agents may be used instead. These drugs are effective in reducing blood pressure; however, long-term clinical trials to show decreased morbidity and mortality have not been performed.

In addition, the therapeutic response to antihypertensives varies among patients of different races. (See Cultural Considerations: *Ethnic differences in drug response,* page 261.) In step three, if needed, the physician increases the drug dosage, substitutes another diuretic or beta-adrenergic blocker, or adds to the initial drug regimen a second antihypertensive agent from a different class. If hypertension remains uncontrolled, step four begins. In this step, the physician adds a second or third antihypertensive agent or a diuretic (if not already prescribed) to the treatment regimen to bring blood pressure under control. (See *Stepped-care approach to antihypertensive therapy,* page 262.)

In nonemergency circumstances, the stepped-care approach to therapy can reduce the blood pressure to an acceptable level while avoiding significant adverse reactions in most patients. If blood pressure remains controlled for at

Classification of blood pressure

Blood pressure is classified into three categories: normal, high normal, and hypertension, as shown below. Hypertension is divided into four stages of increasing risk of cardiovascular or renal disease. A patient's blood pressure is based on the average of two or more readings taken at each of two or more evaluations after an initial screening. If the systolic and diastolic blood pressures fall into two different categories, the higher risk category is used to determine a patient's blood pressure category.

CATEGORY	SYSTOLIC BLOOD PRESSURE (mm Hg)	DIASTOLIC BLOOD PRESSURE (mm Hg)
Normal	below 130	below 85
High normal	130 to 139	85 to 89
Hypertension		
stage 1 (mild)	140 to 159	90 to 99
stage 2 (moderate)	160 to 179	100 to 109
stage 3 (severe)	180 to 209	110 to 119
stage 4 (very severe)	210 or more	120 or more

Source: U.S. Department of Health and Human Services. National Institutes of Health. National Heart, Lung, and Blood Institute. *The Fifth Report of the Joint National Committee on Detection, Evaluation, and Treatment of High Blood Pressure (JNC V).* Washington, D.C.: Government Printing Office, 1992.

least 1 year, as documented by at least four follow-up visits, the physician should decrease the dosage or the number of antihypertensives while the patient continues to follow lifestyle modifications. Complete cessation of an antihypertensive treatment program is not recommended.

Uncontrolled hypertension can lead to hypertensive crisis and malignant hypertension. *Hypertensive crisis* is characterized by a diastolic blood pressure above 140 mm Hg. If left untreated, hypertensive crisis can result in severe tissue and organ damage, such as retinopathy, heart failure, renal failure, and encephalopathy. *Malignant hypertension* is characterized by a diastolic blood pressure above 140 mm Hg and papilledema. Both complications require aggressive parenteral treatment with a potent, rapid-acting vasodilator to reduce the diastolic blood pressure to 100 mm Hg or less. (See *Selected major antihypertensive agents,* pages 263 through 267.)

Drugs covered in this chapter include:

- acebutolol hydrochloride
- amlodipine besylate
- atenolol
- benazepril hydrochloride
- betaxdol hydrochloride
- captopril
- clonidine hydrochloride
- diazoxide
- diltiazem hydrochloride
- doxazosin
- enalapril
- felodipine
- fosinopril sodium
- guanabenz acetate
- guanadrel sulfate
- guanethidine monosulfate
- guaufacine
- hydralazine hydrochloride
- isradipine
- labetolol
- lisinopril
- methyldopa
- minoxidil
- nadolol
- nicardipine hydrochloride
- nifedipine
- nitroprusside sodium
- penbutolol sulfate
- phentolamine
- pindolol
- prazosin hydrochloride
- propranolol hydrochloride
- quinapril hydrochloride
- ramipril
- terazosin
- timolol maleate
- verapamil.

Sympatholytic agents

The sympatholytics include various groups of drugs that reduce blood pressure by inhibiting or blocking motor and secretory action in the sympathetic nervous system. They are classified by their site or mechanism of action and include central-acting sympathetic nervous system inhibitors (clonidine hydrochloride, guanabenz acetate, guanfacine, and methyldopa), beta-adrenergic blocking agents (acebutolol hydrochloride, atenolol, betaxolol hydrochloride, carteolol hydrochloride, metoprolol tartrate, nadolol, penbutolol sulfate, pindolol, propranolol hydrochloride, and timolol maleate), alpha-adrenergic blocking agents (doxazosin mesylate, phentolamine, prazosin hydrochloride, and terazosin), mixed alpha- and beta-adrenergic blocking agents (labetalol), and norepinephrine depletors (guanadrel sulfate, guanethidine monosulfate, and reserpine).

PHARMACOKINETICS

Most sympatholytics are absorbed well from the gastrointestinal (GI) tract, are distributed widely, metabolized in the liver, and excreted primarily in the urine. The pharmacokinetics of phentolamine are unknown. The onset of action, peak concentration levels, and duration of action vary greatly among the sympatholytics.

Route	Onset	Peak	Duration
P.O.	10-90 min	1.5-12 hr	6-24 hr
I.V.	2-5 min	2-60 min	4-8 hr
Transdermal	2-3 days	2-3 days	Days

PHARMACODYNAMICS

All sympatholytic agents inhibit stimulation of the sympathetic nervous system. They perform this function in different ways, but they all produce the same result: decreased blood pressure resulting from peripheral vasodilation or decreased cardiac output.

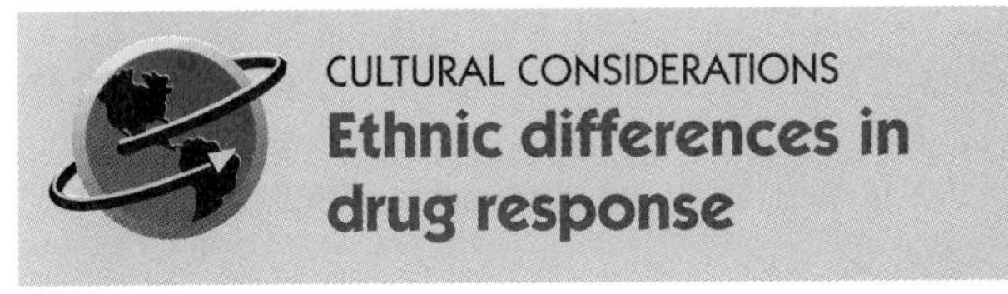

CULTURAL CONSIDERATIONS

Ethnic differences in drug response

Antihypertensive and other cardiac agents display differences in their effectiveness among Black, White, and Asian patients. For example, Black patients respond better to thiazide diuretics; whereas White patients respond better to angiotensin-converting enzyme inhibitors such as captopril. Asian patients are twice as responsive to propranolol's effects on blood pressure and heart rate as White patients.

Plasma renin activity may account for this difference in drug response because it varies by ethnic group. For example, White patients usually have a higher rate of plasma renin activity than Black patients.

PHARMACOTHERAPEUTICS

Sympatholytics typically are used to lower the blood pressure of patients with all stages of hypertension. However, beta-adrenergic blockers along with diuretics are the first drugs of choice for treating hypertension.

Drug interactions

Many different drugs can interact with sympatholytic agents, frequently producing blood pressure changes and other effects.

ADVERSE DRUG REACTIONS

Many sympatholytic agents cause adverse reactions in the central nervous system (CNS) and the cardiovascular system. Additional reactions affecting other body systems vary with each drug.

Central-acting agents typically produce CNS effects, such as sedation, drowsiness, and depression. Other common reactions include forgetfulness, inability to concentrate, and vivid dreams, which usually diminish after 2 to 3 weeks of therapy. Additional adverse reactions include sodium and water retention, edema, hepatic dysfunction, vertigo, paresthesia, weakness, fever, nasal congestion, and dry mouth. These drugs may decrease the libido and result in impotence, limiting their usefulness in males. They also may produce lactation in both sexes.

Other adverse reactions vary according to the specific drug used. For example, clonidine may cause dry mouth or rebound hypertension when the drug is discontinued.

Guanabenz may produce adverse cardiovascular reactions, such as arrhythmias, chest pain, edema, and palpitations. Its other effects may include anxiety, ataxia, blurred vision, nasal congestion, and rebound hypertension (if discontinued suddenly).

Because of their ability to penetrate the blood-brain barrier, beta-adrenergic blockers can produce the same CNS effects as the central-acting agents. Adverse cardiovascular reactions may include bradycardia, hypotension, heart failure, and exacerbation of peripheral vascular disease (PVD). The beta-adrenergic blockers also may reduce high-density lipoprotein levels and increase serum triglyceride, total cholesterol, low-density lipoprotein (LDL), and very-low-density lipoprotein levels.

Other adverse reactions to beta-adrenergic blockers include nausea, vomiting, diarrhea, nightmares, depression, insomnia, hallucinations, dry eyes, paresthesia, transient thrombocytopenia, agranulocytosis, sore throat, fever, and breathing difficulty.

In a patient with intermittent claudication or PVD, beta-adrenergic blockers may produce further symptoms of arterial insufficiency. In an insulin-dependent diabetic patient, beta-adrenergic blockers can mask the early warning signs of hypoglycemia and, rarely, produce hyperglycemia. They also may alter test results for alkaline phosphatase, blood urea nitrogen (BUN), LDL, serum creatinine, serum potassium, serum transaminase, serum triglycerides, serum uric acid, and serum glucose levels.

Alpha-adrenergic blockers tend to produce different adverse reactions than the beta-adrenergic blockers. For example, doxazosin and prazosin produce orthostatic hypotension more commonly than the beta-adrenergic blockers. They also produce first-dose syncope. Terazosin produces a few mild adverse reactions, including orthostatic hypotension and dizziness. Phentolamine can precipitate anginal attacks from rebound tachycardia and may produce hypotension as well as dizziness, weakness, flushing, palpitations, diarrhea, nausea, vomiting, and nasal congestion.

Adverse reactions to the mixed alpha- and beta-adrenergic blocker labetalol resemble those of the beta-adrenergic blockers. Other reactions may include scalp tingling, alopecia, orthostatic hypotension, intermittent claudication, bronchospasm, drug-induced systemic lupus erythematosus (SLE), eye irritation, myalgia, and rash.

Norepinephrine depletors produce a wide range of adverse reactions. The most clinically relevant adverse reaction

Stepped-care approach to antihypertensive therapy

The diagram below illustrates the four-step approach to antihypertensive therapy endorsed by the Joint National Committee on Detection, Evaluation, and Treatment of High Blood Pressure. The progression of therapy is based on the patient's response, defined in two ways: the patient has achieved the target blood pressure set by the physician or the patient is making considerable progress toward this goal.

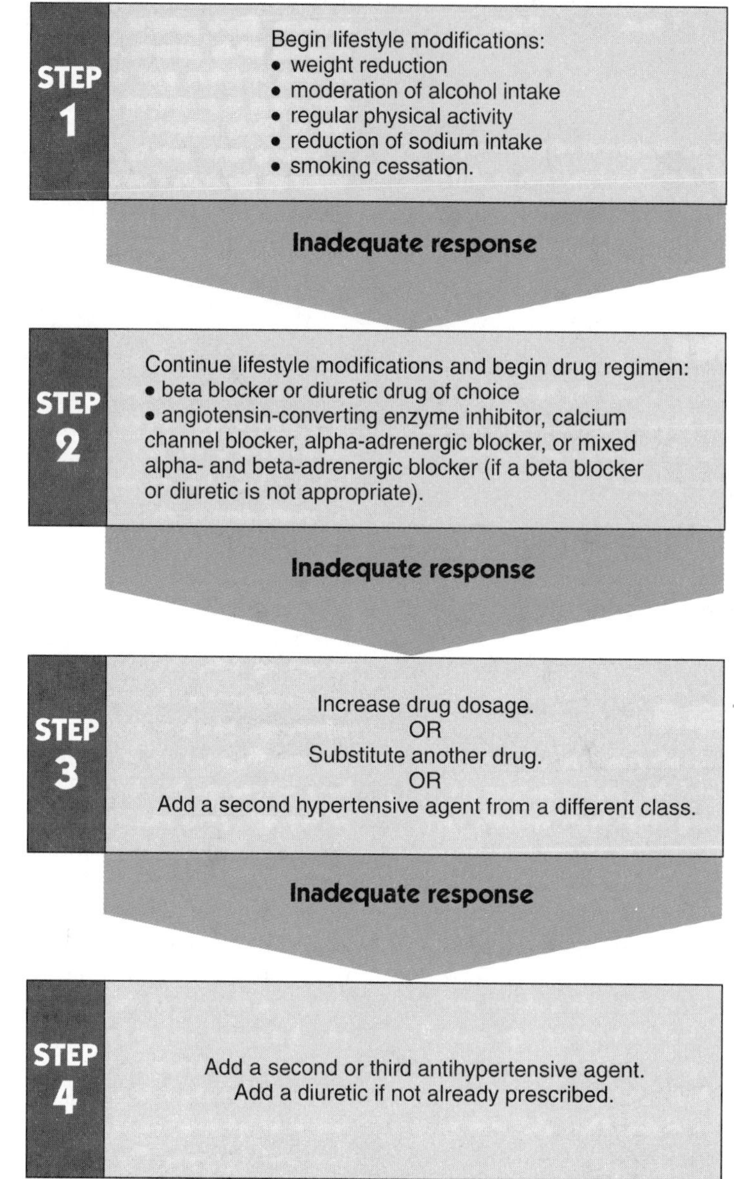

Source: U.S. Department of Health and Human Services. National Institutes of Health. National Heart, Lung, and Blood Institute. *The Fifth Report of the Joint National Committee on Detection, Evaluation, and Treatment of High Blood Pressure (JNC V).* Washington, D.C.: Government Printing Office, 1992.

to guanethidine and guanadrel is orthostatic hypotension, occurring primarily on awakening. Many patients also experience generalized weakness, especially in the beginning of therapy. A patient receiving guanadrel may faint upon exertion or standing and may develop nocturia and dyspnea, especially during the first 8 weeks of treatment.

Guanethidine can produce explosive diarrhea; failure to ejaculate; decreased myocardial contractility; fluid reten-

(Text continues on page 267.)

Selected major antihypertensive agents

This table summarizes the major antihypertensive agents currently in clinical use.

DRUG	MAJOR INDICATIONS AND USUAL DOSAGES	CONTRAINDICATIONS AND PRECAUTIONS
Sympatholytic agents		
Central-acting sympathetic nervous system inhibitors		
clonidine hydrochloride (Catapres, Catapres-TTS)	*Adjunct therapy for mild to moderate hypertension* ADULT: initially, 0.05 to 0.1 mg P.O. b.i.d., increased by 0.1 mg to 0.2 mg/day every 2 to 4 days until the desired response is achieved; for maintenance, 0.1 to 0.2 mg b.i.d. to q.i.d., or up to a maximum of 2.4 mg/day. With a transdermal patch, the usual dose is a 0.1-mg system. If blood pressure has not been reduced sufficiently after 1 or 2 weeks, a second 0.1-mg or larger system is added.	• Oral clonidine has no known contraindications. A transdermal system is contraindicated in a patient with known hypersensitivity to the drug or any ingredient or component in the administration system. • This drug requires cautious use in a pregnant or breast-feeding patient or one with severe coronary insufficiency, recent myocardial infarction (MI), cerebrovascular disease, chronic renal failure, Raynaud's disease, thromboangiitis obliterans, or history of mental depression. • Safety and efficacy in children have not been established.
methyldopa (Aldomet)	*Adjunct therapy for mild to moderate hypertension* ADULT: initially, 250 mg P.O. b.i.d. or t.i.d., increased biweekly to a maintenance dosage of 500 mg to 2 g daily in 2 to 4 divided doses or up to a maximum of 3 g daily PEDIATRIC: 10 mg/kg daily or 300 mg/m^2 given in 2 to 4 divided doses *Hypertensive crisis* ADULT: 250 to 500 mg I.V. in 100 ml of D_5W over 30 to 60 minutes, repeated every 6 hours as necessary	• Methyldopa is contraindicated in a patient with known hypersensitivity, pheochromocytoma, active liver disease, history of methyldopa use associated with liver abnormalities, or direct Coombs' test positive for hemolytic anemia. • This drug requires cautious use in a breast-feeding patient or one with a history of liver disease.
Beta-adrenergic blockers		
metoprolol succinate (Toprol XL), metoprolol tartrate (Lopressor)	*Hypertension* ADULT: initially, 50 to 100 mg P.O. daily in single or divided doses, increased by 50 mg daily every week up to maximum of 400 mg (succinate) or 250 mg (tartrate) daily	• Metoprolol is contraindicated in a patient with sinus bradycardia, heart block greater than first-degree, cardiogenic shock, overt cardiac failure or right ventricular failure secondary to pulmonary hypertension, acute MI in which the heart rate is less than 45 beats/minute, systolic blood pressure less than 100 mm Hg, or moderate to severe cardiac failure. • This drug requires cautious use in a pregnant or breast-feeding patient or one with inadequate myocardial function, bronchospastic disease, diabetes mellitus, hyperthyroidism, impaired hepatic function, or substantial cardiomegaly. Metoprolol also requires cautious use in a patient who is receiving general anesthesia. • Safety and efficacy in children have not been established.
propranolol hydrochloride (Inderal, Inderal LA)	*Hypertension* ADULT: 20 to 40 mg P.O. b.i.d., or 60 to 80 mg sustained-release capsules once daily, increased as needed to a maximum of 640 mg/day PEDIATRIC: 1 to 4 mg/kg P.O. daily given in 2 equally divided doses, up to a maximum of 16 mg/kg daily	• Propranolol is contraindicated in a patient with Raynaud's disease, malignant hypertension, bronchial asthma, sinus bradycardia and heart block greater than first-degree, heart failure (unless failure is secondary to a tachyarrhythmia treatable with propranolol), cardiogenic shock, or myasthenia gravis. • This drug requires cautious use in a pregnant or breast-feeding patient or one with inadequate cardiac function, coronary artery disease, sinus node dysfunction, hyperthyroidism, diabetes mellitus, hypoglycemia, nonallergic bronchospastic disease, or renal or hepatic impairment. Propranolol also requires cautious use in a patient who is undergoing major surgery. • Safety and efficacy of sustained-release capsules, oral solutions, and injections have not been established in children.

(continued)

Selected major antihypertensive agents *(continued)*

DRUG	MAJOR INDICATIONS AND USUAL DOSAGES	CONTRAINDICATIONS AND PRECAUTIONS
Sympatholytic agents *(continued)*		
Alpha-adrenergic blockers		
prazosin hydrochloride (Minipress)	*Hypertension* ADULT: initially, 0.5 to 1 mg P.O. b.i.d. or t.i.d.; for a maintenance dosage, increased gradually to 6 to 15 mg daily in divided doses when given alone or 1 to 2 mg P.O. t.i.d. when combined with a diuretic or another antihypertensive drug	• Prazosin has no known contraindications. • This drug requires cautious use in a pregnant or breast-feeding patient or one with chronic renal failure. • Safety and efficacy in children have not been established.
Mixed alpha- and beta-adrenergic blockers		
labetalol (Normodyne, Trandate)	*Hypertension* ADULT: 100 mg P.O. b.i.d. increased every 2 to 3 days as needed up to a maximum of 400 mg b.i.d. *Hypertensive crisis* ADULT: 20 to 80 mg slow I.V. bolus every 10 minutes or 2 mg/minute by continuous infusion to a maximum of 300 mg	• Labetalol is contraindicated in a patient with bronchial asthma, overt cardiac failure, heart block greater than first-degree, cardiogenic shock, severe bradycardia, or other conditions associated with severe and prolonged hypotension. • This drug requires cautious use in a pregnant or breast-feeding patient or one with inadequate cardiac function, nonallergic bronchospasm, pheochromocytoma, diabetes mellitus, impaired hepatic function, or history of heart failure. • Safety and efficacy in children have not been established.
Norepinephrine depletors		
guanethidine sulfate (Ismelin)	*Adjunct therapy for moderate to severe hypertension* ADULT: initially, 10 mg P.O. daily, increased by 10 to 12.5 mg every 5 to 7 days for the first month and every 2 to 3 weeks thereafter as needed; for maintenance dosage, 25 to 50 mg daily	• Guanethidine is contraindicated in a patient with known or suspected pheochromocytoma, overt heart failure not caused by hypertension, or known hypersensitivity. • This drug requires cautious use in a pregnant or breast-feeding patient or one with impaired renal function, incipient cardiac decompensation, coronary insufficiency, recent MI, cerebrovascular disease, history of bronchial asthma, peptic ulcer, severe heart failure related to hypertension, or chronic disorders that may be aggravated by a relative increase in parasympathetic tone. • Safety and efficacy in children have not been established.
Vasodilating agents		
Direct vasodilators		
hydralazine hydrochloride (Apresoline)	*Adjunct therapy for moderate to severe hypertension* ADULT: 40 mg P.O. daily in divided doses for the first 2 to 4 days, increased to 100 mg daily in divided doses for the rest of the week, then to 200 mg daily in divided doses and up to a maximum of 300 mg daily in four divided doses PEDIATRIC: 0.75 mg/kg or 25 mg/m^2 P.O. daily, given in four divided doses; if necessary, dosage may be increased gradually over 3 to 4 weeks up to 7.5 mg/kg daily *Hypertensive crisis* ADULT: 10 to 20 mg I.V. or 10 to 40 mg I.M. repeated as needed PEDIATRIC: 1.7 to 3.5 mg/kg or 50 to 100 mg/m^2 I.M. or I.V. daily, divided into four to six doses (initial parenteral dose should not exceed 20 mg)	• Hydralazine is contraindicated in a breast-feeding patient or one with rheumatic mitral valve disease or known hypersensitivity. • Hydralazine requires cautious use in a pregnant patient or one with sulfite sensitivity, cerebrovascular accident, severe renal damage, or known or suspected coronary artery disease.

Selected major antihypertensive agents *(continued)*

DRUG	MAJOR INDICATIONS AND USUAL DOSAGES	CONTRAINDICATIONS AND PRECAUTIONS
Vasodilating agents *(continued)*		
Direct vasodilators *(continued)*		
nitroprusside sodium (Nipride)	*Hypertensive crisis* ADULT: initially, 0.25 to 0.3 mcg/kg/minute by I.V. infusion, increased to 0.5 to 10mcg/kg/minute; average dose is 3 mcg/kg/minute PEDIATRIC: Varied according to the patient's need and other factors, such as age and weight	• Nitroprusside sodium is contraindicated in a breast-feeding patient or one with inadequate cerebral circulation (during surgery), compensatory hypertension caused by arteriovenous shunt or coarctation of the aorta, Leber's optic (congenital) atrophy, or tobacco amblyopia. • This drug requires cautious use in a pregnant patient or one with severe renal impairment, hepatic insufficiency, hypothyroidism, hyponatremia, low plasma vitamin B_{12} concentrations, or increased intracranial pressure. It also requires cautious use in a patient who is considered a poor surgical risk.
Calcium channel blockers		
amlodipine besylate (Norvasc)	*Hypertension* ADULT: initially, 2.5 to 5 mg P.O. once daily; increased every 7 to 10 days as needed, up to a maximum of 10 mg P.O. once daily	• Amlodipine is contraindicated in a breast-feeding patient or one with known hypersensitivity. • This drug requires cautious use in a pregnant patient or one with severe aortic stenosis, heart failure, or severe hepatic failure. • Safety and efficacy in children have not been established.
diltiazem (Cardizem SR)	*Hypertension* ADULT: initially, 60 to 120 mg P.O. b.i.d. (sustained-release form), increased as needed to the optimal dosage range of 240 to 360 mg daily	• Contraindications are the same as verapamil. • This drug requires cautious use in a geriatric patient or one with heart failure, severe bradycardia, or a pacemaker in place. May cause transient hypotension when therapy initiated. Negative inotropic effects may exacerbate heart failure. Use cautiously in patients with pacemakers, severe bradycardia. Older adults may require dose reduction.
felodipine (Plendil)	*Hypertension* ADULT: initially, 5 mg P.O. once daily; increased as needed, up to a maximum of 10 mg P.O. once daily	• Felodipine is contraindicated in a breast-feeding patient or one with known hypersensitivity. • This drug requires cautious use in a pregnant or geriatric patient or one with heart failure or compromised ventricular function, especially one who also is receiving a beta blocker. • Safety and efficacy in children have not been established.
isradipine (DynaCirc)	*Hypertension* ADULT: initially, 2.5 mg P.O. b.i.d.; increased by 5 mg daily at 2- to 4-week intervals up to a maximum of 20 mg P.O. daily	• Isradipine is contraindicated in a breast-feeding patient or one with known hypersensitivity. • This drug requires cautious use in a pregnant patient or one with heart failure, especially one who also is receiving a beta blocker. • Safety and efficacy in children have not been established.
nifedipine (Procardia XL)	*Hypertension* ADULT: 30- to 60-mg sustained-release tablets once daily, increased to a maximum of 120 mg daily	• Nifedipine is contraindicated in a patient with known hypersensitivity. • This drug requires cautious use in a pregnant patient or one with heart failure, aortic stenosis, or severe gastrointestinal narrowing.
verapamil hydrochloride (Calan SR, Isoptin SR)	*Hypertension* ADULT: initially, 80 mg P.O. t.i.d., titrated to 40 mg t.i.d. for a patient who responds to a lower dosage; or 240 mg sustained-release form P.O. once daily in the morning	• Verapamil is contraindicated in a patient with sick sinus syndrome, significant hypotension, sinus bradycardia, second- and third-heart block except when a functional ventricular pacemaker in place, or severe heart failure. • This drug requires cautious use in a geriatric patient or one with a small stature.

(continued)

Selected major antihypertensive agents *(continued)*

DRUG	MAJOR INDICATIONS AND USUAL DOSAGES	CONTRAINDICATIONS AND PRECAUTIONS
Angiotensin-converting enzyme (ACE) inhibitors		
benazepril hydrochloride (Lotensin)	*Management of hypertension, alone or as an adjunct with a thiazide diuretic* ADULT: for a patient not receiving a thiazide diuretic, initially, 10 mg P.O. once daily, with maintenance dosage of 20 to 40 mg daily in a single dose or two divided doses; for a patient receiving a thiazide diuretic, 5 mg P.O. once daily	• Benazepril is contraindicated in a pregnant patient in her second or third trimester or in one with known hypersensitivity to the drug or any other angiotensin-converting enzyme (ACE) inhibitor. • This drug requires cautious use in a pregnant patient in her first trimester or one with impaired renal function or a history of angioedema. • Safety and efficacy in children have not been established.
captopril (Capoten)	*Hypertension* ADULT: 25 mg P.O. b.i.d. to t.i.d., increased to 50 mg b.i.d. to t.i.d. after 1 to 2 weeks to a maximum of 450 mg daily	• Captopril is contraindicated in a pregnant patient in her second or third trimester or one with known hypersensitivity to the drug or any other ACE inhibitors. • This drug requires cautious use in a pregnant patient in her first trimester, a breast-feeding patient, a patient receiving dialysis or diuretic therapy, or one with renal impairment, collagen vascular disease, sodium depletion, hypovolemia, coronary or cerebrovascular insufficiency, or heart failure. • Safety and efficacy in children under age 15 have not been established.
enalapril (Vasotec)	*Hypertension* ADULT: 5 mg P.O. daily, increased gradually to a maximum of 40 mg daily as needed to control blood pressure	• Enalapril is contraindicated in a patient with a hypersensitivity to drug or previous angioedema caused by an ACE inhibitor. • This drug requires cautious use in a patient with heart failure, dehydration, or renal impairment or one who is receiving diuretic therapy.
fosinopril sodium (Monopril)	*Management of hypertension, alone or as an adjunct with a thiazide diuretic* ADULT: initially, 10 mg P.O. once daily; for maintenance dosage, 20 to 40 mg daily	• Fosinopril is contraindicated in a pregnant patient in her second or third trimester, a breast-feeding patient, or one with known hypersensitivity to the drug or any other ACE inhibitor or a history of angioedema. • This drug requires cautious use in a pregnant patient in her first trimester or one with impaired renal or hepatic function. • Safety and efficacy in children have not been established.
lisinopril (Prinivil, Zestril)	*Mild to severe hypertension* ADULT: 10 mg P.O. daily, increased up to a maximum of 80 mg daily as needed to control blood pressure	• Lisinopril is contraindicated in a patient with a hypersensitivity to drug or previous angioedema caused by an ACE inhibitor. • This drug requires cautious use in a patient with heart failure, dehydration, or renal impairment or one who is receiving diuretic therapy. • Safety and efficacy in children have not been established.
quinapril hydrochloride (Accupril)	*Management of hypertension, alone or as an adjunct with a thiazide diuretic* ADULT: for a patient not receiving a thiazide diuretic, initially 10 mg P.O. once daily, with maintenance dosage of 20 to 80 mg P.O. daily in single or divided doses; for a patient receiving a thiazide diuretic, initially 5 mg P.O. once daily titrate for response up to 80 mg daily	• Quinapril is contraindicated in a pregnant patient in her second or third trimester or one with known hypersensitivity to the drug or a history of angioedema. • This drug requires cautious use in a pregnant patient in her first trimester, a breast-feeding patient, or one with impaired renal function. • Safety and efficacy in children have not been established.

Selected major antihypertensive agents *(continued)*

DRUG	MAJOR INDICATIONS AND USUAL DOSAGES	CONTRAINDICATIONS AND PRECAUTIONS
Angiotensin-converting enzyme (ACE) inhibitors *(continued)*		
ramipril (Altace)	*Management of hypertension, alone or as an adjunct with a thiazide diuretic* ADULT: for a patient not receiving a thiazide diuretic, initially, 2.5 mg P.O. daily, increased as needed, up to a maximum of 20 mg daily; for a patient receiving a thiazide diuretic, initially 1.25 mg P.O. daily titrated for response up to a maximum of 20 mg daily	• Ramipril is contraindicated in a pregnant or breast-feeding patient or one with known hypersensitivity or a history of angioneurotic edema. • This drug requires cautious use in a patient with impaired liver or renal function. • Safety and efficacy in children have not been established.

tion; increased BUN, aspartate aminotransferase, and alanine aminotransferase levels; and decreased prothrombin time and serum glucose and urine catecholamine levels.

Common adverse reactions to reserpine include drowsiness, sleep pattern disturbances, weight gain, and nasal congestion. Increased GI motility, abdominal cramps, and diarrhea also may occur along with nightmares, depression, uterine contractions, and bronchoconstriction (in a patient with bronchitis). Reserpine also may increase the risk of breast cancer. When given to a breast-feeding patient, it may result in increased respiratory secretions, nasal congestion, and cyanosis in the infant. Reserpine also may interfere with serum glucose and urine glucose test results, and may decrease urinary excretion of catecholamines, 17-hydroxycorticosteroid, 17-ketosteroid levels, and vanillylmandelic acid.

Rare reactions to central-acting agents include anorexia, vomiting, parotid pain, and rash. Pruritus, abdominal discomfort, constipation, diarrhea, nausea, vomiting, and aches in the extremities also may occur. Guanabenz may result in headaches and sexual dysfunction. In rare instances, terazosin may produce diminished hearing, chest pain, insomnia, and GI distress. Reserpine may produce angina, bradycardia, blurred vision, impotence, and decreased libido.

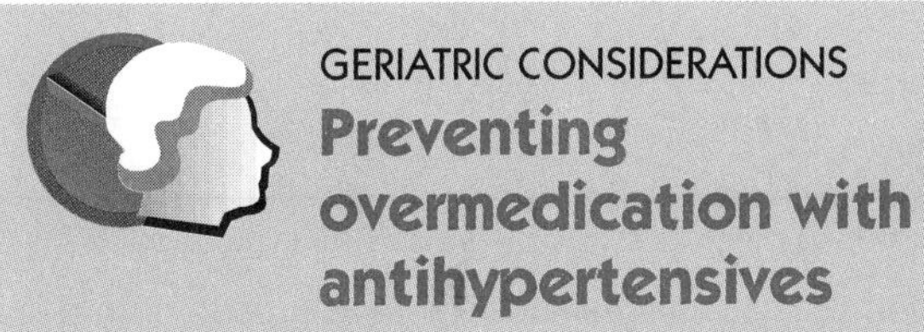

GERIATRIC CONSIDERATIONS

Preventing overmedication with antihypertensives

Geriatric patients commonly experience adverse drug reactions. If the adverse reaction is misinterpreted as a new medical condition, the physician may prescribe a new drug to treat the new "condition." For example, if high-dose therapy with a nonsteroidal anti-inflammatory drug increases the blood pressure in a patient with hypertension, the physician might treat this adverse reaction by changing the patient's antihypertensive agent or increasing its dosage.

To avoid such overmedication, the physician and nurse should review the geriatric patient's use of prescription and over-the-counter drugs and consider their effects on blood pressure.

NURSING PROCESS APPLICATION

The following information assists the nurse in caring for a patient who is receiving a sympatholytic agent. It includes an overview of assessment activities as well as examples of appropriate nursing diagnoses and related interventions. It also highlights the importance of evaluation.

Assessment

Before drug therapy begins, review the patient's history for conditions that contraindicate or require cautious use of the prescribed sympatholytic. Also review the patient's medication history to identify use of drugs that may interact with it. In a geriatric patient, be especially alert for use of drugs that may increase blood pressure. (See Geriatric Considerations: *Preventing overmedication with antihypertensives.*) During therapy, assess the patient for adverse drug reactions and signs of drug interactions. Periodically assess the effectiveness of sympatholytic therapy. (See Drug Interactions: *Sympatholytics,* page 268.) Finally, evaluate the patient's and family's knowledge about the prescribed drug.

Nursing diagnoses

- Risk for injury related to a preexisting condition that contraindicates or requires cautious use of a sympatholytic agent
- Risk for injury related to adverse drug reactions or drug interactions
- Ineffective breathing pattern related to the adverse respiratory effects of the prescribed sympatholytic agent
- Knowledge deficit related to the prescribed sympatholytic agent

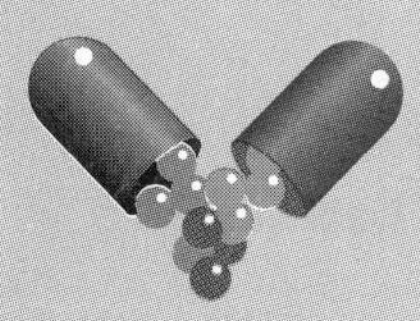

DRUG INTERACTIONS

Sympatholytic agents

Sympatholytics can interact with many drugs to produce blood pressure changes as well as other severe reactions.

DRUG	INTERACTING AGENTS	POSSIBLE EFFECTS	NURSING IMPLICATIONS
Central-acting sympathetic nervous system inhibitors			
clonidine	tricyclic antidepressants	Increased blood pressure	• Avoid concomitant administration.
	central nervous system (CNS) depressants	Additive depressant effects	• Use together with caution. • Monitor the patient for CNS depression.
Mixed alpha- and beta-adrenergic blocking agents			
labetalol	halothane anesthesia	Enhanced hypotensive effects of labetalol	• Monitor the patient's blood pressure frequently.
	cimetidine	Potentiated decrease in blood pressure	• Use concurrently with caution and only if necessary.
Norepinephrine depletors			
guanadrel	sympathomimetics	Inhibited antihypertensive effects of guanadrel	• Monitor the patient's blood pressure frequently.
guanethidine	sympathomimetics, phenothiazines, tricyclic antidepressants, amphetamines	Inhibited antihypertensive effects of guanethidine	• Avoid concomitant administration. • Monitor the patient's blood pressure frequently.
reserpine	levodopa	Depleted dopamine levels, inhibited effect of levodopa	• Avoid giving reserpine to a patient receiving levodopa for Parkinson's disease.
Beta-adrenergic blocking agents			
acebutolol, atenolol, betaxolol, carteolol, metoprolol, nadolol, penbutolol, pindolol, propranolol, timolol	antacids	Delayed drug absorption from gastrointestinal tract	• Administer several hours apart. • Monitor the patient for a decreased therapeutic effect.
	lidocaine	Increased plasma levels of lidocaine (potential toxicity); additive cardiac depressant effects	• Monitor the patient for signs of lidocaine toxicity, such as confusion, restlessness, and tremors.
	insulin, oral hypoglycemic agents	Hypoglycemia or hyperglycemia; masking of tachycardia as a sign of hypoglycemia (diaphoresis and agitation still present)	• Administer these drugs cautiously. • Monitor the patient's blood glucose levels frequently.
	nonsteroidal anti-inflammatory drugs (indomethacin, salicylates)	Decreased hypotensive effects of beta-adrenergic blockers	• Monitor the patient for altered beta-adrenergic blocker effects.
	barbiturates, rifampin	Stimulated metabolism of beta-adrenergic blockers that are metabolized extensively	• Monitor the patient for altered response to beta-adrenergic blockers that are metabolized by the liver (propranolol, metoprolol).

Sympatholytic agents *(continued)*

DRUG	INTERACTING AGENTS	POSSIBLE EFFECTS	NURSING IMPLICATIONS
Beta-adrenergic blocking agents *(continued)*			
acebutolol, atenolol, betaxolol, carteolol, metoprolol, nadolol, penbutolol, pindolol, propranolol, timolol *(continued)*	cardiac glycosides	Additive bradycardia and depression of atrioventricular conduction	• Monitor the patient's blood pressure and heart rate frequently.
	calcium channel blockers	Increased pharmacologic and toxicologic effects of both agents	• Monitor the patient for adverse reactions.
	sympathomimetics (epinephrine, dobutamine, dopamine, isoproterenol, terbutaline, metaproterenol, albuterol, ritodrine)	Hypertension and reflex bradycardia from unopposed alpha effects (vasoconstriction) and increased vagal tone	• Monitor the patient's blood pressure and heart rate frequently.
	cimetidine	Reduced metabolism of beta-adrenergic blockers; enhanced ability of beta-adrenergic blockers to reduce pulse rate	• Monitor the patient for altered response to beta-adrenergic blockers.
	theophyllines	Impaired bronchodilating effects of theophyllines by nonselective beta-adrenergic blockers	• Monitor the patient's therapeutic response.
	clonidine	Attenuated or reversed antihypertensive effects; life-threatening increase in blood pressure	• Monitor the patient's blood pressure closely.

Planning and implementation

- Do not administer a sympatholytic agent to a patient with a condition that contraindicates its use.
- Administer a sympatholytic agent cautiously to a patient at risk because of a preexisting condition.
- Monitor the patient closely for adverse reactions and drug interactions throughout sympatholytic therapy.
- Obtain baseline data before beginning sympatholytic therapy. Assess the patient's blood pressure and pulses in the sitting, standing, and supine positions. Monitor and record the patient's blood pressure and pulse when starting drug therapy, before administering each dose, and during peak concentration times.
- Monitor the patient's vital signs, as instructed. For example, expect to monitor the patient's blood pressure and pulse every 15 to 30 minutes for at least the first 2 hours during initial administration of an alpha-adrenergic blocker.
- Monitor serum electrolyte levels, and correct any imbalances, as prescribed, before administering a norepinephrine depletor.
- Assess the patient's hepatic and renal function before beginning therapy with a beta-adrenergic blocker and at regular intervals. If the BUN or serum creatinine level is elevated, notify the physician.
- Observe the patient closely for syncope when administering the first dose of doxazosin, prazosin, or terazosin. To prevent severe first-dose orthostatic hypotension, have the patient lie down for at least 3 hours after taking the dose. (See Patient Teaching: *Sympatholytics*, page 270.)
- Monitor a diabetic patient's serum glucose level carefully, especially during beta blocker or reserpine therapy.
- Give labetalol, metoprolol, or propranolol between meals. If sedation occurs with a central-acting agent, give the drug in the evening. If the dosage is increased, start with an evening dose to minimize sedative effects.
- Supervise a patient with a history of depression closely, because it may recur during antihypertensive therapy.
- Discontinue guanethidine for 72 hours before elective surgery, as prescribed, to prevent interaction with sympathomimetic agents that may be used during surgery.
- Anticipate gradual discontinuation of a beta-adrenergic blocker over 3 to 14 days. During this time, the patient should avoid vigorous physical activity to prevent overtaxing the heart.

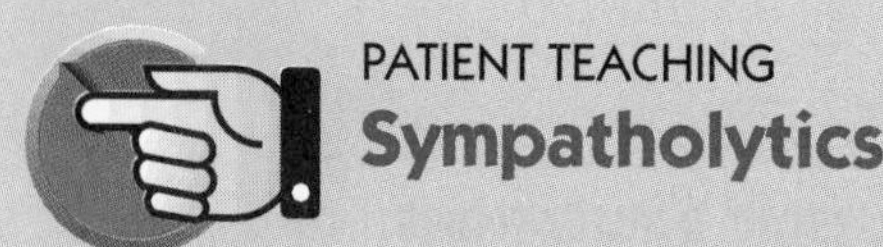

PATIENT TEACHING
Sympatholytics

- Teach the patient and family the name, dose, frequency, action, and adverse effects of the prescribed sympatholytic.
- Review general instructions about use of antihypertensives.
- Inform the patient taking guanadrel of the possibility of fainting on exertion or standing and of developing nocturia and dyspnea, especially during the first 8 weeks of treatment.
- Inform the patient taking clonidine that vivid dreams may occur.
- Reassure the patient receiving a central-acting agent that central nervous system effects usually diminish after 2 to 3 weeks of therapy.
- Advise the patient taking methyldopa that the drug may darken the urine.
- Instruct the patient to take the first dose of doxazosin, prazosin, or terazosin at bedtime or to remain lying down for at least 3 hours after taking it to prevent severe first-dose orthostatic hypotension.
- Teach the patient on reserpine therapy to take the drug with food, milk, or 8 ounces of water to minimize GI distress.
- Instruct the patient and family about possible depression. Describe the early signs of depression, which may not occur until 6 months after therapy begins, and the signs of suicidal behavior if severe depression occurs.
- Instruct the patient to anticipate gradual discontinuation of the prescribed beta-adrenergic blocker and to avoid vigorous physical activity while the drug is being discontinued.
- Alert the patient on a sodium-restricted diet that noncompliance may result in fluid retention and edema.
- Instruct the patient to notify the physician if adverse reactions occur.

• Expect to decrease the guanfacine dosage for a geriatric patient or one with renal impairment; and the atenolol, carteolol, or nadolol dosage for a patient with impaired renal function.
• Do not discontinue clonidine or guanabenz abruptly to prevent rebound hypertension.
• Notify the physician if adverse drug reactions or drug interactions occur or if the drug is ineffective.
Monitor the patient's respiratory rate and pattern before and after administration of each dose and auscultate breath sounds regularly. Continue to monitor the patient closely for respiratory changes, especially noting respiratory depression (with ganglionic blocking agent therapy), breathing difficulty (with beta-adrenergic blocker therapy), bronchospasm (with mixed alpha- and beta-adrenergic blocker or norepinephrine depletor therapy) and bronchoconstriction (with norepinephrine depletor therapy in a patient with bronchitis).
Notify the physician if the patient's breathing pattern changes. Keep emergency respiratory equipment nearby, such as oxygen and bronchodilators. Help the patient into a position that promotes easier breathing.
• Administer prazosin with food.

Evaluation

For each nursing diagnosis, prepare an evaluation statement that describes the patient's or family's response to nursing interventions.

Vasodilating agents

There are two types of vasodilating agents: direct vasodilators and calcium channel blockers. Both types decrease systolic and diastolic blood pressure by relaxing arteriolar smooth muscle, leading to arteriolar dilation and decreasing peripheral resistance.

Direct vasodilators act on arteries, veins, or both. They include diazoxide, hydralazine hydrochloride, minoxidil, and nitroprusside sodium. Hydralazine and minoxidil usually are used to treat resistant or refractory hypertension. Diazoxide and nitroprusside are reserved for use in hypertensive crisis.

Calcium channel blockers produce arteriolar relaxation by preventing the entry of calcium into the cells, thus reducing the mechanical activity of vascular smooth muscle. They include amlodipine besylate, diltiazem hydrochloride, felodipine, isradipine, nicardipine hydrochloride, nifedipine, and verapamil hydrochloride.

PHARMACOKINETICS

Most of these drugs are absorbed rapidly and distributed well. They all are metabolized in the liver, and most are excreted by the kidneys. Vasodilating agents vary widely in their pharmacokinetic processes.

Route	Onset	Peak	Duration
P.O.	20-30 min	2-8 hr	2 hr-5 days
I.V.	Immediate-20 min	5-80 min	1 min-12 hr
I.M.	Unknown	Unknown	3-8 hr

PHARMACODYNAMICS

The direct vasodilators relax peripheral vascular smooth muscles, lowering blood pressure by increasing blood vessel caliber and reducing total peripheral resistance. Calcium channel blockers prevent calcium transport across the cell membrane, reducing the activity of the vascular smooth muscle, thus producing vasodilation and lowering the blood pressure.

PHARMACOTHERAPEUTICS

Vasodilating agents usually are used as adjuncts in treating hypertension. They seldom are used as primary agents.

Drug interactions

Hydralazine and minoxidil produce additive effects when given with other antihypertensive drugs, such as methyldopa or reserpine. They also may produce additive effects when given with nitrates, such as isosorbide dinitrate or nitroglycerin. Few other drug interactions occur with the vasodilating agents. However, diltiazem, felodipine, and verapamil may promote digitalis toxicity when given with digoxin; verapamil may produce a similar interaction with digitoxin. Diltiazem, nicardipine, and verapamil also may interact with drugs that affect the hepatic microsomal system, altering the metabolism of either interacting drug. With concomitant administration, cimetidine may increase felodipine and nicardipine plasma levels. Amlodipine and isradipine have no known drug interactions.

ADVERSE DRUG REACTIONS

Direct vasodilators commonly produce adverse reactions related to reflex activation of the sympathetic nervous system: palpitations, angina, tachycardia, increased myocardial workload, electrocardiogram changes, edema, breast tenderness, fatigue, headache, and rash. Severe pericardial effusions may develop. Alkaline phosphatase, BUN, and creatinine levels may increase. Unlike the other vasodilators, calcium channel blockers do not produce rebound tachycardia or significant edema. Other adverse reactions depend on the specific drug used.

Common adverse reactions to diazoxide include headache, anorexia, nausea, and diaphoresis. The following adverse reactions also may occur and usually require discontinuation of the drug: rash, drug fever, urticaria, polyneuritis, GI hemorrhage, anemia, and pancytopenia. Diazoxide also is especially likely to result in excessive hypotension and reflex sympathetic stimulation. It also may produce hyperglycemia in a diabetic patient.

Hydralazine commonly produces such adverse reactions as headache, diarrhea, constipation, dizziness or light-headedness, orthostatic hypotension, facial flushing, shortness of breath, nasal congestion, urinary hesitancy, lacrimation, conjunctivitis, paresthesia, edema, tremor, and muscle cramps. When hydralazine dosage exceeds 200 mg/day, the patient may develop drug-induced SLE.

Minoxidil commonly produces hypertrichosis (excessive hair growth), especially on the face, arms, and back, 3 to 6 weeks after therapy begins. Minoxidil also is likely to produce reflex tachycardia and fluid retention.

Nitroprusside sodium produces headache, dizziness, nausea, vomiting, and abdominal pain.

The most common adverse reactions to amlodipine are headache and edema. Other adverse reactions include fatigue, nausea, abdominal pain, and somnolence.

The most serious adverse reactions to diltiazem — hypotension and bradycardia — may be extensions of the drug's therapeutic effect. Other reactions may include flushing, palpitations, drowsiness, tremor, insomnia, headache, edema, nausea, rash, and transient elevation of liver enzymes.

The most common adverse reactions to felodipine are headache, peripheral edema, and flushing. Other adverse reactions include dizziness, asthenia, upper respiratory infection, cough, paresthesia, dyspepsia, chest pain, nausea, muscle cramps, palpitations, abdominal pain, constipation, diarrhea, pharyngitis, and back pain.

Most adverse reactions to isradipine are mild and related to its vasodilating effects. They include dizziness, edema, palpitations, flushing, and tachycardia. Other common adverse reactions include headache, fatigue, chest pain, nausea, dyspnea, abdominal discomfort, urinary frequency, weakness, vomiting, and diarrhea.

When used in antihypertensive dosages, nicardipine commonly produces flushing, headache, and facial edema. Less common reactions include palpitations, dizziness, tachycardia, nausea, and somnolence. Allergic reactions are rare.

Nifedipine can produce the same reactions as diltiazem, along with peripheral edema and dizziness or light-headedness.

The most common adverse reaction to verapamil is constipation; other reactions include those listed for diltiazem along with atrioventricular heart block, peripheral edema, dizziness, light-headedness, and fatigue.

Hypersensitivity reactions (urticaria, rash, pruritus, fever, chills, arthralgia, eosinophilia, and, rarely, obstructive jaundice and hepatitis) and blood dyscrasias (leukopenia, agranulocytosis, thrombocytopenia) also may occur with some vasodilating agents.

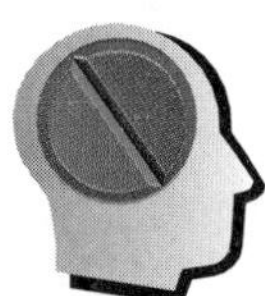

CRITICAL THINKING: To enhance your critical thinking about antihypertensive agents, consider the following situation and its analysis.
Situation: Arlette Naylor, age 52, is in the recovery room after undergoing an appendectomy. Because she was going to have surgery, she did not take her antihypertensive this morning. Now her vital signs are: blood pressure 190/98 mm Hg, pulse 105 beats/minute, and respirations 16 breaths/minute. The physician orders labetalol to control her blood pressure. Why doesn't he order hydralazine instead?
Analysis: Although both antihypertensives can be given intravenously to lower the patient's blood pressure rapidly, labetalol also can decrease her heart rate, whereas hydralazine could increase it. Before any antihypertensive is administered, however, the nurse should assess the patient to ensure that the hypertension is not being caused by post-operative pain, nausea, or other condition. (If it is, the patient might need an analgesic or antiemetic.)

NURSING PROCESS APPLICATION

The following information assists the nurse in caring for a patient who is receiving a vasodilating agent. It includes an overview of assessment activities as well as examples of ap-

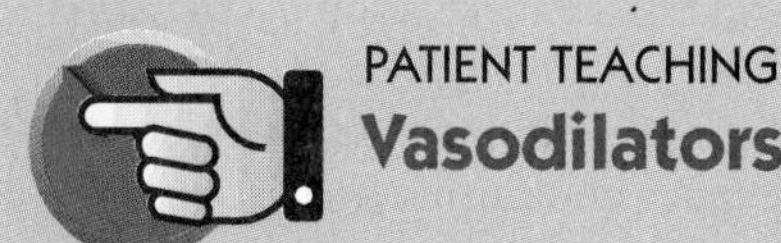

PATIENT TEACHING
Vasodilators

- Teach the patient and family the name, dose, frequency, action, and adverse effects of the prescribed vasodilating agent.
- Provide general information about vasodilator use.
- Advise a patient taking minoxidil that hypertrichosis is likely to occur 3 to 6 weeks after treatment begins. Reassure the patient that the extra hair growth should disappear 1 to 6 months after the drug is discontinued.
- Advise the patient taking felodipine or nifedipine to swallow the capsules whole.
- Instruct the patient to notify the physician if adverse reactions occur.

propriate nursing diagnoses and related interventions. It also highlights the importance of evaluation.

Assessment

Before drug therapy begins, review the patient's history for conditions that contraindicate or require cautious use of the prescribed vasodilating agent. Also review the patient's medication history to identify use of drugs that may interact with it. During therapy, assess the patient for adverse drug reactions and signs of drug interactions. Also, periodically assess the effectiveness of therapy with the prescribed vasodilating agent. Finally, evaluate the patient's and family's knowledge about the prescribed drug. (See Patient Teaching: *Vasodilators.*)

Nursing diagnoses

- Risk for injury related to a preexisting condition that contraindicates or requires cautious use of a vasodilating agent
- Risk for injury related to adverse drug reactions or drug interactions
- Pain related to vasodilating agent-induced headache, angina, or muscle cramps
- Knowledge deficit related to the prescribed vasodilating agent

Planning and implementation

- Do not administer a vasodilating agent to a patient with a condition that contraindicates its use.
- Administer a vasodilating agent cautiously to a patient at risk because of a preexisting condition.
- Monitor the patient closely for adverse reactions and drug interactions throughout vasodilator therapy.
- Obtain baseline blood pressure and pulse rates before diazoxide or hydralazine administration. During administration, monitor the blood pressure and pulse every 5 minutes for the first 30 minutes, and then every 15 minutes for 2 hours after each dose is given and blood pressure stabilizes.
- Monitor the patient's blood pressure continuously during nitroprusside therapy by an arterial line or every 5 minutes if an arterial line is not available.

✱ ***Monitor for signs of cerebral ischemia and impaired renal blood flow. These signs are most likely to occur when vasodilator administration causes a rapid reduction in blood pressure. If any of these signs appear, help the patient into a supine position, elevate the patient's legs, and notify the physician immediately.***

- Monitor the diabetic patient receiving diazoxide therapy for increases in serum glucose levels for up to 1 week after administration.
- Prevent orthostatic hypotension by keeping the patient in a supine position for 15 to 30 minutes after diazoxide or hydralazine administration.
- Observe for early signs of drug-induced SLE, such as myalgia, arthralgia, and pleuritis, when the hydralazine dosage exceeds 200 mg daily.
- Do not crush felodipine tables.
- Monitor the patient for orthostatic hypotension and teach the patient how to manage it.
- Hydralazine should not be administered with food because food increases the drug's plasma level.
- The sustained-release form of verapamil should be given with food.
- Administer diazoxide via a peripheral vein to prevent cardiac arrhythmias.
- Ask the patient to report headache, angina pain, or muscle cramps.
- Notify the physician if the patient's condition does not improve, if adverse reactions or drug interactions occur, or if pain develops.

Evaluation

For each nursing diagnosis, prepare an evaluation statement that describes the patient's or family's response to nursing interventions.

Angiotensin-converting enzyme (ACE) inhibitors

Another class of antihypertensive agents, ACE inhibitors reduce blood pressure by interrupting the renin-angiotensin-aldosterone system. ACE inhibitors discussed include benazepril hydrochloride, captopril, enalapril, fosinopril sodium, lisinopril, quinapril hydrochloride, and ramipril.

PHARMACOKINETICS

The ACE inhibitors are absorbed from the GI tract, distributed to most body tissues, metabolized somewhat in the liver, and excreted by the kidneys. Ramipril also is excreted in the feces.

Benazepril reaches a peak concentration level in 30 to 60 minutes after oral administration; benazeprilat, the active metabolite of benazepril, reaches its peak in 1 to 2 hours. The effective half-life of benazeprilat is 10 to 11 hours.

Captopril reaches a peak concentration level in 30 to 90 minutes and full therapeutic effectiveness in weeks. Its half-life probably is less than 2 hours, and its duration of action ranges from 6 to 12 hours.

Enalapril reaches peak concentration in 30 to 90 minutes after oral administration; enalaprilat, the active metabolite of enalapril, reaches its peak in 3 to 4 hours. The drug produces initial antihypertensive effects in 1 hour and maximal effects in 4 to 8 hours. The estimated half-life of enalaprilat is 11 hours in healthy adults with normal renal function. Enalapril's duration is up to 24 hours.

Fosinopril reaches a peak concentration level approximately 3 hours after oral administration. Its half-life is approximately 12 hours.

Lisinopril begins to act in 1 hour and reaches peak concentration within 6 hours. Its half-life is 12 hours, and its duration is 24 hours.

Quinapril reaches a peak concentration level within 1 hour after oral administration; quinaprilat, the active metabolite of quinapril, in 2 hours. The elimination half-life of quinaprilat is 3 hours.

Ramipril reaches a peak concentration level within 1 hour after oral administration; ramiprilat, the active metabolite of ramipril, in 2 to 4 hours. The plasma concentrations of ramiprilat decline in a triphasic manner: the initial rapid decline has a half-life of 2 to 4 hours; the apparent elimination phase has a half-life of 9 to 18 hours; and the terminal elimination phase has a prolonged half-life of greater than 50 hours.

Route	Onset	Peak	Duration
P.O.	0.5-1 hr	0.5-6 hr	6-24 hr
I.V	<15 min	<4 hr	6 hr

PHARMACODYNAMICS

The ACE inhibitors act by interfering with the renin-angiotensin-aldosterone system. They do so by inhibiting the enzyme that converts angiotensin I to angiotensin II. This inhibition decreases aldosterone release by the adrenal cortex, preventing sodium and water retention. It also reduces peripheral arterial resistance without affecting the heart rate and cardiac output. The result, in a patient with hypertension, is a decreased blood pressure.

PHARMACOTHERAPEUTICS

ACE inhibitors may be used alone or in combination with another agent, such as a thiazide diuretic, to treat hypertension.

Drug interactions

All ACE inhibitors enhance the hypotensive effects of diuretics and other antihypertensives, such as beta-adrenergic blockers. They also can increase serum lithium levels when given concomitantly with lithium, possibly resulting in lithium toxicity. When ACE inhibitors are used concomitantly with potassium-sparing diuretics, potassium supplements, or potassium-containing salt substitutes, hyperkalemia may occur.

Captopril, enalapril, and lisinopril may become less effective when administered with nonsteroidal anti-inflammatory drugs.

Antacids may impair the absorption of fosinopril. Therefore, if concomitant use of these agents is indicated, doses should be separated by 2 hours. Quinapril may reduce the absorption of tetracycline by approximately 28% to 37%; this may be caused by the high magnesium content of quinapril tablets.

ADVERSE DRUG REACTIONS

ACE inhibitors can produce a wide range of mild to severe adverse reactions. Severe adverse reactions, such as proteinuria, neutropenia, agranulocytosis, rash, and loss of taste (dysgeusia), occur most commonly with captopril and may limit its use. Some of these reactions may be dose-related and may disappear during the first few weeks of therapy. The initial dose may cause profound hypotension or a severe allergic reaction. (See Patient Teaching: *Angiotensin-converting enzyme inhibitors,* page 274.)

CNS reactions, which may be related to reduced blood pressure, can occur with all agents. These reactions may include headache, dizziness, fatigue, and syncope. GI reactions, such as abdominal pain, nausea, vomiting, and diarrhea, also can occur.

All ACE inhibitors may cause transient elevations of BUN and serum creatinine levels, especially in patients with hypertension caused by volume depletion or with renal or cardiovascular disease. Increases in serum potassium concentrations commonly occur, especially in patients with reduced renal function.

All ACE inhibitors can produce tickling in the throat and a dry, nonproductive, persistent cough. The cough, which occurs in about 15% of patients receiving ACE inhibitors, usually occurs in the first week of therapy and resolves when the drug is discontinued.

Angioedema may occur with all ACE inhibitors, producing flushing or pallor and swelling of the face, extremities, lips, tongue, glottis, or larynx. If angioedema affects the face, tongue, or glottis or causes laryngeal stridor, the nurse should discontinue the drug, notify the physician, and begin appropriate treatment, as prescribed.

NURSING PROCESS APPLICATION

The following information assists the nurse in caring for a patient who is receiving an ACE inhibitor. It includes an

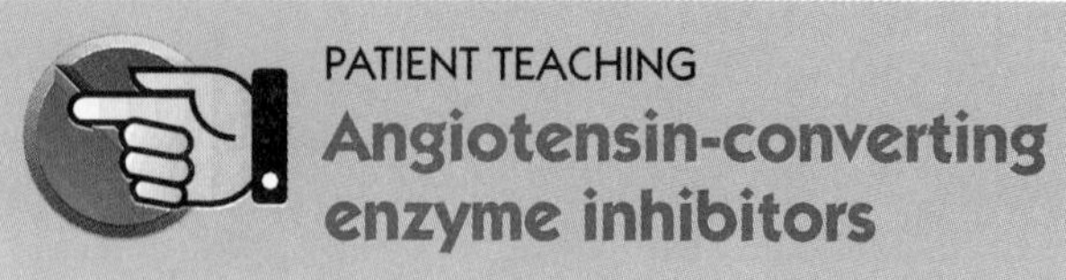

PATIENT TEACHING
Angiotensin-converting enzyme inhibitors

- Teach the patient and family the name, dose, frequency, action, and adverse effects of the prescribed angiotensin-converting enzyme (ACE) inhibitor.
- Provide general information about the use of ACE inhibitors.
- Instruct the patient to notify the physician immediately if signs of angioedema occur.
- Advise the patient to take captopril on an empty stomach, preferably 1 hour before meals, for maximum effectiveness.
- Reassure the patient that adverse reactions to captopril may disappear during the first few weeks of therapy.
- Instruct the patient to notify the physician if adverse reactions occur.

overview of assessment activities as well as examples of appropriate nursing diagnoses and related interventions. It also highlights the importance of evaluation.

Assessment
Before drug therapy begins, review the patient's history for conditions that contraindicate or require cautious use of the prescribed ACE inhibitor. Also review the patient's medication history to identify use of drugs that may interact with it. During therapy, assess the patient for adverse drug reactions and signs of drug interactions. Also, periodically assess the effectiveness of ACE inhibitor therapy. Finally, evaluate the patient's and family's knowledge about the prescribed drug.

Nursing diagnoses
- Risk for injury related to a preexisting condition that contraindicates or requires cautious use of an ACE inhibitor
- Risk for injury related to adverse drug reactions or drug interactions
- Knowledge deficit related to the prescribed ACE inhibitor

Planning and implementation
- Do not administer an ACE inhibitor to a patient with a condition that contraindicates its use.
- Administer an ACE inhibitor cautiously to a patient at risk because of a preexisting condition.
- Monitor the patient closely for adverse reactions and drug interactions.
- Obtain a baseline blood pressure and pulse rate before beginning ACE inhibitor therapy for later use in monitoring the patient. Check the patient for hypotension when an ACE inhibitor is administered for the first time during concomitant diuretic therapy.
- Captopril should not be administered with food, but taken 1 hour before meals.
- Captopril may cause neutropenia, requiring close monitoring of white blood cell counts.
- Monitor the patient's liver function tests and serum BUN, creatinine, and potassium levels before treatment begins and monthly during the first 3 months of therapy.

✱ ***Observe for signs of angioedema, such as flushing or pallor and swelling of the face, extremities, lips, tongue, glottis, or larynx. If angioedema occurs, withhold the drug, notify the physician, and begin emergency treatment, as prescribed.***

- Administer captopril between meals for maximum effectiveness.
- Notify the physician if adverse reactions or drug interactions occur.
- Teach the patient about the prescribed agents.

Evaluation
For each nursing diagnosis, prepare an evaluation statement that describes the patient's or family's response to nursing interventions.

CHAPTER SUMMARY

Chapter 20 discussed sympatholytic agents, vasodilating agents, and ACE inhibitors as they are used to treat hypertension. Here are the highlights of the chapter.

Hypertension is a common disease that may be controlled successfully with drug and nondrug therapies. It is classified into four stages. The higher the blood pressure, the greater the risk of cardiovascular disease.

A stepped-care approach is recommended for treating hypertension. Nondrug therapy should begin as soon as hypertension is diagnosed and should continue throughout the course of treatment. Beta-adrenergic blockers and diuretics are the drugs of choice unless they are contraindicated or unacceptable or unless special considerations are present.

Sympatholytic agents reduce blood pressure by inhibiting or blocking motor and secretory action in the sympathetic nervous system. They are classified by their site or mechanism of action.

Two types of vasodilating agents exist: direct vasodilators and calcium channel blockers. Direct vasodilators act on arteries, veins, or both to reduce blood pressure. Calcium channel blockers prevent calcium transport across the cell membrane, reducing the activity of the vascular smooth muscle, thus producing vasodilation and lowering the blood pressure.

ACE inhibitors reduce blood pressure by interfering with the renin-angiotensin-aldosterone system. They inhibit the enzyme that converts angiotensin I to angiotensin II, a potent vasoconstrictor. ACE inhibitors also reduce peripheral arterial resistance.

Questions to consider

See Appendix 1 for answers.

1. Helga Klemper, age 59, has essential mild hypertension. Despite compliance with the prescribed diet and exercise regimen, her blood pressure remains elevated. The physician prescribes atenolol (Tenormin) 50 mg P.O. daily. Atenolol is classified as which of the following types of sympatholytic agent?
   (a) Ganglionic blocker
   (b) Alpha-adrenergic blocker
   (c) Beta-adrenergic blocker
   (d) Norepinephrine depletor

2. Marshall Woodman, age 68, is beginning atenolol therapy. The nurse should assess Mr. Woodman for which of the following adverse reactions to atenolol?
   (a) Tachycardia
   (b) Hypertension
   (c) Constipation
   (d) Depression

3. Pamela Cohen, age 71, is admitted to the critical care unit with severe hypertension. Her blood pressure ranges from 174/116 mm Hg to 190/150 mm Hg. The physician prescribes nitroprusside sodium 0.5 mcg/kg/minute by I.V. infusion. How does nitroprusside reduce blood pressure?
   (a) It directly relaxes peripheral vascular smooth muscle.
   (b) It inhibits calcium transport during depolarization.
   (c) It depletes norepinephrine stores.
   (d) It inhibits sympathetic activity.

4. The nurse is caring for Daniel Thompson, age 69, who is receiving I.V. nitroprusside. He does not have an arterial line in place. How frequently should the nurse monitor his blood pressure?
   (a) Continuously
   (b) Every 5 minutes
   (c) Every 15 minutes
   (d) Every 30 minutes

5. Mercy Langley, age 74, has secondary hypertension caused by renal disease. The physician prescribes captopril (Capoten) 25 mg P.O. t.i.d. Which of the following drugs may interfere with the effectiveness of captopril?
   (a) Theophyllines
   (b) Nonsteroidal anti-inflammatory drugs
   (c) Tetracyclines
   (d) Cardiac glycosides

6. The nurse is teaching Adam Stern, age 67, about captopril. Which of the following instructions should the nurse include?
   (a) Take captopril on an empty stomach.
   (b) Take captopril with meals.
   (c) Take captopril with milk or a snack.
   (d) Take captopril with an antacid.

21 Diuretic agents

OBJECTIVES

After reading and studying this chapter, the student should be able to:

1. describe the absorption, distribution, metabolism, and excretion of thiazide and thiazide-like, loop, potassium-sparing, and osmotic diuretics.
2. compare the mechanisms of action of the various types of diuretics.
3. identify the major clinical indications for the various types of diuretics.
4. describe the major drug interactions that can occur with the various types of diuretics.
5. describe the fluid and electrolyte imbalances that commonly occur as a result of diuretic therapy.
6. describe how to apply the nursing process when caring for a patient who is receiving a diuretic.

INTRODUCTION

Diuretics are used to increase urine volume and to maximize excretion of solutes and water. The major diuretics discussed in this chapter are classified as thiazide and thiazide-like, loop, potassium-sparing, and osmotic diuretics. Carbonic anhydrase inhibitors are discussed briefly. These agents are used primarily to decrease intraocular pressure. (See *Selected major diuretic agents.*)

Drugs covered in this chapter include:

- acetazolamide
- amiloride
- bendroflumethiazide
- benzthiazide
- bumetanide
- chlorothiazide
- chlorthalidone
- dichlorphenamide
- ethacrynate sodium
- ethacrynic acid
- furosemide
- hydrochlorothiazide
- hydroflumethiazide
- indapamide
- mannitol
- methazolamide
- methyclothiazide
- metolazone
- polythiazide
- quinethazone
- spironolactone
- triamterene
- trichlormethiazide
- urea.

Thiazide and thiazide-like diuretics

Thiazide and thiazide-like diuretics are sulfonamide derivatives that inhibit sodium reabsorption, thereby increasing sodium and water excretion. These diuretics may induce a hypersensitivity reaction similar to that of sulfonamides; they also increase the excretion of chloride, potassium, and bicarbonate ions, which can result in electrolyte imbalances, particularly hypokalemia. The thiazide diuretics include bendroflumethiazide, benzthiazide, chlorothiazide, hydrochlorothiazide, hydroflumethiazide, methyclothiazide, polythiazide, and trichlormethiazide. The thiazide-like diuretics include chlorthalidone, indapamide, metolazone, and quinethazone.

PHARMACOKINETICS

Thiazide diuretics are absorbed rapidly but incompletely from the gastrointestinal (GI) tract after oral administration. The protein binding of thiazide diuretics varies, ranging from 65% for hydrochlorothiazide to 95% for chlorothiazide. Thiazide diuretics cross the placental barrier and are secreted in breast milk. These agents differ in their degree of metabolism and are excreted primarily in the urine. Twenty percent of indapamide's metabolites are excreted in the feces.

Onset of action of the thiazide and thiazide-like diuretics usually occurs within 1 hour of oral administration. However, intravenous (I.V.) chlorothiazide will begin to act within 15 minutes of administration. Optimal antihypertensive effects of these agents, however, usually do not appear until 3 to 4 weeks after therapy begins — but they may appear within 3 or 4 days.

Peak concentration levels of thiazide and thiazide-like diuretics usually occur within 4 to 6 hours. I.V. chlorothiazide, indapamide, and metolazone are the exceptions: I.V. chlorothiazide reaches a peak concentration within 30 minutes; metolazone and indapamide, in 2 hours.

The duration of action of the thiazide and thiazide-like diuretics is 6 to 24 hours, depending on the drug excretion rate. I.V. chlorothiazide, polythiazide, and chlorthalidone are the exceptions. I.V. chlorothiazide has a duration of only 2 hours; polythiazide, of 24 to 48 hours; and chlorthalidone, of 24 to 72 hours.

Selected major diuretic agents

This table summarizes the major diuretic agents currently in clinical use.

DRUG	MAJOR INDICATIONS AND USUAL DOSAGES	CONTRAINDICATIONS AND PRECAUTIONS
Thiazide and thiazide-like diuretics		
chlorothiazide (Diuril)	*Edema* ADULT: 500 mg to 2 g P.O. or I.V. daily or in two divided doses PEDIATRIC: age 6 months and older, 20 mg/kg P.O. or I.V. daily in divided doses; under age 6 months, up to 30 mg/kg P.O. or I.V. daily in divided doses *Hypertension* ADULT: 500 mg to 1 g P.O. or I.V. daily or in divided doses PEDIATRIC: age 6 months and older, 20 mg/kg P.O. or I.V. daily in divided doses; under age 6 months, up to 30 mg/kg P.O. or I.V. daily in divided doses	• Chlorothiazide is contraindicated in a breast-feeding patient or one with anuria, renal decompensation, or known hypersensitivity to this drug or other sulfonamide derivatives. • This drug requires cautious use in a pregnant patient or one with severe renal disease, impaired hepatic function, or progressive liver disease.
hydrochlorothiazide (Esidrix, HydroDIURIL, Oretic)	*Edema* ADULT: 25 to 200 mg P.O. daily or intermittently PEDIATRIC: age 6 months and older, 2.2 mg/kg P.O. daily in two divided doses; under age 6 months, 3.3 mg/kg P.O. daily in two divided doses *Hypertension* ADULT: 25 to 100 mg P.O. daily or in divided doses PEDIATRIC: age 6 months and older, 2.2 mg/kg P.O. daily in two divided doses; under age 6 months, 3.3 mg/kg P.O. daily in two divided doses	• Hydrochlorothiazide is contraindicated in a breast-feeding patient or one with anuria, renal decompensation, or known hypersensitivity to this drug or other sulfonamide derivatives. • This drug requires cautious use in a pregnant patient or one with severe renal disease, impaired hepatic function, or progressive liver disease.
metolazone (Diulo, Zaroxolyn)	*Edema resulting from heart failure* ADULT: 5 to 10 mg P.O. daily *Edema resulting from renal or hepatic disease* ADULT: 5 to 20 mg P.O. daily *Hypertension* ADULT: 2.5 to 5 mg P.O. daily	• Metolazone is contraindicated in a breast-feeding patient, a patient in hepatic coma or precoma, or one with anuria or known hypersensitivity. • This drug requires cautious use in a pregnant patient or one with severe renal impairment. • Safety and efficacy in children have not been established.
Loop diuretics		
bumetanide (Bumex)	*Edema, hypertension* ADULT: initially, 0.5 to 2 mg P.O. in a single daily dose or repeated at 4- to 5-hour intervals up to a total of 10 mg/day; for maintenance dosages given intermittently with 1 to 2 day rest periods, 0.5 to 1 mg I.M. or I.V. given over 1 to 2 minutes; I.V. doses may be repeated every 2 to 3 hours up to a total of 10 mg/day	• Bumetanide is contraindicated in a breast-feeding patient, a patient in hepatic coma or precoma, or one with anuria, severe electrolyte depletion, or known hypersensitivity to this drug or sulfonylureas. • This drug requires cautious use in a pregnant patient, one with severe renal disease, or one receiving another ototoxic agent. • Safety and efficacy in children have not been established.
ethacrynate sodium (Edecrin sodium), ethacrynic acid (Edecrin)	*Acute pulmonary edema* ADULT: 50 to 100 mg of ethacrynate sodium I.V., infused slowly over several minutes *Other forms of edema* ADULT: 50 to 200 mg of ethacrynic acid P.O. once daily after meals or on alternate days; or up to 200 mg b.i.d. to obtain a therapeutic effect PEDIATRIC: 25 mg of ethacrynic acid P.O. daily, gradually increased if needed in 25-mg increments until a therapeutic effect is obtained	• Ethacrynate sodium and ethacrynic acid are contraindicated in an infant, a breast-feeding patient, or one with anuria or known hypersensitivity to these drugs. • These drugs require cautious use in a pregnant patient, one with advanced cirrhosis of the liver, or one receiving another ototoxic agent or a potassium-depleting steroid.

(continued)

Selected major diuretic agents *(continued)*

DRUG	MAJOR INDICATIONS AND USUAL DOSAGES	CONTRAINDICATIONS AND PRECAUTIONS
Loop diuretics *(continued)*		
furosemide (Lasix)	*Acute pulmonary edema* ADULT: 40 mg I.V. injected slowly over several minutes, then repeated every 2 hours as needed PEDIATRIC: 1 mg/kg I.V. or I.M., then repeated every 2 hours as needed to a maximum of 6 mg/kg daily *Other forms of edema* ADULT: 20 to 80 mg P.O. daily or b.i.d. up to 600 mg daily, or 20 to 40 mg I.M. or I.V. with repeated doses of 20 mg every 2 hours until a therapeutic effect is obtained PEDIATRIC: 2 mg/kg P.O. daily with an increase of 1 to 2 mg/kg in 6 to 8 hours if needed, up to 6 mg/kg daily; or 1 mg/kg I.V. or I.M, with repeated doses every 2 hours as needed to a maximum of 6 mg/kg daily *Chronic renal failure* ADULT: 80 mg P.O. daily initially; increased up to 120 mg/day until a therapeutic effect is obtained *Hypertension* ADULT: 20 to 80 mg P.O. daily	• Furosemide is contraindicated in a patient with anuria or known hypersensitivity. • This drug requires cautious use in a pregnant or breast-feeding patient.
Potassium-sparing diuretics		
amiloride (Midamor)	*Hypertension or edema associated with heart failure* ADULT: 5 to 10 mg P.O. daily initially; increased up to 20 mg daily if needed	• Amiloride is contraindicated in a breast-feeding patient, a patient receiving another potassium-sparing drug or potassium supplement, or one with hyperkalemia, impaired renal function, diabetes mellitus, or known hypersensitivity. • This drug requires cautious use in a pregnant patient or a severely ill patient who is prone to respiratory or metabolic acidosis. • Safety and efficacy in children have not been established.
spironolactone (Aldactone)	*Essential hypertension* ADULT: 50 to 100 mg P.O. daily in a single dose or two divided doses PEDIATRIC:1 to 2 mg/kg P.O. b.i.d. *Edema* ADULT: 25 to 200 mg P.O. daily initially, in a single dose or two divided doses, with the total dosage adjusted according to the patient's response PEDIATRIC: initially, 3.3 mg/kg P.O. daily in a single dose or divided doses	• Spironolactone is contraindicated in a breast-feeding patient; a patient receiving another potassium-sparing drug; or one with anuria, acute renal insufficiency, significantly impaired renal excretory function, hyperkalemia, or known hypersensitivity. • This drug requires cautious use in a pregnant patient.
Osmotic diuretics		
mannitol (Osmitrol)	*Oliguria or prevention of acute renal failure* ADULT: 50 to 100 g I.V. of 5% to 25% solution *Increased intracranial or intraocular pressure* ADULT: 1.5 to 2 g/kg I.V. of 15% to 20% solution infused over 30 to 60 minutes; if used as preoperative medication, give 1 to 1.5 hours before surgery *Drug intoxication from secobarbital, imipramine, aspirin, or carbon tetrachloride* ADULT: up to 200 g I.V. of 5% to 10% solution over 24 hours	• Mannitol is contraindicated in a patient with severe pulmonary congestion, severe heart failure, severe dehydration, metabolic edema associated with capillary fragility or membrane permeability, or known hypersensitivity. It also is contraindicated in a patient with anuria caused by severe renal disease or impaired renal function who does not respond to a test dose of mannitol. • This drug requires cautious use in a pregnant or breast-feeding patient. • Safety and efficacy in children under age 12 have not been established.

Route	Onset	Peak	Duration
P.O.	1 hr	4-6 hr	6-24 hr
I.V.	15 min	0.5-2 hr	2-72 hr

PHARMACODYNAMICS

Thiazide and thiazide-like diuretics interfere with the transport of sodium ions across the renal tubular epithelium at the cortical-diluting, or distal, segments of the nephrons. Like the sulfonamides, thiazides create some minor carbonic anhydrase inhibition. These effects result in increased sodium, potassium, chloride, and water excretion with excretion of sodium and chloride in approximately equal amounts and concomitant excretion of magnesium, phosphate, bromide, and iodide. At the same time, the excretion of ammonium, urates, and calcium is decreased. Thiazide diuretics also may decrease the glomerular filtration rate (GFR).

Researchers currently believe that the action of the thiazide and thiazide-like diuretics is linked primarily to increased sodium excretion. Initially, these drugs decrease circulating blood volume, thus decreasing cardiac output. If the therapy is maintained, the cardiac output stabilizes, but extracellular fluid and plasma volume decrease.

PHARMACOTHERAPEUTICS

Thiazide and thiazide-like diuretics may be used alone or in combination with other drugs; they are used primarily to treat hypertension. Although their antihypertensive effects may begin within 3 to 4 days after initiation of therapy, the drugs are most effective after 3 to 4 weeks of continued therapy.

Thiazides also are used primarily to treat the edema associated with mild or moderate heart failure. They are used to treat edema associated not only with heart failure, but also with hepatic disease, renal disease, and corticosteroid and estrogen therapy. Although the thiazide and thiazide-like diuretics usually are not effective if the GFR is less than 20 ml/minute, there is one exception: metolazone, which remains effective even with a decreased GFR.

Because these drugs decrease the urinary calcium level, they also are used alone or with other drugs to prevent the development and recurrence of calcium nephrolithiasis in hypercalciuric and normal calciuric patients.

In patients with diabetes insipidus, thiazides paradoxically decrease urine volume, possibly via sodium depletion and plasma volume reduction.

Drug interactions

Drug interactions related to the thiazide and thiazide-like diuretics result in altered fluid volume, blood pressure, and serum electrolyte levels. When given 30 minutes before a thiazide, thiazide-like, or loop diuretic, metolazone potentiates the diuretic effect. (See Drug Interactions: *Thiazide and thiazide-like diuretics*, page 280.)

ADVERSE DRUG REACTIONS

Numerous adverse reactions are associated with thiazide and thiazide-like diuretics. The most common are blood volume depletion, orthostatic hypotension, hyponatremia, and hypokalemia. Others include glucose intolerance, hypercalcemia, and hypophosphatemia, which may occur with prolonged therapy; hyperuricemia; and GI reactions, such as anorexia, nausea, and pancreatitis.

Hypersensitivity reactions may occur in the form of purpura, photosensitivity, rash, urticaria, necrotizing vasculitis, or blood abnormalities (such as leukopenia, thrombocytopenia, aplastic anemia, or granulocytopenia), especially in patients who are allergic to sulfa-based drugs.

NURSING PROCESS APPLICATION

The following information assists the nurse in caring for a patient who is receiving a thiazide or thiazide-like diuretic. It includes an overview of assessment activities as well as examples of appropriate nursing diagnoses and related interventions. It also highlights the importance of evaluation.

Assessment

Before drug therapy begins, review the patient's history for conditions that contraindicate or require cautious use of the prescribed thiazide or thiazide-like diuretic. Evaluate baseline electrolyte levels, particularly noting the potassium and serum sodium levels. Also review the patient's medication history to identify use of drugs that may interact with it. During therapy, assess the patient for adverse drug reactions and signs of drug interactions. Also, periodically assess the effectiveness of therapy with the thiazide or thiazide-like diuretic. Finally, evaluate the patient's and family's knowledge about the prescribed drug.

Nursing diagnoses

- Risk for injury related to a preexisting condition that contraindicates or requires cautious use of a thiazide or thiazide-like diuretic
- Risk for injury related to adverse drug reactions or drug interactions
- Altered urinary elimination related to the adverse genitourinary effects of the prescribed thiazide or thiazide-like diuretic
- Knowledge deficit related to the prescribed thiazide or thiazide-like diuretic

Planning and implementation

- Do not administer a thiazide or thiazide-like diuretic to a patient with a condition that contraindicates its use.
- Administer a thiazide or thiazide-like diuretic cautiously to a patient at risk because of a preexisting condition.
- Monitor the patient frequently for adverse reactions and drug interactions.

✱ ***Be especially alert for changes in the patient's serum sodium and potassium levels. Also observe for signs and***

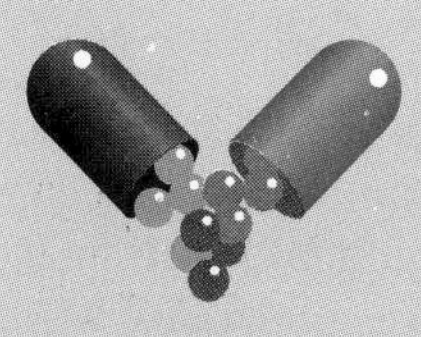

DRUG INTERACTIONS

Thiazide and thiazide-like diuretics

Drug interactions related to thiazide and thiazide-like diuretics may cause severe fluid and electrolyte imbalances and other potentially serious problems. The nurse needs to be aware of these interactions to provide the best possible patient care.

DRUG	INTERACTING AGENTS	POSSIBLE EFFECTS	NURSING IMPLICATIONS
all thiazide and thiazide-like diuretics	oral hypoglycemic agents, insulin	Hyponatremia, thiazide resistance, hyperglycemia	• Monitor the patient's serum sodium and glucose levels. • Monitor the patient for signs and symptoms of hyponatremia, such as dizziness and weakness, and of hyperglycemia, such as polyuria, polydipsia, polyphagia, and weight loss.
	corticosteroids, adrenocorticotropic hormone, amphotericin	Hypokalemia	• Monitor the patient's serum potassium level. • Monitor the patient for the signs and symptoms of hypokalemia, such as weakness and flattened T wave on an electrocardiogram.
	lithium carbonate	Lithium toxicity	• Monitor the patient for signs and symptoms of lithium toxicity, such as ataxia. • Monitor the patient's serum lithium level.
	skeletal muscle relaxants (tubocurarine, gallamine)	Increased responsiveness to the skeletal muscle relaxant	• Monitor the patient for the therapeutic effects of skeletal muscle relaxants. • Expect to adjust the muscle relaxant dosage.
	cardiac glycosides	Digitalis toxicity (as a result of hypokalemia)	• Monitor the patient for signs and symptoms of digitalis toxicity, such as GI, cardiovascular, or neurologic problems. • Monitor the patient's serum digoxin or digitoxin level. • Monitor the patient's serum electrolyte levels.
	probenecid	Decreased renal excretion of uric acid, which may precipitate or worsen gout	• Monitor the patient's fluid intake and output. • Monitor the patient's serum electrolyte levels.
	cholestyramine, colestipol	Decreased therapeutic effect of the diuretic	• Administer the thiazide or thiazide-like diuretic 2 hours before administering cholestyramine or colestipol. • Monitor the patient for the therapeutic effects of the diuretic.
	indomethacin, other nonsteroidal anti-inflammatory drugs	Decreased antihypertensive effect	• Monitor the patient's vital signs, especially noting an increase in blood pressure. • Monitor the patient for the therapeutic effects of the diuretic.

symptoms of hyponatremia, such as anxiety, hypotension, and nausea; and hypokalemia, such as drowsiness, paresthesia, muscle cramps, and hyporeflexia.

• Administer potassium supplements as prescribed to maintain an acceptable serum potassium level. Administer normal or half-normal saline solution I.V. as prescribed to correct hyponatremia.

• Monitor the blood glucose level in a diabetic patient during long-term therapy with a thiazide or thiazide-like diuretic because these agents can cause glucose intolerance.

• Weigh the patient daily under controlled conditions (at the same time each morning, after the patient voids, before the patient eats, with the patient wearing similar clothing each morning, and on the same scale).

• Do not administer chlorothiazide intramuscularly or subcutaneously.

• Expect a delay in urine elimination changes when administering a thiazide or thiazide-like agent to a patient with heart failure, impaired renal function, or any other disorder that reduces renal blood flow.

- Expect to switch the patient to metolazone as prescribed if the patient's GFR falls below 20 ml/minute.
- Document the patient's fluid intake and output to detect alterations in urine elimination.

∗ ***Administer the diuretic in the morning or early afternoon, if permissible, to prevent nocturia from upsetting the patient's normal sleep pattern. Keep a urinal or bedpan within reach for a bedridden patient; ensure that the bathroom is easily accessible for an ambulatory patient.***

- Notify the physician if the patient's condition does not improve or if adverse reactions or drug interactions occur.
- Teach the patient about the prescribed agent. (See Patient Teaching: *Thiazide and thiazide-like diuretics.*)

Evaluation

For each nursing diagnosis, prepare an evaluation statement that describes the patient's or family's response to nursing interventions.

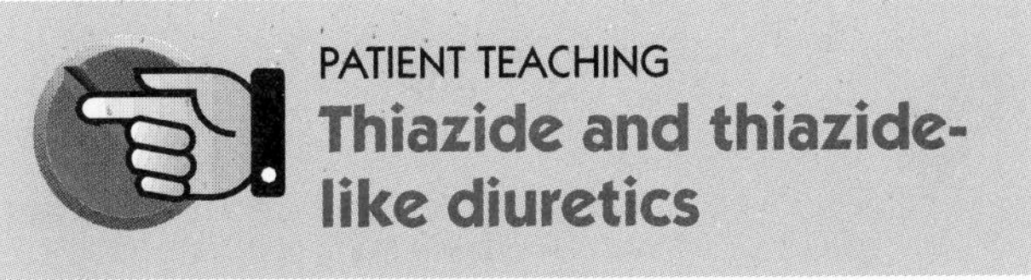

PATIENT TEACHING

Thiazide and thiazide-like diuretics

- ➤ Teach the patient and family the name, dose, frequency, action, and adverse effects of the prescribed thiazide or thiazide-like diuretic.
- ➤ Advise the female patient to tell the physician if she is pregnant or plans to become pregnant during diuretic therapy.
- ➤ Inform the patient that periodic blood tests must be performed to detect imbalances that may be caused by diuretic therapy.
- ➤ Teach the patient to recognize and report to the physician the signs of hypokalemia, such as muscle cramps, paresthesia, or drowsiness.
- ➤ Explain the importance of taking potassium supplements, if prescribed, and eating a potassium-rich diet. Give the patient a list of potassium-rich foods.
- ➤ Teach the patient receiving concomitant cardiac glycoside therapy to identify the signs of digitalis toxicity, such as GI, cardiac, and neurologic disturbances.
- ➤ Instruct the diabetic patient receiving a thiazide or thiazide-like diuretic to monitor blood glucose levels closely. Advise this patient that diabetes treatment may require adjustment during diuretic therapy.
- ➤ Instruct the patient to take the diuretic in the morning or early afternoon, if possible, to avoid nocturia.
- ➤ Teach the patient to obtain a daily weight under the same conditions every time and to notify the physician of any sudden weight gain (greater than 2 lb [0.9 kg] in 1 day), peripheral edema, or shortness of breath.
- ➤ Instruct the patient how to minimize the effects of orthostatic hypotension.
- ➤ Advise the patient to expect an increase in urinary frequency and amount voided.
- ➤ Teach the patient to recognize and report to the physician the signs and symptoms of dehydration.
- ➤ Instruct the patient to notify the physician if adverse reactions occur or if concerns arise about the prescribed diuretic therapy.

Loop diuretics

Loop, or high-ceiling, diuretics are highly potent agents and include bumetanide, ethacrynate sodium, ethacrynic acid, and furosemide.

PHARMACOKINETICS

Loop diuretics usually are absorbed well and distributed rapidly. Extensively protein-bound, these agents undergo partial or complete metabolism in the liver, except for furosemide, which is excreted primarily unchanged. Loop diuretics are excreted primarily by the kidneys. Besides their greater potency, these diuretics have a more rapid onset of action and produce a much greater volume of diuresis than other types of diuretics.

Bumetanide's onset of action occurs within 30 minutes after oral administration, within 40 minutes after intramuscular (I.M.) administration, and within a few minutes after I.V. administration. The peak concentration level is reached within 1.5 to 2 hours after oral administration and within minutes after I.V. administration. The duration of action of bumetanide is from 3.5 to 4 hours, although it may increase to 6 hours with higher doses. Its half-life is 1 to 1.5 hours.

Onset of ethacrynate sodium and ethacrynic acid occurs 30 minutes after oral administration and 5 minutes after I.V. administration. The duration is 6 to 8 hours after oral administration and 2 hours after I.V. administration. As with bumetanide, the duration of ethacrynate sodium and ethacrynic acid may increase with higher doses. The half-life of these drugs is 30 to 70 minutes.

Onset of furosemide occurs within 30 to 60 minutes after oral administration, and 5 minutes after I.V. administration. Peak concentration occurs within 20 to 60 minutes; the drug's duration is about 2 hours after an I.V. dose and 6 hours after an oral dose. The half-life of furosemide usually is 30 to 60 minutes but may increase to 75 to 155 minutes in a patient with renal or hepatic insufficiency and to 20 hours in a patient with renal system dysfunction.

Route	Onset	Peak	Duration
P.O.	30-60 min	1.5-2 hr	3.5-8 hr
I.M.	40 min	Unknown	Unknown
I.V.	Minutes	Up to 60 min	2 hr

PHARMACODYNAMICS

The loop diuretics are the most potent diuretics available, producing the greatest volume of diuresis and having a high potential for causing severe adverse reactions. Producing maximal sodium excretion of 20% to 25% of the filtered load, loop diuretics inhibit sodium and chloride reabsorption in the renal tubules by direct action on the thick ascending limb of the loop of Henle. These drugs also may in-

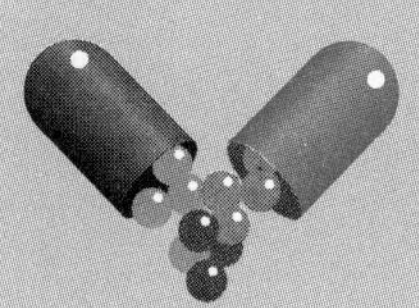

DRUG INTERACTIONS

Loop diuretics

Drug interactions with loop diuretics can alter renal function, cause fluid and electrolyte imbalances, and enhance certain effects of the drug.

DRUG	INTERACTING AGENTS	POSSIBLE EFFECTS	NURSING IMPLICATIONS
bumetanide, ethacrynate sodium, ethacrynic acid, furosemide	oral hypoglycemic agents	Hyperglycemia	• Monitor the patient's serum glucose level. • Monitor the patient for signs and symptoms of hyperglycemia, such as thirst and lethargy.
	aminoglycosides	Increased ototoxicity	• Exercise extreme caution when administering these drugs together. • Monitor the patient's auditory acuity.
	lithium carbonate	Decreased excretion, resulting in lithium toxicity	• Monitor the patient for signs and symptoms of lithium toxicity such as ataxia. • Monitor the patient's serum lithium level.
	cisplatin	Increased ototoxicity	• Monitor the patient's auditory acuity.
	cardiac glycosides	Electrolyte disturbances that may predispose the patient to cardiac glycoside-induced arrhythmias	• Measure the patient's potassium and magnesium serum levels. • Monitor the patient's electrocardiogram and check the pulse rate and rhythm periodically.
furosemide	nonsteroidal anti-inflammatory agents	Inhibited antihypertensive and diuretic effects	• Monitor the patient's fluid intake and output, daily weight, and blood pressure.
	neuromuscular blocking agents	Enhanced neuromuscular blockade	• Monitor for prolonged effects of the neuromuscular blocking agent. • Administer with caution to a patient with decreased renal function.
	phenytoin	Decreased furosemide absorption and effectiveness	• Monitor the patient's response to furosemide.

hibit sodium, chloride, and water reabsorption in the proximal tubule while increasing the excretion of ammonium and titratable acids in the distal tubule. Increased potassium excretion from the distal tubule may result from the accelerated exchange with sodium ions caused by the increased sodium volume delivered to the distal tubule. Ethacrynate sodium and ethacrynic acid bind to sulfhydryl groups in renal cellular protein. Bumetanide, the shorter-acting agent, is 40 times more potent than furosemide.

PHARMACOTHERAPEUTICS

Loop diuretics are used primarily to treat edema associated with heart failure, hepatic or renal disease, or nephrotic syndrome. Loop diuretics also are used to treat hypertension, usually with a potassium-sparing diuretic or a potassium supplement to prevent hypokalemia. Bumetanide also has been used to treat edema related to menstruation and lymphedema. Ethacrynate sodium and ethacrynic acid also are used to treat cancer-related ascites, lymphedema, acute pulmonary edema, nephrogenic diabetes insipidus, and hypercalcemia. Furosemide also is used with mannitol to treat severe cerebral edema.

Drug interactions

Various drugs interact with loop diuretics, causing altered renal function, fluid and electrolyte imbalances, and specific enhanced drug effects. (See Drug Interactions: *Loop diuretics.*)

ADVERSE DRUG REACTIONS

The adverse drug reactions to loop diuretics may be severe because of the potent effects of these drugs. The most severe reactions involve frequently occurring fluid and electrolyte imbalances.

Common adverse drug reactions include volume depletion (especially in geriatric patients), orthostatic hypotension, hypokalemia, hypochloremia, hypochloremic alkalosis, asymptomatic hyperuricemia, hyponatremia, hypocalcemia, and hypomagnesemia. Transient deafness, diarrhea, abdominal discomfort or pain, impaired glucose tolerance, dermatitis, paresthesia, hepatic dysfunction, and thrombocytopenia can also occur. Furosemide toxicity may produce such adverse drug reactions as tinnitus, abdominal pain, sore throat, and fever.

Hypersensitivity reactions include purpura, photosensitivity, rash, pruritus, urticaria, necrotizing angiitis, exfoliative dermatitis, allergic interstitial nephritis, and erythema multiforme. Agranulocytosis also can occur.

NURSING PROCESS APPLICATION

The following information assists the nurse in caring for a patient who is receiving a loop diuretic. It includes an overview of assessment activities as well as examples of appropriate nursing diagnoses and related interventions. It also highlights the importance of evaluation.

Assessment

Before drug therapy begins, review the patient's history for conditions that contraindicate or require cautious use of the prescribed loop diuretic. Evaluate the patient's fluid balance and baseline electrolyte levels to ensure that they are within normal limits before therapy begins. Also review the patient's medication history to identify use of drugs that may interact with it. During therapy, assess the patient for adverse drug reactions (especially fluid and electrolyte imbalances) and signs of drug interactions. Also, periodically assess the effectiveness of loop diuretic therapy. Finally, evaluate the patient's and family's knowledge about the prescribed drug.

Nursing diagnoses

- Risk for injury related to a preexisting condition that contraindicates or requires cautious use of a loop diuretic
- Risk for injury related to adverse drug reactions or drug interactions
- Risk for fluid volume deficit related to use of the prescribed loop diuretic
- Knowledge deficit related to the prescribed loop diuretic

Planning and implementation

- Do not administer a loop diuretic to a patient with a condition that contraindicates its use.
- Administer a loop diuretic cautiously to a patient at risk because of a preexisting condition.
- Monitor the patient frequently for adverse reactions and drug interactions during loop diuretic therapy.

**** Be especially alert for changes in the patient's serum sodium and potassium levels. Also observe for signs and symptoms of hyponatremia, such as anxiety, hypotension, and nausea; and hypokalemia, such as drowsiness, paresthesia, muscle cramps, hyporeflexia, and tachycardia or bradycardia.***

- Administer potassium supplements as prescribed to maintain an acceptable serum potassium level. Administer normal or half-normal saline solution I.V. as prescribed to correct hyponatremia.
- Weigh the patient daily under controlled conditions (at the same time each morning, after the patient voids, before the patient eats, with the patient wearing similar clothing each morning, and on the same scale).
- Carefully monitor a diabetic patient's blood glucose level.
- Check the bumetanide dosage with extreme care; this drug is 40 times more potent than furosemide.
- Do not administer ethacrynate sodium or ethacrynic acid by I.M. or subcutaneous injection, to avoid tissue irritation.
- Administer I.M. furosemide using the Z-track method to minimize tissue irritation.
- Administer an I.V. loop diuretic slowly over 1 to 2 minutes to prevent adverse reactions.
- Store oral furosemide tablets and injectable furosemide in light-resistant containers to prevent discoloration.

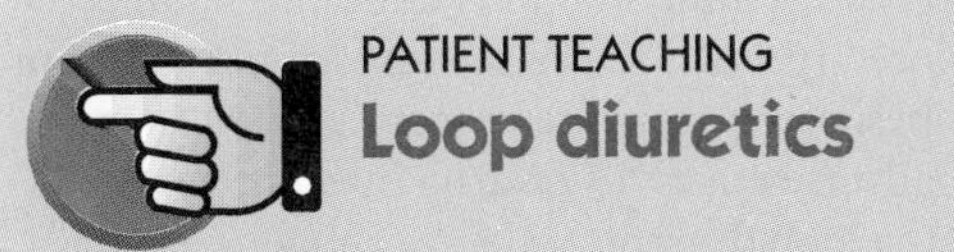

PATIENT TEACHING

Loop diuretics

- Teach the patient and family the name, dose, frequency, action, and adverse effects of the prescribed loop diuretic.
- Advise the female patient to tell the physician if she is pregnant or plans to become pregnant during loop diuretic therapy.
- Inform the patient that periodic blood tests must be performed to detect imbalances caused by loop diuretic therapy.
- Teach the patient to recognize and report to the physician the signs of hypokalemia.
- Explain the importance of taking potassium supplements, if prescribed, and eating a potassium-rich diet. Give the patient a list of potassium-rich foods.
- Teach the patient receiving concomitant cardiac glycoside therapy to identify the signs of digitalis toxicity, such as GI, cardiac, and neurologic disturbances.
- Instruct the diabetic patient receiving a loop diuretic to monitor blood glucose levels closely. Advise this patient that diabetes treatment may require adjustment during loop diuretic therapy.
- Instruct the patient to take the diuretic in the morning or early afternoon, if possible, to avoid nocturia.
- Teach the patient to obtain a daily weight under the same conditions every time and to notify the physician of any sudden weight gain (greater than 2 lb [0.9 kg] in 1 day), peripheral edema, or shortness of breath.
- Teach the patient how to minimize the effects of orthostatic hypotension.
- Advise the patient to expect an increase in urinary frequency and amount voided.
- Instruct the patient taking furosemide to report to the physician any signs of furosemide toxicity, such as tinnitus, abdominal pain, sore throat, and fever.
- Instruct the patient to store furosemide tablets in light-resistant containers to prevent discoloration.
- Instruct the patient to notify the physician if adverse reactions occur or if concerns arise about the prescribed loop diuretic therapy.
- Tell the patient not to discontinue the loop diuretic without consulting the physician.

Refrigerate oral furosemide solutions to ensure stability. Do not use discolored (yellow) injectable furosemide solutions.
• Notify the physician if the patient's condition does not improve or if adverse reactions or drug interactions occur.
• Administer the loop diuretic in the morning or early afternoon, if possible, to prevent nocturia from disturbing the patient's normal sleep pattern.
✱ ***Monitor the patient for signs of dehydration, such as poor skin turgor and dry oral mucous membranes. Check the vital signs to detect signs of hypovolemia, such as tachycardia, hypotension, and dyspnea. If signs are present, notify the physician.***
✱ ***Accurately record the patient's fluid intake and output. If extreme discrepancies occur, notify the physician and expect to decrease the diuretic dosage, as prescribed.***
• Teach the patient about the prescribed agents. (See Patient Teaching: *Loop diuretics,* page 283.)

Evaluation

For each nursing diagnosis, prepare an evaluation statement that describes the patient's or family's response to nursing interventions.

Potassium-sparing diuretics

Potassium-sparing diuretics have weaker diuretic and antihypertensive effects than other diuretics, but they have the advantage of conserving potassium. The potassium-sparing diuretics include amiloride, spironolactone, and triamterene.

PHARMACOKINETICS

Potassium-sparing diuretics are administered orally and are absorbed in the GI tract. They are metabolized in the liver except for amiloride, which is not metabolized, and are excreted primarily in the urine and bile.

These diuretics have a rapid onset of action, and their duration of action increases with multiple doses. The onset of action for amiloride occurs within 2 hours; for spironolactone and triamterene, in 2 to 4 hours. Amiloride reaches a peak concentration level in 3 to 4 hours; spironolactone, in 1 to 2 hours; spironolactone metabolites, in 2 to 4 hours; and triamterene, in 2 to 4 hours. The duration of action of amiloride is 24 hours; of spironolactone, 48 to 72 hours; of triamterene, 12 to 16 hours. For all three drugs, duration may increase with multiple doses and prolonged therapy.

After a single oral dose in a healthy adult, spironolactone has an average half-life of 1.3 to 2 hours. The half-lives of its active metabolites canrenone and 7a-thiomethylspironolactone are 13 to 24 hours and 2.8 hours, respectively. Amiloride's half-life is 6 to 9 hours; triamterene's, 100 to 150 minutes.

Route	Onset	Peak	Duration
P.O.	1-4 hr	1-4 hr	12-72 hr

PHARMACODYNAMICS

The direct action of the potassium-sparing diuretics on the distal renal tubules produces mild diuretic and antihypertensive effects that increase the urinary excretion of sodium, chloride, and calcium ions and reduce the excretion of potassium and hydrogen ions. These effects lead to increased serum potassium levels and urine pH. Amiloride and spironolactone do not depress the GFR, but triamterene does.

Spironolactone is an aldosterone antagonist. When hypovolemia, hyponatremia, hyperkalemia, or renin release leads to aldosterone secretion, metabolic alkalosis and potassium depletion may occur. Spironolactone counteracts these effects by competing with aldosterone for receptor sites and blocking the action of aldosterone on the distal tubules. As a result, sodium, chloride, and water are excreted and potassium is retained.

PHARMACOTHERAPEUTICS

Potassium-sparing diuretics commonly are used with other diuretics to potentiate their action or to counteract their potassium-wasting effects. Potassium-sparing diuretics are used primarily to treat edema (including refractory edema) and diuretic-induced hypokalemia in patients with heart failure, cirrhosis, nephrotic syndrome, or hypertension. Spironolactone also is used to treat hyperaldosteronism and hirsutism, including hirsutism associated with Stein-Leventhal (polycystic ovary) syndrome.

Drug interactions

Few drug interactions are associated with the use of amiloride, spironolactone, and triamterene. Those that do occur are not directly related to the drug, but to its potassium-sparing effects. (See Drug Interactions: *Potassium-sparing diuretics.*)

ADVERSE DRUG REACTIONS

Few adverse drug reactions occur with the potassium-sparing diuretics. However, their potassium-sparing effects can lead to hyperkalemia, especially if a potassium-sparing diuretic is given with a potassium supplement or a high-potassium diet.

Other dose-related reactions to potassium-sparing diuretics include megaloblastic anemia (especially with triamterene), dizziness, orthostatic hypotension, sore throat, dry mouth, nausea, and vomiting.

Amiloride may produce headache, nausea, vomiting, anorexia, diarrhea, muscle cramps, abdominal pain, constipation, impotence, and metabolic disturbances, including volume depletion, hyponatremia, a transient rise in the

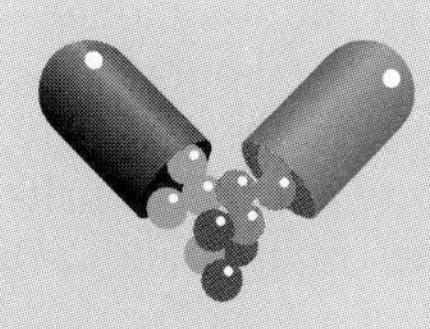

DRUG INTERACTIONS

Potassium-sparing diuretics

The drug interactions that occur with these diuretics may be related to their potassium-sparing effects. The nurse must observe patients receiving potassium-sparing diuretics for signs and symptoms of hyperkalemia.

DRUG	INTERACTING AGENTS	POSSIBLE EFFECTS	NURSING IMPLICATIONS
amiloride, spironolactone, triamterene	potassium supplements, other potassium-sparing diuretics, potassium-based salt substitutes, angiotensin-converting enzyme inhibitors (captopril, enalapril, lisinopril)	Hyperkalemia	• Monitor the patient for signs and symptoms of hyperkalemia. • Advise the patient not to use a potassium-based salt substitute.
spironolactone	cardiac glycosides	Decreased renal excretion of cardiac glycosides	• Monitor the patient for signs and symptoms of digitalis toxicity, such as nausea and yellow vision. • Monitor the patient's serum digoxin or digitoxin level.
	salicylates	Reduced clinical effects of spironolactone	• Monitor the patient's fluid intake and output and serum potassium level.

blood urea nitrogen level, and acidosis. Spironolactone may produce headache, abdominal cramps, diarrhea, gynecomastia in males, breast soreness and menstrual abnormalities in females, and rarely, agranulocytosis.

Hypersensitivity reactions to potassium-sparing diuretics include urticaria, pruritus, erythematous eruptions, rash, photosensitivity, and anaphylaxis.

NURSING PROCESS APPLICATION

The following information assists the nurse in caring for a patient who is receiving a potassium-sparing diuretic. It includes an overview of assessment activities as well as examples of appropriate nursing diagnoses and related interventions. It also highlights the importance of evaluation.

Assessment

Before drug therapy begins, review the patient's history for conditions that contraindicate or require cautious use of the prescribed potassium-sparing diuretic. Also review the patient's medication history to identify use of drugs that may interact with it. During therapy, assess the patient for adverse drug reactions and signs of drug interactions. Also, periodically assess the effectiveness of potassium-sparing diuretic therapy. Finally, evaluate the patient's and family's knowledge about the prescribed drug.

Nursing diagnoses

• Risk for injury related to a preexisting condition that contraindicates or requires cautious use of a potassium-sparing diuretic
• Risk for injury related to adverse drug reactions or drug interactions
• Risk for fluid volume deficit related to the adverse GI effects of the prescribed potassium-sparing diuretic
• Knowledge deficit related to the prescribed potassium-sparing diuretic

Planning and implementation

• Do not administer a potassium-sparing diuretic to a patient with a condition that contraindicates its use.
• Administer a potassium-sparing diuretic cautiously to a patient at risk because of a preexisting condition.
• Monitor the patient frequently for adverse reactions and drug interactions.
**** Monitor the patient for signs and symptoms of hyperkalemia, such as confusion, hyperexcitability, muscle weakness, paresthesia, flaccid paralysis, arrhythmias, abdominal distention, diarrhea, and intestinal colic. Also monitor the patient's serum electrolyte levels for imbalances.***
• Weigh the patient daily under controlled conditions (at the same time each morning, after the patient voids, before the patient eats, with the patient wearing similar clothing each morning, and on the same scale).
• Store spironolactone in a light-resistant container.
• Administer a potassium-sparing diuretic in the morning or early afternoon, if possible, to avoid nocturia.
• Administer amiloride with food.
• Observe the patient with nausea, vomiting, or diarrhea for signs of dehydration.
• Notify the physician if the patient's condition does not improve or if adverse reactions (such as GI distress) or drug interactions occur. Obtain a prescription for an antiemetic or antidiarrheal agent, as needed.
• Teach the patient about the prescribed agent.

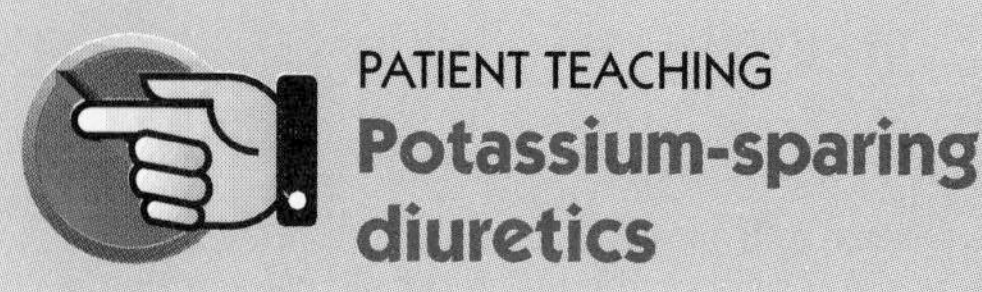

PATIENT TEACHING
Potassium-sparing diuretics

- Teach the patient and family the name, dose, frequency, action, and adverse effects of the prescribed potassium-sparing diuretic.
- Instruct the patient to expect an increase in urinary frequency and amount voided.
- Advise the female patient to tell the physician if she is pregnant or plans to become pregnant during potassium-sparing diuretic therapy.
- Inform the patient that periodic blood tests must be performed to detect imbalances caused by the potassium-sparing diuretic.
- Teach the patient to recognize and report to the physician the signs of hyperkalemia.
- Advise the patient to avoid eating potassium-rich foods because these diuretics conserve potassium.
- Instruct the patient to take the potassium-sparing diuretic in the morning or early afternoon, if possible, to avoid nocturia.
- Teach the patient to obtain a daily weight under the same conditions every time and to notify the physician of any sudden weight gain (greater than 2 lb [0.9 kg] in 1 day), peripheral edema, or shortness of breath.
- Teach the patient how to minimize the effects of orthostatic hypotension.
- Teach the patient how to manage minor adverse reactions, such as dry mouth (by chewing sugarless gum or sucking on sugarless hard candy) and constipation (by increasing fiber intake and exercise).
- Instruct the patient to ask the physician to recommend an analgesic if headaches occur.
- Inform the patient that amiloride-induced impotence may occur but should subside when the drug is discontinued.
- Instruct the patient to notify the physician if adverse reactions occur or if concerns arise about the prescribed therapy.

Evaluation

For each nursing diagnosis, prepare an evaluation statement that describes the patient's or family's response to nursing interventions. (See Patient Teaching: *Potassium-sparing diuretics.*)

Osmotic diuretics

Mannitol and urea are the primary osmotic diuretics used today because they are effective in patients with compromised renal circulation.

PHARMACOKINETICS

After I.V. administration, mannitol and urea are distributed rapidly and are excreted primarily unchanged in the urine.

When used to decrease intraocular pressure, the onset of action of mannitol and urea occurs within 15 minutes. The peak concentration level for mannitol is reached in 30 minutes to 1 hour; of urea, in 1 to 2 hours. The duration of action of mannitol is 4 to 8 hours; of urea, 5 to 6 hours.

When used to reduce intracranial pressure, the duration of mannitol is 3 to 8 hours; of urea, 3 to 10 hours. The half-life of mannitol is from 15 to 100 minutes; of urea, about 70 minutes.

Diuresis occurs in 1 to 3 hours after mannitol administration and in 1 to 2 hours after urea administration.

Route	Onset	Peak	Duration
I.V.	15 min	0.5-2 hr	3-10 hr

PHARMACODYNAMICS

Osmotic diuretics act by increasing the osmolality of the plasma, glomerular filtrates, and tubular fluid. This decreases the reabsorption of fluid and electrolytes, which increases the excretion of water, chloride, and sodium and slightly increases the excretion of potassium.

PHARMACOTHERAPEUTICS

Mannitol and urea primarily are used to reduce intracranial or intraocular pressure and to prevent acute renal failure. They are effective even in a patient with compromised renal circulation.

Drug interactions

No significant drug interactions occur with the use of mannitol or urea.

ADVERSE DRUG REACTIONS

Common adverse reactions to the osmotic diuretics include transient expansion of plasma volume during infusion, (resulting in circulatory overload and tachycardia), electrolyte imbalances, volume depletion, cellular dehydration, headache, nausea, and vomiting. These drugs can produce local irritation at the infusion site if extravasation occurs and may lead to thrombophlebitis. Mannitol may cause rebound increased intracranial pressure 8 to 12 hours after diuresis and angina-like chest pain, blurred vision, rhinitis, thirst, and urine retention. Other adverse reactions to the osmotic diuretics include hypersensitivity reactions and thrombophlebitis.

NURSING PROCESS APPLICATION

The following information assists the nurse in caring for a patient who is receiving an osmotic diuretic. It includes an overview of assessment activities as well as examples of appropriate nursing diagnoses and related interventions. It also highlights the importance of evaluation.

Assessment

Before drug therapy begins, review the patient's history for conditions that contraindicate or require cautious use of the prescribed osmotic diuretic. During therapy, assess the patient for adverse drug reactions. Also, periodically assess the effectiveness of osmotic diuretic therapy. Finally, evaluate the patient's and family's knowledge about the prescribed drug.

Nursing diagnoses

- Risk for injury related to a preexisting condition that contraindicates or requires cautious use of an osmotic diuretic
- Risk for injury related to adverse drug reactions
- Knowledge deficit related to the prescribed osmotic diuretic

Planning and implementation

- Do not administer an osmotic diuretic to a patient with a condition that contraindicates its use.
- Administer an osmotic diuretic cautiously to a patient at risk because of a preexisting condition.
- Monitor the patient closely for adverse reactions, especially electrolyte imbalances.
- Monitor the patient's vital signs hourly during osmotic diuretic therapy.

***** ***Document the patient's fluid intake and output hourly because therapy is based on the hourly urine flow rate. Assess the patient for circulatory overload if the urine output is less than 30 to 50 ml/hour.***

- Administer mannitol 1 to 1.5 hours before surgery when it is used as a preoperative medication.
- Expect to give a test dose of mannitol as prescribed to a patient undergoing a transurethral prostatic resection. Infuse mannitol with sorbitol over 3 to 5 minutes to elicit a urine flow of 30 to 50 ml/hour for urogenital irrigation.
- Redissolve parenteral mannitol, which crystallizes at low temperatures, by warming it in a hot-water bath and shaking the container vigorously. Then let the solution return to room temperature before administering.

***** ***Do not administer crystallized medication. Also, do not add blood products to I.V. lines used for mannitol administration because they are incompatible.***

- Administer mannitol at the prescribed rate using an in-line I.V. filter.
- Store mannitol at 59° to 86° F (15° to 30° C) unless otherwise directed, and do not allow it to freeze.
- Notify the physician if the patient's condition does not improve or if adverse reactions occur.
- Teach the patient about the prescribed agent. (See Patient Teaching: *Osmotic diuretics.*)

Evaluation

For each nursing diagnosis, prepare an evaluation statement that describes the patient's or family's response to nursing interventions.

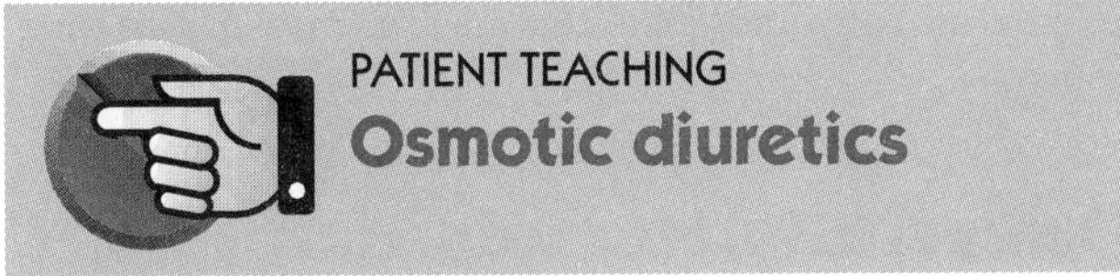

PATIENT TEACHING
Osmotic diuretics

- Teach the patient and family the name, dose, frequency, action, and adverse effects of the prescribed osmotic diuretic.
- Instruct the patient to notify the nurse if angina-like chest pain occurs during mannitol therapy.
- Reassure the patient that blurred vision, rhinitis, and excessive thirst should subside when mannitol is discontinued.
- Advise the patient that vital signs will be checked and the urinary catheter will be drained every hour to monitor the effectiveness of diuretic therapy.
- Explain the need for frequent blood tests to monitor for osmotic diuretic-induced electrolyte imbalances.
- Encourage the patient and family to ask questions about the prescribed osmotic diuretic.
- Instruct the patient to notify the physician if any adverse reactions occur.

Carbonic anhydrase inhibitors

Carbonic anhydrase inhibitors are used to induce diuresis. Sometimes given with miotics, carbonic anhydrase inhibitors (acetazolamide, dichlorphenamide, and methazolamide) primarily are used to decrease the formation of aqueous humor by the ciliary body and thereby to control the excessive intraocular pressure associated with glaucoma. Carbonic anhydrase inhibitors also are used to treat edema related to cardiac disorders, periodic paralysis, and acute mountain sickness.

CHAPTER SUMMARY

Chapter 21 presented thiazide, thiazide-like, loop, potassium-sparing, osmotic, and other diuretic agents as they are used for therapeutic diuresis. Here are the chapter highlights.

Thiazide and thiazide-like diuretics are sulfonamide derivatives that inhibit sodium reabsorption, thereby increasing the excretion of water, chloride, sodium, and potassium. They typically are used to treat hypertension and edema resulting from heart failure and other conditions.

Loop diuretics, the most potent diuretics, are effective in treating edema and hypertension.

Potassium-sparing diuretics are less potent than the other diuretics but have the advantage of conserving potassium. Potassium-sparing diuretics typically are used with other diuretics or antihypertensives.

Osmotic diuretics are used to prevent acute renal failure and to reduce increased intracranial or intraocular pressure.

Carbonic anhydrase inhibitors are used primarily to treat glaucoma.

Questions to consider

See Appendix 1 for answers.

1. Franklin Kane, age 43, needs a diuretic agent, but is allergic to sulfa-based drugs. Which of the following diuretics should he avoid?
   (a) Thiazide and thiazide-like diuretics
   (b) Loop diuretics
   (c) Potassium-sparing duiretics
   (d) Carbonic anhydrase inhibitors

2. Rhonda Lemke, age 51, is not responding well to a benzthiazide. Which of the following diuretics might be prescribed to help potentiate benzthiazide's effect?
   (a) furosemide
   (b) chlorothiazide
   (c) bumetanide
   (d) metolazone

3. Martin Mosler, age 54, is taking the thiazide diuretic hydrochlorothiazide (HydroDIURIL) 25 mg P.O. daily for mild hypertension. During a routine follow-up visit, he reports muscle cramps, paresthesia, and drowsiness. These symptoms may signal which of the following adverse reactions?
   (a) Hyperuricemia
   (b) Hypophosphatemia
   (c) Hypokalemia
   (d) Hypernatremia

4. Laura Perloff, age 37, develops acute renal failure. Which of the following types of diuretics would be the most effective treatment?
   (a) Potassium-sparing
   (b) Thiazide
   (c) Thiazide-like
   (d) Loop

5. The physician orders metolazone for Gladys Mertz, age 65, to treat edema caused by heart failure. The nurse double-checks Ms. Mertz's medication history before administering the metolazone. Which of the following drugs is likely to interact with this diuretic?
   (a) captopril
   (b) aspirin
   (c) penicillin
   (d) lithium

6. Jeff Walters, age 51, has just been prescribed spironolactone 50 mg P.O. daily for hypertension. The nurse informs him that he will need to have his blood checked periodically to detect which of the following adverse reactions to spironolactone?
   (a) Hyperkalemia
   (b) Hypernatremia
   (c) Hyperglycemia
   (d) Hypercalcemia

22 Antilipemic agents

OBJECTIVES

After reading and studying this chapter, the student should be able to:

1. identify the three major classes of antilipemic drugs and give an example of a drug found in each class.
2. explain the mechanisms of action for each of the three major classes of antilipemic agents: bile-sequestering agents, fibric acid derivatives, and cholesterol synthesis inhibitors.
3. identify the major adverse reactions for each of the three major classes of antilipemic drugs.
4. describe how niacin acts as an antilipemic agent, and identify its major adverse reactions.
5. describe how to apply the nursing process when caring for a patient who is receiving an antilipemic agent.

INTRODUCTION

Antilipemic agents are used to lower abnormally high blood levels of **lipids** (fatty substances), when other measures, such as proper diet, weight loss, exercise, and treatment of an underlying disorder causing the lipid abnormality, have failed.

Antilipemic drug classes include bile-sequestering agents, fibric acid derivatives, cholesterol synthesis inhibitors, and miscellaneous drugs. (See *Selected major antilipemic agents,* page 290.)

Drugs covered in this chapter include:

- cholestyramine
- clofibrate
- colestipol hydrochloride
- dextrothyroxine sodium
- ethinyl estradiol
- gemfibrozil
- lovastatin
- nandrolone and other anabolic steroid agents
- neomycin
- niacin
- norethindrone acetate
- pravastatin sodium
- probucol
- simvastatin.

Bile-sequestering agents

The bile-sequestering agents, cholestyramine and colestipol hydrochloride, are anion-exchange resins that remove excess bile acids from the fat depots under the skin.

PHARMACOKINETICS

Because bile-sequestering agents have a high molecular weight, they are not absorbed from the gastrointestinal (GI) tract. Instead, they remain in the GI tract where they combine with bile acids for about 5 hours. Eventually, they are excreted in the feces.

Route	Onset	Peak	Duration
P.O.	1 day-2 wk	1 mo	2-4 wk

PHARMACODYNAMICS

The bile-sequestering agents lower blood levels of low-density **lipoproteins** (LDLs). As these agents form insoluble complexes with the bile acids in the gastrointestinal (GI) tract, the bile acid levels in the gallbladder decrease. This triggers the liver to synthesize more bile acids from their precursor, cholesterol. As cholesterol leaves the bloodstream and other storage areas to replace the lost bile acids, blood cholesterol levels decrease. Because the small intestine needs bile acids to emulsify lipids and form chylomicrons, absorption of all lipids and lipid-soluble drugs decreases until the bile acids are replaced.

PHARMACOTHERAPEUTICS

Bile-sequestering agents are the drugs of choice for treating type IIa **hyperlipoproteinemia** (familial hypercholesterolemia) in patients who do not respond to dietary management. A patient whose blood cholesterol levels indicate a severe risk of coronary artery disease is most likely to require one of these agents to supplement the diet.

Drug interactions

Because bile-sequestering agents are anion-exchange resins, they may bind with acidic drugs in the GI tract, decreasing

Selected major antilipemic agents

This table summarizes the major antilipemic agents currently in clinical use.

DRUG	MAJOR INDICATIONS AND USUAL DOSAGES	CONTRAINDICATIONS AND PRECAUTIONS
Bile-sequestering agent		
cholestyramine (Questran, Questran Light)	*Types IIa and IIb hyperlipoproteinemia (hypercholesterolemia)* ADULT: 4 g of resin P.O. two to four times daily mixed with 120 to 180 ml of fluid, soups, hot cereal, or pulpy fruits	• Cholestyramine is contraindicated in a patient with complete biliary obstruction or known hypersensitivity. • This drug requires cautious use in a pregnant or breast-feeding patient or one with constipation. • Safety and efficacy in children have not been established.
Fibric acid derivative		
gemfibrozil (Lopid)	*Types II, III, IV, and V hyperlipoproteinemia* ADULT: 1,200 mg P.O. daily in two divided doses	• Gemfibrozil is contraindicated in a breast-feeding patient or one with known hypersensitivity, gallbladder disease, or hepatic (including primary biliary cirrhosis) or severe renal dysfunction. • This drug requires cautious use in a pregnant patient or one with peptic ulcer disease or a history of jaundice. • Safety and efficacy in children have not been established.
Cholesterol synthesis inhibitors		
lovastatin (Mevacor)	*Primary types IIa and IIb hyperlipoproteinemia* ADULT: 10 to 80 mg P.O. daily in a single dose or divided doses with meals	• Lovastatin is contraindicated in a pregnant or breast-feeding patient or one with active liver disease, persistent aminotransferase elevations, or known hypersensitivity. • This drug requires cautious use in a patient with high alcohol consumption or a history of liver disease.
pravastatin sodium (Pravachol)	*Adjunct therapy for primary types IIa and IIb hypercholesterolemia* ADULT: initially, 10 or 20 mg P.O. at bedtime, increased as needed, up to a maximum of 40 mg daily	• Pravastatin is contraindicated in a pregnant or breast-feeding patient or one with known hypersensitivity, active liver disease, or unexplained, persistent elevations in liver function tests. • This drug requires cautious use in a patient who consumes a large quantity of alcohol or one with a history of liver disease. • Safety and efficacy in children have not been established.
simvastatin (Zocor)	*Adjunct therapy for hypercholesterolemia or mixed hyperlipidemia* ADULT: 5 to 10 mg P.O. in the evening, increased as needed, up to a maximum of 40 mg daily	• Simvastatin is contraindicated in a pregnant or breast-feeding patient or one with known hypersensitivity, active liver disease, or unexplained, persistent elevations of serum transaminase levels. • This drug requires cautious use in a patient who consumes a large quantity of alcohol or one with a history of liver disease. • Safety and efficacy in children have not been established.

their absorption and effectiveness. (See Drug Interactions: *Bile-sequestering agents.*) Other acidic drugs that are likely to be affected include barbiturates, phenytoin, penicillins, cephalosporins, thyroid hormones, thyroid derivatives, chenodiol, digitoxin, and digoxin. Bile-sequestering agents also may reduce absorption of lipid-soluble vitamins, such as vitamins A, D, E, and K; poor absorption of vitamin K can affect prothrombin times significantly. Many other drugs that normally are absorbed from the GI tract — including tetracyclines — also may have decreased absorption.

ADVERSE DRUG REACTIONS

Short-term adverse reactions to these drugs are relatively mild. More severe reactions can result from long-term use.

With long-term therapy, these drugs commonly produce adverse GI effects, which can be minimized by introducing and titrating the drugs slowly to a maximum dosage. Constipation may occur but usually is not serious. Severe fecal impaction, however, may occur. Other adverse GI effects may include abdominal pain, abdominal distention, flatulence, belching, nausea, vomiting, diarrhea, or hemorhoid

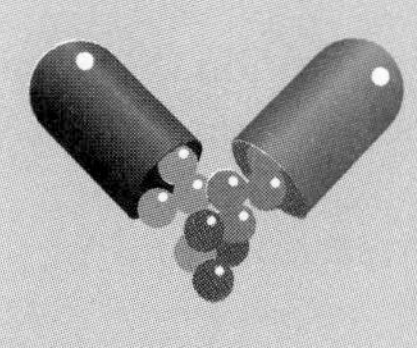

DRUG INTERACTIONS

Bile-sequestering agents

When given concomitantly, bile-sequestering agents will counteract the effects of acidic substances. However, when given concomitantly with beta-adrenergic blockers, cholestyramine will decrease their GI absorption; therefore, the beta-blocker dosage should be adjusted when cholestyramine therapy begins or ends.

DRUG	INTERACTING AGENTS	POSSIBLE EFFECTS	NURSING IMPLICATIONS
cholestyramine, colestipol	oral anticoagulants	Increased risk of clotting	• Administer an oral anticoagulant 1 hour before or 4 to 6 hours after administering a bile-sequestering agent. • Monitor the patient's prothrombin time carefully, and expect to increase the anticoagulant dosage, as needed. • Assess the patient for signs of thromboembolism (pain, swelling, redness in the calf) or of pulmonary embolism (shortness of breath, chest pain, anxiety).
	corticosteroids	Decreased effect of corticosteroids	• Administer a corticosteroid 1 hour before or 4 to 6 hours after administering a bile-sequestering agent as prescribed. • Monitor the patient carefully for therapeutic effects of these drugs and expect to increase the corticosteroid dosage, as needed. • Assess the patient's weight and blood pressure regularly. • Monitor the patient's serum electrolyte levels.
	cardiac glycosides	Decreased effect of glycosides	• Administer cardiac glycosides 1 hour before or 4 to 6 hours after administering a bile-sequestering agent. • Monitor the patient's cardiac glycoside level carefully, and expect to increase the cardiac glycoside dosage, as needed. • Assess the patient for signs of heart failure, such as tachycardia, peripheral edema, and hypotension.
	iron preparations	Reduced serum iron levels	• Administer an iron preparation 1 hour before or 4 to 6 hours after administering a bile-sequestering agent. • Monitor the patient's serum iron and hemoglobin levels, and expect to increase the iron dosage, as needed. • Inform the patient to expect that stools may become black.
	thiazide diuretics	Diminished diuretic effect	• Administer a thiazide diuretic 1 hour before or 4 to 6 hours after administering a bile-sequestering agent. • Monitor the patient carefully for therapeutic effects of these drugs, and expect to increase the thiazide diuretic dosage, as needed. • Assess the patient for peripheral edema. • Monitor the patient's serum electrolyte levels.
	thyroid hormones	Reduced triidothyronine (T_3) and thyroxine (T_4) levels by decreasing absorption of thyroid hormone from the GI tract	• Administer a thyroid hormone 1 hour before or 4 to 6 hours after administering a bile-sequestering agent. • Monitor the patient's T_3 and T_4 levels, and expect to increase thyroid hormone dosage, as needed.
	methotrexate	Decreased absorption of methotrexate from the GI tract	• Administer methotrexate 1 hour before or 4 to 6 hours after administering a bile-sequestering agent.

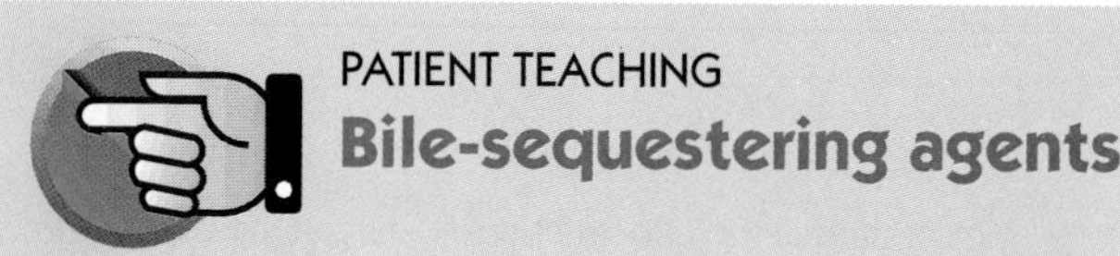

PATIENT TEACHING
Bile-sequestering agents

- Teach the patient and family the name, dose, frequency, action, and adverse effects of the prescribed bile-sequestering agent.
- Advise the patient to have blood cholesterol levels checked every 3 to 6 months to evaluate the effectiveness of therapy.
- Advise the patient not to take the drug in its powder form. Demonstrate how to mix the agent in a suitable liquid, fruit, or other food.
- Advise the patient not to drive or perform activities that require alertness if dizziness or weakness occurs.
- Instruct the patient taking a drug that binds with the prescribed bile-sequestering agent to take it 1 hour before or 4 to 6 hours after taking the bile-sequestering agent.
- Instruct the patient to inform all other physicians of the use of a bile-sequestering agent; the dosages of the other drugs may need to be adjusted.
- Teach the patient how to prevent constipation.
- Reassure the patient that adverse GI effects usually diminish as therapy continues.
- Stress the importance of following the prescribed regimen for the bile-sequestering agent.
- Instruct the patient to notify the physician if adverse reactions occur or if concerns arise about the prescribed bile-sequestering agent therapy.

irritation. Rarely, peptic ulceration and bleeding, cholelithiasis, and cholecystitis occur.

Miscellaneous reactions to bile-sequestering agents include headache, dizziness, anorexia, weakness, and fatigue.

NURSING PROCESS APPLICATION

The following information assists the nurse in caring for a patient who is receiving a bile-sequestering agent. It includes an overview of assessment activities as well as examples of appropriate nursing diagnoses and related interventions. It also highlights the importance of evaluation.

Assessment

Before drug therapy begins, review the patient's history for conditions that contraindicate or require cautious use of the prescribed bile-sequestering agent. Also review the patient's medication history to identify use of drugs that may interact with it. During therapy, assess the patient for adverse drug reactions and signs of drug interactions. Also, periodically assess the effectiveness of therapy with the prescribed bile-sequestering agent. Finally, evaluate the patient's and family's knowledge about the prescribed drug. (See Patient Teaching: *Bile-sequestering agents.*)

Nursing diagnoses

- Risk for injury related to a preexisting condition that contraindicates or requires cautious use of a bile-sequestering agent
- Risk for injury related to adverse drug reactions or drug interactions
- Constipation related to the adverse GI effects of the prescribed bile-sequestering agent
- Knowledge deficit related to the prescribed bile-sequestering agent

Planning and implementation

- Do not administer a bile-sequestering agent to a patient with a condition that contraindicates its use.
- Administer a bile-sequestering agent cautiously to a patient at risk because of a preexisting condition.

*** *Obtain baseline blood cholesterol levels before therapy begins. Then monitor blood cholesterol levels every 3 to 6 months for a patient receiving long-term therapy.***

- Introduce and titrate the bile-sequestering agent slowly as prescribed to minimize adverse GI reactions.
- Monitor the patient regularly for adverse reactions and drug interactions.
- Administer drugs that bind with bile-sequestering agents 1 hour before or 6 hours after giving the agent.
- Mix the powder form with 120 to 180 ml of liquid, such as water, carbonated beverage, or soup, or a pulpy fruit with a high moisture content, such as applesauce. Never administer the dry powder because the patient may inhale it accidentally.
- Notify the physician if adverse reactions or drug interactions occur.
- Monitor the patient's bowel habits throughout therapy to detect constipation.
- Encourage the patient to drink 2 to 3 liters of fluid daily, increase the dietary fiber intake (unless contraindicated), and get plenty of exercise to prevent constipation.
- Notify the physician and request a prescription for a laxative if constipation develops.

Evaluation

For each nursing diagnosis, prepare an evaluation statement that describes the patient's or family's response to nursing interventions.

Fibric acid derivatives

Fibric acid is produced by several fungi. Two derivatives of this acid, clofibrate and gemfibrozil, are used to reduce high triglyceride levels and, to a lesser extent, high cholesterol levels.

PHARMACOKINETICS

Clofibrate and gemfibrozil are absorbed readily from the GI tract and 95% bound to plasma proteins. Clofibrate is hy-

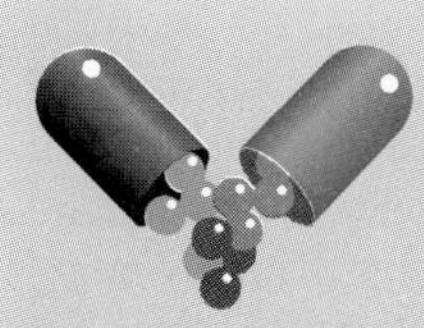

DRUG INTERACTIONS
Fibric acid derivatives

Drug interactions with fibric acid derivatives usually involve acidic drugs, such as oral anticoagulants and sulfonylureas.

DRUG	INTERACTING AGENTS	POSSIBLE EFFECTS	NURSING IMPLICATIONS
clofibrate, gemfibrozil	oral anticoagulants	Increased anticoagulant effect	• Monitor the patient's prothrombin time closely, and expect to adjust the anticoagulant dosage, as needed. • Assess the patient for signs of internal bleeding, such as hematuria and easy bruising. • Monitor the patient for signs of gastrointestinal bleeding, such as hematemesis and melena.
clofibrate	sulfonylureas	Increased hypoglycemic effect	• Monitor the patient's blood glucose level and expect to adjust the sulfonylurea dosage, as needed.

drolyzed while gemfibrozil undergoes extensive metabolism in the liver before both agents are excreted in the urine. Both of these antilipemic agents begin to reduce very-low-density lipoprotein (VLDL) levels in 2 to 5 days. Clofibrate's action peaks in 4 weeks, and its duration of action is unknown. Gemfibrozil's action peaks in 3 weeks and has a 3-week duration. Clofibrate's half-life is 12 to 35 hours; gemfibrozil's is 1.5 hours.

Route	Onset	Peak	Duration
P.O.	2-5 days	3-4 wk	3 wk

PHARMACODYNAMICS

Although the exact mechanism of action for these drugs has not been established, researchers believe that the drugs may reduce cholesterol formation early in the biosynthetic process, mobilize cholesterol from the tissues, increase sterol excretion, decrease lipoprotein synthesis and secretion, and decrease triglyceride synthesis. The decreased triglyceride synthesis probably results from inhibition of lipolysis in adipose tissue.

Gemfibrozil produces two other effects. It increases high-density lipoprotein (HDL) levels in the blood by increasing the synthesis of certain apoproteins (substances derived from proteins), and it increases the serum's capacity to dissolve additional cholesterol.

PHARMACOTHERAPEUTICS

These drugs are used primarily to reduce triglyceride levels — especially very-low-density triglycerides — and secondarily to reduce blood cholesterol levels. Therefore, they should be used primarily in patients with types II, III, IV, and mild type V hyperlipoproteinemia. However, these agents should be used only in patients at severe risk for coronary artery disease who have not responded adequately to diet changes; who have premature coronary artery disease or a family member with the disease; who have hypercholesterolemia or have a family member with the disease; who have marked hypertriglyceridemia; or who smoke or exhibit other risk factors, such as hypertension or obesity. Fibric acid derivatives are most effective for patients with no previous history of coronary artery disease or angina.

In patients with types IIa, IIb, and IV hyperlipoproteinemia, niacin is used as adjunct therapy. Fibric acid derivatives are used with these patients when niacin does not produce an adequate response, is poorly tolerated, or is contraindicated. They also may be added to niacin and bile-sequestering agent therapy if the latter two agents do not produce an adequate response.

Drug interactions

Although no studies have shown that these antilipemic agents displace acidic drugs, such as barbiturates, phenytoin, thyroid derivatives, and cardiac glycosides, the possibility of displacement exists when these drugs are administered concurrently. (See Drug Interactions: *Fibric acid derivatives.*)

ADVERSE DRUG REACTIONS

The most common reactions to fibric acid derivatives are adverse GI effects, which resemble those of the bile-sequestering agents.

Several studies show that these agents increase the incidence of cholelithiasis and the need for cholecystectomy. Clofibrate also is associated with benign and malignant liver tumors in rodents and malignant tumors in humans. This antilipemic can cause other adverse drug reactions, including pancreatitis, cardiac arrhythmias, intermittent claudica-

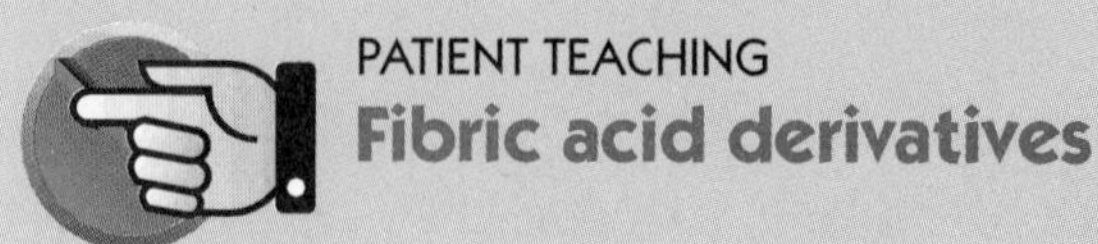

PATIENT TEACHING
Fibric acid derivatives

- Teach the patient and family the name, dose, frequency, action, and adverse effects of the prescribed fibric acid derivative.
- Stress the importance of regular liver function studies and triglyceride and cholesterol level tests. Explain the purpose of these tests and tell the patient that they require a blood sample after fasting from midnight the previous night.
- Teach the patient to recognize the warning signs of cancer and to report them or any other unusual symptoms to the physician.
- Advise the patient that GI disturbances are the most common adverse effect. Teach the patient how to manage GI disturbances. For example, urge the patient to increase fluid and fiber intake and amount of exercise (unless contraindicated) to relieve constipation.
- Instruct the patient who also takes an anticoagulant to notify the physician about fibric acid derivative therapy because the anticoagulant dosage may need to be reduced to prevent bleeding. Teach the patient to take bleeding precautions, such as avoiding cuts and bruises, using a soft toothbrush, and using an electric razor when shaving.
- Instruct the patient with a decreased white blood cell count to prevent infection by avoiding crowds and people who are ill and by getting plenty of rest.
- Advise the patient receiving gemfibrozil to take it in two divided doses, 30 minutes before the morning and evening meals.
- Instruct the patient to notify the physician of biliary colic, which typically appears as abdominal pain or nausea and vomiting that subsides, with or without treatment, after several hours. Explain that diagnostic tests may be needed to check for cholelithiasis.
- Instruct the patient to notify the physician if leg pain occurs when walking or if pain, swelling, or redness develops in either calf. Instruct the patient to go to the nearest emergency department if shortness of breath suddenly develops.
- Tell the patient to notify the physician if adverse reactions occur.

tion, thromboembolic events, angina, flulike symptoms, and an increased creatine phosphokinase (CPK) level.

Fibric acid derivatives may produce a wide range of hypersensitivity reactions. These may include skin rash, alopecia, urticaria, dry skin, brittle hair, hepatomegaly, impotence, decreased libido, leukopenia, weight gain, muscle pain, and abnormal liver function test results.

NURSING PROCESS APPLICATION

The following information assists the nurse in caring for a patient who is receiving a fibric acid derivative. It includes an overview of assessment activities as well as examples of appropriate nursing diagnoses and related interventions. It also highlights the importance of evaluation.

Assessment

Before drug therapy begins, review the patient's history for conditions that contraindicate or require cautious use of the prescribed fibric acid derivative. Also review the patient's medication history to identify use of drugs that may interact with it. During therapy, assess the patient for adverse drug reactions and signs of drug interactions. Also, periodically assess the effectiveness of therapy with the fibric acid derivative. Finally, evaluate the patient's and family's knowledge about the prescribed drug. (See Patient Teaching: *Fibric acid derivatives.*)

Nursing diagnoses

- Risk for injury related to a preexisting condition that contraindicates or requires cautious use of a fibric acid derivative
- Risk for injury related to adverse drug reactions or drug interactions
- Pain related to biliary colic from drug-induced cholelithiasis
- Knowledge deficit related to the prescribed fibric acid derivative

Planning and implementation

- Do not administer a fibric acid derivative to a patient with a condition that contraindicates its use.
- Administer a fibric acid derivative cautiously to a patient at risk because of a preexisting condition.

**** Monitor liver function studies and white blood cell counts, as prescribed, to detect abnormalities. Check blood triglyceride and cholesterol levels, as prescribed, to assess the drug's effectiveness.***

- Monitor the patient regularly for adverse reactions and drug interactions.
- Administer gemfibrozil in two divided doses daily 30 minutes before morning and evening meals, as prescribed.
- Notify the physician if adverse reaction or drug interactions occur.
- Notify the physician if biliary colic occurs, and request a prescription for an analgesic, if needed.
- Teach the patient about the prescribed agent.

Evaluation

For each nursing diagnosis, prepare an evaluation statement that describes the patient's or family's response to nursing interventions.

Cholesterol synthesis inhibitors

This section presents four other antilipemic agents: lovastatin, pravastatin sodium, probucol, and simvastatin. These drugs lower lipid levels by interfering with cholesterol synthesis.

PHARMACOKINETICS

After oral administration, lovastatin is absorbed incompletely and undergoes extensive first-pass metabolism in the liver. Food may increase the drug's systemic absorption. Lovastatin and its major metabolite are more than 95% protein-bound. It is metabolized extensively and excreted in the urine and feces. Lovastatin's half-life is unknown.

Little is known about lovastatin's onset of action, peak concentration level, and duration of action. Usually, lovastatin produces a therapeutic response within 2 weeks. Maximal changes in lipoprotein and cholesterol concentrations occur within 4 to 6 weeks.

Pravastatin is absorbed rapidly but incompletely after oral administration. Although food reduces the systemic bioavailability of the drug, the overall lipid-lowering effects of the drug are similar whether taken with or 1 hour before meals. Pravastatin also undergoes extensive first-pass metabolism in the liver. Approximately 50% of the drug is bound to plasma proteins. Pravastatin is excreted primarily in the feces with a small amount eliminated in the urine. Peak plasma levels are reached within 1 to 1.5 hours after administration. Its onset and duration of action are not known.

Probucol is absorbed poorly from the GI tract; absorption improves somewhat if it is given with food. Probucol is distributed mainly in fatty acid deposits. Although its method of metabolism is unknown, probucol passes through the bile for elimination in the feces.

Probucol begins to produce effects 2 to 4 weeks after therapy begins. The effects peak in 20 to 50 days. When therapy ends, some probucol remains in the body for up to 6 months afterward.

Simvastatin is absorbed incompletely and undergoes extensive first-pass metabolism in the liver. Both simvastatin and its major metabolite are more than 95% protein-bound. It is eliminated primarily in the feces with a small amount eliminated in the urine. The peak concentration level of simvastatin's active metabolite is reached within 1.3 to 2.4 hours after administration. Its onset and duration of action are not known.

Route	Onset	Peak	Duration
P.O.	Variable	1 hr- 50 days	Variable

PHARMACODYNAMICS

Lovastatin lowers blood cholesterol levels by reducing cholesterol biosynthesis. The mechanisms by which lovastatin reduces LDL cholesterol are not understood fully.

Pravastatin produces its lipid-lowering effects in two ways. First, as a consequence of its reversible inhibition of 3-hydroxy-3-methylglutaryl coenzyme A reductase activity, it modestly reduces intracellular pools of cholesterol. This results in an increased number of LDL-receptors on cell surfaces and enhanced receptor-mediated catabolism and clearance of circulating LDLs. Second, pravastatin inhibits LDL production by inhibiting hepatic synthesis of VLDL, the LDL precursor.

Although probucol's exact mechanism of action is unknown, it primarily reduces blood cholesterol levels and LDL levels.

The mechanism of action of the LDL-lowering effect of simvastatin may involve reduction of VLDL cholesterol concentration and induction of LDL receptors, leading to reduced production and increased catabolism of LDL cholesterol. In addition, simvastatin modestly reduces VLDL cholesterol and plasma triglycerides and can produce increases of variable magnitude in HDL cholesterol.

PHARMACOTHERAPEUTICS

The cholesterol synthesis inhibitors are used to treat various types of hyperlipoproteinemia.

Drug interactions

Cholesterol synthesis inhibitors appear to interact with several other drugs. Probucol can produce additive effects when given with clofibrate; pravastatin can produce additive effects when given with gemfibrozil. These interactions prohibit the combined use of these agents. Probucol should not be used with drugs that prolong the QT interval, affect the atrial rate, or produce atrioventricular block because additive effects can occur. When lovastatin, pravastatin, and simvastatin are administered with an immunosuppressant (especially cyclosporine), gemfibrozil, erythromycin, or niacin (in antilipemic dosages), the interaction may increase the risk of myopathy or rhabdomyolysis. Pravastatin and simvastatin may prolong prothrombin time and increase the risk of bleeding when administered concurrently with warfarin. When simvastatin and digoxin are administered concomitantly, simvastatin may increase the digoxin plasma concentration slightly. Cholestyramine and colestipol may decrease the effectiveness of pravastatin when used together.

ADVERSE DRUG REACTIONS

The most common adverse reactions to lovastatin include GI disturbances and headache. Increased liver enzyme levels may occur in patients receiving long-term lovastatin therapy. Other adverse reactions include an elevated CPK level, myalgia, muscle cramps, myopathy, lens opacities, blurred vision, rash, or pruritus.

Adverse reactions with pravastatin and simvastatin usually are mild and transient. The most common adverse reactions reported during clinical trials included headache and GI upset, such as abdominal pain, constipation, diarrhea, nausea, and vomiting. Other adverse reactions reported include myopathy, rhabdomyolysis, arthralgia, dysfunction of certain cranial nerves, vertigo, memory loss, paresthesia, anxiety, insomnia, depression, alopecia, loss of libido, hep-

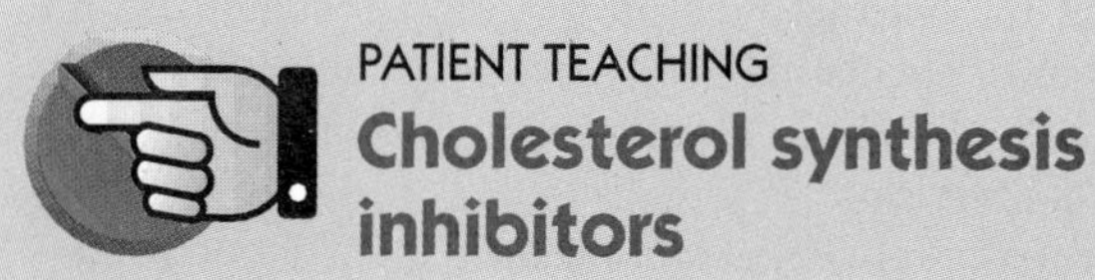

PATIENT TEACHING
Cholesterol synthesis inhibitors

- Teach the patient and family the name, dose, frequency, action, and adverse effects of the prescribed cholesterol synthesis inhibitor.
- Inform the patient that an electrocardiogram must be obtained before and periodically during probucol therapy.
- Inform the patient who must take lovastatin that blood must be drawn for liver function studies before and periodically during lovastatin therapy.
- Inform the patient that the cholesterol level must be checked periodically to assess the drug's effectiveness.
- Advise the patient to take probucol with morning and evening meals or lovastatin with evening meals to enhance absorption.
- Describe the adverse GI reactions to cholesterol synthesis inhibitors. Instruct the patient to notify the physician if these reactions become severe or persistent.
- Instruct the patient to notify the physician of any other adverse reactions.
- Advise the female patient to avoid becoming pregnant for at least 6 months after discontinuation of probucol therapy.

atitis, cirrhosis, and vomiting. Although rare, a hypersensitivity reaction may occur.

In animals, probucol has affected cardiac nerve conduction. It also has prolonged the QT interval of the cardiac cycle. Other adverse reactions to probucol resemble those of the other antilipemic agents. Because the drug's teratogenic effects are unknown, women receiving probucol should not become pregnant for at least 6 months after treatment ends.

NURSING PROCESS APPLICATION

The following information assists the nurse in caring for a patient who is receiving a cholesterol synthesis inhibitor. It includes an overview of assessment activities as well as examples of appropriate nursing diagnoses and related interventions. It also highlights the importance of evaluation.

Assessment

Before drug therapy begins, review the patient's history for conditions that contraindicate or require cautious use of the prescribed cholesterol synthesis inhibitor. Also review the patient's medication history to identify use of drugs that may interact with it. During therapy, assess the patient for adverse drug reactions and signs of drug interactions. Also, periodically assess the effectiveness of therapy with the cholesterol synthesis inhibitor. Finally, evaluate the patient's and family's knowledge about the prescribed drug. (See Patient Teaching: *Cholesterol synthesis inhibitors.*)

Nursing diagnoses

- Risk for injury related to a preexisting condition that contraindicates or requires cautious use of a cholesterol synthesis inhibitor
- Risk for injury related to adverse drug reactions or drug interactions
- Diarrhea related to the adverse GI effects of the prescribed cholesterol synthesis inhibitor
- Knowledge deficit related to the prescribed cholesterol synthesis inhibitor

Planning and implementation

- Do not administer a cholesterol synthesis inhibitor to a patient with a condition that contraindicates its use.
- Administer a cholesterol synthesis inhibitor cautiously to a patient at risk because of a preexisting condition.

* ***Obtain an ECG when probucol treatment begins and after 6 months and 12 months of treatment, as prescribed, to detect any adverse cardiac effects, such as a prolonged QT interval. Obtain liver function tests before lovastatin therapy begins, every 4 to 6 weeks during the first 12 to 15 months of therapy, and periodically thereafter, as prescribed, to detect liver function abnormalities.***

- Monitor the patient's cholesterol level to assess the drug's effectiveness. Also monitor the patient for adverse reactions and drug interactions.
- Administer lovastatin with the evening meal and probucol with morning and evening meals to enhance absorption.
- Administer pravastatin at bedtime to a geriatric patient or one with primary hypercholesterolemia and significant renal or hepatic dysfunction.
- Administer simvastatin in the evening.
- Notify the physician if adverse reactions or drug interactions occur.
- Notify the physician if diarrhea occurs, and request a prescription for an antidiarrheal agent.
- Teach the patient about the prescribed agent.

Evaluation

For each nursing diagnosis, prepare an evaluation statement that describes the patient's or family's response to nursing interventions.

Other antilipemic agents

Several other drugs rarely used to treat hyperlipoproteinemia include ethinyl estradiol, norethindrone acetate, nandrolone and other anabolic steroid agents, and neomycin.

Dextrothyroxine sodium also may be used to treat hypercholesterolemia. Its adverse cardiovascular effects, however, limit its use to pediatric patients with no history of coronary artery disease. One additional agent, niacin, may be used to treat certain kinds of hyperlipoproteinemia. A vitamin, niacin decreases blood levels of LDL, VLDL, and phospholipids and increases the high-density lipoprotein level, especially in types II, III, IV, and V hyperlipoproteinemia. Its adverse reactions, however, also limit its usefulness.

CHAPTER SUMMARY

Chapter 22 discussed the antilipemic agents. Here are the chapter highlights.

Antilipemic agents should be used only when other measures, such as proper diet, weight loss, exercise, and treatment of any disorder causing the lipid abnormality have failed to lower blood lipid levels sufficiently.

The three major classes of antilipemic agents are bile-sequestering agents, fibric acid derivatives, and cholesterol synthesis inhibitors. Niacin also acts as an antilipemic agent.

Questions to consider

See Appendix 1 for answers.

1. Kenneth Young, age 57, has hypercholesterolemia. After 6 months of nonpharmacologic therapy, his cholesterol level has not changed significantly. The physician prescribes the bile-sequestering agent cholestyramine (Questran) 9 grams P.O. q.i.d. Which of the following points should the nurse teach Mr. Young about taking cholestyramine powder?
   (a) Take the powder on an empty stomach.
   (b) Swallow the powder dry for optimal effects.
   (c) Mix the powder in a liquid or semiliquid food.
   (d) Take the powder on a full stomach.

2. Susan Kelly, age 42, has type IV hyperlipoproteinemia, which does not respond to diet restrictions and weight loss. The physician prescribes clofibrate (Atromid-S) 500 mg P.O. q.i.d. Clofibrate administration would have to proceed cautiously if Ms. Kelly is also receiving which of the following drugs?
   (a) A penicillin
   (b) A thiazide diuretic
   (c) An alkalinizing agent
   (d) An oral anticoagulant

3. Wendy Pfeiffer, age 49, is about to begin therapy with the fibric acid derivative clofibrate. Which of the following symptoms is *not* an adverse effect of this drug?
   (a) Migraine headaches
   (b) Pancreatitis
   (c) Intermittent claudication
   (b) Cardiac arrhythmias

4. Arthur Grimes, age 38, has type II hyperlipoproteinemia and takes lovastatin 20 mg P.O. daily. While Mr. Grimes is receiving lovastatin, which of the following parameters should the nurse expect to monitor periodically?
   (a) Liver function test results
   (b) Electrolyte levels
   (c) Results of GI ultrasonography
   (d) Thyroid hormone levels

5. Frances Hurley, age 59, is about to begin antilipemic therapy with lovastatin. To enhance lovastatin absorption, the nurse should advise Ms. Hurley to take the drug at which of the following times?
   (a) With morning and evening meals
   (b) With the evening meal
   (c) Upon arising
   (d) At bedtime

6. John Landesman, age 55, is being discharged after undergoing cardiac catheterization. His physician has advised him to reduce his cholesterol level. Which of the following antilipemic agents could he use without a prescription?
   (a) gemfibrozil
   (b) cholestyramine
   (c) clofibrate
   (d) niacin

UNIT

VII

Drugs affecting the hematologic system

Unit 7 covers drugs that affect red blood cell (RBC) formation, or **erythropoiesis** (**hematinic** agents), alter the coagulation properties of the blood (**anticoagulant** agents), and dissolve thrombi, or blood clots (thrombolytic agents) in acute situations. The unit introduction includes a brief overview of drugs used to control bleeding, whole blood, and blood derivatives.

ERYTHROPOIESIS

Blood is composed of plasma, which is the liquid component, and blood cells, which are formed elements including the RBCs, white blood cells (WBCs), and platelets. An RBC, or erythrocyte, transports oxygen to tissues. A WBC, or leukocyte, defends the body against invading organisms. Platelets aid in hemostasis, stopping bleeding.

Hematinic agents provide essential building blocks for RBC production (erythropoiesis) by increasing **hemoglobin,** the necessary element for oxygen transportation.

Normally, an RBC is small — about 7 microns in diameter. Shaped like a biconcave disk, the RBC has a large surface area relative to its volume. It can change shape as it moves through narrow blood vessels and can withstand the turbulence in small capillaries. RBCs are the most numerous of the formed elements of the blood. Normal RBC count is approximately 5,500,000 per cubic millimeter of blood.

RBCs carry oxygen to cells and exchange it for carbon dioxide. They carry most of these gases in combination with hemoglobin. Each RBC contains 200 to 300 million molecules of hemoglobin. One hemoglobin molecule contains four iron atoms, enabling the molecule to combine with four oxygen molecules and form oxyhemoglobin. The globin (protein) part of the hemoglobin molecule combines with carbon dioxide to form carbaminohemoglobin.

RBC maturation occurs in bone marrow and involves nucleated cells called hemocytoblasts, or stem cells. The stem cells divide by mitosis and evolve through several stages to mature erythrocytes. When an RBC leaves the bone marrow and enters the blood, it contains hemoglobin.

The life span of an RBC is 105 to 120 days, after which time the blood cell breaks down — usually in the capillaries and in the reticuloendothelial cells in the lining of the hepatic blood vessels. Phagocytes in the spleen and bone marrow envelop and destroy the fragments of the RBC, a process known as phagocytosis. During phagocytosis, iron is released from hemoglobin and a pigment called bilirubin is formed. The iron and bilirubin are transported to the liver, where the iron is stored and the bilirubin is excreted in bile. The bone marrow then reuses the stored iron to produce new RBCs. In healthy individuals, the number of RBCs remains constant, with RBC production balancing destruction.

Erythropoiesis becomes more rapid when more RBCs are needed. For example, cell production increases when RBCs are lost in hemorrhage and when tissue hypoxia exists. Hemorrhage and hypoxia stimulate the kidneys to produce the hormone erythropoietin, which accelerates RBC production in the bone marrow.

The bone marrow requires adequate supplies of iron, vitamin B_{12}, amino acids, copper, and cobalt to produce erythrocytes.

Anemia represents a significant decrease in RBC or hemoglobin concentration in the circulating blood. Although many types of anemia exist, the two major types are **microcytic anemia,** from iron deficiency, and **macrocytic anemia,** from vitamin B_{12} or folic acid deficiency.

BLOOD COAGULATION

The pathways involved in blood coagulation include the intrinsic (intravascular) and the extrinsic (extravascular). (See *Coagulation factors,* page 299, and *Coagulation pathways,* page 300.) The intrinsic pathway is activated by injury to the endothelial layer of the blood vessel, disrupting blood flow. The disrupted blood flow initiates a chain of events that forms a thrombus, or clot. Atherosclerotic plaque formation is a condition that activates this type of clotting.

The extrinsic pathway is activated by injury to tissues and vessels, such as surgical wounds or burns, releasing tissue thromboplastin into the circulation. The thromboplastin, a powerful procoagulant, stimulates a chain of events that forms a thrombus.

Coagulation factors

Along with platelets, coagulation factors control clotting. That inhibition significantly affects coagulation. The chart below lists those factors by number, name, and location.

NUMBER	NAME	LOCATION
I	Fibrinogen	Plasma
II	Prothrombin	Plasma
III	Tissue thromboplastin	Tissue cells
IV	Calcium ion	Plasma
V	Labile factor	Plasma
VII	Stable factor	Plasma
VIII	Antihemophilic globulin or antihemophilic factor (AHF)	Plasma
IX	Plasma thromboplastin component or Christmas factor	Plasma
X	Stuart-Prower factor	Plasma
XI	Plasma thromboplastin antecedent	Plasma
XII	Hageman factor	Plasma
XIII	Fibrin stabilizing factor	Plasma

The body also produces blood clots to repair damage in blood vessel walls from normal wear and tear. Platelets adhere to the damaged vessel area and release adenosine diphosphate, which produces platelet stickiness that helps a clot to form. Vasoconstriction in the damaged blood vessel reduces blood flow and produces blood stasis, allowing time for the clot to form.

The body maintains a delicate balance between clot formation (coagulation) and clot destruction (fibrinolysis). Coagulation is inhibited by (1) the liver and reticuloendothelial system, which remove clotting factors from the blood, (2) **antithrombins,** which neutralize **thrombin,** (3) adequate blood flow, which dilutes clotting factors, and (4) the fibrinolytic system, which interferes with the action of thrombin on **fibrinogen.**

Certain diseases are characterized by abnormal coagulation. Thrombus formation can occur in the venous system, causing venothrombosis (such as a pulmonary **embolus**), or in the arterial system, causing arterial **thrombosis** (such as a cerebrovascular thrombosis from a diseased mitral valve). Drugs that are used to treat or prevent thrombotic disorders are known as anticoagulant and **antiplatelet drugs**. They act by inhibiting formation of thrombin and of factors II, VII, IX, and X (oral anticoagulants) and II, Xa, XIa, and XII (heparin) in the liver or by interfering with platelet aggregation.

FIBRINOLYSIS

Conditions such as blood stagnation or blood vessel damage trigger the coagulation mechanism and activate the fibrinolytic system. The fibrinolytic system restricts clot propagation in the general circulation, breaks down thrombi (fibrinolysis), and removes the **fibrin** networks as the injured area heals.

When the fibrinolytic system is activated, tissue plasminogen activator (TPA) is released from stored areas in the endothelium. TPA is released during stress reactions, vigorous exercise, hypoglycemia, and anabolic steroid use. TPA binds to fibrin and converts inactive circulating **plasminogen** to **plasmin,** the proteolytic enzyme that digests fibrin threads, fibrinogen, prothrombin, and factors V, VIII, and XII. The plasmin then can cause clot lysis.

Plasmin normally is inactivated in the circulation by alpha$_2$-antiplasmin, a physiologic inhibitor that prevents too much circulating plasmin, which can cause blood hypocoagulability. However, plasmin bound to fibrin is resistant to alpha$_2$-antiplasmin. Normally, fibrinolysis is restricted to a thrombus area, preventing generalized fibrinolysis and bleeding.

Fibrinolysis of a thrombus produces fibrin degradation products (FDPs). FDPs, which normally are not present in

Coagulation pathways

Various factors can affect coagulation through the intrinsic and extrinsic pathways, illustrated here. A naturally occuring protein, antithrombin III neutralizes thrombin. Heparin increases the thrombin-neutralizing action of antithrombin III, so its effect on coagulation is multiple. Oral anticoagulants diminish the action of vitamin K, responsible for the formation of factors II, VII, IX, and X in the liver.

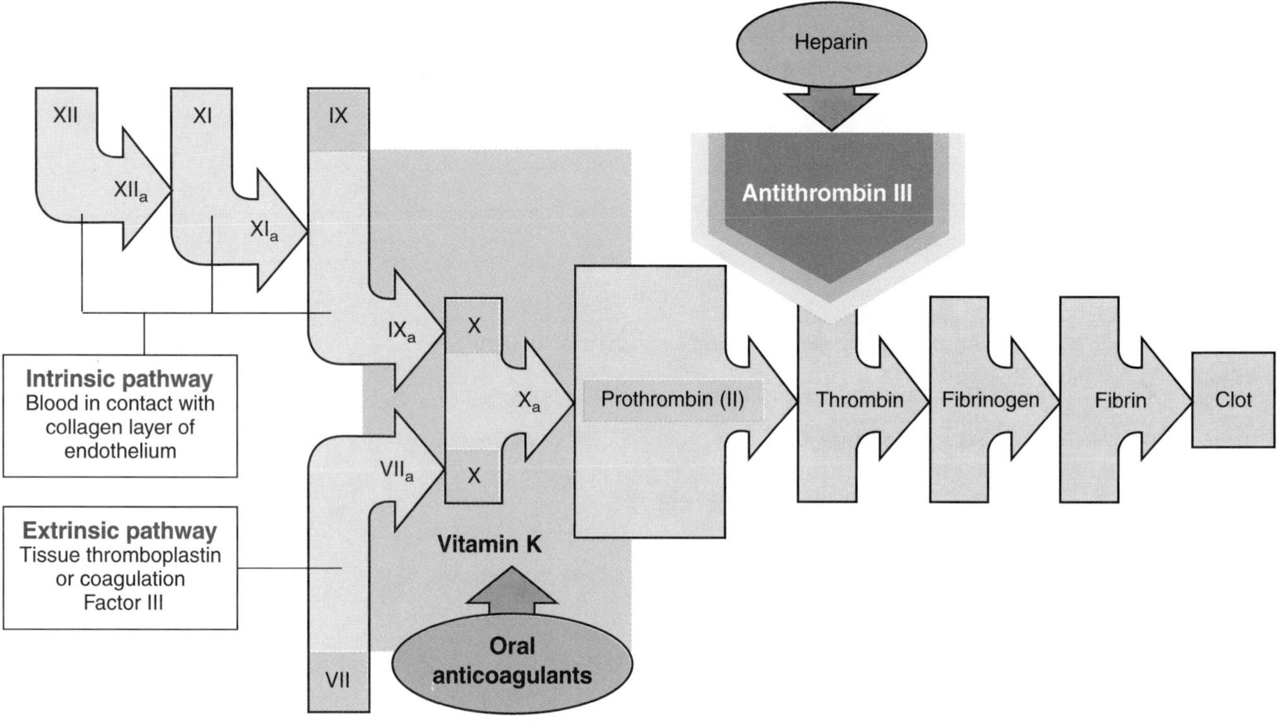

the bloodstream, interfere with platelet aggregation and produce an anticoagulant effect.

AGENTS TO CONTROL BLEEDING

Because bleeding is the major adverse effect of anticoagulant and thrombolytic agents, the nurse must be familiar with the appropriate hemostatic agents. If bleeding results from a deficiency in the body's clotting factors, as in hemophilia, prescribed hemostatic agents, such as antihemophilic factor (factor VIII) and factor IX complex, would be administered. If the patient's bleeding is caused by fibrinolytic therapy, aminocaproic acid (Amicar) might be administered. Excessive bleeding from heparin or oral anticoagulant therapy is treated with protamine sulfate or vitamin K, respectively. Also, several agents can be applied locally to a wound or puncture site to control bleeding and capillary oozing.

WHOLE BLOOD AND BLOOD DERIVATIVES

Whole blood or one of its components may be administered to replace blood volume lost in hemorrhage or to control bleeding. Some components of whole blood that can be separated are packed red cells, plasma, normal serum albumin, plasma protein, and platelets. Using component transfusions provides therapy for specific deficiencies, expands the usefulness of a single blood donation, eases chronic shortages of blood supplies, and reduces the patient's risks of viral hepatitis and exposure to sensitizing agents and drugs. However, some patients will not accept whole blood or derivatives. Blood derivatives are used primarily to provide plasma expanders in patients with hypovolemic shock and other conditions.

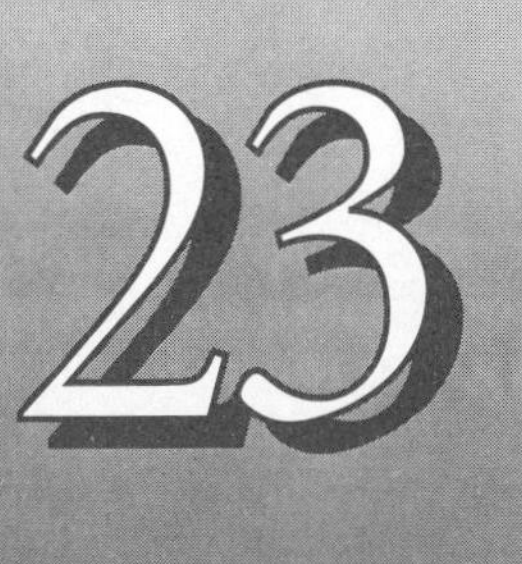

Hematinic agents

OBJECTIVES

After reading and studying this chapter, the student should be able to:
1. discuss the pharmacokinetics of iron, vitamin B_{12}, folic acid, and epoetin alfa preparations.
2. explain the mechanisms of action of the major hematinic agents.
3. discuss the use of iron to treat iron deficiency anemia; the use of vitamin B_{12} and folic acid to treat megaloblastic anemias; and the use of epoetin alfa to treat normocytic anemia caused by chronic renal failure.
4. identify the most common drug interactions and adverse effects of iron, vitamin B_{12}, folic acid, and epoetin alfa.
5. describe how to apply the nursing process when caring for a patient who is receiving a hematinic agent.

INTRODUCTION

Microcytic hypochromic (iron-deficiency) anemia, characterized by small, incompletely hemoglobinized red blood cells (RBCs), results from inadequate dietary intake of iron or excessive blood loss, which may occur with slow, insidious gastrointestinal (GI) bleeding or heavy menstrual bleeding. Macrocytic (megaloblastic) anemia, characterized by abnormally large RBCs, results from inadequate intake or insufficient GI tract absorption of vitamin B_{12} or folic acid. Normocytic anemia, characterized by a decreased number of RBCs, stems from erythropoietin deficiency.

This chapter discusses the **hematinic** agents that are used to treat **microcytic** and **macrocytic anemia:** iron, vitamin B_{12}, and folic acid. It also describes the use of epoetin alfa to treat **normocytic anemia.** (See *Selected major hematinic agents,* page 302.)

Drugs covered in this chapter include:
- cyanocobalamin
- epoetin alfa
- ferrous fumarate, gluconate, and sulfate
- folic acid
- hydroxocobalamin
- iron dextran
- leucovorin calcium.

Iron

Iron preparations are used to treat the most common form of anemia — iron deficiency anemia. Iron preparations discussed in this chapter include ferrous fumarate, ferrous gluconate, ferrous sulfate, and iron dextran.

PHARMACOKINETICS

Iron is absorbed primarily from the duodenum and upper jejunum. The amount of iron absorbed depends partially on the body stores of iron; when body stores are low or **erythropoiesis** is accelerated, iron absorption may increase by 20% to 30%. When total iron stores are large, only about 5% to 10% of iron is absorbed. Enteric-coated preparations decrease iron absorption because the iron is released after it leaves the duodenum. The lymphatic system absorbs the parenteral form after intramuscular (I.M.) injections.

Iron is transported by the blood and bound to transferrin, its carrier plasma protein. About 30% of the iron is stored primarily as hemosiderin or **ferritin** in the reticuloendothelial cells of the liver, spleen, and bone marrow. About two-thirds of the total body iron is contained in **hemoglobin.** Iron is excreted in urine, feces, sweat, and through intestinal cell sloughing, and is secreted in breast milk.

Within 3 days after the patient starts oral iron therapy, the reticulocyte count rises; after 1 week of therapy, the hemoglobin and hematocrit levels increase. The peak concentration level occurs in about 4 weeks. When iron is given by the intravenous (I.V.) or I.M. route, the hemoglobin level rises approximately 1 g/week, with the peak concentration occurring in 4 to 8 weeks.

Route	Onset	Peak	Duration
P.O.	3-7 days	4 wk	Variable
I.V.	1 wk	4-8 wk	Variable
I.M.	1 wk	4-8 wk	Variable

PHARMACODYNAMICS

Although iron serves as a component of myoglobin and various intracellular enzymes (such as cytochrome oxidase, peroxidase, and catalase), its most important role involves the normal production of hemoglobin. About 80% of iron

Selected major hematinic agents

This chart summarizes the major hematinic agents currently in clinical use.

DRUG	MAJOR INDICATIONS AND USUAL DOSAGES	CONTRAINDICATIONS AND PRECAUTIONS
Iron		
ferrous sulfate (Feosol, Feratab, Fer-In-Sol, Fer-Iron, Ferospace, Slow FE)	*Prevention and treatment of iron-deficiency anemia* ADULT: 300 mg to 1.2 g P.O. daily PEDIATRIC: for a child age 2 to 12 years, 3 mg/kg P.O. daily in 3 or 4 divided doses; for a child age 6 to 24 months, up to 6 mg/kg P.O. daily in 3 or 4 divided doses; for a child under age 6 months, 10 to 25 mg P.O. daily in 3 or 4 divided doses	• Ferrous sulfate is contraindicated in a patient with primary hemochromatosis, hemosiderosis, and hemolytic anemias. • This drug requires cautious use in a patient with peptic ulcer, enteritis, ulcerative colitits, or known hypersensitivity.
iron dextran (InFeD)	*Treatment of iron-deficiency anemia in patients who cannot tolerate oral therapy* ADULT: as a test dose, 0.5 ml I.M. or I.V. initially; for a patient under 110 lb (50 kg), 2 ml I.M. daily; for a patient over 110 lb (50 kg), 5 ml I.M. daily, or 2 ml I.V. daily infused slowly at 1 ml/minute PEDIATRIC: as a test dose, 0.5 ml I.M. or I.V.; for an infant under 11 lb (5 kg), 0.5 ml (25 mg) daily; for a child 11 to 20 lb (5 to 9 kg), 1 ml (50 mg) daily; for a child over 20 lb (9 kg), 2 ml daily	• Iron dextran is contraindicated in a patient with any anemia other than iron-deficiency anemia or known hypersensitivity. • This drug requires cautious use in a pregnant or breast-feeding patient or one with severely impaired liver function, significant allergies, asthma, or rheumatoid arthritis.
Vitamin B_{12}		
cyanocobalamin (Crystamine, Cyanoject, Rubesol-1000, Redisol)	*Treatment of vitamin B_{12}-deficiency anemia caused by malabsorption syndrome (as seen in pernicious anemia); GI disease, dysfunction, or surgery; or inadequate dietary intake* ADULT: 100 mcg I.M. or S.C. daily for 10 to 30 days, or 100 mcg daily for 14 days followed by 100 mcg once a month PEDIATRIC: 100 mcg I.M. or S.C. daily for 14 or more days, followed by 60 mcg monthly	• Cyanocobalamin is contraindicated in a patient with early Leber's optic atrophy or known hypersensitivity to vitamin B_{12} or cobalt.
Folic acid		
folic acid (Folacin, Folvite)	*Treatment of megaloblastic anemia resulting from folic acid deficiency* ADULT: 100 to 400 mcg P.O. daily; for severe malabsorption, 1 mg P.O. 1 to 3 times daily PEDIATRIC: 100 to 400 mcg P.O. daily	• Folic acid is contraindicated in a patient with pernicious anemia or other megaloblastic anemia in which vitamin B_{12} is deficient. • This drug requires cautious use in a patient with anemia when the cause has not been determined.
Other hematinic agents		
epoetin alfa (Epogen, Procrit)	*Treatment of normocytic anemia associated with chronic renal failure or other anemias related to malignancies and acquired immunodeficiency syndrome* ADULT: initially, 50 to 100 units/kg I.V. three times weekly in a patient on dialysis (I.V. or S.C. for other patients); then reduced when the target range is reached or the hematocrit level increases more than 4 points in 2 weeks, or increased if hemotocrit level does not increase by 5 or 6 points after 8 weeks and remains below the target range	• Epoetin alfa is contraindicated in a patient with uncontrolled hypertension or known hypersensitivity to mammalian cell-derived albumin or albumin-containing products. • This drug requires cautious use in a pregnant or breast-feeding patient or one with porphyria. • Safety and efficacy in children have not been established.

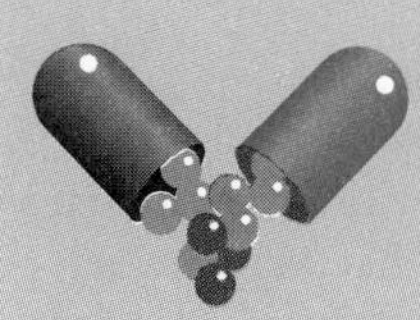

DRUG INTERACTIONS

Iron

Obtain a complete drug and food history to evaluate iron therapy and decrease possible interactions, listed below.

DRUG	INTERACTING AGENTS	POSSIBLE EFFECTS	NURSING IMPLICATIONS
ferrous fumarate, ferrous gluconate, ferrous sulfate	tetracycline, oxytetracycline, methacycline, doxycycline	Decreased absorption of tetracycline and related drugs	• Instruct the patient to take these drugs at least 2 hours apart.
	antacids	Decreased rate or extent of iron absorption	• Do not administer within 2 hours of each other. • Encourage the patient to use foods to buffer adverse gastric effects, such as nausea.
	penicillamine	Decreased penicillamine absorption	• Instruct the patient not to take these drugs together.
	methyldopa	Reduced absorption and inhibited antihypertensive effects of methyldopa	• Do not administer at the same time. • Expect to administer a different antihypertensive if blood pressure control is inadequate.
	vitamin E	Impaired therapeutic response to iron therapy in children	• Monitor the patient's response to iron therapy. • Avoid concurrent use, if possible.
	cholestyramine, colestipol	Reduced serum iron levels	• Administer iron preparation 1 hour before or 6 hours after cholestyramine or colestipol. • Monitor the patient's serum iron and hemoglobin levels.
	cimetidine and other histamine-2 (H_2) blockers	Decreased gastrointestinal absorption of iron	• Administer iron preparation at least 2 hours before or after the H_2 blocker.
	ciprofloxacin, ofloxacin, chloramphenicol	Reduced absorption and serum concentration of antibiotic	• Administer the antibiotic at least 2 hours before an oral iron preparation.
	coffee, tea	Inhibited iron absorption	• Teach the patient to avoid drinking coffee or tea for at least 1 hour after an iron dose.
	eggs, milk	Inhibited iron absorption	• Teach the patient not to use eggs or milk to buffer the adverse gastric effects of iron therapy.

in the plasma goes to the bone marrow, where it is used for erythropoiesis.

PHARMACOTHERAPEUTICS

Oral iron therapy is used to prevent or treat iron deficiency anemia. It also is used to prevent anemias in pediatric patients age 6 months to 2 years because this is a period of rapid growth and development. Pregnant women may need iron supplements to replace the iron used by the developing fetus. Treatment for iron deficiency anemia usually lasts for 6 months.

Parenteral drug therapy is used for patients who cannot absorb oral preparations, are noncompliant with oral therapy, or have bowel disorders (such as ulcerative colitis). The only currently available parenteral form is iron dextran, which builds up iron stores more rapidly than oral preparations but does not correct anemia any faster.

Drug interactions

Few drugs interact with iron, but some antibiotics, antacids, and vitamin preparations, such as ascorbic acid, may alter the absorption rate of iron. Similarly, a few foods may interfere with iron absorption. (See Drug Interactions: *Iron.*)

ADVERSE DRUG REACTIONS

The most common adverse reaction to iron therapy is gastric irritation, which may cause heartburn, anorexia, nausea, vomiting, constipation, and diarrhea. Iron preparations also darken the stool, and liquid ones can stain the teeth.

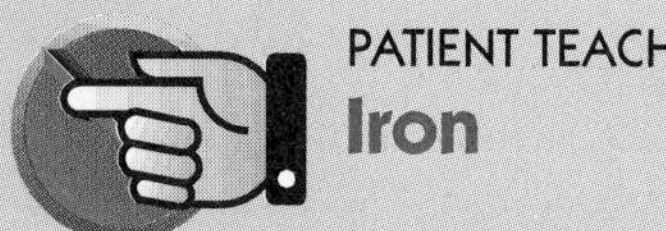

PATIENT TEACHING
Iron

- Teach the patient and family the name, dose, frequency, action, and adverse effects of the prescribed iron preparation.
- Inform the patient of the daily iron requirement.
- Help the patient explore possible causes of anemia, such as inadequate diet or excessive menstrual bleeding, to prevent recurrence.
- Advise the patient to include iron-rich foods in the diet.
- Teach the patient how to prevent accidental poisoning in small children.
- Teach the patient to take liquid preparations with a straw to prevent staining of the teeth.
- Inform the patient that iron preparations normally darken the stool. However, the patient should notify the physician if bloody stool or abdominal cramping or pain occurs.
- Inform the patient receiving intramuscular iron dextran that soreness, inflammation, and skin discoloration may occur at the injection site.
- Advise the patient not to perform activities that require alertness if dizziness or malaise develops.
- Instruct the patient to take an oral iron preparation between meals and to take the oral preparation 2 hours before or after taking a prescribed antacid.
- Tell the patient how to prevent or relieve constipation.
- Instruct the patient who develops seizures to withhold the next iron dose and notify the physician.
- Advise the patient to check with the physician before taking any new prescription or over-the-counter drugs.
- Instruct the patient to notify the physician if adverse reactions occur.

Oral preparations that contain tartrazine yellow may produce allergic reactions, such as bronchospasm, especially in patients with aspirin hypersensitivity.

When iron dextran is given I.M., the patient may experience soreness, inflammation, and brownish skin discoloration at the injection site. Rapid I.V. administration may result in lymphadenopathy, localized phlebitis, and peripheral vascular reddening (flushing) at the injection site.

Iron dextran injection also may cause acute hypersensitivity reactions, including anaphylaxis, dyspnea, urticaria and other rashes, pruritus, arthralgia, myalgia, fever, sweating, and allergic purpura. Therefore, a test dose of iron dextran always should be administered before initiating therapy. Hypotension, seizures, recurrence of arthritis, leukocytosis, headache, backache, dizziness, malaise, transitory paresthesia, and shivering also may occur.

NURSING PROCESS APPLICATION

The following information assists the nurse in caring for a patient who is receiving iron. It includes an overview of assessment activities as well as examples of appropriate nursing diagnoses and related interventions. It also highlights the importance of evaluation.

Assessment

Before drug therapy begins, review the patient's history for conditions that contraindicate or require cautious use of the prescribed iron preparation. Also review the patient's medication history to identify use of drugs that may interact with it. During therapy, assess the patient for adverse drug reactions and signs of drug interactions. Also, periodically assess the effectiveness of iron therapy. Finally, evaluate the patient's and family's knowledge about the prescribed drug. (See Patient Teaching: *Iron.*)

Nursing diagnoses

- Risk for injury related to a preexisting condition that contraindicates or requires cautious use of iron
- Risk for injury related to adverse drug reactions or drug interactions
- Constipation related to the adverse GI effects of iron
- Knowledge deficit related to the prescribed iron preparation

Planning and implementation

- Do not administer iron to a patient with a condition that contraindicates its use.
- Administer iron, especially iron dextran, cautiously to a patient at risk because of a preexisting condition.
- Monitor the patient closely for adverse reactions and drug interactions.
- Regularly monitor the patient's serum iron levels and complete blood count with differential to evaluate the drug's effectiveness. Increased iron and hemoglobin levels indicate effective therapy; a decreased white blood cell count indicates leukocytosis, an adverse reaction.
- Administer oral iron preparations between meals and at least 2 hours before or after giving an antacid.

* ***Closely monitor the patient receiving iron dextran for an acute hypersensitivity reaction, which can be fatal. Keep standard emergency equipment nearby. Give a test dose of iron dextran before beginning therapy as instructed, to assess the patient's response. If no adverse reactions occur within 1 hour, give the total dose.***

* ***Infuse I.V. iron dextran slowly, at a rate of 1 ml/minute. More rapid infusion may cause phlebitis and peripheral vascular reddening (flushing) at the infusion site. Do not administer more than 100 mg I.V. in a single dose. Use only single-dose vials for I.V. therapy. Multidose vials contain the preservative phenol, which can cause serious adverse reactions.***

* ***Administer I.M. iron dextran by the Z-track method to avoid leakage into subcutaneous tissue and to prevent skin discoloration at the injection site. Administer it into a muscle mass on the upper outer buttock.***

- Encourage the patient to drink at least 2 liters of fluid daily (unless contraindicated), increase fiber intake, and exercise regularly to prevent constipation. If constipation occurs, obtain a prescription for a laxative, as needed.

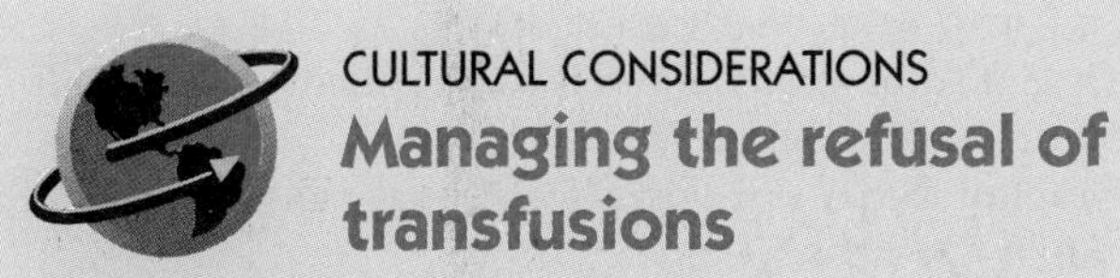

CULTURAL CONSIDERATIONS
Managing the refusal of transfusions

Some groups of people do not accept blood transfusions of whole blood, red blood cells, white blood cells, platelets, or plasma. For example, Jehovah's Witnesses refuse blood and blood products because of their religious beliefs.

When preparing such a patient for surgery, the nurse should assess his or her desire to use alternatives, including blood expanders, fractional blood products (such as albumin and erythropoietin), and blood conservation methods (such as autologous blood collection). Before elective surgery, the nurse should expect to administer an iron supplement to help manage anticipated blood loss.

• Administer iron as prescribed to a patient who refuses transfusions, but needs elective surgery. (See Cultural Considerations: *Managing the refusal of transfusions.*)
• Notify the physician if adverse reactions or drug interactions occur.

Evaluation

For each nursing diagnosis, prepare an evaluation statement that describes the patient's or family's response to nursing interventions.

Vitamin B_{12}

This section discusses the vitamin B_{12} preparations, cyanocobalamin and hydroxocobalamin, used to treat megaloblastic anemia.

PHARMACOKINETICS

Vitamin B_{12} is available in oral and injectable forms. Its absorption depends on an intrinsic factor in the gastric mucosa, and most cases of vitamin B_{12}-deficiency megaloblastic anemia result from the patient's inability to absorb vitamin B_{12}. Therefore, the injectable form most commonly is used to treat this type of anemia.

When cyanocobalamin is injected by the I.M. or subcutaneous (S.C.) route, it is absorbed and binds to transcobalamin II for transport to the tissues. Vitamin B_{12} is transported in the bloodstream to the liver, where 90% of the body's supply is stored. Although hydroxocobalamin is absorbed more slowly from the injection site, its uptake in the liver may be greater than that of cyanocobalamin. With either agent, the liver slowly releases vitamin B_{12} as needed for cellular metabolic functions. It is secreted in breast milk during lactation. About 3 to 8 mcg of vitamin B_{12} are excreted in bile each day and then reabsorbed in the ileum. Within 48 hours after injection of 100 to 1,000 mcg of vitamin B_{12}, 50% to 95% of the dose appears in urine, with the major portion excreted in the first 8 hours.

The onset of action is quite rapid; within 3 days, mature RBCs appear in a blood smear. Patients usually feel better within 24 hours of therapy. The first objective change is the disappearance of the megaloblastic morphology of the bone marrow. The plasma iron concentration dramatically decreases, and the reticulocyte count increases on the second or third day and peaks 6 to 8 days later. By the 10th day, the platelet count is higher than normal, and the granulocyte count reverts to normal within 2 weeks.

Route	Onset	Peak	Duration
I.M.	3 days	6-8 days	2 wk

PHARMACODYNAMICS

When vitamin B_{12} is taken orally or by injection, it replaces vitamin B_{12} that the body normally would absorb from the diet. This vitamin is essential for cell growth and replication and for the maintenance of normal myelin levels throughout the nervous system. Vitamin B_{12} also may be involved in lipid and carbohydrate metabolism.

PHARMACOTHERAPEUTICS

Cyanocobalamin and hydroxocobalamin are used to treat vitamin B_{12}-deficiency anemia. They typically are administered by the I.M. route because this type of anemia usually is related to an inability to absorb dietary sources of vitamin B_{12}.

Drug interactions

Alcohol, aminosalicylic acid, neomycin, and colchicine may decrease the absorption of oral cyanocobalamin. Chloramphenicol may antagonize the hematopoietic effects of cyanocobalamin.

ADVERSE DRUG REACTIONS

No dose-related adverse reactions occur with vitamin B_{12} therapy. However, some rare reactions may occur when vitamin B_{12} is administered parenterally. These include hypersensitivity reactions that could result in anaphylaxis and death; cardiovascular reactions (pulmonary edema, congestive heart failure, and peripheral vascular thrombosis); hematologic reactions (polycythemia vera); hypokalemia; dermatologic reactions (itching, transient exanthema, and urticaria); and GI reactions (mild diarrhea). Severe, swift optic nerve atrophy has been reported in patients with hereditary optic nerve atrophy. Some patients report a feeling of swelling throughout the entire body.

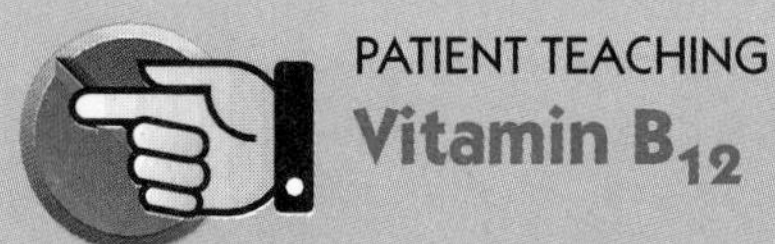

PATIENT TEACHING
Vitamin B_{12}

- Teach the patient and family the name, dose, frequency, action, and adverse effects of the prescribed vitamin B_{12} preparation.
- Explain that the patient should start to feel better 24 hours after therapy begins.
- Inform the patient that initial parenteral therapy with cyanocobalamin requires daily injections for up to 30 days; with hydroxocobalamin, up to 10 days. Also, monthly maintenance therapy is needed until the deficiency resolves, except in the case of pernicious anemia, which requires lifelong therapy.
- Teach the patient and family how to administer vitamin B_{12} subcutaneously or intramuscularly, as prescribed, if long-term therapy is necessary.
- Teach the patient how to store the parenteral drug properly.
- Stress the importance of regular laboratory testing to monitor the effectiveness of therapy or to detect adverse hematologic reactions.
- Emphasize the importance of compliance with the drug regimen.
- Teach the patient that a well-balanced diet can eliminate vitamin deficiencies.
- Instruct the patient to eat vitamin B_{12}-rich foods, such as meat, seafood, milk, eggs, liver, and legumes.
- Reassure the patient with exanthema that it is transient.
- Reassure the patient with diarrhea that it usually remains mild. Tell the patient to ask the physician for a prescription for an antidiarrheal agent, if needed.
- Instruct the patient to notify the physician if adverse reactions occur.

NURSING PROCESS APPLICATION

The following information assists the nurse in caring for a patient who is receiving a vitamin B_{12} preparation. It includes an overview of assessment activities as well as examples of appropriate nursing diagnoses and related interventions. It also highlights the importance of evaluation.

Assessment

Before drug therapy begins, review the patient's history for conditions that contraindicate or require cautious use of the prescribed vitamin B_{12} preparation. During therapy, assess the patient for adverse drug reactions. Also, periodically assess the effectiveness of vitamin B_{12} therapy. Finally, evaluate the patient's and family's knowledge about the prescribed drug. (See Patient Teaching: *Vitamin B_{12}*.)

Nursing diagnoses

- Risk for injury related to a preexisting condition that contraindicates or requires cautious use of vitamin B_{12}
- Risk for injury related to adverse drug reactions
- Noncompliance related to lifelong vitamin B_{12} therapy
- Knowledge deficit related to vitamin B_{12}

Planning and implementation

- Do not administer vitamin B_{12} to a patient with a condition that contraindicates its use.
- Monitor the patient closely for adverse reactions during vitamin B_{12} therapy.
- Monitor appropriate laboratory tests, such as hematocrit and reticulocyte counts, to determine the effectiveness of therapy. Check blood folate levels for a patient who is receiving more than 10 mcg daily of vitamin B_{12}. In such a patient, the hematologic results may seem normal but may mask a folate deficiency, which could be the actual cause of megaloblastic anemia. Monitor the potassium level during the first 48 hours, particularly in a patient with Addisonian pernicious anemia or megaloblastic anemia.

* ***Keep standard emergency equipment readily available because of the risk of anaphylaxis.***

- Expect to administer the injectable form of vitamin B_{12}, as prescribed, to a patient who cannot take vitamin B_{12} orally. Administer a higher dosage of cyanocobalamin, to a critically ill patient with a neurologic or infectious disease or hyperthyroidism. Expect to administer an intradermal test dose, as prescribed, to a patient with cobalt sensitivity.
- Store the parenteral form of the drug in a light-resistant container at room temperature.
- Encourage the patient to eat foods rich in vitamin B_{12}, such as meat, seafood, milk, eggs, and liver.
- Notify the physician if adverse reactions occur.
- Monitor the degree of compliance by reviewing the results of appropriate laboratory tests, especially for the patient who needs lifelong therapy.
- Stress the importance of monthly B_{12} injections for the patient with pernicious anemia.
- Stress the importance of treatment for the patient receiving long-term therapy with I.M. injections because neurologic damage (for example, degenerative spinal cord lesions) can occur as early as 3 months after a vitamin B_{12} deficiency develops.
- Alert the physician if noncompliance occurs.

Evaluation

For each nursing diagnosis, prepare an evaluation statement that describes the patient's or family's response to nursing interventions.

Folic acid

Folic acid and leucovorin calcium are the two folic acid preparations discussed in this section.

PHARMACOKINETICS

Folate absorption requires transport and the action of an enzyme in the duodenal and upper jejunum mucosal cell membranes. Once absorbed, folate is distributed rapidly to all body tissues. Folate supplies are maintained from food and by the enterohepatic cycle. The liver actively reduces and methylates the folate components, which then are transported to bile for resorption by the intestine and subsequently delivered to the tissues. This pathway may provide as much as 200 mcg of folate daily for recirculation to the tissues.

Folates are excreted in urine and feces and secreted in breast milk.

Within 48 hours after the patient starts folic acid therapy, megaloblastic erythropoiesis disappears, the plasma iron level decreases, and erythropoiesis becomes more efficient. The reticulocyte count begins to rise by day 2 and reaches a peak concentration level between days 5 and 7. The hematocrit level begins to rise by week 2.

Route	Onset	Peak	Duration
P.O.	2 days	5-7 days	Variable

PHARMACODYNAMICS

Folic acid is an essential component for normal erythrocyte production and growth. A deficiency results in megaloblastic anemia and low serum and RBC folate levels.

PHARMACOTHERAPEUTICS

Folic acid is used to treat folic acid deficiency. Parenteral folic acid seldom is required except to reverse the effect of folic acid antagonists during oncologic chemotherapy or during a therapeutic trial to determine the hematopoietic response before oral therapy begins. Patients who are pregnant or undergoing treatment for liver disease, hemolytic anemia, alcohol abuse, skin disease, or renal failure will need prophylactic folic acid therapy.

Drug interactions

Folic acid antagonists that inhibit dihydrofolate reductase activity may cause a deficiency of active folate compounds, which can lead to megaloblastic anemia. These drugs include methotrexate (antimetabolite agent), antimalarial agents, triamterene (diuretic), pentamidine (antiprotozoal agent), and trimethoprim (urinary antiseptic agent). Leucovorin calcium may be needed to minimize interference.

In large doses, folic acid may increase seizure activity because it counteracts the effects of anticonvulsants, such as phenytoin, phenobarbital, and primidone. Folic acid may interfere with the antimicrobial action of pyrimethamine. Such drugs as glutethimide, isoniazid, cycloserine, and oral contraceptives may interfere with folic acid absorption.

ADVERSE DRUG REACTIONS

Allergic responses (erythema, rash, itching) have been reported after folic acid and leucovorin calcium administration.

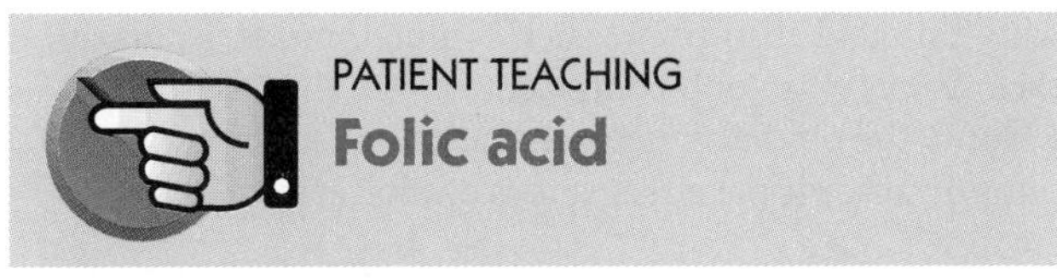

PATIENT TEACHING

Folic acid

- Teach the patient and family the name, dose, frequency, action, and adverse effects of the prescribed folic acid preparation.
- Teach the patient the dietary sources of folate. Instruct the patient not to overcook vegetables because this may destroy folic acid compounds.
- Teach the female patient to inform all personal physicians about folic acid therapy to prevent drug interactions.
- Advise the patient to notify the physician if adverse reactions occur or if signs of megaloblastic anemia recur.

NURSING PROCESS APPLICATION

The following information assists the nurse in caring for a patient who is receiving a folic acid preparation. It includes an overview of assessment activities as well as examples of appropriate nursing diagnoses and related interventions. It also highlights the importance of evaluation.

Assessment

Before drug therapy begins, review the patient's history for conditions that require cautious use of the prescribed folic acid preparation. Also review the patient's medication history to identify use of drugs that may interact with it. During therapy, assess the patient for adverse drug reactions and signs of drug interactions. Also, periodically assess the effectiveness of folic acid therapy. Finally, evaluate the patient's and family's knowledge about the prescribed drug. (See Patient Teaching: *Folic acid.*)

Nursing diagnoses

- Risk for injury related to a preexisting condition that requires cautious use of a folic acid preparation
- Risk for injury related to adverse drug reactions or drug interactions
- Knowledge deficit related to the prescribed folic acid preparation

Planning and implementation

- Administer a folic acid preparation cautiously to a patient at risk because of a preexisting condition.
- Monitor the patient closely for adverse reactions and drug interactions.
- Monitor the effectiveness of folic acid therapy, particularly during the first 2 weeks.

* ***Take seizure precautions in a patient receiving large doses of folic acid during concomitant anticonvulsant therapy.***

- Monitor the patient closely for recurrence of megaloblastic anemia if the patient is also taking a drug that interferes

with folic acid absorption, such as glutethimide, isoniazid, cycloserine, or an oral contraceptive.
• Notify the physician if adverse reactions or drug interactions occur or if the effectiveness of folic acid therapy decreases.
• Teach the patient about the prescribed agent.

Evaluation

For each nursing diagnosis, prepare an evaluation statement that describes the patient's or family's response to nursing interventions.

Other hematinic agents

Epoetin alfa, which stimulates RBC production, is used to treat patients with normocytic anemia caused by chronic renal failure (CRF). It also is used to treat anemia associated with zidovudine therapy in patients with human immunodeficiency virus infection, and appears to decrease transfusion requirements in patients with nonmyeloid malignancies.

PHARMACOKINETICS

After S.C. administration, epoetin alfa reaches its peak plasma level within 24 hours. It has a circulating half-life of 4 to 13 hours. No difference in half-life is apparent in patients on dialysis and patients not on dialysis whose serum creatinine level is greater than 3 mg/dl. Small amounts of the drug have been recovered in plasma and urine after administration. The exact metabolic pathway has not been determined. Clinical response usually occurs in 2 to 6 weeks.

Route	Onset	Peak	Duration
S.C.	Unknown	24 hr	2-4 days

PHARMACODYNAMICS

Erythropoietin is an amino acid polypeptide that stimulates RBC production in the bone marrow. Normally, erythropoietin is formed in the kidneys in response to hypoxia and anemia and stimulates erythropoiesis. Patients with conditions that decrease production of erythropoietin then develop chronic normocytic anemia. Epoetin alfa boosts the production of erythropoietin.

PHARMACOTHERAPEUTICS

Like the other hematinic agents, epoetin alfa is used to replace a substance that is essential to the hematologic system.

Drug interactions

No known drug interactions exist.

ADVERSE DRUG REACTIONS

Hypertension is the most common adverse reaction to epoetin alfa. It may occur even in previously hypotensive patients. Other adverse reactions reported in more than 5% of patients during clinical trials include headache, arthralgia, nausea, edema, fatigue, diarrhea, vomiting, chest pain, skin reactions at the administration site, asthenia, and dizziness. Adverse reactions also include iron deficiency anemia and clotting of atrioventricular fistula. Other significant, but rare, reactions noted during clinical trials include seizures (in 1.1% of patients), cerebrovascular accident or transient ischemic attack (in 0.4% of patients), and myocardial infarction (in 0.4% of patients). Seizures are more likely to occur during the first 90 days of therapy, especially if the patient experiences a rapid rise in the hematocrit level.

NURSING PROCESS APPLICATION

The following information assists the nurse in caring for a patient who is receiving epoetin alfa. It includes an overview of assessment activities as well as examples of appropriate nursing diagnoses and related interventions. It also highlights the importance of evaluation.

Assessment

Before drug therapy begins, review the patient's history for conditions that contraindicate or require cautious use of epoetin alfa. During therapy, assess the patient for adverse drug reactions. Also, periodically assess the effectiveness of epoetin alfa therapy. Finally, evaluate the patient's and family's knowledge about the prescribed drug.

Nursing diagnoses

• Risk for injury related to a preexisting condition that contraindicates or requires cautious use of epoetin alfa
• Risk for injury related to adverse drug reactions
• Knowledge deficit related to epoetin alfa

Planning and implementation

• Do not administer epoetin alfa to a patient with a condition that contraindicates its use.
• Administer epoetin alfa cautiously to a patient at risk because of a preexisting condition.
• Monitor the patient closely for adverse reactions during epoetin alfa therapy. Check the patient's blood pressure regularly to detect hypertension.
* ***Take seizure precautions and monitor the patient's neurologic status closely because of the risk of seizures, especially during the first 90 days of therapy.***
* ***Notify the physician if the patient experiences headache, arthralgia, or chest pain. Obtain a prescription, as needed, to relieve the discomfort. Expect to obtain an electrocardiogram immediately, as prescribed, if chest pain occurs.***
• Evaluate the patient's hemoglobin and hematocrit levels regularly, as prescribed, to monitor the effectiveness of epoetin alfa therapy.

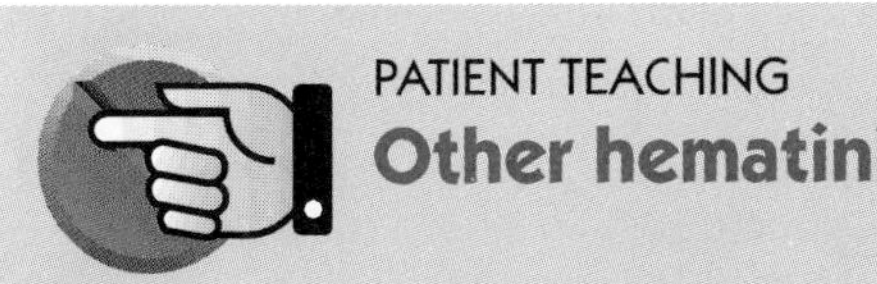

PATIENT TEACHING
Other hematinic agents

- Teach the patient and family the name, dose, frequency, action, and adverse effects of epoetin alfa.
- Inform the patient receiving dialysis that the initial drug dosage will be I.V. epoetin alfa three times weekly, and then a maintenance dosage will be established. Inform all other patients that the initial drug dosage will be I.V. or subcutaneous epoetin alfa three times weekly, and then a maintenance dosage will be established.
- Stress the importance of having blood tests as prescribed to assess the effectiveness of epoetin alfa.
- Inform the patient and family that seizures may occur, especially during the first 90 days of therapy.
- Caution the patient not to perform activities that require alertness if dizziness occurs.
- Advise the patient to have the blood pressure checked regularly.
- Instruct the patient to notify the physician immediately or go to the nearest emergency department if chest pain occurs.
- Instruct the patient to notify the physician if any other adverse reactions occur.

• Expect to decrease the dosage as prescribed when the hematocrit level reaches the target range or rises above 4 points in 2 weeks. Expect to increase the dosage as prescribed if the hematocrit level does not increase by 5 to 6 points after 8 weeks of therapy and remains below the target range of 30% to 33% of blood volume (maximum 36%).
• Do not shake the solution. Shaking may inactivate the drug.
• Do not administer the solution if it is discolored or contains particles.
• Administer only one dose from the single-use vial. Do not mix the solution with other drugs because it does not contain preservatives.
• Notify the physician if adverse reactions occur or if epoetin alfa therapy is ineffective.
• Teach the patient about the prescribed agent. (See Patient Teaching: *Other hematinic agents.*)

Evaluation

For each nursing diagnosis, prepare an evaluation statement that describes the patient's or family's response to nursing interventions.

CHAPTER SUMMARY

Chapter 23 discussed the hematinic agents used to treat certain types of anemias. Here are the highlights of the chapter.

Iron deficiency anemia is correctable with oral administration of an iron preparation, such as ferrous fumarate, ferrous gluconate, or ferrous sulfate. Therapy, which lasts about 6 months, restores normal hemoglobin levels and creates iron stores in the body.

Megaloblastic anemia caused by a vitamin B_{12} deficiency is correctable with replacement therapy. Patients who cannot absorb vitamin B_{12} from their diets will require monthly I.M. injections for life to ensure proper cellular metabolic functioning. Cyanocobalamin and hydroxocobalamin are used in vitamin B_{12} therapy.

Treating megaloblastic anemia caused by a folic acid deficiency with 1 mg of oral folic acid daily will reverse the anemia.

Epoetin alfa, which has no known drug interactions, is used to treat anemia associated with chronic renal failure, malignancies, and acquired immunodeficiency syndrome.

When caring for a patient receiving a hematinic agent, the nurse uses the nursing process. Key aspects of nursing care include observing the patient closely for adverse reactions, minimizing such discomfort as iron-induced constipation, monitoring patient compliance during lifelong therapy, and teaching the patient about hematinic drug administration.

Questions to consider

See Appendix 1 for answers.

1. Bonnie Grant, age 27, is diagnosed with iron deficiency anemia. Because she also has ulcerative colitis that contraindicates the use of oral iron preparations, the physician prescribes iron dextran (InFeD) 0.5 ml I.M. initially, followed by 2 ml I.M. daily. Why should the nurse use the Z-track method when administering this drug?
   (a) To prevent pain
   (b) To prevent necrosis
   (c) To prevent skin discoloration
   (d) To prevent delayed absorption

2. Roy Lee Baker, age 41, is diagnosed with megaloblastic anemia caused by vitamin B_{12} deficiency. His physician prescribes cyanocobalamin 100 mcg I.M. daily. When can Mr. Baker expect to feel better after cyanocobalamin therapy is begun?
   (a) 24 hours
   (b) 72 hours
   (c) 1 week
   (d) 2 weeks

3. Mary Collins, age 57, needs iron therapy to correct iron deficiency anemia. Because she has difficulty swallowing pills, her doctor prescribes a liquid iron preparation. Which of the following instructions should the nurse give Ms. Collins before discharge?
   (a) Mix the liquid with food.
   (b) Use a straw to ingest the preparation.
   (c) Mix the liquid in a glass of juice before drinking it.
   (d) Take the liquid within 30 minutes of the prescribed antacid.

4. Carl McPherson, a critically ill 70-year-old patient with megaloblastic anemia, is receiving cyanocobalamin (vitamin B_{12}) therapy. For this patient, which of the following electrolyte levels should the nurse monitor closely?
   (a) calcium
   (b) sodium
   (c) magnesium
   (d) potassium

5. Margaret Mears, age 52, has megaloblastic anemia caused by folic acid deficiency. Her physician prescribes folic acid replacement therapy. What is the usual adult dosage?
   (a) 3 to 5 mg/day
   (b) 1 to 2 mg/day
   (c) 100 to 400 mcg/day
   (d) 50 to 75 mcg/day

6. Daniel Peters, age 45, is receiving epoetin alfa to treat normocytic anemia caused by chronic renal failure. Which of the following adverse reactions is caused by epoetin alfa?
   (a) Blurred vision
   (b) Hypertension
   (c) Constipation
   (d) Urine retention

24 Anticoagulant and thrombolytic agents

OBJECTIVES

After reading and studying this chapter, the student should be able to:

1. describe how heparin, oral anticoagulants, antiplatelet drugs, and thrombolytic agents produce their effects.
2. discuss the indications for heparin, oral anticoagulants, antiplatelet drugs, and thrombolytic agents.
3. identify adverse reactions associated with heparin, oral anticoagulants, antiplatelet drugs, and thrombolytic agents.
4. describe how to apply the nursing process when caring for a patient who is receiving an anticoagulant or thrombolytic agent.

INTRODUCTION

Anticoagulant agents are used to reduce clotting, and thrombolytic agents are used to dissolve thrombi. Antiplatelet drugs may be used alone or with an oral anticoagulant to disrupt platelet aggregation, thereby reducing arterial thromboembolism. (See *Selected major anticoagulant and thrombolytic agents,* pages 312 and 313.)

Drugs covered in this chapter include:

- alteplase
- anistreplase
- aspirin
- dicumarol
- dipyridamole
- heparin
- streptokinase
- sulfinpyrazone
- ticlopidine
- urokinase
- warfarin sodium.

Heparin

Heparin is prepared commercially from animal tissue for use in preventing clot formation and in treating **thromboembolism.** It does not, however, affect the synthesis of clotting factors and therefore cannot dissolve clots. Low molecular weight heparins, like dalteparin sodium and enoxaparin sodium, have recently been developed for the prevention of deep vein thrombosis in various surgical populations.

PHARMACOKINETICS

Because heparin is not absorbed well from the gastrointestinal (GI) tract, it must be administered parenterally to achieve distribution to the intravascular compartments. Distribution is immediate after intravenous (I.V.) administration, using I.V. bolus or continuous I.V. infusion, but it is much less predictable with a subcutaneous (S.C.) injection. The intramuscular (I.M.) route should be avoided because of the risk of local bleeding. Heparin is metabolized in the liver, and its metabolites are excreted in urine.

Heparin's anticoagulant effect is measured by the **activated partial thromboplastin time** (APTT) test and the **partial thromboplastin time** (PTT) test. Its half-life, approximately 1 to 1.5 hours, is dose-related.

Route	Onset	Peak	Duration
S.C.	20-60 min	2-4 hr	Unknown
I.V.	Immediate	Within minutes	2-6 hr

PHARMACODYNAMICS

Heparin indirectly inactivates **thrombin** by accelerating the interaction between thrombin and **antithrombin III,** a thrombin-inactivating glycoprotein found in the blood. Factors IXa, Xa, XIa, and XIIa also are inactivated. Low heparin doses increase the activity of antithrombin III against factor Xa and thrombin and can inhibit the initiation of clotting. Much larger doses are necessary to inhibit **fibrin** formation once a clot has been formed. This relationship between dose and effect is the rationale for using low-dose heparin to prevent clotting. Whole blood clotting time, **thrombin time,** PTT, and APTT are prolonged during heparin therapy. However, these times may be prolonged only slightly with low or ultra-low prophylactic doses.

PHARMACOTHERAPEUTICS

Heparin is prescribed to prevent or treat venous thromboembolisms, characterized by inappropriate or excessive intravascular activation of blood clotting. It also is used whenever the patient's blood must circulate outside the body through a machine, such as the cardiopulmonary bypass machine or hemodialysis machine. Heparin may be

Selected major anticoagulant and thrombolytic agents

This chart summarizes the major anticoagulant and thrombolytic agents currently in clinical use.

DRUG	MAJOR INDICATIONS AND USUAL DOSAGES	CONTRAINDICATIONS AND PRECAUTIONS
Heparin		
heparin	*Pulmonary embolism or thromboembolism* ADULT: for continuous therapy, 5,000 to 10,000 units I.V. bolus followed by continuous infusion of 1,000 to 2,000 units/hour; for intermittent therapy, 5,000 to 10,000 units every 6 hours; for prophylaxis, 5,000 units S.C. every 8 to 12 hours PEDIATRIC: initially, 50 units/kg by I.V. bolus; followed by 100 units/kg every 4 hours or 20,000 units/m^2 over 24 hours by continuous I.V. infusion	• Heparin is contraindicated in a patient with known hypersensitivity, severe thrombocytopenia (unless coagulation studies can be performed regularly), or uncontrollable active bleeding except when caused by disseminated intravascular coagulation. • This drug requires cautious use in a pregnant patient or one with a disease that carries a high risk of hemorrhage, such as subacute bacterial endocarditis, severe hypertension, hemophilia, thrombocytopenia, some vascular purpuras, ulcerative lesions, or liver disease with impaired hemostasis. Heparin also requires cautious use in a patient undergoing a spinal tap procedure, spinal anesthesia, or major surgery, especially those involving the brain, spinal cord, or eye. It also requires cautious use in a patient with renal failure, allergies, or continuous tube drainage of the stomach or small intestine.
Oral anticoagulants		
warfarin (Coumadin)	*Venous thrombosis after initial treatment with heparin, prevention of deep vein thromboembolism in patients with artificial heart valves, diseased mitral valves, or atrial fibrillation* ADULT: initially, 5 to 10 mg P.O. daily for 2 days, adjusted according to prothrombin time or international normalized ratio results; for maintenance dosage, 2 to 10 mg P.O. daily	• Warfarin is contraindicated in a patient with a condition in which the risk of hemorrhage might be greater than the drug's benefit, such as pregnancy; preeclampsia, eclampsia, or threatened abortion; hemorrhagic tendency or blood dyscrasias; bleeding tendency associated with active ulceration; overt bleeding of the GI, genitourinary (GU), or respiratory tract; cerebrovascular hemorrhage; aneurysm; pericarditis; pericardial effusion; subacute bacterial endocarditis; malignant hypertension; senile dementia or cognitive impairment; alcoholism; or psychosis. It also is contraindicated in a patient who has recently undergone or is undergoing major surgery on the central nervous system or eye or traumatic surgery resulting in large, open surfaces; is undergoing major regional lumbar block anesthesia, spinal puncture, or another procedure that carries a high risk of uncontrollable bleeding; has no access to adequate laboratory facilities; or is unwilling to comply with therapy or regular laboratory testing. • This drug requires cautious use in a breast-feeding patient or one with a condition that increases the risk of hemorrhage or necrosis, such as moderate to severe hepatic or renal insufficiency; infectious disease; intestinal flora disturbance; trauma; moderate to severe hypertension; known or suspected hereditary, familial, or clinical deficiency of protein C; polycythemia vera; vasculitis; severe diabetes; severe allergic response; or anaphylaxis. It also requires cautious use in a patient with an indwelling catheter or large exposed raw surfaces resulting from surgery. • Safety and efficacy in children have not been established.
Antiplatelet drugs		
aspirin	*Prevention of clot formation in arteriovenous shunts in hemodialysis patients* ADULT: 160 mg P.O. daily *Prevention of clot formation in patients with unstable angina* ADULT: 325 mg P.O. daily *Prevention of myocardial infarction (MI)* ADULT: 325 mg P.O. daily *Prevention of transient ischemic attack* ADULT: 325 mg P.O. q.i.d.	• Aspirin is contraindicated in a pregnant patient during the last trimester; a child or adolescent with varicella or influenza (unless prescribed by a physician); or a patient with a bleeding disorder, known hypersensitivity, or a history of acute asthmatic attacks, urticaria, or aspirin-induced rhinitis. • This drug requires cautious use in a breast-feeding patient, one receiving anticoagulant therapy, or one with impaired renal or hepatic function, a history of GI lesions, advanced chronic renal insufficiency, hypoprothrombinemia, vitamin K deficiency, thrombocytopenia, or thrombotic thrombocytopenic purpura. • Highly buffered aspirin preparations require extremely cautious use in a patient with heart failure or any other condition in which high sodium intake is harmful.

Selected major anticoagulant and thrombolytic agents *(continued)*

DRUG	MAJOR INDICATIONS AND USUAL DOSAGES	CONTRAINDICATIONS AND PRECAUTIONS
Antiplatelet drugs *(continued)*		
ticlopidine (Ticlid)	*Reduction of risk of thrombotic stroke in high-risk patients* ADULT: 250 mg P.O. b.i.d. with food	• Ticlopidine is contraindicated in a patient with known hypersensitivity, a hematopoietic disorder such as neutropenia or thrombocytopenia, hemostatic disorder, active pathological bleeding, or severe liver impairment. • This drug requires cautious use in a pregnant or breast-feeding patient. • Safety and efficacy in children under age 18 have not been established.
Thrombolytic agents		
alteplase (Activase)	*Acute MI* ADULT: for patients over 67 kg, 15 mg by I.V. bolus, followed by 50 mg infused over 30 minutes and 35 mg infused over 60 minutes; for patients under 67 kg, 15 mg by I.V. bolus, followed by 0.75 mg/kg infused over the next 30 minutes (to a maximum of 50 mg) and 0.5 mg/kg infused over the next 60 minutes (to a maximum of 35 mg) *Pulmonary embolism* ADULT: 100 mg I.V. infused over 2 hours	• Alteplase is contraindicated in a patient with active internal bleeding, a history of cerebrovascular accident (CVA), intracranial neoplasm, arteriovenous malformation, aneurysm, known bleeding diathesis, severe uncontrolled hypertension, or known hypersensitivity. It also is contraindicated in a patient who has experienced intracranial or intraspinal surgery or trauma within the past 2 months. • This drug requires cautious use in a pregnant patient, a patient over age 75, one who has undergone major surgery in the past 10 days, one receiving concurrent administration of an oral anticoagulant, one who has experienced trauma (including trauma caused by cardiopulmonary resuscitation) in the past 10 days, or one who is at high risk for left heart thrombus. Alteplase also requires cautious use in a patient with cerebrovascular disease, GI or GU bleeding in the past 10 days, hypertension with systolic blood pressure over 180 mm Hg or diastolic blood pressure over 110 mm Hg, subacute bacterial endocarditis, acute pericarditis, hemostatic defects (such as those caused by severe hepatic or renal disease), diabetic hemorrhagic retinopathy or other hemorrhagic ophthalmic condition, significant liver dysfunction, septic thrombophlebitis, occluded arteriovenous cannula at a seriously infected site, or any other condition in which bleeding constitutes a significant hazard or would be difficult to manage because of its location.
anistreplase (Eminase)	*Acute MI* ADULT: 30 units I.V. over 2 to 5 minutes	• Anistreplase is contraindicated in a patient with any of the conditions that contraindicate the use of alteplase. • This drug requires cautious use in a patient with any of the conditions that require cautious use of alteplase (except for significant liver dysfunction).
streptokinase (Kabikinase, Streptase)	*Deep vein thrombosis, arterial thrombosis, arterial emboli* ADULT: 250,000 IU I.V. as a loading dose given over 30 minutes, then 100,000 IU/hour I.V. for up to 72 hours *Pulmonary embolus* ADULT: 250,000 IU I.V. as a loading dose given over 30 minutes, then 100,000 IU/hour I.V. for 24 hours *Acute evolving transmural MI* ADULT: 1,500,000 IU by I.V. infusion over 60 minutes, or 140,000 IU by intracoronary infusion (20,000 IU by I.V. bolus followed by 2,000 IU/minute for 60 minutes) *Clot dissolution in arteriovenous cannula* ADULT: 100,000 to 250,000 IU instilled slowly into the occluded cannula	• Streptokinase is contraindicated in a patient with active internal bleeding, intracranial neoplasm, severe uncontrolled hypertension, or known hypersensitivity or one who has experienced a CVA in the past 2 months or is undergoing intracranial or intraspinal surgery. • This drug requires cautious use in a pregnant patient, one giving birth, a patient over age 75, one undergoing organ biopsy, or one who has undergone major surgery in the past 10 days, has experienced recent trauma (including trauma caused by cardiopulmonary resuscitation) in the past 10 days, or is at high risk for left heart thrombus (as in mitral stenosis with atrial fibrillation). Streptokinase also requires cautious use in a patient with previous puncture of noncompressible vessels, severe GI bleeding, hypertension with systolic blood pressure over 180 mm Hg or diastolic over 110 mm Hg, subacute bacterial endocarditis, hemostatic defects (such as those caused by severe hepatic or renal disease), cerebrovascular disease, diabetic hemorrhagic retinopathy, septic thrombophlebitis, occluded arteriovenous cannula at a seriously infected site, or any other condition in which bleeding constitutes a significant hazard or would be difficult to manage because of its location.

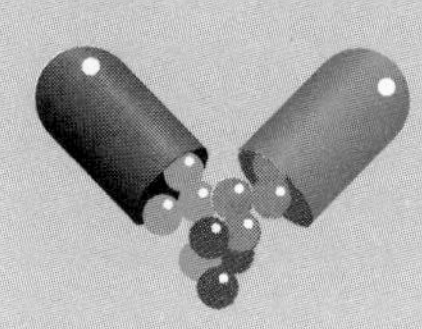

DRUG INTERACTIONS

Heparin

Many interactions involving heparin increase the risk of bleeding or clot formation.

DRUG	INTERACTING AGENTS	POSSIBLE EFFECTS	NURSING IMPLICATIONS
heparin	oral anticoagulants (warfarin, dicumarol)	Increased risk of bleeding	• Monitor the patient's activated partial thromboplastin time (APTT) regularly. • Assess the patient for signs of bleeding in gums, urine, I.V. and other injection sites, nasogastric drainage, and wounds.
	antiplatelet drugs (aspirin, dipyridamole, ticlopidine), nonsteroidal anti-inflammatory drugs (NSAIDs), iron dextran	Increased risk of bleeding	• Teach the patient about the dangers of taking drugs that contain aspirin or NSAIDs during heparin therapy. • Assess the patient for signs of bleeding.
	cardiac gylcosides, quinidine, tetracycline, neomycin, penicillin, phenothiazines, antihistamines	Inactivated heparin if mixed in same solution	• Do not add any of these drugs to heparin solutions. • Administer I.V. forms through separate or flushed I.V. lines.
	nicotine	Inactivated heparin	• Monitor APTT closely if the patient uses tobacco.
	nitroglycerin	Inhibited heparin effect	• Monitor APTT closely if nitroglycerin infusion is added to or withdrawn from the regimen.

used for a patient with disseminated intravascular coagulation when massive clotting is the primary manifestation of this disorder. It also is used to treat arterial clotting and to prevent embolus formation in patients with atrial fibrillation. It may be used in an acute myocardial infarction (MI) to prevent thrombus formation and promote cardiac circulation.

Heparin is used in orthopedic surgery, which in many cases activates the coagulation mechanisms excessively. For orthopedic surgery, heparin is the drug of choice to treat thromboembolism and to prevent clot formation in the venous system because of its immediate anticoagulant effect after I.V. administration.

Drug interactions

Because heparin acts synergistically with all the oral anticoagulants, the risk of patient bleeding increases when both types of drugs are administered concomitantly; the **prothrombin time** (PT), used to monitor the effects of oral anticoagulants, also may be prolonged. Similarly, the risk of bleeding increases when the patient takes an antiplatelet drug, such as aspirin or dipyridamole, while receiving heparin. Drugs that antagonize or inactivate heparin include antihistamines, digitalis compounds, nicotine, phenothiazines, tetracycline hydrochloride, quinidine, neomycin sulfate, and I.V. penicillin. Some of these drugs are incompatible with highly acidic heparin and should not be mixed in the same solution. The nurse should check with the pharmacist for incompatibilities before mixing drugs with heparin. (See Drug Interactions: *Heparin.*)

ADVERSE DRUG REACTIONS

One advantage of heparin is that it produces relatively few adverse reactions, which usually can be prevented if the patient's APTT is maintained within the therapeutic range (1.5 to 2.5 times the control). Bleeding, the most common adverse effect, may lead to more serious consequences if it occurs in the brain (subdural hematoma), at arterial puncture sites, or in or behind the peritoneum (intraperitoneal or retroperitoneal hemorrhage). The effects of heparin can be reversed easily by administering protamine sulfate, which has a specific affinity for heparin and forms a stable salt with it.

Heparin may depress the platelet count, resulting in thrombocytopenia, depending on the type of heparin used. Bovine heparin may have a greater tendency than porcine heparin to produce thrombocytopenia.

Because heparin is procured from animal sources, it can produce hypersensitivity reactions. Hypersensitivity reactions can produce such signs and symptoms as chills, fever, urticaria, rash, and anaphylaxis, which are reversible upon discontinuation of the drug.

Alopecia may occur if therapy lasts more than 6 months. Osteoporosis and spontaneous fractures may occur in patients receiving long-term therapy.

NURSING PROCESS APPLICATION

The following information assists the nurse in caring for a patient who is receiving heparin. It includes an overview of assessment activities as well as examples of appropriate nursing diagnoses and related interventions. It also highlights the importance of evaluation.

Assessment

Before drug therapy begins, review the patient's history for conditions that contraindicate or require cautious use of heparin. Also review the patient's medication history to identify use of drugs that may interact with it. During therapy, assess the patient for adverse drug reactions (such as bleeding) and signs of drug interactions. Also, periodically assess the effectiveness of heparin therapy. Finally, evaluate the patient's and family's knowledge about the prescribed drug. (See Patient Teaching: *Heparin.*)

Nursing diagnoses

- Risk for injury related to a preexisting condition that contraindicates or requires cautious use of heparin
- Risk for injury related to adverse drug reactions or drug interactions
- Knowledge deficit related to heparin

Planning and implementation

- Do not administer heparin to a patient with a condition that contraindicates its use.
- Administer heparin cautiously to a patient at risk because of a preexisting condition.
- Monitor the patient closely for bleeding and other adverse reactions or drug interactions.
- Monitor the patient's APTT, as ordered. Notify the physician if the patient's APTT level exceeds the therapeutic range (1.5 to 2.5 times the control) Check the PTT and platelet count daily, as prescribed. Be aware that use of porcine heparin lowers the risk of heparin-induced thrombocytopenia.
- Observe the patient's vital signs, hemoglobin level, and hematocrit level for indications of bleeding.
- Assess wounds, drainage tubes, and I.V. sites frequently for signs of bleeding. Also observe for purpura, a sign of S.C. bleeding.
- Check the patient's urine, stool, and vomit for occult blood.

* ***Notify the physician immediately if the patient develops neurologic dysfunction, a sign of intracranial bleeding. Expect to withhold the heparin dose to reduce the severity of intracranial bleeding, bleeding at arterial puncture sites, or bleeding in or behind the peritoneum.***

- Administer S.C. heparin as prescribed into the anterior abdominal wall fold above the iliac crest and 2" (5 cm) or more from the umbilicus to avoid risk of bleeding. Do not aspirate or massage the injection site after administering heparin S.C. to prevent the risk of bleeding. Apply gentle pressure to the site for 5 to 10 seconds after the injection.

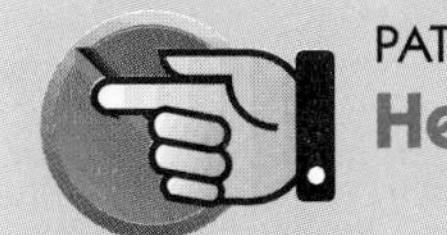

PATIENT TEACHING

Heparin

- ➤ Teach the patient and family the name, dose, frequency, action, and adverse effects of heparin.
- ➤ Teach the patient and family about home care, if appropriate, including how to administer the drug properly and how to observe for signs of bleeding.
- ➤ Help the home care patient schedule necessary activated partial thromboplastin time (APTT) tests. Keep in mind, however, that these tests may not be necessary if the APTT is maintained at the lower end of the therapeutic range (1.5 times the control).
- ➤ Advise the patient that all normal activities of daily living may be performed if the platelet count is normal.
- ➤ Encourage the patient to use an electric razor and a soft toothbrush to avoid the risk of bleeding from cuts or irritated gums.
- ➤ Advise the patient to avoid all over-the-counter drugs, including aspirin preparations and antihistamines, unless the physician or pharmacist is consulted first.
- ➤ Teach the hospitalized patient the signs and symptoms of bleeding and precautions to take after venipuncture.
- ➤ Reassure the patient with alopecia that hair loss is reversible.
- ➤ Instruct the patient and family to notify the physician immediately if bleeding or other adverse reactions occur.

- Do not administer heparin I.M., and avoid other I.M. injections, if possible.
- Expect to administer a trial dose of 1,000 units of heparin to a patient with a history of allergies. During the trial, observe the patient for signs of hypersensitivity.
- Use an infusion pump for continuous I.V. infusion to ensure correct dosage, as prescribed.
- Check the drug label carefully before administering, because heparin is available in different strengths. Keep in mind that heparin is prescribed in units rather than in milligrams.
- Check with the pharmacist before mixing any other drug with a heparin infusion to prevent a drug interaction.
- Do not freeze or refrigerate heparin; it is stable at room temperature.
- Inspect all heparin vials for particulate matter or discoloration. If either is present, discard the vial.

* ***Have the antidote protamine sulfate readily available in case severe bleeding occurs.***

- Notify the physician if adverse reactions or drug interactions occur.
- Teach the patient about the prescribed agent.

Evaluation

For each nursing diagnosis, prepare an evaluation statement that describes the patient's or family's response to nursing interventions.

Oral anticoagulants

The coumarin compounds warfarin sodium and dicumarol are the major oral anticoagulants used in the United States, with warfarin sodium being the most commonly used.

PHARMACOKINETICS

Warfarin is absorbed rapidly and almost completely after oral administration; food decreases the absorption rate but not the total amount absorbed. Dicumarol is absorbed more slowly and erratically. Warfarin and dicumarol are bound extensively to plasma albumin, metabolized in the liver, and excreted in urine.

Oral anticoagulants appear quickly in the plasma after administration. However, therapeutic anticoagulation does not occur until the blood has been depleted of clotting factors. Therefore, maximum anticoagulation and thrombolytic effects may not be achieved for 3 to 5 days after therapy begins. The duration of action of warfarin is 2 to 5 days; of dicumarol, 2 to 10 days. The half-life of the oral anticoagulants varies from 0.5 to 2 days for warfarin and 1 to 2 days for dicumarol.

Route	Onset	Peak	Duration
P.O.	Immediate	1-4 days	2-10 days

PHARMACODYNAMICS

The oral anticoagulants alter the synthesis of vitamin K-dependent clotting factors, including **prothrombin** and factors VII, IX, and X. This alteration does not impede the synthesis of these factors, but makes them dysfunctional. The resulting therapeutic anticoagulant effect does not occur until the already circulating clotting factors are depleted; this takes several hours for factor VII and 2 to 3 days for prothrombin. Thus, optimal PT response is achieved in 1 to 4 days.

PHARMACOTHERAPEUTICS

Oral anticoagulants are prescribed to treat thromboembolism after initial treatment with heparin. Warfarin, however, may be started without heparin in outpatients at high risk for thromboembolism. Oral anticoagulants also are the drugs of choice for the prophylactic therapy of deep vein **thrombosis** and for patients with prosthetic heart valves or diseased mitral valves. They sometimes are combined with an antiplatelet drug, such as dipyridamole, to decrease the risk of arterial clotting.

Drug interactions

Many patients on oral anticoagulant therapy are receiving other drugs. The hazards of serious interactions between oral anticoagulants and other drugs are ever present, and many clinically significant interactions occur. (See Drug Interactions: *Oral anticoagulants*.) Many foods, especially those high in vitamin K, also interact with the oral anticoagulants; however, only a diet containing high amounts of vitamin K is likely to cause problems.

ADVERSE DRUG REACTIONS

The primary adverse reaction to oral anticoagulant therapy is minor bleeding. Severe bleeding, however, may occur in the GI tract, urinary tract, or uterus; it also can occur as intraperitoneal hemorrhage from a ruptured corpus luteum, retroperitoneal hemorrhage, hemopericardium, intracranial hemorrhage, or adrenal hemorrhage. Ecchymoses and hematomas may form at arterial puncture sites (for example, after a blood gas sample is drawn).

Red-orange urine, nausea, vomiting, diarrhea, abdominal cramping, priapism, mouth ulcers, and nephropathy rarely may occur. Other rare adverse reactions to the oral anticoagulants include alopecia, urticaria, dermatitis, skin necrosis, hepatitis, jaundice, fever, hypersensitivity reactions, agranulocytosis, leukopenia, and eosinophilia.

The effects of the oral anticoagulants can be reversed with adequate doses of phytonadione (vitamin K_1).

NURSING PROCESS APPLICATION

The following information assists the nurse in caring for a patient who is receiving an oral anticoagulant. It includes an overview of assessment activities as well as examples of appropriate nursing diagnoses and related interventions. It also highlights the importance of evaluation.

Assessment

Before drug therapy begins, review the patient's history for conditions that contraindicate or require cautious use of the prescribed oral anticoagulant. Also review the patient's medication history to identify use of drugs that may interact with it. During therapy, assess the patient for adverse drug reactions (such as bleeding) and signs of drug interactions. Also, periodically assess the effectiveness of oral anticoagulant therapy. Finally, evaluate the patient's and family's knowledge about the prescribed drug.

Nursing diagnoses

- Risk for injury related to a preexisting condition that contraindicates or requires cautious use of an oral anticoagulant
- Risk for injury related to adverse drug reactions or drug interactions
- Noncompliance related to long-term use of the prescribed oral anticoagulant
- Knowledge deficit related to the prescribed oral anticoagulant

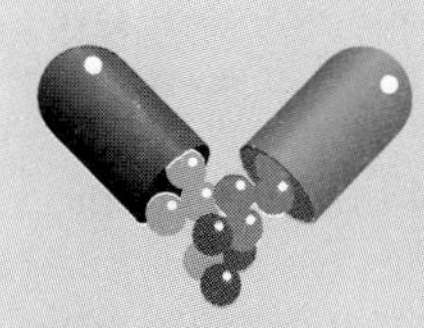

DRUG INTERACTIONS

Oral anticoagulants

This chart illustrates the wide range of potential interactions between oral anticoagulants and other drugs and between oral anticoagulants and food.

DRUG	INTERACTING AGENTS	POSSIBLE EFFECTS	NURSING IMPLICATIONS
warfarin, dicumarol	salicylates, phenylbutazone, sulfinpyrazone, indomethacin, clofibrate, anabolic and androgenic steroids, chloral hydrate, chloramphenicol, disulfiram, heparin, gemfibrozil, meclofenamate, mefenamic acid, metronidazole, miconazole, nalidixic acid, piroxicam, allopurinol, cimetidine, dextrothyroxine, erythromycin, glucagon, co-trimoxazole (sulfamethoxazole-trimethoprim), sulindac, thyroid hormones, influenza vaccine	Increased risk of bleeding	• Monitor the patient's prothrombin time (PT) or international normalized ratio (INR) frequently after any new drug is added to the drug regimen. • Assess the patient for signs of bleeding, such as epistaxis, bleeding gums, hematuria, or bruising. • Advise the patient to avoid using any over-the-counter products containing aspirin.
	barbiturates, glutethimide, ethchlorvynol, griseofulvin, carbamazepine, rifampin, vitamin K, cholestyramine, colestipol, aminoglutethimide, propylthiouracil, methimazole, corticotropin, mercaptopurine, spironolactone	Increased risk of clotting	• Assess the patient for signs of thromboembolism (increased pain, swelling, or redness in calf) and pulmonary embolism (increased shortness of breath, chest pain, or fever). • Monitor the patient's PT or INR frequently after any of these drugs is administered.
	phenytoin	Increased risk of phenytoin toxicity; increased or decreased anticoagulant effect	• Monitor the patient frequently for signs of phenytoin toxicity, such as nystagmus, ataxia, slurred speech, or confusion. • Assess the patient for signs of bleeding or thromboembolism.
	foods high in vitamin K (cabbage, cauliflower, broccoli, asparagus)	Increased clotting	• Obtain a dietary history from the patient to evaluate the amount of vitamin K–rich foods in the daily diet. • Caution the patient against sudden changes in ingestion of vitamin K–rich foods.
	alcohol	Increased risk of clotting with chronic abuse; increased risk of bleeding with acute intoxication	• Obtain a history from the patient and family about the extent of alcohol use. • Monitor the patient for bleeding. • Monitor the patient's PT or INR frequently.

Planning and implementation

- Do not administer an oral anticoagulant to a patient with a condition that contraindicates its use.
- Administer an oral anticoagulant cautiously to a patient at risk because of a preexisting condition.
- Monitor closely for bleeding and other adverse reactions throughout oral anticoagulant therapy, especially in a geriatric patient. Also monitor for drug interactions.
- Monitor PT responses daily for inpatients and every 1 to 4 weeks for outpatients; be aware that for venous thromboembolism, the therapeutic range established by the American College of Chest Physicians and the National Heart, Lung, and Blood Institute is a PT ratio of 1.2 to 1.5 times the control. Also be aware that bleeding can occur even when a patient's PT falls within the therapeutic range. Expect to see a higher PT ratio (1.5 to 2) in a patient with prosthetic heart valves, recurrent embolism, or rheumatic mitral valve disease. (Laboratories may report PT as an international normalized ratio [INR]. The recommended INR is 2 to 4 times the control).

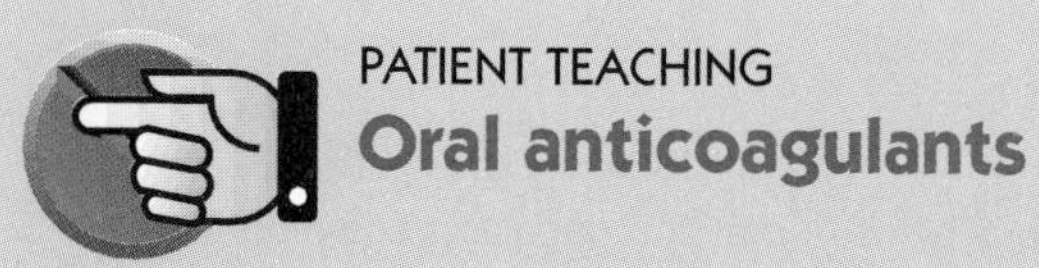

PATIENT TEACHING
Oral anticoagulants

- Teach the patient and family the name, dose, frequency, action, and adverse effects of the prescribed oral anticoagulant.
- Advise the patient to follow the written instructions for dosage; encourage the patient to keep a daily log to reinforce taking the correct dosage.
- Instruct the patient receiving warfarin to take it in the evening and to have blood drawn in the morning for accurate prothrombin time (PT) or international normalized ratio (INR) test results. Teach the patient the importance of having blood drawn for PT or INR tests as prescribed (usually monthly after drug has stabilized the patient's condition).
- Instruct the patient not to take any prescription or over-the-counter drug without first consulting the physician who ordered the anticoagulant therapy. Provide the patient and family members with written information about the interactions between oral anticoagulants and other drugs or food.
- Instruct the patient to avoid increased amounts of green leafy vegetables and all medications containing aspirin.
- Teach the patient the importance of immediately reporting to the physician any bruises, blood in the stool, or blood in the urine.
- Encourage the patient to wear a medical identification bracelet to alert health care personnel in case of trauma or sudden illness.
- Encourage the patient to avoid activities that pose a high risk of physical injury.
- Advise the female patient to inform the physician if she is pregnant or planning to become pregnant.
- Reassure the patient with drug-induced alopecia that hair loss is reversible.
- Instruct the patient to notify the physician if adverse reactions occur.

- Reevaluate the patient's PT as prescribed whenever a drug is added to or removed from the therapeutic regimen to detect drug interactions.
- Check and record the PT results before administering an oral anticoagulant dose. When a patient is switched from heparin to warfarin therapy, expect heparin therapy to continue for several days until warfarin produces therapeutic effects.

***Notify the physician immediately if the patient's PT or INR exceeds the therapeutic range, and withhold the next dose as prescribed.**

- Monitor the patient's vital signs frequently for indications of severe internal bleeding.
- Treat minor bleeding by omitting one or more doses as instructed until the PT or INR returns to the therapeutic range. If minor bleeding continues, administer vitamin K_1 (phytonadione) 1 to 10 mg P.O., as prescribed.

***Administer 5 to 50 mg of vitamin K parenterally, as prescribed, if frank bleeding occurs. Small doses (1 to 15 mg) are recommended to prevent hypercoagulability.**

- Administer 250 to 500 ml of fresh frozen plasma or give commercial factor IX complex, as prescribed, if severe bleeding occurs.
- Notify the physician if adverse reactions or drug interactions occur.
- Stress the importance of adhering to the prescribed oral anticoagulant regimen. (See Patient Teaching: *Oral anticoagulants.*)
- Regularly assess the patient's compliance with oral anticoagulant therapy.
- Notify the physician if noncompliance occurs.

Evaluation

For each nursing diagnosis, prepare an evaluation statement that describes the patient's or family's response to nursing interventions.

Antiplatelet drugs

The antiplatelet drugs have shown some potential for preventing arterial thromboembolism, particularly in patients at risk for MI and cerebrovascular accidents from arteriosclerosis. These drugs have varying mechanisms of action.

PHARMACOKINETICS

The pharmacokinetic properties of the antiplatelet drugs vary. Aspirin is absorbed rapidly in the stomach and upper intestine (more slowly when taken with enteric-coated preparations or food), then is distributed quickly into the bloodstream. After metabolism in the liver, aspirin is eliminated by the excretion of salicylic acid in the kidneys and by the oxidation and conjugation of metabolites.

Dipyridamole is absorbed from the GI tract; it is almost completely plasma protein-bound (91% to 97%). The drug is distributed widely in body tissues and can cross the placental barrier in small amounts. Dipyridamole is metabolized in the liver and excreted in bile. Small amounts may be excreted in the urine.

Sulfinpyrazone is absorbed well after oral administration and is 98% to 99% protein-bound. After rapid but incomplete metabolism in the liver, about 45% of the drug is excreted unchanged in the urine.

Ticlopidine is absorbed rapidly and is about 98% plasma protein-bound. It is metabolized extensively in the liver and excreted in the feces and urine.

Aspirin's onset of action and peak concentration level as an antiplatelet drug still are being investigated. The duration of action of aspirin's platelet-inhibitor effect is the life span of the platelet, approximately 10 days. The half-life of low dosages of aspirin is about 3 hours.

The peak plasma concentration of dipyridamole occurs 2 to 2.5 hours after oral administration.

Sulfinpyrazone's onset, peak concentration, and duration as an antiplatelet drug still are being investigated. The drug may require several days of administration; some effects persist after withdrawal.

Ticlopidine reaches its peak plasma concentration about 2 hours after oral administration. Its average half-life is 12 hours.

Route	Onset	Peak	Duration
P.O.	Variable	1-2 hr	4 hr-2 wk

PHARMACODYNAMICS

The antiplatelet drugs interfere with platelet activity in different drug-specific and dose-related ways. Low dosages of aspirin (325 mg per day) appear to inhibit clot formation by blocking prostaglandin synthase action, which in turn prevents formation of the platelet-aggregating substance thromboxane A_2.

In vitro studies of dipyridamole have shown that this drug can inhibit platelet aggregation. However, in vivo studies have not shown the same effects. Sulfinpyrazone appears to inhibit several platelet functions. At dosages of 400 to 800 mg daily, sulfinpyrazone lengthens platelet survival; dosages of more than 600 mg daily prolong the patency of arteriovenous shunts used for hemodialysis. A single dose produces rapid inhibition of platelet aggregation, suggesting that the drug directly affects circulating platelets.

Ticlopidine inhibits platelet-fibrinogen binding induced by adenosine phosphate as well as subsequent platelet interactions. This inhibits platelet aggregation and the release of platelet granule constituents. It also prolongs bleeding time.

PHARMACOTHERAPEUTICS

Aspirin is used in patients with a previous MI or unstable angina pectoris to reduce the risk of death from these conditions, and in men to reduce the risk of transient ischemic attacks (TIAs).

Dipyridamole is used as an adjunct to a coumarin compound in the prevention of thromboembolic complications after cardiac valve replacement.

After an MI, sulfinpyrazone may be used to decrease the risk of sudden cardiac death. In patients with rheumatic mitral stenosis, it may decrease the risk of systemic embolism.

Ticlopidine is used to reduce the risk of thrombotic stroke in high-risk patients (including those with a history of frequent TIAs) and in patients with a history of thrombotic stroke.

Adverse reactions to some of these drugs may limit their usefulness in preventing arterial clotting. The patient's bleeding time and platelet aggregation studies can measure the effectiveness of the antiplatelet ability of these agents.

Drug interactions

The risk of bleeding increases in patients receiving high dosages of aspirin because aspirin's effect on platelets increases bleeding time. However, the additive effect of dipyridamole with aspirin has been used to prevent thromboembolic disorders in patients with aortocoronary bypass grafts or prosthetic heart valves. Many other drug interactions may occur. (See Drug Interactions: *Antiplatelet drugs*, page 320.)

Because guidelines have not been established for administration of ticlopidine with heparin, oral anticoagulants, aspirin, or fibrinolytic agents, these drugs should be discontinued before ticlopidine therapy begins.

ADVERSE DRUG REACTIONS

In the dosage prescribed to prevent arterial clotting, aspirin most commonly produces adverse GI effects, such as stomach pain, heartburn, nausea, constipation, hematemesis, melena, and slight gastric blood loss. Rarely, it may cause significant GI bleeding or peptic ulcer disease.

Dipyridamole, usually well tolerated, produces minimal adverse reactions that may include headache, dizziness, nausea, flushing, weakness, syncope, and mild GI distress. These disappear when the drug is discontinued.

The major adverse reaction to sulfinpyrazone is epigastric discomfort, which may aggravate or reactivate peptic ulcer disease. Taking the drug with food, milk, or an antacid usually reduces this discomfort.

During clinical trials with ticlopidine, 5% or more of the adult patients developed these adverse reactions: diarrhea, nausea, dyspepsia, rash, and elevated alkaline phosphatase and transaminase levels on liver function tests. About 2.4% of patients developed neutropenia.

Hypersensitivity reactions to the antiplatelet drugs, particularly anaphylaxis, can occur; the most common is the induction of bronchospasm with asthmalike symptoms. Dipyridamole may cause a rash. Other reactions to sulfinpyrazone may include rash, blood dyscrasias (anemia, leukopenia, agranulocytosis, thrombocytopenia, or aplastic anemia), and bronchoconstriction. Some patients have experienced renal dysfunction during sulfinpyrazone therapy, which disappears when the drug is discontinued.

NURSING PROCESS APPLICATION

The following information assists the nurse in caring for a patient who is receiving an antiplatelet drug. It includes an overview of assessment activities as well as examples of appropriate nursing diagnoses and related interventions. It also highlights the importance of evaluation.

Assessment

Before drug therapy begins, review the patient's history for conditions that contraindicate or require cautious use of the prescribed antiplatelet drug. Also review the patient's medication history to identify use of drugs that may interact

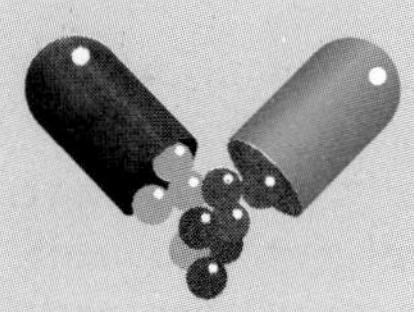

DRUG INTERACTIONS

Antiplatelet drugs

Antiplatelet drugs cause clinically significant interactions with any drugs that may cause bleeding. The chart below discusses some of the most clinically significant drugs.

DRUG	INTERACTING AGENTS	POSSIBLE EFFECTS	NURSING IMPLICATIONS
aspirin	heparin, oral anticoagulants	Increased risk of bleeding	• Monitor the patient's activated partial thromboplastin time, prothrombin time (PT) or international normalized ratio (INR), and bleeding times daily. Report any prolonged results to the physician. • Assess the patient for signs of minor or major bleeding.
	dipyridamole	Increased risk of bleeding	• Assess the patient's bleeding times closely if dipyridamole is added to or deleted from the drug regimen. • Assess the patient for signs of minor or major bleeding.
	methotrexate	Increased risk of methotrexate toxicity	• Do not administer aspirin to a patient receiving methotrexate.
	valproic acid	Increased risk of valproic acid toxicity	• Monitor valproic acid levels closely if aspirin is added to or deleted from the drug regimen. • Assess for signs of valproic acid toxicity, such as nausea, vomiting, sedation, or ataxia.
aspirin, ticlopidine	sulfinpyrazone	Inhibited uricosuric effects of sulfinpyrazone	• Assess the patient for increased signs and symptoms of gout, such as joint pain or swelling.
dipyridamole	aspirin	Increased risk of bleeding	• Assess the patient's bleeding time closely if aspirin is added to or deleted from the drug regimen. • Assess the patient for signs of minor or major bleeding.
sulfinpyrazone	aspirin	Inhibited uricosuric effects of sulfinpyrazone	• Assess the patient for increased signs and symptoms of gout, such as joint pain or swelling.
	oral anticoagulants	Increased risk of bleeding	• Monitor the patient's PT or INR closely if sulfinpyrazone is added to or deleted from the drug regimen. • Assess the patient for signs of minor or major bleeding.
ticlopidine	heparin, oral anticoagulants, aspirin, fibrinolytic agents	Increased risk of bleeding	• Discontinue the interacting drug before ticlopidine therapy begins. • Assess the patient for signs of minor and major bleeding.
	antacids	Reduced plasma levels of ticlopidine	• Do not administer an antacid to a patient receiving ticlopidine.
	cimetidine	Reduced ticlopidine clearance	• Assess the patient regularly for signs of minor and major bleeding when long-term cimetidine therapy coincides with ticlopidine administration.

with it. During therapy, assess the patient for adverse drug reactions and signs of drug interactions. Also, periodically assess the effectiveness of antiplatelet drug therapy. Finally, evaluate the patient's and family's knowledge about the prescribed drug.

Nursing diagnoses

- Risk for injury related to a preexisting condition that contraindicates or requires cautious use of an antiplatelet drug
- Risk for injury related to adverse drug reactions or drug interactions
- Knowledge deficit related to the prescribed antiplatelet drug

Planning and implementation

- Do not administer an antiplatelet drug to a patient with a condition that contraindicates its use.
- Administer an antiplatelet drug cautiously to a patient at risk because of a preexisting condition.
- Monitor the patient closely for adverse reactions and drug interactions throughout antiplatelet therapy.
- Monitor the patient for signs of GI distress, such as stomach pain, heartburn, nausea, constipation, hematemesis, melena, and gastric blood loss (with aspirin); nausea (with dipyridamole); epigastric distress (with sulfinpyrazone); and diarrhea, nausea, and dyspepsia (with ticlopidine).
- Administer aspirin or sulfinpyrazone with milk, food, or an antacid to minimize the GI distress that these drugs commonly produce. If distress persists during aspirin therapy, ask the physician to prescribe enteric-coated tablets.
- Do not administer aspirin if it has a strong vinegar-like odor, which indicates drug deterioration.
- Give dipyridamole 1 hour before meals with 8 oz (240 ml) of water.
- Administer ticlopidine with food or immediately after eating to minimize adverse GI reactions. Do not administer an antacid with ticlopidine because it can reduce the plasma ticlopidine level.
- Monitor the patient's bleeding time and platelet aggregation studies to assess the effectiveness of antiplatelet therapy.
- Obtain a complete blood count and white cell differential every 2 weeks from the second week of ticlopidine therapy through the end of the third month.
- Auscultate the patient's breath sounds regularly, and assess for changes in the patient's respiratory rate or pattern.

**** Observe for bronchospasm, asthmalike symptoms, or bronchoconstriction in a patient receiving aspirin or dipyridamole. If breathing difficulty occurs, place the patient in a high Fowler's position to maximize breathing effectiveness. Prepare to administer oxygen and drugs, as prescribed, to relieve respiratory symptoms of a hypersensitivity reaction.***

- Notify the physician if adverse reactions or drug interactions occur or if antiplatelet therapy is ineffective.
- Teach the patient about the prescribed agent. (See Patient Teaching: *Antiplatelet drugs.*)

PATIENT TEACHING

Antiplatelet drugs

- ➤ Teach the patient and family the name, dose, frequency, action, and adverse effects of the prescribed antiplatelet drug.
- ➤ Instruct the patient taking aspirin or sulfinpyrazone to take it with milk, food, or an antacid and to report any severe gastric pain to the physician. Also tell the patient to take enteric-coated tablets, as prescribed.
- ➤ Instruct the patient not to take aspirin if it has a strong vinegar-like odor, but to purchase new tablets.
- ➤ Advise the patient to take dipyridamole 1 hour before meals and with 8 oz (240 ml) of water.
- ➤ Instruct the patient to take ticlopidine with food or immediately after eating, but never to take the drug with an antacid.
- ➤ Teach the patient taking ticlopidine to report any signs of infection, such as fever, chills, and sore throat, as well as severe or persistent diarrhea, yellow skin or sclera, dark urine, or light-colored stools.
- ➤ Stress the importance of returning for laboratory tests, as instructed, to monitor the effectiveness of therapy or to detect adverse reactions.
- ➤ Teach the patient and family to recognize the signs of bleeding and to report them to the physician.
- ➤ Instruct the patient taking aspirin to consult the physician before taking additional over-the-counter products that contain aspirin.
- ➤ Teach the patient to avoid participating in sports that pose a high risk of injury, which could lead to bleeding.
- ➤ Instruct the patient taking large doses of aspirin to recognize and report signs of salicylism.
- ➤ Advise the patient not to perform activities requiring alertness if dizziness, weakness, or syncope occurs.
- ➤ Instruct the patient to notify the physician immediately if adverse reactions occur.

Evaluation

For each nursing diagnosis, prepare an evaluation statement that describes the patient's or family's response to nursing interventions.

Thrombolytic agents

Alteplase, anistreplase, streptokinase, and urokinase are some of the thrombolytic agents currently used to dissolve existing thrombi in the clinical setting.

PHARMACOKINETICS

After I.V. or intracoronary administration, thrombolytic agents are distributed immediately throughout the circulation, quickly activating **plasminogen.** (See *How alteplase helps restore perfusion,* page 322.) Alteplase is cleared rapidly from circulating plasma primarily by the liver. Anistreplase is metabolized in the plasma. Streptokinase is removed rapidly from the circulation by antibodies and the mononu-

How alteplase helps restore perfusion

When a thrombus forms in an artery, it obstructs the blood supply, causing ischemia and necrosis. Alteplase can dissolve a thrombus made of fibrin strands in a cerebral, coronary, or pulmonary artery, restoring the blood supply to the area beyond the blockage.

OBSTRUCTED ARTERY

A thrombus blocks blood flow through the artery, causing distal ischemia.

Thrombus

Blood flow

Ischemic area

Artery wall

INSIDE THE THROMBUS

Alteplase enters the thrombus, which consists of plasminogen bound to fibrin.

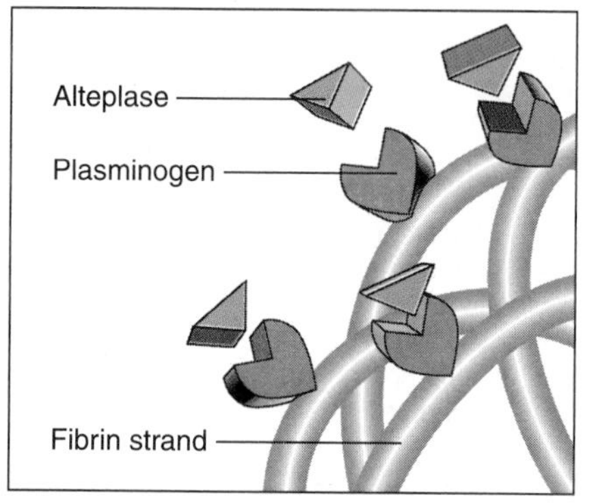

Alteplase binds to the fibrin-plasminogen complex, converting the inactive plasminogen into active plasmin.

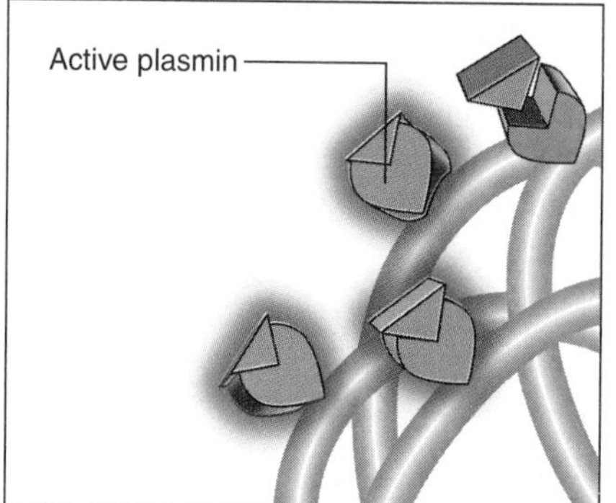

This active plasmin digests the fibrin, dissolving the thrombus.

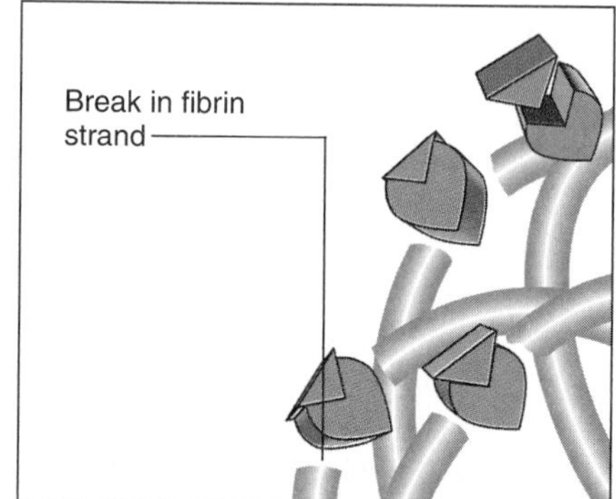

RESTORED BLOOD FLOW

As the thrombus dissolves, blood flow resumes.

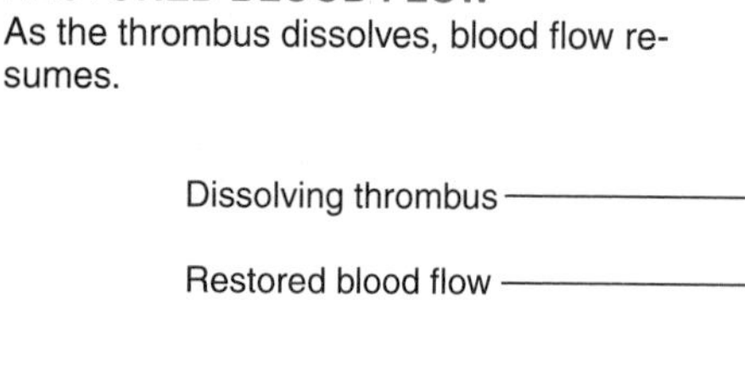

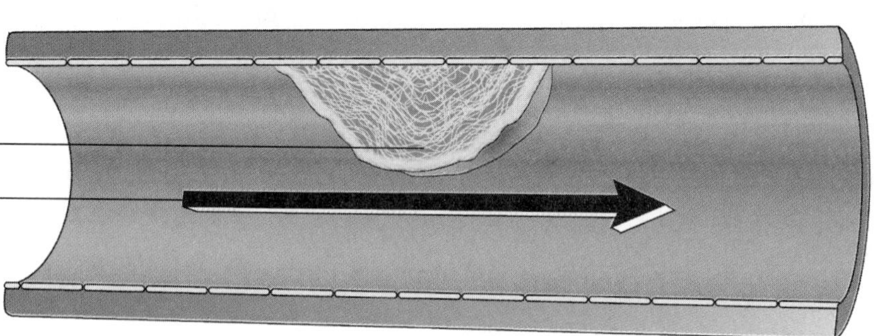

clear phagocytic system (reticuloendothelial system). It does not appear to cross the placental barrier. Urokinase is metabolized rapidly by the liver, and small amounts are excreted in bile and urine. Research has not determined yet if it crosses the placental barrier.

The onset of action of the thrombolytic agents is almost immediate, with rapid plasminogen activation after I.V. or intracoronary administration.

The initial half-life of alteplase is less than 5 minutes; the drug is cleared rapidly from the plasma, with a subsequent half-life of 26.5 minutes. The half-life of the activated fibrinolytic compound of anistreplase is 70 to 120 minutes. In clinical studies, streptokinase demonstrates a biphasic decline in plasma concentration, with an initial half-life of 18 minutes and a subsequent half-life of 83 minutes. The serum half-life of urokinase is 20 minutes.

After therapy is discontinued, the thrombolytic effects of all four thrombolytic agents disappear within a few hours, but the systemic effect on coagulation and the risk of bleeding may persist for 12 to 24 hours.

Route	Onset	Peak	Duration
I.V.	Immediate	Variable	12-24 hr

PHARMACODYNAMICS

The thrombolytic agents convert plasminogen to the enzyme plasmin, which lyses (dissolves) thrombi, fibrinogen, and other plasma proteins.

PHARMACOTHERAPEUTICS

The FDA has approved the thrombolytic agents for treating certain thromboembolic disorders. These drugs also have been used to dissolve thrombi in arteriovenous cannulas to reestablish blood flow. Thrombolytic agents are the drugs of choice to break down newly formed thrombi. They seem most effective when administered immediately after thrombosis and up to 6 hours after the onset of symptoms.

Alteplase is used to treat acute MI, pulmunary embolism, and acute ischemic cerebrovascular accident. Anistreplase is also used in acute MI. Streptokinase is used to treat acute MI, pulmonary embolus, deep vein thrombosis, arterial thrombosis, and arterial embolism as well as to clear an occluded arteriovenous cannula. (See Geriatric Considerations: *Treating acute MI.*) Urokinase is used to treat pulmonary embolus and coronary thrombosis and to clear an occluded I.V. catheter.

Drug interactions

Thrombolytic agents interact with heparin, oral anticoagulants, antiplatelet drugs, and nonsteroidal anti-inflammatory drugs; the patient's risk of bleeding is increased. Aminocaproic acid inhibits streptokinase and can be used to reverse its fibrinolytic effects.

ADVERSE DRUG REACTIONS

The major reactions associated with the thrombolytic agents are bleeding and allergic responses, especially with streptokinase and anistreplase. Thrombolytic agents dissolve fibrin deposits at all sites, not just at the arterial thrombus obstructing coronary or pulmonary circulation. Thus, bleeding can occur at a sutured wound or any puncture site, such as an arterial line or central line catheter site. Major bleeding may occur in some patients, resulting from a systemic bleeding disturbance. Hemorrhaging may occur in the cranium, the GI or urinary tract, the vagina, or behind the peritoneum.

Allergic reactions to streptokinase are common, because most patients possess circulating streptococcal antibodies.

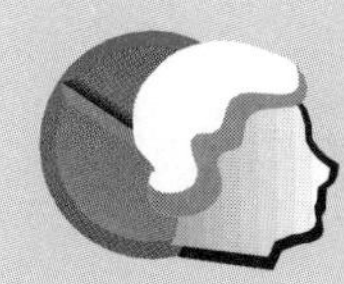

GERIATRIC CONSIDERATIONS

Treating acute MI

A geriatric patient who has had an acute myocardial infarction (MI) is at greater risk of dying from the MI than a younger patient. Fortunately, thrombolytic therapy is just as effective in reducing mortality in older patients as it is in younger ones. Therefore, do not consider advanced age a contraindication to thrombolytic therapy. In fact, expect to use it in your geriatric patients just as you would in younger patients.

Anistreplase and urokinase also have caused allergic reactions; symptoms include urticaria, itching, flushing, nausea, headache, and musculoskeletal pain.

Streptokinase can produce hemorrhagic infarct at the site of myocardial necrosis as well as reperfusion arrhythmias. The reperfusion arrhythmias usually are premature ventricular contractions that require no treatment. (After I.V. administration, alteplase also may cause reperfusion arrhythmias.) Occasionally, more serious arrhythmias, such as complex or grouped premature ventricular contractions, ventricular tachycardia, and fibrillation may occur. Hypotension (unrelated to bleeding or anaphylaxis) also may occur.

Some patients experience fever (an average temperature elevation of 1.5° F [0.56° C]) after receiving a dose, particularly after receiving streptokinase or anistreplase. The cause of this response has not been established.

Anistreplase may cause conduction disorders and hypotension. Less common adverse reactions to anistreplase include chills, sweating, shock, cardiac rupture, chest pain, dyspnea, lung edema, emboli, purpura, nausea, vomiting, thrombocytopenia, elevated transaminase levels, arthralgia, headache, agitation, dizziness, vertigo, paresthesia, and tremor.

An anaphylactic response to streptokinase or anistreplase is a serious, although rare, reaction. Symptoms range from minor breathing difficulties to bronchospasm, periorbital swelling, and angioedema.

CRITICAL THINKING: To enhance your critical thinking about anticoagulant and thrombolytic agents, consider the following situation and its analysis.

Situation: Armand Paulo, age 56, is admitted to the emergency department with an acute MI. The physician orders alteplase (Activase) 100 mg I.V. Coagulation studies must be done before and after the infusion and then every 4 hours for the next 24 hours. For Mr. Paulo, how should the nurse obtain blood specimens for studies, while maintaining thrombolytic precautions?

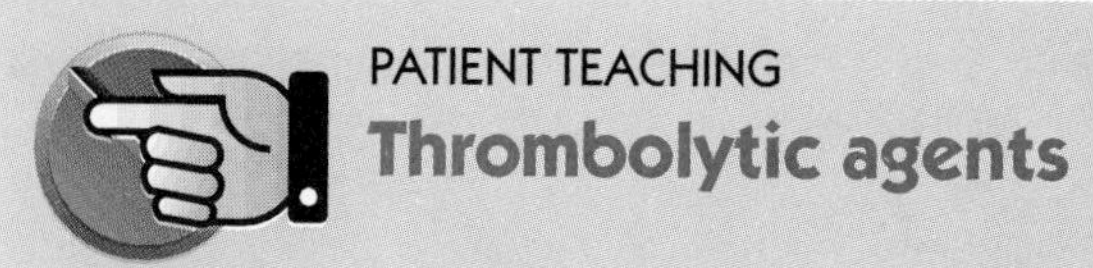

PATIENT TEACHING

Thrombolytic agents

- Teach the patient and family the name, dose, frequency, action, and adverse effects of the prescribed thrombolytic agent.
- Encourage the patient and family to ask questions about the drug regimen.
- Instruct the patient to inform the nurse if adverse reactions occur or if initial symptoms, such as chest pain, improve or worsen.

Analysis: The nurse should observe thrombolytic precautions, such as using a noninvasive blood pressure cuff and avoiding arterial blood sticks, to prevent bleeding. Therefore, the nurse should insert a large-bore (18-gauge) cannula into a large vein and should cap off the cannula with an intermittent infusion port. Then the nurse can draw blood specimens for coagulation studies from this line, which should be flushed with normal saline between uses. The nurse also may use this intermittent port to administer boluses of drugs given intermittently, such as morphine.

NURSING PROCESS APPLICATION

The following information assists the nurse in caring for a patient who is receiving a thrombolytic agent. It includes an overview of assessment activities as well as examples of appropriate nursing diagnoses and related interventions. It also highlights the importance of evaluation.

Assessment

Before drug therapy begins, review the patient's history for conditions that contraindicate or require cautious use of the prescribed thrombolytic agent. Also review the patient's medication history to identify use of drugs that may interact with it. During therapy, assess the patient for adverse drug reactions and signs of drug interactions. Also, periodically assess the effectiveness of thrombolytic therapy. Finally, evaluate the patient's and family's knowledge about the prescribed drug. (See Patient Teaching: *Thrombolytic agents.*)

Nursing diagnoses

- Risk for injury related to a preexisting condition that contraindicates or requires cautious use of a thrombolytic agent
- Risk for injury related to adverse drug reactions or drug interactions
- Knowledge deficit related to the prescribed thrombolytic agent

Planning and implementation

- Do not administer a thrombolytic agent to a patient with a condition that contraindicates its use.
- Administer a thrombolytic agent cautiously to a patient at risk because of a preexisting condition.
- Monitor the patient closely for bleeding and other adverse reactions, especially during concomitant heparin therapy. Also monitor for drug interactions.
- Monitor the patient's coagulation studies during thrombolytic therapy. Coagulation studies are recommended immediately before and 4 hours after the systemic administration of a thrombolytic agent.

* ***Monitor the patient's vital signs frequently to assess for signs of internal bleeding and to detect hypotension, significant pulse or respiratory changes, or fever.***

* ***Treat severe bleeding complications by stopping the infusion of the thrombolytic agent and infusing fresh whole blood, packed red cells, or fresh frozen plasma, as prescribed. Prepare to administer aminocaproic acid, which may be prescribed as an antidote.***

- Continue to assess the patient for bleeding complications for 24 hours after thrombolytic therapy is discontinued.
- Assess the patient's chest pain if the intracoronary route of administration is used; a decrease in pain may signal myocardial reperfusion. Also monitor the patient's electrocardiogram pattern, especially the ST segment, and watch for reperfusion or ventricular arrhythmias or conduction disorders.
- Keep antiarrhythmic drugs, such as lidocaine, and a defibrillator readily accessible at all times.
- Observe the patient for signs of an allergic reaction to streptokinase or anistreplase.

* ***Leave the femoral venous and arterial sheaths in place for 24 hours after intracoronary thrombolytic therapy. Immobilize the patient's entire leg for 24 hours to prevent bleeding. If bleeding occurs at the femoral insertion site, apply direct pressure with a pressure dressing or aminocaproic acid–soaked sponges. Monitor the patient's color, temperature, and femoral, popliteal, and dorsalis pedis pulses every 15 minutes for 1 hour, then every 30 minutes for 8 hours, and then once each shift.***

- Monitor the patient's neurologic status during the infusion. If the patient reports sudden severe headache or develops neurologic deficits during the infusion, stop the infusion and notify the physician. The patient may have developed intracranial bleeding.
- Reposition the patient carefully during and after the infusion to minimize bruising.
- Do not administer I.M. injections or insert new arterial lines during thrombolytic therapy or for 24 hours after it is discontinued.
- Administer other medications through existing I.V. sites, orally, or by nasogastric tube, as prescribed.
- Administer acetaminophen rather than aspirin for fever, as prescribed, to decrease the patient's risk of bleeding.

- Notify the physician immediately if adverse reactions or drug interactions occur.
- Teach the patient about the prescribed agent.

Evaluation

For each nursing diagnosis, prepare an evaluation statement that describes the patient's or family's response to nursing interventions.

CHAPTER SUMMARY

Chapter 24 focused on anticoagulant and thrombolytic agents. Here are the chapter highlights.

Heparin is the drug of choice to treat and prevent venous thromboembolism because of its immediate anticoagulant effect when administered intravenously. Because heparin is synergistic with all oral anticoagulants, the risk of bleeding is increased in patients receiving both drugs. For severe bleeding, protamine sulfate is used to neutralize heparin.

The coumarin compounds, the most commonly used oral anticoagulants in the United States, are the drugs of choice for long-term management of patients with deep vein thrombosis and patients at high risk for thrombus formation, such as those with prosthetic heart valves or diseased mitral valves. The major adverse reactions to oral anticoagulants are bleeding complications. Treatment may include discontinuing the drug, reducing the dosage, or administering oral or parenteral vitamin K, as prescribed. Bleeding times and platelet aggregation studies are the best indicators of the effectiveness of antiplatelet therapy.

The nurse should teach patients receiving anticoagulants about interactions with other drugs and with food, ways to check for signs of bleeding, and the need for having blood drawn for APTT, PT, or INR results as prescribed.

When administering antiplatelet drugs, the nurse should monitor the patient regularly for GI signs and symptoms and hypersensitivity reactions.

Thrombolytic agents activate and convert plasminogen to plasmin, which dissolves thrombi. Thrombolytic agents currently approved for clinical use include alteplase, anistreplase, streptokinase, and urokinase.

When administering thrombolytics, the nurse should assess the patient carefully for signs of bleeding and allergic reactions. The nurse must be prepared to intervene quickly in hemorrhagic or allergic complications and should keep appropriate emergency drugs and equipment available. Aminocaproic acid may be used as an antidote.

Questions to consider

See Appendix 1 for answers.

1. Jorge Valasquez, age 67, is admitted to the coronary care unit with an acute inferior wall MI. Because the pain persists after Mr. Valasquez has received oxygen, I.V. nitroglycerin, and I.V. morphine, his physician prescribes streptokinase 140,000 IU by intracoronary infusion. Which of the following conditions in his medical history would contraindicate the use of streptokinase?
   (a) Acute pulmonary thromboembolism
   (b) History of previous MI
   (c) Cerebrovascular accident in the past 2 months
   (d) Age 60 or older

2. William White, age 38, develops acute thrombophlebitis in his left calf after surgery. His physician orders heparin 5,000 units as an I.V. bolus, followed by continuous I.V. infusion of 1,000 units/hour. If Mr. White starts to bleed excessively during heparin therapy, which of the following drugs is likely to be prescribed as an antidote?
   (a) vitamin K
   (b) factor VIII
   (c) protamine sulfate
   (d) sulfinpyrazone

3. While Joyce Douglass, age 51, is receiving heparin, her physician begins oral anticoagulant therapy with warfarin (Coumadin) 10 mg P.O. daily. Why is heparin administered concurrently with warfarin?
   (a) Warfarin's therapeutic effects do not occur until clotting factors are depleted.
   (b) Heparin activates warfarin.
   (c) Warfarin and heparin have a synergistic effect.
   (d) Heparin hastens warfarin's onset of action.

4. Brenda Frank, age 59, has a history of thrombotic stroke. To prevent future strokes, her physician prescribes ticlopidine (Ticlid) 250 mg P.O. b.i.d. When teaching Ms. Frank about ticlopidine therapy, the nurse should tell her to be alert for which of the following adverse reactions?
   (a) Diarrhea, nausea, and dyspepsia
   (b) Anemia, leukopenia, or thrombocytopenia
   (c) Headache, dizziness, and syncope
   (d) Hemorrhagic infarct and reperfusion arrhythmias

5. After being admitted to the hospital with an acute MI, Gordon Ramsey, age 70, receives alteplase I.V. When the nurse assesses Mr. Ramsey, which of the findings below suggests that his heart is responding to the drug by reperfusing the affected coronary artery?
   (a) Hypotension
   (b) Tingling in the arm
   (c) Oozing around the I.V. site
   (d) Premature ventricular contractions

UNIT

VIII

Drugs to improve respiratory function

Unit 8 discusses pharmacologic agents used to improve respiratory function, including **methylxanthines,** expectorants, **antitussives, mucolytics,** and **decongestants.** These drugs are used to relieve constricted airways, mucosal edema, cough, abnormally **viscid** secretions, and nasal congestion. Other agents that improve respiratory function include pirbuterol acetate, an aerosolized *bronchodilator,* and cromolyn sodium, an agent that can prevent acute asthmatic attacks. (See *Pirbuterol acetate* and *Cromolyn sodium.*)

RESPIRATORY FUNCTION

The respiratory system extends from the nose to the pulmonary capillaries. It oxygenates tissue, removes carbon dioxide, regulates acid-base balance, and provides defense against infection.

Oxygen-carbon dioxide exchange

Air flows into the lungs via the conducting airways (nose to bronchioles) and reaches the alveoli, where gas exchange occurs. Oxygen diffuses from the alveoli into the pulmonary capillaries, where most of the oxygen is bound to the hemoglobin in the red blood cells (RBCs). Only a small percentage is dissolved in the plasma. Then the RBCs are transported to all tissues, where oxygen is diffused from the blood into the cell to be used for cellular metabolism. Carbon dioxide, a by-product of cellular metabolism, is returned to the lungs to be eliminated. After diffusing from the blood into the alveoli, the carbon dioxide is exhaled from the lungs. (See *Normal respiratory anatomy and physiology,* page 328.) Such conditions as mucosal edema, alveolar damage, bronchoconstriction, or a disrupted mucociliary clearance mechanism affect the integrity of the respiratory structures and can alter oxygen-carbon dioxide gas exchange.

Acid-base balance

The respiratory system is a major regulator of acid-base balance; the blood-buffer system and the kidneys are the other regulators. Normal arterial blood pH ranges from 7.35 to 7.45; blood pH can be lowered or raised by the retention or excretion of hydrogen ions and bicarbonate ions. Carbon dioxide and water combine in the presence of carbonic anhydrase (a catalyst) to form carbonic acid, as follows:

$$CO_2 + H_2O = H_2CO_3 = H + HCO_3$$

This reaction, which is reversible, is affected by respiratory and renal function. In patients with compromised respiratory function, carbon dioxide retention increases hydrogen ion levels in the blood, thereby decreasing the blood pH; this state is known as respiratory acidosis. Similarly, carbon dioxide elimination by the respiratory system causes the blood to become more alkaline; this is known as respiratory alkalosis. The alterations in carbon dioxide levels are regulated by breathing frequency and the depth of the breaths, which is measured as minute ventilation. The respiratory system can restore normal arterial blood pH in minutes; however, dysfunction of the system can be the primary cause of an acid-base imbalance.

Pirbuterol acetate

An aerosolized bronchodilator, pirbuterol acetate (Maxair) acts as a beta$_2$-adrenergic receptor agonist. It is used to prevent and reverse bronchospasm in patients with reversible bronchospasm, including that caused by asthma. Pirbuterol may be used alone or with theophylline or steroid therapy.

For adults and children age 12 and older, the usual pirbuterol dosage is two inhalations (0.2 mg each), followed by one or two inhalations repeated every 4 to 6 hours. The patient may use a maximum of 12 inhalations daily. Adverse reactions to pirbuterol include nervousness, tremors, headache, palpitations, tachycardia, chest pain or tightness, nausea, diarrhea, and dry mouth.

Cromolyn sodium

Cromolyn sodium prevents the release of histamine and slow-reacting substances of anaphylaxis by stabilizing the mast cell membrane, thereby reducing the stimulus for bronchospasm and bronchoconstriction.

Cromolyn sodium is used primarily as prophylactic treatment of bronchial asthma. It is not useful, however, in treating acute asthmatic attacks or status asthmaticus.

Cromolyn sodium usually is tolerated well by patients, even with prolonged continuous therapy. Adverse reactions are infrequent and minor. The most frequently seen adverse reactions are bronchospasm, sneezing, wheezing, cough, nasal congestion, and pharyngeal irritation. Dizziness, dysuria, joint swelling, joint pain, nausea, headache, and skin rash also may occur.

Cromolyn sodium is given by inhalation because it is absorbed poorly after oral administration. The drug is not metabolized and is excreted unchanged, 50% in urine and 50% in bile.

Two of the commonly used forms of cromolyn sodium include a metered-dose aerosol inhaler and a turbo inhaler. The aerosol delivers a small dose in a fine white mist. The turbo inhaler delivers a larger dose of dry white powder. Both delivery systems are of equal efficacy. The aerosol requires the patient to synchronize breathing with dose delivery. The turbo inhaler is less likely to be confused with the bronchodilators that are used for acute asthmatic attacks. The two types of devices are illustrated below.

When administering cromolyn sodium, monitor the patient's respiratory patterns and the integrity of the nasal and oral passages before and after therapy. Also inform the patient that throat irritation and cough may be decreased by gargling or drinking after each treatment.

Metered-dose aerosol inhaler

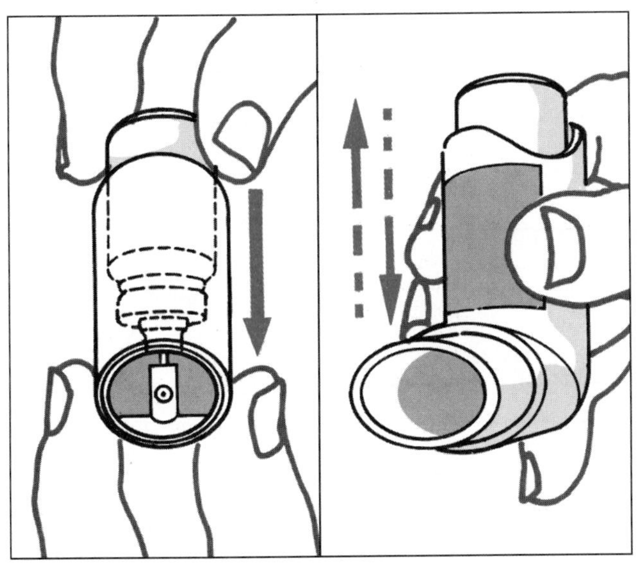

Turbo inhaler

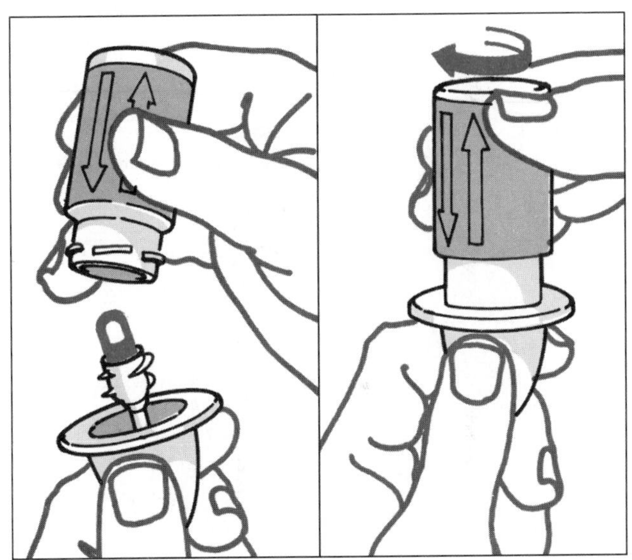

Defense mechanism

The nose filters, humidifies, and warms air during inhalation. It also traps particles in the mucosa to prevent their deposition lower in the respiratory tract. The mucosa and its secretions are influenced by the parasympathetic and sympathetic nervous systems. Sympathetic stimulation causes vasoconstriction of the nasal vascular structures and decreased **mucus** production. Parasympathetic stimulation has the opposite effect: It narrows the airway by vascular engorgement of mucosal tissues and increases mucus production.

Cilia are hairlike projections from the columnar epithelial cells that line the nasal and tracheal passageways. Ciliary undulations project respiratory secretions and particles toward the oropharynx to be coughed out or swallowed. The respiratory tract mucus, produced by the **goblet cells,** contains lysosomes and other elements that fight invading bacteria. The mucus also clears particles via the "mechanical" mucociliary escalator.

The **cough** is a protective mechanism that rapidly expels air and particles from the airways. The sneeze clears the nasal passageway. Should particles evade the mucociliary defense mechanism and reach the lower respiratory tract, alveolar macrophages can phagocytize and detoxify them.

Normal respiratory anatomy and physiology

A knowledge of intrapulmonary blood circulation and gas exchange will help the nurse understand the actions of the drugs discussed in this unit. The respiratory system's major structures are illustrated below. The insert below left, which is an enlargement of an alveolus and the surrounding vessels, shows intrapulmonary blood circulation around the alveolus; the insert below right shows the partial pressures of the carbon dioxide and oxygen exchanged.

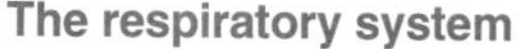

The respiratory system

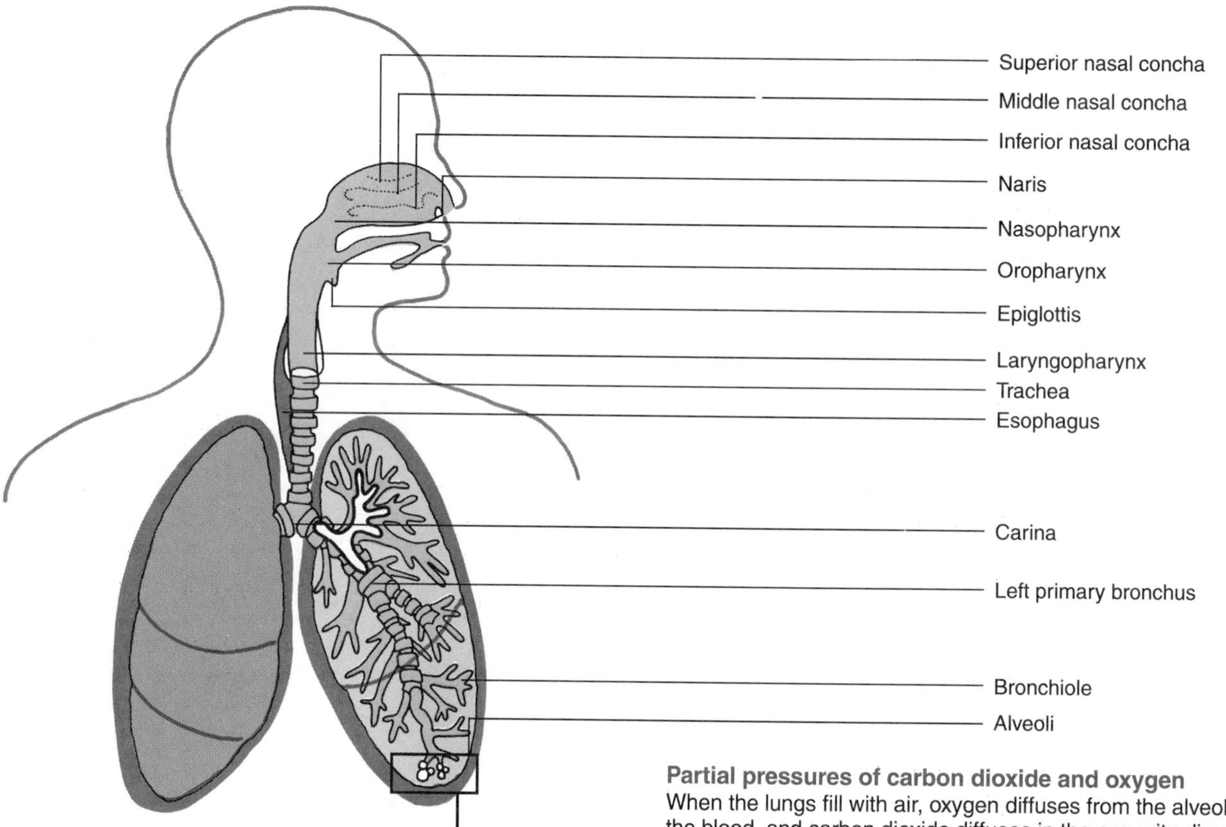

Partial pressures of carbon dioxide and oxygen

When the lungs fill with air, oxygen diffuses from the alveoli into the blood, and carbon dioxide diffuses in the opposite direction. Gas exchange (diffusion) depends on differences in the partial pressures of the gases, which are determined by Dalton's law of partial pressures. This law states that the pressure (tension) exerted by each gas in a mixture is related to its percentage of the total mixture.

Intrapulmonary blood circulation

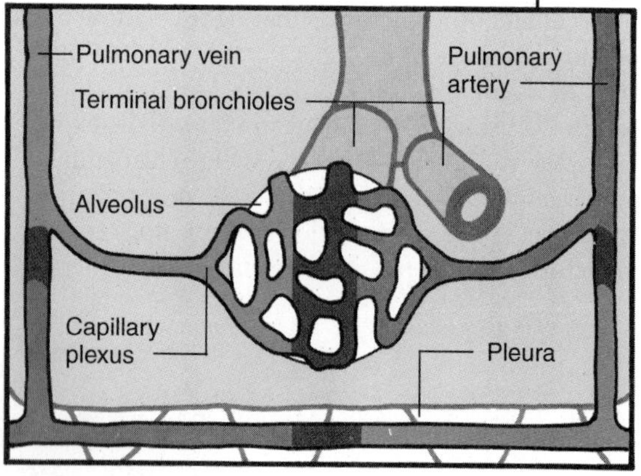

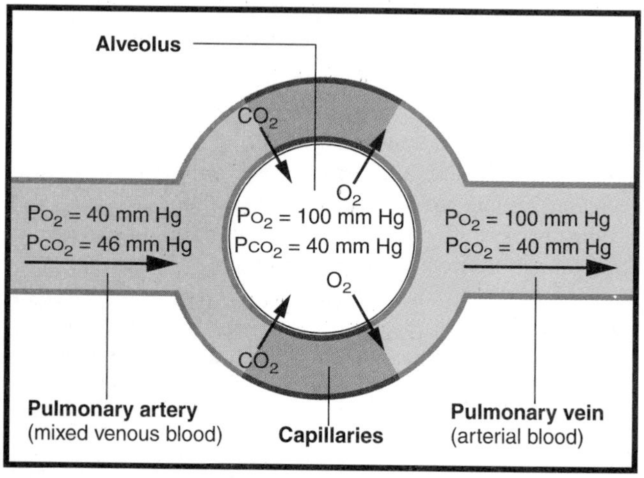

25 Methylxanthine agents

OBJECTIVES

After reading and studying this chapter, the student should be able to:

1. identify the clinical indications for theophylline, its derivatives, and caffeine.
2. describe the pharmacokinetic properties of the various methylxanthine agents, and explain their effects on drug administration.
3. describe the drug interactions and adverse reactions to methylxanthine therapy, including the signs and symptoms of methylxanthine toxicity.
4. describe how to apply the nursing process when caring for a patient who is receiving a methylxanthine agent.

INTRODUCTION

The **methylxanthine** agents (also called xanthines) are used extensively to treat asthma, chronic bronchitis, emphysema, and neonatal apnea. Theophylline, theophylline derivatives, and caffeine are the agents used to treat these disorders. (See *Selected major methylxanthine agents,* page 330.) Chapter 25 focuses on the methylxanthine agents as they are used to treat respiratory diseases.

Drugs covered in this chapter include:

- aminophylline
- anhydrous theophylline
- caffeine
- dyphylline
- oxtriphylline
- theophylline sodium glycinate.

Theophylline, theophylline derivatives, and caffeine

The methylxanthine agents are used primarily to treat asthma, chronic bronchitis, emphysema, and neonatal apnea. (See Cultural Considerations: *Beliefs about asthma treatment,* page 331.) Drugs in this class include anhydrous theophylline, its salts (aminophylline, oxtriphylline, and theophylline sodium glycinate), dyphylline, and caffeine. The nurse should be aware that some controversy exists regarding certain clinical uses for these agents, such as the use of beta$_2$-adrenergic agonists with theophylline to treat acute asthma and the use of intravenous (I.V). theophylline to treat acute asthma.

PHARMACOKINETICS

The pharmacokinetics of methylxanthine agents vary according to the agent administered, its dosage form, and the administration route. When theophylline is given as an oral solution, a rapid-release tablet, or a retention enema, it is absorbed rapidly and completely. However, rectal suppositories are absorbed erratically and are used less frequently. Absorption of some of theophylline's slow-release forms depends on the gastric pH; food can alter absorption of other slow-release forms. Dyphylline is absorbed incompletely after oral or intramuscular (I.M.) administration. Caffeine is absorbed well after oral administration; however, rectal preparations may be absorbed slowly and erratically. Caffeine should not be given intramuscularly because of the irritating effect of the solution.

The volume of distribution for theophylline ranges from 0.3 L/kg to 0.7 L/kg of body weight, averaging 0.5 liter/kg. Because theophylline is not distributed well into adipose tissue, dosage should be based on the patient's ideal or actual body weight, whichever is less. Theophylline is approximately 60% protein-bound in adults and 36% protein-bound in the neonate. It readily crosses the placental barrier, producing similar serum concentrations in the mother and fetus. Theophylline also crosses into breast milk.

No information on dyphylline's distribution and protein-binding capacity is available. Caffeine is distributed rapidly and widely. Less than 20% of a caffeine dose is protein-bound in the plasma. Caffeine readily crosses the blood-brain barrier and the placental barrier, and small amounts are secreted in breast milk.

Theophylline is metabolized primarily in the liver. In adults and children, about 10% of a theophylline dose is excreted unchanged in the urine; in neonates and infants, as much as 50% of a dose may be excreted unchanged in the urine because the immature liver has limited metabolizing ability. Dyphylline is not metabolized; approximately 83% of a dose is excreted unchanged in the urine. Like theophylline, caffeine is metabolized extensively by the liver. In an adult, about 2% of a dose is excreted unchanged in the

Selected major methylxanthine agents

This chart summarizes the major methylxanthine agents currently in clinical use.

DRUG	MAJOR INDICATIONS AND USUAL DOSAGES	CONTRAINDICATIONS AND PRECAUTIONS
anhydrous theophylline (Slo-bid Gyrocaps, Theo-24, Theo-Dur)	*Asthma, chronic bronchitis, emphysema* ADULT: individualized, based on the patient's serum theophylline concentration, response, and occurrence of adverse reactions with the daily dosage divided into 6- or 8-hour doses for rapid-release forms and 8-, 12-, or 24-hour doses for slow-release forms; initial maximum, 13 mg/kg or a total of 600 mg daily, whichever is less; final dosage based on theophylline concentration *Neonatal apnea* PEDIATRIC: initially, 5 mg/kg P.O. or I.V. (if I.V., administered over 20 to 30 minutes) as a loading dose; for maintenance dosage, 2 mg/kg every 12 hours with the final dosage determined by serum theophylline concentrations and patient response *Acute and chronic bronchospasm* PEDIATRIC: highly individualized	• Theophylline is contraindicated in a patient with known hypersensitivity to methylxanthines. • This drug requires cautious use in a neonate; a geriatric, pregnant, or breast-feeding patient; or one with heart failure, severe cardiovascular disease, severe hypoxemia, hypertension, hyperthyroidism, acute myocardial injury, obstructive lung disease, or liver disease.
aminophylline (Aminophyllin)	*Asthma, chronic bronchitis, emphysema* ADULT: individualized, based on theophylline content of the preparation and the patient's serum theophylline concentration, response, and occurrence of adverse reactions with the daily dosage divided into 6- or 8-hour doses for rapid-release forms and 8- or 12-hour doses for slow-release forms; initial loading dose, 5 to 6 mg/kg I.V. given over 20 to 30 minutes; maintenance dosage, 0.4 to 0.7 mg/kg/hour; initial maximum, 13 mg/kg or a total of 600 mg daily, whichever is less; final dosage based on theophylline concentration *Acute and chronic bronchospasm* PEDIATRIC: highly individualized	• Aminophylline is contraindicated in a patient with active peptic ulcer disease, known hypersensitivity to methylxanthines, or concurrent administration of other xanthine preparations. • This drug requires cautious use in a neonate; a pregnant, breast-feeding, or geriatric (especially male) patient; or one with severe cardiac disease, hypertension, hyperthyroidism, acute myocardial injury, cor pulmonale, severe hypoxemia, hepatic impairment, alcoholism, history of peptic ulcer, or heart failure.
oxtriphylline (Choledyl)	*Asthma, chronic bronchitis, emphysema, other similar chronic obstructive pulmonary diseases* ADULT: initially, 200 mg P.O. every 6 to 8 hours, with the specific dosage adjusted, based on the patient's body weight, serum theophylline concentration, response, and occurrence of adverse reactions PEDIATRIC: for children age 2 to 12, 3.7 mg/kg P.O. every 6 hours, with the specific dosage adjusted, based on serum theophylline concentration, patient response, and occurrence of adverse reactions	• Oxtriphylline is contraindicated in a breast-feeding patient or one with active peptic ulcer disease, a seizure disorder (unless the patient is receiving anticonvulsant medication), or known hypersensitivity to oxtriphylline's components. • This drug requires cautious use in a pregnant patient or one with hypoxemia, hypertension, or a history of peptic ulcer.
dyphylline (Dyline, Lufyllin)	*Asthma, chronic bronchitis, emphysema* ADULT: up to 15 mg/kg P.O. every 6 hours, or 250 to 500 mg I.M. up to a maximum of 15 mg/kg every 6 hours PEDIATRIC: 4.4 to 6.6 mg/kg daily in divided doses	• Dyphylline is contraindicated in a patient with known hypersensitivity to dyphylline or related xanthine compounds. • This drug requires cautious use in a pregnant or breast-feeding patient or one with severe cardiac disease, hypertension, hyperthyroidism, acute myocardial injury, or peptic ulcer.

urine; in the neonate, however, about 85% of a dose is excreted unchanged in the urine.

Theophylline's onset and duration of action are related to the patient's serum theophylline concentration level, which in turn depends on the drug's absorption and excretion rates. To treat respiratory disease, a serum concentration level of 10 to 20 mcg/ml is considered therapeutic. To treat neonatal apnea, a serum concentration level of 5 to 10 mcg/ml is required.

Dyphylline's onset and duration of action remain unknown because therapeutic serum concentration levels have not been determined.

Caffeine's onset of action usually occurs within 30 minutes after administration, and concentration levels peak within 1 to 2 hours. Its duration of action depends on the patient's serum concentration levels.

Route	Onset	Peak	Duration
P.O.	15-60 min	1-13 hr	Variable
I.M.	Unknown	1 hr	Unknown
I.V.	15 min	15-30 min	Unknown

PHARMACODYNAMICS

Although methylxanthine agents decrease nonspecific airway reactivity and, in the presence of **bronchospasm,** relax bronchial smooth muscle, their specific mechanism of action in reversible obstructive airway disease, such as asthma, is not understood completely. In nonreversible obstructive airway disease (chronic bronchitis, emphysema, and apnea), methylxanthines appear to increase the central respiratory center's sensitivity to carbon dioxide and to stimulate the respiratory drive. In chronic bronchitis and emphysema, these agents also decrease diaphragmatic fatigue and improve cardiac ventricular function.

PHARMACOTHERAPEUTICS

Theophylline, its salts, and dyphylline are used to treat asthma, chronic bronchitis, and emphysema. Caffeine is used primarily as a central nervous system (CNS) stimulant and appears in many over-the-counter preparations, prescription antihistamines, barbiturates (to offset their sedative effects), and ergot alkaloids (to produce cerebrovascular constriction in treating migraine headaches). Theophylline and sometimes caffeine also are used to treat neonatal apnea, although the Food and Drug Administration has not approved their use for this condition. Dosages of methylxanthine agents should be individualized using the patient's body weight, serum concentration levels, response, and adverse reactions as guides.

Drug interactions

Theophylline and its salts can interact with food or other drugs. (See Drug Interactions: *Theophylline, theophylline derivatives, and caffeine,* page 332.) Smoking cigarettes or marijuana increases theophylline elimination, decreasing its serum concentrations.

Probenecid inhibits renal excretion of dyphylline, increasing its half-life and prolonging its action. Drugs that affect theophylline's excretion also may affect caffeine's excretion. Concomitant administration of adrenergic stimulants or consumption of beverages that contain caffeine may result in additive adverse reactions or signs and symptoms of methylxanthine toxicity.

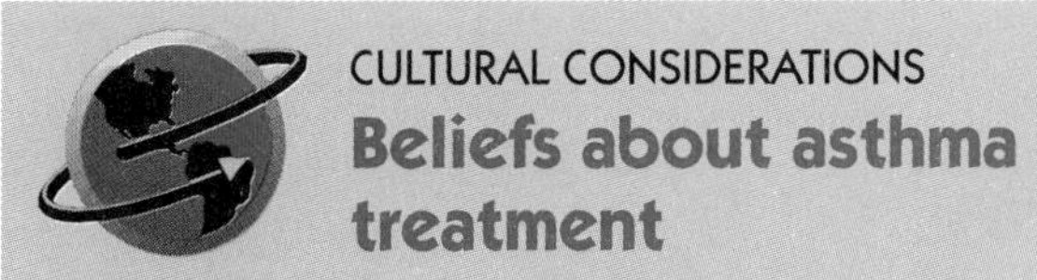

CULTURAL CONSIDERATIONS

Beliefs about asthma treatment

Many Hispanics believe that disorders are cold or hot, and that cold disorders should be treated with hot remedies and vice versa. Those who adhere to such beliefs consider asthma a cold disorder. If your Hispanic patient holds such beliefs and must take an oral methylxanthine for asthma, suggest taking the prescribed drug with hot herbal tea to incorporate these cultural beliefs and promote effective asthma management.

Many Asians use coin rubbing as a form of healing. They believe that this practice will draw out the illness and restore balance in the body. When teaching an asthmatic Asian patient about bronchodilator inhalation therapy (which often accompanies methylxanthine therapy), ask what the coin rubbing practice means to him or her. To enhance compliance, compare coin rubbing with the bronchodilator, emphasizing that it draws out the tightness and wheezing in the chest.

ADVERSE DRUG REACTIONS

The adverse reactions to methylxanthines can be transient or symptomatic of toxicity. Adverse reactions, which may appear shortly after administration of the first dose, can affect the gastrointestinal (GI) tract and the CNS. GI tract irritation and increased gastric acid secretion may cause nausea, vomiting, abdominal cramping, epigastric pain, anorexia, or diarrhea. Adverse CNS effects include headache, irritability, restlessness, anxiety, insomnia, and rarely dizziness.

Methylxanthines also can produce adverse reactions when a dose results in a high serum concentration (for theophylline and caffeine, this concentration usually is above 20 mcg/ml). These reactions include nausea, vomiting, diarrhea, and such CNS effects as irritability, insomnia, anxiety, headache, and seizures (with very high serum concentrations).

Methylxanthines also can irritate the myocardium, producing such cardiovascular symptoms as tachycardia, palpitations, extrasystoles, or arrhythmias. Also, these drugs can cause peripheral vasodilation and hypotension.

Although hypersensitivity reactions can occur, they are extremely rare and typically are associated with the base of the theophylline salt formulations. Shortly after receiving the drug, the patient may display severe signs and symptoms of theophylline toxicity, which include nausea, vomiting, diarrhea, headache, and occasionally anxiety and dizziness; this indicates intolerance.

Because theophylline is secreted in breast milk, the nurse should monitor the neonate for such adverse reactions as tachycardia or vomiting.

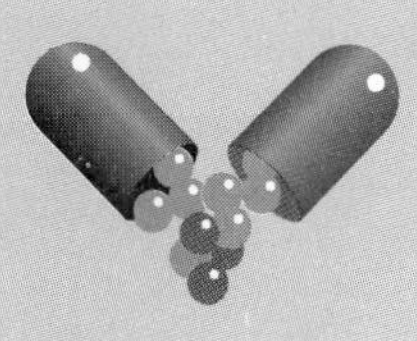

DRUG INTERACTIONS

Theophylline, theophylline derivatives, and caffeine

In many cases, interactions between theophylline and other drugs increase the risk of toxicity or subtherapeutic levels.

DRUG	INTERACTING AGENTS	POSSIBLE EFFECTS	NURSING IMPLICATIONS
anhydrous theophylline, aminophylline, oxtriphylline, theophylline sodium glycinate	cimetidine	Increased theophylline concentration, resulting in a potentially toxic concentration	• Avoid concomitant administration with cimetidine. If a histamine$_2$ receptor is desired, ranitidine or famotidine can be used instead, because they do not alter theophylline's metabolism significantly.
	erythromycin, clarithromycin	Increased theophylline concentration	• Decrease the theophylline dosage by 25%, as prescribed, if administered concomitantly, and monitor the patient for adverse reactions to theophylline.
	troleandomycin	Increased theophylline concentration	• Avoid concomitant administration with theophylline.
	allopurinol (high dose), disulfiram, thiabendazole	Increased theophylline concentration	• Observe the patient for signs and symptoms of theophylline toxicity, such as palpitations and restlessness.
	oral contraceptives	Increased serum theophylline concentration	• Encourage the patient to use an alternative contraceptive method, if possible. • Monitor the theophylline concentration closely when adding or deleting oral contraceptives from the treatment regimen.
	beta-adrenergic blocking agents	Increased theophylline concentration and theophylline bronchodilating effect	• Avoid concomitant administration with theophylline. • Use a cardioselective agent, if a beta-adrenergic blocker is required.
	phenobarbital, phenytoin, rifampin, carbamazepine	Decreased serum theophylline concentration	• Monitor the serum theophylline concentration and expect to adjust the theophylline dosage.
	halothane, enflurane, isoflurane, methoxyflurane	Increased risk of cardiac toxicity	• Administer concomitantly with extreme caution.
	lithium	Increased lithium clearance	• Monitor the serum lithium concentration and expect to adjust the lithium dosage.
	thyroid hormones, antithyroid agents	Decreased theophylline concentration (thyroid hormones); increased theophylline concentration (antithyroid agents)	• Assess for signs and symptoms of theophylline toxicity or ineffectiveness. • Monitor the theophylline concentration closely if initiating thyroid or antithyroid therapy. • Know that hyperthyroidism increases theophylline metabolism and hypothyroidism decreases theophylline metabolism. Correction of either condition may affect the serum theophylline concentration in a patient whose theophylline dosage previously had been stabilized.
	ciprofloxacin, norfloxacin, enoxacin	Increased serum theophylline concentration, resulting in a potentially toxic concentration	• Administer concomitantly with caution. • Observe the patient for signs and symptoms of theophylline toxicity, such as palpitations and restlessness. • Monitor the serum theophylline concentration and expect to adjust the theophylline dosage.
	zileuton	Increased serum theophylline concentration, resulting in a potentially toxic concentration	• Decrease the theophylline dosage by 50% if these drugs must be administered concomitantly. • Monitor the patient for adverse reactions to theophylline.

NURSING PROCESS APPLICATION

The following information assists the nurse in caring for a patient who is receiving a methylxanthine agent. It includes an overview of assessment activities as well as examples of appropriate nursing diagnoses and related interventions. It also highlights the importance of evaluation.

Assessment

Before drug therapy begins, review the patient's history for conditions that contraindicate or require cautious use of the prescribed methylxanthine. Also review the patient's medication history to identify use of drugs that may interact with it. During therapy, assess the patient for adverse drug reactions and signs of drug interactions. Also, periodically assess the effectiveness of methylxanthine therapy. Finally, evaluate the patient's and family's knowledge about the prescribed drug. (See Patient Teaching: *Theophylline, theophylline derivatives, and caffeine.*)

Nursing diagnoses

- Risk for injury related to a preexisting condition that contraindicates or requires cautious use of a methylxanthine
- Risk for injury related to adverse drug reactions or drug interactions
- Risk for fluid volume deficit related to the adverse GI effects of the prescribed methylxanthine
- Knowledge deficit related to the prescribed methylxanthine

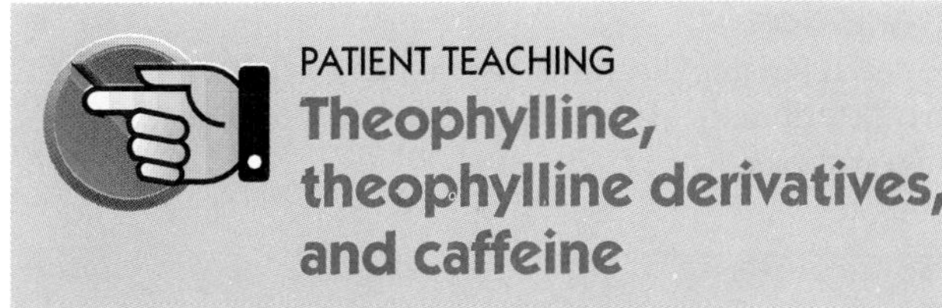

PATIENT TEACHING

Theophylline, theophylline derivatives, and caffeine

- ➤ Teach the patient and family the name, dose, frequency, action, and adverse effects of the prescribed methylxanthine.
- ➤ Stress the importance of returning for drug level testing, as prescribed, to detect toxicity or ineffectiveness (except with dyphylline therapy).
- ➤ Advise the patient to withhold the drug and consult the physician if an adverse reaction occurs.
- ➤ Instruct the patient to inform all personal physicians about methylxanthine therapy to prevent drug interactions.
- ➤ Teach the patient who misses a dose to consult the physician before increasing the next scheduled dose.
- ➤ Instruct the patient to take a mild analgesic, as prescribed, for methylxanthine-induced headache.
- ➤ Advise the patient that intramuscular aminophylline produces severe pain at the injection site.
- ➤ Instruct the patient to take an oral preparation with 8 oz of water and preferably on an empty stomach. Advise the patient taking a sustained-release product not to chew or crush it.
- ➤ Advise the patient to avoid using products that contain methylxanthine during methylxanthine therapy. The additional agents may not contribute to the therapy's effectiveness and may cause adverse reactions.

Planning and implementation

- Do not administer a methylxanthine agent to a patient with a condition that contraindicates its use.
- Administer a methylxanthine agent with caution to a patient at risk because of a preexisting condition.
- Monitor for adverse CNS, cardiovascular, and GI effects, especially when the serum theophylline or caffeine concentration exceeds 20 mcg/ml, when therapy is initiated or restarted, or when the dosage is changed. Also, monitor for drug interactions.
- Withhold the drug and ask the physician about a dosage alteration, if adverse reactions occur.
- Monitor the patient's serum theophylline concentration level during theophylline treatment or the serum caffeine concentration during caffeine treatment. When theophylline is administered to a neonate, monitor serum theophylline and caffeine concentration levels because theophylline is metabolized to caffeine in the neonate.

∗ *Consult the physician before repeating a dose of an oral methylxanthine preparation if vomiting occurs shortly after administration. If the patient misses a dose, do not increase or double subsequent doses without first consulting the physician.*

- Mix the loading dose for I.V. aminophylline in dextrose 5% in water or normal saline solution; administer it over 20 to 30 minutes. Administer the I.V. maintenance dosage by constant infusion, using an infusion pump. Use a standard concentration, and do not vary the volume administered unless the patient is volume-restricted.
- When switching a patient from I.V. to oral theophylline or dyphylline, stop the infusion when starting the oral drug as prescribed.
- Do not administer the I.V. caffeine and sodium benzoate solution to a neonate, because benzoate displaces bound bilirubin.
- Do not administer a rectal preparation or suppository if rectal irritation or infection is present.
- Encourage the patient receiving a theophylline enema or rectal preparation to retain it as long as possible.
- Administer an oral preparation with a full glass of water on an empty stomach or with a small amount of food. Open bead-filled capsules and scatter their contents on small amounts of soft food for a patient who cannot swallow tablets. Slow-release products should not be chewed or crushed.
- Notify the physician if adverse reactions or drug interactions occur or if the methylxanthine is ineffective.
- Assess the patient with adverse GI reactions for signs of fluid volume deficit, such as poor skin turgor, dry mucous membranes, and decreased urine volume. Request a prescription for an antiemetic or antidiarrheal agent, as needed.
- Teach the patient about the prescribed agent. Incorporate the patient's cultural beliefs, when possible, in your teaching.

Evaluation

For each nursing diagnosis, prepare an evaluation statement that describes the patient's or family's response to nursing interventions.

CHAPTER SUMMARY

Chapter 25 covered the methylxanthine agents used clinically in the United States, including theophylline and its salts, dyphylline, and caffeine. Here are the highlights of the chapter.

Theophylline, its salts, and dyphylline are prescribed to treat asthma, chronic bronchitis, and emphysema. Theophylline and sometimes caffeine are used to treat neonatal apnea.

Dosages of methylxanthines should be individualized based on serum drug concentration level, patient response, and occurrence of adverse reactions.

Drug interactions involving methylxanthine agents can result in toxicity or reduced effectiveness. Adverse reactions to methylxanthine agents may affect the GI tract, the CNS, and the cardiac system.

When caring for a patient receiving a methylxanthine agent, the nurse applies the nursing process and focuses on monitoring the patient closely for adverse reactions, administering the methylxanthine carefully, protecting the patient from injury, and teaching the patient and family about the prescribed drug.

Questions to consider

See Appendix 1 for answers.

1. Andy Kellerman, age 62, is diagnosed with emphysema. His physician prescribes anhydrous theophylline 200 mg P.O. every 8 hours. Which of the following factors is most important for the physician to consider when calculating the theophylline dosage?
   (a) Blood count
   (b) Weight
   (c) Age
   (d) Sex

2. Andrea Winkler, age 58, is receiving anhydrous theophylline to treat her emphysema. She admits to being a heavy smoker. In which of the following ways can smoking cigarettes interact with anhydrous theophylline?
   (a) It may decrease theophylline absorption.
   (b) It may increase theophylline elimination.
   (c) It may inhibit theophylline metabolism.
   (d) It may produce additive effects.

3. Which of the following serum theophylline levels represents the therapeutic range for treating asthma?
   (a) 1 to 5 mcg/ml
   (b) 5 to 10 mcg/ml
   (c) 10 to 20 mcg/ml
   (d) 20 to 25 mcg/ml

4. Jane Robinson, age 25, comes to the emergency department with shortness of breath caused by chronic asthma. She has been using her albuterol inhaler every hour for the past 6 hours, but it has not completely relieved her shortness of breath. She has taken beclomethasone 4 puffs b.i.d. for the past few days. Ms. Robinson also has a prescription for sustained-release theophylline 300 mg b.i.d. However, she takes it only when she feels her asthma is getting worse. She has taken theophylline b.i.d. for the past two days. How should the nurse proceed with Ms. Robinson's theophylline therapy?
   (a) Tell her to take sustained-release theophylline, 300 mg b.i.d.
   (b) Ask the physician to switch the patient to I.V. theophylline.
   (c) Discontinue the theophylline immediately.
   (d) Obtain a theophylline level stat.

5. Howard Dunn, age 49, develops acute respiratory insufficiency. As part of his treatment, he receives I.V. anhydrous theophylline. After Mr. Dunn's condition stabilizes, the physician switches him to oral anhydrous theophylline. When should the nurse discontinue I.V. administration of this drug?
   (a) When oral therapy begins
   (b) 24 hours before oral therapy begins
   (c) 24 hours after oral therapy begins
   (d) After administering three oral doses

26 Expectorant, antitussive, mucolytic, and decongestant agents

OBJECTIVES

After reading and studying this chapter, the student should be able to:
1. compare the pharmacokinetic properties of expectorant, antitussive, mucolytic, and decongestant agents.
2. differentiate among the different actions of expectorants, antitussives, mucolytics, and decongestants.
3. identify adverse reactions associated with expectorants, antitussives, mucolytics, and decongestants.
4. describe how to apply the nursing process when caring for a patient who is receiving an expectorant, antitussive, mucolytic, or decongestant agent.

INTRODUCTION

This chapter discusses the expectorant and **mucolytic** agents, which purport to enhance **mucokinesis** (**mucus** removal), and drugs that act to suppress **cough,** the narcotic and nonnarcotic **antitussives.** It also discusses the **decongestant** agents that relieve the swelling in clogged nasal passages associated with the common cold. Primarily synthetic versions of epinephrine, most decongestants are termed sympathomimetic in action and are used systemically or topically. (See *Selected major expectorant, antitussive, mucolytic, and decongestant agents,* page 336.)

Drugs covered in this chapter include:

- acetylcysteine
- benzonatate
- codeine
- dextromethorphan hydrobromide
- ephedrine
- epinephrine
- guaifenesin
- hydrocodone bitartrate
- naphazoline
- oxymetazoline
- phenylephrine
- phenylpropanolamine
- propylhexedrine
- pseudoephedrine
- tetrahydrozoline
- xylometazoline.

Expectorants

Expectorants facilitate mucokinesis. They help remove mucus by liquefying **viscid** secretions and thereby promoting the mobilization and evacuation of secretions. The most commonly used expectorant is guaifenesin. Potassium iodide also is an expectorant; however, it is rarely used because of its potentially toxic effects.

PHARMACOKINETICS

Guaifenesin is absorbed through the gastrointestinal (GI) tract and metabolized by the liver. Its excretion is primarily renal. Guaifenesin's onset of action is relatively short (up to 30 minutes). Data remain unavailable on its peak concentration, duration, and half-life.

Route	Onset	Peak	Duration
P.O.	30 min	Unknown	Unknown

PHARMACODYNAMICS

Expectorants are thought to increase mucus by acting on the bronchial glands or by reducing the adhesiveness and surface tension of the mucus. They also may provide a soothing demulcent effect on respiratory tract mucosa.

PHARMACOTHERAPEUTICS

Guaifenesin is used for the symptomatic relief of cough from colds, as well as for minor bronchial irritations, bronchitis, influenza, sinusitis, bronchial asthma, emphysema, and other respiratory disorders. This drug also is used to relieve a dry, hacking cough and is safe if taken as directed. It can be used alone or with antitussives, analgesics, or antihistamines.

Drug interactions

Guaifenesin administered with anticoagulants may increase the risk of bleeding.

ADVERSE DRUG REACTIONS

Adverse reactions to guaifenesin rarely or infrequently occur. However, the drug may produce vomiting if taken in doses larger than necessary for the expectorant action. Diarrhea, drowsiness, nausea, vomiting, and abdominal pain also may occur. Guaifenesin also may interfere with urinary 5-hydroxyindoleacetic acid (5-HIAA) and urinary vanillylmandelic acid (VMA) tests, resulting in falsely increased determinations.

Selected major expectorant, antitussive, mucolytic, and decongestant agents

The following chart summarizes the major expectorant, antitussive, mucolytic, and decongestant agents currently in clinical use.

DRUG	MAJOR INDICATIONS AND USUAL DOSAGES	CONTRAINDICATIONS AND PRECAUTIONS
Expectorant		
guaifenesin (Breonesin, Robitussin)	*Cough associated with common cold and upper respiratory tract infection* ADULT: 200 to 400 mg P.O. every 4 hours, not to exceed 2.4 grams daily PEDIATRIC: for children age 12 and older, 200 to 400 mg P.O. every 4 hours, not to exceed 2.4 grams daily; for children age 6 to 12, 100 to 200 mg P.O. every 4 hours, not to exceed 1.2 grams daily; for children age 2 to 6, 50 to 100 mg P.O. every 4 hours, not to exceed 600 mg daily; for children under age 2, dosage must be individualized	• Guaifenesin is contraindicated in a patient with known hypersensitivity or chronic cough associated with emphysema, asthma, or chronic bronchitis. • This drug requires cautious use in a pregnant or breast-feeding patient or one with an ineffective cough reflex or respiratory insufficiency.
Antitussives		
codeine	*Nonproductive cough* ADULT: 10 to 20 mg P.O. every 4 to 6 hours, not to exceed 120 mg daily PEDIATRIC: for children age 12 and older, 10 to 20 mg P.O. every 4 to 6 hours, not to exceed 120 mg daily; for children age 6 to 12, 5 to 10 mg P.O. every 4 to 6 hours, not to exceed 60 mg daily; for children age 2 to 6, 1 mg/kg P.O. daily given in four equally divided doses every 4 to 6 hours	• Codeine is contraindicated in a pregnant or breast-feeding patient, one with a productive cough or known hypersensitivity, or one who can benefit from coughing, such as a postoperative patient. • This drug requires cautious use in a debilitated patient, one who has undergone thoracotomy or laparotomy, or one with a history of drug or alcohol abuse. • Safety and efficacy in children under age 2 have not been established.
dextromethorphan hydrobromide (Robitussin-DM, St. Joseph's Cough Suppressant)	*Nonproductive cough* ADULT: 10 to 20 mg P.O. every 4 hours or 30 mg every 6 to 8 hours, not to exceed 120 mg daily; for a long-acting preparation, 60 mg P.O. every 12 hours PEDIATRIC: for children age 12 and older, 10 to 20 mg P.O. every 4 hours or 30 mg every 6 to 8 hours, not to exceed 120 mg daily; for children age 6 to 12, 5 to 10 mg P.O. every 4 hours or 15 mg every 6 to 8 hours, not to exceed 60 mg daily; for children age 2 to 6, 2.5 to 5 mg P.O. every 4 hours or 7.5 mg every 6 to 8 hours, not to exceed 30 mg daily; for children less than age 2, dosage must be individualized	• Dextromethorphan is contraindicated in a patient with a productive cough, persistent or chronic cough, or known hypersensitivity to the drug; one who is receiving a monoamine oxidase (MAO) inhibitor; or one who can benefit from coughing, such as a postoperative patient. • This drug requires cautious use in a pregnant or breast-feeding patient or one with prostatic hypertrophy.
Mucolytics		
acetylcysteine (Mucomyst)	*Bronchopulmonary diseases (chronic bronchitis, emphysema, bronchiectasis, pneumonia, atelectasis, cystic fibrosis)* ADULT: for nebulization, 3 to 5 ml (20% solution), t.i.d. or q.i.d., or 6 to 10 ml (10% solution) t.i.d. or q.i.d.; for direct instillation, 1 to 2 ml of a 10% to 20% solution every hour	• Acetylcysteine is contraindicated in a patient with known hypersensitivity. • This drug requires cautious use in an asthmatic, pregnant, or breast-feeding patient or a geriatric or debilitated patient with severe respiratory insufficiency.
Decongestants		
Systemic decongestants (sympathomimetic amines)		
phenylpropanolamine (Propagest, Rhindecon, Sucrets Cold Decongestant Formula)	*Nasal congestion associated with acute or chronic rhinitis, sinusitis, the common cold, hay fever, or other allergies* ADULT: 25 mg P.O. every 4 hours or 75 mg P.O. of the sustained-release form every 12 hours, not to exceed 150 mg P.O. daily	• Systemic decongestants are contraindicated in a pregnant or breast-feeding patient, a patient receiving an MAO inhibitor, or one with porphyria, severe coronary artery disease, cardiac arrhythmias, acute angle-closure glaucoma, psychoneurosis, or known

Selected major expectorant, antitussive, mucolytic, and decongestant agents *(continued)*

DRUG	MAJOR INDICATIONS AND USUAL DOSAGES	CONTRAINDICATIONS AND PRECAUTIONS
Decongestants *(continued)*		
Systemic decongestants (sympathomimetic amines) *(continued)*		
phenylpropanolamine (Propagest, Rhindecon, Sucrets Cold Decongestant Formula) *(continued)*	PEDIATRIC: for children age 6 to 12, 10 to 12.5 mg P.O. every 4 hours, up to a maximum of 75 mg daily; for children age 2 to 6, 6.25 mg P.O. every 4 hours, up to a maximum of 37.5 mg daily; for children under age 2, dosage must be individualized	hypersensitivity to systemic decongestants. • This drug requires cautious use in a geriatric patient or one with hypertension, hyperthyroidism, cardiovascular disease, or prostatic hypertrophy.
pseudoephedrine (Efidac/24, Novafed, Sudafed)	ADULT: 60 mg P.O. every 4 to 6 hours, or 120 mg P.O. of the sustained-release preparation every 12 hours, not to exceed 240 mg daily PEDIATRIC: for children age 12 and older, 60 mg P.O. every 4 to 6 hours, or 120 mg P.O. of the sustained-release form every 12 hours, up to a maximum of 240 mg daily; for children age 6 to 12, 30 mg P.O. every 4 to 6 hours, up to a maximum of 120 mg daily; for children age 2 to 6, 15 mg P.O. every 4 to 6 hours, up to a maximum of 60 mg daily; alternatively, 4 mg/kg or 125 mg/m^2 P.O. daily in four divided doses	• Pseudophedrine is contraindicated in a breast feeding patient, one with severe coronary artery disease, or one receiving MAO inhibitors; extended-release preparations are contraindicated in children under age 12. • This drug requires cautious use in a patient with hypertension, cardiac disease, diabetes, glaucoma, hyperthyroidism, and prostatic hyperplasia.
Topical decongestants (local vasoconstrictors)		
naphazoline (Privine)	*Nasal congestion associated with acute or chronic rhinitis, sinusitis, the common cold, hay fever, or other allergies* ADULT: 2 drops or sprays of 0.05% solution in each nostril, repeated every 3 to 6 hours PEDIATRIC: for children age 12 and older, 2 drops or sprays of 0.05% solution in each nostril, repeated every 3 to 6 hours as needed; for children age 6 to 12, 1 or 2 drops or sprays of 0.025% solution in each nostril, repeated every 3 to 6 hours as needed	• Naphazoline is contraindicated in a pregnant patient, in one with acute angle-closure glaucoma or known hypersensitivity to topical decongestants, or for more than 3 to 5 days of use. • This drug requires cautious use in a breast-feeding patient or one with hypertension, diabetes mellitus, cardiovascular disease, hyperthyroidism, or prostatic hypertrophy.
oxymetazoline (Afrin, Duration, Dristan Long Lasting)	ADULT: 2 or 3 drops or 1 or 2 sprays of 0.05% solution in each nostril every 10 to 12 hours PEDIATRIC: for children age 6 and older, 2 or 3 drops or 1 or 2 sprays of 0.05% solution in each nostril every 10 to 12 hours; for children age 2 to 6, 2 or 3 drops of 0.025% solution or drops in each nostril every 10 to 12 hours	• Oxymetazoline is contraindicated in a patient with known hypersensitivity. • This drug requires cautious use in a patient with hyperthyroidism, cardiac disease, hypertension, or diabetes mellitus.
phenylephrine (Neo-Synephrine, Nostril, Vicks Sinex)	ADULT: 2 or 3 sprays or drops in each nostril, repeated every 4 hours PEDIATRIC: for children age 12 and older, 2 or 3 sprays or drops of a 0.25 to 0.5% solution in each nostril, repeated every 4 hours; for children age 6 to 12, 2 or 3 sprays or drops of a 0.25% solution in each nostril, repeated every 4 hours	• Phenylephrine is contraindicated in patients with severe hypertension or ventricular tachycadia and hypersensitivity. • This drug requires cautious use in a geriatric patient or one with heart disease, hyperthyroidism, severe atherosclerosis, bradycardia, partial heart block, or sulfite sensitivity.

NURSING PROCESS APPLICATION

The following information assists the nurse in caring for a patient who is receiving guaifenesin. It includes an overview of assessment activities as well as examples of appropriate nursing diagnoses and related interventions. It also highlights the importance of evaluation.

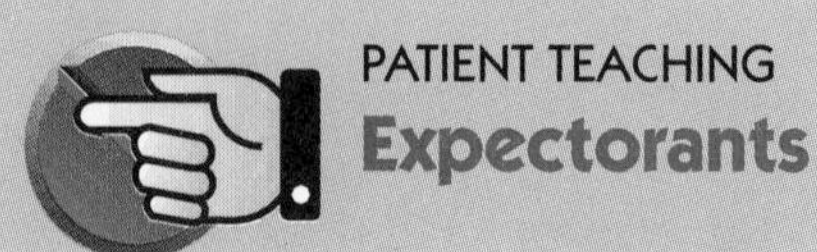

PATIENT TEACHING
Expectorants

- Teach the patient and family the name, dose, frequency, action, and adverse effects of guaifenesin.
- Stress the importance of taking the drug exactly as prescribed.
- Advise family members purchasing guaifenesin for a child to check with the pharmacist or physician if the pediatric dosage is unclear to them.
- Instruct the patient to avoid activities that require alertness if drowsiness occurs.
- Encourage the patient to increase fluid intake to eight to thirteen 8-oz (240-ml) glasses per day.
- Teach the patient to perform deep-breathing exercises and change positions frequently to help increase mucokinesis.
- Instruct the patient to notify the physician if adverse reactions occur or guaifenesin is ineffective.

Assessment

Before drug therapy begins, review the patient's history for conditions that contraindicate or require cautious use of guaifenesin. Also review the patient's medication history to identify use of drugs that may interact with it. During therapy, assess the patient for adverse drug reactions and signs of drug interactions. Also, periodically assess the effectiveness of guaifenesin therapy. Finally, evaluate the patient's and family's knowledge about the prescribed drug.

Nursing diagnoses

- Risk for injury related to a preexisting condition that contraindicates or requires cautious use of guaifenesin
- Risk for injury related to adverse drug reactions or drug interactions
- Knowledge deficit related to guaifenesin

Planning and implementation

- Do not administer guaifenesin to a patient with a condition that contraindicates its use.
- Administer guaifenesin cautiously to a patient at risk because of a preexisting condition.
- Monitor the patient closely for adverse reactions or drug interactions during guaifenesin therapy.

*** *Monitor the patient for dyspnea or ineffective cough. Keep suction equipment readily available during expectorant therapy.***

- Interpret 5-HIAA and VMA tests cautiously because guaifenesin may cause falsely elevated determinations.
- Notify the physician if adverse reactions or drug interactions occur.
- Teach the patient about the prescribed agent. (See Patient Teaching: *Expectorants.*)

Evaluation

For each nursing diagnosis, prepare an evaluation statement that describes the patient's or family's response to nursing interventions.

Antitussives

An antitussive is any agent that suppresses or inhibits coughing. The major antitussives include benzonatate, codeine, dextromethorphan hydrobromide, and hydrocodone bitartrate.

PHARMACOKINETICS

Antitussives are absorbed well through the GI tract, metabolized in the liver, and excreted in the urine.

The onset of action for codeine occurs in 30 minutes. Codeine and hydrocodone bitartrate reach peak concentrations in about 1 hour. Duration of action varies; codeine lasts about 4 hours, and hydrocodone bitartrate lasts between 4 and 6 hours. Codeine has a half-life of 2.5 to 3 hours; hydrocodone bitartrate, of 4 hours.

Benzonatate's and dextromethorphan's onset of action occurs in about 15 to 30 minutes. The duration of action for benzonatate ranges from 3 to 8 hours. For conventional dosage forms of dextromethorphan, it ranges from 3 to 6 hours; for sustained-release forms, up to 12 hours.

Route	Onset	Peak	Duration
P.O.	15-30 min	1 hr	3-12 hr

PHARMACODYNAMICS

Benzonatate, the peripherally acting antitussive, acts by anesthetizing cough receptors of vagal afferent fibers throughout the bronchi, alveoli, and pleura. Codeine, dextromethorphan, and hydrocodone bitartrate suppress the cough reflex by directly affecting the sensitivity of the cough center in the medulla to incoming stimuli.

PHARMACOTHERAPEUTICS

Antitussives are used to treat a serious, nonproductive cough that interferes with a patient's ability to rest or carry out activities of daily living.

Benzonatate, a nonnarcotic antitussive, relieves cough associated with such respiratory conditions as pneumonia, bronchitis, and the common cold, as well as with such chronic pulmonary diseases as emphysema. It also can be used as adjunctive treatment during bronchial diagnostic tests, such as bronchoscopy, when the patient must avoid coughing during the procedure.

The nonnarcotic antitussive dextromethorphan is the most widely used cough suppressant in the United States. Some data suggest that dextromethorphan may provide better antitussive activity than codeine. The popularity of dextromethorphan also may stem from the fact that the drug produces few adverse reactions. The narcotic antitussives are reserved for treating intractable cough, usually associated with lung cancer.

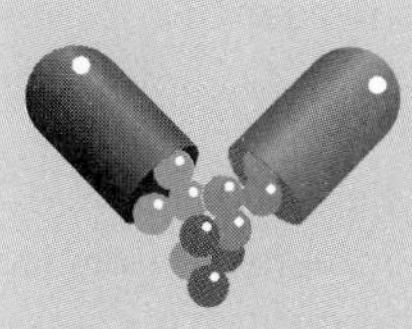

DRUG INTERACTIONS

Antitussives

Drug interactions involving centrally acting antitussives can be serious. The nurse must give special attention to patient teaching to prevent problems.

DRUG	INTERACTING AGENTS	POSSIBLE EFFECTS	NURSING IMPLICATIONS
codeine, hydrocodone bitartrate	monoamine oxidase (MAO) inhibitors (isocarboxazid, phenelzine, tranylcypromine)	Excitation, hypertension or hypotension, coma	• Instruct the patient to avoid concomitant use of these drugs.
codeine	central nervous system (CNS) depressants (alcohol, barbiturates, sedative-hypnotics, phenothiazines)	Increased CNS depressant effects (drowsiness, lethargy, stupor, respiratory depression, coma, death)	• Monitor the patient closely for CNS depression. • Instruct the patient to avoid concomitant use of these drugs.
dextromethorphan	MAO inhibitors (isocarboxazid, phenelzine, tranylcypromine)	Excitation, hyperpyrexia, hypotension, coma	• Instruct the patient to avoid concomitant use of these drugs.

Drug interactions

Benzonatate produces no significant drug interactions. Dextromethorphan may cause excitation and hyperpyrexia when taken with monoamine oxidase (MAO) inhibitors. The narcotic antitussives potentiate the depressant effects of MAO inhibitors, alcohol, and other central nervous system (CNS) depressants. (See Drug Interactions: *Antitussives.*)

ADVERSE DRUG REACTIONS

Benzonatate can cause dizziness, sedation, headache, nasal congestion, burning in the eyes, nausea, GI upset, constipation, and skin rash. "Chilly" sensations, skin eruptions, pruritus, and numbness in the chest also have been reported.

At recommended doses, adverse reactions rarely occur with dextromethorphan. Patients most commonly complain of drowsiness and GI upset.

Toxic doses of the narcotic antitussives can produce miosis, bradycardia, tachycardia, hypotension, narcosis, seizures, circulatory collapse, and respiratory arrest.

Antitussive doses of codeine seldom cause respiratory depression. However, the patient may experience an impaired ability to perform activities that require alertness or coordination. Repeated doses of codeine increase the risk of nausea, vomiting, constipation, dizziness, sedation, palpitations, pruritus, excessive perspiration, and agitation. Long-term use of codeine may result in physical dependence.

Usual oral antitussive doses of hydrocodone bitartrate do not produce adverse reactions in most cases. However, ambulatory patients may experience dizziness, sedation, nausea, and vomiting more so than nonambulatory patients. Rash, pruritus, constipation, euphoria, and dysphoria also can occur with hydrocodone bitartrate use.

Hypersensitivity reactions to benzonatate, codeine, and dextromethorphan are rare; however, urticaria, pruritus, rash, and facial swelling can result from codeine use. Hypersensitivity reactions to hydrocodone bitartrate can occur.

NURSING PROCESS APPLICATION

The following information assists the nurse in caring for a patient who is receiving an antitussive. It includes an overview of assessment activities as well as examples of appropriate nursing diagnoses and related interventions. It also highlights the importance of evaluation.

Assessment

Before drug therapy begins, review the patient's history for conditions that contraindicate or require cautious use of the prescribed antitussive. Also review the patient's medication history to identify use of drugs that may interact with it. During therapy, assess the patient for adverse drug reactions and signs of drug interactions. Also, periodically assess the effectiveness of antitussive therapy. Finally, evaluate the patient's and family's knowledge about the prescribed drug. (See Patient Teaching: *Antitussives,* page 340.)

Nursing diagnoses

- Risk for injury related to a preexisting condition that contraindicates or requires cautious use of an antitussive
- Risk for injury related to adverse drug reactions or drug interactions
- Constipation related to the adverse GI effects of the prescribed antitussive
- Knowledge deficit related to the prescribed antitussive

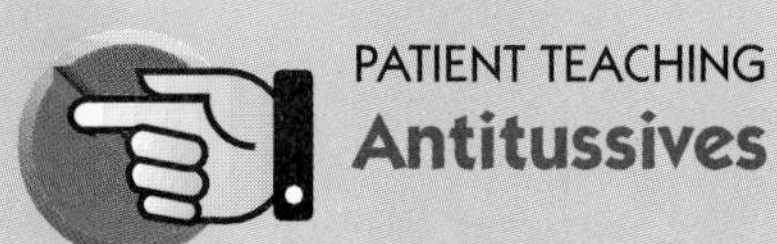

PATIENT TEACHING
Antitussives

- Teach the patient and family the name, dose, frequency, action, and adverse effects of the prescribed antitussive.
- Stress the importance of taking the antitussive exactly as prescribed. Tell the patient not to exceed the prescribed or recommended dosage to prevent toxicity.
- Caution the patient not to perform activities that require alertness if sedation or dizziness occurs.
- Instruct the patient to take a mild analgesic, as prescribed, if headache results from benzonatate use.
- Inform the patient that prolonged use of codeine can cause physical dependence.
- Teach the patient to recognize the signs of toxicity and, if these signs appear, to withhold the drug and notify the physician.
- Instruct the patient to swallow benzonatate capsules whole; the patient should not chew these capsules because the release of benzonatate in the mouth can anesthetize the oral mucosa.
- Instruct the patient to report persistent cough (lasting longer than 7 days) or a cough that changes from nonproductive to productive.
- Advise the patient to keep the antitussive out of the reach of children.
- Warn the patient about the potentially fatal additive effects of central nervous system depressants, such as alcohol, when combined with an antitussive.
- Teach the patient how to prevent constipation.
- Instruct the patient to notify the physician if adverse reactions occur or if the antitussive is ineffective.

Planning and implementation

- Do not administer an antitussive to a patient with a condition that contraindicates its use.
- Administer an antitussive cautiously to a patient at risk because of a preexisting condition.
- Monitor the patient closely for adverse reactions and drug interactions during antitussive therapy.

∗ ***Administer codeine with caution to a patient who also is receiving a CNS depressant; this combination can be fatal. Closely monitor the patient's level of consciousness to detect increased CNS depression.***

∗ ***Monitor for signs of respiratory depression, such as decreased respiratory rate, depth of respiration, and level of consciousness, in a patient receiving codeine.***

- Monitor for hypersensitivity reactions and toxic effects of narcotics in a patient taking codeine or hydrocodone bitartrate.
- Periodically assess the effectiveness of the prescribed antitussive.
- Notify the physician if adverse reactions or drug interactions occur or if the antitussive is ineffective.
- Encourage the patient to drink eight to thirteen 8-oz (240-ml) glasses of fluid daily, increase dietary fiber intake, and exercise regularly to prevent constipation.
- Obtain a prescription for a laxative, as needed, if constipation occurs.

Evaluation

For each nursing diagnosis, prepare an evaluation statement that describes the patient's or family's response to nursing interventions.

Mucolytics

The two types of mucolytics include thiol compounds and proteolytic enzymes. Acetylcysteine is the only thiol compound used clinically in the United States to treat patients with abnormal, viscid, or **inspissated** mucus. It also is used to treat acetaminophen overdose. Health care professionals rarely use the proteolytic enzymes because the expense and toxicity of these enzymes outweigh their minor therapeutic benefits.

PHARMACOKINETICS

Acetylcysteine is absorbed from the pulmonary epithelium and metabolized in the liver. Researchers do not know if acetylcysteine is secreted in breast milk.

The onset of action of acetylcysteine occurs 1 minute after inhalation and immediately after direct application or instillation. Maximal effect occurs in 5 to 10 minutes after inhalation. Additional data about peak concentration levels, duration of action, and half-life remain unavailable.

Route	Onset	Peak	Duration
Inhalation	1 min	5-10 min	Unknown

PHARMACODYNAMICS

Acetylcysteine decreases the viscosity of respiratory tract secretions by altering the molecular composition of mucus. The mechanism of action that occurs when acetylcysteine is used for acetaminophen (acetylcysteine metabolite) overdose has not been determined fully.

PHARMACOTHERAPEUTICS

Mucolytics are used as adjunctive therapy to treat patients with abnormal, viscid, or inspissated mucus secretions. Mucolytic therapy may benefit patients with bronchitis, emphysema, or pulmonary complications related to cystic fibrosis, as well as patients who develop atelectasis secondary to mucus obstruction, as may occur in pneumonia, bronchiectasis, or chronic bronchitis. Mucolytics also may be used to prepare patients for bronchograms and other bronchial studies. Acetylcysteine is the antidote for acetaminophen overdose; however, it does not provide full protection from hepatic damage caused by the overdose. This drug also is used for tracheostomy care.

Drug interactions

Acetylcysteine is incompatible with the following drugs: amphotericin B, chlortetracycline hydrochloride, erythromycin lactobionate, oxytetracycline hydrochloride, ampicillin sodium, tetracycline hydrochloride, iodized oil, hydrogen peroxide, chymotrypsin, and trypsin. The nurse should not administer any of these drugs during acetylcysteine therapy.

Activated charcoal decreases acetylcysteine's effectiveness. Therefore, in acetaminophen overdose, activated charcoal should be removed by gastric lavage before the oral administration of acetylcysteine.

ADVERSE DRUG REACTIONS

Acetylcysteine provides a wide margin of safety; however, its "rotten egg" odor during administration may lead to nausea. With prolonged or persistent use, acetylcysteine may produce stomatitis, nausea, vomiting, drowsiness, and severe rhinorrhea.

Hypersensitivity reactions rarely occur; however, a rash can develop with prolonged or frequent exposure to acetylcysteine. Patients may have **bronchorrhea,** which may cause increased airway obstruction for those who cannot expectorate effectively. **Bronchospasm** can occur, particularly in asthmatic patients. The frequency of this adverse reaction increases with the 20% solution. Because bronchospasm can occur unpredictably, the nurse must monitor patients closely during inhalation therapy.

NURSING PROCESS APPLICATION

The following information assists the nurse in caring for a patient who is receiving acetylcysteine. It includes an overview of assessment activities as well as examples of appropriate nursing diagnoses and related interventions. It also highlights the importance of evaluation.

Assessment

Before drug therapy begins, review the patient's history for conditions that contraindicate or require cautious use of acetylcysteine. Also review the patient's medication history to identify use of drugs that may interact with it. During therapy, assess the patient for adverse drug reactions and signs of drug interactions. Also, periodically assess the effectiveness of acetylcysteine therapy. Finally, evaluate the patient's and family's knowledge about the prescribed drug.

Nursing diagnoses

- Risk for injury related to a preexisting condition that contraindicates or requires cautious use of acetylcysteine
- Risk for injury related to adverse drug reactions or drug interactions
- Altered oral mucous membrane related to acetylcysteine-induced stomatitis
- Knowledge deficit related to acetylcysteine

Planning and implementation

- Do not administer acetylcysteine to a patient with a condition that contraindicates its use.
- Administer acetylcysteine cautiously to a patient at risk because of a preexisting condition.
- Monitor the patient closely for adverse reactions and drug interactions during acetylcysteine therapy.
- Prepare the patient for the drug's "rotten egg" smell, which may cause nausea.
- Administer acetylcysteine via nebulizer. Because acetylcysteine reacts with iron, copper, and rubber, frequently monitor the patient's nebulizer equipment for reactive effects. The drug does not react with glass, plastic, aluminum, or stainless steel.

*** *Be prepared to administer a beta$_2$-adrenergic agonist by aerosol, as prescribed, if the patient experiences bronchospasm.***

- Use 10% and 20% acetylcysteine solutions undiluted, as prescribed. If further dilution is needed, use normal saline solution or sterile water for injection. During continuous nebulization with dry gas, when three-fourths of the initial volume has been nebulized, dilute the remaining solution with an equal volume of sterile water for injection.
- Avoid contamination of the solution and refrigerate an opened vial; acetylcysteine does not contain an antimicrobial agent. Discard opened vials after 96 hours.
- Assess the patient's respiratory status before and after administration of each dose, particularly noting any breathing difficulty, ineffective cough, or dyspnea. Follow acetylcysteine administration with chest physiotherapy and postural drainage, as prescribed, and encourage coughing and deep breathing to facilitate removal of respiratory secretions. Suction the patient as needed.
- Have the patient gargle after administration to relieve the unpleasant odor and dryness; wash the patient's face to eliminate stickiness caused by the drug.
- Remove previously administered activated charcoal by gastric lavage before administering acetylcysteine when treating acetaminophen overdose, as prescribed. If the patient vomits within 1 hour of acetylcysteine administration, repeat the dose.
- Notify the physician if adverse reactions or drug interactions occur.
- Monitor the patient closely for signs of stomatitis, such as swollen, tender gums that bleed easily, papulovesicular ulcers in the mouth and throat, malaise, irritability, and fever.
- Rinse the patient's mouth with warm, water-based mouth solutions if stomatitis occurs. Avoid antiseptic mouthwashes, which are irritating. Obtain a prescription for a topical anesthetic to relieve mouth ulcer pain, as needed. Change the patient's diet to a bland or liquid diet until symptoms subside.
- Notify the physician if stomatitis occurs; acetylcysteine therapy may need to be discontinued.

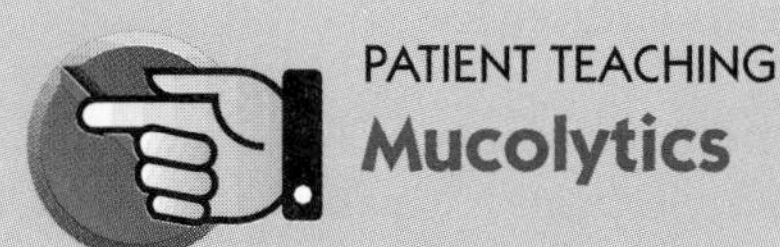

PATIENT TEACHING
Mucolytics

- Teach the patient and family the name, dose, frequency, action, and adverse effects of acetylcysteine.
- Advise the patient not to perform activities that require alertness if drowsiness occurs.
- Show the patient how to use and maintain the nebulizer.
- Teach the patient and family how to avoid contamination of the solution. Tell them that acetylcysteine may discolor to a light purple, but is still usable. Instruct the patient and family to refrigerate an opened vial and to discard it after 96 hours.
- Stress the importance of gargling after treatment to relieve odor; also inform the patient about effective coughing before and after each treatment. Teach the patient and family to perform chest physiotherapy and postural drainage after acetylcysteine administration, if prescribed.
- Teach the patient to recognize signs of stomatitis and, if they occur, to manage symptoms appropriately.
- Instruct the patient to seek medical help if the respiratory condition becomes progressively worse or if adverse reactions occur.

• Teach the patient about the prescribed agent. (See Patient Teaching: *Mucolytics.*)

Evaluation

For each nursing diagnosis, prepare an evaluation statement that describes the patient's or family's response to nursing interventions.

Decongestants

Decongestants may be classified as systemic decongestants or topical decongestants. As sympathomimetic amines, systemic decongestants activate the sympathetic division of the autonomic nervous system. The three major systemic decongestants are ephedrine, phenylpropanolamine, and pseudoephedrine. Topical decongestants are powerful **vasoconstrictors** and provide immediate relief from nasal congestion and swollen mucous membranes when applied directly to the nasal mucosa. Topical decongestants include sympathomimetic amines (ephedrine, epinephrine, phenylephrine, and propylhexedrine) and imidazoline derivatives of sympathomimetic amines (naphazoline, oxymetazoline, tetrahydrozoline, and xylometazoline).

PHARMACOKINETICS

The systemic decongestants discussed in this chapter are absorbed readily from the GI tract after oral intake. They are distributed widely throughout the body into various tissues and fluids, including the cerebrospinal fluid, placenta, and breast milk. Slowly and incompletely metabolized by the liver, they are excreted largely unchanged in the urine within 24 hours after oral administration.

After oral administration of the systemic decongestants, the onset of nasal decongestion is 15 to 30 minutes, peaking within 60 to 90 minutes. The duration of action is 3 to 6 hours for tablets and syrups, and 8 to 12 hours for sustained-release capsules and tablets. For ephedrine and pseudoephedrine, respectively, the half-life is 3 hours with a urine pH of 5, and about 6 hours with a pH of 6.3. Phenylpropanolamine has a half-life of 3 to 4 hours.

Topical decongestants act directly on the alpha receptors of the nasal vascular smooth muscle, thereby constricting arterioles and reducing blood flow in the edematous membranes. As a result of this direct vasoconstriction, vascular absorption becomes negligible.

Onset of action rapidly follows the application of topical decongestants. Drug action then peaks quickly. Sympathomimetic agents provide symptomatic relief within seconds, peaking in 2 to 4 minutes with a 30-minute to 2-hour duration of action. Imidazoline derivatives of the sympathomimetic amines provide relief from nasal congestion within 5 to 10 minutes after application. Their effects last 3 to 10 hours, depending on the preparation.

Route	Onset	Peak	Duration
P.O.	15-30 min	60-90 min	3-12 hr
Topical	Seconds	2-10 min	0.5-10 hr

PHARMACODYNAMICS

The systemic decongestants, ephedrine, phenylpropanolamine, and pseudoephedrine act directly and indirectly. When taken orally, the drugs act directly on alpha-adrenergic receptors in the nasal mucosa and elsewhere, causing contraction of urinary and GI sphincters, mydriasis, and decreased pancreatic beta cell secretion. The major activity of these drugs, however, occurs indirectly and results in norepinephrine release from storage sites in the body. The release of norepinephrine, a catecholamine, together with the direct action on receptors, produces vasoconstriction and nasal decongestion.

Topical decongestants stimulate alpha-adrenergic receptors in nasal vascular smooth muscle, which results in increased alpha-adrenergic activity and vasoconstriction. The subsequent reduction in nasal mucosal blood flow, together with decreased capillary permeability, decreases the edema associated with inflammation. The action of topical decongestants also helps drain sinuses, clear nasal passages, and open eustachian tubes, temporarily improving aeration.

PHARMACOTHERAPEUTICS

Systemic decongestants are indicated for the symptomatic relief of swollen nasal membranes resulting from hay fever, allergic rhinitis, vasomotor rhinitis, acute coryza, sinusitis, and the common cold. Ephedrine, phenylpropanolamine,

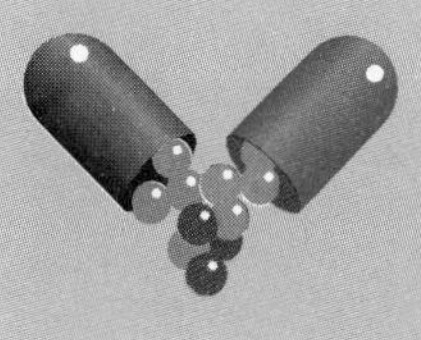

DRUG INTERACTIONS
Decongestants

Systemic decongestants potentiate the effect of sympathetic nervous system–stimulating drugs and interact with monoamine oxidase (MAO) inhibitors, releasing large amounts of stored norepinephrine. Drug interactions associated with topical decongestants are few but can cause major problems for the patient.

DRUG	INTERACTING AGENTS	POSSIBLE EFFECTS	NURSING IMPLICATIONS
Systemic decongestants			
ephedrine, phenylpropanolamine, pseudoephedrine	other sympathomimetic amines, including epinephrine, norepinephrine, dopamine, dobutamine, isoproterenol, metaproterenol, terbutaline, phenylephrine, tyramine	Increased central nervous system (CNS) stimulation	• Do not administer drugs concurrently because the interaction can be life-threatening.
	MAO inhibitors	Severe hypertension or hypertensive crisis	• Do not administer drugs concurrently because the interaction can be life-threatening.
pseudoephedrine	alkalinizing agents	Decreased urinary excretion of pseudoephedrine	• Monitor the patient for signs of increased pseudoephedrine effect, such as excessively dry nasal passages.
Topical decongestants			
ephedrine, epinephrine, naphazoline, oxymetazoline, phenylephrine, propylhexedrine, tetrahydrozoline, xylometazoline	MAO inhibitors	Increased CNS stimulation, increased hypertension, hypertensive crisis	• Do not administer drugs concurrently.
	beta-adrenergic blockers, methyldopa, reserpine, guanethidine, tricyclic antidepressants	Decreased hypotensive drug action	• Do not administer drugs concurrently. • Monitor the patient for changes in blood pressure control.

and pseudoephedrine are administered orally, frequently with other drugs, such as antihistamines, antimuscarinics, antipyretic-analgesics, caffeine, and antitussives. The topical decongestants serve as alternatives to these systemic drugs. They provide two major advantages: minimal adverse reactions and rapid relief of symptoms.

Drug interactions

When given concurrently with other drugs, systemic decongestants may result in one of three different types of drug interactions. The first type of interaction may occur with the simultaneous administration of two or more drugs having opposing effects. Under these circumstances, the effects of one drug override the intended effects of the second.

A second type of interaction between drugs occurs when systemic decongestants are administered with other sympathomimetic amines. This interaction causes additive or cumulative drug effects, and potentiates the adverse effects of both drugs.

The third type of drug interaction occurs with concurrent administration of drugs that interfere with the excretion of sympathomimetic amines. Because the excretion of pseudoephedrine and ephedrine sulfate depends on urine acidity, the nurse needs to monitor drugs that alter urine pH. In the presence of alkaline urine, renal tubular reabsorption of these sympathomimetic amines increases.

Because of the topical drug route and vasoconstrictor action, which decrease drug absorption, drug interactions involving topical decongestants seldom occur. (See Drug Interactions: *Decongestants.*)

ADVERSE DRUG REACTIONS

The incidence and severity of adverse drug reactions depends primarily on the patient's sensitivity to decongestants and, with topical decongestants, on the duration of action and frequency of drug use as well. Patients hypersensitive to other sympathomimetic amines may also be hypersensitive to decongestants.

For nonsensitive patients, the incidence of adverse reactions with systemic decongestants is low. The most common adverse reactions result from CNS stimulation and in-

Patient positioning for instilling nasal and sinus drops

Obtain a box of tissues and the ordered medication. After identifying the patient and explaining the procedure and medication, help the patient assume the appropriate position. The illustrations below show proper head positioning based on the area of congestion. For drops, place the patient in the head low or supine position with the head supported by a pillow. With incorrect patient positioning, the drops will run down the back of the throat and be ineffective. When instilling sprays, the patient should be upright. For drops, place the dropper ⅓" to ½" (0.8 to 1.3 cm) inside the nostril, being careful to avoid touching the dropper to the nostril. Squeeze the dropper bulb to deliver the prescribed number of drops. Instruct the patient to remain in this position for 5 minutes to prevent the medication from running out of the nostrils. Repeat on the opposite side if necessary.

Eustachian tubes. Have the patient turn the head laterally to the affected side.

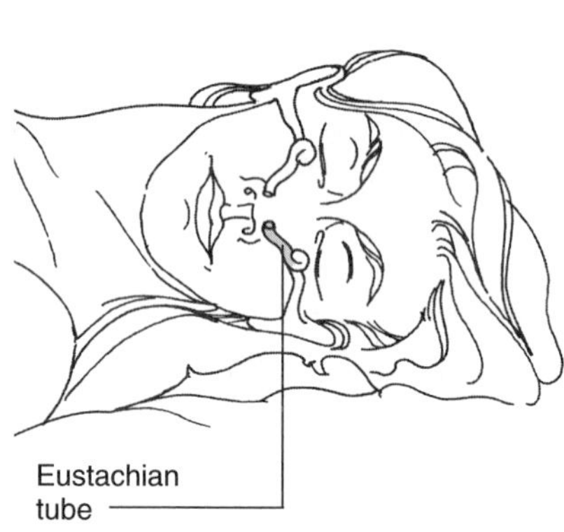

Sphenoid or ethmoid sinuses. Have the patient hyperextend the neck over a pillow.

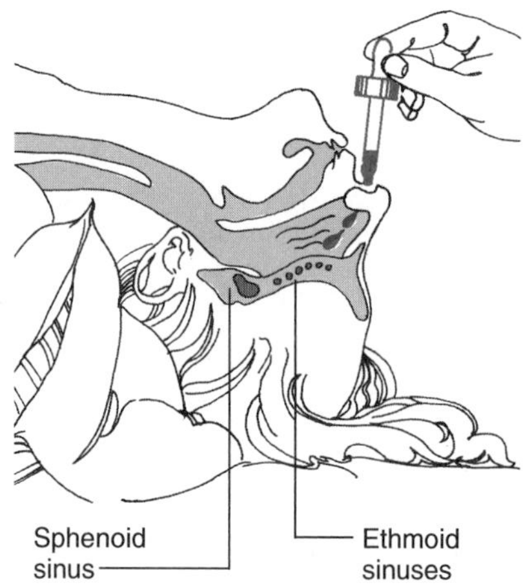

Maxillary and frontal sinuses. Have the patient rotate the head laterally after hyperextension.

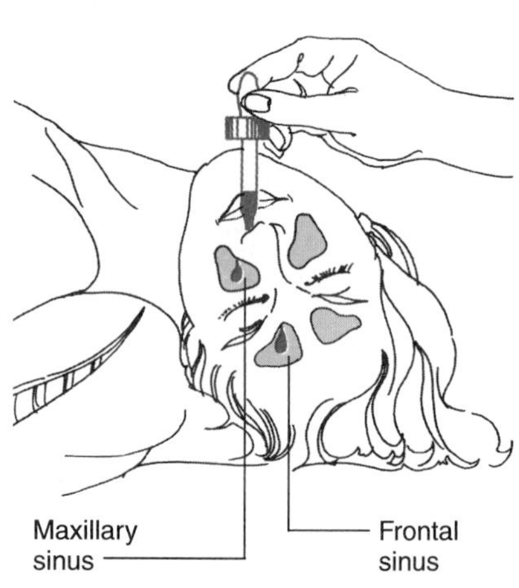

clude nervousness, restlessness, and insomnia. Nausea, palpitations, increased difficulty in urinating, and dose-related elevations in blood pressure occasionally occur.

The most commonly reported adverse reaction associated with prolonged use (more than 3 to 5 days) of topical decongestants is rebound nasal congestion. (See *Patient positioning for instilling nasal and sinus drops.*) The disorder is characterized by hyperemia of the nasal mucosa, which appears red, boggy, and swollen. The rebound nasal congestion usually resolves spontaneously within a few days after discontinuation of the topical decongestant.

The second most frequent adverse reaction is a transient burning and stinging of the nasal mucosa upon application. Patients also report sneezing and mucosal dryness or ulceration.

Less common adverse reactions result from CNS stimulation and include nervousness, restlessness, and insomnia. Occasionally, nausea, palpitations, increased difficulty in urinating, and dose-related elevations in blood pressure occur. These effects more commonly are associated with administration of epinephrine, ephedrine, phenylephrine, and propylhexedrine.

Other adverse reactions to systemic and topical decongestants may include first-time drug hypersensitivity reactions, irregular heartbeat or tachycardia, feeling of tightness in the chest, hallucinations, seizures, headache, greatly elevated blood pressure, and teratogenic effects.

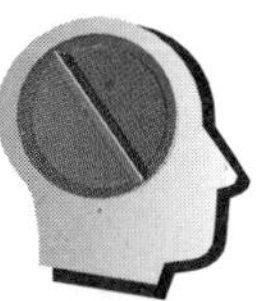

CRITICAL THINKING: To enhance your critical thinking about expectorant, antitussive, mucolytic, and decongestant agents, consider the following situation and its analysis.

Situation: For the past 2 days, Alice Thompson, age 63, has had a productive cough that interferes with her sleep. Ms. Thompson asks her nurse practitioner what type of cough preparation to take that will let her "get some sleep." She says that there are so many cough products in the drug store that she doesn't know what to buy. How should the nurse respond?

Analysis: The nurse could tell Ms. Thompson to try an over-the-counter product that contains guaifenesin, such as Robitussin, to help liquefy her respiratory secretions. The nurse should advise her to take this medication throughout the day as directed on the label. Alternatively, the nurse may suggest that Ms. Thompson take a combination product that contains guaifenesin and dextromethorpan, such as Robitussin DM. The dextromethorpan in this preparation will help to depress the cough center during the night. Also, the nurse should remind the patient to increase her fluid intake to 2 to 3 liters per day to further help liquefy her respiratory secretions.

NURSING PROCESS APPLICATION

The following information assists the nurse in caring for a patient who is receiving a decongestant. It includes an overview of assessment activities as well as examples of appropriate nursing diagnoses and related interventions. It also highlights the importance of evaluation.

Assessment

Before drug therapy begins, review the patient's history for conditions that contraindicate or require cautious use of the prescribed decongestant. Also review the patient's medication history to identify use of drugs that may interact with it. During therapy, assess the patient for adverse drug reactions and signs of drug interactions. Also, periodically assess the effectiveness of decongestant therapy. Finally, evaluate the patient's and family's knowledge about the prescribed drug. (See Patient Teaching: *Decongestants.*)

Nursing diagnoses

- Risk for injury related to a preexisting condition that contraindicates or requires cautious use of a decongestant
- Risk for injury related to adverse drug reactions or drug interactions
- Urinary retention related to the adverse genitourinary effects of the prescribed systemic decongestant
- Impaired tissue integrity related to mucosal dryness and ulcerations caused by the prescribed topical decongestant
- Knowledge deficit related to the prescribed decongestant

Planning and implementation

- Do not administer a decongestant to a patient with a condition that contraindicates its use.
- Administer a decongestant cautiously to a patient at risk because of a preexisting condition.
- Monitor the patient closely for adverse reactions and drug interactions during decongestant therapy.
- Discourage the use of over-the-counter decongestants in a patient who is hypersensitive to other sympathomimetic amines. Such a patient also may be hypersensitive to decongestants.

***** ***Monitor the patient's blood pressure, pulse, and electrocardiogram, as instructed, particularly noting hypertension and an irregular heartbeat or tachycardia.***

***** ***Take seizure precautions during decongestant therapy.***

- Notify the physician if the patient uses drugs that alter urine pH because alkaline urine increases renal tubular reabsorption of sympathomimetic amines.
- Do not administer an MAO inhibitor, a beta-adrenergic blocker, methyldopa, reserpine, or guanethidine concomitantly with a topical decongestant.
- Warn the patient that transient burning and stinging of the nasal mucosa may occur during administration of the topical decongestant.

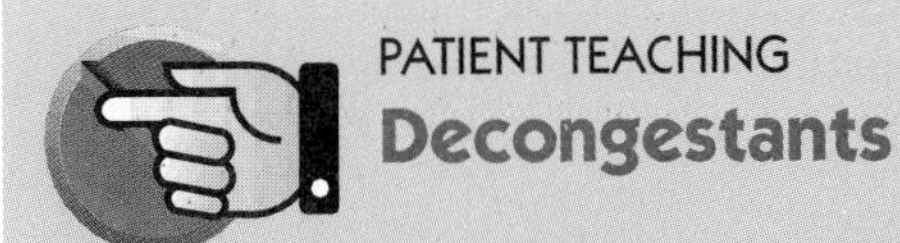

PATIENT TEACHING

Decongestants

- Teach the patient and family the name, dose, frequency, action, and adverse effects of the prescribed decongestant.
- Teach the patient to recognize and report to the physician any adverse reactions because a dosage change may be needed.
- Remind the patient not to exceed the recommended amount, frequency, and duration of use because rebound nasal congestion may occur after the vasoconstrictor effect subsides. Warn the patient that increasing the amount or frequency of decongestant use may increase the severity or frequency of adverse reactions or worsen rebound nasal congestion. Caution the patient about taking other over-the-counter products that may interact with the decongestant.
- Encourage avoidance of decongestants if the patient is pregnant or breast-feeding (only with systemic decongestants) or has a condition that contraindicates their use. Such a patient should ask the physician to recommend an appropriate decongestant.
- Inform the patient that a decongestant may interfere with sleep, and suggest taking the drug a few hours before bedtime to minimize insomnia.
- Instruct the patient to use the drug in its complete form when taking sustained-release capsules or long-acting tablets. The patient should not break, cut, crush, or chew the capsule or tablet.
- Teach the patient receiving a topical decongestant to minimize central nervous system–stimulating effects through proper administration: in the lateral head low position for drops, in the upright position for sprays. Instruct the patient who is using a decongestant to relieve blocked eustachian tubes to instill the drops by lying supine with the head turned 15 degrees toward the affected ear. Explain that the drops instilled in the affected nasal passage should be allowed to flow along the floor of the nose to the low point, where they will collect. The low point marks the entrance of the eustachian tube. Instruct the patient to remain in this position for 5 minutes. When both sides require treatment, advise the patient to repeat the procedure on the second side after the 5-minute wait.
- Instruct the patient to use a humidifier if nasal dryness occurs, and to discontinue the drug if mucosal ulceration occurs.

- Inspect the patient receiving a topical decongestant for signs of rebound nasal congestion, such as red, swollen, boggy nasal mucosa. If rebound nasal congestion occurs, withhold the drug and notify the physician. Obtain a prescription for normal saline nasal spray, as needed.
- Administer topical decongestant drops correctly.
- Notify the physician if adverse reactions or drug interactions occur.
- Encourage the patient taking a decongestant to report difficulty urinating, which is especially common in patients with prostatic hypertrophy.
- Palpate the bladder after the patient voids to detect urine retention.
- Notify the physician if the patient develops urine retention.

- Inspect the patient's oral and nasal mucosa regularly for ulceration, if a topical decongestant is being used.
- Encourage the patient to use a humidifier if nasal dryness occurs.
- Withhold the topical decongestant if the patient's tissue integrity becomes impaired.
- Notify the physician if the patient's tissue integrity becomes impaired.

Evaluation

For each nursing diagnosis, prepare an evaluation statement that describes the patient's or family's response to nursing interventions.

CHAPTER SUMMARY

Chapter 26 focused on expectorants, antitussives, mucolytics, and decongestants. Here are the chapter highlights.

The expectorant, guaifenesin, is administered to patients who experience difficulty expectorating sputum or who retain respiratory tract secretions.

Narcotic and nonnarcotic antitussives are used to treat a nonproductive cough that is irritating and exhausting. The most widely used antitussive in the United States is dextromethorphan.

The mucolytic, acetylcysteine, is used to facilitate sputum expectoration and to unblock airways that are plugged with mucus. Acetylcysteine is also the antidote for acetaminophen overdose.

Decongestants may be classified according to their route of administration: systemic or topical. As sympathomimetic amines, systemic decongestants activate the sympathetic division of the autonomic nervous system; they are administered orally. Topical decongestants are powerful vasoconstrictors and include sympathomimetic amines and imidazoline derivatives of sympathomimetic amines.

When caring for a patient receiving an expectorant, antitussive, mucolytic, or decongestant, the nurse should apply the nursing process. Appropriate care includes observing the patient for adverse drug reactions and providing comprehensive information to the patient and family about the prescribed drug.

Questions to consider

See Appendix 1 for answers.

1. James Lewis, age 48, has influenza. His physician prescribes guaifenesin (Breonesin) 200 mg P.O. every 4 hours. The nurse cautions Mr. Lewis not to exceed the dosage prescribed. Which of the following adverse reactions can occur if guaifenesin is taken in larger doses than necessary?
   (a) Bronchospasm
   (b) Vomiting
   (c) Insomnia
   (d) Constipation

2. The nurse has just finished teaching Martin Lemaine, age 42, about using guaifenesin. Which of the following statements by this patient indicates that he understands what he was taught?
   (a) I should sip the medication whenever I need it — every hour, if necessary.
   (b) I should drink at least 2 qt (2 L) of fluid every day.
   (c) I should make sure that I don't drink more than a pint of fluid each day.
   (d) I should rinse my mouth after each dose so the drug doesn't discolor my teeth.

3. Donna Ortiz, age 33, has a nonproductive cough that awakens her at night. Which of the following antitussive agents is the physician most likely to order for her?
   (a) codeine
   (b) hydrocodone
   (c) benzonatate
   (d) dextromethorphan

4. Rhonda Goldstein, age 36, is taking an antitussive product that contains dextromethorphan. Which of the following medications should she avoid when taking dextromethorphan?
   (a) acetaminophen
   (b) guaifenesin
   (c) phenelzine
   (d) oxymetazoline hydrochloride

5. William Elkins, age 64, has emphysema. His physician prescribes acetylcysteine (Mucomyst) via nebulizer. Acetylcysteine also may be used to treat which of the following other conditions?
   (a) Acetaminophen overdose
   (b) Severe rhinorrhea
   (c) Hepatic tumor
   (d) Stomatitis

6. Kim Luk, age 27, has chronic rhinitis. Her physician prescribes 2 sprays of oxymetazoline 0.0.5% solution in each nostril b.i.d. Which of the following adverse reactions most commonly occurs with a decongestant like oxymetazoline?
   (a) Nausea
   (b) Dizziness
   (c) Epistaxis
   (d) Rebound nasal congestion

UNIT IX

Drugs to improve gastrointestinal function

The gastrointestinal (GI) tract has three major functions: digestion of foods and fluids, absorption of foods and fluids, and excretion of metabolic waste. In the GI tract, various hormones and enzymes break down food into particles that are small enough to permeate cell membranes and be used for cellular energy. The GI tract itself helps prevent infection by maintaining mucous membrane integrity, secreting immunoglobulins, and destroying pathogens.

Many GI disorders disrupt activities of daily living, interrupt work schedules, and lead to hospital admissions. They may result from such diseases as benign or malignant tumors, peptic ulcer disease, gastroesophageal reflux, regional ileitis (Crohn's disease), ulcerative colitis, malabsorption, intestinal obstruction, or diverticulosis, or they may stem from stress or other psychological problems. No matter what the cause, however, GI disorders usually produce similar signs and symptoms that typically are so vague and nonspecific that many patients delay seeking treatment.

Common signs and symptoms of GI tract disorders include anorexia, dysphagia, nausea, vomiting, dyspepsia, epigastric or abdominal pain, abdominal distention, flatulence, diarrhea, constipation, and rectal bleeding. These findings may suggest many possible causes. GI tract disorders may cause fluid and electrolyte imbalances with resultant cardiac arrhythmias and hypovolemia, extended areas of inflammation or infection, abscesses or fistulas, malnutrition, perforated structures with resultant peritonitis, and altered body image.

Medical management of GI disorders is usually conservative, symptomatic, and supportive. Initial treatment typically consists of diet therapy, rest, and stress management. If these measures prove ineffective, drug therapy or surgery may be used. There are two general categories of drug therapy: (1) treatment of such specific diseases as digestive enzyme deficiencies, hepatic encephalopathy, acute toxic poisoning, peptic ulcer disease, and gastroesophageal reflux; and (2) control of symptoms of specific diseases, such as **nausea, vomiting, epigastric pain, dyspepsia, flatulence, diarrhea,** and **constipation.**

Various drugs are used to treat these diseases and symptoms. **Antacids**, histamine$_2$–receptor antagonists, and other **peptic ulcer agents** are used to treat peptic **ulcers.** These agents neutralize acid in the GI tract, reduce acid secretion, bind to and protect ulcers, or block the mechanism that maintains gastric acidity in the parietal cells.

Adsorbents are used to help manage poisonings. By binding with toxins in the intestinal lumen, they inhibit absorption from the GI tract. **Antiflatulents** are prescribed to treat conditions associated with excess gas, such as functional gastric bloating or diverticulitis. They act by dispersing and preventing the formation of gas pockets. Digestive agents (**digestants**) aid digestion in patients who lack one or more of the specific substances that naturally digest food. They achieve this effect by mimicking the action of these body substances.

Antidiarrheal agents correct diarrhea in various ways. **Laxatives** and **cathartics,** prescribed to treat constipation and to evacuate the bowel, increase the water content of the feces and movement of intestinal materials.

Antiemetics act in various ways to relieve nausea and vomiting from motion sickness, chemotherapy, and other causes. **Emetics** are used primarily to induce vomiting in poisonings. They do this by stimulating the vomiting center in the brain.

Many of the drugs in these categories are available over the counter, so self-medication is common.

27 Peptic ulcer agents

OBJECTIVES

After reading and studying this chapter, the student should be able to:

1. differentiate among the ways in which antacids, histamine$_2$ (H_2)-receptor antagonists, and other agents decrease peptic ulcer formation.

2. discuss the use of antibiotics in the treatment of peptic ulcers.

3. discuss which peptic ulcer agents are the treatment of choice for both duodenal and gastric ulcers.

4. discuss the adverse reactions associated with antacids, H_2-receptor antagonists, antibiotics, and other peptic ulcer agents.

5. describe how to apply the nursing process when caring for a patient who is receiving a peptic ulcer agent.

INTRODUCTION

The treatment of peptic **ulcers** is directed at the imbalance between acid and **pepsin** secretion and the gastrointestinal (GI) mucosal defense mechanisms or toward the eradication of the *Helicobacter pylori* bacteria. Peptic ulcer agents include **antacids, H_2-receptor antagonists, antibiotics,** and other peptic ulcer agents, such as misoprostol, omeprazole, lansoprazole and sucralfate. (See *Selected major peptic ulcer agents.*)

Drugs covered in this chapter include:

- aluminum hydroxide with simethicone
- amoxicillin
- bismuth citrate
- bismuth subsalicylate
- calcium carbonate
- cimetidine
- clarithromycin
- famotidine
- lansoprazole
- magaldrate or aluminum-magnesium complex
- magnesium hydroxide
- metronidazole
- misoprostol
- nizatidine
- omeprazole
- ranitidine
- sucrafate
- tetracycline.

Antibiotics

H. pylori is a gram-negative bacteria that is thought to be a major causative factor in gastritis and in the formation of duodenal and gastric ulcers. Successful treatment involves the use of antibiotics either alone or in combination. (See *Common drug regimens to eradicate* Helicobacter pylori, page 351.) Eradication of the bacteria promotes ulcer healing and decreases their recurrence.

PHARMACOKINETICS

Metronidazole, tetracycline, clarithromycin, and amoxicillin are systemic antibiotics. All are absorbed from the GI tract to varying extent, but sufficiently to produce serum concentrations effective against *H. pylori.* Food, especially dairy products, will decrease the absorption of tetracycline, but does not significantly delay the absorption of the other antibiotics. All of these antibiotics are distributed widely and are excreted primarily in the urine.

The bismuth component of bismuth subsalicylate and bismuth citrate is relatively insoluble and not absorbed from the GI tract. The salicylate is well absorbed with plasma levels similar to that seen in aspirin. Both agents produce their anti-infective activity locally, so absorption is neither necessary nor desired. These drugs are distributed throughout the GI tract and are eliminated in the feces.

PHARMACODYNAMICS

The antibiotics act by treating the *H. pylori* infection. They are usually combined with an H_2-receptor antagonist or an acid pump inhibitor to decrease stomach acidity and promote healing. Bismuth provides a protective coating that prevents back diffusion of gastric acid in ulcer disease as well as provides a direct antibacterial action against *H. pylori.*

PHARMACOTHERAPEUTICS

Various combinations of antimicrobial drugs with either an H_2-receptor antagonist or an acid pump inhibitor have been studied. Regimens that have included the 1- to 2-week administration of at least two antimicrobial drugs that are active against *H. pylori* have been successful in eradicating

Selected major peptic ulcer agents

The following chart summarizes the major peptic ulcer agents currently in clinical use.

DRUG	MAJOR INDICATIONS AND USUAL DOSAGES	CONTRAINDICATIONS AND PRECAUTIONS
Antacids		
magaldrate or aluminum-magnesium complex (Riopan, Riopan Plus); magnesium hydroxide and aluminum hydroxide with simethicone (Maalox-Plus, Mylanta-II, Gelusil-II) calcium carbonate (TUMS, Alka-mints)	*Symptomatic and therapeutic treatment of peptic ulcer disease* ADULT: 15 to 60 ml of suspension P.O. with water, 1 to 3 hours after meals and h.s. *Treatment of heartburn, acid indigestion* ADULT: 500 mg P.O. t.i.d. with meals.	• Magnesium-containing antacids are contraindicated in a patient with renal failure. • Aluminum-containing antacids require cautious use in a patient with renal failure. • Calcium carbonate should be used with caution in individuals with renal calculi and in conditions of hypercalcemia or hypophosphatemia. • Calcium carbonate should be used with caution in patients taking digitalis preparations. • Aluminum-containing antacids require cautious use in a patient with renal failure.
Histamine$_2$–receptor antagonists		
cimetidine (Tagamet)	*Treatment and prevention of peptic ulcer disease* ADULT: 800 mg P.O. daily h.s. or 300 mg P.O. or I.V. every 6 to 8 hours, up to a maximum of 2.4 g in 24 hours for 4 to 8 weeks; maintenance dosage, 400 mg P.O. h.s. PEDIATRIC: 20 to 40 mg/kg P.O. or I.V. daily in divided doses *Treatment of heartburn, acid indigestion* ADULT: 200 mg P.O. p.r.n.; maximum of 400 mg in 24 hours	• Cimetidine is contraindicated in a breast-feeding patient or one with known hypersensitivity. • This drug requires cautious use in a pregnant or geriatric patient or one with impaired renal or hepatic function. • Cimetidine should not be administered to children under age 16 unless the anticipated benefits outweigh the potential risks.
famotidine (Pepcid)	*Treatment and prevention of peptic ulcer disease* ADULT: 20 mg P.O. b.i.d. with the second dose h.s., 40 mg P.O. h.s., or 20 mg I.V. every 12 hours; maintenance dosage, 20 m P.O. h.s. *Treatment of heartburn, acid indigestion* ADULT: 10 mg P.O. p.r.n.; maximum of 20 mg in 24 hours	• Famotidine is contraindicated in a breast-feeding patient or one with known hypersensitivity. • This drug requires cautious use in a pregnant patient. • Safety and efficacy in children have not been established.
nizatidine (Axid)	*Treatment and prevention of peptic ulcer disease* ADULT: 300 mg P.O. h.s. or 150 mg P.O. b.i.d.; maintenance dosage, 150 mg P.O. h.s. *Treatment of heartburn, acid indigestion* ADULT: 75 mg P.O. p.r.n.; maximum of 150 mg in 24 hours	• Nizatidine is contraindicated in a breast-feeding patient or one with known hypersensitivity to this drug or other histamine$_2$–receptor antagonists. • This drug requires cautious use in a pregnant patient or one with impaired renal function. • Safety and efficacy in children have not been established.
ranitidine (Zantac)	*Treatment and prevention of peptic ulcer disease* ADULT: 150 mg P.O. b.i.d. with the second dose h.s., 300 mg P.O. h.s., or 50 mg I.V. or I.M. every 6 to 8 hours; maintenance dosage, 150 mg P.O. h.s. *Treatment of heartburn, acid indigestion* ADULT: 75 mg P.O. once or twice daily	• Ranitidine is contraindicated in a patient with known hypersensitivity. • This drug requires cautious use in a pregnant or breast-feeding patient or one with hepatic dysfunction. • Safety and efficacy in children under age 12 have not been established.
Other peptic ulcer agents		
bismuth subsalicylate (Pepto Bismol)	*Treatment of Helicobacter pylori* ADULT: 2 tablets (262 mg) or 30 ml suspension P.O. q.i.d. PEDIATRIC: 1 tablet or 15 ml suspension P.O. q.i.d.	• Contraindicated in presence of viral infections in children age 18 or under and in patients with aspirin allergy. • Use cautiously in infants and debilitated patients.

(continued)

Selected major peptic ulcer agents *(continued)*

DRUG	MAJOR INDICATIONS AND USUAL DOSAGES	CONTRAINDICATIONS AND PRECAUTIONS
Other peptic ulcer agents *(continued)*		
lansoprazole (Prevacid)	*Treatment of duodenal ulcer* ADULT: 15 mg once daily for 4 weeks *Treatment of erosive esophagitis* ADULT: 30 mg once daily for up to 8 weeks; may repeat for 8 more weeks; maintenance is 15 mg once daily *Treatment of hypersecretory conditions* ADULT: initially, 60 mg once daily; maximum is 90 mg twice daily; dosage of this drug should be reduced cases of hepatic impairment	• Lansoprazole is contraindicated in patients with known hypersensitivity. • Use cautiously in patients with hepatic impairment. • Safety and efficacy in children have not been established.
misoprostol (Cytotec)	*Prevention of nonsteroidal anti-inflammatory drug–induced gastric ulcers* ADULT: 200 mcg P.O. q.i.d. with food or, if the patient cannot tolerate this dosage, 100 mcg P.O. q.i.d.	• Misoprostol is contraindicated in a pregnant or breast-feeding patient or one with a history of allergies to prostaglandins. • Safety and efficacy in children have not been established.
omeprazole (Prilosec)	*Treatment of severe erosive or symptomatic esophagitis* ADULT: 20 mg P.O. daily for 4 to 8 weeks *Treatment of pathologic hypersecretory conditions* ADULT: initially, 60 mg P.O. daily, with dosage adjusted based on the severity of the condition *Treatment of gastric ulcers* ADULT: 40 mg once daily for 4 to 8 weeks *Treatment of duodenal ulcer* ADULT: 20 mg once daily for 4 weeks; may continue for 4 more weeks	• Omeprazole is contraindicated in a patient with known hypersensitivity to this drug or any of its components. • This drug requires cautious use in a pregnant or breast-feeding patient. • Safety and efficacy in children have not been established.
sucralfate (Carafate)	*Short-term treatment and prevention of duodenal ulcers* ADULT: 1 g P.O. q.i.d. for 4 to 8 weeks; maintenance dosage, 1 g P.O. b.i.d.	• Sucralfate requires cautious use in a pregnant or breast-feeding patient or one with chronic renal failure. • Safety and efficacy in children have not been established.

the organism in 60% to 90% of patients. Clarithromycin as a single antibiotic plus omeprazole, followed by 2 or more weeks of omeprazole, is equally effective. The bismuth agents promote healing and also are effective in treatment of gastroesophageal reflux and diarrhea.

Drug interactions

Tetracycline and metronidazole can interact with many other medications. Clarithromycin may decrease the metabolism and increase the serum concentration of the nonsedating antihistamines terfenadine and astemizole, which may lead to serious ventricular arrhythmias.

ADVERSE DRUG REACTIONS

Metronidazole, clarithromycin, and tetracycline commonly cause mild GI disturbances. Clarithromycin may also cause taste disturbances. Amoxicillin may cause diarrhea. Bismuth subsalicylate temporarily turns the tongue and stool black and may cause tinnitus. Bismuth toxicity can cause encephalopathy and osteodystrophy.

NURSING PROCESS APPLICATION

The following information assists the nurse in caring for a patient who is receiving antibiotics or bismuth products for the treatment of peptic ulcers. It includes an overview of assessment activities as well as examples of appropriate nurs-

Common drug regimens to eradicate *Helicobacter pylori*

This chart shows four common oral regimens used to treat *Helicobactor pylori* infections.

REGIMEN	DOSAGE	DURATION
1. Bismuth subsalicylate metronidazole tetracycline ranitidine	525 mg q.i.d. 250 mg q.i.d. 500 mg q.i.d. 150 mg b.i.d.	2 weeks
2. First, clarithromycin and omeprazole	500 mg t.i.d. 40 mg daily	2 weeks
Then omeprazole alone	20 mg daily	2 weeks
3. Clarithromycin omeprazole (or lansoprazole 15 mg b.i.d.) metronidazole (or amoxicillin 1 g b.i.d.)	500 mg b.i.d. 20 mg b.i.d. 500 mg b.i.d. 500 mg b.i.d.	10 days
4. First, ranitidine bismuth citrate and clarithromycin	400 mg b.i.d. 500 mg t.i.d.	2 weeks
Then ranitidine bismuth citrate alone	400 mg b.i.d.	2 weeks

ing diagnoses and related interventions. It also highlights the importance of evaluation.

Assessment

When bismuth salicylate is prescribed, review the patient's current history for use of salicylates. Also review the medication history to identify use of drugs that may interact with prescribed antibiotics. If clarithromycin is prescribed, assess for use of nonsedating antihistamines, whose concurrent use may lead to ventricular arrhythmia. Assessment of treatment efficacy and drug adverse effects should be performed on an ongoing basis as well as evaluation of the patient's and family's knowledge of the prescribed drugs.

Nursing diagnoses

- Risk for injury related to preexisting conditions that contraindicate use of antibiotics or bismuth products
- Risk for injury related to adverse drug effects or drug interactions
- Altered nutrition less than body requirements due to taste disturbances with use of clarithromycin
- Knowledge deficit related to prescribed antibiotic regimen

Planning and implementation

- Concurrent medications should be administered 2 hours prior to dose of bismuth subsalicylate.

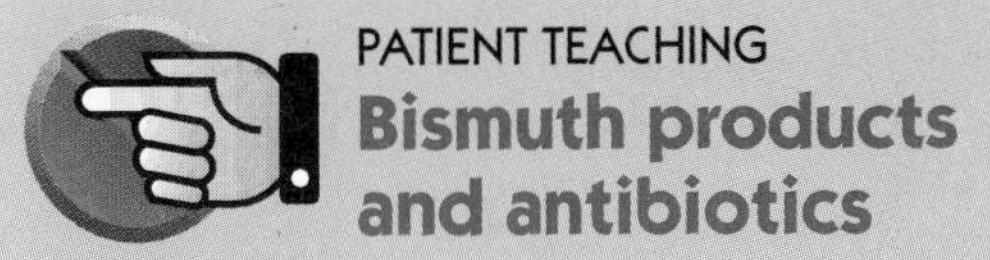

PATIENT TEACHING

Bismuth products and antibiotics

Bismuth products

- Teach the patient and family the name, dose, frequency, action, and adverse effects of the prescribed bismuth product.
- If the patient is age 18 or younger, teach the patient and family to discontinue the medication and notify the primary physician if symptoms of a viral infection are present.
- Teach the patient that the mouth, tongue, and stools may become blackened and that this is a temporary condition.
- Teach the patient and family that if tinnitus occurs, they should notify their primary physician.
- Teach the patient to avoid aspirin products when taking bismuth products.

Antibiotics

- Teach the patient that the absorption of tetracycline can be inhibited by food, especially dairy products.
- Warn the patient taking clarithromycin that it can cause disturbances in taste.
- Advise the patient that if diarrhea, nausea, or vomiting occur, the primary physician should be notified.

- Avoid concurrent use of salicylates such as aspirin (See Patient Teaching: *Bismuth products and antibiotics*).
- Tell patients to expect changes in the color of their tongue and stool if bismuth salicylate is used.
- Monitor the patient closely for adverse reactions and for effects from drug interactions.
- Monitor for bismuth toxicity, including signs of tinnitus, encephalopathy, and osteodystrophy.
- Monitor for signs of salicylate toxicity in elderly patients or patients with compromised renal function.
- Notify primary health care provider if adverse reactions occur.

Evaluation

For each nursing diagnosis, prepare an evaluation statement that describes the patient's or family's response to nursing interventions.

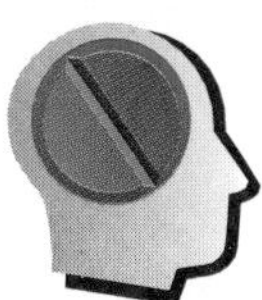

CRITICAL THINKING. To enhance your critical thinking about peptic ulcer agents, consider the following situation and its analysis.

Situation: Kay Jones, 35, has had *H. pylori* duodenal ulcer disease diagnosed and is being treated with the regimen of bismuth subsalicylate, metronidazole, tetracycline, and ranitidine for 2 weeks. She has been treated for ulcers in the past with long-term H_2-receptor antagonists and is very happy to find that she only needs 2 weeks of therapy.

Ms. Jones returns after 1 week of therapy and is concerned. She tells you that when she was first diagnosed with her ulcer, she had black tarry stools, which she was told

were associated with her GI bleeding. Her stools became normal after her treatment with H_2-receptor antagonists, but now she has developed the same black stools. How valid are her concerns?
Analysis: Ms. Jones is correct to be concerned, as black stools can indicate upper GI bleeding. However, in this case, it most likely is due to the bismuth compound. She should have been counseled to expect this common adverse reaction. You discuss this with her and allay her fears. You also point out that she did the right thing by coming to her primary care provider with this question because, in another situation, it could have been symptomatic of a problem.

Antacids

Antacids are over-the-counter medications used alone or with other drugs to treat peptic ulcer disease. The subject of extensive advertising, antacids sometimes are used indiscriminately by the public for a wide variety of conditions. Antacids discussed in this chapter include magnesium hydroxide and aluminum hydroxide with simethicone, magaldrate or aluminum-magnesium complex, and calcium carbonate.

PHARMACOKINETICS

The action of antacids takes place in the stomach. Absorption is neither necessary nor desired. Antacids are distributed throughout the GI tract and are eliminated primarily in the feces.

Route	Onset	Peak	Duration
P.O.	Immediate	Immediate-15 min	1 hr (empty stomach)-3 hr (full stomach)

PHARMACODYNAMICS

The acid-neutralizing action of antacids reduces the total acid load in the GI tract, which allows peptic ulcers to heal. Because pepsin acts more effectively in an acid medium, antacids also reduce its activity. Antacids do not coat peptic ulcers or the lining of the GI tract.

PHARMACOTHERAPEUTICS

Antacids are used alone or with other drugs primarily to relieve pain and promote healing in peptic ulcer disease. Antacids also are used to relieve symptoms of gastroesophageal reflux disease, acid indigestion, heartburn, and dyspepsia. During times of severe physical stress in critically ill patients, antacids are used to prevent stress ulcers and GI bleeding. Calcium carbonate antacids are prescribed to control hyperphosphatemia in renal failure because the calcium cation binds with phosphate in the GI tract, thus preventing phosphate absorption.

Drug interactions

All antacids can interfere with the absorption of concomitantly administered oral drugs. Some antacids also increase urine pH, which in turn increases the excretion of weakly acidic drugs and decreases the excretion of weakly alkaline drugs. However, aluminum and magnesium antacids do not affect urine pH. (See Drug Interactions: *Antacids.*)

ADVERSE DRUG REACTIONS

The most common adverse reactions to antacids occur in the GI tract. Diarrhea and constipation commonly result from long-term antacid use. Aluminum hydroxide is particularly constipating. Constipation can be severe and, if accompanied by dehydration or fluid restriction, may lead to intestinal obstruction. Hemorrhoids, rectal fissures, and fecal impaction may occur from hard stools. Conversely, magnesium-containing antacids produce a laxative effect and with frequent use can produce diarrhea and electrolyte abnormalities. Aluminum hydroxide and magnesium-containing antacids usually are prescribed in combination, which typically produces a mild laxative effect.

Most antacid products have been reformulated to decrease their sodium content. Furthermore, all antacids that contain more than 0.2 mEq of sodium per dose must be labeled with the amount. Some antacids also may have a high potassium content, so patients on a potassium-restricted diet should note the product label.

If used in patients with renal failure, aluminum-containing antacids may produce hyperaluminemia, in which aluminum accumulates in bones, lungs, and nerve tissue. Osteomalacia and dementia may occur. Hypophosphatemia, characterized by anorexia, malaise, and muscle weakness, also may occur from prolonged administration of aluminum-containing antacids.

Hypermagnesemia (characterized by hypotension, nausea, vomiting, electrocardiogram changes, respiratory or mental depression, and coma) has occurred in patients with renal failure taking magnesium-containing antacids.

Calcium-containing antacids usually are not recommended to treat peptic ulcer disease, but are recommended for short-term therapy for other GI conditions. When calcium carbonate is used, gastric hypersecretion and acid rebound occur. Calcium carbonate also may cause milk-alkali syndrome, characterized by hypercalcemia, metabolic alkalosis, and renal impairment.

All adverse reactions to antacids are dose related. No hypersensitivity reactions occur.

NURSING PROCESS APPLICATION

The following information assists the nurse in caring for a patient who is receiving an antacid. It includes an overview of assessment activities as well as examples of appropriate nursing diagnoses and related interventions. It also highlights the importance of evaluation.

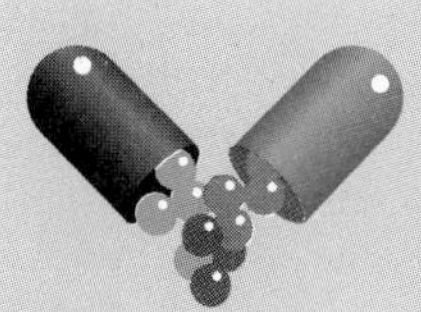

DRUG INTERACTIONS
Antacids

The nurse should be aware of the following drug interactions involving antacids, the possible effects of the interactions, and the nursing implications.

DRUG	INTERACTING DRUGS	POSSIBLE EFFECTS	NURSING IMPLICATIONS
antacids	digoxin, digitoxin, iron salts, isoniazid, quinolones, tetracyclines	Decreased rate or extent of absorption of digoxin and other drugs	• Do not administer the drugs within 2 hours of each other. • Monitor the patient for decreased therapeutic effects. • Monitor the patient's digoxin or digitoxin concentration level.
	amphetamines, quinidine	Increased urine pH; decreased excretion of weakly alkaline drugs, such as amphetamines and quinidine	• Do not administer the drugs within 1 hour of each other. • Monitor the patient for increased therapeutic effects. • Monitor the patient's quinidine concentration level.
	salicylates	Increased urine pH; increased excretion of weakly acidic drugs such as salicylates	• Monitor the patient for decreased salicylate effects or decreased salicylate concentration level.

Assessment
Before drug therapy begins, review the patient's history for conditions that contraindicate or require cautious use of the prescribed antacid. Also review the patient's medication history to identify use of drugs that may interact with it. During therapy, assess the patient for adverse drug reactions and signs of drug interactions. Also, periodically assess the effectiveness of antacid therapy. Finally, evaluate the patient's and family's knowledge about the prescribed drug.

Nursing diagnoses
- Risk for injury related to a preexisting condition that contraindicates or requires cautious use of an antacid
- Risk for injury related to adverse drug reactions or drug interactions
- Constipation related to the adverse GI effects of aluminum hydroxide
- Knowledge deficit related to the prescribed antacid

Planning and implementation
- Do not administer an antacid to a patient with a condition that contraindicates its use.
- Administer an antacid cautiously to a patient at risk because of a preexisting condition.
- Monitor the patient closely for GI and other adverse reactions and for drug interactions during antacid therapy. (See Patient Teaching: *Antacids,* page 354.)

∗ Avoid administering calcium carbonate for long-term treatment of peptic ulcer disease because gastric hypersecretion and acid rebound may occur.

- Monitor for signs of hyperaluminemia (which can result in osteomalacia and dementia) in a patient with renal failure who is receiving an aluminum-containing antacid.
- Monitor for symptoms of hypophosphatemia, such as anorexia, malaise, and muscle weakness, in a patient on long-term therapy with an aluminum-containing antacid. If hypophosphatemia is suspected, withhold the drug and notify the patient's primary health care provider.
- Shake the suspension well and give with a small amount of water. Have the patient drink 6 to 8 oz (175 to 240 ml) of water after swallowing the suspension.

∗ Do not give other oral medications within 1 to 2 hours of antacid administration because antacids impair the absorption of many other drugs.

- Separate the administration of antacids and enteric-coated drugs by 1 hour because antacids may cause premature release of enteric-coated drugs in the stomach.
- Notify the physician or primary health care provider if adverse reactions occur or if the antacid is ineffective.

∗ Monitor the patient for constipation, which may become severe, especially with aluminum hydroxide use.

- Place the patient on a high-fiber diet, and encourage to drink eight to thirteen 8-oz (240-ml) glasses of fluid a day (unless contraindicated) to help prevent constipation.
- Request a prescription for a laxative, as needed, if constipation occurs.

∗ Expect to discontinue the drug if constipation occurs in a dehydrated patient or one who must restrict fluids. Such a patient is at increased risk for intestinal obstruction.

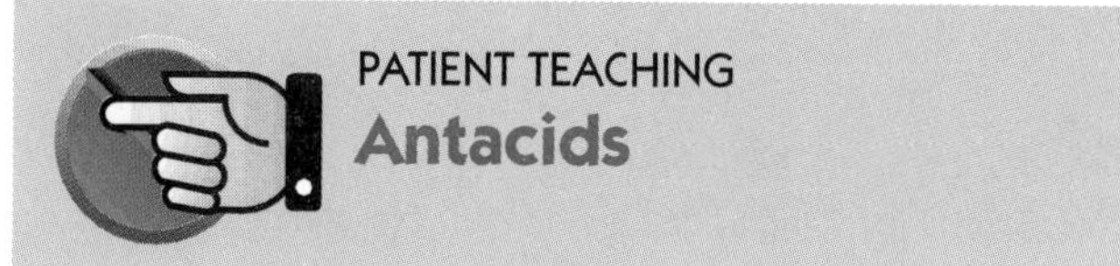

PATIENT TEACHING
Antacids

- Teach the patient and family the name, dose, frequency, action, and adverse effects of the prescribed antacid.
- Reassure the patient that antacid therapy normally makes stools appear speckled or whitish.
- Teach the patient when and how to take the antacid.
- Stress the importance of taking the antacid exactly as prescribed for maximum effectiveness.
- Instruct the patient with renal failure not to take a magnesium-containing antacid to prevent hypermagnesemia.
- Advise the patient who must restrict sodium intake to avoid antacids with a high sodium content (greater than 0.2 mEq of sodium) because sodium and fluid retention may occur or increase.
- Instruct the patient who must restrict potassium intake to read antacid labels carefully because some antacids have a high potassium content.
- Teach the patient how to prevent constipation during antacid therapy.
- Instruct the patient to notify the physician if adverse reactions occur.

Evaluation

For each nursing diagnosis, prepare an evaluation statement that describes the patient's or family's response to nursing interventions.

Histamine$_2$-receptor antagonists

The H_2-receptor antagonists are commonly prescribed antiulcer drugs in the United States. The H_2-receptor antagonists available in the United States include cimetidine, famotidine, nizatidine, and ranitidine.

PHARMACOKINETICS

Cimetidine, nizatidine, and ranitidine are absorbed rapidly and completely from the GI tract; famotidine is not completely absorbed. Cimetidine reaches peak effect in 1 to 2 hours. Food and antacids may impair the absorption of H_2-receptor antagonists. These drugs are distributed widely throughout the body and metabolized by the liver. The H_2-receptor antagonists are excreted primarily in the urine.

Route	Onset	Peak	Duration
P.O.	<30 min-1 hr	40 min-3 hr	4-13 hr
I.M.	Unknown	Unknown	<13 hr
I.V.	Immediate-1 hr	Immediate-20 min	10-12 hr

PHARMACODYNAMICS

The H_2-receptor antagonists block the stimulant action of histamine on the acid-secreting parietal cells of the stomach. (See *How cimetidine reduces gastric acid.*)

Acid secretion in the stomach depends on the binding of gastrin, acetylcholine, and histamine to their respective receptors on the parietal cells. If the binding of any one of these substances is blocked, acid secretion is reduced. Thus, by binding with H_2 receptors, the H_2-receptor antagonists reduce acid secretion.

PHARMACOTHERAPEUTICS

The H_2-receptor antagonists promote healing of duodenal and gastric ulcers. These drugs also are used for long-term treatment of pathologic GI hypersecretory conditions, such as **Zollinger-Ellison syndrome**. The H_2-receptor antagonists also are prescribed to reduce gastric acid output and prevent stress ulcers in severely ill patients and in those with reflux esophagitis or upper GI bleeding. Although antacids may be used with the H_2-receptor antagonists to control pain, their addition does not appear to increase ulcer healing.

Oral administration of an H_2-receptor antagonist usually is as effective as parenteral administration; however, the parenteral route may be preferred for hospitalized patients with pathologic hypersecretory conditions, intractable ulcers, or an inability to take oral medication. Experimental trials have shown that an intravenous (I.V.) loading dose followed by an I.V. infusion is somewhat more effective than I.V. bolus injections alone for treatment of active gastric bleeding.

Drug interactions

The H_2-receptor antagonists may interact with antacids and various other drugs. (See Drug Interactions: *Histamine$_2$-receptor antagonists,* page 356.)

ADVERSE DRUG REACTIONS

Cimetidine and ranitidine may produce headache, dizziness, malaise, myalgia, nausea, diarrhea or constipation, rashes, pruritus, loss of libido, and impotence; cimetidine, however, is more likely to produce these adverse reactions. Famotidine and nizatidine produce few adverse reactions, with headache being the most common (about 2% of patients), followed by constipation or diarrhea and rash. Reversible confusion, agitation, depression, and hallucinations also may occur. These adverse reactions are more common in patients receiving cimetidine, especially in severely ill or older patients with decreased renal function.

How cimetidine reduces gastric acid

These illustrations show how the H_2-receptor antagonist cimetidine reduces the release of gastric acid.

To stimulate gastric acid secretion, certain endogenous agents — primarily histamine, but also acetylcholine and gastrin — attach to receptors on the parietal cell surface. These agents activate the enzyme adenyl cyclase, which converts adenosine triphosphate (ATP) to the intracellular catalyst cyclic adenosine monophosphate (cAMP).

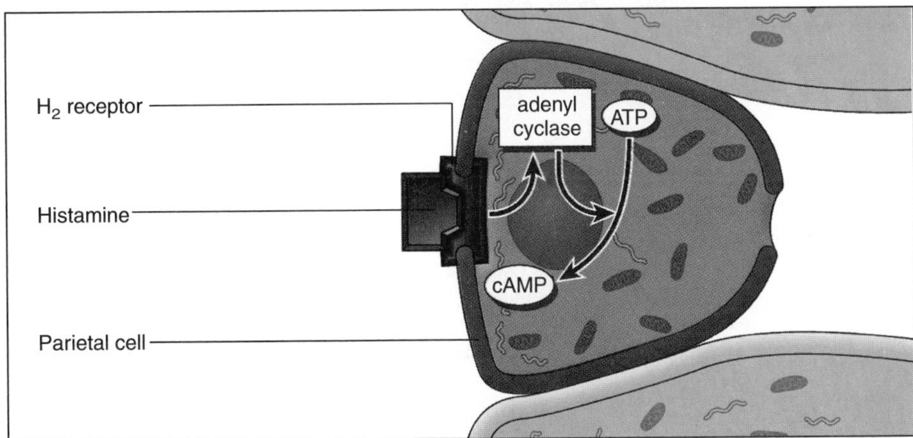

The cAMP ultimately stimulates proton pump (H/K ATPase) activity. The pump catalyzes the exchange of extracellular potassium (K) ions for intracellular hydrogen (H) ions. When the H^+ ions combine with extracellular chloride (Cl) ions excreted by the gastric cell at a different site, the result is hydrochloric acid (HCl), or gastric acid.

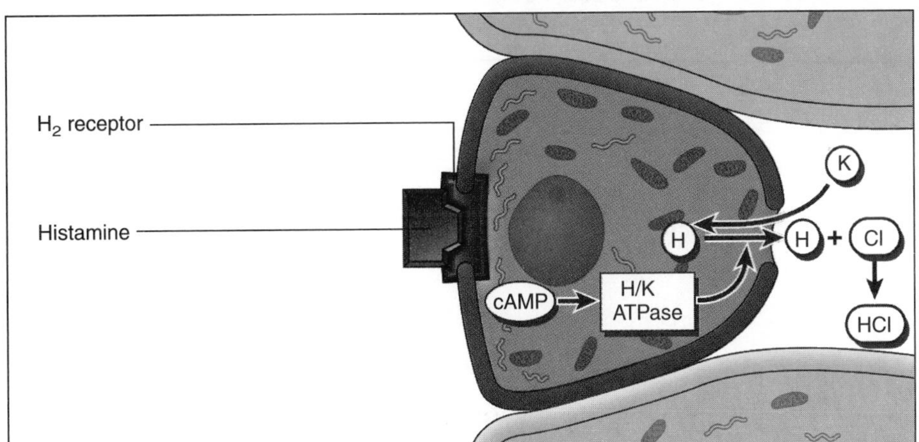

Cimetidine competitively binds to H_2-receptor sites on the parietal cell surface, inhibiting the common pathway that histamine and the other agents must travel to stimulate proton pump activity and promote gastric acid secretion.

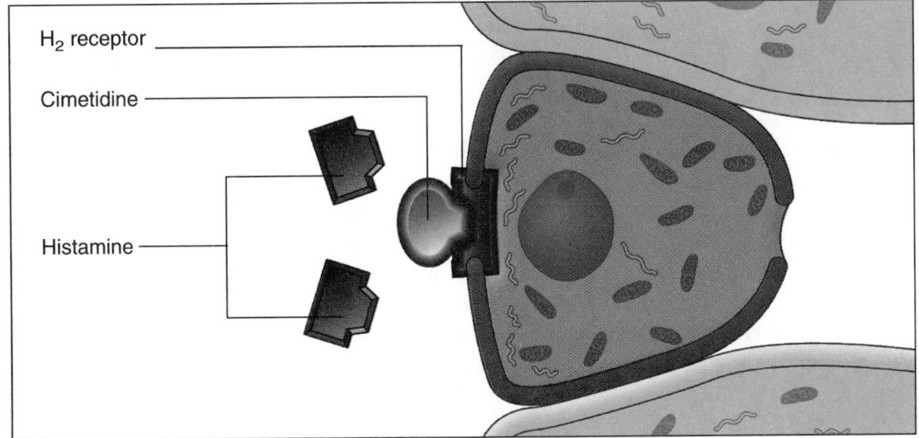

When given by rapid I.V. injection, H_2-receptor antagonists can produce profound bradycardia and other cardiotoxic effects. Pain at the injection site occasionally occurs.

The H_2-receptor antagonists seldom cause hypersensitivity reactions. Some patients develop increased hepatic enzyme levels, but this reaction also is rare. Cimetidine has been associated with adverse hematologic effects, such as thrombocytopenia and granulocytopenia, and seizures if drug accumulation occurs.

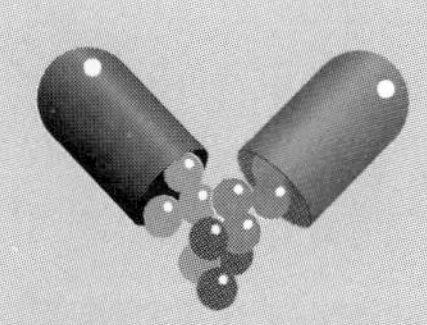

DRUG INTERACTIONS

Histamine$_2$-receptor antagonists

The following chart contains information about drug interactions involving histamine-2 (H_2)-receptor antagonists, the possible effects from the interactions, and important nursing implications.

DRUG	INTERACTING DRUGS	POSSIBLE EFFECTS	NURSING IMPLICATIONS
cimetidine, famotidine, nizatidine, ranitidine	antacids	Inhibited H_2-receptor antagonist absorption	• Do not administer within 1 hour of one another. • Monitor the patient for decreased therapeutic effects.
cimetidine	oral anticoagulants, propranolol, possibly other beta-adrenergic blockers, benzodiazepines, tricyclic antidepressants, theophylline, procainamide, quinidine, lidocaine, phenytoin, calcium channel blockers, cyclosporine, carbamazepine, narcotic analgesics	Inhibited hepatic enzyme metabolism of these drugs, resulting in increased levels and effects	• Avoid concurrent administration, if possible. • Monitor the patient for increased sedative effects with benzodiazepines. Oxazepam, lorazepam, and temazepam are eliminated differently and are not affected by cimetidine. • Monitor the patient for drug toxicity. • Monitor the patient's concentration levels of procainamide, phenytoin, quinidine, lidocaine, theophylline, and cyclosporine. • Monitor the patient's prothrombin time, as prescribed, when beginning or discontinuing cimetidine therapy during concomitant oral anticoagulant therapy.
	carmustine	Increased bone marrow toxicity	• Monitor the patient's blood cell counts carefully if concomitant use is necessary.
	ethyl alcohol	Increased alcohol absorption, decreased metabolism	• Caution the patient about the risk of increased alcohol effects.

NURSING PROCESS APPLICATION

The following information assists the nurse in caring for a patient who is receiving an H_2-receptor antagonist. It includes an overview of assessment activities as well as examples of appropriate nursing diagnoses and related interventions. It also highlights the importance of evaluation.

Assessment

Before drug therapy begins, review the patient's history for conditions that contraindicate or require cautious use of the prescribed H_2-receptor antagonist. Also review the patient's medication history to identify use of drugs that may interact with it. During therapy, assess the patient for adverse drug reactions and signs of drug interactions. Also, periodically assess the effectiveness of therapy with the H_2-receptor antagonist. Finally, evaluate the patient's and family's knowledge about the prescribed drug.

Nursing diagnoses

• Risk for injury related to a preexisting condition that contraindicates or requires cautious use of an H_2-receptor antagonist
• Risk for injury related to adverse drug reactions or drug interactions
• Sexual dysfunction related to the adverse genitourinary (GU) effects of cimetidine or ranitidine
• Knowledge deficit related to the prescribed H_2-receptor antagonist

Planning and implementation

• Do not administer an H_2-receptor antagonist to a patient with a condition that contraindicates its use.
• Administer an H_2-receptor antagonist cautiously to a patient at risk because of a preexisting condition.
• Monitor the patient closely for adverse reactions and drug interactions during H_2-receptor antagonist therapy.
* ***Do not give an antacid within 1 hour of H_2-receptor antagonist administration because decreased absorption of the H_2-receptor antagonist may occur.*** (See Patient Teaching: *Histamine$_2$-receptor antagonists.*)
• Monitor the patient for profound bradycardia and other cardiotoxic effects when giving an H_2-receptor antagonist rapidly by I.V. injection.
• Evaluate the results of hematologic studies for signs of abnormalities, such as thrombocytopenia and granulocytopenia, in a patient receiving cimetidine.
• Take seizure precautions if cimetidine accumulation occurs.
• Expect to administer an I.V. H_2-receptor antagonist as prescribed to a critically ill patient to prevent GI bleeding.

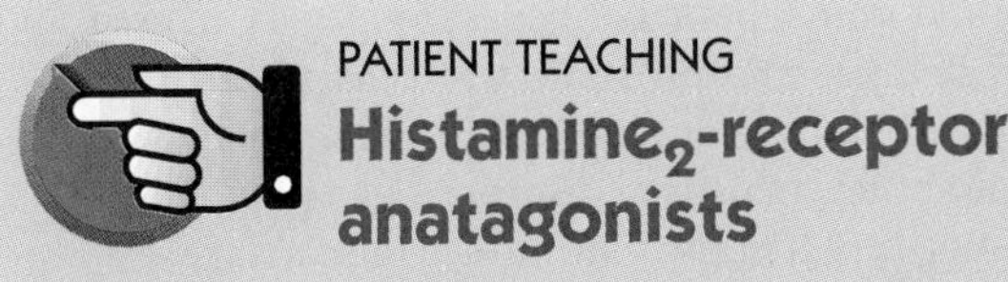

PATIENT TEACHING

Histamine$_2$-receptor anatagonists

- Teach the patient and family the name, dose, frequency, action, and adverse effects of the prescribed histamine-2 (H_2)-receptor antagonists.
- Instruct the patient not to take an antacid within 1 hour of taking the prescribed H_2-receptor antagonist.
- Advise the patient to avoid any activity that requires alertness if dizziness or such mental changes as confusion occur.
- Teach the patient how to avoid constipation.
- Stress the importance of having laboratory studies done as instructed.
- Instruct the patient to take the H_2-receptor antagonist as prescribed, without regard to meals.
- Inform the patient that sexual dysfunction may occur as an adverse reaction to cimetidine or ranitidine.
- Advise the patient to notify the physician if adverse reactions occur.

• Administer an H_2-receptor antagonist as prescribed without regard to meals; expect to administer the final daily dose at bedtime.

∗ ***Dilute cimetidine, famotidine, and ranitidine before I.V. administration.*** Dilute cimetidine in at least 50 ml, famotidine in at least 100 ml, and ranitidine in at least 20 ml of a compatible I.V. solution, such as normal saline, dextrose 5% or 10% in water (and combinations of these), lactated Ringer's, or 5% sodium bicarbonate. ***Do not use sterile water for injection as a diluent.***

• Notify the physician if adverse reactions occur.

• Encourage the patient receiving cimetidine or ranitidine to express concerns about adverse GU effects, such as loss of libido and impotence.

• Consult with the physician or primary health care provider if the patient experiences sexual dysfunction. The patient may need to be changed to a different H_2-receptor antagonist.

Evaluation

For each nursing diagnosis, prepare an evaluation statement that describes the patient's or family's response to nursing interventions.

Other peptic ulcer agents

Besides antacids and H_2-receptor antagonists, misoprostol, omeprazole, lansoprazole, and sucralfate may be used as peptic ulcer agents. Other agents currently are being investigated for their usefulness in treating peptic ulcer disease.

PHARMACOKINETICS

The pharmacokinetics of misoprostol, omeprazole, lansoprazole, and sucralfate differ. After oral administration, misoprostol is absorbed extensively and rapidly. It is metabolized by de-esterification to misoprostol acid, which is clinically active. Misoprostol acid is 90% protein-bound and is excreted primarily in the urine.

Omeprazole and lansoprazole, which are known as acid pump inhibitors, utilize enteric coating to bypass the stomach because they are highly acid labile. Absorption is rapid once the medications reach the small intestine. Both medications are highly protein bound and both are extensively metabolized by the liver to inactive compounds, which are eliminated by the kidney.

Sucralfate is absorbed minimally from the GI tract, is distributed minimally to other areas of the body, and is excreted in the feces.

Route	Onset	Peak	Duration
P.O.	30 min-1 hr	12 min-2 hr	3-72 hr

PHARMACODYNAMICS

Misoprostol's antiulcer activity may result from increased bicarbonate and mucus production in the GI tract or by inhibition of gastric acid secretion. Omeprazole is an acid pump inhibitor that blocks the action of H^+/K^+ adenosine triphosphatase in the parietal cells of the stomach. Sucralfate exerts its effects locally, rapidly reacting with hydrochloric acid in the GI tract to form a highly condensed, viscous, adhesive, pastelike substance that adheres to the gastric mucosa and especially to ulcer sites. By binding to the ulcer site, sucralfate protects the ulcer from the damaging effects of acid and pepsin and permits healing.

PHARMACOTHERAPEUTICS

Misoprostol has been approved to prevent nonsteroidal anti-inflammatory drug (NSAID)–induced gastric ulcers in patients at high risk for complications resulting from gastric ulcers. It is under study for other uses, including the treatment and prevention of peptic ulcers.

Omeprazole and lansoprazole are indicated for short-term treatment of active benign gastric ulcer, active duodenal ulcer, erosive esophagitis, and refractory symptomatic gastroesophageal reflux disease. They may be used in combination with antibiotics for the treatment of active peptic ulcers associated with *H. pylori* infection. They are indicated for maintenance of healing erosive esophagitis and for long-term treatment of pathologic hypersecretory states such as Zollinger-Ellison syndrome, multiple endocrine adenomas, and systemic mastocytosis.

Sucralfate is used for short-term treatment (up to 8 weeks) of duodenal ulcers. Sucralfate also has been used successfully for the short-term treatment of gastric ulcers

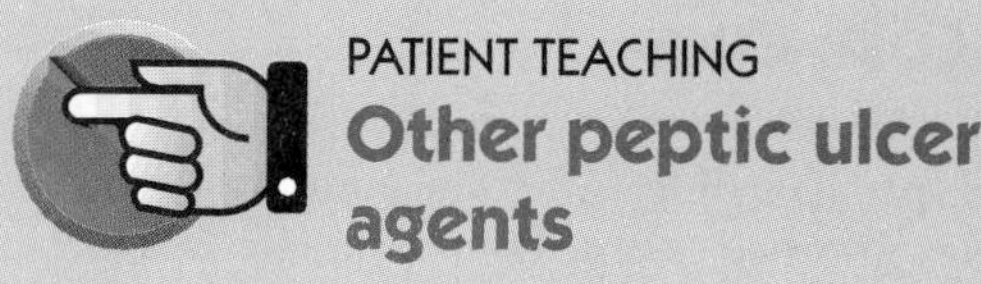

PATIENT TEACHING
Other peptic ulcer agents

- Teach the patient and family the name, dose, frequency, action, and adverse effects of the prescribed peptic ulcer agent.
- Instruct the patient how to manage adverse reactions such as constipation, diarrhea, and dry mouth.
- Advise the patient not to perform any activity that requires alertness if dizziness, sleepiness, or vertigo occurs.
- Instruct the patient not to take an antacid with sucralfate or misoprostol.
- Instruct the patient to take sucralfate 2 hours before or after cimetidine.
- Teach the patient when and how to take the prescribed peptic ulcer agent.
- Alert the patient that nausea and a metallic taste may accompany sucralfate use.
- Provide verbal and written warnings to a woman of childbearing age that misoprostol may induce miscarriage. Advise such a patient to obtain a serum pregnancy test 2 weeks before beginning therapy, to use effective contraceptive methods during treatment, and to notify her physician if she is pregnant or plans to become pregnant. If pregnancy is suspected, misoprostol should be discontinued immediately.
- Instruct the patient to notify the physician if adverse reactions occur.

and may be prescribed to prevent recurrent ulcers, NSAID-induced ulcers, and stress ulcers.

Drug interactions

Concomitant antacid administration may bind with misoprostol or decrease its absorption, reducing the amount of misoprostol available for conversion to misoprostol acid. However, this effect does not appear to be clinically significant.

Omeprazole and lansoprazole may interfere with the metabolism of diazepam, phenytoin, and warfarin, causing increased half-lives and elevated plasma concentrations of these agents. Omeprazole and lansoprazole also may interfere with the absorption of drugs that depend on gastric pH for absorption, such as ketoconazole, ampicillin esters, and iron salts. Therefore, concomitant use should be avoided.

When given orally with sucralfate, some drugs bind with it in the GI tract, which decreases their absorption. Antacids, which increase the pH of the GI tract, display decreased activity when administered with sucralfate. Because sucralfate decreases the bioavailability of cimetidine, the nurse should give sucralfate 2 hours before or after the cimetidine dose.

ADVERSE DRUG REACTIONS

Misoprostol commonly causes adverse GI reactions. Diarrhea occurs in up to 40% of patients. It may be followed by abdominal pain, flatulence, dyspepsia, nausea, and vomiting. Because misoprostol is a prostaglandin, it also may affect the uterus, causing spotting, cramps, hypermenorrhea, and other menstrual disorders. In a pregnant patient, misoprostol therapy may induce miscarriage.

Omeprazole and lansoprazole usually are tolerated well even in the higher dosages used to treat hypersecretory conditions. The most common adverse reactions are diarrhea and headaches.

Usually, sucralfate is well tolerated. Although typically minor, adverse reactions may become bothersome for the patient. Constipation is the most common dose-related adverse reaction, occurring in about 2% of all patients. Nausea and a metallic taste also may accompany the use of sucralfate. Less common reactions to this drug include diarrhea, indigestion, dry mouth, back pain, dizziness, sleepiness, and vertigo. Rarely, sucralfate may cause rash and pruritus. (See Patient Teaching: *Other peptic ulcer agents.*)

NURSING PROCESS APPLICATION

The following information assists the nurse in caring for a patient who is receiving misoprostol, omeprazole, lansoprazole or sucralfate. It includes an overview of assessment activities as well as examples of appropriate nursing diagnoses and related interventions. It also highlights the importance of evaluation.

Assessment

Before drug therapy begins, review the patient's history for conditions that contraindicate or require cautious use of the prescribed peptic ulcer agent. Also review the patient's medication history to identify use of drugs that may interact with it. During therapy, assess the patient for adverse drug reactions and signs of drug interactions. Also, periodically assess the effectiveness of therapy with the peptic ulcer agent. Finally, evaluate the patient's and family's knowledge about the prescribed drug.

Nursing diagnoses

- Risk for injury related to a preexisting condition that contraindicates or requires cautious use of a peptic ulcer agent
- Risk for injury related to adverse drug reactions or drug interactions
- Diarrhea related to the adverse GI effects of the prescribed peptic ulcer agent
- Knowledge deficit related to the prescribed peptic ulcer agent

Planning and implementation

- Do not administer a peptic ulcer agent to a patient with a condition that contraindicates its use.
- Administer a peptic ulcer agent cautiously to a patient at risk because of a preexisting condition.
- Monitor the patient closely for GI disturbances and other adverse reactions and for drug interactions during peptic ulcer agent therapy.

- Do not administer an antacid with sucralfate or misoprostol; antacids decrease the activity of these peptic ulcer agents.

*** Sucralfate should be administered 2 hours before or after all other medications, as it binds with other medication.***
***** Administer omeprazole cautiously during concomitant therapy with diazepam, phenytoin, or warfarin. Omeprazole may interfere with the metabolism of these agents, thus causing elevated plasma concentrations.***

- Monitor the effectiveness of ketoconazole, ampicillin esters, and iron salts during concomitant omeprazole or lansoprazole therapy; omeprazole or lansoprazole may interfere with their absorption.
- Administer misoprostol with food.
- Administer sucralfate at least 1 hour before meals and at bedtime for best results.
- Notify the physician if adverse reactions occur.
- Monitor the patient's bowel function for diarrhea, especially during misoprostol therapy.
- Monitor hydration if the patient develops diarrhea. Obtain a prescription for an antidiarrheal agent, as needed.
- Consult the physician or primary health care provider about discontinuing the peptic ulcer agent if diarrhea becomes severe.

Evaluation

For each nursing diagnosis, prepare an evaluation statement that describes the patient's or family's response to nursing interventions.

CHAPTER SUMMARY

Chapter 27 discussed peptic ulcer drugs. Here are the highlights of the chapter:

Eradication of *H. pylori* infections will promote ulcer healing and prevent recurrence.

Antacids treat peptic ulcer disease safely and effectively. However, the frequent doses required make their use as the first choice in treating peptic ulcer disease less attractive than the H_2-receptor antagonists.

H_2-receptor antagonists, with possible adjunctive antacid therapy for pain, are treatment alternatives for duodenal and gastric ulcers.

Misoprostol is a synthetic prostaglandin used to prevent NSAID-induced gastric ulcers in patients at high risk for complications from gastric ulcers.

Omeprazole and lansoprazole are acid pump inhibitors approved for short-term use in treating severe erosive or symptomatic esophagitis and pathologic hypersecretory conditions.

Sucralfate binds to the ulcer site and produces a protective barrier. This agent is used for short-term treatment of duodenal and gastric ulcers.

When caring for a patient receiving a peptic ulcer agent, the nurse must monitor closely for adverse drug reactions and teach the patient about the prescribed agent.

Questions to consider

See Appendix 1 for answers.

1. Kia Sawyer is interested in buying an over-the-counter medication for occasional heartburn and acid indigestion. Which of the following drugs would *not* be appropriate for her?
   (a) omeprazole 20 mg P.O. daily
   (b) magaldrate antacid 15 to 30 ml P.O. with water as needed
   (c) ranitidine 75 mg P.O. once or twice daily
   (d) cimetidine 200 mg P.O. as needed to a maximum of 400 mg/day

2. When. Raymond Allen takes cimetidine, how does it exert its therapeutic effects?
   (a) By increasing the absorption of stomach acid
   (b) By decreasing the effectiveness of stomach alkalies in buffering acids
   (c) By blocking the stimulant action of histamine on acid-secreting cells in the stomach
   (d) By inhibiting the gastrocolic reflex, which is necessary for gastrin secretion

3. Which of the following instructions should the nurse give Xu Li about administration of cimetidine and an antacid?
   (a) Take both drugs with meals.
   (b) Take both drugs 1 to 3 hours after meals.
   (c) Take both drugs between meals with water.
   (d) Take the antacid at least 1 hour before or after taking cimetidine.

4. Ira Lang, age 45, takes large doses of an NSAID for rheumatoid arthritis. Her physician prescribes misoprostol 200 mcg P.O. q.i.d. with food for the prevention of NSAID-induced ulcers. Which of the following is a common dose-related adverse reaction to misoprostol?
   (a) Dyspepsia
   (b) Diarrhea
   (c) Headache
   (d) Tinnitus

28 Adsorbent, antiflatulent, and digestive agents

OBJECTIVES

After reading and studying this chapter, the student should be able to:

1. explain how an adsorbent works to treat acute poisoning.
2. describe the action of antiflatulents in the gastrointestinal (GI) tract.
3. identify the purpose of each of the major groups of digestive agents.
4. identify adverse reactions associated with digestive agents.
5. describe how to apply the nursing process when caring for a patient who is receiving an adsorbent, antiflatulent, or digestive agent.

INTRODUCTION

Natural and synthetic **adsorbents** are used when toxins have been ingested. Toxins that may cause poisoning or overdose include such drugs as amphetamines, aspirin, barbiturates, cocaine, morphine, opium, and tricyclic antidepressants. Poisonous mushrooms also produce toxins when ingested.

Two major disturbances of digestion in the GI tract include gastric bloating with or without flatulence and inadequate or incomplete digestion. **Antiflatulents** commonly are indicated for patients with functional gastric bloating. (See *Selected major adsorbent, antiflatulent, and digestive agents.*)

Digestive agents (**digestants**) used in clinical situations involving incomplete digestion include dehydrocholic acid, a bile acid that is used to treat biliary stasis that is not caused by mechanical obstruction of the hepatic or common bile duct, and pancreatic enzymes for conditions that decrease pancreatic juice production (pancreatitis or cystic fibrosis).

Drugs covered in this chapter include:

- activated charcoal
- dehydrocholic acid
- pancreatin
- pancrelipase
- simethicone.

Adsorbent agents

An adsorbent is an agent that attracts molecules of a liquid, gas, or dissolved substance to its surface. Adsorbents are prescribed in acute situations to prevent the absorption of drugs or toxins from the GI tract. The adsorbent most commonly used clinically is activated charcoal, a black powder residue obtained from the distillation of various organic materials.

PHARMACOKINETICS

Activated charcoal, which is not absorbed or metabolized by the body, is excreted unchanged in the feces. Activated charcoal must be administered soon after poison ingestion because it only can bind with drugs or toxins that have not been absorbed from the GI tract. Duration of action depends on the poison's transit time through the intestines and the resultant contact time for adsorption to occur. After initial absorption, some poisons move back into the intestines, where they are reabsorbed. Activated charcoal may be administered repeatedly to break this cycle. The particle size of the charcoal also influences its duration. Activated charcoals composed of small particles are the most effective because the small particles provide a larger total surface area for the toxin to adhere to.

Route	Onset	Peak	Duration
P.O.	Immediate	Unknown	Variable

PHARMACODYNAMICS

Adsorbents attract and bind toxins in the intestinal lumen, thus inhibiting toxin absorption from the GI tract. This nonspecific GI binding delays or blocks further absorption of the poison, but does not alter systemic toxicity caused by earlier absorption of the toxin.

PHARMACOTHERAPEUTICS

Activated charcoal is a general-purpose antidote used for many types of acute oral poisoning. It is not indicated in acute poisoning from cyanide, ethanol, methanol, iron, sodium chloride alkalies, inorganic acids, or organic solvents.

Selected major adsorbent, antiflatulent, and digestive agents

The following chart summarizes the major adsorbents, antiflatulents, and digestants currently in clinical use.

DRUG	MAJOR INDICATIONS AND USUAL DOSAGES	CONTRAINDICATIONS AND PRECAUTIONS
Adsorbents		
activated charcoal (Charcocaps)	*Acute toxic poisoning* ADULT: 5 to 10 times the estimated weight of the drug or chemical ingested, or a minimum dose of 30 g P.O. mixed in 250 ml of water PEDIATRIC: same as adult	• Activated charcoal is contraindicated in a patient who has ingested a corrosive agent or petroleum distillate. • Agent is not effective for ingestion of iron salts, ethanol, or methanol
Antiflatulents		
simethicone (Mylicon)	*Excess gastrointestinal tract gas* ADULT: 160 to 500 mg P.O. daily in divided doses, given after each meal and h.s.; not to exceed 500 mg daily PEDIATRIC: highly individualized, based on severity of the condition and the surface area of the patient rather than on body weight; usual dose is: infants, 20 mg P.O. q.i.d; children under age 12, 40 mg P.O. q.i.d.	• Simethicone is contraindicated in a patient with known hypersensitivty to the drug. • The drug is not recommended for treatment of infant colic.
Digestants		
dehydrocholic acid (Decholin, Cholan-HMB)	*Insufficient bile production and temporary relief of constipation* ADULT: 244 to 500 mg P.O. t.i.d. after meals for 4 to 6 weeks, not to exceed 1.5 g in 24 hours.	• Dehydrocholic acid is contraindicated in a patient with biliary obstruction, profound cholecystitis, in the presence of jaundice, nausea, or abdominal pain.
pancreatin (Dizymes, Entozyme, Donazyme, Hi-Vegi-Lip)	*Insufficient pancreatic enzyme production* ADULT: 1 to 3 tablets P.O. after meals	• Pancreatin is contraindicated in a patient with known hypersensitivity to swine protein. • This drug requires cautious use in a pregnant or breast-feeding patient. • Safety and efficacy in children have not been established.
pancrelipase (Cotazym, Ilozyme, Pancrease, Viokase)	*Insufficient pancreatic enzymes, steatorrhea* ADULT: 1 to 3 capsules or tablets P.O. before or with meals and 1 capsule or tablet P.O. with snacks; or 0.7 g of powder P.O. before meals and snacks	• Pancrelipase is contraindicated in a patient with known hypersensitivity to swine protein. • This drug requires cautious use in a pregnant or breast-feeding patient.

Drug interactions

Do not administer activated charcoal simultaneously with ipecac syrup; the activated charcoal will adsorb the ipecac syrup, rendering it inactive. Give emetics, such as ipecac, and allow emesis to occur before administering activated charcoal because emesis enhances the effectiveness of the activated charcoal by decreasing the amount of toxin in the GI tract to be adsorbed. The result is more complete toxin removal.

ADVERSE DRUG REACTIONS

Adverse reactions to activated charcoal administration include black stools and constipation. A laxative, such as sorbitol, usually is given with activated charcoal to prevent constipation. No known hypersensitivity reactions exist.

NURSING PROCESS APPLICATION

The following information assists the nurse in caring for a patient who is receiving activated charcoal. It includes an overview of assessment activities as well as examples of appropriate nursing diagnoses and related interventions. It also highlights the importance of evaluation.

Assessment

Before drug therapy begins, review the patient's history for conditions that contraindicate the use of activated charcoal.

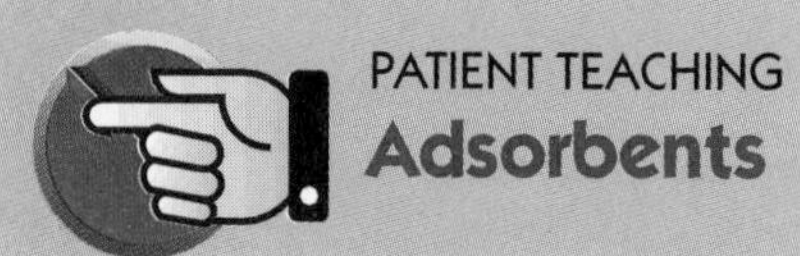

PATIENT TEACHING
Adsorbents

- ➤ Teach the patient and family the name, dose, frequency, action, and adverse effects of activated charcoal.
- ➤ Advise the patient to avoid drinking milk or eating ice cream or sherbet because these substances decrease the adsorbent capacity of the drug.
- ➤ Caution the patient to anticipate black stools from the activated charcoal.

During therapy, assess the patient for adverse drug reactions and signs of drug interactions. Also, periodically assess the effectiveness of activated charcoal therapy. Finally, evaluate the patient's and family's knowledge about the prescribed drug. (See Patient Teaching: *Adsorbents*.)

Nursing diagnoses

- Risk for injury related to adverse drug reactions and drug interactions
- Constipation related to the adverse GI effects of activated charcoal
- Knowledge deficit related to activated charcoal regimen

Planning and implementation

- Do not administer activated charcoal to a patient with a condition that contraindicates its use.
- Expect to administer large doses of activated charcoal to treat the poisoning if food is present in the patient's stomach.
- Add grape juice to the charcoal and water mixture to make it more palatable.

*** *Administer activated charcoal within 30 minutes of the poisoning for maximum effect.***

- Prepare to administer activated charcoal every 2 hours to treat poisoning by drugs that undergo enterohepatic recycling or are resecreted into the stomach.

*** *Do not administer activated charcoal simultaneously with ipecac syrup. Allow ipecac syrup–induced emesis to occur before administering activated charcoal.***

- Expect to administer a laxative such as sorbitol to prevent adsorbent-induced constipation.

*** *Do not administer activated charcoal to a child under age 12 months.***

- Do not mix activated charcoal with milk, ice cream, or sherbert.
- Know that excessive doses of pancrelipase may cause nausea, abdominal cramping, or diarrhea.

Evaluation

For each nursing diagnosis, prepare an evaluation statement that describes the patient's or family's response to nursing interventions.

Antiflatulent agents

Antiflatulents disperse gas pockets in the GI tract. They are available alone or in combination with antacids. This section discusses the major antiflatulent agent simethicone.

PHARMACOKINETICS

Antiflatulents are not absorbed from the GI tract. They are distributed only in the intestinal lumen and are eliminated intact in the feces. Their onsets of action are immediate, with a duration of approximately 3 hours.

Route	Onset	Peak	Duration
P.O.	Immediate	Immediate	3 hr

PHARMACODYNAMICS

Antiflatulents provide defoaming action in the GI tract. By producing a film in the intestines that can collapse gas bubbles, simethicone disperses and helps prevent the formation of mucus-enclosed gas pockets.

PHARMACOTHERAPEUTICS

Antiflatulents are prescribed to treat conditions in which excess gas is a problem, such as functional gastric bloating, postoperative gaseous bloating, diverticular disease, spastic or irritable colon, air swallowing, and peptic ulcer.

Drug interactions

Simethicone does not interact significantly with other drugs.

ADVERSE DRUG REACTIONS

Simethicone does not cause any known adverse reactions.

NURSING PROCESS APPLICATION

The following information assists the nurse in caring for a patient who is receiving simethicone. It includes an overview of assessment activities as well as examples of appropriate nursing diagnoses and related interventions. It also highlights the importance of evaluation.

Assessment

Periodically assess the effectiveness of simethicone therapy and evaluate the patient's and family's knowledge about the prescribed drug.

Nursing diagnoses

- Knowledge deficit related to use of simethicone

Planning and implementation

- Periodically assess the patient's degree of GI discomfort.

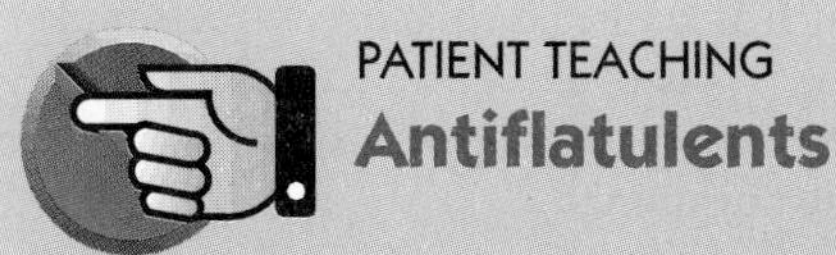

PATIENT TEACHING
Antiflatulents

- Teach the patient and family the name, dose, frequency, and action of simethicone.
- Instruct the patient to take simethicone after meals and at bedtime.
- Teach the patient to shake the simethicone suspension before preparing the dose for administration.
- Advise the patient that chewable tablets must be chewed thoroughly before swallowing.
- Encourage a patient with functional gastric bloating to increase physical activity and exercise, unless contraindicated.
- Instruct the patient to notify the physician if simethicone is ineffective.
- Advise the patient not to exceed the recommended dose.

- Shake the antiflatulent suspension before administering to ensure adequate mixing. (See Patient Teaching: *Antiflatulents.*)
- Use a calibrated dropper to administer the liquid medication.
- Administer simethicone after each meal and at bedtime for maximum effectiveness.
- Notify the physician or primary health care provider if simethicone is ineffective.

Evaluation
For each nursing diagnosis, prepare an evaluation statement that describes the patient's or family's response to nursing interventions.

Digestive agents

Digestive agents (digestants) aid digestion in patients who lack one or more of the specific substances that naturally digest food. This section discusses digestants that function in the GI tract, liver, and pancreas; they include dehydrocholic acid, pancreatin, and pancrelipase.

PHARMACOKINETICS
The digestants are absorbed, distributed, metabolized, and excreted as they would be if they were produced by the patient rather than taken therapeutically. The onset of action, peak concentration level, and duration of action of the digestants resemble those of the body substances they replace. Onset and duration depend on the type and amount of food ingested.

Route	Onset	Peak	Duration
P.O.	Variable	Variable	Variable

PHARMACODYNAMICS
The action of digestants resembles the action of the body substances they replace. Dehydrocholic acid, a bile acid, increases bile output without increasing the amount of solids in it.

The pancreatic enzymes pancreatin and pancrelipase replace the normal exocrine pancreatic enzymes. These agents digest proteins via trypsin, carbohydrates via amylase, and fats via lipase.

PHARMACOTHERAPEUTICS
Bile acids may be administered to provide temporary relief from constipation or to replace the natural substances in patients with conditions in which the bile component concentration in the small intestine is low.

Pancreatic enzymes are used in clinical situations characterized by an insufficiency of pancreatic enzymes (specifically, pancreatitis and cystic fibrosis). Pancreatic enzymes also are used to treat steatorrhea, a disorder related to fat metabolism.

Drug interactions
No significant drug interactions occur with the administration of dehydrocholic acid. However, antacids negate the effects of pancreatin and pancrelipase. Therefore, concomitant administration of these agents should be avoided.

ADVERSE DRUG REACTIONS
Dehydrocholic acid can produce abdominal cramping and diarrhea. If a dislodged gallstone is obstructing a biliary duct, the choleretic bile acids can produce biliary colic.

Administration of the pancreatic enzymes typically causes nausea and diarrhea.

NURSING PROCESS APPLICATION
The following information assists the nurse in caring for a patient who is receiving a digestant. It includes an overview of assessment activities as well as examples of appropriate nursing diagnoses and related interventions. It also highlights the importance of evaluation.

Assessment
Before drug therapy begins, review the patient's history for conditions that contraindicate or require cautious use of the prescribed digestant. Also review the patient's medication history to identify use of antacids that may interact with a pancreatic enzyme. During therapy, assess the patient for adverse drug reactions and signs of drug interactions. Also, periodically assess the effectiveness of digestant therapy. Finally, evaluate the patient's and family's knowledge about the prescribed drug.

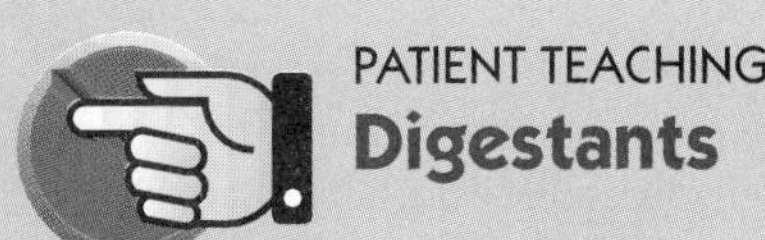

PATIENT TEACHING
Digestants

- Teach the patient and family the name, dose, frequency, action, and adverse effects of the prescribed digestant.
- Instruct the patient taking a pancreatic enzyme to balance fat, protein, and carbohydrate intake to avoid indigestion.
- Instruct the patient not to crush enteric coated forms. Capsules that contain enteric-coated microspheres may be opened and sprinkled on a small quantity of cooled, soft food (not protein in nature). Stress the importance of swallowing the drug immediately without chewing, following with a glass of water or juice.
- Warn the patient not to inhale the powder form or powder from capsules; this may cause irritation to the skin and mucous membranes.
- Instruct patients not to change brands without consulting their physician.
- Inform the patient that the number of bowel movements will decrease during digestant therapy and that the stool consistency will improve when therapy reaches a therapeutic level. Advise the patient to report diarrhea to the physician.
- Advise the patient not to take a pancreatic enzyme with an antacid.
- Stress the importance of taking the digestant before, with, or after meals, as prescribed, to enhance effectiveness.

Nursing diagnoses

- Risk for injury related to adverse drug reactions or drug interactions
- Knowledge deficit related to use of the prescribed digestant

Planning and implementation

- Do not administer a digestant to a patient with a condition that contraindicates its use.
- Monitor the patient frequently for adverse reactions and drug interactions during digestant therapy. (See Patient Teaching: *Digestants.*)
- Administer the digestant before, with, or after meals, as prescribed.
- Do not administer antacids with pancreatin or pancrelipase because antacids negate the effects of these agents.

Evaluation

For each nursing diagnosis, prepare an evaluation statement that describes the patient's or family's response to nursing interventions.

CHAPTER SUMMARY

Chapter 28 discussed adsorbents, antiflatulents, and digestants. Here are the chapter highlights.

An adsorbent, such as activated charcoal, attracts molecules of a liquid, gas, or dissolved substance to its surface. Adsorbents are used to prevent drug or toxin absorption in the GI tract in acute poisonings.

Antiflatulents, such as simethicone, prevent the formation of mucus-enclosed gas pockets in the GI tract.

Specific digestants include dehydrocholic acid, pancreatin, and pancrelipase. Digestants aid digestion in the patient who lacks one or more of the specific digestive substances produced by the body.

Questions to consider

See Appendix 1 for answers.

1. Angela Barron, age 42, is taking simethicone tablets 320 mg P.O. daily for excess GI tract gas caused by diverticular disease. How does simethicone relieve GI tract gas?
   (a) It disperses and prevents gas pocket formation.
   (b) It facilitates expulsion of gas pockets.
   (c) It neutralizes gastric contents and reduces gas.
   (d) It absorbs gas bubbles.

2. George Hillman, age 30, is admitted to the emergency department with an amphetamine overdose. The physician orders immediate administration of activated charcoal. Which of the following calculations is used to estimate the dose of activated charcoal?
   (a) 2 to 5 times the patient's weight
   (b) 5 to 10 times the patient's weight
   (c) 5 to 10 times the weight of the drug ingested
   (d) 10 to 15 times the weight of the drug ingested

3. Amy Collins, age 15 months, is given pancrelipase with meals. Which of the following methods is the best for administering this drug to Amy?
   (a) Mix with milk in a cup or bottle
   (b) Sprinkle on cereal and milk
   (c) Mix with her meat
   (d) Sprinkle on applesauce

4. In the case of substance ingestion, it is important to find out what substance was ingested before selecting a treatment. Using activated charcoal as an adsorbent would be acceptable for which of the following substances?
   (a) petroleum distillates
   (b) aspirin
   (c) ethanol
   (d) iron salts

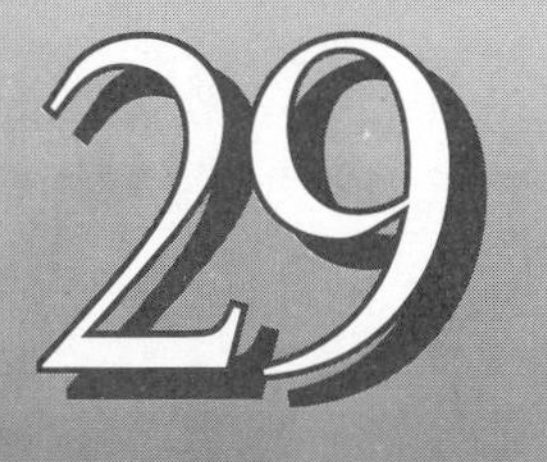

Antidiarrheal and laxative agents

OBJECTIVES

After reading and studying this chapter, the student should be able to:

1. identify the antidiarrheal agents indicated for acute, nonspecific diarrhea and chronic diarrhea.
2. discuss the potential adverse effects of opium tincture, paregoric, difenoxin, diphenoxylate, loperamide, and kaolin and pectin.
3. identify the contraindications and precautions the nurse should be aware of when administering antidiarrheals.
4. describe the mechanism of action of laxatives.
5. compare the clinical indications for hyperosmolar, bulk-forming, emollient, stimulant, and lubricant laxatives.
6. describe how to apply the nursing process when caring for a patient who is receiving an antidiarrheal or laxative agent.

INTRODUCTION

Diarrhea and **constipation** represent the two major symptoms related to disturbances of the large intestine. **Antidiarrheals** act systemically or locally. Opium tincture, paregoric, loperamide, difenoxin, and diphenoxylate are systemic agents. The combination of kaolin and pectin is a local agent.

Laxatives and **cathartics** include various drugs that stimulate defecation. The major classes of laxatives include hyperosmolar agents, dietary fiber and related bulk-forming substances, **emollients,** stimulants, and lubricants. The U.S. Food and Drug Administration Advisory Review Panel for Over-the-Counter Drugs has approved various laxative-cathartic agents as nonprescription drugs. (See *Selected major antidiarrheal and laxative agents,* pages 366 and 367.)

Drugs covered in this chapter include:

- bisacodyl
- diphenoxalate
- docusate sodium
- glycerin
- kaolin and pectin mixtures
- loperamide
- mineral oil
- paregoric
- psyllium
- saline compounds
- sodium biphosphate.

Opium preparations

Opium tincture and paregoric (camphorated opium tincture) are effective in treating acute, nonspecific diarrhea.

PHARMACOKINETICS

Opium tincture and paregoric have similar pharmacokinetic properties. Both are absorbed systemically, metabolized by the liver, and excreted by the kidneys.

Route	Onset	Peak	Duration
P.O.	1 hr	2-3 hr	4 hr

PHARMACODYNAMICS

These drugs exert an antidiarrheal effect by (1) slowing the effects of the mesenteric plexus of the intestine, (2) inhibiting intestinal peristalsis by direct central action on the brain, (3) decreasing expulsive contractions, (4) enhancing anal sphincter tone, and (5) enhancing ileocecal valve tone.

PHARMACOTHERAPEUTICS

Opium tincture and paregoric are used to treat acute, nonspecific diarrhea; however, they should not be used for diarrhea caused by toxic chemicals or pathogens. They commonly are used with kaolin, pectin, and bismuth salts because these three drugs offer adsorbent and protective effects. Also, opium tincture may be added to enteral feeding preparations to prevent the diarrhea that they typically cause.

Drug interactions

Opium tincture and paregoric can enhance the depressant effects of alcohol, barbiturates, tranquilizers, and other central nervous system (CNS) depressants. The drugs have an additive effect of constipation when used with anticholinergic drugs.

Selected major antidiarrheal and laxative agents

The following chart summarizes the major antidiarrheals and laxatives currently in clinical use.

DRUG	MAJOR INDICATIONS AND USUAL DOSAGES	CONTRAINDICATIONS AND PRECAUTIONS
Antidiarrheals		
diphenoxylate (with atropine) (Lomotil)	*Acute, nonspecific diarrhea* ADULT: initially, 5 mg P.O. q.i.d.; with dosage adjusted to individual response PEDIATRIC: 0.3 to 0.4 mg/kg P.O. daily, given in divided doses for children over age 2 (liquid form only); dosage may be reduced to as low as one-fourth the initial dose as soon as initial symptoms have been controlled	• Diphenoxylate is contraindcated in a patient with known hypersensitivity, jaundice, antibiotic-induced diarrhea, pseudomembranous colitis, or diarrhea caused by certain infections. • This drug requires cautious use in a pregnant or breast-feeding patient or one with advanced hepatorenal disease, abnormal liver function, narcotic dependence, or benign prostatic hyperplasia.
kaolin and pectin mixtures (Kapectolin)	*Mild to moderate nonspecific diarrhea* ADULT: 60 to 120 ml regular strength suspension or 45 to 90 ml concentrated suspension P.O. after each loose bowel movement, maximum of 8 doses daily PEDIATRIC: for children ages 3 to 5, 15 to 30 ml P.O. of regular suspension or 15 ml P.O. concentrated suspension; for children ages 6 to 11, 30 to 60 ml P.O. of regular suspension or 30 ml of concentrated suspension after each loose bowel movement	• Kaolin and pectin have no known contraindications or precautions.
loperamide (Imodium)	*Acute, nonspecific diarrhea* ADULT: initially, 4 mg P.O., then 2 mg after each unformed stool; up to a maximum of 16 mg daily PEDIATRIC: initially, 1 mg P.O. (liquid form only) t.i.d. for children ages 2 to 5; 2 mg P.O. b.i.d. for ages 6 to 8; 2 mg P.O. t.i.d. for ages 6 to 12 with weight above 66 lb (30 kg); after first day, 0.1 mg/kg after each loose stool *Chronic diarrhea* ADULT: initially, 4 mg P.O., then 2 mg after each unformed stool	• Loperamide is contraindicated in a patient with known hypersensitivity, antibiotic-induced pseudomembranous colitis or diarrhea, diarrhea caused by infection with certain organisms, or a condition in which constipation must be avoided. • This drug requires cautious use in a pregnant or breast-feeding patient or one with benign prostatic hyperplasia, renal dysfunction, or narcotic dependence. • Safety and efficacy in children under age 2 have not been established.
paregoric (camphorated opium tincture)	*Acute, nonspecific diarrhea* ADULT: 5 to 10 ml P.O. up to q.i.d. until acute diarrhea subsides PEDIATRIC: 0.25 to 0.5 ml/kg P.O. up to q.i.d. until diarrhea subsides	• Paregoric is contraindicated in a patient with diarrhea caused by toxic chemicals or pathogens or known hypersensitivity to it or atropine sulfate. • This drug requires cautious use in a pregnant or breast-feeding patient or one with asthma, severe prostatic hyperplasia, narcotic dependence, or liver or renal dysfunction.
Hyperosmolar laxatives		
glycerin	*Constipation* ADULT AND CHILDREN AGE 6 AND OVER: 2 to 3 g as a rectal suppository or 5 to 15 ml as an enema CHILDREN AGE 2 TO 5: 1 to 1.7 g as a rectal suppository or 2 to 5 ml as an enema	• Glycerin has no known contraindications or precautions when used as a laxative.
saline compounds—magnesium salts (Milk of Magnesia), sodium biphosphate (Fleet Enema), sodium phosphate	*Prompt and complete bowel evacuation* ADULT: 10 to 15 g of magnesium sulfate P.O. in a glass of water; 240 ml of magnesium citrate P.O. h.s.; 20 to 30 ml P.O. of oral sodium phosphate or sodium biphosphate solution mixed with a glass of water; or 120 ml (4 oz) of sodium phosphate or sodium biphosphate as an enema PEDIATRIC: highly individualized according to age and compound used	• Saline compounds are contraindicated in a patient with congenital megacolon, imperforate anus, or heart failure. • These drugs require cautious use in a patient who has a colostomy or one with renal impairment, cardiac disease, electrolyte imbalances, or a condition or treatment regimen that predisposes the patient to electrolyte imbalances.

Selected major antidiarrheal and laxative agents *(continued)*

DRUG	MAJOR INDICATIONS AND USUAL DOSAGES	CONTRAINDICATIONS AND PRECAUTIONS
Bulk-forming laxative		
psyllium hydrophilic mucilloid (Metamucil, Syllact, Konsyl)	*Treatment of constipation* ADULT: 1 to 2 teaspoons or 1 packet P.O. dissolved in a glass of water b.i.d. or t.i.d., followed by a second glass of water PEDIATRIC: for children age 12 and older, 1 to 2 teaspoons or 1 packet P.O. dissolved in a glass of water b.i.d. or t.i.d., followed by a second glass of water; for children ages 6 to 11, up to 15 g P.O. daily given in divided doses of 2.5 to 3.75 g per dose	• Psyllium hydrophilic mucilloid is contraindicated in a patient with known hypersensitivity, intestinal obstruction, or fecal impaction.
Emollient laxative		
docusate sodium (Colace, Correctol, Doxinate, Regutol)	*Stool softening for patients who should not strain during defecation* ADULT: 50 to 500 mg P.O. daily until bowel movements are normal PEDIATRIC: for children age 13 and older, 50 to 360 mg P.O. daily until bowel movements are normal; for children ages 2 to 12, 50 to 150 mg P.O. daily until bowel movements are normal; for children under age 2, 25 mg P.O. daily until bowel movements are normal	• Docusate sodium has no known contraindications. • This drug requires cautious use in a pregnant or breast-feeding patient.
Stimulant laxative		
bisacodyl (Dulcolax)	*Chronic constipation* ADULT: 5 to 15 mg P.O. in the evening or before breakfast, or 10 mg as a rectal suppository or 1.25 oz as an enema PEDIATRIC: for children age 12 and older, 5 to 15 mg P.O. in the evening or before breakfast, or 10 mg as a rectal suppository or 1.25 oz as an enema; for children ages 4 to 6, 5 to 10 mg P.O. in the evening or before breakfast; for children ages 2 to 12, 5 to 10 mg as a rectal suppository *Bowel evacuation before delivery, surgery, or rectal or bowel examination* ADULT: up to 30 mg P.O.	• Bisacodyl is contraindicated in a breast-feeding patient or one with intestinal obstruction or an acute abdominal condition that requires immediate surgery. • This drug requires cautious use in a pregnant patient.
Lubricant laxative		
mineral oil (Agoral Plain, Fleet Mineral Oil Enema)	*Constipation or maintenance of soft stools when the patient should not strain during defecation* ADULT: 15 to 30 ml P.O., usually h.s., or 4 oz as an enema PEDIATRIC: for children age 12 and older, 15 to 30 ml P.O. daily, or 4 oz as an enema; for children ages 6 to 11, 5 to 15 ml P.O. daily, or 1 to 2 oz as an enema; for children ages 2 to 5, 1 to 2 oz as an enema	• Oral mineral oil is contraindicated in a geriatric, debilitated, or pregnant patient or one with esophageal or gastric retention, dysphagia, or hiatal hernia.

ADVERSE DRUG REACTIONS

Some adverse reactions to opium tincture and paregoric occur. However, reactions to usual doses typically are mild. Dose-related reactions to opium tincture and paregoric include nausea, vomiting, dizziness, dysphoria, constipation, and increased biliary tract pressure.

Hypersensitivity reactions include allergic reactions, such as urticaria and contact dermatitis. Anaphylactoid reactions

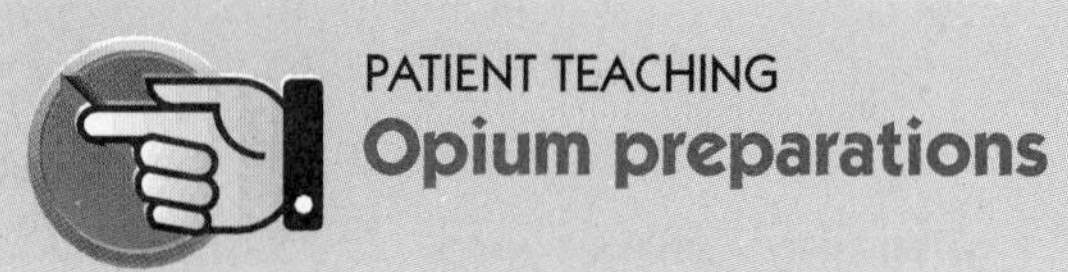

PATIENT TEACHING

Opium preparations

- ➤ Teach the patient and family the name, dose, frequency, action, and adverse effects of the prescribed opium preparation.
- ➤ Advise the patient to take the drug as prescribed to avoid dependence.
- ➤ Instruct the patient to notify the physician if diarrhea lasts longer than 48 hours or if fever and abdominal pain develop during treatment.
- ➤ Instruct the patient to drink additional fluids to replace those lost through diarrhea.
- ➤ Advise the patient to avoid activities that may require mental alertness if dizziness occurs.
- ➤ Inform the patient that paregoric normally appears milky when added to water.
- ➤ Instruct the patient to notify the physician if adverse reactions occur.

are rare. Patients over age 60 experience more frequent allergic reactions.

NURSING PROCESS APPLICATION

The following information assists the nurse in caring for a patient receiving an opium preparation. It includes an overview of assessment activities, appropriate nursing diagnoses, and related interventions.

Assessment

Before drug therapy begins, review the patient's history for conditions that contraindicate or require cautious use of the prescribed antidiarrheal, and to identify use of drugs that may interact with it. During therapy, monitor for adverse drug reactions and signs of drug interactions. Periodically assess the effectiveness of antidiarrheal therapy. Finally, evaluate the patient's and family's knowledge about the drug. (See Patient Teaching: *Opium preparations.*)

Nursing diagnoses

- Risk for injury related to adverse drug reactions or drug interactions
- Constipation related to the adverse gastrointestinal (GI) effects of the opium preparation
- Knowledge deficit related to the prescribed opium preparation

Planning and implementation

- Do not administer an opium preparation to a patient with a condition that contraindicates its use. Also do not administer an opium preparation to treat diarrhea caused by toxic chemicals or pathogens.
- Administer an opium preparation cautiously to a patient at risk because of a preexisting condition.
- Monitor the patient closely for adverse reactions and drug interactions during treatment with an opium preparation.

**** Do not interchange opium tincture with paregoric because the opium content of opium tincture is 25 times greater.***

- Expect a milky fluid to form when paregoric is added to water.
- Notify the physician or primary health care provider if adverse reactions occur.

**** Monitor for enhanced CNS depression if the patient is also receiving another CNS depressant.***

- Consult with the primary health care provider if the patient's diarrhea lasts longer than 48 hours or if fever and abdominal pain develop during therapy.
- Monitor for constipation, especially if the patient is also receiving an anticholinergic drug.
- Notify the health care provider if constipation occurs.

Evaluation

For each nursing diagnosis, prepare an evaluation statement that describes the patient's or family's response to nursing interventions.

Difenoxin, diphenoxylate, and loperamide

Difenoxin, diphenoxylate, and loperamide are antidiarrheal agents that decrease peristalsis in the intestines.

PHARMACOKINETICS

Difenoxin and diphenoxylate have better absorption, a faster onset of action, and a shorter duration of action than loperamide.

At the usual dosage, difenoxin and diphenoxylate are absorbed readily from the GI tract; loperamide is not absorbed well after oral administration. These medications are distributed in the serum, and metabolism occurs with the detoxification process in the liver. Diphenoxylate is metabolized to difenoxin, its biologically active major metabolite. All three drugs are excreted primarily in the feces.

Route	Onset	Peak	Duration
P.O.	30-60 min	40 min-5 hr	3-24 hr

PHARMACODYNAMICS

Difenoxin, diphenoxylate, and loperamide decrease GI motility by depressing the circular and longitudinal muscle action in the large and small intestines. These drugs also decrease expulsive contractions throughout the entire colon. Difenoxin and diphenoxylate are combined with the anticholinergic agent atropine to discourage abuse of these agents.

PHARMACOTHERAPEUTICS

Difenoxin, diphenoxylate, and loperamide are used to treat acute, nonspecific diarrhea. Loperamide also is used to treat chronic diarrhea.

Drug interactions

Difenoxin, diphenoxylate, and loperamide may enhance the depressant effects of barbiturates, alcohol, narcotics, tranquilizers, and sedatives.

ADVERSE DRUG REACTIONS

The adverse reactions to difenoxin, diphenoxylate, and loperamide include nausea, vomiting, abdominal discomfort or distention, drowsiness, fatigue, CNS depression, tachycardia, hypoperistalsis, and paralytic ileus. Allergic responses, such as rash and urticaria, also may occur as hypersensitivity reactions.

Adverse reactions to atropine include flushing, diminished secretions, hyperthermia, tachycardia, urine retention, miosis, nystagmus, and blurred vision.

NURSING PROCESS APPLICATION

The following information assists the nurse in caring for a patient who is receiving difenoxin, diphenoxylate, or loperamide. It includes an overview of assessment activities as well as examples of appropriate nursing diagnoses and related interventions. It also highlights the importance of evaluation.

Assessment

Before drug therapy begins, review the patient's history for conditions that contraindicate or require cautious use of the prescribed antidiarrheal. Also review the patient's medication history to identify use of drugs that may interact with it. During therapy, assess the patient for adverse drug reactions and signs of drug interactions. Also, periodically assess the effectiveness of antidiarrheal therapy. Finally, evaluate the patient's and family's knowledge about the prescribed drug.

Nursing diagnoses

- Risk for injury related to a preexisting condition that contraindicates or requires cautious use of difenoxin, diphenoxylate, or loperamide
- Risk for injury related to adverse drug reactions or drug interactions
- Urinary retention related to the adverse genitourinary effects of atropine in difenoxin or diphenoxylate
- Knowledge deficit related to the prescribed antidiarrheal

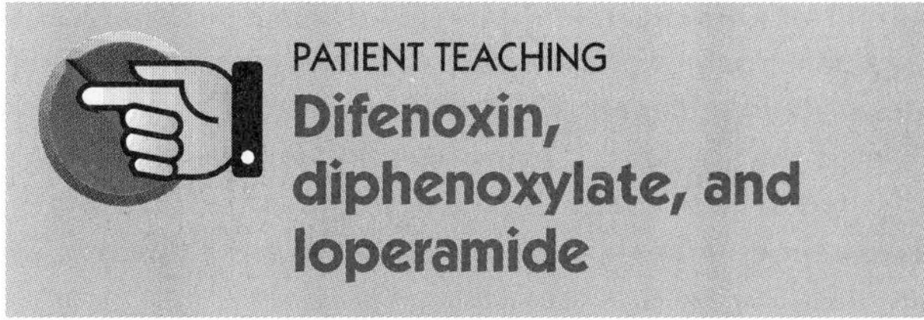

PATIENT TEACHING

Difenoxin, diphenoxylate, and loperamide

- ➤ Teach the patient and family the name, dose, frequency, action, and adverse effects of the prescribed antidiarrheal.
- ➤ Advise the patient not to use alcohol or any other central nervous system depressant during difenoxin, diphenoxylate, or loperamide therapy.
- ➤ Teach the patient taking difenoxin or diphenoxylate with atropine to recognize and report the signs of atropine toxicity, which may require a dosage reduction.
- ➤ Instruct the patient to be alert for early warning signs of hypoperistalsis (nausea and anorexia) and toxic megacolon (abdominal distention). If these signs occur, tell the patient to notify the physician before taking the next dose of the prescribed antidiarrheal.
- ➤ Encourage the patient to drink eight to thirteen 8-oz (240-ml) glasses of fluid daily to replace lost fluids.
- ➤ Caution the patient to avoid any activity that requires mental alertness if drowsiness occurs.
- ➤ Teach the patient taking difenoxin or diphenoxylate with atropine to recognize and report signs or symptoms of urine retention.
- ➤ Instruct the patient to consult the physician if acute nonspecific diarrhea does not improve in 48 hours or if chronic diarrhea does not improve after 10 days.

Planning and implementation

- Do not administer difenoxin, diphenoxylate, or loperamide to a patient with a condition that contraindicates its use.
- Administer difenoxin, diphenoxylate, or loperamide cautiously to a patient at risk because of a preexisting condition.
- Monitor the patient closely for adverse reactions to the prescribed antidiarrheal agents and for drug interactions. (See Patient Teaching: *Difenoxin, diphenoxylate, and loperamide.*)

* ***Observe for signs of atropine toxicity during difenoxin or diphenoxylate therapy, and reduce the dosage as prescribed.***

- Observe for signs of hypoperistalsis, and consult a physician if it occurs.

* ***Withhold the drug and consult the physician if the patient shows signs of abdominal distention, which may indicate toxic megacolon, especially if a patient has ulcerative colitis.***

* ***Withhold the drug and consult the physician if the patient with acute nonspecific diarrhea shows no improvement in 48 hours or if the patient with chronic diarrhea shows no improvement after 10 days.***

- Notify the physician if adverse reactions occur.

Monitor for urine retention regularly in a patient receiving difenoxin or diphenoxylate with atropine, especially if the patient has benign prostatic hyperplasia.

• Notify the physician if urine retention is suspected. Be prepared to catheterize the patient as prescribed. Expect to reduce the antidiarrheal dosage or administer a different antidiarrheal agent as prescribed.

Evaluation

For each nursing diagnosis, prepare an evaluation statement that describes the patient's or family's response to nursing interventions.

Kaolin and pectin

Kaolin and pectin mixtures, which are locally acting antidiarrheals, are sold over the counter.

PHARMACOKINETICS

Kaolin and pectin are not absorbed and, therefore, not distributed throughout the body. Up to 90% of a dose is metabolized in the GI tract. The drugs and their metabolites are excreted in the feces.

Route	Onset	Peak	Duration
P.O.	30 min	Unknown	4-6 hr

PHARMACODYNAMICS

Kaolin and pectin act as adsorbents, binding with bacteria, toxins, and other irritants on the intestinal mucosa. Pectin decreases the pH in the intestinal lumen and provides a soothing demulcent effect on the irritated mucosa.

PHARMACOTHERAPEUTICS

Kaolin and pectin are used to relieve mild to moderate acute diarrhea. They also may be used to relieve chronic diarrhea temporarily until the cause has been determined and definitive treatment instituted.

Drug interactions

Kaolin and pectin mixtures interfere with lincomycin absorption if administered within 2 hours before or 3 to 4 hours after lincomycin. These antidiarrheals also can interfere with absorption of digoxin or other drugs from the intestinal mucosa if administered concurrently.

ADVERSE DRUG REACTIONS

Kaolin and pectin mixtures cause few adverse reactions. Constipation may occur, especially in a geriatric or debilitated patient or with overdose and prolonged use, but the constipation usually is mild and transient. Rarely, fecal impaction occurs in infants and debilitated patients.

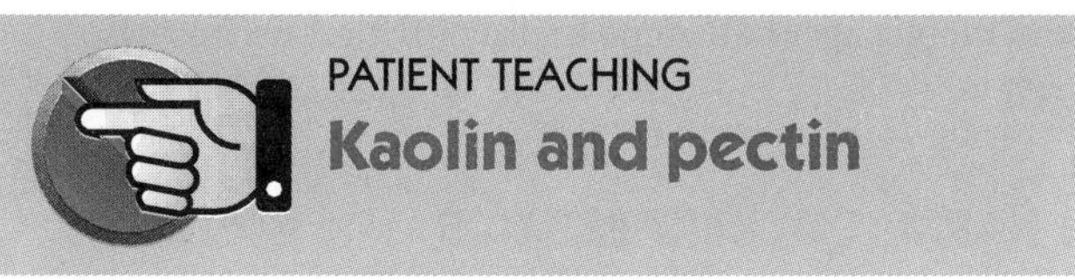

PATIENT TEACHING

Kaolin and pectin

- Teach the patient and family the name, dose, frequency, action, and adverse effects of kaolin and pectin.
- Advise the patient to avoid self-medication for longer than 48 hours. Instruct the patient to consult a physician if diarrhea persists.
- Instruct the patient taking other medications to consult the physician because kaolin and pectin can interfere with the absorption of other drugs, making them less effective.
- Instruct the patient to drink eight to thirteen 8-oz (240-ml) glasses of fluid daily to replace lost fluids.
- Instruct the patient to take kaolin and pectin as prescribed; for example, a dose of kaolin and pectin after each loose bowel movement, but not more than eight doses per day. The patient who experiences more than eight bowel movements in 1 day should consult the physician.

NURSING PROCESS APPLICATION

The following information assists the nurse in caring for a patient who is receiving a kaolin and pectin mixture. It includes an overview of assessment activities as well as examples of appropriate nursing diagnoses and related interventions. It also highlights the importance of evaluation.

Assessment

Before drug therapy begins, review the patient's medication history to identify use of drugs that may interact with kaolin and pectin mixtures. During therapy, assess the patient for adverse drug reactions and signs of drug interactions. Also, periodically assess the effectiveness of kaolin and pectin therapy. Finally, evaluate the patient's and family's knowledge about the prescribed drug.

Nursing diagnoses

• Risk for injury related to adverse drug reactions or drug interactions

• Constipation related to the adverse GI effects of kaolin and pectin

• Knowledge deficit related to kaolin and pectin

Planning and implementation

• Monitor the patient for adverse reactions and signs of drug interactions.

• Notify the physician if adverse reactions or drug interactions occur.

Monitor the patient closely for constipation during kaolin and pectin therapy. Be aware that fecal impaction can result from severe constipation, especially in an infant or debilitated patient.

• Withhold kaolin and pectin if the patient develops constipation, and notify the physician. (See Patient Teaching: *Kaolin and pectin.*)

Evaluation

For each nursing diagnosis, prepare an evaluation statement that describes the patient's or family's response to nursing interventions.

Hyperosmolar laxatives

Hyperosmolar laxatives include glycerin, lactulose, and saline compounds (magnesium salts, sodium biphosphate, sodium phosphate, and polyethylene glycol and electrolytes).

PHARMACOKINETICS

Glycerin is introduced into the large intestine and is not absorbed systemically. Lactulose enters the GI tract and is absorbed only to a minor degree; thus, the drug is distributed only in the intestine. Lactulose is metabolized by the intestinal microflora and is excreted in the feces. Once the saline compounds are introduced into the GI tract, some absorption of its component ions occurs. It is excreted in the urine.

Glycerin usually causes bowel evacuation 15 to 30 minutes after administration. Bowel evacuation should occur 1 to 2 days after administration of lactulose. Saline cathartics produce a watery stool evacuation within 1 to 3 hours after administration.

Polyethylene glycol (PEG) is a virtually nonabsorbable solution that acts as an osmotic agent but does not alter electrolyte balance. Bowel evacuation begins in 30 to 60 minutes and usually subsides in 3 to 4 hours.

Route	Onset	Peak	Duration
P.O.	15 min-2 days	Variable	Variable
P.R.	30 min-48 hr	Variable	Variable

PHARMACODYNAMICS

The hyperosmolar laxatives produce bowel evacuation by drawing water into the intestine. Distention of the bowel from fluid accumulation promotes peristalsis and bowel movement.

PHARMACOTHERAPEUTICS

Glycerin is helpful in bowel retraining. Lactulose is used to treat chronic constipation and to reduce ammonia production and absorption from the intestines in liver disease. Saline compounds are used when prompt and complete bowel evacuation is required.

Drug interactions

Hyperosmolar laxatives do not interact significantly with other drugs.

It is important to note that oral medication given 1 hour before initiating treatment with PEG will be flushed from the GI tract unabsorbed.

ADVERSE DRUG REACTIONS

The adverse reactions to hyperosmolar laxatives involve fluid and electrolyte imbalances. Glycerin administration also may cause weakness and fatigue; rarely, severe diarrhea and hypovolemia may occur.

Adverse reactions to lactulose include abdominal distention, flatulence, and abdominal cramps in approximately 20% of patients taking full doses. Other adverse reactions include nausea, vomiting, diarrhea, hypokalemia, hypovolemia, increased blood glucose level in patients with impaired glucose tolerance, and increased hepatic encephalopathy in patients with severe liver dysfunction.

Adverse reactions to saline compounds include weakness, lethargy, dehydration from hypernatremia and resultant hypovolemia, hypermagnesemia, hyperphosphatemia, hypocalcemia, cardiac arrhythmias from electrolyte imbalances, and hypovolemic shock.

The most common adverse reactions associated with PEG include nausea, abdominal fullness, and bloating.

NURSING PROCESS APPLICATION

The following information assists the nurse in caring for a patient who is receiving a hyperosmolar laxative. It includes an overview of assessment activities as well as examples of appropriate nursing diagnoses and related interventions. It also highlights the importance of evaluation.

Assessment

Before drug therapy begins, review the patient's history for conditions that contraindicate or require cautious use of the prescribed hyperosmolar laxative. During therapy, assess the patient for adverse drug reactions. Also, periodically assess the effectiveness of therapy with the hyperosmolar laxative. Finally, evaluate the patient's and family's knowledge about the prescribed drug.

Nursing diagnoses

• Risk for injury related to adverse reactions
• Risk for fluid volume deficit related to hypovolemia caused by lactulose or a saline compound
• Knowledge deficit related to the prescribed hyperosmolar laxative

Planning and implementation

• Do not administer a hyperosmolar laxative to a patient with a condition that contraindicates its use.
• Administer a hyperosmolar laxative cautiously to a patient at risk because of a preexisting condition.

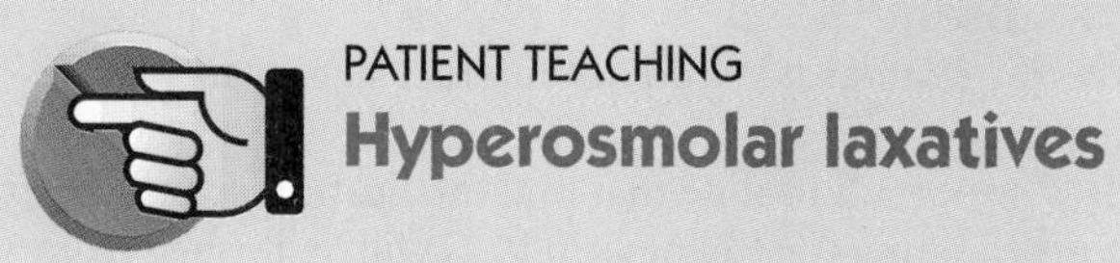

PATIENT TEACHING
Hyperosmolar laxatives

- Teach the patient and family the name, dose, frequency, action, and adverse effects of the prescribed hyperosmolar laxative.
- Describe the proper use of laxatives and caution the patient about laxative dependence.
- Discuss additional measures the patient can take to prevent constipation.
- Teach the patient with chronic constipation about bowel retraining, if prescribed.
- Stress the importance of taking the hyperosmolar laxative exactly as prescribed to help prevent fluid and electrolyte imbalances.
- Teach the patient to recognize the signs of fluid and electrolyte imbalances and, if they occur, to withhold the drug and notify the physician.
- Advise the patient to avoid activities that require mental alertness if weakness, drowsiness, or lethargy occurs.
- Instruct the patient with impaired glucose tolerance to be alert for signs of hyperglycemia and to monitor blood glucose levels regularly during lactulose therapy.
- Instruct the patient to drink at least 64 oz (2 L) of fluid with saline compound therapy.
- Instruct the patient who experiences diarrhea to withhold the agent, notify the physician, and increase fluid intake (unless contraindicated).
- Advise the patient to notify the physician if adverse reactions occur or if the prescribed hyperosmolar laxative is ineffective.
- Advise the patient that oral medications should be taken more than 1 hour before taking polyethylene glycol (PEG) or they will not be absorbed.
- Advise the patient that PEG is best tolerated chilled; if signs of hypothermia occur, the physician should be contacted.

• Monitor the patient for signs of adverse reactions to hyperosmolar laxative therapy.
***Monitor the patient closely for fluid and electrolyte imbalances.**
***Perform a neurologic assessment regularly to detect the CNS effects of an electrolyte imbalance.**
***Monitor blood glucose levels once every shift or as prescribed for a patient with impaired glucose tolerance who is receiving lactulose. Also observe for signs and symptoms of hyperglycemia, such as polyuria, polydipsia, polyphagia, and weakness.**
• Dilute lactulose with water or unsweetened juice before administration to reduce the sweetness and prevent nausea.
• Store lactulose below 86° F (30° C), but do not allow the drug to become frozen.
• Encourage the patient to drink eight to thirteen 8-oz (240-ml) glasses of fluid daily (unless contraindicated) during saline compound therapy. (See Patient Teaching: *Hyperosmolar laxatives.*)
• Periodically monitor the patient's bowel patterns throughout therapy to assess the drug's effectiveness or detect diarrhea.
• Notify the physician if adverse reactions occur or if the hyperosmolar laxative is ineffective.
• Monitor hydration for the patient with nausea, vomiting, or diarrhea. Obtain a prescription for an antiemetic agent as needed. Also expect to decrease the dosage or discontinue the hyperosmolar laxative as prescribed. Replace fluids as prescribed.
• Prepare the PEG solution with tap water and shake vigorously to dissolve the powdered drug. Store the solution under refrigeration for up to 48 hours.
• Administer PEG after a fast of at least 3 to 4 hours.
• Encourage the patient to drink the prescribed 4 L of PEG solution rapidly (240 ml every 10 minutes) rather than drinking small amounts continuously.
• Use caution in administering chilled PEG solution. Although chilling does enhance the flavor, hypothermia has been reported after ingestion of a large amount of chilled solution.

Evaluation

For each nursing diagnosis, prepare an evaluation statement that describes the patient's or family's response to nursing interventions.

Dietary fiber and related bulk-forming laxatives

A high-fiber diet is the most natural way to prevent or treat constipation. Dietary fiber refers to the amount of plant food that is not digested in the small intestine. The bulk-forming laxatives, which resemble dietary fiber, contain natural and semisynthetic polysaccharides and cellulose. These laxatives include methylcellulose, polycarbophil, and psyllium hydrophilic mucilloid.

PHARMACOKINETICS

Dietary fiber and bulk-forming laxatives are not absorbed systemically. The polysaccharides in these agents are metabolized by intestinal bacterial flora into osmotically active metabolites. Dietary fiber and bulk-forming laxatives are excreted in the feces.

Route	Onset	Peak	Duration
P.O.	12-24 hr	3-4 days	Variable

PHARMACODYNAMICS

Dietary fiber and bulk-forming laxatives increase stool mass and water content, thereby promoting peristalsis.

PHARMACOTHERAPEUTICS

Bulk-forming laxatives are used to treat simple cases of constipation, especially constipation resulting from a low-fiber or low-fluid diet. These agents also are indicated for patients recovering from acute myocardial infarction (MI) or cerebral aneurysms who need to avoid **Valsalva's maneuver** and maintain soft feces. Bulk-forming laxatives also may be used to manage patients with irritable bowel syndrome and diverticulosis.

Drug interactions

No significant drug interactions occur with the use of dietary fiber or bulk-forming laxatives.

ADVERSE DRUG REACTIONS

Adverse reactions include flatulence, a sensation of abdominal fullness, intestinal obstruction, fecal impaction, esophageal obstruction (if sufficient liquid has not been administered with the agent), and severe diarrhea. Hypersensitivity reactions rarely occur.

NURSING PROCESS APPLICATION

The following information assists the nurse in caring for a patient who is receiving dietary fiber or a bulk-forming laxative. It includes an overview of assessment activities as well as examples of appropriate nursing diagnoses and related interventions. It also highlights the importance of evaluation.

Assessment

Before drug therapy begins, review the patient's history for conditions that contraindicate the use of dietary fiber or the prescribed bulk-forming laxative. During therapy, assess the patient for adverse drug reactions. Also, periodically assess the effectiveness of therapy with dietary fiber or a bulk-forming laxative. Finally, evaluate the patient's and family's knowledge about the prescribed drug.

Nursing diagnoses

- Risk for injury related to adverse drug reactions
- Diarrhea related to the adverse GI effects of dietary fiber or the prescribed bulk-forming laxative
- Knowledge deficit related to dietary fiber or the prescribed bulk-forming laxative

Planning and implementation

- Do not administer dietary fiber or a bulk-forming laxative to a patient with a condition that contraindicates its use.
- Monitor the patient closely for adverse GI effects. (See Patient Teaching: *Dietary fiber and related bulk-forming laxatives.*)
- Evaluate the effects of dietary fiber intake or the bulk-forming laxative on the patient's bowel pattern. Notify the physician if these measures are ineffective.

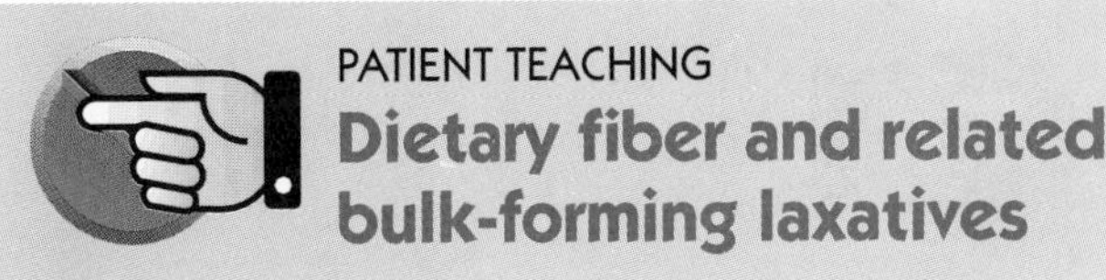

PATIENT TEACHING

Dietary fiber and related bulk-forming laxatives

- Teach the patient and family the name, dose, frequency, action, and adverse effects of the prescribed bulk-forming laxative.
- Inform the patient and family about dietary sources of fiber, such as bran, whole grain cereals, fresh fruits and vegetables, and legumes. Tell the patient to consume 6 to 11 servings (around 25 mg) of dietary fiber daily to prevent constipation, but to increase consumption slowly to minimize GI upset.
- Advise the patient with restricted sugar and salt intake against the frequent use of bulk-forming laxatives because most of these agents contain sugar and salt. Recommend sugar-free laxatives to a diabetic patient.
- Teach the patient to take each dose of a bulk-forming laxative with an 8-oz (240-ml) glass of water and to increase fluid intake during the day to prevent fecal impaction. Also tell the patient to follow each dose of psyllium hydrophilic mucilloid with a second 8-oz glass of water.
- Inform a patient with chronic constipation to use additional measures to correct constipation.
- Explain that the patient may experience flatulence or a sensation of abdominal fullness when taking dietary fiber or a bulk-forming laxative.
- Instruct the patient to tell the physician if adverse reactions occur or if the dietary fiber or laxative is ineffective.

**** Administer a bulk-forming laxative with an 8-oz (240-ml) glass of water to prevent esophageal obstruction. Ensure that the patient follows each dose of psyllium hydrophilic mucilloid with a second 8-oz glass of water.***
**** Monitor the patient for diarrhea, which may become severe. Also monitor for laxative dependence.***
**** Monitor hydration if the patient develops diarrhea, and withhold dietary fiber or the bulk-forming laxative until the physician has been notified.***

Evaluation

For each nursing diagnosis, prepare an evaluation statement that describes the patient's or family's response to nursing interventions.

Emollient laxatives

Emollients also are known as stool softeners. Emollients include the calcium, potassium, and sodium salts of docusate and poloxamer 188.

PHARMACOKINETICS

Administered orally, emollients are absorbed and excreted through bile in the feces. After oral administration, the on-

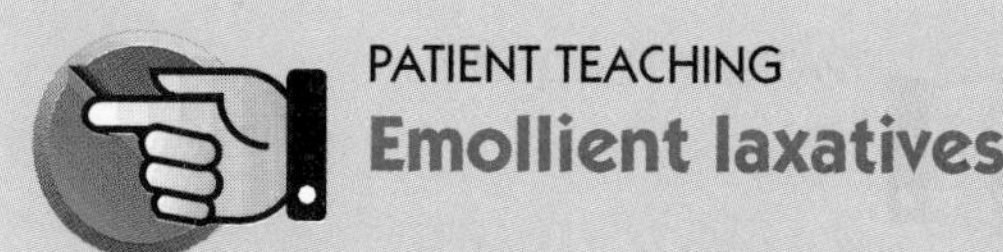

PATIENT TEACHING
Emollient laxatives

- Teach the patient and family the name, dose, frequency, action, and adverse effects of the prescribed emollient laxative.
- Discuss additional measures the patient can take to prevent constipation.
- Instruct the patient how to store and take the emollient laxative. For example, caution the patient to swallow the emollient capsules and not to chew or open them.
- Tell the patient to notify the physician if adverse reactions occur or if the prescribed emollient laxative is ineffective.

set of action occurs within 12 to 72 hours for docusate salts and within 3 to 5 days for poloxamer 188.

Route	Onset	Peak	Duration
P.O.	12 hr-5 days	Variable	Variable

PHARMACODYNAMICS

Emollients soften the stool and ease defecation by emulsifying the fat and water components of feces in the small and large intestines. This detergent action allows water and lipids to penetrate the fecal material, thereby producing net fluid accumulation. Emollients also stimulate electrolyte and fluid secretion from intestinal mucosal cells.

PHARMACOTHERAPEUTICS

Emollients are the drugs of choice for softening stool in patients who should avoid straining during defecation. Such patients include those who recently have had an MI or surgery and those with a disease of the anus or rectum, increased intracranial pressure (ICP), or hernias. Children with hard, dry stools can receive emollients safely. Emollients also may be given before rectal cathartics to treat fecal impaction.

Drug interactions

The nurse should not administer oral emollients with oral mineral oil because they enhance the systemic absorption of mineral oil and may result in tissue deposits. Because emollients may enhance the absorption of many oral drugs, the nurse should not administer them concurrently with oral drugs that have low therapeutic indexes.

ADVERSE DRUG REACTIONS

Although adverse reactions to emollients seldom occur, they may include a bitter taste, diarrhea, throat irritation, and mild, transient abdominal cramping.

NURSING PROCESS APPLICATION

The following information assists the nurse in caring for a patient who is receiving an emollient laxative. It includes an overview of assessment activities as well as examples of appropriate nursing diagnoses and related interventions. It also highlights the importance of evaluation.

Assessment

Before drug therapy begins, review the patient's history for conditions that require cautious use of the prescribed emollient laxative. Also review the patient's medication history to identify use of drugs that may interact with it. During therapy, assess the patient for adverse drug reactions and signs of drug interactions. Also, periodically assess the effectiveness of therapy with the emollient laxative. Finally, evaluate the patient's and family's knowledge about the prescribed drug.

Nursing diagnoses

- Risk for injury related to adverse drug reactions or drug interactions
- Knowledge deficit related to the prescribed emollient laxative

Planning and implementation

- Administer an emollient laxative cautiously to a patient at risk because of a preexisting condition.
- Monitor the patient closely for adverse reactions and drug interactions during emollient laxative therapy. (See Patient Teaching: *Emollient laxatives.*)
- Store the emollient laxative at 59° to 86° F (15° to 30° C). Protect liquid preparations from light.
- Give a liquid emollient in milk or fruit juice to mask the bitter taste.

* ***Monitor hydration and notify the physician if the patient develops diarrhea. Replace fluid and electrolytes lost through diarrhea as prescribed.***

Evaluation

For each nursing diagnosis, prepare an evaluation statement that describes the patient's or family's response to nursing interventions.

Stimulant laxatives

Stimulant laxatives, also known as irritant cathartics, include bisacodyl, cascara sagrada, castor oil, phenolphthalein, and senna.

PHARMACOKINETICS

Stimulant laxatives are absorbed slightly and metabolized in the liver. The metabolites are excreted in the urine or feces. Bisacodyl and phenolphthalein produce evacuation within 6 to 8 hours after oral administration and within 15 minutes to 1 hour after rectal administration. The duration of a single dose of phenolphthalein may be several days. Cascara sagrada and senna produce an onset of action within 6 to 12 hours after oral administration and within 30 minutes to 2 hours after rectal administration. Castor oil acts more quickly, with loose bowel movements occurring 2 to 3 hours after oral administration.

Route	Onset	Peak	Duration
P.O.	2-12 hr	Variable	Variable
P.R.	15-60 min	Variable	Variable

PHARMACODYNAMICS

Stimulant laxatives stimulate peristalsis and induce defecation by irritating the intestinal mucosa or stimulating nerve endings of the intestinal smooth muscle. Castor oil and phenolphthalein increase the peristaltic activity of the small intestine as well.

PHARMACOTHERAPEUTICS

Stimulant laxatives are the preferred drugs for emptying the bowel before general surgery, sigmoidoscopic or proctoscopic procedures, and radiologic procedures, such as barium studies of the GI tract. Stimulant laxatives also are used to treat constipation caused by prolonged bed rest, neurologic dysfunction of the colon, and constipating drugs such as narcotics.

Drug interactions

No significant drug interactions occur with the stimulant laxatives. However, because stimulant laxatives produce increased intestinal motility, they reduce the absorption of concomitantly administered oral drugs, especially sustained-release forms of oral drugs.

ADVERSE DRUG REACTIONS

Adverse reactions to stimulant laxatives include weakness, nausea, abdominal cramps, and mild proctitis. Rectal administration of bisacodyl can produce a burning sensation. Phenolphthalein can cause a reddish discoloration in alkaline urine. Cascara sagrada and senna cause a reddish pink or brown discoloration of urine. Castor oil may cause pelvic congestion in menstruating women.

With long-term use or overdose, stimulant laxatives may cause electrolyte imbalances, including hypokalemia, hypocalcemia, metabolic alkalosis, or metabolic acidosis. Malabsorption and weight loss also may occur. Habitual use may lead to cathartic colon with **atony** and dilation.

Stimulant laxatives can cause hypersensitivity reactions, such as rash and pruritus. Phenolphthalein allergy may result in renal, cardiac, and respiratory dysfunction.

PATIENT TEACHING
Stimulant laxatives

- Teach the patient and family the name, dose, frequency, action, and adverse effects of the prescribed stimulant laxative.
- Alert the patient that phenolphthalein may cause a reddish discoloration in alkaline urine and that cascara sagrada and senna may cause a reddish pink or brown discoloration of urine.
- Instruct the patient to take the stimulant laxative exactly as prescribed, to prevent dependence, chronic use, and cathartic colon with atony and dilation.
- Advise the patient to discontinue the laxative and notify the physician if a rash or pruritus occurs.
- Teach the patient how to administer and store the prescribed stimulant laxative.
- Instruct the patient not to chew bisacodyl tablets because they are coated to prevent GI irritation. Also advise the patient not to take them with antacids.
- Discuss additional measures the patient can take to prevent constipation.
- Advise the patient to notify the physician if adverse reactions occur or if the prescribed stimulant laxative is ineffective.

NURSING PROCESS APPLICATION

The following information assists the nurse in caring for a patient who is receiving a stimulant laxative. It includes an overview of assessment activities as well as examples of appropriate nursing diagnoses and related interventions. It also highlights the importance of evaluation.

Assessment

Before drug therapy begins, review the patient's history for conditions that contraindicate or require cautious use of the prescribed stimulant laxative. During therapy, assess the patient for adverse drug reactions. Also, periodically assess the effectiveness of therapy with the stimulant laxative. Finally, evaluate the patient's and family's knowledge about the prescribed drug.

Nursing diagnoses

- Risk for injury related to adverse drug reactions
- Knowledge deficit related to the prescribed stimulant laxative

Planning and implementation

- Do not administer a stimulant laxative to a patient with a condition that contraindicates its use.

• Administer a stimulant laxative cautiously to a patient at risk because of a preexisting condition.
• Monitor the patient closely for adverse reactions during stimulant laxative therapy.
***** *Monitor the patient's fluid and electrolyte levels, and notify the physician if an imbalance occurs.***
• Monitor the patient's bowel evacuation pattern, and notify the physician if the stimulant laxative is ineffective.
***** *Discontinue the drug and notify the physician if the patient develops a rash or pruritus.***
• Administer castor oil on an empty stomach for best results.
• Mix castor oil with juice or a carbonated beverage to mask the preparation's oily taste. Tell the patient to hold ice in the mouth before taking castor oil to help decrease the taste. (See Patient Teaching: *Stimulant laxatives,* page 375.)
• Store castor oil below 104° F (40° C), but do not freeze; shake well before administering.

Evaluation

For each nursing diagnosis, prepare an evaluation statement that describes the patient's or family's response to nursing interventions.

Lubricant laxatives

Mineral oil is the main lubricant laxative in current clinical use.

PHARMACOKINETICS

In its nonemulsified form, mineral oil is absorbed minimally; in the emulsified form, about half is absorbed. Absorbed mineral oil is distributed to the mesenteric lymph nodes, intestinal mucosa, liver, and spleen. Mineral oil is metabolized by the liver and excreted in the feces.

Route	Onset	Peak	Duration
P.O.	6-8 hr	Variable	Variable
P.R.	30 min-2 hr	Variable	Variable

PHARMACODYNAMICS

Mineral oil lubricates the feces and the intestinal mucosa by preventing water reabsorption from the lumen of the bowel. The increased fluid content of the feces increases peristalsis. Rectal administration via an enema also produces laxation by physical distention.

PHARMACOTHERAPEUTICS

Mineral oil is used to treat constipation and maintain soft stools when straining is contraindicated (after recent MI to avoid Valsalva's maneuver, after eye surgery to prevent increased intraocular pressure, and after cerebral aneurysm repair to avoid increased ICP). Administered orally or by enema, this lubricant laxative also is used to treat patients with fecal impaction.

Drug interactions

Mineral oil may impair the absorption of many oral medications, including fat-soluble vitamins, oral contraceptives, and anticoagulants. Mineral oil also may interfere with the antibacterial activity of nonabsorbable sulfonamides.

ADVERSE DRUG REACTIONS

Mineral oil may produce nausea, vomiting, diarrhea, and abdominal cramping. Seepage from the rectum after rectal administration may result in anal irritation, pruritus ani, infection, and impaired healing of lesions in the area. Chronic oral use of nonemulsified mineral oil may impair absorption of fat-soluble vitamins (A, D, E, and K), causing vitamin deficiencies. Lipid pneumonitis may result from aspiration of oral mineral oil.

Systemic absorption of emulsified mineral oil can lead to granulomatous reactions in the mesenteric lymph nodes, liver, and spleen.

NURSING PROCESS APPLICATION

The following information assists the nurse in caring for a patient who is receiving mineral oil. It includes an overview of assessment activities as well as examples of appropriate nursing diagnoses and related interventions. It also highlights the importance of evaluation.

Assessment

Before drug therapy begins, review the patient's history for conditions that contraindicate the use of mineral oil. Also review the patient's medication history to identify use of drugs that may interact with it. During therapy, assess the patient for adverse drug reactions and signs of drug interactions. Also, periodically assess the effectiveness of mineral oil therapy. Finally, evaluate the patient's and family's knowledge about the prescribed drug.

Nursing diagnoses

• Risk for injury related to adverse reactions or drug interactions
• Altered nutrition: less than body requirements related to impaired absorption of nutrients and fat-soluble vitamins caused by long-term use of mineral oil
• Knowledge deficit related to mineral oil

Planning and implementation

• Do not administer mineral oil to a patient with a condition that contraindicates its use.
• Administer mineral oil cautiously to prevent aspiration.
• Monitor the patient closely for adverse reactions and drug interactions. (See Patient Teaching: *Lubricant laxatives.*)

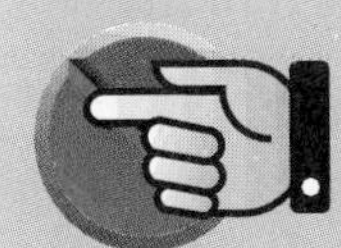

PATIENT TEACHING
Lubricant laxatives

- Teach the patient and family the name, dose, frequency, action, and adverse effects of mineral oil.
- Stress the importance of taking mineral oil exactly as prescribed. Long-term use can cause fat-soluble vitamin deficiencies. Review the signs of vitamin deficiencies with the patient as needed.
- Advise the female patient taking an oral contraceptive that mineral oil can interfere with absorption of the oral contraceptive, thus reducing the drug's effectiveness.
- Teach the patient how to take mineral oil to disguise its taste.
- Instruct the patient not to take mineral oil with or shortly after meals or other medications.
- Discuss additional measures the patient can take to prevent constipation.
- Advise the patient to notify the physician if adverse reactions occur or if mineral oil is ineffective.

* ***Monitor hydration, withhold the next dose of mineral oil, and notify the physician if the patient develops nausea, vomiting, or diarrhea.***
* ***Avoid administering mineral oil with other oral medications because it impairs the absorption of many of these medications.***
- Monitor the patient for decreased effectiveness of fat-soluble vitamins, anticoagulants, and nonabsorbable sulfonamides during concomitant mineral oil therapy.
- Mix mineral oil with fruit juice or a carbonated beverage to disguise its taste. (See Geriatric Considerations: *Mineral oil.*)
- Notify the physician if adverse reactions occur or if mineral oil is ineffective.
* ***Monitor the patient on long-term mineral oil therapy for early signs of fat-soluble vitamin deficiencies: night blindness (vitamin A deficiency); profuse sweating, restlessness, and irritability (vitamin D deficiency); muscle weakness or intermittent claudication (vitamin E deficiency); or abnormal bleeding tendency (vitamin K deficiency).***
* ***Withhold mineral oil and notify the physician if fat-soluble vitamin deficiency is suspected.***
* ***Do not administer mineral oil with or shortly after meals or with fat-soluble vitamins because it can interfere with vitamin absorption.***

Evaluation

For each nursing diagnosis, prepare an evaluation statement that describes the patient's or family's response to nursing interventions.

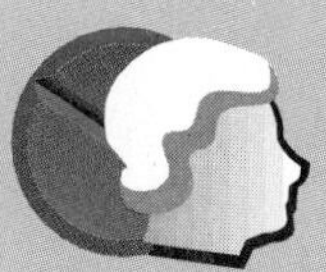

GERIATRIC CONSIDERATIONS
Mineral oil

Do not administer mineral oil at bedtime to an older patient because of the increased risk of aspiration. Mineral oil is best administered at a time when the patient is awake, alert and, preferably, ambulatory. Although many older patients are accustomed to taking mineral oil at bedtime, this is not a prudent practice while hospitalized. The patient may think that the treatment isn't effective unless it is given in the evening. Explain the rationale for changing the patient's routine if he is accustomed to taking mineral oil at bedtime.

CRITICAL THINKING. To enhance your critical thinking about antidiarrheal and laxative agents, consider the following situation and its analysis.

Situation: Ms. Evelyn Mills, age 87, was transferred from the hospital to a skilled-care facility for intensive physical therapy following a hip fracture. She tells you that she is constipated and that she has always had a problem with constipation. At home she took a dose of mineral oil at bedtime. During hospitalization, she was found to have hypertension and diabetes mellitus and is taking a number of medications, including a diuretic, an oral antidiabetic agent, and a vitamin supplement. She also developed a urinary tract infection and is finishing a course of sulfonamides. Standing orders from the physician at the skilled-care facility allow the nurse to choose a laxative agent for Ms. Mills. What should the nurse administer and why?

Analysis: Because lubricant laxatives such as mineral oil have the potential to cause a number of drug interactions for Ms. Mills, especially with the bedtime dose of sulfonamide, and because of the potential for aspiration of mineral oil, the nurse should offer Ms. Mills a dose of milk of magnesia to alleviate the current problem. The nurse should then plan to administer a bulk-forming laxative that would be acceptable for a diabetic patient. During this period of inactivity, because of her age and because she suffers from chronic constipation, a bulk-forming laxative is a reasonable alternative. Explain to Ms. Mills that mineral oil will interfere with the action of her sulfonamide by reducing the bacterial activity of the drug. A bulk-forming laxative should help prevent constipation because it retains fluid and helps to keep the stool soft. Ms. Mills should be encouraged to drink at least 8 oz (240 ml) of fluid with the laxative and increase her overall fluid intake during the day.

CHAPTER SUMMARY

Chapter 29 covered information about the antidiarrheal and laxative agents. Here are the highlights of the chapter.

Antidiarrheals are used to treat acute, nonspecific diarrhea or chronic diarrhea. They can cause nausea, vomiting, and constipation as well as other adverse reactions.

When caring for a patient receiving an antidiarrheal, the nurse must monitor the patient's GI response to these drugs. Fluids and electrolytes should be replaced as needed.

The major classes of laxatives include the hyperosmolar agents, dietary fiber and related bulk-forming laxatives, emollients, stimulants, and lubricants.

The excessive use of laxatives may result in severe problems, such as habitual dependence, fluid and electrolyte imbalances, acid-base abnormalities, dehydration, and cardiac arrhythmias. For habitual users of laxatives, the nurse should institute bowel retraining and teach how to prevent chronic constipation.

Questions to consider

See Appendix 1 for answers.

1. Jack Rogers, age 29, develops diarrhea caused by an intestinal virus. His physician tells him to take kaolin and pectin 60 ml after each loose bowel movement. Mr. Rogers's physician should provide which of the following important instructions about the administration of this antidiarrheal?
   (a) Take it on a full stomach.
   (b) Take it on an empty stomach.
   (c) Take it immediately before other drugs.
   (d) Take it up to eight times a day, as needed.

2. Hannah Blumberg, age 67, is recovering from cataract surgery. To prevent Ms. Blumberg from straining during defecation, the physician is most likely to prescribe which of the following laxatives?
   (a) docusate sodium
   (b) magnesium citrate
   (c) bisacodyl
   (d) lactulose

3. Rita Schmidt, age 47, is scheduled for a proctoscopy. To prepare her for this procedure, which of the following laxatives is most likely to be prescribed?
   (a) psyllium hydrophilic mucilloid
   (b) polyethylene glycol
   (c) bisacodyl
   (d) loperamide

4. Jason Anderson, age 58, is admitted to the coronary care unit with an acute MI. His physician orders mineral oil 15 ml P.O. at bedtime to maintain soft stools. When administering mineral oil, the nurse should be alert for which of the following adverse reactions?
   (a) Abdominal cramping
   (b) Leukocytosis
   (c) Rash or urticaria
   (d) Hypocalcemia

30 Antiemetic and emetic agents

OBJECTIVES

After reading and studying this chapter, the student should be able to:

1. compare the pharmacokinetic and pharmacodynamic properties of the various antiemetic agents.
2. describe the clinical indications for the antiemetic agents.
3. discuss drug interactions that may occur with antiemetic agents.
4. identify the adverse reactions associated with antiemetic agents.
5. describe the fundamental pharmacologic properties of ipecac syrup, an emetic.
6. describe how to apply the nursing process when caring for a patient who is receiving an antiemetic or emetic agent.

INTRODUCTION

The **antiemetics** and **emetics** represent two groups of drugs with opposing actions. The emetic drugs, which are derived from plants, produce **vomiting** upon administration. The antiemetic drugs decrease **nausea** and hence, the urge to vomit. For more information on drug names, major indications, dosages, contraindications, and precautions, see *Selected major antiemetic and emetic agents,* pages 380 and 381.

Drugs covered in this chapter include:

- benzquinamide hydrochloride
- buclizine hydrochloride
- chlorpromazine hydrochloride
- cyclizine hydrochloride
- dimenhydrinate
- diphenhydramine hydrochloride
- diphenidol
- dronabinol
- granisetron
- hydroxyzine hydrochloride
- hydroxyzine pamoate
- ipecac syrup
- meclizine hydrochloride
- metroclopramide hydrochloride
- ondansetron
- perphenazine
- prochlorperazine maleate
- promethazine hydrochloride
- scopolamine
- thiethylperazine maleate
- trimethobenzamide hydrochloride

Antihistamine, phenothiazine, and serotonin receptor antagonist antiemetics

The major antiemetics include antihistamines, phenothiazines, and serotonin receptor antagonists. The antihistamine antiemetics discussed in this chapter include dimenhydrinate, diphenhydramine hydrochloride, buclizine hydrochloride, cyclizine hydrochloride, hydroxyzine hydrochloride, hydroxyzine pamoate, meclizine hydrochloride, and trimethobenzamide hydrochloride. The phenothiazines most commonly used for their antiemetic effect include chlorpromazine hydrochloride, perphenazine, prochlorperazine maleate, promethazine hydrochloride, and thiethylperazine maleate. The serotonin receptor antagonists include ondansetron and granisetron.

PHARMACOKINETICS

Antihistamine antiemetics are absorbed well from the GI tract when administered orally and are metabolized primarily by the liver. Their inactive metabolites are excreted in the urine. Phenothiazine antiemetics and serotonin receptor antagonists are absorbed well, extensively metabolized by the liver, and excreted in the urine and feces. Dimenhydrinate produces its effects within 40 minutes.

Route	Onset	Peak	Duration
P.O.	Immediate-40 min	1-2 hr	4-24 hr
I.M.	15-60 min	1-2 hr	6-24 hr

PHARMACODYNAMICS

The mechanism of action that produces the antiemetic effect of antihistamines remains unclear. Phenothiazines produce their antiemetic effect by blocking the dopaminergic receptors in the chemoreceptor trigger zone in the brain. These drugs may also directly depress the vomiting center. The serotonin receptor antagonists block serotonin stimulation and subsequent vagal afferent discharge, which induces vomiting.

Selected major antiemetic and emetic agents

The following chart summarizes the major antiemetics and emetics currently in clinical use.

DRUG	MAJOR INDICATIONS AND USUAL DOSAGES	CONTRAINDICATIONS AND PRECAUTIONS
Antiemetics		
dimenhydrinate (Dramamine)	*Prevention of motion sickness* ADULT: 50 to 100 mg P.O. every 4 to 6 hours up to a maximum of 400 mg daily PEDIATRIC: for children ages 6 to 12, 25 to 50 mg P.O. every 6 to 8 hours, up to a maximum of 150 mg daily; for children ages 2 to 5, 12.5 to 25 mg P.O. every 6 to 8 hours, up to a maximum of 75 mg daily	• Dimenhydrinate is contraindicated in a neonate, a breast-feeding patient, or one with known hypersensitivity. • This drug requires cautious use in a pregnant patient or one with a seizure disorder, acute angle-closure glaucoma, prostatic hyperplasia, bronchial asthma, or cardiac arrhythmias.
granisetron (Kytril)	*Prevention of nausea and vomiting associated with chemotherapy and radiotherapy* ADULT AND PEDIATRIC (age 2 to 16): 10 mcg/kg I.V. infused over 5 minutes within 30 minutes of initiation of chemotherapy.	• Granisetron is used with caution in pregnant or breast-feeding women. • Drug is contraindicated in patients with known hypersensitivity to drug. • Safety and efficacy of drug in children under age 2 have not been established.
meclizine (Antivert, Bonine)	*Prevention of motion sickness* ADULT: 25 to 50 mg P.O. daily at least 1 hour before travel	• Meclizine is contraindicated in a patient with known hypersensitivity. • This drug requires cautious use in a pregnant patient or one with asthma, glaucoma, or prostatic hyperplasia. • Safety and efficacy in children have not been established.
ondansetron (Zofran)	*Prevention of nausea and vomiting associated with chemotherapy and radiotherapy* ADULT: three 0.15 mg/kg I.V. doses, with the first infused over one-half hour before chemotherapy treatment and subsequent doses given 4 and 8 hours after the first infusion. For P.O. dosage: 8 mg P.O. every 8 hours for two doses beginning 30 minutes before chemotherapy, then 8 mg P.O. every 12 hours for 1 to 2 days after chemotherapy is completed. Dosages in radiotherapy are dependent upon dose and location of the radiation. PEDIATRIC: for children ages 4 to 18, three 0.15 mg/kg I.V. doses, with the first infused over 15 minutes one-half hour before chemotherapy treatment and subsequent doses given 4 and 8 hours after the first infusion; P.O. dosage for children under age 4, see literature; for children ages 4 to 11, 4 mg P.O. every 4 hours for three doses beginning 30 minutes before chemotherapy, then 4 mg every 8 hours for 1 to 2 days after chemotherapy completion *Prevention of postoperative nausea and vomiting* ADULT: 16 mg P.O. 1 hour before induction of anesthesia or 4 mg I.V. as single dose immediately before anesthesia, or shortly postoperative if nausea and vomiting occur PEDIATRIC: for children over age 2 (<40 kg), 0.1mg/kg; for children over 40 kg, 4 mg; give as a single I.V. dose immediately before anesthesia or shortly postoperative if nausea or vomiting occur; infuse over	• Ondansetron is contraindicated in a patient with known hypersensitivity. • This drug requires cautious use in a pregnant or breast-feeding patient. • Safety and efficacy in children age 2 and under have not been established.

Selected major antiemetic and emetic agents *(continued)*

DRUG	MAJOR INDICATIONS AND USUAL DOSAGES	CONTRAINDICATIONS AND PRECAUTIONS
Antiemetics *(continued)*		
prochlorperazine maleate (Compazine)	2 to 5 minutes *Prevention and treatment of severe nausea and vomiting from various causes* ADULT: 5 to 10 mg P.O. or I.M. t.i.d. or q.i.d., or 25 mg P.R. b.i.d. PEDIATRIC: for a child who weighs 20 to 29 lb (9 to 13 kg), 2.5 mg P.O. or P.R. once or twice daily; for a child who weighs 30 to 39 lb (14 to 18 kg), 2.5 mg b.i.d. or t.i.d.; for a child who weighs 40 to 85 lb (19 to 39 kg), 2.5 mg P.O. or P.R. t.i.d. or 5 mg b.i.d.; for I.M. administration, 0.132 mg/kg as needed	• Prochlorperazine is contraindicated in a pediatric patient who is undergoing surgery, a patient in a coma, or one with known hypersensitivity, central nervous system (CNS) depression, bone marrow depression, Reye's syndrome, or brain damage. • This drug requires cautious use in a geriatric, debilitated, or pregnant patient or one with hepatic disease, cardiovascular disease, respiratory disorder, hypocalcemia, seizure disorder, suspected brain tumor, intestinal obstruction, glaucoma, or prostatic hyperplasia. Prochlorperazine maleate also requires cautious use in a patient who has experienced a severe reaction to insulin or electroconvulsive therapy or one who has been exposed to extreme heat or cold.
promethazine (Phenergan)	*Prevention and treatment of severe nausea and vomiting from various causes* ADULT: 12.5 to 25 mg P.O., I.M., or P.R. every 4 to 6 hours, as needed PEDIATRIC: 0.25 to 0.5 mg/kg P.R. or 12.5 to 25 mg P.O. every 4 to 6 hours, as needed	• Promethazine is contraindicated in a pediatric patient who is undergoing surgery, a patient in a coma, or one with known hypersensitivity, CNS depression, bone marrow depression, Reye's syndrome, or brain damage. • This drug requires cautious use in a geriatric, debilitated, or pregnant patient or one with hepatic disease, cardiovascular disease, respiratory disorder, hypocalcemia, seizure disorder, suspected brain tumor, intestinal obstruction, glaucoma, or prostatic hyperplasia. Promethazine requires cautious use in a patient who has experienced a severe reaction to insulin or electroconvulsive therapy or one who has been exposed to extreme heat or cold.
trimethobenzamide (Tigan)	*Prevention and treatment of mild to moderate nausea and vomiting* ADULT: 250 mg P.O. t.i.d. or q.i.d. or 200 mg I.M. or P.R.t.i.d. or q.i.d. PEDIATRIC: for children who weigh 31 to 88 lb (14 to 40 kg), 100 to 200 mg P.O. or P.R. t.i.d. or q.i.d.; for children who weigh less than 31 lb (14 kg), 100 mg P.R. t.i.d. or q.i.d.	• Trimethobenzamide is contraindicated in a patient with known hypersensitivity. • This drug requires cautious use in the treatment of vomiting in children.
Emetics		
ipecac syrup	*Emesis of ingested poisons* ADULT: 15 to 30 ml P.O. followed by 7 to 10 oz (200 to 300 ml) of water, dose may be repeated in 30 minutes if vomiting does not occur PEDIATRIC: for children age 1 and older, 15 ml P.O. followed by 7 oz (200 ml) of water or other clear liquid; for children under age 1, 5 to 10 ml P.O. followed by 3.5 oz (100 ml) of water or other clear liquid; dose may be repeated in 30 minutes if vomiting does not occur	• Ipecac syrup is contraindicated in an inebriated, semicomatose, or unconscious patient or one with petroleum distillate or caustic substance poisoning, bulimia, anorexia nervosa, seizures, shock, or absent gag reflex. • This drug requires cautious use in a pregnant or breast-feeding patient or one with impaired cardiac function or sclerotic or other pathologic changes in blood vessels.

PHARMACOTHERAPEUTICS

With the exception of trimethobenzamide, the antihistamines are antiemetics specifically used for nausea and vomiting caused by inner ear stimulation. As a consequence, these drugs prevent or treat motion sickness. They usually prove most effective when given prophylactically before activities that produce motion sickness; they are much less effective when nausea or vomiting has already begun.

Phenothiazine antiemetics and serotonin receptor antagonists control severe nausea and vomiting from various causes. They are the drugs of choice when vomiting becomes severe and potentially hazardous, such as in postoperative nausea and vomiting and nausea and vomiting caused by viral illnesses. Both categories of agents are prescribed extensively to control the nausea and vomiting resulting from cancer chemotherapy and radiotherapy.

Drug interactions

Antiemetics can produce an additive effect when they interact with other drugs that also produce an anticholinergic effect. (See Drug Interactions: *Antihistamine and phenothiazine antiemetics.*)

ADVERSE DRUG REACTIONS

Antihistamine and phenothiazine antiemetics produce some drowsiness. Paradoxical central nervous system (CNS) stimulation has occurred with antihistamine antiemetics, in more children than adults. Symptoms of paradoxical CNS stimulation may range from restlessness, insomnia, and euphoria to tremors and even seizures. Other adverse CNS effects associated with antihistamine antiemetics include dizziness, headache, and lassitude. Adverse CNS effects associated with phenothiazine and serotonin receptor antagonist antiemetics include confusion, anxiety, euphoria, agitation, depression, headache, insomnia, restlessness, and weakness.

The anticholinergic effect of the antiemetics may cause constipation, dry mouth and throat, dysuria, urine retention, impotence, and visual and auditory disturbances (such as blurred vision or tinnitus).

Antihistamine antiemetics themselves may cause mild nausea, epigastric distress, or anorexia. Hypotension and orthostatic hypotension with tachycardia, syncope, and dizziness are common adverse reactions to the phenothiazine antiemetics.

Trimethobenzamide and the phenothiazine antiemetics also may produce extrapyramidal symptoms, such as acute dystonia and dyskinesia, that require discontinuation of the prescribed drug.

Hypersensitivity reactions, manifested by rashes and photosensitivity, may occur with antihistamine antiemetics but rarely occur with phenothiazine antiemetics. Rarely, such blood dyscrasias as granulocytopenia, hemolytic anemia, leukopenia, thrombocytopenia, and pancytopenia also may occur. Rare cases of rashes have been reported with serotonin receptor antagonists.

NURSING PROCESS APPLICATION

The following information assists the nurse in caring for a patient who is receiving an antihistamine, phenothiazine or serotonin receptor antagonist antiemetic. It includes an overview of assessment activities as well as examples of appropriate nursing diagnoses and related interventions. It also highlights the importance of evaluation.

Assessment

Before drug therapy begins, review the patient's history for conditions that contraindicate or require cautious use of the prescribed antiemetic. Also review the patient's medication history to identify use of drugs that may interact with it. During therapy, assess the patient for adverse drug reactions and signs of drug interactions. Also, periodically assess the effectiveness of antiemetic therapy. Finally, evaluate the patient's and family's knowledge about the prescribed drug.

Nursing diagnoses

- Risk for injury related to adverse drug reactions or drug interactions
- Sensory/perceptual alterations (visual, auditory) related to the anticholinergic effects of the prescribed antiemetic
- Knowledge deficit related to the prescribed antiemetic regimen

Planning and implementation

- Do not administer an antiemetic to a patient with a condition that contraindicates its use.
- Administer an antiemetic cautiously to a patient at risk because of a preexisting condition.
- Monitor the patient closely for adverse reactions to the prescribed antiemetic and for drug interactions. (See Patient Teaching: *Antihistamine, phenothiazine, and serotonin receptor antagonist antiemetics,* page 384.)
- Take seizure precautions when administering a phenothiazine antiemetic to a patient who is predisposed to seizures because these drugs can lower the threshold for seizures.
- Monitor a pediatric patient for signs of paradoxical CNS stimulation during antihistamine antiemetic therapy. Notify the physician if paradoxical CNS stimulation occurs.
- Observe the patient for extrapyramidal symptoms during trimethobenzamide or phenothiazine therapy.
- Evaluate the patient's hematologic studies for signs of blood dyscrasias. Alert the physician if abnormalities occur.
- Avoid skin contact with oral solutions and injections when preparing or administering these drugs because they can cause dermatologic effects.
- Administer an antihistamine antiemetic with food or milk to minimize nausea or epigastric distress.
- Administer I.M. injections deep in the upper outer quadrant of the gluteus muscle.
- Consult the physician about giving a rectal suppository or intramuscular injection if the patient vomits before drug administration.

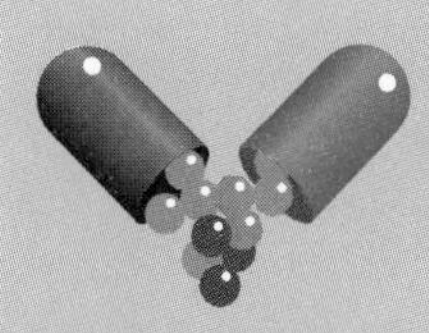

DRUG INTERACTIONS

Antihistamine and phenothiazine antiemetics

This chart presents important drug interactions for major antihistamine and phenothiazine antiemetics discussed in this chapter. No significant interactions are known for serotonin receptor antagonist antiemetics.

DRUG	INTERACTING DRUGS	POSSIBLE EFFECTS	NURSING IMPLICATIONS
Antihistamine antiemetics			
buclizine, cyclizine, dimenhydrinate, diphenhydramine, hydroxyzine pamoate, meclizine, trimethobenzamide	Central nervous system (CNS) depressants (including barbiturates, tranquilizers, alcohol, opioids)	Additive CNS depression	• Use caution when administering concurrently to avoid excessive CNS depression or sedation. • Inform ambulatory patients of the possible additive effect.
	anticholinergic drugs (including tricyclic antidepressants, phenothiazines, antiparkinsonian drugs)	Additive anticholinergic effects	• Assess for signs of increased anticholinergic activity, such as constipation, dry mouth, visual disturbances, and urine retention.
	ototoxic medications	Masked signs and symptoms of ototoxicity	• Monitor the patient for signs of hearing loss and conduct an audiometric test weekly or biweekly.
Phenothiazine antiemetics			
chlorpromazine, perphenazine, prochlorperazine maleate, promethazine, thiethylperazine	guanethidine	Inhibited uptake of guanethidine	• Frequently monitor the patient's blood pressure. • Expect to increase the guanethidine dosage or replace guanethidine with another antihypertensive agent, as prescribed.
	amphetamines, nonamphetamine anorexigenic agents	Inhibited effects of both drugs	• Do not administer these drugs concurrently.
	anticholinergics	Increased anticholinergic effects; decreased antiemetic effects	• Do not administer together routinely. If these drugs must be given concurrently, assess the patient for signs of reduced phenothiazine effects, such as continued vomiting. • Perform abdominal assessments to monitor the patient for diminished or absent bowel sounds, abdominal pain, constipation, and other abdominal problems.
	barbiturates	Increased CNS depressant effects; increased phenothiazine metabolism	• Observe the patient for erratic therapeutic effects, such as intermittent nausea and vomiting, and for increased CNS depressant effects, such as stupor.
	levodopa	Reduced antiparkinsonian effects of levodopa	• Avoid concurrent administration, if possible. • Monitor the patient for increased signs of parkinsonism.
	lithium	Increased risk of neurotoxicity, seizures, delirium, and encephalopathy in manic patients; respiratory depression and hypotension	• Monitor the patient for reduced phenothiazine response and changes in neurologic status. • Frequently monitor the patient's vital signs.
	droperidol	Increased risk of extrapyramidal effects	• Monitor the patient for tremor.

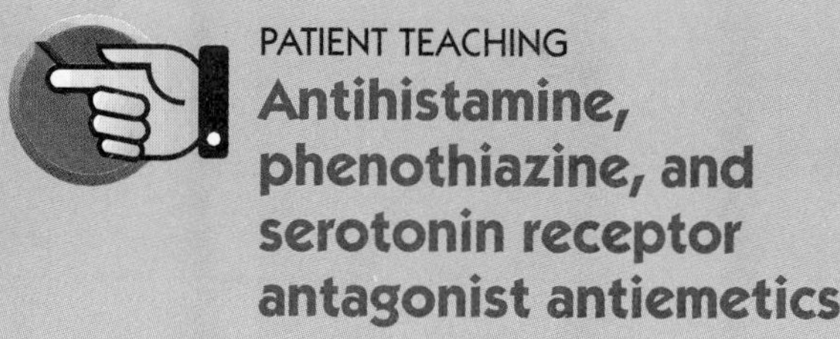

PATIENT TEACHING

Antihistamine, phenothiazine, and serotonin receptor antagonist antiemetics

- Teach the patient and family the name, dose, frequency, action, and adverse effects of the prescribed antiemetic.
- Tell the patient about the drug's sedative effects, and advise the patient not to drive or participate in other activities that require mental alertness. Advise the patient not to drink alcohol or take other central nervous system (CNS) depressants because doing so can result in additive sedative effects.
- Teach the patient how to relieve the anticholinergic effects, such as constipation and dry mouth, caused by these agents.
- Reassure the patient that visual and auditory disturbances are dose-related and should disappear when the drug is discontinued.
- Inform the male patient that impotence may occur.
- Instruct the patient to avoid prolonged exposure to sunlight or to wear protective clothing and a sunscreen because the antiemetic may cause photosensitivity.
- Advise the patient to notify the physician if urinary frequency and a sense of fullness in the lower abdomen occurs.
- Advise family members that paradoxical CNS stimulation may occur in a child receiving an antihistamine antiemetic.
- Instruct the patient to notify the primary health care provider if anorexia or a weight loss of more than 3 lb (1.4 kg) in 1 week occurs during long-term antihistamine antiemetic therapy.
- Instruct the patient to take the prescribed antihistamine antiemetic with milk or food to minimize adverse gastrointestinal effects.
- Advise the patient to ingest an antihistamine antiemetic 30 to 60 minutes before the activity that might produce motion sickness.
- Advise the patient that phenothiazine antiemetics are not effective for motion sickness.
- Inform the patient about the possibility of hypotension with phenothiazine antiemetics, and instruct the patient to remain recumbent for 30 to 60 minutes after receiving the drug.
- Explain that phenothiazine antiemetics may make the patient's urine pink or reddish brown in color but that this discoloration is harmless.
- Inform the seizure-prone patient that a phenothiazine antiemetic can lower the seizure threshold. Instruct the patient to notify the physician if a seizure occurs because the drug may need to be discontinued.
- Advise the patient to discontinue trimethobenzamide or a phenothiazine antiemetic and to notify the physician if the patient develops extrapyramidal symptoms, such as slow, involuntary movements of large muscles in the limbs, trunk, and neck.
- Advise the patient to notify the physician if adverse reactions occur or if the prescribed antiemetic is ineffective.
- Advise the patient that serotonin receptor antagonist antiemetics may cause a taste disorder. If this occurs to the point that appetite is effected, the patient should notify the physician.

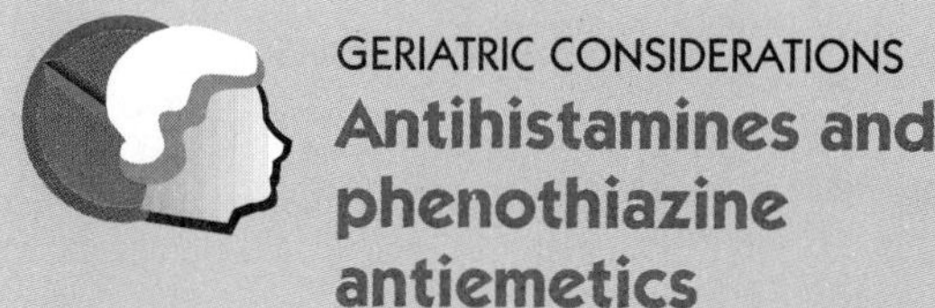

GERIATRIC CONSIDERATIONS

Antihistamines and phenothiazine antiemetics

Older patients should be closely monitored for adverse reactions and sensitivities to the usual adult dose for antihistamine or phenothiazine antiemetics. If sensory or perceptual alterations occur, safety precautions should be taken. For example, put the patient's bed in the low position, keep the side rails up, and supervise the patient's ambulation. Notify the doctor if visual or auditory disturbances worsen or severely affect the patient's ability to carry out activities of daily living.

- Notify the physician if adverse reactions occur or if the prescribed antiemetic is ineffective.
- Assess the patient regularly for visual and auditory disturbances. (See Geriatric Considerations: *Antihistamine and phenothiazine antiemetics.*)

Evaluation

For each nursing diagnosis, prepare an evaluation statement that describes the patient's or family's response to nursing interventions.

Other antiemetics

Other drugs, unrelated to antihistamines, phenothiazines, or serotonin receptor antagonists, also act effectively to prevent and treat nausea and vomiting.

Benzquinamide hydrochloride is used to prevent or treat nausea and vomiting associated with anesthesia and surgery. This drug may be preferred in some circumstances because it does not produce CNS or respiratory depression. Furthermore, benzquinamide does not produce the extrapyramidal effects or hypotension associated with the phenothiazines.

Scopolamine has been used for years to prevent motion sickness. However, its use is limited because of its sedative and anticholinergic effects. One scopolamine transdermal preparation, Transderm-Scōp, provides highly effective action without producing the drug's usual adverse effects. (See *Facts about scopolamine patches.*)

Metoclopramide hydrochloride is used to manage GI motility disorders. Used for many years in Europe to prevent motion sickness, metoclopramide currently is being used in the United States to prevent cancer chemotherapy–induced nausea and vomiting.

Diphenidol effectively prevents vertigo in addition to preventing or treating generalized nausea and vomiting. However, its use is limited because of the auditory and visual hallucinations, confusion, and disorientation that may occur.

Facts about scopolamine patches

Instruct the patient to apply the transdermal scopolamine patch behind the ear. For optimal effect, advise the patient to apply the patch at least 4 hours before it is needed. Also advise the patient to remove the patch after it no longer is needed or after 72 hours.

Why the transdermal route for motion sickness?

- The nerve fibers in the vestibular apparatus of the inner ear help people maintain balance. But for some, motion increases the activity of these fibers, causing dizziness, nausea, and vomiting. The transdermal scopolamine patch helps reduce the activity of these inner ear fibers.
- The patch releases minute amounts of scopolamine that permeate the intact skin at a programmed rate, minimizing adverse reactions. Scopolamine is absorbed directly into the bloodstream, quickly achieving and maintaining an optimal dose for up to 72 hours, which prevents the nausea and vomiting of motion sickness.
- The patch is a flexible, adhesive disk of four layers, as shown in the illustration.
- The priming dose of scopolamine rapidly achieves the required steady-state blood concentration. Over the 3-day lifetime of the patch, the drug is delivered at a nearly constant rate.
- The drug passes by diffusion through the membrane from the higher concentration inside the reservoir in the patch to the lower concentration outside the reservoir.
- The amount of drug delivered through diffusion is regulated by the membrane thickness, the surface area and composition of the patch, and the drug concentration on each side of the membrane.

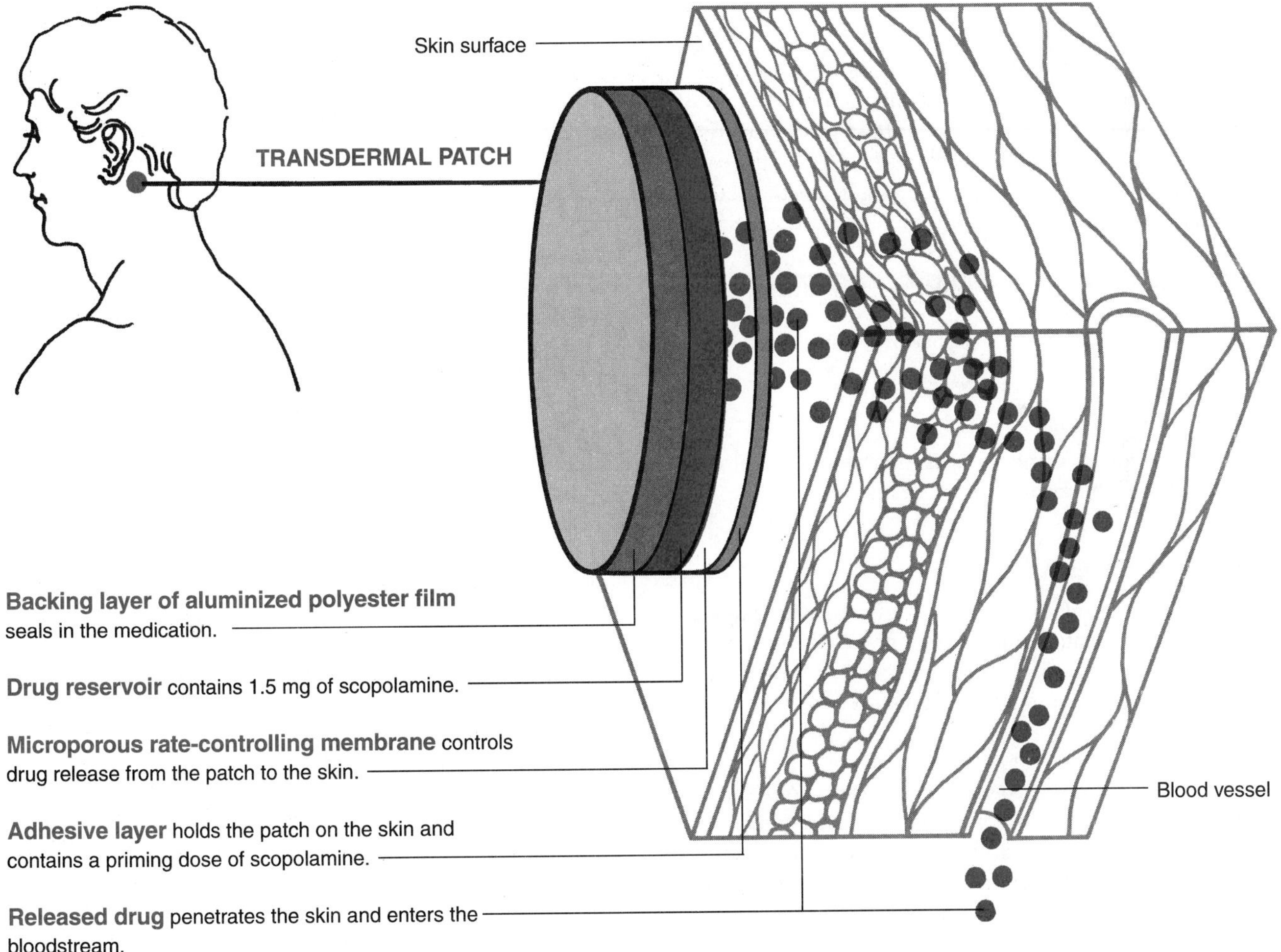

Dronabinol is a schedule II drug, used to treat the nausea and vomiting resulting from cancer chemotherapy in patients who do not respond adequately to conventional antiemetics. It also has been used to stimulate appetite in patients with acquired immunodeficiency syndrome. However, dronabinol can accumulate in the body, and the patient can develop tolerance or physical and psychological dependence.

Emetics

Emetics are used to induce vomiting after the ingestion of toxic substances. Although many substances were used in the past to induce vomiting, ipecac syrup is considered the emetic of choice because it is the most effective and is less likely to cause problems than other emetics (such as apomorphine hydrochloride) or mechanical stimulation. Household emetics such as sodium chloride (salt) solutions can result in fatalities from electrolyte imbalances (hypernatremia). Researchers have not determined the safety and efficacy of soaps and detergents as emetics. Studies of mechanically stimulated vomiting, such as placing a finger or spoon in the throat to stimulate the gag reflex, have shown this method to be much less effective than the administration of ipecac syrup.

PHARMACOKINETICS

Little information exists concerning the absorption, distribution, and excretion of ipecac syrup. After administration of ipecac syrup, a delay of approximately 10 minutes usually occurs before the onset of vomiting. About 50% of the patients receiving ipecac will begin vomiting in less than 20 minutes; about 90% will vomit within 30 minutes.

Route	Onset	Peak	Duration
P.O.	20-30 min	Unknown	20-25 min

PHARMACODYNAMICS

Ipecac syrup induces vomiting by stimulating the vomiting center located in the medulla of the brain.

PHARMACOTHERAPEUTICS

Ipecac syrup is considered the therapy of choice for emptying the stomach because of its effectiveness and low incidence of adverse effects. It can be purchased without a prescription and can be stored in the home for emergencies.

Drug interactions

Because ipecac syrup is used only in acute situations, drug interactions rarely occur. If poisoning results from ingestion of a phenothiazine, the phenothiazine's antiemetic effect may decrease the emetic effect of ipecac syrup. The administration of activated charcoal should be delayed until emesis has occurred because activated charcoal may be vomited or become bound with the ipecac syrup, thereby inactivating it.

ADVERSE DRUG REACTIONS

Ipecac syrup rarely produces adverse reactions when used in the recommended dosages. Adverse reactions may include prolonged vomiting for more than 1 hour or repeated vomiting involving more than six episodes in 1 hour, lethargy, and diarrhea. Ipecac contains a specific toxin that, in high doses, may cause cardiac arrhythmias or fatal myocarditis. Heart failure usually is the cause of death after ipecac overdose.

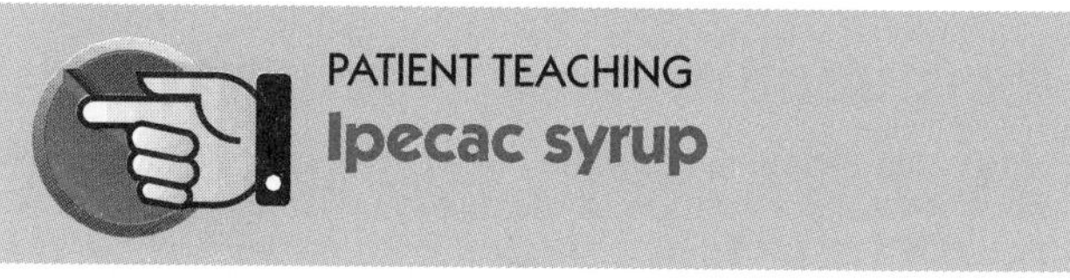

PATIENT TEACHING
Ipecac syrup

- Teach the patient and family the name, dose, frequency, action, and adverse effects of ipecac syrup.
- Teach family members not to administer ipecac syrup to a child unless advised by a poison control center or other qualified health care personnel.
- Explain that the patient may resume eating several hours after ipecac syrup administration.
- Encourage the patient and family to ask questions as concerns about therapy arise.

NURSING PROCESS APPLICATION

The following information assists the nurse in caring for a patient who is receiving ipecac syrup. It includes an overview of assessment activities as well as examples of appropriate nursing diagnoses and related interventions. It also highlights the importance of evaluation.

Assessment

Before drug therapy begins, review the patient's history for conditions that contraindicate or require cautious use of ipecac syrup. Also review the patient's medication history to identify use of drugs that may interact with it. During therapy, assess the patient for adverse drug reactions and signs of drug interactions. Also, periodically assess the effectiveness of ipecac syrup therapy. Finally, evaluate the patient's and family's knowledge about the prescribed drug.

Nursing diagnoses

- Risk for injury related to adverse drug reactions or drug interactions
- Risk for fluid volume deficit related to prolonged vomiting caused by ipecac syrup
- Knowledge deficit related to use of ipecac syrup

Planning and implementation

- Do not administer ipecac syrup to a patient with a condition that contraindicates its use.
- Administer ipecac syrup cautiously to a patient at risk because of a preexisting condition.
- Monitor the patient closely for adverse reactions and drug interactions. (See Patient Teaching: *Ipecac syrup.*)

- Follow administration of ipecac syrup with the proper amount of water or other clear liquid based on the patient's age.
- Induce early emesis after drug administration by moving an adult or gently bouncing a child.
- Repeat the initial dose of ipecac syrup as prescribed, if vomiting does not occur within 30 minutes. If the second dose does not produce emesis, prepare to take other measures as prescribed, such as gastric lavage or activated charcoal administration.
- Frequently inform the physician about the patient's condition.
- Notify the physician if adverse reactions occur.
- Monitor hydration if the patient experiences prolonged vomiting or diarrhea and continue to do so until vomiting or diarrhea ceases.
- Prepare to replace lost fluid and electrolytes as prescribed if a fluid volume deficit occurs.

Evaluation

For each nursing diagnosis, prepare an evaluation statement that describes the patient's or family's response to nursing interventions.

CHAPTER SUMMARY

Chapter 30 discussed the antiemetics and emetics. Here are the highlights of the chapter.

The four basic groups of antiemetics include the antihistamines, the phenothiazines, the serotonin receptor antagonists, and others such as scopolamine. Some antiemetics control nausea and vomiting resulting from inner ear disturbances; others control generalized nausea and vomiting that arise from other causes.

Antihistamine antiemetics and scopolamine commonly are used to prevent motion sickness. However, these drugs usually are not effective after the nausea has begun.

For a patient receiving an antiemetic, the nurse should monitor the drug's effectiveness as well as fluid and electrolyte levels to detect serious imbalances.

Ipecac syrup has become the emetic of choice because of its effectiveness in evacuating the stomach and relatively low incidence of adverse reactions. The nurse should teach safe home use of the drug and instruct the family to contact the poison control center, physician, or other qualified health care professional before any use of the drug.

When caring for a patient receiving ipecac syrup, the nurse should monitor the drug's effectiveness to prevent damage from the ingested toxin.

Questions to consider

See Appendix 1 for answers.

1. Fred Miller has severe nausea and vomiting from radiotherapy he is receiving for metastatic prostate cancer. Which of the following antiemetics would probably be the best for Mr. Miller?
   (a) chlorpromazine hydrochloride
   (b) trimethobenzamide
   (c) ondansetron
   (d) meclazine hydrochloride

2. Amy Morrison, age 25, is planning a vacation to Mexico. Because Ms. Morrison experiences motion sickness whenever she flies, she asks the physician to prescribe an antiemetic. Which of the following antiemetic agents would probably be best for Ms. Morrison?
   (a) chlorpromazine hydrochloride
   (b) dronabinol
   (c) benzquinamide hydrochloride
   (d) dimenhydrinate

3. Virginia Alber, age 23, is brought to the emergency department by her family. She is confused and disoriented. Her mother tells the nurse that she found an empty bottle of ibuprofen by her daughter's bed. The physician orders an emetic for Ms. Alber. When is an emetic contraindicated?
   (a) When the patient is a child
   (b) When the patient is elderly
   (c) When a caustic substance has been ingested
   (d) When ingestion occurred less than 1 hour ago

4. Janine Brown, age 37, is recovering from a hysterectomy. To control postoperative nausea, her physician prescribes the phenothiazine agent promethazine 12.5 mg P.O. every 6 hours. The nurse should monitor Ms. Brown for which of the following adverse reactions?
   (a) Hypotension
   (b) Extrapyramidal effects
   (c) Myocarditis
   (d) Diarrhea

UNIT X

Drugs to prevent or treat infection

Attempts to treat systemic microbial infections with chemicals date back to the 16th century when mercury was used to treat syphilis. Other organometallic compounds, such as arsenic and bismuth, were introduced during the 1920s to treat syphilis, malaria, and other parasitic diseases. Compounds containing arsenic and antimony are still used to treat protozoa and other parasites. With the introduction of sulfonamides in 1936, a new era in treating infectious diseases began. In 1941, penicillin was introduced as the first antimicrobial that could be mass-produced, making it available to treat a wide patient population. Since then, numerous other antimicrobials have been introduced.

ANTIMICROBIAL SPECTRUM

The currently available antimicrobial drugs vary in their degree of effectiveness against different microorganisms. A drug's spectrum *of activity* refers to the number and type of organisms vulnerable to its action. Broad-spectrum antimicrobials affect a wide variety of pathogens, and narrow-spectrum drugs affect a few. Antimicrobials tend to affect pathogens with similar biochemical characteristics.

The most common method used to distinguish among various microorganisms is the Gram stain, which uses laboratory dyes to stain organisms; the reactions reveal chemical differences in the cell wall. Organisms that are stained by the Gram stain are called gram-positive; those that are not are called gram-negative.

For some bacteria, Gram staining is not a useful diagnostic tool. Some of these organisms, such as mycobacteria, can be stained with carbolfuchsin, then decolorized with ethyl alcohol and hydrochloric acid. They are classified as acid-fast if they retain the stain.

Spirochetes can be visualized only by special techniques such as dark-field examination. Other important stains used to identify bacteria include Gimenez stain for *Rickettsia,* Giemsa and Wright's stains for parasites and intracellular microorganisms, and fluorescent antibody for various organisms.

Organisms with similar staining properties tend to be susceptible to the same antimicrobial agents. Therefore, a drug's antimicrobial spectrum may be described by its activity against gram-negative, gram-positive, or acid-fast bacilli. (See *Gram-negative, gram-positive, and acid-fast organisms.*)

Organisms also are classified as aerobes — those organisms that can live and grow in the presence of oxygen — or as anaerobes — those that can live or grow without oxygen.

DRUG SELECTION

Selecting an appropriate antimicrobial agent to treat a specific infection involves several important factors. First the microorganism must be isolated and identified. Then its susceptibility to various drugs must be determined. The lowest antimicrobial concentration that prevents visible growth after an 18- to 24-hour incubation is known as the minimal inhibitory concentration (MIC). The minimal bactericidal concentration (MBC) is defined as the lowest antimicrobial concentration that totally suppresses growth after overnight incubation. Because culture and sensitivity results take 48 hours, treatment usually is initiated on clinical assessment and then reevaluated when test results are complete.

Another important factor in choosing an antimicrobial is the location of the infection. For antimicrobial therapy to be effective, an adequate concentration of the drug must be delivered to the infection site. That means the local antimicrobial concentration should equal at least the MIC for the infecting organism. Other factors in selecting an antimicrobial are the relative cost of the drug, its potential adverse effects, and patient allergies.

Mixed infections (those caused by two or more organisms, each of which may be sensitive to different drugs) respond best to treatment with a selected combination of antimicrobial agents. Examples are peritoneal or pelvic infections caused by mixed bowel flora and foot infections in diabetic patients.

Gram-negative, gram-positive, and acid-fast organisms

Knowing which organisms are gram-negative, gram-positive, or acid-fast helps the nurse understand the therapeutic use of selected agents. An antibacterial agent that is effective against one gram-negative bacterium may be effective against other bacteria in that group. The same principle applies to the gram-positive group. In contrast, the bacilli in the acid-fast group must be treated individually with drugs that are effective against that specific organism.

GRAM-NEGATIVE BACTERIA

Acinetobacter calcoaceticus
Bacteroides asaccharolyticus
Bacteroides distasonis
Bacteroides fragilis
Bacteroides melaninogenicus
Bacteroides ovatus
Bacteroides thetaiotaomicron
Bacteroides vulgatus
Bartonella bacilliformis
Bordetella pertussis
Branhamella catarrhalis
Brucella abortus
Brucella canis
Brucella melitensis
Brucella suis
Calymmatobacterium granulomatis
Campylobacter coli
Campylobacter fetus
Campylobacter jejuni
Chlamydia trachomatis
Citrobacter diversus
Citrobacter freundii
Enterobacter aerogenes
Enterobacter cloacae
Escherichia coli
Francisella tularensis
Fusobacterium nucleatum
Haemophilus ducreyi
Haemophilus influenzae
Haemophilus parahemolyticus
Haemophilus parainfluenzae
Klebsiella pneumoniae
Legionella micdadei
Legionella pneumophila
Moraxella catarrhalis
Morganella morganii
Mycoplasma pneumoniae
Neisseria gonorrhoeae
Neisseria meningitidis
Pasteurella multocida
Proteus mirabilis
Proteus morganii
Proteus vulgarisi
Providencia rettgeri
Providencia stuartii
Pseudomonas aeruginosa
Salmonella choleraesuis
Salmonella enteritidis
Salmonella sendai
Salmonella typhimurium
Salmonella typhi
Serratia marcescens
Shigella boydii
Shigella dysenteriae
Shigella flexneri
Shigella sonnei
Streptobacillus moniliformis
Ureaplasma urealyticum
Veillonella
Vibrio alginolyticus
Vibrio cholerae
Vibrio mimicus
Vibrio parahaemolyticus
Vibrio vulnificus
Yersinia enterocolitica

GRAM-POSITIVE BACTERIA

Actinomyces israelii
Arachnia propionica
Bacillus anthracis
Bacillus cereus
Clostridium botulinum
Clostridium butyricum
Clostridium difficile
Clostridium perfringens
Clostridium septicum
Clostridium sordellii
Clostridium tetani
Corynebacterium diphtheriae
Erysipelothrix rhusiopathiae
Eubacterium alactolyticum
Listeria monocytogenes
Nocardia asteroides
Peptococcus
Peptostreptococcus
Propionibacterium acnes
Staphylococcus aureus
Staphylococcus epidermidis
Streptococcus bovis
Streptococcus faecalis
Streptococcus pneumoniae
Streptococcus pyogenes
Streptococcus sanguis
Streptococcus viridans

ACID-FAST BACILLI

Mycobacterium avium
Mycobacterium bovis
Mycobacterium chelonei
Mycobacterium fortuitum
Mycobacterium intracellulare
Mycobacterium kansasii
Mycobacterium leprae
Mycobacterium marinum
Mycobacterium scrofulaceum
Mycobacterium tuberculosis
Mycobacterium xenopi

The patient's clinical condition determines when antimicrobial therapy is started and how it is administered. If the patient is stable, therapy may be delayed until culture and sensitivity test results are available. Unstable patients usually are treated immediately with broad-spectrum agents. Patients with serious infections usually need higher and more predictable blood concentration levels, necessitating intravenous therapy. In less severe infections, intramuscular or oral therapy can be used.

PREVENTION OF RESISTANCE

One factor limits the usefulness of antimicrobial agents: Pathogens may develop resistance to a drug's action. *Resistance* is the ability of a microorganism to live and grow in the presence of an antibacterial agent that usually is bactericidal or bacteriostatic. Resistance usually results from genetic events that develop mutant strains of the microorganism. These mutant strains resist a drug's activity by enhancing the action of specific enzymes that break down the chemical structure of the drug, restricting uptake of the drug, or altering critical cellular target sites.

Antimicrobial drugs should not be used indiscriminately, because unnecessary exposure of organisms to these agents encourages emergence of resistant strains. The drugs should be reserved for patients with infections caused by susceptible organisms and should be used in high enough dosages and for an appropriate duration of therapy. Administration of subtherapeutic dosages may allow resistant mutant strains to proliferate. New antimicrobial agents should be reserved for severely ill patients with serious infections that do not respond to conventional drugs.

ANTIMICROBIAL AGENTS

The chapters in Unit 10 explore the agents used to prevent or treat infections; they include antibacterial, antiviral, antitubercular, antimycotic (antifungal), anthelmintic, antimalarial, other antiprotozoal, and urinary antiseptic agents.

Antibacterial agents are used to treat systemic bacterial infections, such as respiratory tract infections, septicemia, and Lyme disease. Antiviral agents are prescribed to prevent or treat viral infections, including human immunodeficiency virus and cytomegalovirus infections. Antitubercular agents are used to treat tuberculosis. Antimycotic agents are used to treat fungal infections, which range from the common (such as athlete's foot) to the rare (such as sporotrichosis). Anthelmintic agents destroy parasitic worms, including roundworms, tapeworms, and flukes. Antiprotozoal agents are used to treat protozoal diseases, such as malaria, amebiasis, and giardiasis. Urinary antiseptic agents provide antibacterial effects that are limited to the urine.

All antimicrobials can produce beneficial and adverse reactions in a patient. The adverse reactions can be classified as direct toxic effects on such organs as the gastrointestinal tract, kidneys, and liver or the auditory, optic, and peripheral nerves; allergic reactions and other kinds of hypersensitivity reactions affecting the skin and other organs and structures, including the bone marrow and blood; and superinfections resulting from drug-induced overgrowths of resistant bacterial strains or fungal organisms.

31 Antibacterial agents

OBJECTIVES

After reading and studying this chapter, the student should be able to:

1. identify the different types of antibacterial agents used to treat systemic bacterial infections.
2. describe the adverse reactions associated with the aminoglycosides.
3. compare the antibacterial activity of the four types of penicillins: natural penicillins, penicillinase-resistant penicillins, aminopenicillins, and extended-spectrum penicillins.
4. describe the differences among the first-, second-, and third-generation cephalosporins.
5. identify the adverse reactions to tetracyclines.
6. discuss the pharmacokinetics of chloramphenicol.
7. explain the pharmacodynamics of lincomycin and clindamycin.
8. discuss the pharmacotherapeutic uses of the various macrolides.
9. describe the **hypotension** reaction associated with vancomycin administration.
10. discuss why imipenem and cilastatin have been combined to make a new antibacterial drug.
11. discuss the antibacterial spectrum of aztreonam.
12. describe how to apply the nursing process when caring for a patient who is receiving an antibacterial agent.

INTRODUCTION

This chapter describes drugs used mainly to treat systemic bacterial **infections.** The **antibacterial** classes discussed include aminoglycosides, penicillins, cephalosporins, tetracyclines, chloramphenicol, clindamycin and lincomycin, macrolides, vancomycin, carbapenems, and monobactams. (See *Selected major antibacterial agents,* pages 392 to 395.)

Drugs covered in this chapter include:

- amikacin
- ampicillin
- axetil
- azithromycin
- azlocillin
- aztreonam
- carbenicillin
- cefaclor
- cefadroxil
- cefixime
- cefoperaxone
- cefprozil
- ceftriaxone
- cefuroxime
- cephalexin
- cephradine
- chloramphenicol sodium succinate
- chlortetracycline
- clarithromycin
- clindamycin hydrochloride
- clindamycin palmitate hydrochloride
- clindamycin phosphate
- demeclocycline
- doxycycline
- erythromycin
- erythromycin ethyl succinate
- erythromycin gluceptate
- erythromycin lactobionate
- erythromycin stearate
- gentamicin
- imipenem-cilastin
- kanamycin
- loracarbef
- meropenem
- methacycline
- mezlocillin
- minocycline
- nafcillin
- neomycin
- netilmicin
- oxacillin
- oxytetracycline
- paramomycin
- penicillin G
- pipercillin
- streptomycin
- ticaracillin
- tobramycin
- vancomycin.

Aminoglycosides

The aminoglycosides provide effective **bactericidal** activity against aerobic gram-negative **bacilli,** some aerobic gram-positive **bacteria, mycobacteria,** and some **protozoa.** Currently used aminoglycosides include amikacin sulfate, gentamicin sulfate, kanamycin sulfate, neomycin sulfate, netilmicin sulfate, paromomycin sulfate, streptomycin sulfate, and tobramycin sulfate. (See Drug Interactions: *Aminoglycosides,* pages 396.)

PHARMACOKINETICS

After oral administration, aminoglycosides are absorbed poorly from the gastrointestinal (GI) tract. However, after intravenous (I.V.) or intramuscular (I.M.) administration, aminoglycoside absorption is complete and rapid. Aminoglycosides are distributed widely in extracellular fluid. When administered in therapeutic dosages, they readily cross the placental barrier but do not cross the blood-brain barrier. Aminoglycosides are not metabolized. They are ex-

(Text continues on page 396.)

Selected major antibacterial agents

This chart summarizes the major antibacterial agents currently in clinical use.

DRUG	MAJOR INDICATIONS AND USUAL DOSAGES	CONTRAINDICATIONS AND PRECAUTIONS
Aminoglycosides		
gentamicin (Garamycin)	*Infections caused by sensitive* Pseudomonas aeruginosa, Escherichia coli, *indole-positive and indole-negative* Proteus, Providencia, Klebsiella, Serratia, Enterobacter, Citrobacter, Staphylococcus, *and other gram-negative aerobic bacteria* ADULT: 1 to 1.75 mg/kg I.V. or I.M. every 8 hours; dosage adjustment is required for patients with renal impairment PEDIATRIC: for children ages 6 weeks to 12 years, 2 to 2.5 mg/kg I.V. or I.M. every 8 hours or 3 to 3.75 mg/kg I.M. or I.V. every 12 hours	• Gentamicin is contraindicated in a patient with known hypersensitivity to the drug or other aminoglycosides. • This drug requires cautious use in a pregnant, breast-feeding, or geriatric patient or one with a neuromuscular disorder or renal impairment.
Penicillins		
ampicillin (Omnipen)	*Respiratory tract infection* ADULT: 250 to 500 mg P.O. every 6 hours or 1 to 3 g I.M. or I.V. every 6 hours PEDIATRIC: 50 to 100 mg/kg P.O. daily in divided doses every 6 hours or 100 to 200 mg/kg I.M. or I.V. daily in divided doses every 6 hours *Urinary tract infection (UTI)* ADULT: 500 mg P.O. every 6 hours PEDIATRIC: 50 to 100 mg/kg P.O. daily in divided doses every 6 hours or 100 to 200 mg/kg I.M. or I.V. daily in divided doses every 6 hours *Meningitis* ADULT: 8 to 14 g or 150 to 200 mg/kg I.M. or I.V. daily in equally divided doses every 3 to 4 hours (initially, doses should be given I.V. for at least 3 days) PEDIATRIC: up to 300 mg/kg I.V. daily in divided doses every 4 hours	• Ampicillin is contraindicated in a patient with known hypersensitivity to any penicillin. • This drug requires cautious use in a breast-feeding patient, one with allergies to other drugs (especially cephalosporins), or one with mononucleosis.
penicillin G aqueous	*Meningitis, septicemia, pericarditis, endocarditis, severe pneumonia, and other serious infections* ADULT: 600,000 to 5,000,000 U I.V. or I.M. every 4 to 6 hours PEDIATRIC: 100,000 to 250,000 U/kg I.V. or I.M. daily in divided doses every 4 hours	• Penicillin G aqueous is contraindicated in a breast-feeding patient or one with known hypersensitivity to any penicillin. • This drug requires cautious use in a pregnant patient or one with a history of significant allergies or asthma.
ticarcillin disodium (Ticar)	*Uncomplicated UTI* ADULT: 1 g I.M. or I.V. every 6 hours PEDIATRIC: for children over age 1 month who weigh less than 88 lb (40 kg), 50 to 100 mg/kg I.M. or I.V. daily in divided doses every 6 to 8 hours; for children who weigh 88 lb (40 kg) or more, 1 g I.M. or I.V. every 6 hours *Complicated UTI* ADULT: 3 g I.V. every 4 to 6 hours PEDIATRIC: for children over age 1 month who weigh less than 88 lb (40 kg), 150 to 200 mg/kg I.V. daily in divided doses every 4 to 6 hours; for children who weigh 88 lb or more, 3 g I.V. every 4 to 6 hours *Septicemia* ADULT: 3 g I.V. every 3 to 6 hours PEDIATRIC: for children over age 1 month who weigh less than 88 lb (40 kg), 200 to 300 mg/kg I.V. daily in divided doses every 4 to 6 hours; for children who weigh 88 lb or more, 3 g I.V. every 3 to 6 hours	• Ticarcillin is contraindicated in a patient with known hypersensitivity to any penicillin. • This drug requires cautious use in a patient who must restrict sodium intake or one with allergies to other drugs (especially cephalosporins), a hemorrhagic condition, or hypokalemia.

Selected major antibacterial agents *(continued)*

DRUG	MAJOR INDICATIONS AND USUAL DOSAGES	CONTRAINDICATIONS AND PRECAUTIONS
Cephalosporins		
ceftizoxime (Cefizox)	*Infections caused by gram-negative aerobic organisms (except* P. aeruginosa*) and gram-positive organisms (except enterococci) and anaerobes (such as* Bacteroides fragilis) ADULT: 1 to 2 g I.V. or I.M. every 8 to 12 hours PEDIATRIC: for children over age 6 months, 50 mg/kg I.V. every 6 to 8 hours	• Ceftizoxime is contraindicated in a patient with hypersensitivity to any cephalosporin. • This drug requires cautious use in a pregnant or breast-feeding patient or one with a history of allergies (especially to such drugs as penicillin) or gastrointestinal (GI) disease (particularly colitis).
cefaclor (Ceclor)	*Respiratory tract infections, otitis media* ADULT: 250 to 500 mg P.O. every 8 hours PEDIATRIC: 20 mg/kg P.O. daily in divided doses every 8 hours	• Cefaclor is contraindicated in a patient with hypersensitivity to any cephalosporin. • This drug requires cautious use in a pregnant or breast-feeding patient or one with a history of allergies or GI disease (particularly colitis).
cefprozil (Cefzil)	*Mild to moderate tonsillitis, pharyngitis, secondary bacterial infection of acute bronchitis, acute bacterial exacerbation of chronic bronchitis, or uncomplicated skin and skin-structure infections caused by susceptible organisms* ADULT: 250 to 500 mg P.O. every 12 hours for 10 days; for upper respiratory tract infections, 500 mg P.O. every 24 hours *Otitis media* ADULT: 250 to 500 mg P.O. every 12 hours for 10 days PEDIATRIC: for children ages 6 months to 12 years, 15 mg/kg P.O. every 12 hours	• Cefprozil is contraindicated in a patient with known hypersensitivity to any cephalosporin. • This drug requires cautious use in a pregnant or breast-feeding patient, one receiving a potent diuretic, or one with penicillin hypersensitivity, impaired renal function, or history of GI disease (particularly colitis). • Safety and efficacy in children under age 6 months have not been established.
loracarbef (Lorabid)	*Mild to moderate infections caused by susceptible strains of designated microorganisms* ADULT: 200 to 400 mg P.O. b.i.d. for 7 to 10 days, depending on the infection being treated PEDIATRIC: for children age 13 and over, 200 to 400 mg P.O. b.i.d. for 7 to 10 days, depending on the infection; for children ages 6 months to 12 years, 15 to 30 mg/kg P.O. daily in two divided doses	• Loracarbef is contraindicated in a patient with known hypersensitivity to the drug or any other cephalosporin or one with diarrhea suspected to be caused by pseudomembranous colitis. • This drug requires cautious use in a pregnant or breast-feeding patient. • Safety and efficacy in children under age 6 months have not been established.
Tetracyclines		
minocycline (Minocin)	*Infections caused by sensitive gram-negative and gram-positive organisms,* Chlamydia trachomatis, *or amebiasis* ADULT: initially, 200 mg P.O. or I.V.; for maintenance dosage, 100 mg every 12 hours or 50 mg P.O. every 6 hours PEDIATRIC: for children over age 8, initially, 4 mg/kg P.O. or I.V.; for maintenance dosage, 2 mg/kg P.O. daily in divided doses every 12 hours *Meningococcal carrier state* ADULT: 100 to 200 mg P.O. every 12 hours for 5 days *Uncomplicated urethral, endocervical, or rectal infection caused by* C. trachomatis *or* U. urealyticum ADULT: 100 mg P.O. b.i.d. for at least 7 days *Uncomplicated gonococcal urethritis in males* ADULT: 100 mg P.O. b.i.d. for 7 days	• Minocycline is contraindicated in a pediatric patient age 8 or under, a pregnant or breast-feeding patient, or one with known hypersensitivity to any tetracycline. • This drug requires cautious use in a patient with impaired renal or hepatic function.
doxycycline (Vibramycin)	*Infections caused by* C. trachomatis, Ureaplasma urealyticum, Neisseria gonorrhoeae *or in syphilis as an alternative to penicillin G* ADULT: 100 mg P.O. b.i.d. for 7 days; for treatment of syphilis, 100 mg P.O. b.i.d. for 2 to 4 weeks.	• Doxycycline is contraindicated in a patient age 8 or under, a pregnant or breast-feeding patient, or one with known hypersensitivity to any tetracycline. • This drug requires cautious use in a patient with impaired renal or hepatic function.

(continued)

Selected major antibacterial agents *(continued)*

DRUG	MAJOR INDICATIONS AND USUAL DOSAGES	CONTRAINDICATIONS AND PRECAUTIONS
Tetracyclines *(continued)*		
tetracycline (Achromycin, Sumycin)	*Infections caused by sensitive gram-negative and gram-positive organisms,* Rickettsia, *or* Mycoplasma ADULT: 250 to 500 mg P.O. every 6 hours; 250 mg I.M. daily; 150 mg I.M. every 12 hours; or 250 to 500 mg I.V. every 8 to 12 hours (use only hydrochloride salt form in I.M. and I.V. administration) PEDIATRIC: for children over age 8, 25 to 50 mg/kg P.O. daily in divided doses every 6 hours; 15 to 25 mg/kg (up to a maximum of 250 mg) I.M. daily as a single dose or in divided doses every 8 to 12 hours; or 10 to 20 mg/kg I.V. daily in divided doses every 12 hours *Uncomplicated urethral, endocervical, or rectal infection caused by* C. trachomatis ADULT: 500 mg P.O. every 6 hours for at least 7 days *Brucellosis* ADULT: 500 mg P.O. every 6 hours for 3 weeks with 1 g streptomycin I.M. every 12 hours in week 1 and daily in week 2 *Syphilis in a patient hypersensitive to penicillin* ADULT: 30 to 50 g P.O. total in equally divided doses over 10 to 15 days *Acne* ADULT: initially, 250 mg P.O. every 6 hours; for maintenance dosage, 125 to 500 mg P.O. daily or every other day PEDIATRIC: for adolescent, same as adult dosage *Lyme disease* ADULT: 500 mg P.O. b.i.d. for 10 to 30 days	• Tetracycline is contraindicated in a pediatric patient age 8 or under, a pregnant or breast-feeding patient, or one with hypersensitivity to any tetracycline. • This drug requires cautious use in a patient with impaired renal or hepatic function.
Chloramphenicol		
chloramphenicol (Chloromycetin)	*Serious infections caused by many gram-positive and gram-negative aerobic and some anaerobic organisms* ADULT: 50 to 100 mg/kg I.V. daily in divided doses every 6 hours PEDIATRIC: for neonates under age 2 weeks, 25 mg/kg I.V. once daily; for children over age 2 weeks, up to 50 mg/kg I.V. in divided doses every 6 hours	• Chloramphenicol is contraindicated in a patient with known hypersensitivity, history of toxic reactions to it, or a trivial infection or condition in which it is not specifically indicated. It also is contraindicated for the prevention of bacterial infections. • This drug requires cautious use in an infant, a pregnant patient who is at term or in labor, a breast-feeding patient, or one with impaired renal or hepatic function.
Clindamycin		
clindamycin phosphate (Cleocin Phosphate)	*Serious infections caused by aerobic gram-positive cocci and anaerobes* ADULT: 300 to 600 mg I.V. or I.M. every 6 to 8 hours PEDIATRIC: for children over age 1 month, 3.75 to 10 mg I.M. or I.V. every 6 hours, or 5 to 13.3 mg/kg I.M. or I.V. every 8 hours	• Clindamycin is contraindicated in a pregnant or breast-feeding patient or one with known hypersensitivity to clindamycin or lincomycin. • This drug requires cautious use in a patient with a history of GI disease (particularly colitis), severe renal or hepatic impairment, or multiple allergies.
Macrolides		
erythromycin (E-Mycin, Ery-Tab, Ilotycin)	*Infections caused by many gram-positive and gram-negative bacteria, including* Acinetobacter, Mycobacterium, Treponema, Mycoplasma, Rickettsia, *and* Chlamydia ADULT: 250 mg P.O. every 6 hours PEDIATRIC: 7.5 to 25 mg/kg P.O. every 6 hours, 15 to 50 mg/kg P.O. every 12 hours, or 500 mg P.O. every 12 hours	• Erythromycin is contraindicated in a patient with known hypersensitivity. • This drug requires cautious use in a breast-feeding patient or one with impaired hepatic function or biliary excretion.

Selected major antibacterial agents *(continued)*

DRUG	MAJOR INDICATIONS AND USUAL DOSAGES	CONTRAINDICATIONS AND PRECAUTIONS
Macrolides		
azithromycin (Zithromax)	*Treatment of streptococcal pharyngitis and chlamydial cervicitis and urethritis* ADULT: 250 to 500 mg P.O. daily	• Azithromycin is contraindicated in a patient with known hypersensitivity to the drug, erythromycin, or any other macrolide. • This drug requires cautious use in a pregnant or breast-feeding patient or one with impaired renal or hepatic function. • Safety and efficacy in children under age 16 have not been established.
clarithromycin (Biaxin)	*Treatment of upper and lower respiratory tract infections (including sinusitis, pharyngitis, tonsillitis, pneumonia, and bronchitis) and uncomplicated skin infections caused by susceptible organisms* ADULT: 250 to 500 mg P.O. b.i.d.	• Clarithromycin is contraindicated in a pregnant patient unless no alternative therapy is appropriate or in a patient with known hypersensitivity to the drug, erythromycin, or any other macrolide. • This drug requires cautious use in a breast-feeding patient or one with severe renal impairment. • Safety and efficacy in children under age 12 have not been established.
Vancomycin		
vancomycin hydrochloride (Vancocin)	*Serious staphylococcal infections when other antibacterials are ineffective or contraindicated* ADULT: 500 mg I.V. every 6 hours or 1 g I.V. every 12 hours; daily dosage should not exceed 2 g PEDIATRIC: 44 mg/kg I.V. daily in divided doses; for neonates, 10 mg/kg I.V. daily every 6 to 12 hours	• Vancomycin is contraindicated in a pregnant patient, one with known hypersensitivity, or one with hearing loss. • This drug requires cautious use in a breast-feeding patient or one with impaired renal function.
Carbapenems		
imipenem-cilastatin (Primaxin)	*Infections caused by gram-positive, gram-negative, and anaerobic organisms* ADULT: 250 mg imipenem and 250 mg cilastatin via intermittent I.V. every 6 hours; for more serious infections, 500 mg imipenem and 500 mg cilastatin via intermittent I.V. every 6 hours or 500 mg or 750 mg I.M. every 6 to 12 hours; dosage depends on severity of infection and patient's renal function PEDIATRIC: for children age 12 and over, 250 mg imipenem and 250 mg cilastatin via intermittent I.V. every 6 hours; for more serious infections, 500 mg imipenem and 500 mg cilastatin via intermittent I.V. every 6 hours or 500 mg or 750 mg I.M. every 6 to 12 hours; dosage depends on severity of infection and patient's renal function	• Imipenem-cilastatin is contraindicated in a pregnant patient or one with known hypersensitivity to the drug or any of its ingredients. • This drug requires cautious use in a breast-feeding patient, one with impaired renal function, or one with known hypersensitivity to penicillins. • Safety and efficacy in children under age 12 have not been established.
Monobactams		
aztreonam (Azactam)	*Urinary tract infections* ADULT: 500 mg to 1 g I.M. or I.V. every 8 to 12 hours *Moderate to severe systemic infections caused by a wide range of gram-negative aerobic organisms, including* Pseudomonas aeruginosa ADULT: 1 to 2 g I.M. or I.V. every 8 to 12 hours *Severe systemic or life-threatening infections* ADULT: 2 g I.V. every 6 to 8 hours	• Aztreonam is contraindicated in a patient with known hypersensitivity. • This drug requires cautious use in a patient with impaired renal or hepatic function or a history of immediate type I hypersensitivity reaction to penicillins or cephalosporins. • Safety and efficacy in children have not been established.

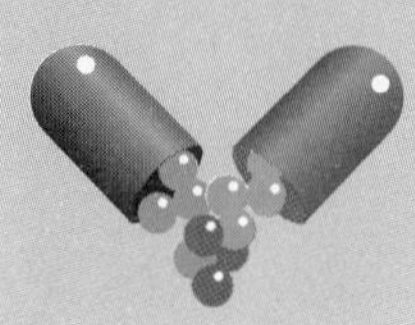

DRUG INTERACTIONS

Aminoglycosides

This chart summarizes significant interactions between aminoglycosides and other drugs. The nurse should be familiar with these interactions before administering an aminoglycoside.

DRUG	INTERACTING DRUGS	POSSIBLE EFFECTS	NURSING IMPLICATIONS
all aminoglycosides	antiemetics	Masked vestibular ototoxicity	• Monitor the patient for hearing loss.
	loop diuretics	Increased ototoxicity	• Monitor the patient for hearing loss.
	methoxyflurane	Increased nephrotoxicity and neurotoxicity	• Do not administer together. • Make sure the anesthesiologist knows that the patient is receiving an aminoglycoside.
amikacin, gentamicin, kanamycin, neomycin, netilmicin, streptomycin, tobramycin	neuromuscular blockers	Increased neuromuscular blockade	• Administer calcium and anticholinesterase agents as prescribed. • Administer the aminoglycoside cautiously during surgery and during the postoperative period.
	carbenicillin, ticarcillin, azlocillin, mezlocillin, piperacillin	Decreased effect of aminoglycoside	• Never mix these two types of antibacterials; if the patient must receive concomitant therapy, administer the doses at least 1 hour apart.
amikacin, gentamicin, kanamycin, netilmicin, tobramycin	amphotericin B, cephalosporins, acyclovir	Increased nephrotoxicity	• Monitor renal function tests frequently for the patient on combination therapy.
	cyclosporines	Increased nephrotoxicity	• Do not administer an aminoglycoside to a patient receiving a cyclosporine. • Monitor the patient's blood urea nitrogen and creatinine levels.

creted primarily via the kidneys; therefore, decreased renal function can increase the serum half-life from the normal 2 to 3 hours to between 50 and 60 hours in uremic patients.

Route	Onset	Peak	Duration
I.M.	Rapid	30-120 min	4-6 hr
I.V.	Rapid	30 min after infusion ends	4-6 hr

PHARMACODYNAMICS

The aminoglycosides act as bactericidal agents against susceptible organisms by binding irreversibly to their ribosomal subunits, thus inhibiting the protein synthesis required for maintaining the bacterial cell.

Bacterial **resistance** to an aminoglycoside may be related to failure of the drug to cross the cell membrane, altered binding to **ribosomes,** or destruction of the drug by bacterial enzymes. Some gram-positive **cocci** (enterococci) resist aminoglycoside transport across the cell membrane. When penicillin is used with aminoglycoside therapy, the cell wall is altered, enabling the aminoglycoside to penetrate the bacterial cell.

PHARMACOTHERAPEUTICS

Aminoglycosides are most useful in treating infections caused by aerobic gram-negative bacilli. They also are valuable in treating serious **nosocomial** infections, such as gram-negative **bacteremia,** peritonitis, and pneumonia, in critically ill patients. Urinary tract infections (UTIs) caused by enteric bacilli that are resistant to less toxic **antibiotics,** such as penicillins and cephalosporins, commonly respond to aminoglycosides. Infections of the central nervous system (CNS) and the eye require local instillation. Streptomycin is active against many strains of mycobacteria, including *Mycobacterium tuberculosis,* and against gram-positive bacteria *Nocardia* and *Erysipelothrix.* Amikacin, gentamicin, netilmicin, and tobramycin are active against *Acinetobacter, Citrobacter, Enterobacter, Klebsiella, Proteus* (indole-positive and indole-negative), *Providencia, Serratia, Escherichia coli,* and *Pseudomonas aeruginosa.* Because the susceptibility of these organisms to the particular aminoglycoside varies with time and clinical setting, a culture and sensitivity test should be performed before beginning and periodically during therapy. Against gram-positive organisms, aminoglycosides are used as synergistic combinations with penicillins to treat staphylococcal or enterococcal infections. Aminoglycosides are inactive against anaerobic bacteria.

Drug interactions

Aminoglycosides can interact with other antibiotics, such as extended-**spectrum** penicillins and cephalosporins as well as with a variety of other drugs.

ADVERSE DRUG REACTIONS

Serious adverse reactions limit the use of aminoglycosides, all of which display the same spectrum of **toxicity;** the total dosage and duration of therapy contribute to toxicity. The most notable adverse reactions are **ototoxicity** and nephrotoxicity. These most commonly occur in older patients, dehydrated patients, those with renal impairment, and those receiving concomitant therapy with an ototoxic or nephrotoxic drug.

Aminoglycosides can produce irreversible damage to cranial nerve VIII. High-frequency hearing loss usually occurs before clinical hearing loss. These drugs can induce vestibular symptoms, such as dizziness, nystagmus, vertigo, and ataxia.

Aminoglycosides can produce renal tubular necrosis, resulting in elevated serum creatinine and blood urea nitrogen (BUN) levels. Nephrotoxicity is related to high drug concentrations that accumulate in the renal cortex. Renal tubular damage usually is reversible after discontinuation of the drug.

Aminoglycosides can produce neuromuscular reactions that range from peripheral nerve toxicity to neuromuscular blockade. Reactions commonly occur after local, peritoneal, pleural, or wound instillation. Neuromuscular reactions also can occur when aminoglycosides are administered to patients immediately after surgery. Neomycin and netilmicin produce the most potent neuromuscular reactions.

The most common adverse reactions to orally administered aminoglycosides are nausea, vomiting, and diarrhea.

Allergic reactions to aminoglycosides are rare. Rash, urticaria, stomatitis, pruritus, generalized burning, fever, and eosinophilia occasionally occur.

NURSING PROCESS APPLICATION

The following information assists the nurse in caring for a patient who is receiving an aminoglycoside. It includes an overview of assessment activities as well as examples of appropriate nursing diagnoses and related interventions (under "Planning and implementation"). It also highlights the importance of evaluation.

Assessment

Before drug therapy begins, review the patient's history for conditions that contraindicate or require cautious use of the prescribed aminoglycoside. Also review the patient's medication history to identify use of drugs that may interact with it. During therapy, assess the patient for adverse drug reactions, such as nephrotoxicity and ototoxicity, and signs of drug interactions. Periodically assess the effectiveness of aminoglycoside therapy. Finally, evaluate the patient's and family's knowledge about the prescribed drug.

Serum aminoglycoside levels

Periodic assessment of aminoglycoside serum peak and trough concentration levels is needed to assess therapeutic efficacy and toxicity. This is especially important in patients with altered renal function and in those on concomitant therapy with an extended-spectrum penicillin. The goal is to obtain a peak serum concentration between 4 and 8 mcg/ml for gentamicin or tobramycin, 4 and 10 mcg/ml for netilmicin, or 15 and 30 mcg/ml for kanamycin or amikacin. These therapeutic peak concentrations will vary with the pathogen and the infection site. Serum trough concentrations for gentamicin, tobramycin, and netilmicin generally are lower than 2 mcg/ml; for amikacin and kanamycin, lower than 5 mcg/ml. High trough concentrations correlate with nephrotoxicity; high peak concentrations, with ototoxicity and nephrotoxicity.

Blood for serum aminoglycoside trough concentrations should be obtained within 30 minutes before the next dose. Blood for peak concentrations should be obtained 1 hour after the administration of an intramuscular dose and 30 minutes after the end of a 30-minute infusion. Each specimen must be dated and timed.

Nursing diagnoses

- Risk for injury related to adverse drug reactions or drug interactions
- Sensory/perceptual alterations (auditory) related to ototoxicity caused by the adverse effects of the prescribed aminoglycoside
- Knowledge deficit related to the prescribed aminoglycoside regimen

Planning and implementation

- Do not administer an aminoglycoside to a patient with a condition that contraindicates its use.
- Administer an aminoglycoside cautiously to a patient at risk because of a preexisting condition.
- Monitor the patient for adverse reactions and drug interactions during aminoglycoside therapy.
- Regularly monitor the serum aminoglycoside level. (See *Serum aminoglycoside levels.*)

***** ***Immediately after drawing a serum aminoglycoside sample, place it on ice and transport it to the laboratory to prevent inactivation of the aminoglycoside. Notify the physician if the peak or trough levels do not fall within the expected range for the prescribed aminoglycoside.***

- Collect appropriate specimens (blood, urine, sputum, and wound) for culture and sensitivity tests before beginning aminoglycoside therapy.
- Make sure the patient is well hydrated before beginning therapy (unless contraindicated) in order to decrease the risk of nephrotoxicity.
- Monitor the serum creatinine level to help detect changes in renal function. The serum creatinine level should be

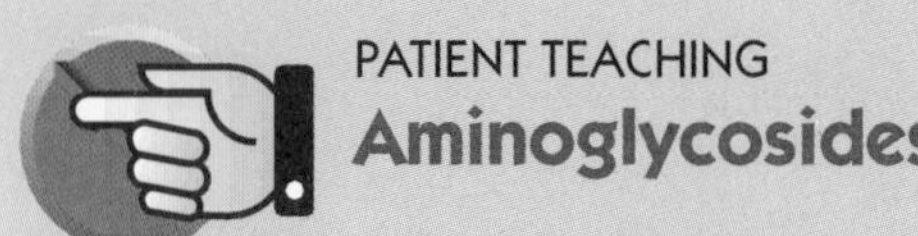

PATIENT TEACHING
Aminoglycosides

- Teach the patient and family the name, dose, frequency, action, and adverse effects of the prescribed aminoglycoside.
- Stress the importance of completing the course of aminoglycoside therapy.
- Instruct the female patient to alert the physician if pregnancy is suspected or confirmed during aminoglycoside therapy.
- Stress the importance of having blood tests to monitor the serum aminoglycoside level and renal function in order to determine the effectiveness of therapy or detect any increased risk of adverse reactions.
- Instruct the patient to notify the nurse immediately if breathing difficulty or irregular heartbeat occurs, because neuromuscular blockade may be present.
- Caution the patient with vestibular toxicity not to perform any activity that requires alertness. Also instruct the patient to notify the physician if dizziness, nystagmus, vertigo, or ataxia occurs.
- Advise the patient receiving an oral aminoglycoside to notify the physician if nausea, vomiting, or diarrhea occurs and to request a prescription for an antiemetic or antidiarrheal as needed.
- Instruct the patient to notify the physician at once if changes in hearing occur.
- Instruct the patient to notify the physician if other adverse reactions occur or if the infection persists or worsens.

monitored at least every other day in a patient with unstable renal function and at least once a week in a patient with normal renal function.

- Notify the physician if routine urinalysis indicates casts or protein in the urine. These findings may indicate aminoglycoside-induced renal damage.
- Refrigerate prepared I.V. aminoglycoside solution until use; infuse the I.V. solution over at least 30 minutes.
- Do not mix an aminoglycoside in a solution containing extended-spectrum penicillins; the aminoglycoside may be inactivated.
- Administer an aminoglycoside and an extended-spectrum penicillin or cephalosporin at least 2 hours apart to prevent a decrease in the therapeutic aminoglycoside level and half-life in a patient with normal renal function.
- Notify the physician if adverse reactions or drug interactions occur.
- Monitor for ototoxicity in a patient receiving an aminoglycoside. Prepare the patient for audiometric testing as indicated, because high-frequency loss usually occurs before clinical hearing loss. (See Patient Teaching: *Aminoglycosides.*)
- Expect to discontinue the prescribed aminoglycoside and initiate another type of antibacterial therapy if ototoxicity is suspected.

Evaluation

For each nursing diagnosis, prepare an evaluation statement that describes the patient's or family's response to nursing interventions.

Penicillins

Penicillins remain one of the most important and useful antibacterials, despite the availability of numerous others. The penicillins can be divided into four groups: natural penicillins, penicillinase-resistant penicillins, aminopenicillins, and extended-spectrum penicillins. (See *Penicillins and their uses.*)

PHARMACOKINETICS

After oral administration, the penicillins are absorbed mainly in the duodenum and the upper jejunum. The extent of absorption of oral dosage forms varies and depends on such factors as the particular penicillin used, the patient's gastric and intestinal pH, and the presence of food in the GI tract.

Penicillins are distributed widely to most areas of the body, including the lungs, liver, kidneys, muscle, bone, and placenta. High concentrations also appear in the urine, making penicillins useful in treating UTIs.

Penicillins are metabolized, to a limited extent, in the liver to inactive metabolites and are excreted 60% unchanged by the kidneys. Nafcillin also is excreted in bile. Because excretion into the urine is rapid, they have a short half-life, ranging from less than 30 minutes for penicillin G to 72 minutes for carbenicillin.

Route	Onset	Peak	Duration
P.O.	Unknown	30-120 min	Variable
I.M.	Unknown	Variable	Variable
I.V.	Immediate	Immediate	Immediate

PHARMACODYNAMICS

Penicillins usually are bactericidal in action. Although the exact mechanism of action of penicillins is not understood, research has shown that they bind reversibly to several enzymes outside the bacterial cytoplasmic membrane. These enzymes, known as penicillin-binding proteins (PBPs), are involved in cell wall synthesis and cell division. Interference with these processes increases internal osmotic pressure and ruptures the cell.

PHARMACOTHERAPEUTICS

No other class of antibacterial agents provides as wide a spectrum of antimicrobial activity as the penicillins. Natural penicillins and their derivatives are used to treat many common infections.

Penicillins and their uses

Natural or semisynthetic derivatives of the *Penicillium* fungus, penicillins are prepared by chemically modifying a natural penicillin. The resulting drugs are classified according to their antimicrobial spectrum of activity.

DRUG	ANTIMICROBIAL SPECTRUM
Natural penicillins	
penicillin G benzathine, penicillin G potassium, penicillin G procaine, penicillin G sodium, penicillin V potassium	Gram-positive organisms: *Actinomyces israelii*; *Staphylococcus aureus* (non-penicillinase-producing strains); *Streptococcus* (groups A, B, C, and D); *Streptococcus viridans*; *Streptococcus faecalis*; Beta-hemolytic *Streptococcus*; *Streptococcus bovis*; *Streptococcus pneumoniae*; *Eubacterium*; *Bacillus anthracis*; *Peptostreptococcus*; *Clostridium tetani*; *Clostridium perfringens*; *Listeria monocytogenes* Gram-negative organisms: *Bacteroides* (all species except for many strains of *Bacteroides fragilis*); *Neisseria gonorrhoeae*; *Neisseria meningitidis*; *Pasteurella multocida*; *Streptobacillus moniliformis* Anaerobic organisms: *Treponema pallidum*; *Treponema pertenue*; *Borrelia recurrentis*; *Leptospira icterohaemorrhagiae*
Penicillinase-resistant penicillins	
cloxacillin, dicloxacillin, methicillin, nafcillin, oxacillin	Gram-positive organisms: *Staphylococcus aureus*; *Staphylococcus epidermidis*; *Streptococcus* (some species)
Aminopenicillins	
amoxicillin, ampicillin, bacampicillin	Gram-positive organisms: *Staphylococcus* (non-penicillinase-producing strains); *Streptococcus* (some species) Gram-negative organisms: *Escherichia coli*; *Haemophilus influenzae*; *Neisseria gonorrhoeae*; *Proteus mirabilis*; *Salmonella*; *Shigella*
Extended-spectrum penicillins	
carbenicillin, mezlocillin, piperacillin, ticarcillin	Gram-positive and gram-negative organisms that natural penicillins and aminopenicillins are active against, plus: *Pseudomonas aeruginosa*; *Proteus* (indole-positive); *Providencia*; *Enterobacter*; *Citrobacter*; *Serratia*; *Acinetobacter*; *Veillonella*

I.M. administration is indicated primarily when compliance with an oral regimen is inconvenient or questionable. Because long-acting preparations of penicillin G (penicillin G benzathine and penicillin G procaine) are relatively insoluble, they must be administered by the I.M. route.

Concurrent administration of probenecid increases the penicillin serum concentration by 50% to 100%, because probenecid blocks tubular secretion of penicillin. Combined probenecid-penicillin therapy is used to treat bacterial endocarditis and acute gonorrhea.

Drug interactions

High dosages of penicillin G and extended-spectrum penicillins (azlocillin, carbenicillin, mezlocillin, piperacillin, and ticarcillin) inactivate aminoglycosides. This interaction is clinically relevant in patients with poor renal function because elevated blood concentrations of both agents may exist simultaneously. Penicillins should not be mixed in the same I.V. solutions with aminoglycosides.

Inactivation of aminoglycosides by penicillins depends on the penicillin concentration, the temperature of the patient's blood, and the duration of contact between the two drugs. When the serum aminoglycoside level is measured, the sample should be kept on ice while being transported to the laboratory and should be stored in the laboratory until the assay can be made. The presence of penicillins in the serum samples may result in falsely decreased aminoglycoside concentrations. (See Drug Interactions: *Penicillins, page 400.*)

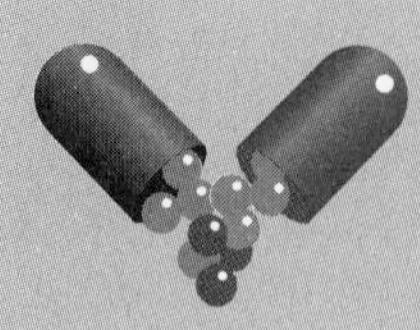

DRUG INTERACTIONS
Penicillins

This chart summarizes significant interactions between penicillins and other drugs. The nurse should be familiar with these interactions before administering any penicillin.

DRUG	INTERACTING DRUGS	POSSIBLE EFFECTS	NURSING IMPLICATIONS
all penicillins	probenecid	Increased plasma penicillin concentration	• May be used to enhance antibiotic efficacy.
	methotrexate	Decreased renal tubular secretion of methotrexate	• Monitor the patient for enhanced methotrexate action and possible methotrexate toxicity.
	tetracyclines, chloramphenicol	Decreased bactericidal action of penicillin	• Administer doses of these drugs several hours apart if they are used together.
penicillin G (high doses), extended-spectrum penicillins (azlocillin, carbenicillin, mezlocillin, piperacillin, ticarcillin)	aminoglycosides	Decreased effect of aminoglycoside	• Do not mix these drugs; administer doses at least 1 hour apart.
penicillin V	neomycin	Decreased absorption of penicillin V	• Administer doses at least 1 hour apart.
penicillin V, ampicillin	oral contraceptives	Altered gastrointestinal flora, increased risk of decreased contraceptive efficacy and breakthrough bleeding	• Advise the patient to use an alternative contraceptive method during antibacterial therapy and for 1 week after the antibacterial is discontinued.

ADVERSE DRUG REACTIONS

Hypersensitivity reactions are the major adverse reactions to penicillins. Anaphylactic reactions, **serum sickness,** drug fever, or various skin rashes may occur. Large dosages, prolonged therapy, or parenteral administration also may lead to allergic reactions.

Certain extended-spectrum penicillins (carbenicillin and ticarcillin) are administered as disodium salts. The increased sodium or potassium intake resulting from the use of these drugs may pose a problem for patients with cardiac disease or decreased renal function.

Penicillins can produce adverse hematologic effects. A positive Coombs' test for hemolytic anemia can occur in patients receiving high dosages of I.V. penicillin G (more than 10 million units a day in uremic patients or 40 million units a day in patients with normal renal function). Discontinuing the penicillin usually returns the hemoglobin to the baseline normal value. Penicillins (especially carbenicillin and ticarcillin) may induce platelet dysfunction, causing prolonged bleeding time. Platelet function returns to normal when the drug is discontinued.

Hepatotoxicity has occasionally developed during oxacillin therapy. Adverse GI reactions, such as glossitis, nausea, vomiting, and diarrhea, are usually associated with oral use; they occur most commonly in ampicillin therapy. The aminopenicillins and extended-spectrum penicillins can produce pseudomembranous colitis.

Seizures or coma caused by direct CNS irritation can occur with penicillin G in dosages greater than 20 million units daily in patients with decreased renal function.

Renal failure and interstitial nephritis may occur in patients receiving large parenteral dosages of penicillin G or methicillin. Usually, these reactions begin within 5 to 10 days after therapy is initiated. Signs and symptoms may include fever, eosinophilia, hematuria, proteinuria, or pyuria.

Some patients may experience an allergic reaction to tartrazine, a dye contained in certain penicillin preparations.

NURSING PROCESS APPLICATION

The following information assists the nurse in caring for a patient who is receiving a penicillin. It includes an overview of assessment activities as well as examples of appropriate nursing diagnoses and related interventions. It also highlights the importance of evaluation.

Assessment

Before drug therapy begins, review the patient's history for conditions that contraindicate or require cautious use of the prescribed penicillin. Also review the patient's medication history to identify use of drugs that may interact with it. During therapy, assess the patient for adverse drug reactions and signs of drug interactions. Also, periodically assess the effectiveness of penicillin therapy. Finally, evaluate the patient's and family's knowledge about the prescribed drug.

Nursing diagnoses

- Risk for injury related to adverse drug reactions or drug interactions
- Risk for injury related to platelet dysfunction caused by the prescribed penicillin
- Knowledge deficit related to the prescribed penicillin regimen

Planning and implementation

- Do not administer a penicillin to a patient with a condition that contraindicates its use.
- Administer a penicillin cautiously to a patient with a preexisting condition.
- Monitor the patient closely for adverse reactions and drug interactions during penicillin therapy. Keep in mind that the patient may become sensitized to penicillin through exposure.
- Obtain a complete patient history to assess the risk of allergic reaction whenever penicillin therapy is considered.
- Discontinue the prescribed penicillin at once if the patient develops anaphylactic shock (exhibited by rapidly developing dyspnea and hypotension). Notify the physician and prepare to administer immediate treatment, such as epinephrine, corticosteroids, antihistamines, and other resuscitative measures, as indicated. (See Patient Teaching: *Penicillins.*)
- Monitor the patient's temperature for a sudden elevation that may indicate drug fever. Notify the physician if a fever occurs.
- Monitor for decreased level of consciousness or seizures in a patient with decreased renal function who is receiving more than 20 million units of penicillin G daily. Take seizure precautions during therapy.
- Observe for signs of renal failure or interstitial nephritis, such as fever, eosinophilia, hematuria, proteinuria, or pyuria, which usually occur 5 to 10 days after therapy begins, in a patient receiving large parenteral dosages of penicillin G or methicillin. Notify the physician if any of these signs occur, and expect to discontinue the drug. Corticosteroids may need to be administered to improve renal function.
- Observe for signs and symptoms of pseudomembranous colitis, such as abdominal pain or diarrhea, in a patient receiving an aminopenicillin or extended-spectrum penicillin. If signs or symptoms occur, notify the physician before giving the next dose.

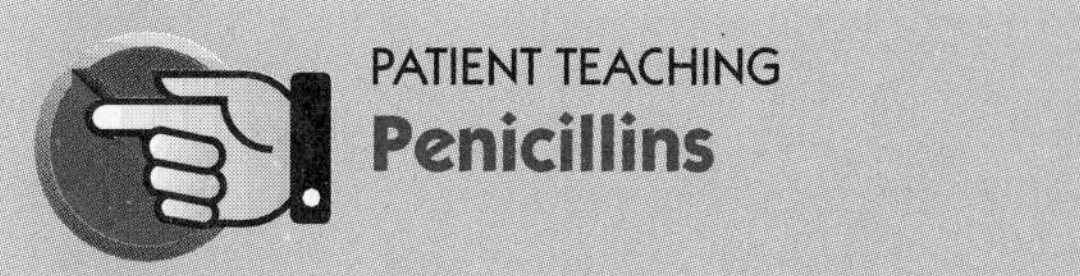

PATIENT TEACHING

Penicillins

- Teach the patient and family the name, dose, frequency, action, and adverse effects of the prescribed penicillin.
- Advise the patient to complete the course of penicillin therapy.
- Advise the patient to take an oral penicillin 1 hour before or 2 hours after meals to ensure an optimal serum concentration.
- Review the signs and symptoms of allergic reactions with the patient. Instruct the patient to withhold the drug and notify the physician if such a reaction occurs. If an anaphylactic reaction occurs, instruct the family to seek emergency treatment immediately.
- Advise the patient who is allergic to penicillins to wear a medical identification necklace or bracelet stating this information.
- Encourage the patient to have prescribed blood or urine tests completed and to keep follow-up appointments.
- Instruct the patient to notify the physician if the infection persists or worsens or if adverse reactions occur.
- Describe the risk of elevated serum sodium or potassium levels to a patient with cardiac disease or decreased renal function who is taking carbenicillin or ticarcillin. Teach the patient to recognize and report signs and symptoms of sodium and potassium imbalances.

- Monitor for adverse GI reactions in a patient receiving an oral penicillin, especially ampicillin. If nausea, vomiting, diarrhea, or glossitis occurs, monitor the patient's hydration and request a prescription for an antiemetic or antidiarrheal as needed. If the GI reactions are severe, expect the drug to be discontinued or replaced with a parenteral form.
- Do not mix an aminoglycoside with an extended-spectrum penicillin or a high dose of penicillin G. This prevents inactivation of the aminoglycoside.
- Administer oral penicillin 1 hour before or 2 hours after meals to ensure an optimal serum concentration.
- Administer penicillin G benzathine and procaine by the I.M. route only.
- Notify the physician if adverse reactions or drug interactions occur.
- Monitor the patient for bleeding tendencies, such as easy bruising, bleeding gums, or blood in the urine or stool.
- Monitor the patient's platelet count during penicillin therapy. Prolonged bleeding time is most likely to occur in a patient with uremic or hepatic disease who is receiving carbenicillin or ticarcillin. Expect to discontinue the drug if this occurs.

Evaluation

For each nursing diagnosis, prepare an evaluation statement that describes the patient's or family's response to nursing interventions.

Cephalosporins

Most of the antibacterial agents introduced for clinical use in recent years have been cephalosporins. Loracarbef is a synthetic beta-lactam antibiotic that belongs to a new class of drugs known as the carbacephen antibiotics. Because it is similar to second-generation cephalosporins, it is included with cephalosporins. Because penicillins and cephalosporin molecules have a beta-lactam structure, some cross-sensitivity occurs. Cephalosporins are categorized into groups called generations, based on their antimicrobial spectra of activity. (See *Antimicrobial activity of cephalosporins.*)

PHARMACOKINETICS

Many cephalosporins are administered parenterally because they are not absorbed from the GI tract. Cephalosporins absorbed from the GI tract and administered orally include cefprozil, cephradine, cephalexin, cefadroxil, cefaclor, cefuroxime axetil, cefixime, and loracarbef. Food usually delays the absorption of the oral cephalosporins.

After absorption, cephalosporins are distributed widely, although most are not distributed in the CNS. Cefuroxime (second generation); cefotaxime, ceftizoximine, ceftriaxone, and ceftazidime (third generation), however, *do* cross the blood-brain barrier. Many cephalosporins, including loracarbef, are not metabolized at all. Cephalothin sodium, cephapirin sodium, and cefotaxime sodium are metabolized to the nonacetyl forms and provide less antibacterial activity than the parent compounds. To a small extent, ceftriaxone is metabolized in the intestines to inactive metabolites, which are excreted via the biliary system. All cephalosporins are excreted primarily unchanged by the kidneys with the exception of cefoperazone and ceftriaxone, which are excreted in the feces via bile.

After I.V. administration of 1 g, the peak concentration is 50 to 100 mcg/ml for most cephalosporins. The higher concentration of cefazolin sodium given I.V. or I.M. is a considerable advantage over other first-generation cephalosporins. After I.M. administration, the onset is usually delayed. The peak concentration achieved is about 50% of that achieved after I.V. administration.

Route	Onset	Peak	Duration
P.O.	Immediate-30 min	1-2 hr	30 min-10 hr
I.V.	Rapid	≤1 hr	30 min-10 hr
I.M.	15-60 min	30 min-4 hr	30 min-10 hr

PHARMACODYNAMICS

Cephalosporins inhibit cell wall synthesis by binding to bacterial enzymes located on the cell membrane. These enzymes, which have been classified as PBPs, are important for the biosynthesis of bacterial cell wall components. The antibacterial action of cephalosporins depends on their ability to penetrate the bacterial cell wall and bind with proteins in the cytoplasmic membrane. Once the drug damages the cell wall by binding with the PBPs, the body's natural defense mechanisms destroy the bacteria. (See *How cephalosporins attack bacteria,* page 404.)

PHARMACOTHERAPEUTICS

Cephalosporins are classified into one of three generations based on their spectra of activity. First-generation cephalosporins, which act primarily against gram-positive organisms, can be used as alternative therapy in patients allergic to penicillin. They also are used to treat staphylococcal and streptococcal infections, including pneumonia, cellulitis, and osteomyelitis. Second-generation cephalosporins are used to treat polymicrobial infections, such as foot ulcers in diabetic patients, nosocomial aspiration pneumonia, and pelvic and intra-abdominal infections. Third-generation cephalosporins, which act primarily against gram-negative organisms, are the drugs of choice for infections caused by *Enterobacter, P. aeruginosa,* and anaerobic organisms.

Drug interactions

Patients receiving cefamandole, cefoperazone, or moxalactam who drink alcoholic beverages concurrently or up to 72 hours after taking a dose may experience acute alcohol intolerance, with signs and symptoms similar to a disulfiram reaction. Patients may experience headache, flushing, dizziness, nausea, vomiting, or abdominal cramps within 30 minutes of alcohol ingestion.

Concomitant use of cephalosporins and imipenem-cilastatin can antagonize the antibacterial activity of the beta-lactam cephalosporins.

Uricosurics, such as probenecid and sulfinpyrazone, can block the renal tubular secretion of some cephalosporins, including loracarbef. Probenecid is used therapeutically to increase and prolong cephalosporin plasma concentrations.

ADVERSE DRUG REACTIONS

Hypersensitivity reactions are the most common systemic adverse reactions to cephalosporins. Allergic reactions range in severity from mild to life-threatening. Usually, allergic reactions appear as urticaria, pruritus or morbilliform eruptions, and serum sickness. Anaphylaxis is rare.

Because of the similarities between penicillins and cephalosporins, a 5% to 10% cross-sensitivity may occur. Patients with a history of penicillin reactions are at risk for developing an allergic reaction to cephalosporins.

I.M. administration of cephalothin and cefoxitin commonly produces pain, induration, and tenderness at the injection site. Thrombophlebitis is associated most commonly with I.V. cephalothin.

In patients with impaired renal function who are receiving high dosages of cephalosporins, the most common reactions are confusion and seizures. Seizures associated with high dosages of cefazolin also can occur.

Serious bleeding related to hypoprothrombinemia, thrombocytopenia, or platelet dysfunction can occur in patients receiving moxalactam or cefoperazone. This coagulation disorder is a problem in geriatric and poorly nourished patients and in those with renal failure.

Orally administered cephalosporins commonly cause nausea, vomiting, and diarrhea, which may be alleviated by administering the drug with food. Antibiotic-associated pseudomembranous colitis caused by *Clostridium difficile* may occur during cephalosporin therapy or after it is stopped, especially with the third-generation cephalosporins.

Cephalosporins may produce nephrotoxicity. High dosages of cephalothin can lead to acute tubular necrosis, and the usual daily dosage of 8 to 12 g can be nephrotoxic in patients with renal disease. Concomitant therapy with cephalothin and an aminoglycoside (such as gentamicin) can be nephrotoxic.

Use of the cephalosporins may lead to **superinfection,** producing such problems as diarrhea, sore mouth (oral **thrush**), and vaginal itching.

All cephalosporins, except cefotaxime, can cause false-positive results on urine glucose tests using cupric sulfate solution, such as Benedict's test and Clinitest. However, they do not affect the results of glucose oxidase tests, such as glucose enzymatic test strip and Clinistix.

Antimicrobial activity of cephalosporins

This chart shows three generations of cephalosporins and the basis for those generations — their antimicrobial spectrum of activity.

DRUG	ANTIMICROBIAL SPECTRUM
First-generation	
cefadroxil **cefazolin** **cefprozil** **cephalexin** **cephalothin** **cephapirin** **cephradine** **loracarbef**	Gram-positive organisms— *Staphylococcus* (most species) Groups A and B hemolytic streptococci *Streptococcus* (most species) Gram-negative organisms— *Escherichia coli* *Klebsiella* *Proteus mirabilis* *Haemophilus influenzae*
Second-generation	
cefaclor **cefamandole** **cefmetazole** **cefonicid** **ceforanide** **cefotetan** **cefoxitin** **cefuroxime**	All of the above, plus: Gram-negative organisms— *Neisseria gonorrhoeae* *Neisseria meningitidis* *Proteus* (indole-positive) *Providencia* *Enterobacter* *Citrobacter* Anaerobic organisms— *Clostridium* *Peptococcus* *Peptostreptococcus* *Fusobacterium* *Bacteroides*
Third-generation	
cefixime **cefoperazone** **cefotaxime** **ceftazidime** **ceftizoxime** **ceftriaxone** **moxalactam**	All organisms susceptible to first- and second-generation cephalosporins, plus: Gram-negative organisms— *Pseudomonas aeruginosa* *Serratia* *Acinetobacter* (some strains)

NURSING PROCESS APPLICATION

The following information assists the nurse in caring for a patient who is receiving a cephalosporin. It includes an overview of assessment activities as well as examples of appropriate nursing diagnoses and related interventions. It also highlights the importance of evaluation.

Assessment

Before drug therapy begins, review the patient's history for conditions that contraindicate or require cautious use of the prescribed cephalosporin. Also review the patient's medication history to identify use of drugs that may interact with it. During therapy, assess the patient for adverse drug reactions and signs of drug interactions. Also, periodically assess the effectiveness of cephalosporin therapy. Finally, evaluate the patient's and family's knowledge of the prescribed drug.

Nursing diagnoses

- Risk for injury related to adverse drug reactions or drug interactions
- Risk for fluid volume deficit related to the adverse GI effects of an oral cephalosporin
- Knowledge deficit related to the prescribed cephalosporin regimen

Planning and implementation

- Do not administer a cephalosporin to a patient with a condition that contraindicates its use.
- Administer a cephalosporin cautiously to a patient with a preexisting condition.
- Monitor the patient for adverse reactions and drug interactions during cephalosporin therapy. Keep in mind that toxicity increases from the first to the third generation of cephalosporins.

How cephalosporins attack bacteria

The antibacterial action of cephalosporins depends on their ability to penetrate the bacterial wall and bind with proteins on the cytoplasic membrane, as shown here.

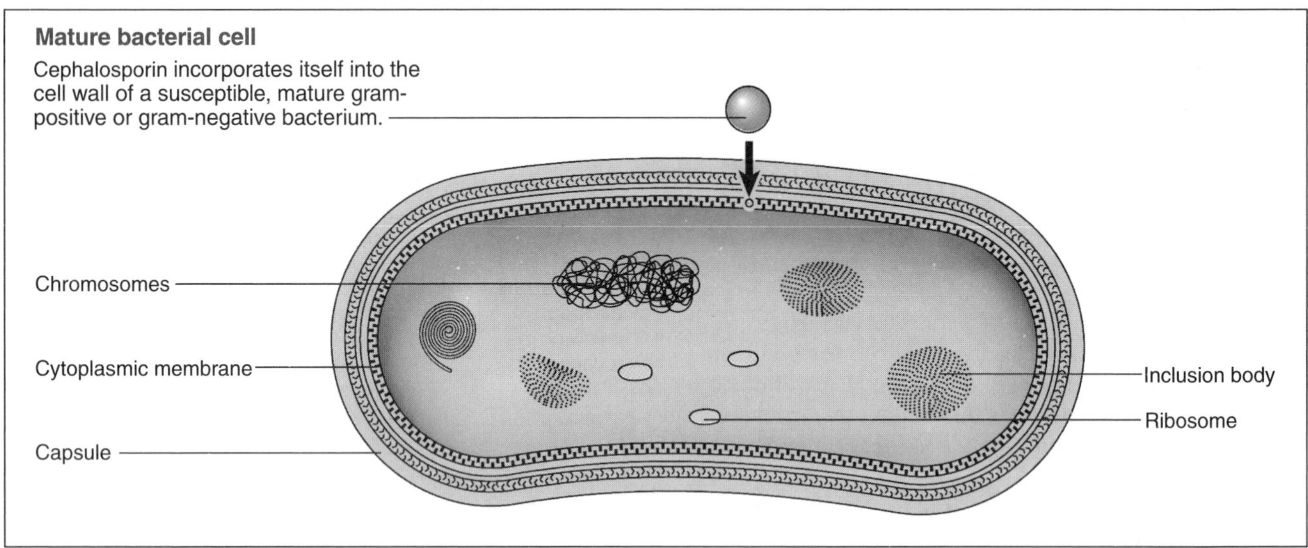

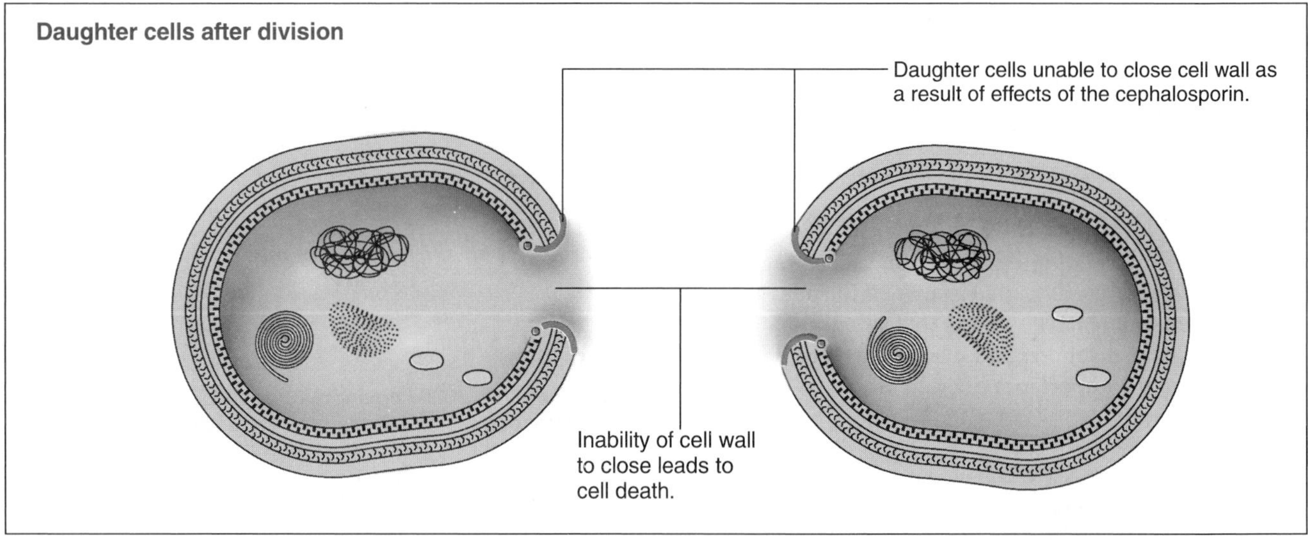

• Observe the patient for hypersensitivity reactions. Keep standard emergency equipment readily available. If a hypersensitivity reaction occurs, withhold the drug and notify the physician.
• Avoid administering a cephalosporin to a patient who recently has experienced a severe, immediate reaction to a penicillin or cephalosporin. Obtain a thorough drug history, and screen the patient for possible allergy and cross-sensitivity with cephalosporins.
• Expect to adjust the dosage, as prescribed, in a patient with renal insufficiency receiving a cephalosporin (except for cefoperazone or ceftriaxone).
• Infuse all I.V. cephalosporins over 30 minutes to minimize pain and irritation at the injection site.
• Routinely monitor the I.V. site for signs of thrombophlebitis, such as localized redness, swelling, and pain.
• Reconstitute cefoxitin or ceftriaxone with a 0.5% to 1% lidocaine injection, as prescribed, to decrease pain at the injection site during I.M. administration.

• Notify the physician if adverse reactions or drug interactions occur.
• Administer the prescribed cephalosporin with food to prevent or minimize GI upset. Loracarbef however, should be administered at least 1 hour before or at least 2 hours after meals. (See Patient Teaching: *Cephalosporins.*)
• Monitor hydration if the patient experiences nausea, vomiting, or diarrhea. If these adverse reactions persist or worsen, notify the physician, request a prescription for an antiemetic or antidiarrheal agent as needed, and expect to change the oral form to a parenteral equivalent.
• Monitor the patient—especially one receiving a third-generation cephalosporin—for signs of pseudomembranous colitis (such as abdominal pain and diarrhea) during cephalosporin therapy and after it is stopped.

Evaluation

For each nursing diagnosis, prepare an evaluation statement that describes the patient's or family's response to nursing interventions.

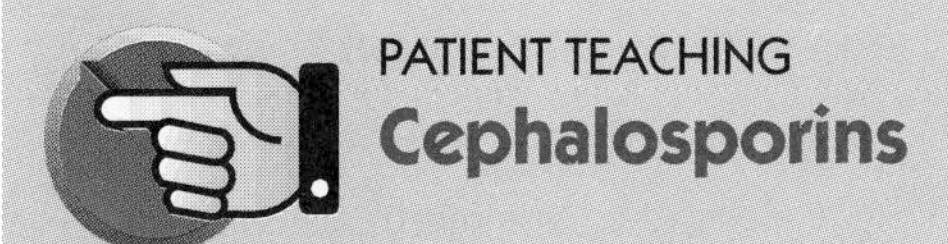

PATIENT TEACHING
Cephalosporins

- Teach the patient and family the name, dose, frequency, action, and adverse effects of the prescribed cephalosporin.
- Teach the patient to recognize and immediately report the signs and symptoms of a hypersensitivity reaction.
- Review with the patient the signs and symptoms of a superinfection.
- Advise the patient to ingest yogurt or buttermilk, which replenishes normal gastrointestinal (GI) flora, to prevent intestinal superinfection.
- Instruct the patient to take a prescribed oral cephalosporin with food to prevent GI upset.
- Inform the patient that an intramuscular cephalosporin injection may cause pain, inflammation, or tenderness at the injection site.
- Advise the patient to avoid taking moxalactam, cefoperazone, cefamandole, or cefotetan with alcohol or medications that contain alcohol (elixirs).
- Advise the diabetic patient taking a cephalosporin to test urine glucose levels with glucose enzymatic test strip or Clinistix (not Clinitest).
- Instruct the patient to complete the full course of therapy.
- Stress the importance of keeping follow-up appointments and having laboratory tests done to evaluate drug effectiveness or detect adverse reactions.
- Advise the patient receiving moxalactam or cefoperazone to take bleeding precautions, such as using an electric razor when shaving, avoiding cuts and bruises, using a soft toothbrush, and wearing shoes at all times.
- Instruct the patient to notify the physician if adverse reactions occur or if the condition persists or worsens.

Tetracyclines

The tetracycline analogues are classified as (1) short-acting compounds (chlortetracycline hydrochloride, oxytetracycline hydrochloride, and tetracycline hydrochloride), (2) intermediate-acting compounds (demeclocycline hydrochloride and methacycline hydrochloride), and (3) long-acting compounds (doxycycline hyclate and minocycline hydrochloride). Doxycycline and minocycline provide a broader spectrum of activity than the other antibacterials.

PHARMACOKINETICS

Tetracyclines are absorbed from the duodenum after oral administration. Absorption is impaired by intake of dairy products (not true for doxycycline and minocycline), iron preparations, and concomitant administration of antacids that contain calcium, magnesium, or aluminum salts. Tetracyclines are distributed widely into body tissues and fluids, concentrated in bile, and excreted primarily by the kidneys. However, researchers believe that doxycycline is excreted in the feces; minocycline undergoes enterohepatic recirculation; and the excretion of chlortetracycline is unknown. With usual dosages, the serum concentration achieved after I.M. administration is lower than that after oral administration.

Route	Onset	Peak	Duration
P.O.	30 min	1-4 hr	Unknown

PHARMACODYNAMICS

All tetracyclines are primarily **bacteriostatic.** The tetracyclines penetrate the interior of the bacterial cell by an energy-dependent process. Once within the cell, the tetracyclines reversibly bind primarily to a subunit of the ribosome, thereby inhibiting access of transfer ribonucleic acid (RNA)–amino acid complexes to the messenger RNA–ribosome complex. This action prevents the addition of new amino acids to the peptide chain of the bacteria.

PHARMACOTHERAPEUTICS

The tetracyclines provide a broad spectrum of activity against gram-positive, gram-negative, aerobic, and anaerobic bacteria as well as spirochetes, mycoplasmas, rickettsiae, chlamydiae, and some protozoa. Doxycycline and minocycline typically provide more action against various organisms than other tetracyclines. Tetracyclines are used to treat Rocky Mountain spotted fever, Q fever, Lyme disease, brucellosis, and tularemia. They are the drugs of choice for treating nongonococcal urethritis caused by *Chlamydia* and *Ureaplasma urealyticum.*

Tetracycline or erythromycin is the drug of choice for treating *Mycoplasma pneumoniae* infections. Combination therapy with a tetracycline and streptomycin is the most effective treatment for brucellosis. The tetracyclines effective-

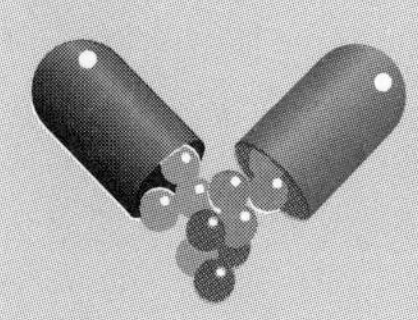

DRUG INTERACTIONS

Tetracyclines

This chart summarizes significant interactions between the tetracyclines and other drugs. The nurse should be familiar with these interactions before administering any tetracycline.

DRUG	INTERACTING DRUGS	POSSIBLE EFFECTS	NURSING IMPLICATIONS
chlortetracycline, demeclocycline, doxycycline, methacycline, minocycline, oxytetracycline, tetracycline	antacids with divalent or trivalent cations, such as aluminum and magnesium	Inhibited oral absorption of tetracyclines	• Administer doses 1 to 2 hours apart.
	methoxyflurane	Nephrotoxicity	• Avoid tetracycline use in patients who are to receive anesthesia with methoxyflurane.
doxycycline, methacycline, oxytetracycline, tetracycline	iron salts, bismuth subsalicylate, zinc sulfate	Decreased gastrointestinal (GI) absorption of tetracyclines	• Administer these agents 3 hours before or 2 hours after tetracyclines.
doxycycline	barbiturates, carbamazepine, phenytoin	Increased doxycycline metabolism	• Avoid concurrent use. • Use a tetracycline other than doxycycline if barbiturate, phenytoin, or carbamazepine therapy is required, or expect to increase the doxycycline dosage.
tetracycline	oral contraceptives	Altered GI bacterial flora, leading to decreased contraceptive efficacy and breakthrough bleeding	• Advise the patient to use an alternative contraceptive method during tetracycline therapy and for 1 week after it is discontinued.
all tetracyclines	penicillin	Decreased bactericidal action of penicillin	• Administer doses several hours apart.

ly treat acne because they can decrease the fatty acid content of sebum; low-dosage tetracycline therapy (250 mg twice daily) is used for this condition.

Drug interactions

The nurse should be aware of the numerous significant interactions between tetracyclines and other drugs. (See Drug Interactions: *Tetracyclines.*) These drugs, with the exception of doxycycline and minocycline, may also interact with milk and milk products, which bind with the drugs and prevent their absorption.

ADVERSE DRUG REACTIONS

Tetracyclines produce many of the same adverse reactions as other antibacterials, such as superinfection (overgrowth of tetracycline-resistant organisms) and GI disturbances.

Adverse GI reactions resulting from oral administration include nausea, vomiting, abdominal distress and distention, and diarrhea. The diarrhea usually subsides when the drug is stopped; however, prolonged symptoms from pseudomembranous colitis may occur.

Photosensitivity reactions (red rash on areas exposed to sunlight) are most common in patients receiving demeclocycline and doxycycline. However, photosensitivity reactions can occur with any tetracycline.

Tetracyclines cause permanent gray-brown to yellow discoloration of the teeth when administered during tooth formation. The tetracyclines should not be administered to pregnant patients or to children under age 8 (the period when tooth enamel is forming) because bone deposition of tetracycline temporarily halts bone growth in the fetus or the child.

Hepatotoxic reactions to tetracyclines, which include lipid infiltration of the liver, are associated primarily with I.V. tetracyclines. Nephrotoxicity can develop in patients with renal failure; the antianabolic effects of tetracyclines may increase BUN and serum creatinine levels. Fanconi-like syndrome (nephrotoxicity) can also occur if the patient receives outdated tetracycline.

CNS toxicity, which includes vestibular disturbances, occurs primarily with minocycline. Light-headedness, loss of balance, dizziness, and tinnitus usually begin on the 2nd or

3rd day of minocycline therapy. Symptoms are reversible several days after discontinuation of the drug.

As with any antibiotic, superinfection commonly develops during tetracycline therapy. Overgrowth of yeast typically occurs, and oral or vaginal moniliasis requires specific therapy. Staphylococcal enterocolitis caused by tetracycline-resistant staphylococci can lead to severe diarrhea, dehydration, and possible circulatory collapse.

Although uncommon, hypersensitivity reactions to tetracyclines include anaphylaxis, urticaria, periorbital edema, fixed drug eruptions, and morbilliform rashes.

NURSING PROCESS APPLICATION

The following information assists the nurse in caring for a patient who is receiving a tetracycline. It includes an overview of assessment activities as well as examples of appropriate nursing diagnoses and related interventions. It also highlights the importance of evaluation.

Assessment

Before drug therapy begins, review the patient's history for conditions that contraindicate or require cautious use of the prescribed tetracycline. Also review the patient's medication history to identify use of drugs that may interact with it. During therapy, assess the patient for adverse drug reactions and signs of drug interactions. Also, periodically assess the effectiveness of tetracycline therapy. Finally, evaluate the patient's and family's knowledge of the prescribed drug.

Nursing diagnoses

- Risk for injury related to adverse drug reactions or drug interactions
- Risk for injury related to development of a superinfection caused by the prescribed tetracycline
- Knowledge deficit related to the prescribed tetracycline regimen

Planning and implementation

- Do not administer a tetracycline to a patient with a condition that contraindicates its use.
- Administer a tetracycline cautiously to a patient with a preexisting condition.
- Monitor the patient periodically for adverse reactions and drug interactions during tetracycline therapy.
- Observe the patient closely for hypersensitivity reactions. Although anaphylaxis is rare, have standard emergency equipment nearby. If a hypersensitivity reaction occurs, notify the physician and expect to discontinue the drug.
- Administer doxycycline or minocycline with food to minimize GI irritation. Administer any other tetracycline on an empty stomach, 1 hour before or 2 hours after meals.
- Do not administer a tetracycline, except doxycycline or minocycline, with milk or milk products because dairy foods can bind with the tetracycline, preventing its absorption. (See Patient Teaching: *Tetracyclines.*)

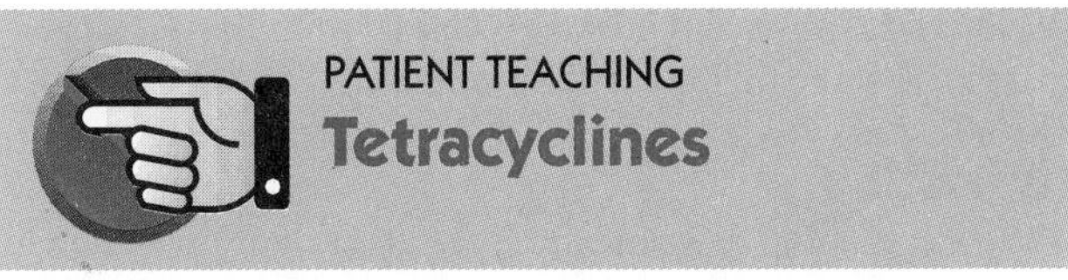

PATIENT TEACHING
Tetracyclines

- Teach the patient and family the name, dose, frequency, action, and adverse effects of the prescribed tetracycline.
- Advise the patient experiencing a hypersensitivity reaction to withhold the drug and notify the physician.
- Advise the patient not to ingest milk, milk products, or drugs containing calcium, magnesium, aluminum, or iron at the same time as the prescribed tetracycline because these products prevent tetracycline absorption.
- Advise the patient to take the prescribed tetracycline on an empty stomach (except for doxycycline or minocycline, which should be taken with food to minimize gastrointestinal irritation).
- Advise the patient who experiences esophageal irritation to take tetracycline with 8 oz (240 ml) of water.
- Warn the patient receiving oxytetracycline intramuscularly that the injection will be painful.
- Inform the patient that chlortetracycline may stain clothing.
- Inform the patient with minocycline-induced central nervous system toxicity that the symptoms should disappear several days after the drug is discontinued.
- Advise the patient to avoid direct sunlight, cover exposed skin, or use a sunscreen with a sun protective factor of 15 or higher during tetracycline therapy.
- Teach the patient the importance of completing the course of tetracycline therapy.
- Advise the female patient taking an oral contraceptive to use an alternative means of contraception during tetracycline therapy and for 1 week after therapy is discontinued.
- Instruct the patient to notify the physician if adverse reactions occur.

- Do not administer a tetracycline with drugs that contain calcium, magnesium, aluminum, or iron. These drugs can bind with the tetracycline, preventing its absorption.
- Dilute an I.V. preparation in a large volume of fluid and administer it by continuous slow drip.
- Monitor for thrombophlebitis at the I.V. site in a patient receiving parenteral tetracycline or oxytetracycline.
- Double-check any prescription for an I.M. injection because I.M. administration usually is not recommended. If I.M. injections must be administered, inject oxytetracycline deeply into a large muscle.
- Notify the physician if adverse reactions or drug interactions occur.
- Monitor the patient regularly for signs of superinfection, such as oral thrush, GI disturbance, or worsening of signs and symptoms of the systemic infection.
- Inspect the patient's mouth regularly for signs of oral moniliasis, such as cream-colored or bluish white pseudomembranous patches on the tongue, mouth, or pharynx. Encourage the female patient to report unusual vaginal discharge.

• Notify the physician if oral or vaginal moniliasis is suspected; specific therapy will be required.

Evaluation

For each nursing diagnosis, prepare an evaluation statement that describes the patient's or family's response to nursing interventions.

Chloramphenicol

Drug-induced aplastic anemia, a serious adverse reaction, has limited chloramphenicol's clinical usefulness. The drug is usually reserved for treating serious infections or those with ampicillin-resistant *Haemophilus influenzae.* It is available as chloramphenicol sodium succinate.

PHARMACOKINETICS

Chloramphenicol is absorbed rapidly and completely from the GI tract and is not impaired by the concomitant administration of food or antacids. After absorption, chloramphenicol is distributed widely to body fluids and tissue, including breast milk. In patients with normal hepatic function, chloramphenicol is metabolized primarily in the liver and excreted in the urine.

Route	Onset	Peak	Duration
I.V.	Immediate	1-4 hr	3-8 hr

PHARMACODYNAMICS

Chloramphenicol, which inhibits protein synthesis of susceptible organisms, also inhibits protein synthesis in cells that proliferate rapidly, such as bone marrow cells. This can lead to bone marrow suppression. Chloramphenicol overcomes enzymatic acetylation, the major mechanism of resistance in gram-negative bacilli other than *P. aeruginosa,* which is plasmid-mediated. *P. aeruginosa* and some strains of *Proteus* and *Klebsiella* resist chloramphenicol via nonenzymatic mechanisms, including an induced block that prevents chloramphenicol from entering the bacterial cell; larger doses may be needed.

PHARMACOTHERAPEUTICS

Chloramphenicol is active against various organisms, including bacteria, spirochetes, rickettsiae, chlamydiae, and mycoplasmas. It is used specifically to treat serious infections and *H. influenzae* infections resistant to ampicillin. Chloramphenicol is extremely active against anaerobic bacteria, including *Bacteroides fragilis.* It is the drug of choice for treating ampicillin-resistant typhoid fever and other systemic *Salmonella* infections. It also is effective for brain abscesses and certain types of bacterial **meningitis.** Topical chloramphenicol is used to treat eye and external ear infections.

Drug interactions

Chloramphenicol may inhibit the metabolism of oral hypoglycemic agents (such as chlorpropamide and tolbutamide), anticonvulsants (such as phenytoin), and oral anticoagulants (such as dicumarol). This inhibited metabolism can lead to hypoglycemia, phenytoin toxicity, or hemorrhage. During concomitant therapy, the dosage of the oral hypoglycemic, anticonvulsant, or anticoagulant may need to be decreased.

Concomitant administration of chloramphenicol and other drugs causing bone marrow suppression should be avoided because additive toxicity can occur.

ADVERSE DRUG REACTIONS

The use of chloramphenicol is limited by its potential toxicities. Gray syndrome, a potentially fatal adverse reaction associated with excessive chloramphenicol serum concentrations, is most common in neonates. Initial manifestations include abdominal distention, vomiting, anorexia, tachypnea, cyanosis, green stools, lethargy, and an ashen color. These reactions are followed by circulatory collapse and death.

Bone marrow suppression is the most toxic reaction to chloramphenicol. Signs of bone marrow suppression include granulocytopenia, reticulocytopenia, anemia, leukopenia, and thrombocytopenia. These signs correlate with daily dosages of 4 g or more, relatively long duration of treatment, and serum concentrations exceeding 25 mcg/ml. Bone marrow suppression is reversible when chloramphenicol is discontinued.

Aplastic anemia, which is usually irreversible, may occur after chloramphenicol is discontinued; peripheral blood studies will show pancytopenia. Aplastic anemia occurs in about 1 in 40,000 or more patients taking chloramphenicol. Its mortality rate is greater than 50%.

Hypersensitivity reactions, including fever, macular and vesicular rashes, angioedema, urticaria, and anaphylaxis, have been reported.

NURSING PROCESS APPLICATION

The following information assists the nurse in caring for a patient who is receiving chloramphenicol. It includes an overview of assessment activities as well as examples of appropriate nursing diagnoses and related interventions. It also highlights the importance of evaluation.

Assessment

Before drug therapy begins, review the patient's history for conditions that contraindicate or require cautious use of

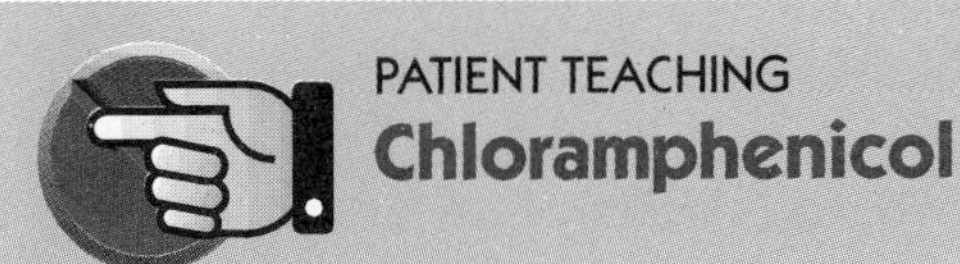

- Teach the patient and family the name, dose, frequency, action, and adverse effects of chloramphenicol.
- Instruct the patient to withhold the drug and notify the physician if a hypersensitivity reaction occurs.
- Advise the patient to notify the physician if fever, sore throat, fatigue, unusual bleeding, or bruising occurs.
- Teach the patient the importance of returning for regular blood tests to detect adverse reactions.
- Warn the patient about the unpleasant taste of oral chloramphenicol.
- Instruct the patient to notify the nurse or physician if adverse reactions occur.
- Instruct the patient to complete the course of chloramphenicol therapy.

chloramphenicol. Also review the patient's medication history to identify use of drugs that may interact with it. During therapy, assess the patient for adverse drug reactions, such as aplastic anemia, and signs of drug interactions. Also, periodically assess the effectiveness of chloramphenicol therapy. Finally, evaluate the patient's and family's knowledge of the prescribed drug.

Nursing diagnoses

- Risk for injury related to adverse drug reactions or drug interactions
- Risk for injury related to chloramphenicol-induced bone marrow suppression
- Knowledge deficit related to chloramphenicol regimen

Planning and implementation

- Do not administer chloramphenicol to a patient with a condition that contraindicates its use.
- Administer chloramphenicol cautiously to a patient with a preexisting condition.
- Monitor the patient periodically for adverse reactions such as aplastic anemia and drug interactions during chloramphenicol therapy.
- Regularly monitor the patient's complete blood counts.
- Screen the patient for a history of chloramphenicol hypersensitivity before initiating therapy. Throughout therapy, monitor the patient for hypersensitivity reactions. Have standard emergency equipment nearby. If a hypersensitivity reaction occurs, withhold the drug and notify the physician.
- Continue to observe the patient for signs and symptoms of aplastic anemia, such as anemia, infection, or bleeding, after chloramphenicol has been discontinued. (See Patient Teaching: *Chloramphenicol.*)
- Notify the physician if adverse reactions or drug interactions occur.
- Monitor the patient's serum chloramphenicol concentration closely for values that exceed 25 mcg/ml. If the concentration exceeds 25 mcg/ml, take bleeding precautions and infection-control measures because bone marrow suppression may occur.
- Consult the physician about decreasing the dosage or substituting another antibiotic if bone marrow suppression occurs.

Evaluation

For each nursing diagnosis, prepare an evaluation statement that describes the patient's or family's response to nursing interventions.

Clindamycin and lincomycin

Clindamycin hydrochloride, clindamycin palmitate hydrochloride, clindamycin phosphate, and lincomycin hydrochloride are antibacterials with similar spectra of activity. Clindamycin is usually more effective than lincomycin, which is seldom used.

PHARMACOKINETICS

After oral administration, clindamycin is absorbed well and distributed widely in the body. Lincomycin is absorbed poorly. Clindamycin and lincomycin are eliminated primarily via hepatic metabolism and renal and biliary excretion.

Route	Onset	Peak	Duration
P.O.	Unknown	1-4 hr	Unknown
I.V.	Immediate	Immediate	Unknown
I.M.	Unknown	30 min-3 hr	Unknown

PHARMACODYNAMICS

Clindamycin and lincomycin inhibit bacterial protein synthesis; they also may inhibit the binding of bacterial ribosomes. At therapeutically attainable concentrations, clindamycin and lincomycin are primarily bacteriostatic against most organisms.

PHARMACOTHERAPEUTICS

Because of its greater activity, enhanced absorption properties, and smaller potential for toxicity, clindamycin is preferred over lincomycin. However, because of its potential for serious toxicity and pseudomembranous colitis, clindamycin is limited to a few clinical indications where safer alternative antibacterials are not available.

Clindamycin is more potent than lincomycin against most aerobic gram-positive organisms, including *Staphylococcus, Streptococcus* (except *Enterococcus faecalis*), and pneumococci. Clindamycin is effective against most of the clinically important anaerobes and is used primarily to treat anaerobic intra-abdominal or pleuropulmonary infections caused by *B. fragilis.* It also is used as an alternative to peni-

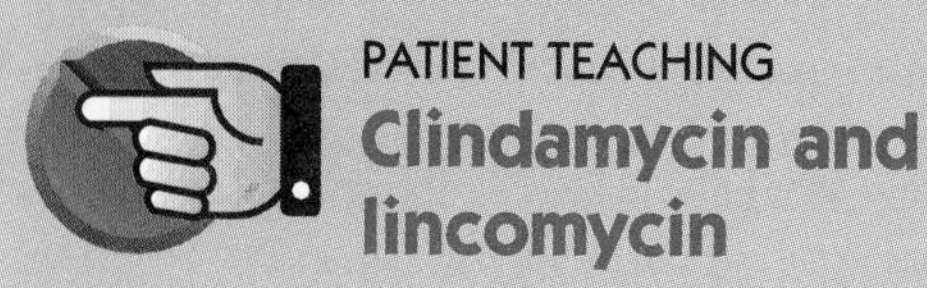

PATIENT TEACHING
Clindamycin and lincomycin

- ➤ Teach the patient and family the name, dose, frequency, action, and adverse effects of clindamycin or lincomycin.
- ➤ Instruct the patient to complete the course of clindamycin or lincomycin therapy.
- ➤ Warn the patient receiving clindamycin intramuscularly that the injection may be painful.
- ➤ Instruct the patient receiving clindamycin intravenously to notify the nurse if discomfort is felt at the infusion site.
- ➤ Teach the patient the importance of notifying the nurse if adverse reactions, such as gastrointestinal upset (especially diarrhea), pseudomembranous colitis, or hypersensitivity reactions, occur.

cillin in treating *Clostridium perfringens* infections. In addition, it may be used as an alternative to penicillin in treating staphylococcal infections in a patient with penicillin allergy.

Drug interactions

Clindamycin and lincomycin may block neuromuscular transmission and may enhance the action of neuromuscular blockers. Clindamycin phosphate in a solution is incompatible with ampicillin, aminophylline, calcium gluconate, and magnesium sulfate. Concomitant use with kaolin and pectin mixtures reduces lincomycin absorption by 90%. The presence of food in the GI tract decreases the rate and extent of lincomycin absorption as well.

ADVERSE DRUG REACTIONS

During clindamycin therapy, diarrhea occurs in about 80% of patients and is most common with oral administration. Persistent diarrhea also may occur with lincomycin. Oral administration of clindamycin or lincomycin may also produce stomatitis, nausea, and vomiting.

Pseudomembranous colitis, characterized by severe diarrhea, abdominal pain, fever, and mucus and blood in the stools, may occur with clindamycin or lincomycin. This syndrome, which can be fatal, requires prompt discontinuation of the antibacterial.

When administered I.V., clindamycin can damage tissue. I.M. administration of clindamycin may produce pain, induration, and sterile abscess. I.V. lincomycin can cause pain and phlebitis at the infusion site.

Hypersensitivity reactions in the form of rashes occur in approximately 10% of patients treated with clindamycin or lincomycin. The rashes resemble those seen in patients receiving ampicillin.

Stevens-Johnson syndrome has occurred rarely, and a few instances of anaphylactic reactions have also occurred.

NURSING PROCESS APPLICATION

The following information assists the nurse in caring for a patient who is receiving clindamycin or lincomycin. It includes an overview of assessment activities as well as examples of appropriate nursing diagnoses and related interventions. It also highlights the importance of evaluation.

Assessment

Before drug therapy begins, review the patient's history for conditions that contraindicate or require cautious use of clindamycin or lincomycin. Also review the patient's medication history to identify use of drugs that may interact with them. During therapy, assess the patient for adverse drug reactions and signs of drug interactions. Also, periodically assess the effectiveness of clindamycin or lincomycin therapy. Finally, evaluate the patient's and family's knowledge about the prescribed drug. (See Patient Teaching: *Clindamycin and lincomycin.*)

Nursing diagnoses

- Risk for injury related to adverse drug reactions or drug interactions
- Impaired tissue integrity related to pseudomembranous colitis caused by clindamycin or lincomycin
- Knowledge deficit related to clindamycin or lincomycin regimen

Planning and implementation

- Do not administer clindamycin or lincomycin to a patient with a condition that contraindicates its use.
- Administer clindamycin or lincomycin cautiously to a patient with a preexisting condition.
- Monitor the patient periodically for adverse reactions and drug interactions during clindamycin or lincomycin therapy.
- Have standard emergency equipment nearby to treat anaphylactic reactions that may occur, although they are rare.
- Inspect the I.V. infusion site regularly for signs and symptoms of thrombophlebitis. If signs and symptoms occur, switch the infusion to another site.
- Observe clindamycin I.M. injection sites regularly for signs of irritation, such as induration or sterile abscess.
- Do not refrigerate reconstituted oral clindamycin palmitate hydrochloride solution because it thickens and becomes difficult to measure accurately. The solution remains stable for 2 weeks at room temperature.
- Notify the physician if adverse reactions or drug interactions occur.
- Monitor the patient for signs of pseudomembranous colitis, such as severe diarrhea, abdominal pain, fever, and mucus and blood in the stools. If this occurs, promptly discontinue the drug and notify the physician.
- Do not administer an antiperistaltic drug because it can aggravate pseudomembranous colitis.
- Expect to administer vancomycin or metronidazole orally for 10 days to treat pseudomembranous colitis.

Evaluation

For each nursing diagnosis, prepare an evaluation statement that describes the patient's or family's response to nursing interventions.

Macrolides

Macrolides are used to treat a number of common infections. They include erythromycin derivatives, such as erythromycin, erythromycin estolate, erythromycin ethylsuccinate, erythromycin gluceptate, erythromycin lactobionate, and erythromycin stearate, and two new macrolides, azithromycin and clarithromycin.

PHARMACOKINETICS

Erythromycin is transported intact to the small intestine, where it is absorbed. The type of tablet used and the patient's food intake affect how well it is absorbed. It is distributed to most tissues and body fluids (except for cerebrospinal fluid) and is metabolized by the liver. Erythromycin is excreted in bile in high concentrations and small amounts are excreted in the urine; it also crosses the placental barrier and is secreted in breast milk.

Route	Onset	Peak	Duration
P.O.	Unknown	1-4 hr	Unknown
I.V.	Immediate	Immediate	Unknown

PHARMACODYNAMICS

Macrolides inhibit protein synthesis much like chloramphenicol, clindamycin, and lincomycin do. Acting on the ribosomal subunit, macrolides inhibit RNA-dependent protein synthesis by blocking translocation of peptides.

PHARMACOTHERAPEUTICS

Erythromycin provides a broad spectrum of antimicrobial activity against gram-positive and gram-negative bacteria, including *Mycobacterium, Treponema, Mycoplasma, Rickettsia,* and *Chlamydia.* Erythromycin also is effective against pneumococci and group A streptococci. Most clinical isolates of *Staphlococcus aureus* are sensitive to erythromycin; however, resistant strains may emerge during therapy. Erythromycin is the drug of choice for treating *M. pneumoniae* infections. It also is the preferred drug for treating pneumonia caused by *Legionella pneumophila.* In patients who are allergic to penicillin, erythromycin is effective for infections produced by group A beta-hemolytic streptococci or *Streptococcus pneumoniae.* It also may be used to treat gonorrhea and syphilis in patients who cannot tolerate penicillin G or the tetracyclines. Erythromycin may also be used to treat minor cutaneous staphylococcal infections.

Azithromycin provides a broad spectrum of antimicrobial activity against gram-positive and gram-negative bacteria, including *Mycobacterium, Treponema, Mycoplasma,* and *Chlamydia.* It also is effective against pneumococci and groups C, F, and G streptococci, and it may be used to treat *S. aureus* and *H. influenzae.*

Clarithromycin is a broad-spectrum antibacterial agent that has been shown to be active against gram-positive aerobes, such as *S. aureus, S. pneumoniae,* and *Streptococcus pyogenes;* gram-negative aerobes, such as *H. influenzae* and *Moraxella catarrhalis;* and other aerobes such as *M. pneumoniae.*

Drug interactions

Concurrent use of erythromycin, azithromycin, or clarithromycin in patients receiving high dosages of theophylline can decrease theophylline clearance and increase theophylline concentrations. The theophylline dosage may have to be decreased to avoid toxicity.

The antibacterial spectrum of activity of chloramphenicol, clindamycin, and lincomycin may be affected by erythromycin, azithromycin, or clarithromycin because of competition for common binding sites.

Erythromycin lactobionate is incompatible with vitamin B complex, vitamin C, cephalothin, tetracycline, heparin, colistimethate sodium, furosemide, metaraminol bitartrate, and metoclopramide hydrochloride. When combined in a solution, the drugs form a precipitate, which renders both drugs ineffective.

Clarithromycin has been shown to increase the concentration of carbamazepine when used together; this may necessitate monitoring of the serum carbamazepine level.

ADVERSE DRUG REACTIONS

Few adverse reactions are associated with erythromycin. Dose-related GI reactions (epigastric distress, nausea, vomiting, and diarrhea) are most common, especially with large doses. Stomatitis, heartburn, anorexia, and melena may also occur.

Although rare, reversible sensorineural hearing loss may occur with I.V. erythromycin lactobionate. This reaction is most likely to occur in patients with renal failure who are receiving high dosages of erythromycin. Venous irritation and thrombophlebitis can occur after I.V. administration of erythromycin gluceptate or erythromycin lactobionate.

Allergic reactions, including rashes, fever, eosinophilia, and anaphylaxis, also can occur.

Although rare, the most serious toxicity is cholestatic hepatitis, which is most commonly associated with erythromycin estolate and erythromycin ethylsuccinate. This syndrome is characterized by nausea, vomiting, and abdominal pain followed by jaundice, fever, and abnormal liver function test results that are consistent with cholestatic hepatitis. These reactions sometimes are accompanied by rash, leukocytosis, and eosinophilia. The syndrome may represent a hypersensitivity reaction to the specific structure of

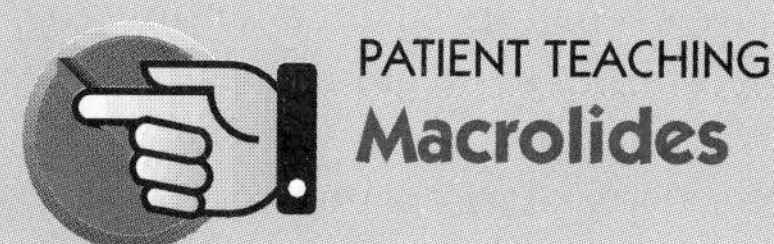

PATIENT TEACHING
Macrolides

- Teach the patient and family the name, dose, frequency, action, and adverse effects of the prescribed macrolide.
- Instruct the patient to complete the course of macrolide therapy.
- Instruct the patient not to take erythromycin stearate with food.
- Instruct the patient to take azithromycin at least 1 hour before or 2 hours after a meal.
- Instruct the patient receiving intravenous erythromycin lactobionate to notify the nurse if changes in hearing occur.
- Review the signs and symptoms of cholestatic hepatitis with the patient receiving erythromycin estolate or erythromycin ethylsuccinate. Advise the patient to notify the physician if they appear.
- Teach the patient on long-term macrolide therapy the importance of having routine liver function studies done.
- Instruct the patient to notify the physician if adverse reactions occur.

the estolate compound. The cholestatic jaundice and hepatocellular necrosis may resolve within days or a few weeks after discontinuation of the drug.

The most common adverse reactions to azithromycin include GI disturbances, such as nausea, vomiting, diarrhea, and abdominal pain. However, azithromycin appears to cause fewer adverse GI reactions than erythromycin. Other adverse reactions include palpitations, chest pain, vaginal moniliasis, nephritis, dizziness, headache, vertigo, somnolence, fatigue, rash, and photosensitivity. Rare but potentially serious adverse reactions include angioedema and cholestatic jaundice. (See Patient Teaching: *Macrolides.*)

The most commonly reported adverse reactions to clarithromycin include diarrhea, nausea, abnormal taste, dyspepsia, abdominal pain or discomfort, and headache. Like azithromycin, clarithromycin also appears to cause fewer adverse GI reactions than erythromycin.

NURSING PROCESS APPLICATION

The following information assists the nurse in caring for a patient who is receiving a macrolide. It includes an overview of assessment activities as well as examples of appropriate nursing diagnoses and related interventions. It also highlights the importance of evaluation.

Assessment

Before drug therapy begins, review the patient's history for conditions that contraindicate or require cautious use of the prescribed macrolide. Also review the patient's medication history to identify use of drugs that may interact with it.

During therapy, assess the patient for adverse drug reactions and signs of drug interactions. Also, periodically assess the effectiveness of macrolide therapy. Finally, evaluate the patient's and family's knowledge of the prescribed drug.

Nursing diagnoses

- Risk for injury related to adverse drug reactions or drug interactions
- Risk for injury related to erythromycin-induced cholestatic hepatitis
- Knowledge deficit related to the prescribed macrolide regimen

Planning and implementation

- Do not administer a macrolide to a patient with a condition that contraindicates its use.
- Administer a macrolide cautiously to a patient with a preexisting condition.
- Monitor the patient periodically for adverse reactions and drug interactions during macrolide therapy.
- Observe the patient for allergic reactions and have standard emergency equipment nearby. If allergic reactions occur, withhold further doses of the prescribed macrolide and notify the physician.
- Monitor for hearing changes in a patient receiving I.V. erythromycin lactobionate, especially in an older patient or one with renal insufficiency.
- Do not mix I.V. erythromycin lactobionate with vitamin B complex, vitamin C, cephalothin, tetracycline, heparin, colistimethate sodium, furosemide, metaraminol bitartrate, or metoclopramide hydrochloride because they are incompatible.
- Reconstitute erythromycin solutions in normal saline solution or dextrose 5% in water and administer the solution within 4 hours after preparation.
- Observe the I.V. site for thrombophlebitis when administering erythromycin gluceptate or erythromycin lactobionate.
- Do not administer erythromycin stearate with food.
- Administer azithromycin at least 1 hour before or 2 hours after a meal.
- Do not administer erythromycin by I.M. injection; the injection is painful and may cause abscess or local tissue necrosis.
- Notify the physician if adverse reactions or drug interactions occur.
- Monitor the patient for hepatic dysfunction. Patients on long-term therapy should undergo frequent liver function tests and physical assessment for signs of liver failure.
- Monitor for signs and symptoms of cholestatic hepatitis, such as nausea, vomiting, abdominal pain, jaundice, rash, leukocytosis, and eosinophilia, in a patient receiving erythromycin estolate or erythromycin ethylsuccinate.
- Expect to discontinue erythromycin if cholestatic hepatitis occurs.

Evaluation
For each nursing diagnosis, prepare an evaluation statement that describes the patient's or family's response to nursing interventions.

Vancomycin

Vancomycin hydrochloride and vancomycin hydrochloride pulvules are used increasingly to treat methicillin-resistant *S. aureus,* which has become a major concern in the United States and other parts of the world. Recent emergence of vancomycin-resistant enterococcus requires that vancomycin is used judiciously.

PHARMACOKINETICS
Vancomycin is absorbed poorly from the GI tract. Therefore, to treat systemic infections, vancomycin is administered I.V. Vancomycin diffuses well into pleural, pericardial, synovial, and ascitic fluids. The metabolism of vancomycin is unknown. Approximately 85% of the dose is excreted unchanged in urine within 24 hours. A small amount may be eliminated via the liver and biliary tract.

Route	Onset	Peak	Duration
P.O.	Unknown	1-2 hr	4-6 hr
I.V.	Immediate	Immediate	4-6 hr

PHARMACODYNAMICS
Vancomycin inhibits biosynthesis of peptidoglycan, the major structural component of the bacterial cell wall. When the bacterial cell wall is damaged, the body's natural defenses can attack the organism.

PHARMACOTHERAPEUTICS
Vancomycin is active against gram-positive organisms, such as *S. aureus, Staphylococcus epidermidis, S. pyogenes,* and *S. pneumoniae.* I.V. vancomycin is the therapy of choice for patients with serious staphylococcal infections; methicillin-, oxacillin-, nafcillin-, or cephalosporin-resistant organisms; or intolerance to those drugs.

Vancomycin, when used with an aminoglycoside, is also the treatment of choice for *E. faecalis* endocarditis in patients who are allergic to penicillin. Orally administered, vancomycin is the drug of choice for treating seriously ill patients with antibiotic-associated *C. difficile* colitis.

Drug interactions
Vancomycin may increase the possibility of toxicity when administered concurrently with other nephrotoxic or ototoxic drugs, such as aminoglycosides, amphotericin B, cisplatin, bacitracin, colistin, and polymyxin B.

ADVERSE DRUG REACTIONS
Parenteral vancomycin must be administered I.V. only, and care must be taken to avoid extravasation. Pain and thrombophlebitis may occur after I.V. administration. I.M injection is not recommended because it causes pain and tissue necrosis at the injection site.

Ototoxicity is the most serious reaction to parenteral vancomycin. It is most likely to occur in patients with renal impairment and those receiving long-term, high-dosage I.V. therapy. Vancomycin may damage the auditory branch of cranial nerve VIII; permanent deafness can occur. Tinnitus may precede deafness and necessitates drug discontinuation. Hearing loss occasionally improves when the drug is discontinued, but in many cases it deteriorates further.

Occasionally, mild hematuria, proteinuria, casts in the urine, and azotemia may occur. A higher incidence of nephrotoxicity occurs when vancomycin is administered concurrently with an aminoglycoside.

A hypotensive reaction associated with rapid I.V. administration of vancomycin may be severe and may be accompanied by a maculopapular or erythematous rash on the face, neck, chest, and arms. The reaction usually begins a few minutes after the infusion is started and resolves spontaneously several hours after the infusion is discontinued. It is commonly called the "red man syndrome."

Hypersensitivity reactions occur in 5% to 10% of patients receiving vancomycin. Anaphylactic reactions, eosinophilia, and drug fever may occur. Neutropenia, which is rapidly reversible after discontinuation, may also occur.

NURSING PROCESS APPLICATION
The following information assists the nurse in caring for a patient who is receiving vancomycin. It includes an overview of assessment activities as well as examples of appropriate nursing diagnoses and related interventions. It also highlights the importance of evaluation.

Assessment
Before drug therapy begins, review the patient's history for conditions that contraindicate or require cautious use of vancomycin. Also review the patient's medication history to identify use of drugs that may interact with it. During therapy, assess the patient for adverse drug reactions and signs of drug interactions. Periodically assess the effectiveness of vancomycin therapy. Finally, evaluate the patient's and family's knowledge of the prescribed drug.

Nursing diagnoses
- Risk for injury related to adverse drug reactions or drug interactions
- Sensory/perceptual alterations (auditory) related to ototoxicity caused by vancomycin
- Knowledge deficit related to vancomycin regimen

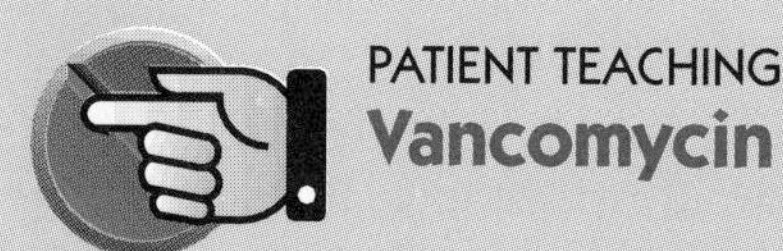

PATIENT TEACHING
Vancomycin

- ➤ Teach the patient and family the name, dose, frequency, action, and adverse effects of vancomycin.
- ➤ Instruct the patient to report tinnitus or hearing loss.
- ➤ Teach the patient the importance of having laboratory studies performed regularly.
- ➤ Instruct the patient to alert the nurse if pain is felt at the intravenous infusion site.
- ➤ Advise the patient to notify the physician if adverse reactions occur or if symptoms persist or worsen.

Planning and implementation

- Do not administer vancomycin to a patient with a condition that contraindicates its use.
- Administer vancomycin cautiously to a patient with a preexisting condition.
- Monitor the patient periodically for adverse reactions and drug interactions during vancomycin therapy; have standard emergency equipment nearby. (See Patient Teaching: *Vancomycin.*)
- Assess the patient's renal status before beginning vancomycin therapy. Monitor serum vancomycin concentrations (peak and trough levels) and the serum creatinine level if the patient is receiving another ototoxic or nephrotoxic drug.
- Do not administer vancomycin by I.M. injection because it is painful and can produce tissue necrosis.
- Do not administer vancomycin by rapid I.V. injection. It should be infused slowly over 30 to 60 minutes in a large volume of fluid to avoid a hypotensive reaction.
- Do not mix vancomycin with other drugs in the same I.V. solution.
- Notify the physician if adverse reactions or drug interactions occur.
- Monitor closely for signs of ototoxicity, especially in a patient with renal impairment or one receiving long-term, high-dosage I.V. therapy.
- Request a baseline audiogram, if possible, before initiating vancomycin therapy. Ask the patient about tinnitus or hearing loss during vancomycin therapy.
- Withhold vancomycin and notify the physician if tinnitus or hearing loss occurs. Expect to discontinue vancomycin and initiate a different antibiotic as prescribed.

Evaluation

For each nursing diagnosis, prepare an evaluation statement that describes the patient's or family's response to nursing interventions.

Carbapenems

A fixed combination, imipenem-cilastatin sodium is the first of a class of beta-lactam antibacterials called carbapenems. Recently, meropenem was released for general use as well. The antibacterial spectrum of activity for imipenem-cilastatin is broader than that of any other antibacterial studied to date.

PHARMACOKINETICS

Imipenem must be given with cilastatin because imipenem alone would be hydrolyzed rapidly in the brush border of the renal tubules, rendering it ineffective. After parenteral administration, imipenem-cilastatin is absorbed well and distributed widely. It is metabolized by several mechanisms and excreted primarily in the urine.

Within 25 minutes of a single 500-mg dose of imipenem-cilastatin, the plasma concentration level is 45.1 mcg/ml for the I.V. form of the drug, compared to 6 mcg/ml for the I.M. form. However, after 2 hours, the plasma concentration is approximately the same for both forms of the drug.

Within 30 minutes of a single I.V. 500-mg dose of meropenem, the plasma concentration is about 23 mcg/ml and 49 mcg/ml following a 1 g dose. Approximately 70% of the I.V. dose is recovered in the urine over 12 hours as unchanged drug.

Route	Onset	Peak	Duration
I.V.	Immediate	≤1 hr	Unknown
I.M.	Unknown	Within 2 hr	90 min-2 hr

PHARMACODYNAMICS

Imipenem and meropenem usually are bactericidal. They exert antibacterial activity by inhibiting mucopeptide synthesis in the bacterial cell wall.

PHARMACOTHERAPEUTICS

Imipenem has a broader spectrum of activity than that of other currently available beta-lactam antibiotics. It displays excellent in vitro activity against aerobic gram-positive species, such as *Streptococcus, S. aureus,* and *S. epidermidis.* Most *Enterobacter* species are inhibited by imipenem concentrations of 1 mcg/ml or less. Imipenem also inhibits *P. aeruginosa* (including strains resistant to piperacillin and ceftazidime) and most anaerobic species, including *B. fragilis.* It also may be used alone for mixed aerobic and anaerobic infections, as therapy for serious nosocomial infections or infections in immunocompromised hosts, and as treatment for infections that normally require combinations of antibiotics.

Meropenem generally is more active in vitro against Enterobacteriaceae and less active against gram-positive bacteria when compared to imipenem. It is indicated in the treatment of intra-abdominal infections as monotherapy as well as for management of bacterial meningitis caused by susceptible organisms.

Drug interactions

Concomitant administration of probenecid, imipenem-cilastatin, and meropenem produces a higher and prolonged serum concentration of cilastatin, but only slightly higher serum concentration of imipenem. Consequently, concomitant use of these drugs is not recommended.

The combination of imipenem-cilastatin and an aminoglycoside acts synergistically against *E. faecalis*, but is not effective against most strains of *P. aeruginosa*. Chloramphenicol can decrease the bactericidal activity of imipenem against *Klebsiella pneumoniae.*

ADVERSE DRUG REACTIONS

The most common adverse reactions to imipenem-cilastatin and meropenem are nausea, vomiting, and diarrhea. Geriatric patients and patients with a history of seizures, underlying CNS disease, or renal insufficiency may experience seizures; this is not as common with meropenem. In some instances, nausea is related to rapid infusion and is reduced by increasing the administration time. Pseudomembranous colitis caused by *C. difficile* also may occur.

Phlebitis, thrombophlebitis, and pain at the I.V. infusion site may occur. Pain also can occur at the injection site when the drug is administered I.M. Transient elevations in liver function values (aspartate aminotransferase [AST], alanine aminotransferase [ALT], and lactate dehydrogenase [LD]) may occur.

Hypersensitivity reactions, such as rashes, have occurred in clinical trials and have been reported in patients with known hypersensitivity to penicillins.

NURSING PROCESS APPLICATION

The following information assists the nurse in caring for a patient who is receiving imipenem-cilastatin or meropenem. It includes an overview of assessment activities as well as examples of appropriate nursing diagnoses and related interventions. It also highlights the importance of evaluation.

Assessment

Before drug therapy begins, review the patient's history for conditions that contraindicate or require cautious use of imipenem-cilastatin. Also review the patient's medication history to identify use of drugs that may interact with it. During therapy, assess the patient for adverse drug reactions and signs of drug interactions. Periodically assess the effectiveness of therapy. Finally, evaluate the patient's and family's knowledge of the prescribed drug. (See Patient Teaching: *Carbapenems.*)

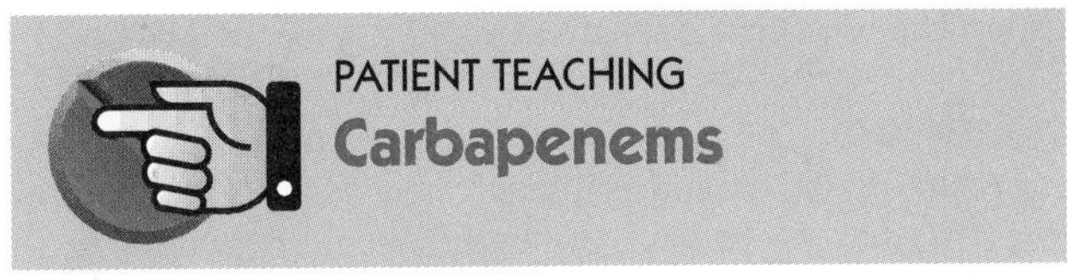

PATIENT TEACHING
Carbapenems

- Teach the patient and family the name, dose, frequency, action, and adverse effects of imipenem-cilastatin or meropenem.
- Instruct the patient receiving intravenous (I.V.) imipenem-cilastatin or meropenem to alert the nurse if nausea is experienced.
- Instruct the patient to inform the nurse if pain is felt at the I.V. infusion site.
- Teach the patient and family to take seizure precautions during imipenem-cilastatin or meropenem therapy, especially in an older patient or one with a history of seizures, an underlying central nervous system disease, or renal insufficency.
- Encourage the patient and family to express concerns or ask questions about imipenem-cilastatin or meropenem therapy as they arise.
- Instruct the patient to notify the physician if adverse reactions occur.

Nursing diagnoses

- Risk for injury related to adverse drug reactions or drug interactions
- Risk for trauma related to imipenem-cilastatin–induced seizures
- Knowledge deficit related to imipenem-cilastatin or meropenem regimen

Planning and implementation

- Do not administer imipenem-cilastatin or meropenem to a patient with a condition that contraindicates its use.
- Administer imipenem-cilastatin or meropenem cautiously to a patient with a preexisting condition.
- Monitor the patient periodically for adverse reactions and drug interactions during therapy.
- Monitor the patient's liver function studies regularly for transient elevations in AST, ALT, and LD.
- Verify that appropriate specimens have been obtained for culture and sensitivity testing before beginning therapy.
- Do not administer imipenem-cilactatin or meropenem concomitantly with probenecid.
- Do not mix imipenem-cilastatin or meropenem with or add it to other antibiotics.
- Administer imipenem-cilastatin or meropenem by intermittent I.V. infusion over 30 minutes. Administer I.M. imipenem-cilastatin deeply into a large muscle mass, such as the gluteal muscle or lateral part of the thigh.
- Notify the physician if adverse reactions or drug interactions occur.
- Take seizure precautions throughout imipenem-cilastatin or meropenem therapy.

***** ***Be especially alert for seizure activity in an older patient or one with a history of seizures, underlying CNS disease, or renal insufficiency.***

- Alert the physician if seizures occur.

Evaluation
For each nursing diagnosis, prepare an evaluation statement that describes the patient's or family's response to nursing interventions.

Monobactams

Aztreonam is the first member of a new class of monobactam antibiotics. It is a synthetic monobactam with a narrow spectrum of activity that includes many gram-negative aerobic bacteria.

PHARMACOKINETICS
After parenteral administration, aztreonam is absorbed completely and rapidly, distributed widely, metabolized partially, and excreted primarily in the urine as unchanged drug.

Route	Onset	Peak	Duration
I.M.	Unknown	0.6-1.3 hr	1.5-2 hr
I.V.	Immediate	Immediate	1.5-2 hr

PHARMACODYNAMICS
Aztreonam's bactericidal activity results from inhibition of mucopeptide synthesis in the bacterial cell wall. It preferentially binds to the PBPs of susceptible gram-negative bacteria. As a result, division of the cell wall is inhibited and lysis occurs.

PHARMACOTHERAPEUTICS
Aztreonam exhibits activity against a wide variety of gram-negative aerobic organisms, including *P. aeruginosa*. It is effective in clinical infections against most strains of the following organisms: *E. coli, Enterobacter, K. pneumoniae, Klebsiella oxytoca, Proteus mirabilis, Serratia marcescens, H. influenzae,* and *Citrobacter.*

Aztreonam also is used to treat complicated and uncomplicated UTIs, septicemia, and lower respiratory tract, skin and skin-structure, intra-abdominal, and gynecologic infections caused by susceptible gram-negative aerobic bacteria. Aztreonam should not be used alone for empiric therapy in seriously ill patients if the infection may be caused by gram-positive bacteria or if a mixed aerobic-anaerobic bacterial infection is suspected. Aztreonam does not induce beta-lactamase activity and usually is active against gram-negative aerobic organisms that are resistant to antibiotics hydrolyzed by beta-lactamases.

Drug interactions
Concomitant use of aztreonam and probenecid may prolong the tubular secretion rate of aztreonam. Synergistic or additive effects occur when aztreonam is used concomitantly with aminoglycosides or other beta-lactam antibiotics such as azlocillin, cefoperazone, cefotaxime, clindamycin, metronidazole, moxalactam, or piperacillin. Potent inducers of beta-lactamase production (cefoxitin, imipenem) may inactivate aztreonam. Chloramphenicol antagonizes aztreonam's effects; the two drugs must be given several hours apart. Use with clavulanic acid may be synergistic or antagonistic, depending on the organism involved. Furosemide increases the serum aztreonam concentration, but this is not a clinically significant interaction.

ADVERSE DRUG REACTIONS
The most common GI reactions include diarrhea, nausea, and vomiting. Less common GI reactions include GI bleeding, abdominal cramps, bloating, a transient unusual taste during or after I.V. infusion, numbness of the tongue, oral ulceration, and halitosis. *C. difficile* diarrhea may also occur.

Hematologic reactions are varied and may include transient eosinophilia, leukopenia, neutropenia, thrombocytopenia, pancytopenia, anemia, leukocytosis, and thrombocytosis.

Transient increases in serum AST, ALT, and alkaline phosphatase concentrations have occurred in 2% to 40% of patients receiving aztreonam. They return to pretreatment concentrations shortly after aztreonam is discontinued. Hepatitis, jaundice, and other manifestations of hepatotoxicity are rare.

Hypotension and transient electrocardiogram changes, including ventricular bigeminy and premature ventricular contractions, may occur. Seizures, confusion, insomnia, dizziness, paresthesia, weakness, fatigue, and headache also may occur as adverse CNS effects.

Thrombophlebitis may occur in patients receiving I.V. aztreonam. Discomfort, pain, and swelling at the injection site also may occur with patients receiving I.M. aztreonam, although the drug is generally well tolerated when administered by this route.

Hypersensitivity and dermatologic reactions also may occur; they include anaphylaxis, urticaria, pruritus, erythema multiforme, and exfoliative dermatitis.

NURSING PROCESS APPLICATION
The following information assists the nurse in caring for a patient who is receiving aztreonam. It includes an overview of assessment activities as well as examples of appropriate nursing diagnoses and related interventions. It also highlights the importance of evaluation.

Assessment
Before drug therapy begins, review the patient's history for conditions that contraindicate or require cautious use of

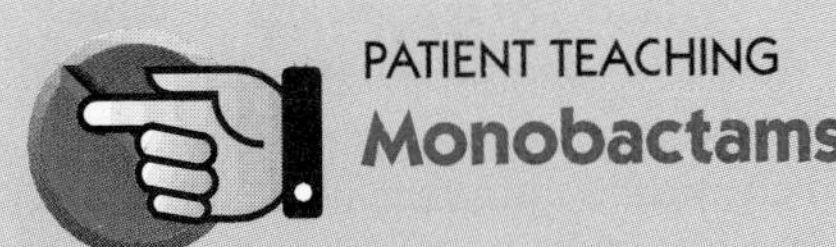

PATIENT TEACHING
Monobactams

- Teach the patient and family the name, dose, frequency, action, and adverse effects of aztreonam.
- Warn the patient receiving intramuscular aztreonam that pain may occur at the injection site. Advise the patient receiving intravenous aztreonam to report pain at the infusion site.
- Teach the patient the importance of having blood studies done periodically to detect adverse hematologic or hepatic reactions.
- Instruct the patient to notify the nurse before getting out of bed if he or she experiences dizziness.
- Teach the patient how to manage mouth ulcers and how to perform frequent mouth care.
- Instruct the patient with thrombocytopenia to take bleeding precautions, such as avoiding cuts and bruises, using a soft toothbrush, and using an electric razor when shaving.
- Review appropriate infection-control measures with the patient and family if leukopenia is present.
- Teach the patient with anemia to stagger activities and to rest frequently.
- Instruct the patient to alert the nurse or physician if adverse reactions occur.

aztreonam. Also review the patient's medication history to identify use of drugs that may interact with it. During therapy, assess the patient for adverse drug reactions and signs of drug interactions. Also, periodically assess the effectiveness of aztreonam therapy. Finally, evaluate the patient's and family's knowledge of the prescribed drug. (See Patient Teaching: *Monobactams.*)

Nursing diagnoses

- Risk for injury related to adverse drug reactions or drug interactions
- Risk for injury related to the adverse hematologic effects of aztreonam
- Knowledge deficit related to aztreonam regimen

Planning and implementation

- Do not administer aztreonam to a patient with a condition that contraindicates its use.
- Administer aztreonam cautiously to a patient with a preexisting condition.
- Monitor the patient periodically for adverse reactions and drug interactions during aztreonam therapy.
- Monitor the patient closely for hypersensitivity reactions. If a hypersensitivity reaction occurs, withhold aztreonam, notify the physician, and expect to switch the patient to a different antibiotic. Have standard emergency equipment nearby.
- Obtain specimens for culture and sensitivity testing before administering the first dose of aztreonam. Notify the physician if results reveal organisms that are resistant to aztreonam.
- Take seizure precautions throughout aztreonam therapy.
- Take safety precautions if the patient experiences confusion, dizziness, or other adverse CNS reactions.
- Notify the physician if adverse reactions or drug interactions occur.
- Monitor the patient's complete blood count and liver function studies for abnormalities.
- Take infection-control measures if leukocytopenia occurs.
- Take bleeding precautions if thrombocytopenia occurs.
- Stagger the patient's activities and provide frequent rest periods if anemia occurs.
- Notify the physician if adverse hematologic or hepatic reactions occur.

Evaluation

For each nursing diagnosis, prepare an evaluation statement that describes the patient's or family's response to nursing interventions.

CHAPTER SUMMARY

Chapter 31 described the clinically important antibacterial drugs used to treat systemic infections. Here are the chapter highlights.

Aminoglycosides are used primarily to treat gram-negative bacterial infections. Amikacin, gentamicin, netilmicin, and tobramycin are the most commonly prescribed aminoglycosides.

Penicillins remain one of the most important and useful antibacterial groups available for clinical use. Because penicillins have a low incidence of serious toxicities and are relatively inexpensive, they are the drugs of choice to treat susceptible organisms in nonallergic patients.

Cephalosporins, which also are commonly prescribed, are classified into three generations based on their spectra of activity.

Tetracyclines, among the most commonly prescribed antibacterials in the world, are primarily bacteriostatic.

Drug-induced aplastic anemia has limited the use of chloramphenicol.

Clindamycin is more effective than lincomycin against susceptible bacteria. Clindamycin remains particularly important in treating certain anaerobic infections.

Macrolides are used to treat a number of common infections. Erythromycin is the drug of choice to treat *M. pneumoniae* infections as well as *L. pneumophila.*

Vancomycin is being used more to treat methicillin-resistant *S. aureus.*

Imipenem-cilastatin and meropenem are new classes of beta-lactam antibacterials called carbapenems. The antibacterial spectrum of activity of imipenem-cilastatin and meropenem is broader than that of any other antibacterial studied to date.

Aztreonam is the first member of a new class of monobactams. It has a narrow spectrum of activity that includes many aerobic gram-negative bacteria.

Before administering an antibacterial agent, the nurse should ensure that specimens have been obtained for culture and sensitivity testing. During antibacterial therapy, the nurse should monitor the patient closely for adverse reactions, especially hypersensitivity ones.

Questions to consider

See Appendix 1 for answers.

1. Willie Jones, age 59, is admitted to the hospital with pneumonia. The physician prescribes cefazolin sodium (a first-generation cephalosporin) 1 g I.V. every 8 hours. After receiving cefazolin for 5 days, Mr. Jones develops oral thrush. This probably is a sign of which of the following adverse reactions?
   (a) Superinfection
   (b) Allergic reaction
   (c) Cefoxitin toxicity
   (d) Bone marrow suppression

2. Tonya Brown, age 10, has been diagnosed as having streptococcal pharyngitis (strep throat). To treat this condition, the physician prescribes amoxicillin 250 mg P.O. every 8 hours. During penicillin therapy, the nurse should assess for which of the following major adverse drug reactions?
   (a) Hepatotoxicity
   (b) Serum sickness
   (c) Blood dyscrasias
   (d) CNS irritation

3. James Howard, age 39, develops a staphylococcal infection. The physician prescribes I.V. erythromycin lactobionate. Knowing that erythromycin causes drug interactions, the nurse questions Mr. Howard about his current and past drug history. Erythromycin lactobionate is incompatible with which of the following drugs?
   (a) folic acid
   (b) aspirin
   (c) acetaminophen
   (d) furosemide

4. Wilhimina Jobes, age 30, is admitted to the hospital with a serious UTI. The physician prescribes aztreonam 500 mg I.V. every 12 hours. Aztreonam is a member of which of the following antibacterial classes?
   (a) Carbapenems
   (b) Penicillins
   (c) Cephalosporins
   (d) Monobactams

5. Jennifer Adams, age 15, takes tetracycline orally as prescribed to treat acne. This drug should not be administered to children under age 8. Why not?
   (a) It is absorbed erratically from the GI tract.
   (b) It has a high incidence of adverse reactions.
   (c) It may darken permanent teeth and disrupt bone growth.
   (d) It is metabolized poorly and may result in toxicity.

6. Janine Albright, age 22, is receiving chloramphenicol for *H. influenzae* meningitis. Which of the following adverse reactions limits the use of this drug to treatment of severe infections only?
   (a) Ototoxicity
   (b) Nephrotoxicity
   (c) Aplastic anemia
   (d) Bone marrow suppression

32 Antiviral agents

OBJECTIVES

After reading and studying this chapter, the student should be able to:

1. discuss the pharmacokinetics and mechanisms of action of the antiviral agents in this chapter.
2. identify the clinical indications for antiviral agents.
3. discuss the adverse reactions associated with antiviral agents.
4. describe how to apply the nursing process when caring for a patient who is receiving an antiviral agent.

INTRODUCTION

Antiviral agents are drugs used to prevent or treat viral **infections.** This chapter discusses major antiviral agents: acyclovir, ganciclovir, foscarnet, amantadine hydrochloride, zidovudine, didanosine, and zalcitabine. It also includes information on the new category of agents, the protease inhibitors. This chapter also focuses primarily on systemic therapy. (See *Selected major antiviral agents,* pages 420 and 421.)

Drugs covered in this chapter include:

- acyclovir
- amantadine hydrochloride
- didanosine
- foscarnet
- ganciclovir
- indinavir sulfate
- ribavarin
- ritonavir
- saquinavir mesylate
- zalcitabine
- zidovudine.

Acyclovir and ganciclovir

The herpesvirus agent acyclovir sodium produces marked antiviral activity and minimal cellular **toxicity.** A derivative of acyclovir, ganciclovir has been shown to have potent antiviral activity against herpes simplex **virus** (HSV) and cytomegalovirus (CMV).

PHARMACOKINETICS

Although gastrointestinal (GI) absorption of acyclovir is slow and only 15% to 30% complete, serum concentration levels of the drug are therapeutic. Acyclovir is distributed throughout the body. Metabolism of acyclovir is complex and is completed in the liver and infected cells. The drug is excreted primarily in the urine.

Ganciclovir is administered intravenously (I.V.) because it is absorbed poorly from the GI tract. Distribution into human body tissues has not been elucidated fully. More than 90% is excreted by the kidneys unchanged

Route	Onset	Peak	Duration
P.O.	Unknown	1.7 hr	2-3.5 hr
I.V.	Immediate	Immediate	2-3.5 hr

PHARMACODYNAMICS

To be effective, acyclovir and ganciclovir must be metabolized to their active form in cells infected by the herpes virus. Acyclovir enters virus-infected cells, where it is changed through a series of steps to acyclovir triphosphate. Acyclovir triphosphate inhibits virus-specific deoxyribonucleic acid (DNA) polymerase, an enzyme necessary for viral growth, and disrupts viral replication.

Upon entry into host cells, ganciclovir is converted to ganciclovir triphosphate. Ganciclovir triphosphate is thought to produce its antiviral activity by inhibiting viral DNA synthesis.

PHARMACOTHERAPEUTICS

Acyclovir is used to treat herpes viruses, including HSV types 1 and 2 and the varicella-zoster virus. Oral acyclovir is used primarily to treat initial and recurrent genital HSV infections. Parenteral acyclovir is used to treat severe initial genital HSV infections in patients with normal immune systems, initial and recurrent mucocutaneous HSV infections (types 1 and 2) in immunocompromised patients, herpes zoster infections (shingles) caused by the varicella-zoster virus in immunocompromised patients, disseminated varicella-zoster virus in immunocompromised patients, and varicella infections (chickenpox) caused by varicella-zoster virus in immunocompromised patients.

Ganciclovir is used to treat CMV retinitis in immunocompromised patients, including those with acquired immunodeficiency syndrome (AIDS). It is also used for other CMV infections such as encephalitis.

Selected major antiviral agents

This chart summarizes the major antiviral agents currently in clinical use.

DRUG	MAJOR INDICATIONS AND USUAL DOSAGES	CONTRAINDICATIONS AND PRECAUTIONS
acyclovir (Zovirax)	*Primary genital herpes simplex virus (HSV) infection* ADULT: 200 mg P.O. every 4 hours while awake five times a day for 10 days; 5 mg/kg I.V. every 8 hours (infused over 1 hour) for 5 to 7 days in patients with a creatinine clearance greater than 50 ml/minute *Recurrent genital HSV infection* ADULT: 200 mg P.O. five times a day for 5 days *Varicella-zoster infection* ADULT: 5 to 10 mg/kg I.V. every 8 hours (infused over 1 hour) for 5 days *Herpes simplex encephalitis* ADULT: 10 mg/kg I.V. every 8 hours (infused over 1 hour) for at least 10 days	• Acyclovir is contraindicated in a patient with known hypersensitivity to the drug or intolerance of any of the components of the formulation. • This drug requires cautious use in a pregnant or breast-feeding patient or one with renal impairment.
ganciclovir (Cytovene)	*Cytomegalovirus (CMV) retinitis in immunocompromised patients, including those with acquired immunodeficiency syndrome (AIDS)* ADULT: initially, 5 mg/kg I.V. infused over 1 hour every 12 hours for 14 to 21 days; for maintenance dosage, 5 mg/kg I.V. infused over 1 hour daily or 6 mg/kg I.V. once daily for 5 out of 7 days a week. P.O.: 1 g t.i.d. with food after I.V. induction course or 500 mg every 3 hours with food after I.V. induction course.	• Ganciclovir is contraindicated in a patient with known hypersensitivity to the drug or intolerance of any of the components of the formulation. • This drug requires cautious use in a pregnant or breast-feeding patient or one with renal impairment
foscarnet (Foscavir)	*CMV retinitis in patients with AIDS* ADULT: 60 mg/kg I.V. every 8 hours for 2 to 3 weeks, depending on clinical response; for maintenance dosage, 60 to 120 mg/kg I.V. daily	• Foscarnet is contraindicated in a patient with known hypersensitivity. • This drug requires cautious use in a pregnant or breast-feeding patient or one with renal impairment. • Safety and efficacy in children have not been established.
zidovudine (Retrovir)	*Patients with AIDS or AIDS-related complex who have a history of* Pneumocystis carinii *pneumonia or a T lymphocyte count below 200/mm³* ADULT: 100 mg P.O. every 4 hours five to six times daily or 200 mg every 8 hours PEDIATRIC: for children over age 12, 200 mg P.O. every 4 hours around the clock; for children ages 3 months to 12 years, 180 mg/m² P.O. every 6 hours around the clock *Symptomatic human immunodeficiency virus (HIV) infection* ADULT: 1 mg/kg I.V. every 4 hours six times a day around the clock *Asymptomatic HIV infection* ADULT: 1 mg/kg every 4 hours while awake (five times a day)	• Zidovudine is contraindicated in a breast-feeding patient or one with known hypersensitivity to the drug or any components of the formulation. • This drug requires cautious use in a pregnant patient or one with impaired hepatic or renal function.
didanosine (Videx)	*Advanced HIV infection in patients who cannot tolerate zidovudine or who have demonstrated significant or immunologic deterioration during zidovudine therapy* ADULT: 125 to 200 mg P.O. tablet form every 12 hours or 167 to 375 mg P.O. powdered form b.i.d. (higher dose used for adults who weigh over 132 lb [60 kg]; lower dose used for adults who weigh less than 60 kg) PEDIATRIC: 90 to 120 mg/m² P.O. daily every 12 hours; use lower dose if used in combination with zidovudine	• Didanosine is contraindicated in a breast-feeding patient or one with known hypersensitivity to the drug or any of its components. • This drug requires cautious use in a pregnant patient or one with impaired hepatic function or phenylketonuria.

Selected major antiviral agents *(continued)*

DRUG	MAJOR INDICATIONS AND USUAL DOSAGES	CONTRAINDICATIONS AND PRECAUTIONS
zalcitabine (Hivid)	*Adjunct therapy with zidovudine to treat advanced HIV infection (a CD4+ cell count < 200 cells/mm³) in adults with significant clinical or immunologic deterioration* ADULT: 0.75 mg P.O. administered with 200 mg zidovudine every 8 hours *HIV Infection* ADULT: (in combination with nucleoside analogue) 200 mg capsules P.O. taken t.i.d. within 2 hours after a full meal	• Zalcitabine is contraindicated in a breast-feeding patient or one with known hypersensitivity to the drug or any of its components. • This drug requires cautious use in a pregnant patient or one with renal or hepatic impairment. • Safety and efficacy in children under age 13 have not been established.
saquinavir mesylate (Invirase)	*HIV infection* ADULT: 600 mg P.O. every 12 hours with food. If nausea is present, then escalate dose (for example, 300 mg b.i.d. for 1 day; 400 mg b.i.d. for 1 day, and so on until 600 mg b.i.d. is reached)	• Saquinavir mesylate is contraindicated in patients with known hypersensitivity to the drug or any of its components. • This drug requires cautious use in a pregnant woman. • Use drug cautiously in a patient with impaired liver function. • Cautious use in breast-feeding women is advised because it is not known whether the drug is present in breast milk. • Safety and efficacy in children under age 12 have not been established.
indinavir sulfate (Crixivan)	*HIV infection* ADULT: 800 mg P.O. every 8 hours. In patients with cirrhosis, dosage is reduced to 600 mg every 8 hours.	• Indinavir sulfate should not be administered concurrently with terfenadine, astemizole, cispapride, triazolam, or midazolam. • Use cautiously in a patient with mild to moderate liver disease. • Indinavir sulfate should be used in a pregnant patient only if the potential benefits outweigh the risk. • Use in breast-feeding women is not recommended because the drug is present in breast milk. • Safety and efficacy in children have not been established.
nelfinavir mesylate (Agouron)	*HIV infection* ADULT: 750 mg P.O. t.i.d. in combination with nucleoside analogues PEDIATRIC: ages 2 to 13, 30 to 30 mg/kg/dose t.i.d.	• Nelfinavir mesylate is used cautiously in a patient with hepatic impairment. • Cautious use in breast-feeding patients is advised because it is not known whether the drug is present in breast milk. • This drug requires cautious use in a pregnant patient.

Drug interactions

Acyclovir and ganciclovir may interact with several different types of drugs. (See Drug Interactions: *Acyclovir and ganciclovir,* page 422.)

ADVERSE DRUG REACTIONS

Local reactions at the injection site, particularly with inadvertent extravasation, are the most common adverse reactions to parenteral acyclovir; they include irritation, phlebitis, inflammation, and pain. Reversible renal impairment occurs in patients receiving parenteral acyclovir by rapid I.V. injection or infusion.

Headache is common with oral acyclovir, in addition to such GI reactions as nausea, vomiting, and diarrhea. Other reactions include vertigo and hematuria.

Oral or parenteral acyclovir occasionally causes diaphoresis, fatigue, insomnia, irritability, depression, and hypotension. Rarely, patients have reported muscle cramps and leg pain.

Other rare reactions to acyclovir include thrombocytosis, thrombocytopenia, transient lymphopenia, transient leukopenia, and bone marrow hypoplasia. Hypersensitivity reactions, which include fever, rash, arthralgia, sore throat, lymphadenopathy, and inguinal adenopathy, may occur.

During clinical trials, the most common adverse reactions to ganciclovir were granulocytopenia and thrombocytope-

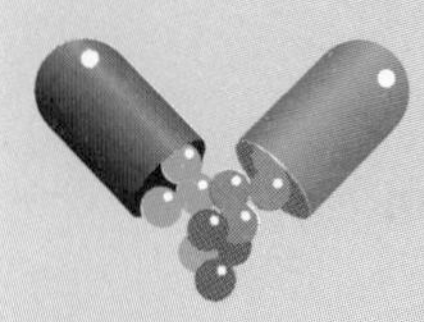

DRUG INTERACTIONS

Acyclovir and ganciclovir

The nurse should be aware of the following drug interactions involving acyclovir and ganciclovir, the possible effects of the interactions, and the nursing implications.

DRUG	INTERACTING DRUGS	POSSIBLE EFFECTS	NURSING IMPLICATIONS
acyclovir, ganciclovir	probenecid and other drugs that inhibit renal tubular secretion or resorption	Decreased renal clearance and increased plasma concentration of ganciclovir	• Monitor the patient's renal function. • Keep the patient well hydrated. • Watch for signs of drug toxicity.
acyclovir	nephrotoxic agents	Increased risk of renal dysfunction	• Monitor the patient's renal function. • Keep the patient well hydrated.
ganciclovir	cytotoxic drugs, such as dapsone, pentamidine isethionate, flucytosine, vincristine, vinblastine, doxorubicin, amphotericin B, and trimethoprim-sulfa combinations	Inhibited replication of rapidly dividing cells in bone marrow, gastrointestinal tract, skin, and spermatogonia; additive toxicity	• Administer these drugs concomitantly only if the potential benefits are thought to outweigh the risks. • Monitor the patient closely for toxicity.
	imipenem-cilastatin	Increased risk of seizures	• Avoid concomitant use.
	zidovudine	Granulocytopenia	• Avoid concomitant use.

nia. Anemia, fever, rash, and abnormal liver function tests also were reported. The following reactions occurred in less than 1% of patients: arrhythmias, hypertension, hypotension, abnormal thoughts and dreams, ataxia, headache, coma, confusion, dizziness, nervousness, paresthesia, psychosis, somnolence, tremor, nausea, vomiting, anorexia, diarrhea, hemorrhage, abdominal pain, alopecia, pruritus, urticaria, hematuria, increased serum creatinine and blood urea nitrogen levels, decreased blood glucose level, chills, edema, infections, malaise, and inflammation, pain, and phlebitis at the injection site.

NURSING PROCESS APPLICATION

The following information assists the nurse in caring for a patient who is receiving acyclovir or ganciclovir. It includes an overview of assessment activities as well as examples of appropriate nursing diagnoses and related interventions. It also highlights the importance of evaluation.

Assessment

Before drug therapy begins, review the patient's history for conditions that contraindicate or require cautious use of acyclovir or ganciclovir. Review the patient's medication history to identify use of drugs that may interact with them. During therapy, assess the patient for adverse drug reactions and signs of drug interactions. Periodically assess the effectiveness of acyclovir or ganciclovir. Finally, evaluate the patient's and family's knowledge of the drug.

Nursing diagnoses

- Risk for injury related to adverse drug reactions or drug interactions
- Altered protection related to the adverse hematologic effects of acyclovir or ganciclovir
- Knowledge deficit related to acyclovir or ganciclovir regimen

Planning and implementation

- Do not administer acyclovir or ganciclovir to a patient with a condition that contraindicates its use.
- Administer acyclovir or ganciclovir cautiously to a patient with a preexisting condition.
- Monitor the patient periodically for adverse reactions and drug interactions during acyclovir or ganciclovir therapy.
- Closely monitor the patient's renal function, especially the serum creatinine level, during parenteral therapy.
- Expect to adjust the dosage as prescribed for a patient with decreased renal function, especially during parenteral therapy.
- Administer an I.V. infusion of acyclovir or ganciclovir slowly (over 60 minutes or as prescribed) to prevent drug crystals from precipitating in the renal tubules.
- Infuse prepared I.V. acyclovir or ganciclovir solution only into veins with adequate blood flow to avoid phlebitis; ganciclovir infusions have a high pH.
- Keep the patient well hydrated during parenteral therapy to ensure good urine output.
- Avoid inhalation or direct skin contact when administering ganciclovir because of its carcinogenic potential.
- Notify the physician if adverse reactions or drug interactions occur.
- Know that photosensitivity can occur.

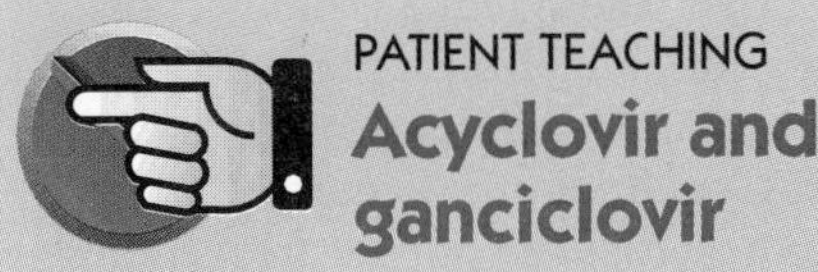

PATIENT TEACHING
Acyclovir and ganciclovir

- Teach the patient and family the name, dose, frequency, action, and adverse effects of acyclovir or ganciclovir.
- Instruct the patient to report pain or discomfort at the intravenous infusion site to the nurse.
- Advise the patient to take a mild analgesic at home if acyclovir or ganciclovir causes a headache.
- Advise a patient of childbearing age to use effective contraception during ganciclovir therapy and for at least 90 days after it is discontinued because of the drug's mutagenic potential.
- Advise the female patient to discontinue breast-feeding during ganciclovir therapy and not to resume it for at least 72 hours after taking the last ganciclovir dose.
- Caution the patient to avoid activities that require alertness if vertigo occurs.
- Teach the patient how to minimize adverse central nervous system effects at home.
- Stress the importance of returning for regular blood tests. If leukopenia occurs, teach the patient about infection-control measures; if thrombocytopenia occurs, teach the patient about taking bleeding precautions.
- Instruct the patient to notify the physician if adverse reactions occur.

- Monitor the patient's complete blood count (CBC) regularly during acyclovir or ganciclovir therapy. Also monitor neutrophil and platelet counts every 2 days during twice-daily therapy and at least weekly during maintenance therapy when administering ganciclovir. (See Patient Teaching: *Acyclovir and ganciclovir.*)
- Closely monitor for signs of infection if the patient develops leukopenia. Take infection-control measures until the patient's white blood cell (WBC) count returns to normal.
- Closely monitor for signs of bleeding if the patient develops thrombocytopenia, which is especially likely to occur with ganciclovir therapy. Test urine, feces, and vomitus for occult blood. Take bleeding precautions until the thrombocyte level returns to normal.
- Stagger the patient's activities and provide frequent rest periods if anemia occurs.
- Notify the physician of abnormalities in blood test results, especially the CBC.

Evaluation

For each nursing diagnosis, prepare an evaluation statement that describes the patient's or family's response to nursing interventions.

Foscarnet

The antiviral agent foscarnet is used to treat CMV retinitis in patients with AIDS.

PHARMACOKINETICS

Foscarnet is approximately 15% bound to plasma protein. In patients with normal renal function, 80% to 90% of foscarnet is excreted unchanged in the urine.

Route	Onset	Peak	Duration
I.V.	Immediate	Immediate	3 hr

PHARMACODYNAMICS

Foscarnet prevents viral replication by selectively inhibiting pyrophosphate binding to virus-specific DNA polymerases and reverse transcriptases.

PHARMACOTHERAPEUTICS

Foscarnet is used to treat CMV retinitis in patients with AIDS. All dosages should be based on the patient's renal function.

Drug interactions

Hypocalcemia from foscarnet and I.V. pentamidine administration has been reported in several patients during clinical trials. Concomitant use of foscarnet and other drugs that alter serum calcium levels may result in hypocalcemia. Because foscarnet can impair renal function, concomitant therapy with nephrotoxic drugs should be avoided.

ADVERSE DRUG REACTIONS

Adverse drug reactions reported in 5% or more of patients during clinical trials include fever, fatigue, rigors, asthenia, malaise, pain, infection, **sepsis,** headache, paresthesia, dizziness, involuntary muscle contractions, hypoesthesia, neuropathy, seizures, anorexia, nausea, vomiting, diarrhea, abdominal pain, anemia, granulocytopenia, leukopenia, mineral and electrolyte imbalances, depression, confusion, anxiety, coughing, dyspnea, rash, increased sweating, altered renal function, vision disturbances, and death.

NURSING PROCESS APPLICATION

The following information assists the nurse in caring for a patient who is receiving foscarnet. It includes an overview of assessment activities as well as examples of appropriate nursing diagnoses and related interventions. It also highlights the importance of evaluation.

Assessment

Before drug therapy begins, review the patient's history for conditions that contraindicate or require cautious use of foscarnet. Also review the patient's medication history to identify use of drugs that may interact with it. During therapy, assess the patient for adverse drug reactions and signs of drug interactions. Also, periodically assess the effective-

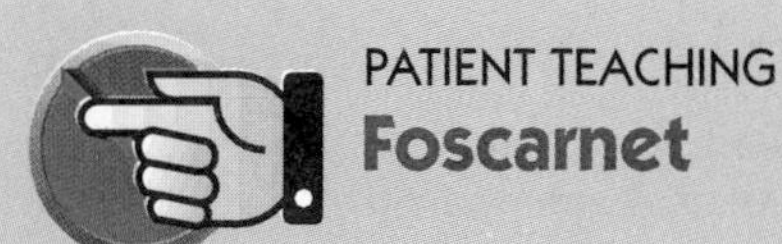

PATIENT TEACHING
Foscarnet

- ➤ Teach the patient and family the name, dose, frequency, action, and adverse effects of foscarnet.
- ➤ Instruct the patient to report pain or discomfort at the intravenous infusion site to the nurse.
- ➤ Inform the pregnant patient that foscarnet use during pregnancy is indicated only if the potential benefit to the patient justifies the potential risk to the fetus.
- ➤ Tell the female patient who is breast-feeding that foscarnet's secretion into breast milk is unverified. She should therefore discuss the safety of breast-feeding with her physician.
- ➤ Caution the patient to seek assistance in walking and getting out of bed if vision disturbances occur.
- ➤ Tell the patient to report immediately any symptoms of hypocalcemia, such as perioral tingling, numbness in the extremities, and paresthesia.
- ➤ Advise the patient that foscarnet does not cure cytomegalovirus-induced retinitis and that retinitis may progress during or after treatment.
- ➤ Instruct the patient to notify the nurse if adverse reactions occur.

ness of foscarnet therapy. Finally, evaluate the patient's and family's knowledge of the prescribed drug.

Nursing diagnoses

- Risk for injury related to adverse drug reactions or drug interactions
- Altered protection related to adverse hematologic effects of foscarnet
- Knowledge deficit related to foscarnet regimen

Planning and implementation

- Do not administer foscarnet to a patient with a condition that contraindicates its use.
- Administer foscarnet cautiously to a patient with a preexisting condition.
- Monitor the patient periodically for adverse reactions or drug interactions during foscarnet therapy. (See Patient Teaching: *Foscarnet*.)
- Closely monitor the patient's renal function, especially the serum creatinine level, during therapy. Because foscarnet can cause renal dysfunction, the dosage must be adjusted to changes in renal function.
- Do not administer foscarnet by rapid I.V. or bolus infusion because high plasma levels are associated with toxicity. An infusion pump is recommended.
- Avoid administering drugs via I.V. piggyback with foscarnet.
- Closely monitor serum electrolyte levels because transient changes may increase the risk of cardiac disturbances and seizures.
- Notify the physician if adverse reactions or drug interactions occur.
- Regularly monitor the patient's CBC during therapy.
- Closely monitor for signs and symptoms of infection, such as fever, chills, cough, and purulent drainage, if the patient develops leukopenia. Take infection-control measures until the patient's WBC count returns to normal.
- Stagger the patient's activities and provide frequent rest periods if anemia occurs.
- Notify the physician of abnormalities in blood test results, especially the CBC.

Evaluation

For each nursing diagnosis, prepare an evaluation statement that describes the patient's or family's response to nursing interventions.

Amantadine

Amantadine hydrochloride was the first oral antiviral drug available for clinical use. It is used to prevent or treat influenza A infections.

PHARMACOKINETICS

After oral administration, amantadine is absorbed well in the GI tract; distributed to saliva, cerebrospinal fluid, nasal secretions, breast milk, and lung tissue; and eliminated primarily in the urine.

Route	Onset	Peak	Duration
P.O.	Unknown	2-4 hr	11-15 hr

PHARMACODYNAMICS

Although the exact mechanism of action of amantadine is unknown, the drug appears to inhibit an early stage of viral replication, such as prevention of virus penetration into the host cell or inhibition of the uncoating of the virus particle.

PHARMACOTHERAPEUTICS

Amantadine is used to prevent and treat respiratory tract infections caused by strains of the influenza A virus. It can protect patients undergoing immunization during the 2 weeks needed for immunity to develop or patients who cannot take the influenza vaccine because of hypersensitivity. When used to treat patients with influenza A infections, amantadine reduces the severity and duration of fever and other symptoms.

Amantadine is also used to treat parkinsonism and drug-induced extrapyramidal reactions.

Drug interactions

Additive anticholinergic effects may occur when amantadine is given with large dosages of anticholinergic drugs. The patient must be monitored closely if the drugs are used concomitantly. Amantadine given concurrently with hydrochlorothiazide/triamterene results in decreased urine excretion of amantadine with a resultant increased plasma concentration of the drug.

ADVERSE DRUG REACTIONS

The most common adverse reactions to amantadine are nausea, anorexia, nervousness, fatigue, depression, irritability, insomnia, psychosis, anxiety, confusion, forgetfulness, and hallucinations. Other central nervous system (CNS) reactions include headache, dizziness, light-headedness, slurred speech, ataxia, tremor, and a sense of drunkenness. Patients with seizure disorders are more prone to seizures while receiving amantadine.

Other less common adverse drug reactions include heart failure, orthostatic hypotension, edema, leukopenia, dermatitis, photosensitivity, dry mouth, rash, urine retention, constipation, and vomiting. Amantadine may also cause hypersensitivity reactions.

NURSING PROCESS APPLICATION

The following information assists the nurse in caring for a patient who is receiving amantadine. It includes an overview of assessment activities as well as examples of appropriate nursing diagnoses and related interventions. It also highlights the importance of evaluation.

Assessment

Before drug therapy begins, review the patient's history for conditions that contraindicate or require cautious use of amantadine. Also review the patient's medication history to identify use of drugs that may interact with it. During therapy, assess the patient for adverse drug reactions and signs of drug interactions. Also, periodically assess the effectiveness of amantadine therapy. Finally, evaluate the patient's and family's knowledge of the prescribed drug.

Nursing diagnoses

- Risk for injury related to adverse drug reactions or drug interactions
- Knowledge deficit related to amantadine regimen

Planning and implementation

- Do not administer amantadine to a patient with a condition that contraindicates its use.
- Administer amantadine cautiously to a patient with a preexisting condition.
- Administer amantadine cautiously to a patient receiving concomitant therapy with an anticholinergic agent.
- Closely monitor the patient for excessive anticholinergic effects. (See Patient Teaching: *Amantadine.*)
- Monitor the patient for adverse reactions or drug interactions during amantadine therapy.
- If the patient experiences insomnia with amantadine use, give it early in the day to prevent sleep loss.
- Take seizure precautions when administering amantadine to a patient with a history of seizures.

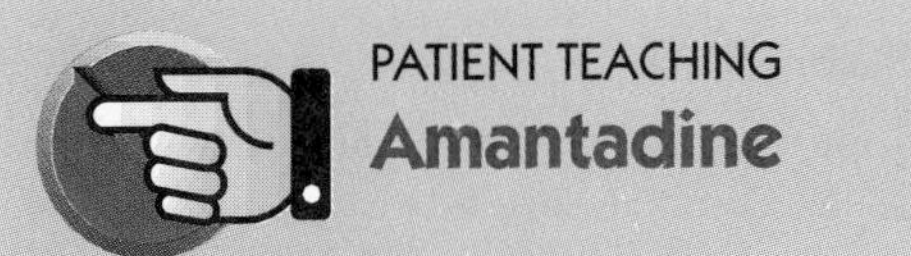

PATIENT TEACHING
Amantadine

- Teach the patient and family the name, dose, frequency, action, and adverse effects of amantadine.
- Instruct the patient to take the drug after meals for maximum absorption.
- Advise an older patient to take the drug in two daily doses rather than a single dose to avoid adverse neurologic reactions.
- Instruct the patient with insomnia to take the drug several hours before bedtime.
- Instruct the patient to stand or change positions slowly if orthostatic hypotension occurs.
- Instruct the patient to report adverse reactions, especially signs of central nervous system (CNS) disturbances (dizziness, depression, anxiety, and nausea) and renal impairment (change in urine itself or in urine elimination pattern).
- Caution the patient not to perform activities that require alertness or physical coordination if adverse CNS reactions occur.
- Teach the patient to use infection-control measures, such as staying away from crowds or people with infections, if leukopenia occurs.
- Advise the patient to be alert for excessive anticholinergic effects during concomitant therapy with an anticholinergic agent.
- Teach the patient how to handle such adverse reactions as dry mouth or constipation.
- Instruct the patient to limit salt and fluid intake if fluid retention occurs.
- Instruct the patient to notify the physician if adverse reactions or drug interactions occur.

- Closely monitor the patient with a history of heart failure for exacerbation or recurrence of heart failure as evidenced by shortness of breath, tachycardia, jugular vein distention, or crackles in the lungs.
- Expect to reduce the dosage as prescribed in a patient with renal impairment or a history of seizures.
- Notify the physician if adverse reactions or drug interactions occur.

Evaluation

For each nursing diagnosis, prepare an evaluation statement that describes the patient's or family's response to nursing interventions.

Ribavirin

Ribavirin currently is available only to treat respiratory syncytial virus (RSV) infections in children. It is administered by aerosol inhalation only, using a small particle aerosol generator such as the Viratek Model 2.

PHARMACOKINETICS

Ribavirin is administered via nasal or oral inhalation and is absorbed well. It has a limited, specific distribution, with the highest concentration level found in the pulmonary tract and in erythrocytes. Ribavirin is metabolized in the liver and by erythrocytes. The main route of excretion is via the kidneys, with some of it excreted in the feces.

Route	Onset	Peak	Duration
Inhalation	Immediate	Immediate	9 hr

PHARMACODYNAMICS

The mechanism of action of ribavirin is not known completely, but the drug's metabolites inhibit viral DNA and ribonucleic acid synthesis, subsequently halting viral replication.

PHARMACOTHERAPEUTICS

Ribavirin therapy is indicated in infants and young children who have severe lower respiratory tract infections caused by RSV.

Drug interactions

Ribavirin has been shown to antagonize the antiviral activity of zidovudine in vitro; the patient should be monitored closely if both drugs are used concomitantly. Because concomitant use of these drugs also may cause hematologic toxicity, blood counts should be monitored routinely.

Concomitant use of ribavirin and a digitalis glycoside, such as digoxin or digitoxin, can cause digitalis intoxication, producing such effects as GI distress, CNS abnormalities, and cardiac arrhythmias. These effects have not yet been fully evaluated.

ADVERSE DRUG REACTIONS

Adverse reactions to ribavirin include worsening of respiratory function, ventilator dependence, pneumothorax, apnea, cardiac arrest, and hypotension. Reticulosis also has been reported. Other adverse reactions include rash, conjunctivitis, and erythema of the eyelids.

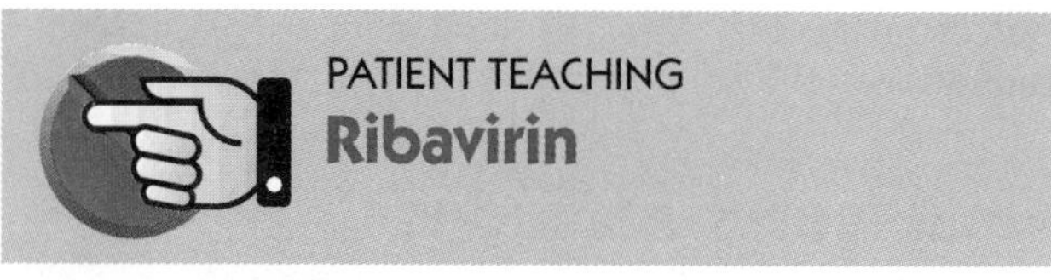

PATIENT TEACHING
Ribavirin

- Teach the patient and family the name, dose, frequency, action, and adverse effects of ribavirin. (Remember to tailor your remarks according to the child's comprehension.)
- Encourage the patient and family to ask questions throughout ribavirin therapy.

NURSING PROCESS APPLICATION

The following information assists the nurse in caring for a patient who is receiving ribavirin. It includes an overview of assessment activities as well as examples of appropriate nursing diagnoses and related interventions. It also highlights the importance of evaluation.

Assessment

Before drug therapy begins, review the patient's history for conditions that contraindicate or require cautious use of ribavirin. Also review the patient's medication history to identify use of drugs that may interact with it. During therapy, assess the patient for adverse drug reactions and signs of drug interactions. Also, periodically assess the effectiveness of ribavirin therapy. Finally, evaluate the patient's and family's knowledge of the prescribed drug.

Nursing diagnoses

- Risk for injury related to adverse drug reactions or drug interactions
- Impaired gas exchange related to worsening of respiratory function caused by ribavirin
- Knowledge deficit related to ribavirin regimen

Planning and implementation

- Do not administer ribavirin to a patient with a condition that contraindicates its use.
- Do not administer ribavirin to a patient who requires mechanical ventilation; the drug can precipitate in the ventilatory apparatus, jeopardizing adequate ventilation.
- Administer ribavirin cautiously to a patient with a preexisting condition.
- Monitor the patient closely for adverse reactions and drug interactions during ribavirin therapy.
- Monitor the patient's cardiac status throughout ribavirin therapy. Notify the physician if hypotension or cardiac dysfunction occurs. Have standard emergency equipment nearby and be prepared to begin cardiopulmonary resuscitation if cardiac arrest occurs.
- Ensure that ribavirin solution is prepared by diluting 6 g of ribavirin powder in 50 to 100 ml of sterile water. The solution should be transferred to an Erlenmeyer flask (which serves as the reservoir for the small particle aerosol generator) and diluted further to a volume of 300 ml.
- Administer ribavirin with the small particle aerosol generator. Do not use any other aerosol-generating device.
- When reconstituting ribavirin powder, use sterile water for injection, not **bacteriostatic** water that may contain antimicrobial agents.
- Discard solutions placed in the small particle aerosol generator at least every 24 hours before adding newly reconstituted solutions.
- Reconstituted solutions can be stored at room temperature for 24 hours; discard after 24 hours.

• Perform a complete respiratory assessment *every hour* throughout ribavirin therapy. Monitor arterial blood gas values and be prepared to support the patient's ventilation if the patient's respiratory condition worsens. Notify the physician immediately of any change in the patient's respiratory status. (See Patient Teaching: *Ribavirin.*)

Evaluation

For each nursing diagnosis, prepare an evaluation statement that describes the patient's or family's response to nursing interventions.

Zidovudine, didanosine, and zalcitabine

Zidovudine was the first drug to receive Food and Drug Administration (FDA) approval for treating AIDS or AIDS-related complex (ARC). Didanosine and zalcitabine are new drugs used to treat advanced human immunodeficiency virus (HIV) infections.

PHARMACOKINETICS

Zidovudine is absorbed well from the GI tract, distributed widely, metabolized by the liver, and excreted by the kidneys. Its duration of action is 4 hours.

Because didanosine is degraded rapidly at gastric pH, didanosine tablets and powder contain a buffering agent to increase pH. The exact route of metabolism has not been determined. Approximately 50% of an absorbed dose is excreted in the urine.

Oral zalcitabine is absorbed well from the GI tract when administered on an empty stomach; absorption is reduced when administered with food. Zalcitabine penetrates the blood-brain barrier.

zidovudine

Route	Onset	Peak	Duration
P.O.	Unknown	0.5-2 hr	2-6 hr
I.V.	Immediate	1.5 hr	3 hr

PHARMACODYNAMICS

Zidovudine is converted by cellular enzymes to an active form, zidovudine triphosphate. The metabolite prevents viral DNA from replicating. Didanosine and zalcitabine also undergo cellular enzyme conversion to their active antiviral metabolites, which block HIV replication. (See *How zidovudine works.*)

PHARMACOTHERAPEUTICS

Zidovudine I.V. has been used to help patients with AIDS and ARC who have a history of *Pneumocystis carinii* pneu-

How zidovudine works

Zidovudine can inhibit replication of human immunodeficiency virus (HIV). The first two illustrations show how HIV invades cells and then replicates itself. The bottom illustration shows how zidovudine blocks viral transformation.

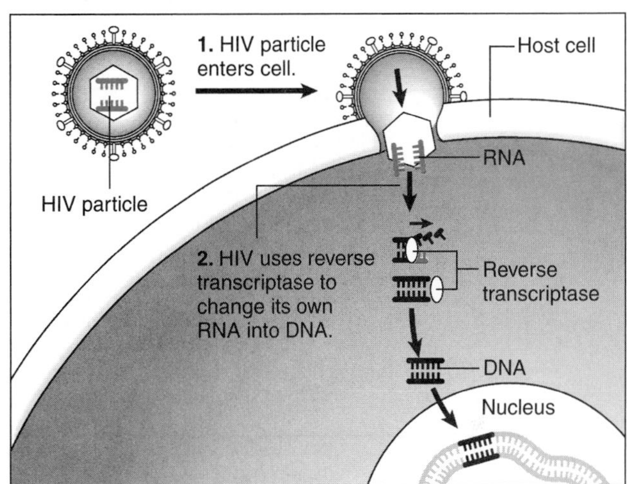

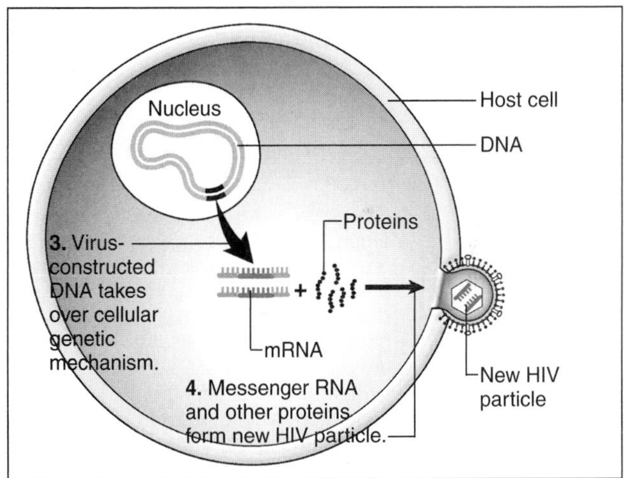

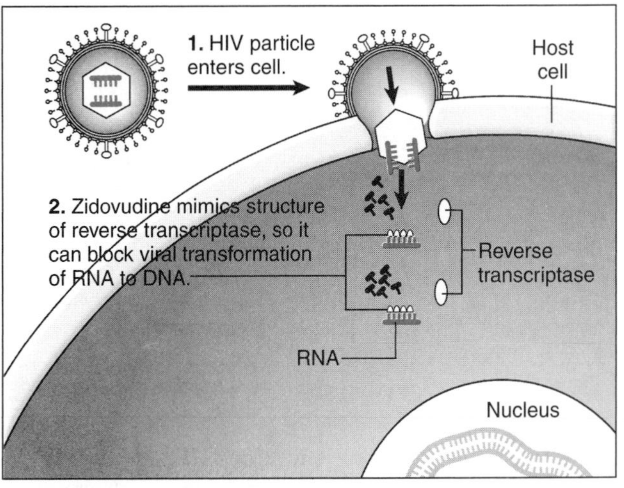

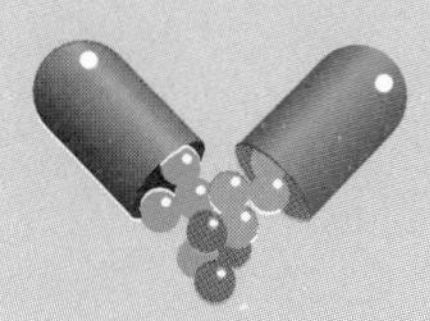

DRUG INTERACTIONS

Zidovudine, didanosine, and zalcitabine

Zidovudine, didanosine, and zalcitabine may interact with various drugs, producing toxic and other adverse effects.

DRUG	INTERACTING DRUGS	POSSIBLE EFFECTS	NURSING IMPLICATIONS
zidovudine	dapsone, pentamidine isethionate, flucytosine, vincristine, vinblastine, doxorubicin, interferon, ganciclovir	Increased nephrotoxic and cytotoxic effects	• Avoid concurrent administration if possible; if not, closely monitor the patient's blood count and renal function.
	probenecid, aspirin, acetaminophen, indomethacin, cimetidine, lorazepam	Inhibited zidovudine metabolism, increased risk of toxicity for either drug	• Avoid concurrent use if possible; if not, use with extreme caution.
	acyclovir	Profound drowsiness and lethargy	• Monitor the patient closely during concomitant therapy.
didanosine	tetracyclines	Decreased absorption of tetracyclines	• Avoid concurrent administration if possible.
	drugs whose absorption is pH-dependent, such as ketoconazole and dapsone	Altered absorption of pH-dependent drugs	• Administer pH-dependent drugs at least 2 hours before didanosine.
didanosine (formulations that contain magnesium or aluminum, such as chewable buffered tablets or oral suspension)	quinolone antibiotics	Decreased plasma concentrations of some quinolone antibiotics	• Administer quinolone antibiotics at least 2 hours before didanosine.
zalcitabine	amphotericin B, foscarnet, aminoglycosides, chloramphenicol, cisplatin, dapsone, disulfiram, ethionamide, glutethimide, gold salts, hydralazine, iodoquinol, isoniazid, metronidazole, nitrofurantoin, phenytoin, ribavirin, vincristine	Increased risk of peripheral neuropathy or nephrotoxicity	• Avoid concurrent administration if possible; if not, monitor the patient closely for signs and symptoms of peripheral neuropathy and monitor laboratory studies for evidence of significant change in renal function that would require a dosage adjustment.
	pentamidine isethionate	Increased risk of fulminant pancreatitis	• Avoid concurrent use. If pentamidine isethionate must be given, treatment with didanosine or zalcitabine must be interrupted.
	magnesium/aluminium antacids	25% decrease in zalcitabine absorption	• Do not administer simultaneously.

monia or a T lymphocyte count lower than 200 cells/mm^3 and to prevent maternal-fetal HIV transmission. Oral zidovudine has been used as initial treatment in patients with a CD4$^+$ T-cell count less than 500 cells/mm^3 or in children younger than age 3 months with HIV-related symptoms or with laboratory values suggesting HIV-related immunosuppression.

Didanosine is used to treat advanced HIV infection in adults and pediatric patients (over age 6 months) who cannot tolerate zidovudine or who have demonstrated significant clinical or immunologic deterioration during zidovudine therapy. Zalcitabine is used in combination with zidovudine to treat advanced HIV infection (a CD4$^+$ T-cell count less than 300 cells/mm^3) in adults who have significant clinical or immunologic deterioration.

Drug interactions

Many drug interactions occur with zidovudine, didanosine, and zalcitabine. (See Drug Interactions: *Zidovudine, didanosine, and zalcitabine.*)

ADVERSE DRUG REACTIONS

The most common adverse reactions to zidovudine are hematologic. Significant anemia occurs 4 to 6 weeks after therapy is initiated, and granulocytopenia appears within 6 to 8 weeks.

Headache has been reported in up to 50% of patients who have received zidovudine. Other CNS reactions include dizziness, agitation, restlessness, and insomnia. Nausea, vomiting, abdominal pain, diarrhea, dyspepsia, and anorexia are the most common GI reactions. Myalgia, diaphoresis, dyspnea, fever, rash, and unusual taste in the mouth also may occur.

Adverse reactions to didanosine reported in 5% or more of adult patients during clinical trials include headache, diarrhea, peripheral neuropathy, asthenia, nausea, vomiting, insomnia, rash, pruritus, abdominal pain, CNS depression, constipation, stomatitis, myalgia, arthritis, loss of taste, unusual taste in the mouth, dry mouth, pancreatitis, alopecia, and dizziness.

Adverse reactions to zalcitabine reported in more than 5% of patients during clinical trials include peripheral neuropathy, mouth ulcers, nausea, rash, headache, myalgia, and fatigue.

NURSING PROCESS APPLICATION

The following information assists the nurse in caring for a patient who is receiving zidovudine, didanosine, or zalcitabine. It includes an overview of assessment activities as well as examples of appropriate nursing diagnoses and related interventions. It also highlights the importance of evaluation.

Assessment

Before drug therapy begins, review the patient's history for conditions that contraindicate or require cautious use of zidovudine, didanosine, or zalcitabine. Also review the patient's medication history to identify use of drugs that may interact with them. During therapy, assess the patient for adverse drug reactions and signs of drug interactions. Also, periodically assess the effectiveness of zidovudine, didanosine, or zalcitabine therapy. Finally, evaluate the patient's and family's knowledge of the prescribed drug.

Nursing diagnoses

- Risk for injury related to adverse drug reactions or drug interactions
- Knowledge deficit related to zidovudine, didanosine, or zalcitabine regimen

Planning and implementation

- Do not administer zidovudine, didanosine, or zalcitabine to a patient with a condition that contraindicates its use.
- Administer zidovudine, didanosine, or zalcitabine cautiously to a patient with a preexisting condition.
- Monitor the patient periodically for adverse reactions and drug interactions to the prescribed drug.

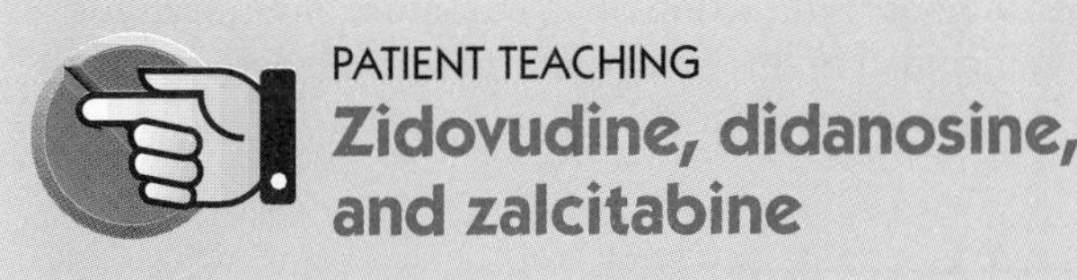

PATIENT TEACHING

Zidovudine, didanosine, and zalcitabine

- Teach the patient and family the name, dose, frequency, action, and adverse effects of zidovudine, didanosine, or zalcitabine.
- Instruct the patient taking zidovudine to take the drug every 4 hours around the clock, even though it means interrupting sleep.
- Inform the patient that zidovudine, didanosine, and zalcitabine do not reduce the risk of transmitting the human immunodeficiency virus to others through sexual contact or blood contamination.
- Caution the patient to avoid over-the-counter medications and to check with the physician, pharmacist, or nurse before taking any.
- Instruct the patient to take didanosine or zalcitabine on an empty stomach.
- Tell the patient receiving didanosine or zalcitabine to immediately report signs and symptoms of pancreatitis, such as abdominal pain and vomiting. Also tell the patient to report numbness, tingling, or pain in hands or feet because didanosine may also cause peripheral neuropathy.
- Caution the patient with phenylketonuria who is receiving didanosine that the drug contains phenylalanine.
- Stress the importance of returning regularly for blood tests.
- Caution the patient not to perform activities that require alertness if adverse central nervous system reactions such as dizziness occur.
- Instruct the patient to notify the physician if adverse reactions occur.

- Monitor the patient's red blood cell count and WBC count, as prescribed, for the patient receiving zidovudine or zalcitabine.
- Monitor the patient closely for pancreatitis and peripheral neuropathy when administering didanosine or zalcitabine. Be aware that pancreatitis may be fatal. If pancreatitis is suspected, expect to discontinue didanosine or zalcitabine immediately. (See Patient Teaching: *Zidovudine, didanosine, and zalcitabine.*)
- Administer didanosine and zalcitabine on an empty stomach.
- Notify the physician if adverse reactions or drug interactions occur.

Evaluation

For each nursing diagnosis, prepare an evaluation statement that describes the patient's or family's response to nursing interventions.

Protease inhibitors

Protease inhibitors are agents that prevent cleavage of the viral polyprotein through inhibition of viral protease. This results in the production of an immature, noninfectious cell. Included in this group are saquinavir mesylate, ritonavir, and indinavir sulfate.

PHARMACOKINETICS

Saquinavir mesylate partitions into the tissues, with up to 98% of it binding to plasma proteins. It is metabolized by the liver and excreted mainly by the kidneys.

Ritonavir is metabolized by the liver and broken down into at least five metabolites. It is mainly excreted in the feces, with some elimination through the kidneys.

Indinavir sulfate is rapidly absorbed and 60% binds to plasma proteins. Seven metabolites have been identified. The drug is excreted mainly through feces.

Route	Onset	Peak	Duration
P.O.	Unknown	20 min-4 hr	< 8 hr

PHARMACODYNAMICS

All of the agents are synthetic peptide-like substrate analogs that inhibit the activity of HIV protease and prevent the cleavage of viral polyproteins. Ritonavir is a petidomimetic inhibitor of both HIV-1 and HIV-2 proteases.

PHARMACOTHERAPEUTICS

Protease inhibitors are indicated for use in combination with nucleoside analogs for treatment of HIV infection.

Drug interactions

Protease inhibitors may interact with various drugs. (See Drug interactions: *Protease inhibitors.*)

ADVERSE DRUG REACTIONS

Most adverse reactions to saquinavir mesylate are of mild intensity. The most commonly reported are diarrhea, abdominal discomfort, and nausea. During clinical trials, the following were rare occurrences: confusion, ataxia, weakness, acute myeloblastic leukemia, hemolytic anemia, Stevens-Johnson syndrome, seizures, severe cutaneous reaction associated with increased liver function tests, isolated elevation of transaminases and thromboplebitis, headache and thrombocytopenia, exacerbation of chronic liver disease with grade 4 elevated liver function tests, jaundice, ascites, and right and left upper quadrant abdominal pain.

The most common clinical adverse events in clinical trials with ritonavir include asthenia and GI and neurologic disturbances, such as nausea, diarrhea, vomiting, anorexia, abdominal pain, taste perversion, and circumoral and peripheral paresthesia.

The most common adverse reactions (occurring in 2% or more of patients) in trials of indinavir sulfate include abdominal pain, asthenia and fatigue, flank pain, malaise, nausea, diarrhea, vomiting, acid regurgitation, anorexia, dry mouth, headache, insomnia, dizziness, sleeplessness, taste perversion, and back pain.

NURSING PROCESS APPLICATION

The following information assists the nurse in caring for a patient who is receiving protease inhibitors. It includes an overview of assessment activities as well as examples of appropriate nursing diagnoses and related interventions. It also highlights the importance of evaluation.

Assessment

Before drug therapy begins, review the patient's history for conditions that contraindicate or require cautious use of protease inhibitors. Also review the patient's medication history to identify use of drugs that may interact with them. During therapy, assess the patient for adverse drug reactions and signs of drug interactions. Also, periodically assess the effectiveness of therapy with protease inhibitors. Finally, evaluate the patient's and family's knowledge of the prescribed drug.

Nursing diagnoses

- Risk for injury related to adverse drug reactions or drug interactions
- Knowledge deficit related to protease inhibitor regimen

Planning and implementation

- Do not administer protease inhibitors to a patient with a condition that contraindicates its use.
- Administer protease inhibitors cautiously to a patient with a preexisting condition.
- Monitor the patient periodically for adverse reactions and drug interactions to the prescribed drug.
- Warn patients on saquinavir mesylate that they should avoid exposure to ultraviolet light, as photosensitization may occur.
- Use caution in administering protease inhibitors to patients with impaired liver function, as these drugs are metabolized by the liver.
- Safe use of saquinavir mesylate in children younger than age 16 has not been established.
- Because it is not known whether saquinavir mesylate is excreted in the breast milk, breast-feeding is not encouraged.
- Indinavir sulfate is excreted in breast milk; it is recommended that breast-feeding be ceased when drug administration begins.
- Advise patients that saquinavir mesylate should be taken within 2 hours after a full meal. (See Patient Teaching: *Protease inhibitors,* page 432.)
- Advise patients that ritonavir should be taken with food.
- For optimum absorption, indinavir sulfate should be taken without food and with a full glass of water at least 1 hour before a meal.
- Notify the primary physician if adverse reactions or drug interactions occur.

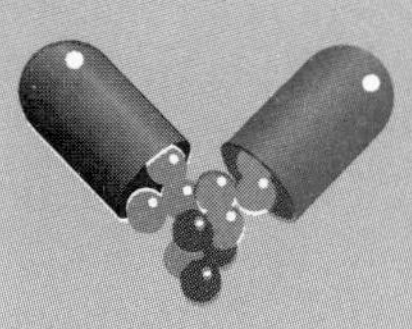

DRUG INTERACTIONS

Protease inhibitors

Protease inhibitors may interact with various drugs, producing toxic and other adverse effects.

DRUG	INTERACTING DRUGS	POSSIBLE EFFECTS	NURSING IMPLICATIONS
saquinavir	rifamycins, phenobarbital, phenytoin, dexamethasone, carbamazepine	Decreased action of saquinavir	• Avoid concurrent administration if possible; if not, closely monitor the patient's serum levels and cardiac function.
	terfenadine, astemizole	Possible prolonged QT intervals leads to serious adverse cardiovascular events	• Avoid concurrent use if possible; if not, use with extreme caution. • Monitor the patient closely during concomitant therapy.
ritonavir	alpha blockers, antiarrhythmics, antidepressants, antiemetics, antifungals, antihyperlipidemics, antimalarials, antineoplastics, beta blockers, calcium channel blockers, cimetidine, corticosteroids, erthyromycin, immunosuppressants, methylphenidiate, pentoxifylline, phenothiazines, warfarin	Ritonavir may increase the pharmaceutical effects of these drugs	• Avoid concurrent administration if possible; if not, monitor the patient closely.
	atovaquone, clofibrate, daunorubicin, diphenoxylate, metoclopramide, sedatives, hypnotics	These agents may have decreased pharmaceutical effects	• Avoid concurrent administration if possible; if not, monitor the patient closely.
indinavir sulfate	astemizole, cisapride, midazolam, terfenadine, triazolam	Use of these drugs with indinavir could result in potentially fatal events such as cardiac arrhythmias	• Avoid concurrent administration if possible; if not, monitor the patient closely.
	zidovudine, rifabutin, clarithromycin, isoniazide, trimethporim, stavudine	The effects of these agents are potentiated	• Avoid concurrent administration; if possible; if not, monitor the patient closely.
	didanosine	Buffering agents in didanosine decrease optimum gastric absorption of indinavir sulfate	• Administer at least 1 hour apart on an empty stomach.
	rifampin	Rifampin is a potent inducer of P450, which will markedly reduce indinavir sulfate plasma concentrations	• Avoid concurrent use.
	nelfinavir	Results in major decrease (82%) plasma decrease in nelfinavir levels	• Do not co-administer nelfinavir and rifampin.
	rifabutin	Results in major increases in serum plasma levels of rifabutin (207%)	• It is recommended that the rifabutin dose be reduced to one-half of usual.
	terfenadine	Interferes with metabolism of terfenadine; possible life-threatening cardiac arrhythmias	• Avoid concurrent administration.
	oral contraceptives	Decreases effectiveness of contraceptive therapy	• Use alternative or additional contraceptive methods.

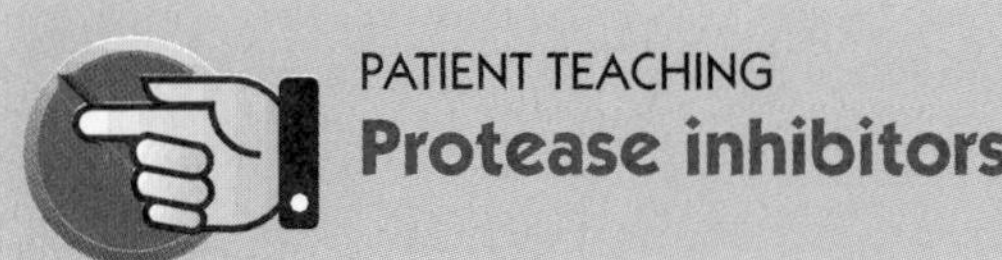

PATIENT TEACHING
Protease inhibitors

- Teach the patient and family the name, dose, frequency, action, and adverse effects of the protease inhibitor that is prescribed.
- Advise the patient that none of the agents have been shown to reduce the risk of transmitting human immunodeficiency virus through sexual contact or blood contamination.
- Instruct the patient taking saquinavir mesylate that he should avoid exposure to ultraviolet light because photosensitization may occur.
- Advise the patient that saquinavir mesylate should be taken within 2 hours after a full meal.
- Advise the patient that ritonavir should be taken with food.
- Teach the patient that indinavir sulfate should be taken without food and with a full glass of water at least 1 hour before a meal.
- Tell the patient taking ritonavir or indinavir sulfate that it should be taken every day as prescribed. If a dose is missed, the next dose should be taken as soon as possible, but if a dose is skipped, a double dose should not be taken.
- Advise the patient that the taste of ritonavir may be improved by mixing it with chocolate milk, Ensure, or Advera within 1 hour of dosing.
- Advise the patient that indinavir capsules are sensitive to moisture; they should be stored in the original container with the desiccant.
- Advise the breast-feeding patient to avoid breast-feeding while on protease inhibitors because of their possible excretion in breast milk.
- Inform the patient that ritonavir should be stored in a refrigerator, but can be unrefrigerated for up to 30 days.

Evaluation

For each nursing diagnosis, prepare an evaluation statement that describes the patient's or family's response to nursing interventions.

CHAPTER SUMMARY

Chapter 32 discussed the antiviral agents available today. Here are the chapter highlights.

Acyclovir is used to treat herpesvirus infections; its derivative, ganciclovir, is used to treat HSV and CMV infections.

Foscarnet is an antiviral agent used to treat CMV retinitis in patients with AIDS.

Amantadine is an oral antiviral drug used to prevent or treat influenza A viral infections.

Ribavirin, the only therapeutic agent available to treat RSV in children, is available in aerosol form only.

Zidovudine was the first drug to receive FDA approval for treating AIDS or ARC. Didanosine is used to treat advanced HIV infections in patients who cannot tolerate zidovudine or who have demonstrated significant clinical or immunologic deterioration during zidovudine therapy. Zalcitabine is prescribed in combination with zidovudine to treat advanced HIV infection in adults with a CD4+ T-cell count less than 200 cells/mm^3 who have significant clinical or immunologic deterioration. Finally, the new class of agents, the protease inhibitors indinavir, ritonavir, and saquinavir, are being used in patients who are HIV-positive.

The nurse must monitor the patient closely for adverse reactions to the prescribed antiviral agent because reactions can be serious.

Questions to consider

See Appendix 1 for answers.

1. John Doant is a 60-year-old male diagnosed with AIDS. The physician has ordered retrovir 200 mg P.O. every hour around the clock. Which of the following drugs is commonly used as an adjunct when the CD4+ T-cell count is less than 200 cells/mm^3?
   (a) didanosine
   (b) cimetidine
   (c) ganciclovir
   (d) zalcitabine

2. Toynesia Johnson, age 32, is diagnosed with an HSV-2 infection. The physician prescribes oral acyclovir. Which of the following is the most common adverse reaction to oral acyclovir?
   (a) Dizziness
   (b) Leg pain
   (c) Headache
   (d) Blurred vision

3. Zidovudine is ordered every 4 hours, but Kim Lee Hoe wants to know if he can take twice as much every 8 hours. Which of the following statements is the best answer?
   (a) Yes, twice as much will last twice as long.
   (b) No, the physician wants you to awaken at night and reposition yourself.
   (c) Yes, as long as you take it on an empty stomach.
   (d) No, because the duration of action is only 4 hours.

4. Sonny Walker, age 24, is hospitalized with an advanced HIV infection. The physician prescribes didanosine 125 mg P.O. twice daily. Which of the following instructions should the nurse give Mr. Walker about didanosine therapy?
   (a) Take didanosine with meals.
   (b) Take didanosine on an empty stomach.
   (c) Take didanosine every 4 hours around the clock.
   (d) Take over-the-counter medications to treat minor adverse reactions.

33 Antitubercular agents

OBJECTIVES

After reading and studying this chapter, the student should be able to:
1. identify the first-line agents employed in treating tuberculosis (TB).
2. identify the genetic factors that can affect the actions of these agents.
3. identify drug interactions associated with antitubercular agents.
4. identify the major adverse reactions to these agents and intervene appropriately.
5. teach the patient with a mycobacterial infection about the disease and its drug therapy.
6. describe how to apply the nursing process when caring for a patient who is receiving an antitubercular agent.

INTRODUCTION

Antitubercular agents are used to treat TB, which is caused by *Mycobacterium tuberculosis.* These agents also are effective against less common mycobacterial infections caused by *M. kansasii, M. avium-intracellulare, M. fortuitum,* and related organisms. Not always curative, these agents can halt the progression of a mycobacterial infection.

Unlike most antibiotics, agents may need to be administered over many months. This creates problems, such as patient noncompliance, the development of bacterial resistance, and drug toxicity. To help the patient during long-term therapy, the nurse must be aware of these and other problems. (See *Selected major antitubercular agents,* page 434.)

Drugs covered in this chapter include:
- aminosalicyclic acid
- capreomycin sulfate
- cycloserine
- ethambutol
- ethionamide
- fluroquinolones
- isoniazid
- pyrazinamide
- rifampin
- streptomycin sulfate.

Antitubercular agents

Since 1984, dramatic changes in TB morbidity trends have threatened the control of this disease. A significant increase in the number of reported cases and the emergence of multiple drug-resistant TB strains, particularly in the human immunodeficiency virus–infected population, have necessitated new treatment recommendations.

Traditionally, isoniazid, rifampin, and ethambutol were the mainstays of multidrug TB therapy and successfully prevented the emergence of drug resistance. Because of the current incidence of drug-resistant strains, however, a four-drug regimen with isoniazid, rifampin, pyrazinamide and streptomycin or ethambutol is now recommended for initial treatment. These agents should be modified if local susceptibility testing demonstrates resistance to one or more of these agents. If local outbreaks of TB resistant to isoniazid and rifampin are occurring in institutions (for example, health-care and correctional facilities), then five-drug or six-drug regimens are recommended as initial therapy. (See *Regimen options for initial treatment of TB in children and adults,* page 435.)

PHARMACOKINETICS

Antitubercular agents almost exclusively are administered orally; isoniazid, capreomycin, streptomycin, kanamycin, and amikacin are commercially available parenterally. When administered orally, they are absorbed well from the gastrointestinal (GI) tract and distributed widely throughout the body. The drugs are metabolized primarily in the liver and excreted by the kidneys.

About 75% to 80% of an oral dose of ethambutol is absorbed rapidly from the GI tract. The drug is distributed widely into most body tissues and fluids; about twice as much appears in erythrocytes as appears in plasma. (The erythrocytes may serve as a reservoir, slowly releasing the drug into the circulation.) Ethambutol crosses the placenta. It appears in breast milk in concentrations roughly equal to those of plasma concentrations. The liver metabolizes up to 15% of ethambutol, and the kidneys excrete almost all of it, primarily as unchanged drug.

Isoniazid is absorbed well from the GI tract and intramuscular (I.M.) injection sites and is distributed into all body tissues and fluids, readily crossing the blood-brain barrier and the placenta. It is distributed into breast milk in

Selected major antitubercular agents

The following chart summarizes the first-line agents used to treat mycobacterial infections. Effective therapy usually combines these drugs with each other or with second-line agents.

DRUG	MAJOR INDICATIONS AND USUAL DOSAGES	CONTRAINDICATIONS AND PRECAUTIONS
Antitubercular agents		
ethambutol (EMB)	*Uncomplicated pulmonary tuberculosis (TB), infections caused by* Mycobacterium bovis *and most strains of* M. kansasii ADULT: 15 to 25 mg/kg P.O. once daily for 60 days; dosage decreased to 15 mg/kg P.O. once daily if previously treated PEDIATRIC: for ages 6 and older, 10 to 15 mg/kg P.O. daily. Although the manufacturer does not recommend EMB for pediatric use, many physicians use this drug dosage for pediatric patients.	• EMB is contraindicated in a patient with known optic neuritis or hypersensitivity to the drug, unless clinical judgment determines that it may be used. • Administer with caution to a pregnant patient.
isoniazid	*Treatment of TB; prevention of TB* ADULT: (treatment) 5 to 15 mg/kg P.O. or I.M. once daily, up to a maximum of 300 mg/day for at least 1 year; (prevention) 300 mg P.O. once daily for 6 months to 1 year PEDIATRIC: 10 to 20 mg/kg P.O. or I.M. once daily, depending on the severity of the disease, up to a maximum of 500 mg daily	• Know that isoniazid is contraindicated in a patient with known hypersensitivity to the drug; a history of severe adverse reactions to isoniazid, such as drug fever, chills, or arthritis; or acute liver disease of any etiology. • Administer with caution to a pregnant or breast-feeding patient; one with current chronic liver disease, severe renal dysfunction, or daily alcohol use; or one who is receiving phenytoin concurrently.
rifampin	*Treatment of TB* ADULT: 10 mg/kg to maximum 600 mg P.O. once daily, 1 hour before or 2 hours after a meal PEDIATRIC: for neonates under age 1 week, up to 10 mg/kg P.O. or I.V. once daily; for older children, 10 to 20 mg/kg P.O. or I.V. once daily, up to a maximum of 600 mg daily *Asymptomatic* Neisseria meningitidis *carriers* ADULTS: 600 mg P.O. once daily 1 hour before or 2 hours after a meal for 4 days, or 600 mg P.O. b.i.d. for 2 days PEDIATRIC: 10 to 20 mg/kg to maximum of 600 mg P.O. once daily 1 hour before or 2 hours after a meal for 4 days	• Rifampin is contraindicated in a breast-feeding patient, one with a history of hypersensitivity to any of the rifamycins, or in the treatment of meningococcal disease. • Administer with extreme caution to a pregnant patient.
pyrazinamide	*Treatment of TB* ADULTS: 15 to 30 mg/kg P.O. daily for patients for 6 months (9 months for patients infected with human immunodeficiency virus). Alternatively, 50 to 70 mg/kg (maximum 4 g) P.O. may be given twice weekly, or 50 to 70 mg/kg (maximum 3 g) P.O. given three times weekly.	• Administer with caution to a pregnant or breast-feeding patient or one with current chronic liver disease, severe renal dysfunction, or daily alcohol use. • Safe use of pyrazinamide in children under age 12 has not definitely been established. While the manufacturer does not recommend its use in children, the Centers for Disease Control and Prevention recommends that pyrazinamide be dosed the same in children as in adults.

concentration levels similar to those of the maternal plasma. Isoniazid is metabolized almost completely by enzymatic acetylation and hydrolysis in the liver. The rate of acetylation, however, is determined by race-linked genetic factors. Although these genetic factors can produce significant variations in the rate of isoniazid elimination, the drug still is effective when administered two or three times a week. Its effectiveness is reduced for some patients (fast acetylators), however, when administered once weekly. From 75% to 95% of isoniazids excreted in the urine as

Regimen options for the initial treatment of TB in children and adults

There are three regimen options for the initial treatment of TB in patients not infected with human immunodeficiency virus (HIV), as shown below. For the treatment of TB in patients infected with HIV, options 1, 2, or 3 can be used, although treatment regimens should continue for a minimum of 9 months, including at least 6 months beyond culture conversion.

TB WITHOUT HIV INFECTION

Option 1

Administer daily isoniazid, rifampin, and pyrazinamide for 8 weeks, followed by 16 weeks of isoniazid and rifampin daily or two to three times weekly* in areas where the isoniazid resistance rate is not documented to be less than 4%. Ethambutol or streptomycin should be added to the initial regimen until susceptibility to isoniazid and rifampin is demonstrated. Continue treatment for a minimum of 6 months, including 3 months beyond culture conversion. Consult a TB medical expert if the patient is symptomatic or if a smear or culture is positive after 3 months.

Option 2

Administer daily isoniazid, rifampin, pyrazinamide, and streptomycin or ethambutol for 2 weeks, followed by two times weekly* administration of the same drugs for 6 weeks (by directly observed therapy [DOT]) and, subsequently, with twice weekly administration of isoniazid and rifampin for 16 weeks (by DOT). Consult a TB medical expert if the patient is symptomatic or if a smear or culture is positive after 3 months.

Option 3

Treat by DOT, three times weekly* with isoniazid, rifampin, pyrazinamide, and ethambutol or streptomycin for 6 months.**

Consult a TB medical expert if the patient is symptomatic or if a smear or culture is positive after 3 months.

*All regimens administered at two or three times weekly should be monitored by direct observation for the duration of therapy.
**The strongest evidence from clinical trials is the effectiveness of all four drugs administered for the full 6 months. There is weaker evidence that streptomycin can be discontinued after 4 months if the isolate is susceptible to all drugs. The evidence for stopping pyrazinamide before the end of 6 months is equivocal for the three times/week regimen, and there is no evidence on the effectiveness of this regimen with ethambutol for less than the full 6 months.

metabolites and unchanged drug within 24 hours after administration. Small amounts are excreted in the saliva, sputum, and feces.

Rifampin also is absorbed well from the GI tract, although food in the stomach can reduce its rate and extent of absorption. The drug diffuses freely into most body tissues and fluids, including the cerebrospinal fluid, in concentrations that are 10% to 20% of plasma concentrations. It crosses the placenta and appears in breast milk. After metabolism in the liver, it is excreted primarily in the feces but also in urine and bile.

Although pyrazinamide is well absorbed and widely distributed into body tissues and fluids, the compound is devoid of antimycobacterial activity at physiologic pH. However, in acidic environments such as those found in TB lesions and macrophages, pyrazinamide has a sterilizing action against *M. tuberculosis,* and is synergistic with isoniazid. pyrazinamide is hydrolyzed in the liver to pyrazinoic acid, the major active metabolite. Approximately 70% of a pyrazinamide dose is excreted in the urine in a 24-hour period.

Route	Onset	Peak	Duration
P.O.	Unknown	1-4 hr	10-24 hr
I.M.	Unknown	1-2 hr	Unknown

PHARMACODYNAMICS

Antitubercular agents are specific for mycobacteria. At usual doses, ethambutol and isoniazid are tuberculostatic, inhibiting growth of *M. tuberculosis* bacteria. In contrast, rifampin is tuberculocidal, destroying the bacteria. Because bacterial resistance to isoniazid and rifampin can develop rapidly, however, they usually are used with other antitubercular agents.

Ethambutol is most active against *M. tuberculosis* but acts, to varying degrees, against all mycobacteria. Although mycobacteria rapidly take up ethambutol, the drug does not inhibit their growth significantly for approximately 24 hours. Its exact mechanism of action remains unclear but may be related to inhibition of cell metabolism, arrest of multiplication, and cell death. Ethambutol acts only against replicating bacteria.

Although isoniazid's exact mechanism of action is not known, evidence suggests that the drug inhibits the synthesis of mycolic acids, important components of the mycobacterium cell wall. This inhibition alters the acid-fastness of the cell and disrupts the cell wall. Because mycolic acid synthesis is unique to mycobacteria, this mechanism explains the high degree of specificity of isoniazid. Only

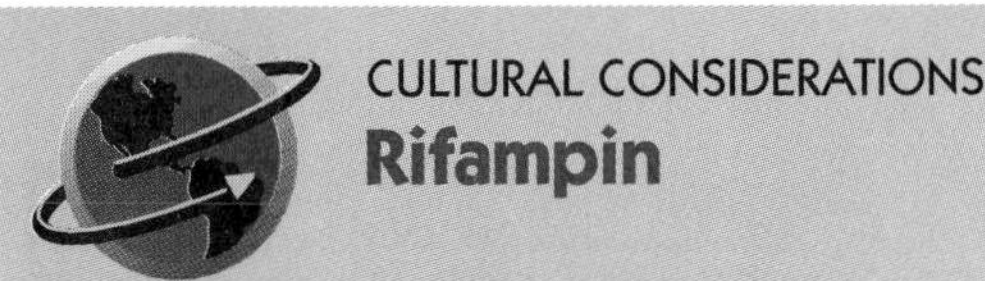

CULTURAL CONSIDERATIONS

Rifampin

The rate of acetylation and dehydrazation of rifampin is genetically determined. Approximately 50% of Blacks and Whites are considered "slow inactivators." The majority of Inuit and Asian peoples, on the other hand, are considered "rapid inactivators." Slow acetylation may lead to higher blood levels of rifampin and an increased risk of toxic reaction.

isoniazid-sensitive bacteria take up the drug, and only replicating, not resting, bacteria appear to be inhibited.

Rifampin inhibits ribonucleic acid (RNA) synthesis in susceptible organisms by acting on the beta subunit of the enzyme RNA polymerase. The drug is effective primarily in replicating bacteria, but may have some effect on resting bacteria as well. (See Cultural Considerations: *Rifampin.*)

The exact mechanism of action of pyrazinamide is not known, but the antimycobacterial activity appears to be linked to the agent's conversion to the active metabolite pyrazinoic acid.

Pyrazinamide is currently recommended as a first-line TB agent in combination with ethambutol, rifampin, and isoniazid. Pyrazinamide is a highly specific agent and only active against *M. tuberculosis.* Natural and acquired resistance to pyrazinamide have been demonstrated and develop rapidly when pyrazinamide is used alone. However, there is no evidence of cross-resistance between pyrazinamide and other available antitubercular agents.

PHARMACOTHERAPEUTICS

Isoniazid usually is used with ethambutol, rifampin, or streptomycin. This is because combination therapy for TB and other mycobacterial infections can prevent or delay the development of bacterial resistance to the drug regimen.

Ehtambutol is used with isoniazid and rifampin to treat uncomplicated pulmonary TB in a patient who lives in a geographic area noted for a high incidence of bacterial resistance or who previously has been treated with antitubercular agents. The drug also is used to treat infections resulting from *Mycobacterium bovis* and most strains of *M. kansasii.*

Although isoniazid is the most important drug for treating TB, bacterial resistance develops rapidly if it is used alone. However, resistance does not pose a problem when isoniazid is used alone to prevent TB in individuals who have been exposed to the disease, and no evidence exists of cross-resistance between isoniazid and other antitubercular agents. Although isoniazid may be given either I.M. or orally (P.O.), I.M. administration offers no special advantages. Experiments with continuous and intermittent therapy eventually may lead to revision of current dosages and regimens.

Rifampin is a first-line agent for treating pulmonary TB and is particularly effective when combined with isoniazid or another antitubercular agent. This drug combats many gram-positive and some gram-negative bacteria but seldom is used for nonmycobacterial infections because bacterial resistance develops rapidly. It is used to treat asymptomatic carriers of *Neisseria meningitidis* when the risk of meningitis is high, but it is not used to treat *N. meningitidis* infections because of the potential for bacterial resistance.

Pyrazinamide is currently recommended as a first-line TB agent in combination with ethambutol, rifampin, and isoniazid. Pyrazinamide is a highly specific agent and only active against *M. tuberculosis.* Natural and acquired resistance to pyrazinamide have been demonstrated and develop rapidly when pyrazinamide is used alone. However, there is no evidence of cross-resistance betweenpyrazinamide and other available antitubercular agents.

Drug interactions

Antitubercular drugs may interact with a number of other drugs. Some evidence suggests that isoniazid, cycloserine, and ethionamide may produce additive central nervous system (CNS) effects. Aluminum hydroxide can significantly decrease the GI absorption of isoniazid. Aminosalicylic acid may inhibit rifampin adsorption. (See Drug Interactions: *Antitubercular agents.*)

ADVERSE DRUG REACTIONS

Adverse reactions to antitubercular agents primarily occur in the GI tract, the peripheral nervous system, and the hepatic system. Fortunately, these reactions seldom are severe enough to necessitate interruption of TB therapy.

Optic neuritis is the only significant adverse reaction to ethambutol. Signs and symptoms include decreased visual acuity, loss of red-green color discrimination, visual field constriction, and central and peripheral scotomas (areas of depressed vision in the visual field). This adverse reaction occurs in only 0.8% of patients receiving 15 mg/kg, but its incidence increases in patients who receive higher dosages or who have renal dysfunction. Discontinuing ethambutol usually reverses the optic neuritis, but if vision impairment is severe, recovery may be incomplete. Pruritus, joint pain, GI distress, malaise, headache, dizziness, and confusion also have been reported with ethambutol therapy. Occasionally, ethambutol therapy increases serum uric acid levels and precipitates an acute gout episode.

The most common hypersensitivity reactions to ethambutol are rash (in 10.5% of patients) and fever (in 0.3%). Hypersensitivity reactions rarely occur with ethambutol and when they do they tend to be mild. Leukopenia, anaphylaxis, and peripheral neuritis with paresthesia of the extremities have been reported.

Peripheral neuritis occurs in 20% of the patients receiving 6 mg/kg of isoniazid daily, and higher doses increase the incidence of this reaction. Usually preceded by paresthesia of the feet and hands, peripheral neuritis is more likely to

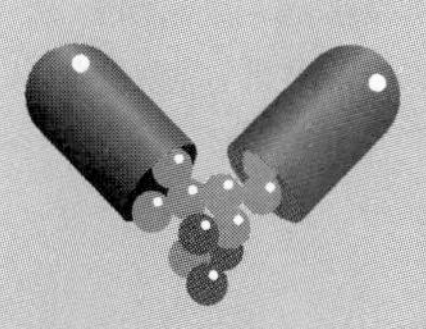

DRUG INTERACTIONS

Antitubercular agents

The following chart presents the important drug interactions for the major antitubercular agents discussed in this chapter.

DRUG	INTERACTING DRUGS	POSSIBLE EFFECTS	NURSING IMPLICATIONS
ethambutol	aluminum hydroxide or other aluminum salts	Decreased gastrointestinal absorption	• Avoid administering ethambutol with antacids.
isoniazid	cycloserine, and ethionamide	Additive central nervous system effects (drowsiness, dizziness, headache, lethargy, depression, tremor, anxiety, confusion, and tinnitus)	• Administer cautiously in combination.
	phenytoin	Increases plasma concentrations of phenytoin	• Decrease dosage of phenytoin as prescribed; monitor for phenytoin toxicity.
	aluminum hydroxide	Significantly decreases isoniazid absorption	• Administer isoniazid at least 1 hour before aluminum antacids.
	corticosteroids	Decreases isoniazid's effects and increases the corticosteroid's effects	• Avoid concomitant use.
	disulfiram	Psychotic episodes and difficulty with coordination	• Avoid concomitant use.
	oral contraceptives, ketoconazole, quinidine, cyclosporine, chloramphenicol, estrogens, corticosteroids, methadone, oral hypoglycemics, warfarin, digitalis glycosides, and dapsone.	Decreased plasma concentration of these drugs	• Dosages of these drugs may need to be increased during rifampin therapy.
rifampin	aminosalicylic acid	Inhibits rifampin absorption	• Avoid concomitant use.

affect an alcoholic, diabetic, or malnourished individual or one who is predisposed to peripheral neuritis. Typically, it produces muscle twitching, dizziness, ataxia, stupor, and paresthesia. Daily administration of 10 to 50 mg of pyridoxine (vitamin B_6) may prevent this reaction. During the first 6 months of therapy, transient elevations occur in levels of the enzymes alanine aminotransferase (ALT) and aspartate aminotransferase (AST) and in bilirubin concentrations in 10% to 20% of patients receiving isoniazid. This drug also may produce hepatitis, especially in elderly patients and usually in the first 4 to 8 weeks of therapy. Isoniazid may precipitate seizures in a patient with a seizure disorder. It also may produce optic neuritis and atrophy, mental abnormalities (such as euphoria and memory impairment), and sedation or incoordination.

While hypersensitivity reactions to isoniazid seldom occur, they produce fever, skin eruptions (morbilliform, maculopapular, purpuric, or exfoliative), lymphadenopathy, and vasculitis. These reactions usually appear 3 to 7 weeks after therapy begins.

The most common adverse reactions to rifampin include epigastric pain, nausea, vomiting, abdominal cramps, flatulence, anorexia, and diarrhea. Joint pain and muscle aches and cramps also may occur. All these reactions, which are most likely to occur during the first 2 weeks of therapy, may subside as biliary excretion of rifampin increases and its half-life decreases; interruption of therapy seldom is necessary. Rifampin can elevate ALT, AST, bilirubin, and alkaline phosphatase levels, possibly leading to eventual discontinuation of the drug. Transient asymptomatic jaundice and red-orange discoloration of sweat, tears, saliva, urine, and feces also may occur but do not necessitate discontinuation of drug therapy.

Large (900- to 1,200-mg) intermittent doses of rifampin produce hypersensitivity reactions in about 1% of patients so treated. This reaction appears as a flulike syndrome characterized by dyspnea with or without wheezing, purpura as-

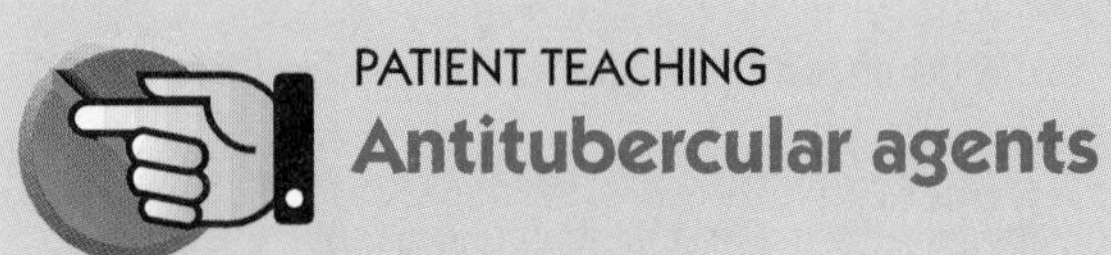

PATIENT TEACHING
Antitubercular agents

- Teach the patient and family the name, dose, frequency, action, and adverse effects of the antitubercular agent.
- Instruct the patient of the importance of adhering to the drug regimen for the full course of the treatment.
- Teach the patient to take rifampin 1 hour before or 2 hours after a meal because food affects the rate and extent of absorption.
- Instruct the patient to take isoniazid at least 1 hour before taking an aluminum antacid to prevent a drug interaction.
- Teach the patient to take pyridoxine concurrently with isoniazid, as prescribed, to prevent peripheral neuritis.
- Instruct the patient taking isoniazid to consult the physician if signs and symptoms of hepatic dysfunction appear, such as nausea, vomiting, fatigue, weakness, and anorexia.
- Instruct the patient taking isoniazid or ethambutol to report any visual changes immediately.
- Advise the patient that rifampin may produce red-orange urine, tears, sputum, sweat, and feces that stain clothes, linen, and soft contact lenses.
- Advise the female patient who is taking rifampin and an oral contraceptive to use an alternate form of birth control.
- Reassure the patient who experiences adverse reactions early in rifampin therapy that most of them will subside with continued treatment.
- Teach the patient the importance of having periodic blood studies performed as instructed.
- Advise the patient to take a mild analgesic (unless contraindicated) for joint pain, muscle aches or cramps, or headache.
- Caution the patient not to perform activities that require mental alertness or motor coordination if adverse central nervous system reactions occur.
- Instruct the patient to notify the physician if adverse reactions occur.

sociated with thrombocytopenia, leukopenia and, rarely, anaphylaxis. A patient with this reaction probably will be able to tolerate a reduced rifampin dosage (only 3% of all patients require discontinuation of this drug).

Hepatotoxicity has been the major limiting adverse effect of pyrazinamide, but this is not as common when the drug is not employed with other hepatoxic agents such as ethionamide. Pyrazinamide is generally well tolerated when used in short-course therapies. Hepatotoxicity appears to be dose-related and can occur anytime during therapy. Renal excretion of urates is inhibited by pyrazinamide, which can result in hyperuricemia and precipitation of gout in predisposed patients. GI disturbances, including nausea, vomiting, and anorexia, have also occurred in patients receiving the drug.

NURSING PROCESS APPLICATION

The following information assists the nurse in caring for a patient who is receiving an antitubercular agent. It includes an overview of assessment activities as well as examples of appropriate nursing diagnoses and related interventions. It also highlights the importance of evaluation.

Assessment

Review the patient's history for a preexisting condition that contraindicates the use of an antitubercular agent, such as known hypersensitivity to the drug or optic neuritis. Also review the patient's history for a preexisting condition that requires cautious use of an antitubercular agent, such as pregnancy, lactation, chronic liver disease, severe renal dysfunction, daily alcohol use, or concomitant phenytoin therapy. Assess the patient for adverse reactions to the prescribed antitubercular agent, such as GI distress, peripheral neuritis, hepatic dysfunction, optic neuritis, or hypersensitivity reactions. Review the patient's medication history to identify the use of drugs that may interact with the prescribed antitubercular agent, such as cycloserine, aluminum hydroxide, phenytoin, oral contraceptives, corticosteroids, or warfarin. Assess the effectiveness of the prescribed antitubercular agent periodically. Evaluate the patient's and family's knowledge about the prescribed antitubercular agent.

Nursing diagnoses

- Risk for injury related to a preexisting condition that requires cautious use of an antitubercular agent
- Risk for injury related to adverse drug reactions
- Sensory/perceptual alterations (tactile, visual) related to peripheral or optic neuritis caused by isoniazid or ethambutol
- Knowledge deficit related to the prescribed antitubercular agent regimen

Planning and implementation

- Do not administer an antitubercular agent to a patient with a condition that contraindicates its use.
- Administer an antitubercular agent cautiously to a patient at risk because of a preexisting condition.
- Monitor the patient for adverse reactions during therapy with an antitubercular agent.
- Assess the patient for sensory deficits when administering ethambutol or isoniazid.
- Monitor the patient closely for hypersensitivity reactions. Keep standard emergency equipment nearby.
- Monitor the patient's liver function tests during isoniazid, pyrazinamide, or rifampin therapy; serum uric acid levels during ethambutol therapy; and white blood cell count during rifampin and ethambutol therapy.
- Monitor hydration if the patient experiences nausea, vomiting, anorexia, or diarrhea during rifampin, pyrazinamide, or ethambutol therapy. Obtain a prescription for an antiemetic or antidiarrheal agent, as needed.
- Instruct the patient of the importance of adhering to the drug regimen for the full course of the treatment. (See Patient Teaching: *Antitubercular agents.*)

- Administer an analgesic as prescribed if the patient experiences a headache during ethambutol therapy or joint pain or muscle aches or cramps during rifampin therapy.
- Take safety measures if the patient experiences adverse CNS reactions, such as confusion or incoordination. For example, place the patient's bed in the lowest position, keep the bed rails raised, and supervise ambulation.
- Take seizure precautions when administering isoniazid to a patient with a seizure disorder.
- Administer rifampin 1 hour before or 2 hours after a meal because food affects the rate and extent of absorption.
- Administer isoniazid at least 1 hour before administering an aluminum antacid to prevent a drug interaction.
- Monitor the patient for additive CNS effects, such as drowsiness, dizziness, headache, lethargy, and depression, during concomitant therapy with isoniazid and cycloserine or ethionamide.
- Expect to increase the dosage of such drugs as oral contraceptives, corticosteroids, and warfarin because rifampin is known to accelerate their metabolism.
- Notify the physician if adverse reactions or drug interactions occur.
- Monitor the patient for peripheral neuritis (exhibited initially by paresthesia of the hands and feet followed by muscle twitching, dizziness, ataxia, and stupor) when administering 6 mg/kg of isoniazid daily or higher.
- Administer pyridoxine concurrently with isoniazid as prescribed, to prevent peripheral neuritis.

*** *Monitor the patient for optic neuritis when administering isoniazid or 15 mg/kg or higher of ethambutol.***

- Test the patient's visual acuity before isoniazid or ethambutol therapy begins and monthly thereafter when the ethambutol dose exceeds 15 mg/kg and throughout isoniazid therapy.
- Notify the physician if visual disturbances occur.

Evaluation

For each nursing diagnosis, prepare an evaluation statement that describes the patient's or family's response to nursing interventions.

Other antitubercular agents

Several other drugs are used as antitubercular agents in combination with first-line agents. Because these drugs have a greater incidence of toxicity, they are used primarily when resistance or allergies to less toxic agents exist.

Aminosalicylic acid (para-aminosalicylic acid) is a tuberculostatic agent that acts like a sulfonamide by decreasing bacterial synthesis of folic acid. The drug is absorbed readily, distributed widely, metabolized rapidly by the liver, and excreted by the kidneys. Its half-life is about 1 hour. The potential for severe GI disturbances limits the use of aminosalicylic acid.

Capreomycin sulfate is a polypeptide antibiotic whose mechanism of action is unknown. Because it is not absorbed well from the GI tract, it must be given I.M. Its half-life is 4 to 6 hours, and it is excreted primarily unchanged in the urine.

Cycloserine is an antibiotic derived from the *Streptomyces* genus. Cycloserine acts against many strains of mycobacteria by inhibiting cell wall synthesis. After oral administration, cycloserine is absorbed well, distributed widely, and excreted primarily by the kidneys. It has a half-life of 10 hours. It is used with other antitubercular agents, but its neurotoxicity and the rapid development of bacterial resistance limit its use.

Ethionamide is a derivative of isonicotinic acid used to treat TB. Its mechanism of action is unknown. Ethionamide is absorbed well after oral administration and is distributed widely. It is metabolized extensively and is excreted in the urine. The plasma half-life is approximately 3 hours. GI disturbances are the most common adverse reactions to the drug.

Fluoroquinolones have demonstrated excellent in vitro and clinical activity against *M. tuberculosis.* Clinical treatment programs have included both ciprofloxacin and ofloxacin. Of these two agents, ofloxacin (300 mg. P.O. daily) is more potent and may be an initial choice in retreatment. These agents are administered P.O. and exhibit favorable adverse reaction profiles. GI adverse reactions are most commonly reported. However, resistance to fluoroquinolones develops rapidly when these agents are used alone or in insufficient doses.

Streptomycin was the first agent recognized as effective in treating TB. Streptomycin is administered I.M. only. It appears to enhance the activity of oral antitubercular agents and is of greatest value in the early weeks to months of therapy. However, I.M. administration limits its usefulness in long-term therapy. Rapidly absorbed from the I.M. injection site, streptomycin is excreted primarily by the kidneys as unchanged drug. Most patients tolerate streptomycin well, but those receiving large doses may exhibit eighth cranial nerve toxicity.

CHAPTER SUMMARY

Chapter 33 covered the antitubercular agents as they are used to treat various mycobacterial infections. Here are the chapter highlights.

Various chemically unrelated agents are used to treat mycobacterial infections. Although these agents show relatively high mycobacterial specificity and inhibition, *M. tuberculosis* infections typically require long-term treatment. In almost all compliant patients, however, combinations of antitubercular agents can control these diseases successfully.

Ethambutol, isoniazid, rifampin, and pyrazinamide serve as the first-line agents for treating TB. Although these drugs vary in terms of specific regimens and length of treatment required, they produce similar therapeutic results.

Antitubercular agents have a favorable benefit-to-risk ratio. Significant adverse reactions do occur, however, usually producing neurotoxic or hepatotoxic effects.

Although the development of bacterial resistance to these drugs is a constant threat, aggressive combination therapy can minimize it greatly.

The nurse must instruct the patient and family in the administration, effects of, and possible adverse reactions to agents; to monitor the patient throughout therapy; and to notify the physician if adverse reactions occur.

Questions to consider

See Appendix 1 for answers.

1. A physician prescribes isoniazid 300 mg P.O. once daily, rifampin 600 mg P.O. once daily, pyridoxine 10 mg P.O. once daily, ethambutol 400 mg P.O. once daily, and pyrazinamide 1.5 g P.O. once daily for a patient with TB. Which of the following best describes the rationale for administering these drugs concurrently in treating active TB?
   (a) They are second-line agents and only effective together.
   (b) Rifampin increases the activity of isoniazid.
   (c) The drugs are bacteriostatic in usual doses.
   (d) Combination therapy can prevent or delay bacterial resistance.

2. Arlene Jones is on a regimen of isoniazid 300 mg P.O. once daily, rifampin 600 mg P.O. once daily, pyridoxine 10 mg P.O. once daily, ethambutol 400 mg P.O. once daily, and pyrazinamide 1.5 g P.O. once daily. She also is taking oral contraceptives. Which of the following instructions should be given to Mrs. Jones about oral contraceptives?
   (a) Oral contraceptive therapy should be discontinued during use of these drugs.
   (b) These drugs, particularly pyrazinamide, increase the effectiveness of oral contraceptives and the dosage should be decreased.
   (c) These drugs, particularly rifampin, decrease the effectiveness of oral contraceptives, and other methods should be used in conjunction.
   (d) Combination therapy can either increase or decrease the effectiveness of oral contraceptives, depending on the individual's metabolism of the drugs.

3. Anetta Hampson is on a regimen of phenytoin when she is diagnosed with TB. She is placed on a treatment regimen that includes isoniazid Which of the following factors should the nurse keep in mind?
   (a) Isoniazid does not interfere with metabolism of phenytoin, but other drugs usually administered with isoniazid may.
   (b) Isoniazid potentiates the effects of phenytoin through unknown mechanisms.
   (c) None of the antitubercular agents affect phenytoin metabolism.
   (d) Isoniazid increases plasma concentration of phenytoin.

4. Ethambutol has an unusual adverse condition that needs specific monitoring, especially when the drug is given in large doses of 15 mg/kg. If this dose is given, which of the following effects should the patient be monitored for?
   (a) Decreased visual acuity and visual field constriction
   (b) Hearing loss, especially high frequency ranges
   (c) Acute aplastic anemia
   (d) Migraine headaches

34 Antimycotic (antifungal) agents

OBJECTIVES

After reading and studying this chapter, the student should be able to:
1. describe the antimycotic agents used to treat systemic fungal infections: amphotericin B, ketoconazole, fluconazole, flucytosine, and miconazole.
2. describe the antimycotic agents used to treat topical fungal infections: nystatin, clotrimazole, griseofulvin, ketoconazole, and miconazole.
3. identify significant interactions between the antimycotic agents and other drugs.
4. identify the adverse reactions caused by these agents, and describe ways to prevent or treat them.
5. describe how to apply the nursing process when caring for a patient who is receiving an antimycotic agent.

INTRODUCTION

Antimycotic, or antifungal, agents include many drugs that are used to treat fungal **infections.** This chapter covers the major systemic antimycotic agents and includes information on major topical antimycotic agents.

Antimycotic agents are categorized in five basic groups: polyene antimycotics, which include amphotericin B and nystatin; the antimetabolite antimycotic agent flucytosine; the synthetic triazole antifungal fluconazole; imidazole agents, which include miconazole, ketoconazole, and clotrimazole; and superficial antimycotic agents, which include griseofulvin and various topical drugs. Because the pharmacotherapeutics and nursing implications of amphotericin B and nystatin are so different, this chapter discusses them separately. (See *Selected major antimycotic agents,* page 442.)

Drugs in this chapter include:

- amphotericin B
- butenafine
- butoconazole nitrate
- ciclopirox olamine
- clioguinol
- clotrimazole
- econazole nitrate
- fluconazole
- flucytosine
- grisofulvin
- haloprogin
- ketoconazole
- miconazole nitrate
- naftifine
- nsytatin
- oxiconazole
- sulconazole
- terbinafine
- tioconazole
- tolnaftate
- triacetin
- undecylenic acid.

Amphotericin B

This drug's potency has made it the most widely used antimycotic agent for severe systemic fungal infections.

PHARMACOKINETICS

After intravenous (I.V.) administration, amphotericin B is distributed throughout the body and excreted by the kidneys. Its metabolic fate has not been demonstrated conclusively

Route	Onset	Peak	Duration
I.V.	Immediate	Unknown	1-15 days

PHARMACODYNAMICS

The irreversible binding of amphotericin B to **sterols** in the membranes of amphotericin B–sensitive fungal cells seems to produce pores or channels that increase cell membrane permeability. This permeability allows leakage of intracellular components, which prevents the fungal cell membrane from functioning normally as a barrier. Amphotericin B usually acts as a **fungistatic** agent but can become **fungicidal** if it reaches high concentrations in the fungi.

PHARMACOTHERAPEUTICS

Amphotericin B usually is administered to treat severe systemic fungal infections and **meningitis** caused by fungi sensitive to the drug. For example, it usually is considered the drug of choice for severe infections caused by *Candida, Paracoccidioides brasiliensis, Blastomyces dermatitidis, Coccidioides immitis, Cryptococcus neoformans,* and *Sporothrix schenckii.* It is also effective against *Aspergillus fumigatus, Histoplasma capsulatum, Microsporum audouini, Rhizopus, Torulopsis glabrata, Trichophyton,* and *Rhodotorula.* It is used to treat aspergillosis; North American blastomycosis; pulmonary, disseminated, or meningeal coccidioidomycosis; disseminated candidiasis;

Selected major antimycotic agents

The following chart summarizes the major antimycotic agents currently in clinical use.

DRUG	MAJOR INDICATIONS AND USUAL DOSAGES	CONTRAINDICATIONS AND PRECAUTIONS
amphotericin B (Fungizone)	*Life-threatening systemic fungal infections and meningitis* ADULT: 0.25 to 1 mg/kg I.V. daily infused over 4 to 6 hours; may give 1.5 mg/kg every other day *Candidal infection of the bladder* ADULT: 50 mg in 1 L sterile water continuously or intermittently instilled into the bladder *Coccidioidal meningitis, cryptococcal meningitis* ADULT: 0.025 to 1 mg intrathecally two or three times a week	• Amphotericin B is contraindicated in a breast-feeding patient or one with known hypersensitivity. • This drug requires cautious use in a pregnant patient. • Safety and efficacy in children have not been established.
nystatin (Mycostatin, Nilstat)	*Oral or esophageal candidiasis* ADULT: 500,000 U of oral suspension, gargled in both sides of the mouth and then swallowed, t.i.d. or q.i.d., or 500,000 U in tablet form, dissolved in the mouth, t.i.d. or q.i.d. for 10 days or until 48 hours after overt symptoms have subsided PEDIATRIC: 400,000 to 600,000 U of oral suspension q.i.d. (with one-half of dose in each side of mouth retained as long as possible before swallowing); for infants, 200,000 U of oral suspension q.i.d. (with one-half of dose in each side of mouth) *Vaginal candidiasis* ADULT: 100,000 U inserted vaginally once or twice daily for 14 days or more *Intestinal candidiasis* ADULT: 500,000 to 1,000,000 U in tablet form t.i.d. or q.i.d.	• Nystatin is contraindicated in a patient with known hypersensitivity. • This drug has no precautions.
flucytosine (Ancobon)	*Fungal infections caused by* Candida *or* Cryptococcus; *used in combination with amphotericin B* ADULT: 50 to 150 mg/kg P.O. daily in four equally divided doses and administered every 6 hours PEDIATRIC: for children who weigh 110 lb (50 kg) or more, 50 to 150 mg/kg P.O. daily in four equally divided doses and administered every 6 hours; for children who weigh under 110 lb, 1.5 to 4.5 g/m^2 P.O. daily	• Flucytosine is contraindicated in a breast-feeding patient or one with known hypersensitivity. • This drug requires cautious use in a pregnant patient or one with impaired renal function or bone marrow suppression.
ketoconazole (Nizoral)	*Systemic, subcutaneous, and superficial fungal infections* ADULT: 200 to 400 mg P.O. daily for 1 week to 12 months, depending on the organism and the infection site	• Ketoconazole is contraindicated in a breast-feeding patient or one with known hypersensitivity. • This drug requires cautious use in a pregnant patient. • Safety and efficacy in children have not been established. • Do not use with terfenadine or astemizole; can cause severe cardiovascular events.
fluconazole (Diflucan)	*Oropharyngeal candidiasis* ADULT: initially, 200 mg P.O. or I.V. on the 1st day, followed by 100 mg daily for 2 weeks *Esophageal candidiasis* ADULT: initially, 200 mg P.O. or I.V. on the 1st day, followed by 100 mg for at least 3 weeks and for at least 2 weeks after resolution of symptoms *Systemic candidiasis* ADULT: initially, 400 mg P.O. or I.V. on the 1st day, followed by 200 mg daily for at least 4 weeks *Cryptococcal meningitis* ADULT: initially, 400 mg P.O. or I.V. on the 1st day, followed by 200 mg daily for 10 to 12 weeks after the cerebrospinal fluid culture becomes negative	• Fluconazole is contraindicated in a patient with known hypersensitivity to the drug or any of its components. • This drug requires cautious use in a pregnant or breast-feeding patient. • Safety and efficacy in children have not been established.

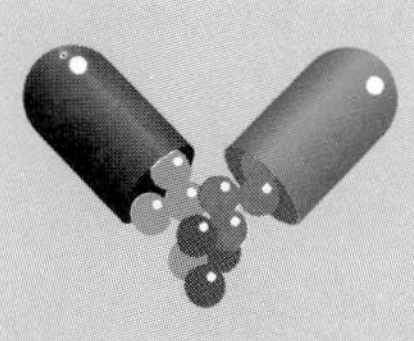

DRUG INTERACTIONS
Amphotericin B

When given with the drugs listed below, amphotericin B may cause significant drug interactions. Some may be severe, such as nephrotoxicity and hypokalemia. Thus, a patient receiving concomitant therapy will need to be monitored closely.

DRUG	INTERACTING DRUGS	POSSIBLE EFFECTS	NURSING IMPLICATIONS
amphotericin B	aminoglycosides, cyclosporine, acyclovir	Increased nephrotoxicity	• Monitor the patient's renal function by monitoring blood urea nitrogen and serum creatinine levels and intake and output patterns.
	corticosteroids	Increased hypokalemia, possibly leading to cardiac dysfunction	• Monitor the patient's serum potassium level. • Monitor the patient for signs and symptoms of cardiac dysfunction, such as palpitations, tachycardia, and hypotension.
	extended-spectrum penicillins	Increased hypokalemia	• Monitor the patient's serum potassium level.
	digitalis glycosides	Increased hypokalemia, possibly causing digitalis toxicity	• Monitor the patient's serum potassium level. • Monitor the patient for signs and symptoms of hypokalemia, such as hypotension, muscle weakness, and confusion.
	nondepolarizing skeletal muscle relaxants (pancuronium bromide)	Increased muscle relaxant effects	• Monitor the patient's serum potassium level. • Monitor the patient for muscle weakness and respiratory insufficiency. • Have emergency equipment nearby.
	electrolyte solutions	Precipitation and inactivation of amphotericin B colloid	• Do not dilute amphotericin B in electrolyte solutions; use only dextrose 5% in water or sterile water that does not contain bacteriostatic agents.

pulmonary or disseminated cryptococcosis; and pulmonary or disseminated histoplasmosis as well.

Amphotericin B therapy usually begins with a test dose that is increased daily until the desired dosage is reached. Duration of therapy depends on the maturity and severity of the infection. Because the drug is highly toxic, its use must be limited to patients who have a definitive diagnosis of life-threatening infections and who are under close medical supervision.

Drug interactions

Amphotericin B can have significant interactions with many drugs. Because of the synergistic effects between flucytosine and amphotericin B, these two drugs commonly are combined in therapy for candidal or cryptococcal infections, especially for cryptococcal meningitis. (See Drug Interactions: *Amphotericin B.*)

ADVERSE DRUG REACTIONS

Amphotericin B probably is the most toxic of the **antibiotics** currently in use today. Almost all patients receiving I.V. amphotericin B experience chills, fever, nausea, vomiting, anorexia, muscle and joint pain, headache, abdominal pain, weight loss, and dyspepsia, especially at the beginning of low-dosage therapy. As therapy continues and the dosage is increased to the optimum level, these reactions usually subside. Most patients also develop normochromic or normocytic anemia that significantly decreases hematocrit.

Up to 80% of patients receiving amphotericin B may develop some degree of nephrotoxicity, causing the kidneys to lose their concentrating ability. This promotes losses of renal stores of potassium, bicarbonate, water, and phosphate. Nephrotoxicity usually disappears within 3 months after the drug is discontinued, but it sometimes leads to permanent renal impairment.

Up to 25% of patients receiving amphotericin B may develop hypokalemia, which can become severe and lead to extreme muscle weakness and electrocardiogram changes. Distal renal tubular acidosis commonly occurs, contributing to the development of hypokalemia.

Other adverse reactions to I.V. amphotericin B therapy include phlebitis and thrombophlebitis. Rarely, hypotension, hypertension, flushing, paresthesia, and seizures may occur.

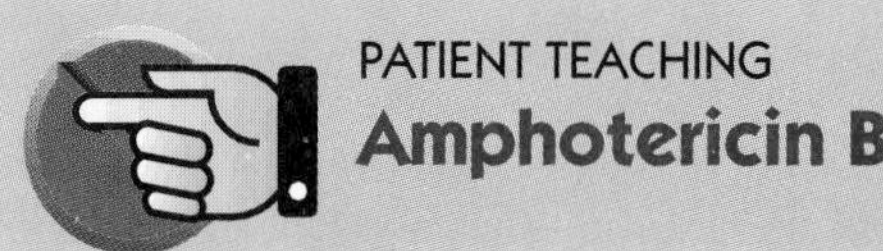

PATIENT TEACHING
Amphotericin B

- Teach the patient and family the name, dose, frequency, action, and adverse effects of amphotericin B.
- Stress the importance of returning for regular blood studies and follow-up appointments.
- Teach the patient how to apply topical amphotericin B.
- Instruct the patient using topical amphotericin B to report such adverse reactions as dry skin, erythema, pruritus, or skin discoloration. Warn the patient that the drug may stain clothing.
- Inform the patient receiving intravenous amphotericin B that chills, fever, gastrointestinal upset, muscle and joint pain, headache, abdominal pain, weight loss, and dyspepsia probably will occur, but that these reactions usually subside with continued therapy.
- Teach the patient which adverse reactions may occur with intrathecal use of amphotericin B.
- Instruct the patient to report oliguria, hematuria, cloudy urine, lack of urine output, or any other adverse reactions.

Intrathecal administration may cause headache, leg and back pain, paresthesia, peripheral neuropathies, sensory loss, and urine retention. Topical application may result in pruritus, skin thickening and discoloration, dry skin, erythema, and contact dermatitis. Less common reactions to amphotericin B include blurred or double vision, ventricular arrhythmias, thrombocytopenia, leukopenia, granulocytopenia, tinnitus, and hearing loss. Rarely, amphotericin B causes anaphylaxis or liver failure.

NURSING PROCESS APPLICATION

The following information assists the nurse in caring for a patient who is receiving amphotericin B. It includes an overview of assessment activities as well as examples of appropriate nursing diagnoses and related interventions. It also highlights the importance of evaluation.

Assessment

Before drug therapy begins, review the patient's history for conditions that contraindicate or require cautious use of amphotericin B. Also review the patient's medication history to identify use of drugs that may interact with it. During therapy, assess the patient for adverse drug reactions and signs of drug interactions. Also, periodically assess the effectiveness of amphotericin B therapy. Finally, evaluate the patient's and family's knowledge about the prescribed drug.

Nursing diagnoses

- Risk for injury related to adverse drug reactions or drug interactions
- Altered urinary elimination related to nephrotoxicity caused by amphotericin B
- Knowledge deficit related to amphotericin B regimen

Planning and implementation

- Do not administer amphotericin B to a patient with a condition that contraindicates its use.
- Administer amphotericin B cautiously to a patient with a preexisting condition.
- Monitor the patient regularly for adverse reactions and drug interactions during amphotericin B therapy. (See Patient Teaching: *Amphotericin B.*)
- Monitor the patient's serum electrolyte levels, particularly watching for changes in potassium, magnesium, calcium, and phosphorus levels.
- Monitor the patient's vital signs during I.V. infusion. Note that a fever may occur, but usually will subside within 4 hours after the infusion is discontinued. To relieve the fever and chills associated with the infusion, expect to administer an antihistamine or antipyretic, as prescribed. Antiemetics sometimes are used to relieve other signs and symptoms, such as nausea and vomiting.
- Check the I.V. site for phlebitis. To reduce phlebitis, rotate the site routinely and add small doses of heparin or corticosteroids to the infusion, as prescribed. Expect to use alternate-day therapy if phlebitis becomes severe. The patient may receive amphotericin B via a central line, which permits greater drug dilution in the blood and decreases the severity of the phlebitis.
- Refrigerate amphotericin B until it is used.

*** *Dilute amphotericin B for infusion or injection in a dextrose 5% in water solution with a pH greater than 4.2 or in sterile water. The drug is not compatible with electrolyte solution.***

- Shake the vial vigorously for at least 3 minutes before administration to assure particle dispersion.

*** *Do not administer the solution if it contains precipitate.***

- Use an in-line filter with a mean pore diameter of 1 micron or greater for I.V. administration. Smaller filters will remove appreciable amounts of the drug from the solution.
- Infuse other antibiotics separately; do not infuse them through the I.V. line used to administer amphotericin B.
- Notify the primary health care provider if adverse reactions or drug interactions occur.
- Monitor the patient's blood urea nitrogen (BUN) and serum creatinine levels before beginning therapy, every other day during initial therapy, and once a week after the optimal dosage is reached. Expect to administer a reduced dosage or to use alternate-day therapy as prescribed if the patient's serum creatinine level approaches 3 mg/dl.
- Monitor the patient's fluid intake and output, and observe for signs of nephrotoxicity.
- Notify the primary health care provider if nephrotoxicity is suspected.

Evaluation

For each nursing diagnosis, prepare an evaluation statement that describes the patient's or family's response to nursing interventions.

Nystatin

Nystatin is used only topically or orally to treat local infections because it is extremely toxic when administered parenterally.

PHARMACOKINETICS

Oral nystatin undergoes little or no absorption, distribution, or metabolism. It is excreted unchanged in the feces. Topical nystatin is not absorbed through the skin or mucous membranes, and the blood concentration level is not measurable at therapeutic doses.

Because nystatin is not absorbed systemically, its onset of action, peak concentration, and duration of action are not significant.

PHARMACODYNAMICS

Nystatin binds to sterols in fungal cell membranes and alters the permeability of the membranes, leading to loss of essential cell components. Nystatin can act as a fungicidal or fungistatic agent, depending on the organism present.

PHARMACOTHERAPEUTICS

Nystatin is used primarily to treat fungal skin infections. The drug is effective against *Candida albicans, C. guilliermondii,* and other *Candida.*

Different forms of nystatin are available for treating different types of candidal infections. Topical nystatin is used to treat cutaneous or mucocutaneous candidal infections, such as oral **thrush,** diaper rash, vulvovaginitis, and intertriginous candidiasis. Oral nystatin is used to treat intestinal candidiasis and may be used as an adjunct to vaginal application in treating vulvovaginitis. Oral nystatin also is used to prevent fungal infection in a patient with neutropenia who is receiving immunosuppressive therapy.

Drug interactions

Nystatin does not interact significantly with other drugs.

ADVERSE DRUG REACTIONS

Reactions to nystatin, which seldom occur, include diarrhea, nausea, vomiting, and abdominal pain, especially with high dosages (greater than 5 million units); some patients also have reported a bitter taste. Topical nystatin also may cause skin irritation. A hypersensitivity reaction may occur with oral or topical administration.

NURSING PROCESS APPLICATION

The following information assists the nurse in caring for a patient who is receiving nystatin. It includes an overview of assessment activities as well as examples of appropriate nursing diagnoses and related interventions. It also highlights the importance of evaluation.

Assessment

Before drug therapy begins, review the patient's history for conditions that contraindicate or require cautious use of nystatin. During therapy, assess the patient for adverse drug reactions. Also, periodically assess the effectiveness of nystatin therapy. Finally, evaluate the patient's and family's knowledge of the prescribed drug.

Nursing diagnoses

- Risk for injury related to adverse drug reactions
- Knowledge deficit related to nystatin regimen

Planning and implementation

- Do not administer nystatin to a patient with a condition that contraindicates its use.
- Monitor the patient periodically for adverse reactions during nystatin therapy.

*** *Monitor for diarrhea, nausea, vomiting, and abdominal pain in a patient receiving high dosages of nystatin.***

- Inspect the patient's skin regularly for signs of irritation. Expect to discontinue the drug if skin irritation occurs. (See Patient Teaching: *Nystatin.*)

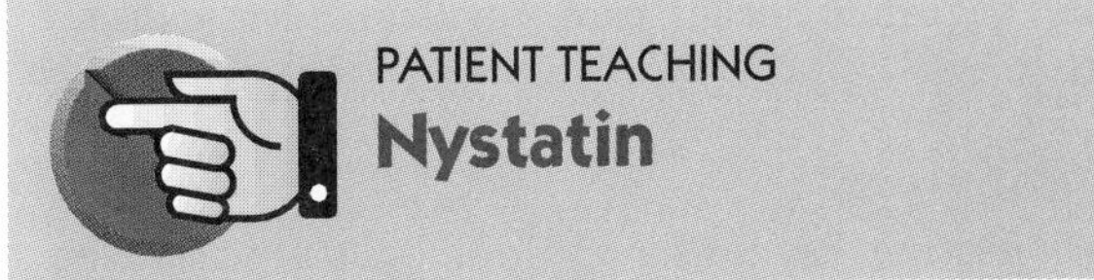

PATIENT TEACHING
Nystatin

- Teach the patient and family the name, dose, frequency, action, and adverse effects of nystatin.
- Instruct the patient taking the suspension form for oral candidiasis to divide the dose in half, place one-half in each side of the mouth, swish the suspension in the mouth for as long as possible, and then swallow it.
- Instruct the patient taking tablets for oral candidiasis to dissolve the tablet in the mouth. Emphasize that the patient must not chew it or swallow it whole.
- Advise the patient receiving topical nystatin to report signs of a hypersensitivity reaction, such as redness or skin irritation.
- Teach the patient how to apply topical nystatin properly. Also emphasize the importance of compliance with therapy and good hygiene.
- Instruct the patient to insert the vaginal nystatin tablets high in the vagina. Also inform the patient that vaginal drainage from the tablets may stain clothing.
- Instruct the patient to avoid using occlusive dressings during therapy with nystatin ointment or cream because they provide a favorable environment for fungal growth.
- Advise the patient with a foot infection to apply nystatin topical powder to shoes and socks as a preventive measure.
- Instruct the patient to take the drug for the length of time prescribed — usually 14 days — even though symptomatic relief may occur in 14 to 72 hours.
- Instruct the patient to notify the physician if adverse reactions occur.

• Notify the primary health care provider if adverse reactions occur.

Evaluation

For each nursing diagnosis, prepare an evaluation statement that describes the patient's or family's response to nursing interventions.

Flucytosine

Flucytosine is the only antimetabolite with antimycotic activity. It is used primarily with another antimycotic agent, such as amphotericin B, to treat systemic fungal infections.

PHARMACOKINETICS

After oral administration, flucytosine is absorbed well from the gastrointestinal (GI) tract and distributed widely. It undergoes little metabolism and is excreted primarily by the kidneys.

Route	Onset	Peak	Duration
P.O.	Unknown	2-4 hr	2.4-4.8 hr

PHARMACODYNAMICS

Flucytosine penetrates fungal cells where it is converted to its active metabolite fluorouracil, a metabolic antagonist. Fluorouracil then is incorporated into the ribonucleic acid of the fungal cells, altering their protein synthesis and causing cell death.

PHARMACOTHERAPEUTICS

Administered orally, flucytosine is used in combination therapy to treat systemic fungal infections caused by *Candida* and *Cryptococcus.* Although amphotericin B is effective in treating candidal and cryptococcal meningitis, flucytosine is given with amphotericin B to reduce the dosage and the risk of **toxicity.** This combination therapy is the treatment of choice for cryptococcal meningitis. Flucytosine can be used alone to treat lower urinary tract *Candida* infections because it reaches a high urinary concentration. It also is used effectively to treat infections caused by *T. glabrata, Phialophora, Aspergillus,* and *Cladosporium.*

Drug interactions

Cytarabine may antagonize antifungal activity of flucytosine, possibly by competitive inhibition.

ADVERSE DRUG REACTIONS

Bone marrow suppression typically occurs when the flucytosine serum concentration exceeds 100 mcg/ml and may lead to leukopenia, thrombocytopenia, anemia, pancytopenia, or granulocytopenia.

Adverse GI reactions to flucytosine include nausea, vomiting, abdominal distention, diarrhea, and anorexia. Rarely, bowel perforation and hepatotoxicity may occur.

Azotemia, increased BUN and creatinine levels, crystalluria, and renal failure may also occur.

Flucytosine may produce unpredictable adverse reactions, including confusion, headache, somnolence, vertigo, hallucinations, dyspnea, respiratory arrest, and rash.

NURSING PROCESS APPLICATION

The following information assists the nurse in caring for a patient who is receiving flucytosine. It includes an overview of assessment activities as well as examples of appropriate nursing diagnoses and related interventions. It also highlights the importance of evaluation.

Assessment

Before drug therapy begins, review the patient's history for conditions that contraindicate or require cautious use of flucytosine. During therapy, assess the patient for adverse drug reactions. Also, periodically assess the effectiveness of flucytosine therapy. Finally, evaluate the patient's and family's knowledge of the prescribed drug.

Nursing diagnoses

• Risk for injury related to adverse drug reactions
• Risk for fluid volume deficit related to the adverse GI effects of flucytosine
• Knowledge deficit related to flucytosine regimen

Planning and implementation

• Do not administer flucytosine to a patient with a condition that contraindicates its use.
• Administer flucytosine cautiously to a patient with a preexisting condition.
• Monitor the patient periodically for adverse reactions and drug interactions during flucytosine therapy.
• Monitor the patient's hematologic values, liver function tests, and BUN and creatinine levels. Notify the primary health care provider if test results are abnormal.
**** Monitor the patient's fluid intake and output. Notify the primary health care provider if the patient develops azotemia, crystalluria, or decreased urine output, all of which may indicate renal failure.***
• Regularly inspect the patient's skin for a rash, which may suggest a hypersensitivity reaction to flucytosine. (See Patient Teaching: *Flucytosine.*)
• Regularly monitor the flucytosine blood level during long-term therapy; therapeutic serum concentrations range from 25 to 120 mcg/ml.
• Notify the primary health care provider if adverse reactions occur.

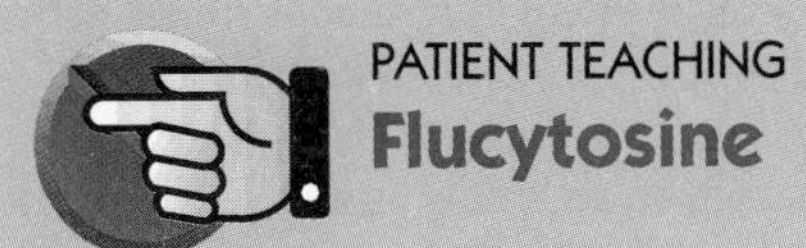

PATIENT TEACHING
Flucytosine

- Teach the patient and family the name, dose, frequency, action, and adverse effects of flucytosine.
- Emphasize to the patient the importance of completing the course of therapy.
- Teach the patient the importance of returning for blood tests.
- Instruct the patient about infection-control measures or bleeding precautions as needed.
- Instruct the patient to report sore throat, fever, easy bruising, bleeding, unusual fatigue or weakness, changes in urine output, severe nausea, vomiting, or skin rash.
- Advise the patient to take a flucytosine dose consisting of several capsules over 15 minutes to minimize nausea or vomiting.
- Instruct the patient to take a missed dose as soon as possible, but not to take a double dose. Explain that missing a dose is safer than overmedicating with a double dose.
- Caution the patient against performing activities that require mental alertness if adverse central nervous system reactions such as dizziness occur.
- Instruct the patient to notify the physician if adverse reactions occur.

• Monitor for fluid volume deficit if the patient experiences anorexia, nausea, vomiting, or diarrhea. Administer an antiemetic or antidiarrheal agent as prescribed.
• Notify the primary health care provider if adverse GI reactions persist or worsen.

Evaluation

For each nursing diagnosis, prepare an evaluation statement that describes the patient's or family's response to nursing interventions.

Ketoconazole

Ketoconazole is an effective oral antimycotic agent with a broad **spectrum** of activity.

PHARMACOKINETICS

After oral administration, ketoconazole is absorbed variably and distributed widely. It undergoes extensive hepatic metabolism and is excreted through the bile and feces.

Route	Onset	Peak	Duration
P.O.	Unknown	1-2 hr	2-8 hr (biphasic)

PHARMACODYNAMICS

Within the fungal cells, ketoconazole interferes with sterol synthesis, damaging the cell membrane and increasing its permeability. This leads to a loss of essential intracellular elements and inhibition of cell growth. Ketoconazole usually produces fungistatic effects, but also can produce fungicidal effects under certain conditions.

PHARMACOTHERAPEUTICS

Ketoconazole is used to treat topical and systemic infections caused by susceptible fungi, which include dermatophytes and most other fungi. Ketoconazole also is active in vitro against some gram-positive **bacteria,** including *Staphylococcus epidermis, S. aureus, Nocardia, Actinomadura,* and enterococci, although it is not usually used against these organisms.

Drug interactions

Use of ketoconazole with drugs that decrease gastric acidity, such as cimetidine, ranitidine, famotidine, antacids, and anticholinergic drugs, may decrease its absorption and antimycotic effects. Concomitant therapy with ketoconazole and phenytoin may alter metabolism and blood levels of both drugs. Concomitant use of ketoconazole and theophylline may decrease the serum theophylline level. Use of ketoconazole with other hepatotoxic drugs may increase the risk of liver disease. Ketoconazole combined with cyclosporine therapy may increase cyclosporine and serum creatinine levels. Concomitant use with an oral anticoagulant can cause hemorrhage from the increased anticoagulant effect. Ketoconazole should not be given concurrently with rifampin because serum ketoconazole concentrations can be decreased.

ADVERSE DRUG REACTIONS

The most common reactions to ketoconazole are nausea and vomiting. Other reactions, which have been reported in less than 1% of patients, include pruritus, rash, dermatitis, urticaria, headache, insomnia, dizziness, vivid dreams, lethargy, paresthesia, diarrhea, flatulence, abdominal pain, and endocrine reactions, such as gynecomastia and breast pain. Hepatotoxicity, although rare, is reversible upon drug discontinuation. Rarely, ketoconazole also can cause anaphylaxis, arthralgia, chills, fever, tinnitus, impotence, and photophobia.

NURSING PROCESS APPLICATION

The following information assists the nurse in caring for a patient who is receiving ketoconazole. It includes an overview of assessment activities as well as examples of appropriate nursing diagnoses and related interventions. It also highlights the importance of evaluation.

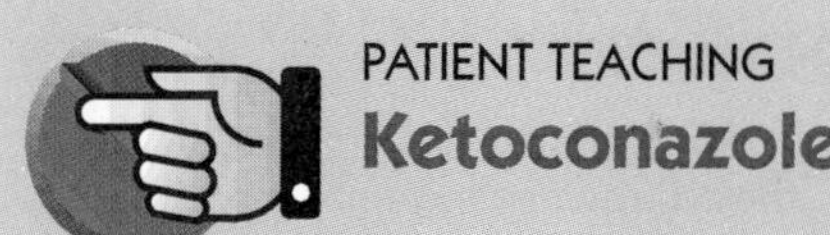

PATIENT TEACHING
Ketoconazole

- Teach the patient and family the name, dose, frequency, action, and adverse effects of ketoconazole.
- Inform the patient when to expect therapeutic results from ketoconazole therapy. Mucosal infections respond in days, skin infections in weeks, and nail infections in months.
- Instruct the patient to notify the primary health care provider if signs and symptoms of hepatotoxicity, such as dark or amber-colored urine, pale stools, abdominal pain, unusual fatigue, or yellowing of the eyes or skin, develop during therapy.
- Advise the patient to report breast enlargement, breast pain, or rash.
- Caution the patient not to perform activities that require mental alertness if dizziness or drowsiness occurs.
- Advise the patient when to take ketoconazole if the patient also is taking other drugs that decrease gastric acidity.
- Teach the patient relaxation techniques if insomnia occurs. Advise the patient with persistent insomnia to request a prescription for a sedative from the physician.
- Advise the patient to take ketoconazole on an empty stomach. However, instruct the patient experiencing adverse GI reactions to take ketoconazole with food and to notify the physician if the reactions persist or worsen.
- Instruct the patient to report adverse reactions to the physician.

Assessment

Before drug therapy begins, review the patient's history for conditions that contraindicate or require cautious use of ketoconazole. Also review the patient's medication history to identify use of drugs that may interact with it. During therapy, assess the patient for adverse drug reactions and signs of drug interactions. Also, periodically assess the effectiveness of ketoconazole therapy. Finally, evaluate the patient's and family's knowledge of the prescribed drug.

Nursing diagnoses

- Risk for injury related to adverse drug reactions or drug interactions
- Risk for fluid volume deficit related to the adverse GI effects of ketoconazole
- Knowledge deficit related to ketoconazole regimen

Planning and implementation

- Do not administer ketoconazole to a patient with a condition that contraindicates its use.
- Administer ketoconazole cautiously to a patient with a preexisting condition.
- Monitor the patient periodically for adverse reactions and drug interactions during ketoconazole therapy.
- Monitor the patient's liver function tests. Expect to discontinue the drug if test results show persistent elevations and the patient displays signs of hepatotoxicity. (See Patient Teaching: *Ketoconazole.*)
- Monitor the serum level of phenytoin, theophylline, or cyclosporine when used concomitantly with ketoconazole. Expect to adjust the dosage as prescribed.
- Administer ketoconazole on an empty stomach, if possible, to promote absorption. If the patient experiences GI distress, however, administer the drug with food.
- Do not administer ketoconazole with drugs that decrease gastric acidity, such as antacids and anticholinergic drugs. If these drugs must be used, administer ketoconazole at least 2 hours before administering the other drugs.
- Do not administer ketoconazole with astemizole or terfenadine because serious cardiovascular effects could result.
- Notify the primary health care provider if adverse reactions or drug interactions occur.
- Monitor for fluid volume deficit if the patient experiences nausea, vomiting, or diarrhea.
- Administer an antiemetic or antidiarrheal agent as needed.
- Notify the primary health care provider if adverse GI reactions persist or worsen.

Evaluation

For each nursing diagnosis, prepare an evaluation statement that describes the patient's or family's response to nursing interventions.

Fluconazole

Fluconazole is a class of synthetic, broad-spectrum bistriazole antimycotic agents.

PHARMACOKINETICS

After oral administration, fluconazole is about 90% absorbed. Fluconazole is distributed into all body fluids and over 80% of the drug is excreted unchanged in the urine.

Route	Onset	Peak	Duration
P.O.	Unknown	1-2 hr	30 hr
I.V.	Immediate	Immediate	Unknown

PHARMACODYNAMICS

A selective inhibitor of fungal cytochrome P-450 and sterol C-14 alpha-demethylation, fluconazole causes fungal cells to lose normal sterols, thereby promoting cell death.

PHARMACOTHERAPEUTICS

Fluconazole is used to treat oropharyngeal and esophageal candidiasis and serious systemic candidal infections, including urinary tract infections, peritonitis, and pneumonia. It also is used to treat cryptococcal meningitis.

Drug interactions

Use of fluconazole with warfarin may increase prothrombin time. Fluconazole may increase levels of phenytoin and cyclosporine in combination therapy. Glyburide and glipizide metabolism may decrease when fluconazole is part of the treatment regimen, resulting in increased blood levels and hypoglycemia. Concomitant use with rifampin and cimetidine enhances fluconazole metabolism, possibly requiring increased fluconazole dosage. Fluconazole can increase the activity of zidovudine. (See Patient Teaching: *Fluconazole*.)

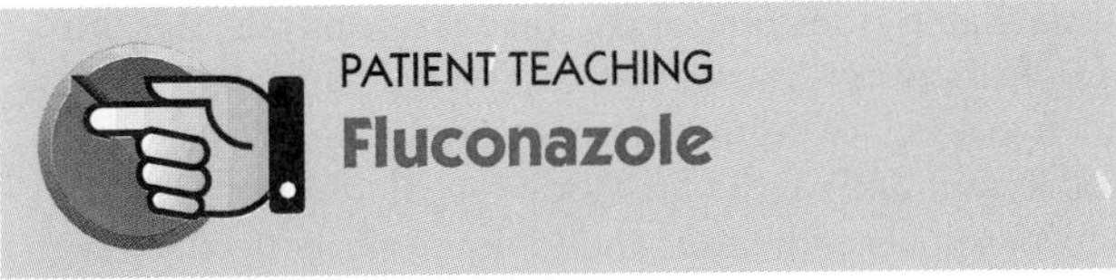

PATIENT TEACHING

Fluconazole

- Teach the patient and family the name, dose, frequency, action, and adverse effects of fluconazole.
- Teach the patient the importance of having routine blood tests performed when also taking drugs known to interact with fluconazole.
- Instruct the patient to take bleeding precautions during concomitant therapy with warfarin, which may increase the prothrombin time.
- Instruct the diabetic patient to monitor the blood glucose level regularly and to watch for signs and symptoms of hypoglycemia (profuse sweating, nervousness, irritability, headache) when taking glyburide or glipizide concomitantly with fluconazole.
- Teach the patient the importance of completing the course of therapy.
- Instruct the patient to report adverse reactions to the physician.

ADVERSE DRUG REACTIONS

In clinical trials, 5% to 7% of patients receiving fluconazole experienced transient elevations in aspartate aminotransferase (AST), alanine aminotransferase (ALT), alkaline phosphatase, and bilirubin levels. About 2% developed dizziness, and more than 1% experienced nausea, vomiting, abdominal pain, diarrhea, rash, and headache. Hypokalemia and increased BUN and creatinine levels also have been reported.

NURSING PROCESS APPLICATION

The following information assists the nurse in caring for a patient who is receiving fluconazole. It includes an overview of assessment activities as well as examples of appropriate nursing diagnoses and related interventions. It also highlights the importance of evaluation.

Assessment

Before drug therapy begins, review the patient's history for conditions that contraindicate or require cautious use of fluconazole. Also review the patient's medication history to identify use of drugs that may interact with it. During therapy, assess the patient for adverse drug reactions and signs of drug interactions. Also, periodically assess the effectiveness of fluconazole therapy. Finally, evaluate the patient's and family's knowledge about the prescribed drug.

Nursing diagnoses

- Risk for injury related to adverse drug reactions or drug interactions
- Risk for fluid volume deficit related to the adverse GI effects of fluconazole
- Knowledge deficit related to fluconazole regimen

Planning and implementation

- Do not administer fluconazole to a patient with a condition that contraindicates its use.
- Administer fluconazole cautiously to a patient with a preexisting condition.
- Monitor the patient periodically for adverse reactions and drug interactions during fluconazole therapy.
- Monitor the patient's laboratory test results to detect elevations in AST, ALT, alkaline phosphatase, bilirubin, BUN, and creatinine levels. Notify the primary health care provider of abnormal results.
- Monitor the patient who develops a rash; be prepared to discontinue fluconazole if symptoms continue.
- Do not administer an I.V. infusion of fluconazole greater than 200 mg/hour by continuous infusion.
- Notify the primary health care provider if adverse reactions or drug interactions occur.
- Monitor hydration if the patient experiences nausea, vomiting, or diarrhea. Administer an antiemetic or antidiarrheal agent as needed.
- Notify the primary health care provider if adverse GI reactions persist or worsen.

Evaluation

For each nursing diagnosis, prepare an evaluation statement that describes the patient's or family's response to nursing interventions.

Other antimycotic agents

Several other antimycotic agents offer alternative forms of treatment for topical fungal infections.

An imidazole derivative, clotrimazole is used topically to treat dermatophyte and *C. albicans* infections, orally to treat oral candidiasis, and vaginally to treat vaginal candidiasis.

Griseofulvin is used to treat fungal infections of the skin on the body (tinea corporis), feet (tinea pedis), groin (tinea cruris), and beard area of the face and neck (tinea barbae) and infections of the nails (tinea unguium) and scalp (tinea capitis). To prevent a relapse, griseofulvin therapy must continue until the fungus is eradicated and the infected skin or nails are replaced.

Available as miconazole or miconazole nitrate, this imidazole derivative is used to treat systemic fungal infections, such as coccidioidomycosis, paracoccidioidomycosis, cryptococcosis, and candidiasis; local fungal infections such as vulvovaginal candidiasis; and topical fungal infections such as chronic mucocutaneous candidiasis. The drug may be administered I.V. or intrathecally to treat fungal meningitis, I.V. or in bladder irrigations to treat fungal bladder infections, locally to treat vaginal infections, and topically to treat topical infections.

Ciclopirox olamine, econazole nitrate, haloprogin, butoconazole nitrate, naftifine, tioconazole, terconazole, tolnaftate, butenafine, terbinafine, sulconazole, oxiconazole, clioquinol, triacetin, and undecylenic acid are available only as topical agents.

CHAPTER SUMMARY

Chapter 34 covered antimycotic (antifungal) agents. Here are the chapter highlights.

Amphotericin B is the most widely used antimycotic for severe systemic fungal infections. Certain adverse reactions, however, limit its parenteral use. These include nephrotoxicity, phlebitis, hematologic effects, electrolyte imbalances, and immediate reactions, such as fever, chills, nausea, vomiting, anorexia, muscle and joint pain, headache, weight loss, and dyspepsia.

Nystatin is administered in tablet or suspension form to treat oral, vaginal, and intestinal candidiasis.

Flucytosine, an oral antimycotic agent, is given with amphotericin B to treat systemic fungal infections.

Ketoconazole is used to treat topical and systemic fungal infections.

Fluconazole is a class of synthetic, broad-spectrum bistriazole antifungal agents. It is used to treat oropharyngeal and esophageal candidiasis and serious systemic candidal infections.

Other antimycotic agents briefly discussed in the chapter included clotrimazole, griseofulvin, and miconazole.

When caring for a patient receiving an antimycotic agent, the nurse should monitor closely for adverse reactions, which may be severe. The nurse also should teach the patient how to administer the specific drug and form prescribed.

Questions to consider

See Appendix 1 for answers.

1. Amos Johnson, age 72, is to receive amphotericin B for a cryptococcal meningitis infection. To reduce amphotericin B dosage and toxicity, the physician may prescribe which of the following antimycotic agents along with amphotericin B?
   (a) nystatin
   (b) flucytosine
   (c) ketoconazole
   (d) griseofulvin

2. Gloria Hatley, age 32, has acquired immunodeficiency syndrome and developed oral candidiasis. Her physician prescribed oral nystatin tablets. Which of the following instructions should the nurse give Ms. Hatley about nystatin administration?
   (a) Swallow the tablet whole.
   (b) Chew the tablet thoroughly.
   (c) Dissolve the tablet in the mouth.
   (d) Dissolve the tablet in warm water and drink it.

3. Juanita Mendez, age 32, is taking ketoconazole for tinea unguium. What is the usual duration of ketoconazole therapy for this indication?
   (a) Hours
   (b) Days
   (c) Weeks
   (d) Months

4. Bruce Brown, age 48, is receiving I.V. amphotericin B for a severe systemic fungal infection. Which of the following adverse reactions do most patients experience when receiving I.V. amphotericin B?
   (a) Anuria
   (b) Coagulation defects
   (c) Peripheral neuropathies
   (d) Normochromic or normocytic anemia

35 Anthelmintic agents

OBJECTIVES

After reading and studying this chapter, the student should be able to:
1. identify the antinematode, anticestode, and antitrematode agents.
2. explain how the pharmacokinetics of these anthelmintic agents relates to their effectiveness.
3. describe the actions of the various anthelmintic agents.
4. discuss the common adverse reactions to anthelmintic agents.
5. describe how to apply the nursing process when caring for a patient who is receiving an anthelmintic agent.

INTRODUCTION

Anthelmintic agents destroy **helminths** — parasitic worms that infect humans. They are divided into three groups: **nematodes** (roundworms); and two groups of flatworms, the **cestodes** (tapeworms) and the **trematodes** (flukes). Thus, the anthelmintic agents are classified as antinematode, anticestode, and antitrematode agents.

This chapter discusses anthelmintic agents currently used in North America, grouped according to the particular helminth group they combat most effectively. (See *Selected major anthelmintic agents*, pages 452 and 453.)

Drugs covered in this chapter include:
- albendazole
- ivermectin
- mebendazole
- oxamniquine
- paromomycin sulfate
- piperazine citrate
- praziquantel
- pyrantel pamoate
- thiabendazole.

Antinematode agents

The drugs with specific antiparasitic action against nematodes, or roundworms, are mebendazole, piperazine citrate, pyrantel pamoate, thiabendazole, ivermectin, and albendazole.

PHARMACOKINETICS

Less than 10% of an oral mebendazole dose is absorbed from the gastrointestinal (GI) tract; the remainder is excreted unchanged in the feces. The absorbed drug is distributed well, metabolized by the liver, and excreted unchanged in the urine.

Piperazine is absorbed readily after oral administration and distributed widely. Approximately 25% is metabolized in the liver, but most of a piperazine dose is excreted unchanged in the urine within 24 hours. Plasma concentration of piperazine after oral administration is unknown.

Like mebendazole, pyrantel pamoate is absorbed poorly from the GI tract. The absorbed drug is metabolized partially in the liver with approximately 50% of an oral dose excreted unchanged in the feces and about 7% excreted in the urine.

Thiabendazole is absorbed rapidly and almost completely from the GI tract. It is distributed widely in the body, metabolized rapidly by the liver, and excreted by the kidneys.

Route	Onset	Peak	Duration
P.O.	Unknown	0.5-7 hr	2.8-16 hr

PHARMACODYNAMICS

The pharmacodynamic effects of the antinematode agents are diverse and include several mechanisms of action, most of which are not fully understood. Antinematode agents immobilize or kill roundworms by impairing their ability to use energy from available sources or by interfering with their nervous systems. Then the immobilized or dead roundworms are eliminated from the GI tract by peristalsis.

PHARMACOTHERAPEUTICS

The rule of thumb in treating nematode **infections** is to continue using the drug of choice for the particular invading organism until the organism is eradicated or the drug clearly has failed to eradicate it. Alternative choices are usually more toxic to the patient. Repeat treatment is commonly necessary because of patient noncompliance or reinfection.

Because mebendazole and piperazine stay in the GI tract, they are particularly effective against roundworms that infect the intestines.

Selected major anthelmintic agents

This chart summarizes the major anthelmintic agents currently in clinical use.

DRUG	MAJOR INDICATIONS AND USUAL DOSAGES	CONTRAINDICATIONS AND PRECAUTIONS
Antinematode agents		
mebendazole (Vermox)	Ascaris *(roundworm)*, Trichuris *(whipworm), and* Necator *(hookworm) infections* ADULT: 100 mg P.O. b.i.d. for 3 days; may be repeated in 2 to 3 weeks PEDIATRIC: for children age 2 and over, 100 mg P.O. b.i.d. for 3 days; may be repeated in 2 to 3 weeks Enterobius *(pinworm) infection* ADULT: 100 mg P.O. as a single dose; may be repeated in 2 to 3 weeks PEDIATRIC: for children age 2 and older, 100 mg P.O. as a single dose; may be repeated in 2 to 3 weeks	• Mebendazole is contraindicated in a pregnant patient or one with known hypersensitivity. • This drug requires cautious use in a breast-feeding patient. • Dosages for children under age 2 have not been established.
thiabendazole (Mintezol)	Strongyloides stercoralis *(threadworm) infection* ADULT: 25 mg/kg (up to a maximum of 3 g daily) P.O. b.i.d. for 2 days, or 1.5 g P.O. b.i.d. for patients who weigh 155 lb (70 kg) or more PEDIATRIC: 25 mg/kg (up to a maximum of 3 g daily) P.O. b.i.d. for 2 days	• Thiabendazole is contraindicated in a breast-feeding patient or one with known hypersensitivity. • This drug requires cautious use in a pregnant patient or one with hepatic or renal dysfunction.
ivermectin (Stromectol)	*Use in strongyloidiasis and onchocerciasis* ADULT: 200 mcg/kg P.O. in a single oral dose PEDIATRIC: for children weighing 33 lb (15 kg) or more, 200 mcg/kg P.O. in a single dose.	• Ivermectin should not be used in a pregnant patient. • Safety and efficacy in children weighing less than 33 lb have not been established.
albendazole (Albenza)	*Hydatid disease* ADULT: weight less than 133 lb (60 kg): 15 mg/kg/day in divided doses twice a day with meals; 28-day cycle followed by a 14-day hiatus for a total of three cycles; weight greater than 133 lb: 400 mg twice a day with meals; 28-day cycle followed by a 14-day hiatus for a total of three cycles PEDIATRIC: weight less than133 lb (60 kg): 15 mg/kg/day in divided doses twice a day with meals; 28-day cycle followed by a 14-day hiatus for a total of three cycles; weight greater than 60 kg: see adult dosing *Neurocysticercosis* ADULT: weight less than133 lb (60 kg): 15 mg/kg/day in divided doses twice a day with meals for 8 to 30 days; weight greater than 133 lb: 400 mg twice a day with meals for 8 to 30 days. PEDIATRIC: weight less than 133 lb (60 kg): 15 mg/kg/day in divided doses twice a day with meals for 8 to 30 days; weight greater than 133 lb: see adult dosing	• Begin treatment with albendazole in a female patient of childbearing years only with result of a negative pregnancy test.
Anticestode agents		
paromomycin (Humatin)	*Tapeworm (fish, beef, pork, dog)* ADULT: 1 g P.O. every 15 minutes for four doses PEDIATRIC: 11 mg/kg P.O. every 15 minutes for four doses *Dwarf tapeworm* ADULT AND PEDIATRIC: 45 mg/kg P.O. daily for 5 to 7 days	• Paromomycin is contraindicated in a patient with known hypersensitivity and in one with impaired renal function or intestinal obstruction. • This drug requires cautious use in a breast-feeding patient or one with ulcerative bowel lesions.

Selected major anthelmintic agents *(continued)*

DRUG	MAJOR INDICATIONS AND USUAL DOSAGES	CONTRAINDICATIONS AND PRECAUTIONS
Antitrematode agents		
praziquantel (Biltricide)	Schistosoma *infections* ADULT: 20 mg/kg P.O. t.i.d. for 1 day PEDIATRIC: for children age 4 and over, 20 mg/kg P.O. t.i.d. for 1 day Paragonimus *infections* ADULT: 25 mg/kg P.O. t.i.d. for 2 days PEDIATRIC: for children age 4 and over, 25 mg/kg P.O. t.i.d. for 2 days Clonorchis *infections* ADULT: 25 mg/kg P.O. t.i.d. for 1 day PEDIATRIC: for children age 4 and over, 25 mg/kg P.O. t.i.d. for 1 day	• Praziquantel is contraindicated in a breast-feeding patient or one with ocular cysticercosis or known hypersensitivity. • This drug requires cautious use in a pregnant patient.

Mebendazole has broad anthelmintic activity and is the drug of choice against infection with *Trichuris trichiura* (whipworm), *Enterobius vermicularis* (pinworm), *Necator americanus* (hookworm), and *Ascaris lumbricoides* (giant intestinal roundworm). Mebendazole has been used with some success in patients with hydatid disease (systemic infection) from *Echinococcus granulosus,* a liver tapeworm.

Piperazine is used primarily as an alternative to mebendazole in patients with large *Ascaris* infections that cause intestinal blockage.

Pyrantel pamoate is an alternative drug of choice for treating a number of nematode infections, including giant intestinal roundworm, hookworm, and pinworm infections.

Thiabendazole is the drug of choice to treat threadworm infection and also acts as an anti-inflammatory agent in trichinosis (caused by the nematode *Trichinella spiralis*).

Ivermectin is indicated in infestations *of Strongyloides stercoralis* and *Onchocerca volvulus.* Albendazole is used in treating neurocysticercosis and hydatid disease.

Drug interactions

When piperazine and pyrantel pamoate are used together, they can cancel each other's effect. In high concentrations, piperazine may increase extrapyramidal effects and the potential for seizures in patients also receiving phenothiazines. Because carbamazepine and phenytoin may increase mebendazole metabolism, other anticonvulsants should be considered for use in patients receiving mebendazole for extraintestinal infections. Cimetidine inhibits mebendazole metabolism, thus increasing plasma concentration. Thiabendazole may interfere with the hepatic metabolism of theophylline. Albendazole levels were increased when administered with dexamethasone, praziquantel and cimethidine.

ADVERSE DRUG REACTIONS

Almost all of the antinematode agents cause adverse GI reactions, which range from abdominal pain to nausea, vomiting, and diarrhea. Other adverse reactions are less common. For example, mebendazole rarely causes leukopenia, and piperazine occasionally causes headache, vertigo, and loss of coordination. Piperazine also may lower a patient's seizure threshold. Pyrantel pamoate and thiabendazole sometimes cause headache, dizziness, drowsiness, and weakness; thiabendazole also may cause rash and hallucinations and, rarely, tinnitus and seizures. Ivermectin has been associated with Mazzotti reaction (pruritus, skin edema and papular rash, and lymph node enlargement and tenderness) as well as ophthalmic symptoms (punctate opacity and conjunctivitis). The most common adverse effects of albendazole were nausea, vomiting, and abdominal pain.

NURSING PROCESS APPLICATION

The following information assists the nurse in caring for a patient who is receiving an antinematode agent. It includes an overview of assessment activities as well as examples of appropriate nursing diagnoses and related interventions. It also highlights the importance of evaluation.

Assessment

Before drug therapy begins, review the patient's history for conditions that contraindicate or require cautious use of the prescribed antinematode agent. Also review the patient's medication history to identify use of drugs that may interact with it. During therapy, assess the patient for adverse drug reactions and signs of drug interactions. Also, periodically assess the effectiveness of therapy with the antinematode agent. Finally, evaluate the patient's and family's knowledge of the prescribed drug.

Nursing diagnoses

- Risk for injury related to adverse drug reactions or drug interactions
- Risk for fluid volume deficit related to the adverse GI effects of the prescribed antinematode agent

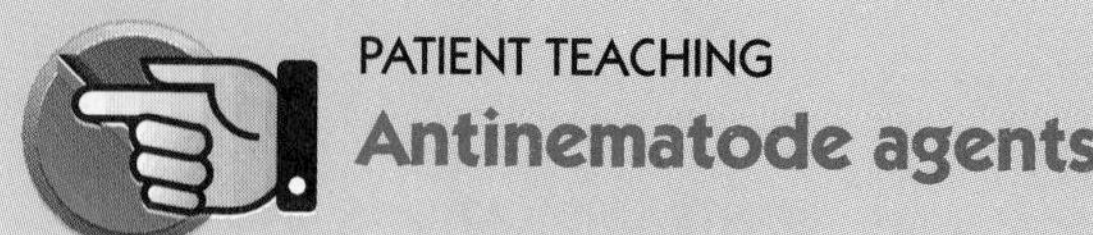

PATIENT TEACHING
Antinematode agents

- Teach the patient and family the name, dose, frequency, action, and adverse effects of the prescribed antinematode agent.
- Instruct the patient receiving mebendazole or thiabendazole tablets to chew them for greatest effectiveness.
- Instruct the patient to change and wash underclothes and bedding daily until the nematodes are eradicated. Explain that washing the perineal area daily and the hands and fingernails after each bowel movement also will reduce the risk of reinfection.
- Instruct the patient to take thiabendazole immediately after meals to minimize gastrointestinal distress.
- Inform the patient that thiabendazole may make urine smell like asparagus but that the odor has no medical significance.
- Teach the patient the importance of completing the course of therapy to prevent treatment failure.
- Caution the patient not to perform activities that require mental alertness or physical coordination if adverse central nervous system reactions, such as dizziness or drowsiness, occur.
- Instruct the patient to notify the physician if adverse reactions occur.
- Instruct a female patient of childbearing age receiving albendazole that she should not become pregnant during the treatment regimen or within a month after treatment.
- Instruct the patient that albendazole should be taken with food.

• Knowledge deficit related to the prescribed antinematode agent regimen

Planning and implementation

• Do not administer an antinematode agent to a patient with a condition that contraindicates its use.
• Administer an antinematode agent cautiously to a patient with a preexisting condition.
• Monitor the patient for adverse reactions and signs of drug interactions during antinematode therapy.
• Ensure that all family members are treated because pinworm and other nematode infections otherwise may recur.
• Shake the container well before administering pyrantel pamoate or thiabendazole to ensure even dispersion of the agent in the suspension.
• Notify the physician if adverse reactions or drug interactions occur.
• Monitor hydration if the patient experiences nausea, vomiting, or diarrhea. Obtain a prescription for an antiemetic or antidiarrheal as needed.
• Notify the physician if adverse GI effects persist or worsen.
• Albendazole may cause fetal harm; therefore treatment should begin only after a negative pregnancy test result is obtained in a female patient of childbearing age.
• Expect to see oral or intravenous corticosteroids administered with albendazole during the first week of treatment for neurocysticercosis to prevent cerebral hypertensive episodes. (See Patient Teaching: *Antinematode agents.*)

Evaluation

For each nursing diagnosis, prepare an evaluation statement that describes the patient's or family's response to nursing interventions.

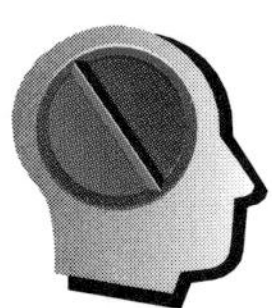

CRITICAL THINKING. To enhance your critical thinking about anthelmintic agents, consider the following situation and its analysis.
Situation: Mrs. Harrison comes to the outpatient department for the 3rd consecutive week. She is frustrated and informs you that no matter how much medicine she takes she cannot get rid of "the worms." She has no other significant past medical history. On her last visit, the physician noted "active *Enterobius vermicularis* infection" as the diagnosis. Social history reveals that Mrs. Harrison is divorced and has a 3-year-old child. You ask Mrs. Harrison what she knows about how the infection is transmitted and what she knows about the medication. Mrs. Harrison informs you that she has had mebendazole dosing twice and still has perianal itching. She has changed all of the linen in the house and now notices that her child is scratching. The toddler is "potty trained," and they share the bathroom facility. What is your next question?
Analysis: You should ask if the child has been treated by her pediatrician. Mrs. Harrison states that she has not been, as "I just saw her scratching the other day and didn't think anything of it at the time." What do you do now?

You inform the physician of the child's symptoms and suggest that the child be treated. You inform Mrs. Harrison that the treatment will not be successful until everyone in the house is treated simultaneously. Allow her to express her feelings of frustration, and encourage her to change and wash linen again and be fairly sure that this extra step should mean the end of the cycle.

Anticestode agents

Anticestode agents include mebendazole and paromomycin sulfate. Paromomycin's use as an anticestode, however, is considered experimental by the Food and Drug Administration (FDA). A third agent, praziquantel, currently is used to treat trematode (fluke) infections, but is gaining wider use for treating tapeworms. The FDA, however, considers this use investigational.

PHARMACOKINETICS

Less than 10% of an oral mebendazole dose is absorbed from the GI tract; the remainder is excreted unchanged in the feces. The absorbed drug is distributed well, metabolized by the liver, and excreted unchanged in the urine.

Paromomycin is absorbed negligibly from the GI tract and excreted in the feces. Its onset of action, peak concentration, and duration of action varies greatly among individuals.

Praziquantel is absorbed readily (over 80%) after oral administration and distributed widely. It undergoes hepatic metabolism, and its metabolites are excreted in the urine.

Route	Onset	Peak	Duration
P.O.	Varies	0.5-7 hr	0.8-9 hr

PHARMACODYNAMICS

Mebendazole interferes with the microtubule system of the tapeworm, thus preventing glucose uptake and distribution. As a result, the tapeworm depletes its energy stores and is immobilized or dies. Paromomycin is thought to inhibit the protein synthesis in the tapeworm by causing misreading of messenger ribonucleic acid. Praziquantel is thought to dislodge the worms from the intestines by impairing their ability to attach themselves to the intestinal wall.

PHARMACOTHERAPEUTICS

Mebendazole is used experimentally to treat hydatid disease caused by *E. granulosus.* Praziquantel is similarly effective against all varieties of tapeworm infection. Paromomycin is an alternative choice if the patient cannot tolerate praziquantel.

Drug interactions

Carbamazepine and phenytoin may increase mebendazole metabolism and decrease its efficacy. Phenytoin may decrease serum praziquantel levels, leading to possible treatment failure. No significant drug interactions involving paromomycin are known to occur.

ADVERSE DRUG REACTIONS

Adverse reactions to mebendazole include transient abdominal pain, diarrhea and, rarely, neutropenia or leukopenia.

The primary adverse reactions to paromomycin include anorexia, nausea, vomiting, cramps, and diarrhea. Secondary infection of the intestinal tract may also occur.

Praziquantel has caused transient dizziness, headache, malaise, abdominal pain or distention, and nausea in about 90% of patients. Drowsiness and fatigue also have been reported. In 3% to 27% of patients, praziquantel produces mild to moderate elevation of aspartate aminotransferase (AST) and alanine aminotransferase (ALT) levels. The drug also may cause macular rash with pruritus.

NURSING PROCESS APPLICATION

The following information assists the nurse in caring for a patient who is receiving an anticestode agent. It includes an overview of assessment activities as well as examples of appropriate nursing diagnoses and related interventions. It also highlights the importance of evaluation.

Assessment

Before drug therapy begins, review the patient's history for conditions that contraindicate or require cautious use of the prescribed anticestode agent. If the patient is receiving mebendazole, also review the patient's medication history to identify use of drugs that may interact with it. During therapy, assess the patient for adverse drug reactions and signs of drug interactions. Also, periodically assess the effectiveness of therapy with the anticestode agent. Finally, evaluate the patient's and family's knowledge of the prescribed drug.

Nursing diagnoses

- Risk for injury related to adverse drug reactions or drug interactions
- Knowledge deficit related to the prescribed anticestode agent regimen

Planning and implementation

- Do not administer an anticestode agent to a patient with a condition that contraindicates its use.
- Administer an anticestode agent cautiously to a patient with a preexisting condition.
- Monitor the patient periodically for adverse reactions and drug interactions during anticestode therapy.
- Monitor hydration if the patient experiences adverse GI reactions, such as nausea, vomiting, and diarrhea. Obtain a prescription for an antiemetic or antidiarrheal agent as needed. Notify the physician if adverse GI reactions persist or worsen. (See Patient Teaching: *Anticestode agents.*)
- Monitor the complete blood count regularly for a patient on high-dosage mebendazole therapy to detect neutropenia.
- Inspect the patient's skin for a rash during niclosamide or praziquantel therapy. Notify the physician if a rash is pre-

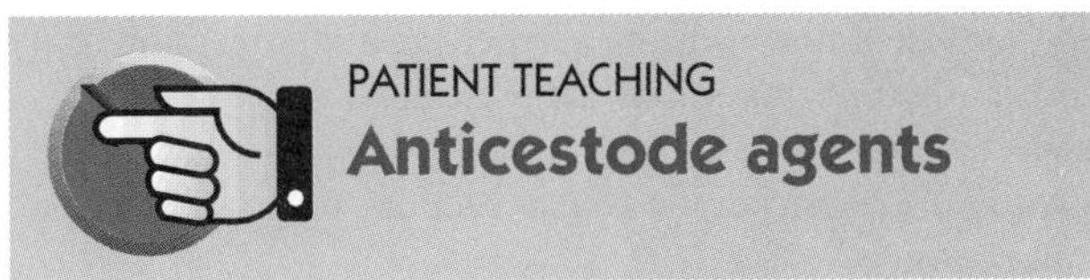

PATIENT TEACHING

Anticestode agents

- Teach the patient and family the name, dose, frequency, action, and adverse effects of the prescribed anticestode agent.
- Instruct the patient to take praziquantel tablets with meals to minimize adverse gastrointestinal reactions. Explain that the tablets are bitter and should be swallowed quickly to prevent gagging or vomiting.
- Teach the patient the importance of completing the course of therapy to prevent treatment failure.
- Advise the patient not to perform activities that require mental alertness if adverse central nervous system (CNS) reactions, such as dizziness, drowsiness, or vertigo, occur.
- Instruct the patient to notify the physician if nausea, vomiting, abdominal pain, rash, or CNS reactions occur.
- Instruct the patient to alert the physician if symptoms persist or worsen despite treatment.

sent because it may indicate a hypersensitivity reaction that requires discontinuation of the prescribed anticestode agent.
• Notify the physician if adverse reactions or drug interactions occur.

Evaluation
For each nursing diagnosis, prepare an evaluation statement that describes the patient's or family's response to nursing interventions.

Antitrematode agents

The two drugs available to treat fluke infections are oxamniquine and praziquantel.

PHARMACOKINETICS
After oral administration, oxamniquine is absorbed well from the GI tract, although the presence of food in the stomach interferes with the rate and amount of absorption. Oxamniquine is metabolized primarily by the intestinal mucosa or lumen and is excreted by the kidneys. The distribution of oxamniquine into body tissues and fluids has not been determined.

After oral administration, praziquantel is absorbed readily (over 80%), distributed widely, and metabolized in the liver. Its metabolites are excreted in the urine.

The antitrematode agents act locally. Therefore, their onsets of action, peak concentrations, and durations of action, which relate to systemic absorption, do not indicate their therapeutic effect.

PHARMACODYNAMICS
Oxamniquine's known anticholinergic activity does not explain its antitrematode action. The drug is known, however, to induce **schistosomes** (adult blood flukes) to migrate from the mesenteric veins into the liver, where they eventually die. Praziquantel causes spastic paralysis of the fluke's musculature, which eventually leads to disintegration.

PHARMACOTHERAPEUTICS
Oxamniquine no longer is the drug of choice to treat fluke infections as it is effective only against *Schistosoma mansoni*. Praziquantel has become the drug of choice for all fluke infections because of its broad **spectrum** of activity.

Drug interactions
The only significant drug interaction with this class of drugs involves the interaction between these two antitrematode agents. Concomitant use may enhance their effectiveness against *S. mansoni*.

ADVERSE DRUG REACTIONS
Oxamniquine and praziquantel have a low human **toxicity** compared to their effects on target flukes. However, some patients may experience a hypersensitivity reaction to these drugs.

Oxamniquine has produced mild, transient dizziness, drowsiness, and headache in 30% to 50% of patients. It has caused adverse GI reactions, such as nausea, vomiting, and abdominal pain, in a smaller percentage of patients. However, the most significant adverse reaction to oxamniquine is rare central nervous system (CNS) stimulation that leads to behavioral changes, seizures, or hallucinations. (The seizures usually occur in patients with a history of epilepsy.) Oxamniquine also causes orange-red urine that has no clinical significance but may alarm the patient and interfere with laboratory tests based on spectrometry or color reactions.

Up to 90% of patients receiving praziquantel have experienced dizziness, headache, malaise, drowsiness, fatigue, and GI disturbances, such as nausea and abdominal pain or discomfort. From 3% to 27% of patients display a mild to moderate, transient increase in AST and ALT levels. Praziquantel also may cause macular rash with pruritus.

NURSING PROCESS APPLICATION
The following information assists the nurse in caring for a patient who is receiving an antitrematode agent. It includes an overview of assessment activities as well as examples of appropriate nursing diagnoses and related interventions. It also highlights the importance of evaluation.

Assessment
Before drug therapy begins, review the patient's history for conditions that contraindicate or require cautious use of the prescribed antitrematode agent. During therapy, assess the patient for adverse drug reactions. Also, periodically assess the effectiveness of therapy with the antitrematode agent. Finally, evaluate the patient's and family's knowledge of the prescribed drug.

Nursing diagnoses
• Risk for injury related to adverse drug reactions
• Knowledge deficit related to the prescribed antitrematode agent regimen

Planning and implementation
• Do not administer an antitrematode agent to a patient with a condition that contraindicates its use.
• Administer an antitrematode agent cautiously to a patient with a preexisting condition.
• Monitor the patient periodically for adverse reactions during antitrematode therapy.
***** ***Note on laboratory slip for urine tests that the patient is receiving oxamniquine because the drug may interfere***

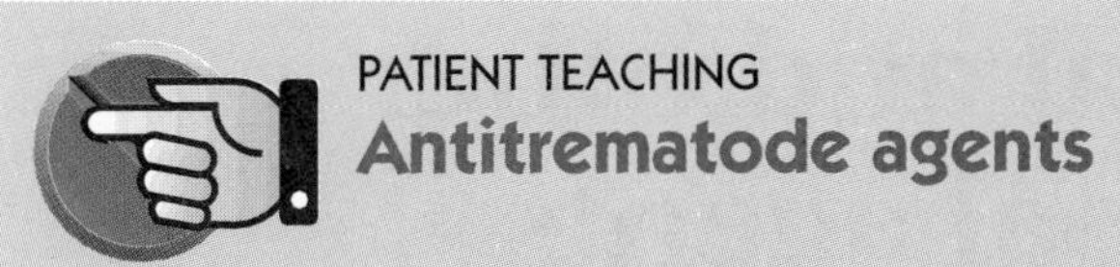

PATIENT TEACHING
Antitrematode agents

- Teach the patient and family the name, dose, frequency, action, and adverse effects of the prescribed antitrematode agent.
- Inform the patient that oxamniquine may turn the urine a harmless orange-red.
- Caution the patient taking oxamniquine or praziquantel that drowsiness and dizziness may occur, necessitating curtailment of activities on the day of and day after treatment.
- Instruct the patient to take praziquantel with meals to minimize adverse gastrointestinal reactions. Explain that the tablet is bitter and should be swallowed rapidly to avoid gagging or vomiting.
- Instruct the patient to report any adverse reactions to the physician.

with laboratory tests based on spectrometry or color reactions.

- Give oxamniquine as a single dose after meals to help prevent adverse GI reactions.
- Take safety measures if the patient experiences adverse CNS effects. For example, place the bed in the lowest position, keep the bed rails raised, and supervise the patient's activities. Also take these safety measures for a patient who is receiving oxamniquine and has a history of epilepsy.
- Notify the physician if adverse reactions occur. (See Patient Teaching: *Antitrematode agents.*)

Evaluation

For each nursing diagnosis, prepare an evaluation statement that describes the patient's or family's response to nursing interventions.

CHAPTER SUMMARY

Chapter 35 discussed the anthelmintic agents as they are used to treat nematode (roundworm), cestode (tapeworm), and trematode (fluke) infections. Here are the chapter highlights.

Anthelmintic agents are categorized according to the helminth groups they combat most effectively. The three major classes of anthelmintic agents are antinematode (antiroundworm), anticestode (antitapeworm), and antitrematode (antifluke) agents.

Two anthelmintic agents are used to treat more than one type of helminth infection: Mebendazole is used to treat roundworm infections and a systemic tapeworm infection (hydatid disease), and praziquantel is becoming the drug of choice for all tapeworm infections as well as trematode infections.

The nurse should instruct the patient and family about the administration, therapeutic effects, and possible adverse effects of anthelmintic agents; monitor the patient throughout therapy; and notify the primary health care provider if adverse reactions occur.

Questions to consider

See Appendix 1 for answers.

1. George Milson, age 9, is diagnosed with a tapeworm infection. The physician orders mebendazole 100 mg P.O. b.i.d. for 3 days. Which of the following instructions should George and his mother be given?
   (a) Mebendazole must be given with antacid to potentiate its effects.
   (b) Mebendazole should be chewed to allow greatest effect.
   (c) Mebendazole must be swallowed whole to achieve greatest effect.
   (d) Mebendazole should be crushed and stirred in water for greatest effect.

2. Xing Xu is being treated for strongyloidiasis with ivermectin. She comes back to the office to report that within a week of taking the medication her skin is itching and swollen and she has a rash. Upon examination, the nurse notices that her inguinal nodes are swollen and tender. Which of the following understandings should the nurse keep in mind about the patient's drug therapy?
   (a) Invermectin may cause a Mazzotti reaction, which includes these symptoms.
   (b) Invermectin may worsen underlying symptoms of Hodgkin's disease.
   (c) Ivermectin is not associated with these conditions, therefore a full laboratory work-up will need to be performed.
   (d) Invermectin may cause lymphatic stasis and swollen lymph nodes.

3. While on vacation, Andy Piper, age 42, is diagnosed with schistosomiasis, a trematode infection. His physician prescribes oxamniquine. Which of the following is the most significant adverse reaction to oxamniquine?
   (a) Hepatotoxicity
   (b) GI distress
   (c) Renal failure
   (d) CNS stimulation

36 Antimalarial and other antiprotozoal agents

OBJECTIVES

After reading and studying this chapter, the student should be able to:

1. discuss the major indications for antimalarial and the other antiprotozoal agents.
2. describe potential interactions between antimalarial or antiprotozoal agents and other drugs.
3. discuss the most common adverse effects of antimalarial and antiprotozoal agents and explain how to minimize them during therapy.
4. describe how to apply the nursing process when caring for a patient who is receiving an antimalarial or other antiprotozoal agent.

INTRODUCTION

This chapter discusses the most commonly used **antimalarial** and **antiprotozoal** drugs and their indications. (See *Selected major antimalarial and other antiprotozoal agents.*)

Drugs covered in this chapter include:

- amphotericin B
- atovaquone
- chloroquine hydrochloride
- chloroquine phosphate
- co-trimoxazole
- dehydroemetine
- diloxanide furoate
- eflornithine
- furazolidone
- hydroxychloroquine sulfate
- iodoquinol
- mefloquine hydrochloride
- melarsoprol
- metronidazole
- nifurtimox
- paromomycin
- pentamidine isethionate
- primaquine phosphate
- pyrimethamine
- quinidine gluconate
- quinine sulfate
- suramin sodium.
- trimetraxate.

Antimalarial agents

The major agents used to prevent and treat **malaria** are the 4-aminoquinoline derivatives (chloroquine hydrochloride, chloroquine phosphate, and hydroxychloroquine sulfate), mefloquine hydrochloride, the 8-aminoquinoline primaquine phosphate, pyrimethamine, quinidine gluconate, and quinine sulfate. The sulfonamides, sulfones, and tetracyclines also may be used in combination with these agents.

PHARMACOKINETICS

After oral administration, the antimalarial agents are absorbed well and distributed widely throughout the body. The extent of metabolism among these agents varies, and excretion occurs primarily in the urine. Peak effect times vary. Chloroquine for instance, reaches peak effect in 1 to 2 hours.

Route	Onset	Peak	Duration
P.O.	Unknown	1-24 hr	8 hr-24 days

PHARMACODYNAMICS

Chloroquine and hydroxychloroquine are thought to disrupt protein synthesis in the **parasite.** Also, these drugs may concentrate in the digestive vacuoles of the parasite, increasing pH and interfering with utilization of hemoglobin.

Primaquine appears to affect the parasite's mitochondria, eventually disrupting cellular metabolism.

Pyrimethamine selectively inhibits the enzyme dihydrofolate reductase, which impedes folic acid reduction and ultimately disrupts parasitic reproduction. Sulfadoxine competitively inhibits dihydrofolic acid synthesis which is necessary to convert para-aminobenzoic acid to folic acid.

Quinine's antimalarial action may result from incorporation into the deoxyribonucleic acid (DNA) of the parasite, rendering it ineffective. Its action also may result from depression of oxygen uptake and carbohydrate metabolism in the parasite. In addition, quinine acts as a skeletal muscle relaxant, a local anesthetic, an antipyretic, and an analgesic, thus relieving malarial symptoms.

The exact mechanism of mefloquine's antimalarial effects remain unknown. Because it is a structural analogue of quinine, it may have similar pharmacodynamic effects.

PHARMACOTHERAPEUTICS

Chloroquine remains the oral drug of choice to prevent and treat all malaria strains, except chloroquine-resistant or multidrug-resistant strains of *Plasmodium falciparum.* Hydroxychloroquine serves as an alternative when chloroquine is not available.

Selected major antimalarial and other antiprotozoal agents

This table summarizes the major antimalarial and other antiprotozoal agents currently in clinical use.

DRUG	MAJOR INDICATIONS AND USUAL DOSAGES	CONTRAINDICATIONS AND PRECAUTIONS
Antimalarial agents		
chloroquine hydrochloride (Aralen HCl), chloroquine phosphate (Aralen)	*Malaria prevention in areas of low risk of exposure to chloroquine-resistant* Plasmodium falciparum *malaria* ADULT: 300 mg base P.O. once a week beginning 1 week before exposure and continuing 4 weeks after exposure PEDIATRIC: 5 mg base/kg P.O. weekly, up to a maximum of 300 mg base *Malaria prevention in areas of higher risk of exposure to chloroquine-resistant* P. falciparum *malaria* ADULT: 300 mg base P.O. once a week beginning 1 week before exposure and continuing 4 weeks after exposure, plus pyrimethamine and sulfadoxine, if needed PEDIATRIC: 5 mg base/kg P.O. weekly, up to a maximum of 300 mg base *Treatment of all malaria except chloroquine-resistant* P. falciparum *malaria* ADULT: initially, 600 mg base P.O., then 300 mg base P.O. at 6, 24, and 48 hours PEDIATRIC: 10 mg base/kg P.O. (600 mg maximum base)	• Chloroquine is contraindicated in a pregnant patient, one with retinal or visual field changes or known hypersensitivity or for long-term therapy in children. • This drug requires cautious use in a patient taking another hepatotoxic agent or one with hepatic disease, glucose-6-phosphate dehydrogenase (G6PD) deficiency, or a history of psoriasis or porphyria.
pyrimethamine plus sulfadoxine (Fansidar) [one tablet equals 25 mg pyrimethamine and 500 mg sulfadoxine]	*Treatment of chloroquine-resistant* P. falciparum *malaria* ADULT: 3 tablets at once on last day of quinine therapy PEDIATRIC: the following doses are taken on the last day of quinine therapy: less than age 1, ¼ tablet P.O.; ages 1 to 3, ½ tablet P.O.; ages 4 to 8, 1 tablet P.O.; ages 9 to 14, 2 tablets P.O. *Self-treatment of febrile illness in areas of risk of exposure to chloroquine-resistant* P. falciparum *when medical care is not available* ADULT: 3 tablets P.O. in combination with chloroquine prophylactic therapy PEDIATRIC: for children less than age 1, ¼ tablet P.O.; for children ages 1 to 3, ½ tablet P.O.; for children ages 4 to 8, 1 tablet P.O.; for children ages 9 to 14, 2 tablets P.O.	• Pyrimethamine is contraindicated in a patient with documented megaloblastic anemia due to folate deficiency or known hypersensitivity. • This drug requires cautious use in a pregnant or breast-feeding patient or one with a history of seizures, impaired renal or hepatic function, folate deficiency, or bronchial asthma.
quinine sulfate (Quinamm, Strema)	*Treatment of chloroquine-resistant* P. falciparum *malaria* ADULT: 650 mg P.O. t.i.d. for 3 to 7 days in combination with pyrimethamine and sulfadoxine PEDIATRIC: 25 mg/kg P.O. daily in divided doses every 8 hours for 3 to 7 days *Malaria prevention in chloroquine-resistant areas* ADULT: 250 mg P.O. once a week beginning 1 week before travel and continuing 4 weeks after exposure. PEDIATRIC: 33 to 43 lb (15 to 19 kg), ¼ tablet P.O.; 44 to 67 lb (20 to 30 kg), ½ tablet P.O.; 68 to 99 lb (31 to 45 kg): ¾ tablet P.O.; over 99 lb: 1 tablet P.O.	• Quinine is contraindicated in a pregnant patient or one with G6PD deficiency, thrombocytopenic purpura, tinnitus, backwater fever, optic neuritis, or known hypersensitivity. • This drug requires cautious use in a breast-feeding patient or one with atrial fibrillation.
mefloquine (Lariam)	*Treatment of chloroquine-resistant* P. falciparum *malaria* ADULT: 750 mg P.O. then 500 mg P.O. in 6 to 8 hours once PEDIATRIC: 25 mg/kg once for children weighing less than 99 lb (45 kg)	• Mefloquine is contraindicated in patients with a known hypersensitivity. • Use during pregnancy only if the potential benefit justifies the potential risk to the fetus. • Women taking mefloquine should not breast-feed. • The safety and efficacy of mefloquine use in children has not been established.

(continued)

Selected major antimalarial and other antiprotozoal agents *(continued)*

DRUG	MAJOR INDICATIONS AND USUAL DOSAGES	CONTRAINDICATIONS AND PRECAUTIONS
Other antiprotozoal agents		
atovaquone (Mepron)	*Mild to moderate* Pneumocystis carinii *pneumonia in patients who cannot tolerate co-trimoxazole therapy* ADULT: 750 mg P.O. with food t.i.d. for 21 days	• Atovaquone is contraindicated in a patient with known hypersensitivity. • This drug requires cautious use in a breast-feeding or pregnant patient or a patient over age 65. • Safety and efficacy in children have not been established.
metronidazole (Flagyl, Metryl)	*Acute intestinal amebiasis, acute amoebic hepatic abscess* ADULT: 750 mg P.O. t.i.d. 10 days PEDIATRIC: 35 to 50 mg/kg P.O. daily in three divided doses for 10 days *Amoebic hepatic abscess* ADULT: 500 to 750 mg P.O. t.i.d. for for 10 days PEDIATRIC: 35 to 50 mg/kg P.O. daily given in three divided doses daily for 10 days *Vaginal trichomoniasis* ADULT: 2 g P.O. once, or 250 mg P.O. t.i.d. for 7 days, or 375 mg P.O. b.i.d. for 7 days	• Metronidazole is contraindicated in a pregnant patient in her first trimester, a breast-feeding patient, or one with hypersensitivity to the drug or any nitroimidazole derivative. • This drug requires cautious use in a patient with severe hepatic disease.
pentamidine isethionate (Pentam 300, NebuPent)	*Treatment of* P. carinii *pneumonia* ADULT: 3 to 4 mg/kg I.V. once daily for 14 to 21 days PEDIATRIC: 3 to 4 mg/kg I.V. once daily for 14 to 21 days *Prevention of* P. carinii *pneumonia* ADULT: 300 mg inhaled via a Respirgard II nebulizer once every 4 weeks *African trypanosomiasis* ADULT: 4 mg/kg I.M. daily for 10 days PEDIATRIC: 4 mg/kg I.M. daily for 10 days *Visceral leishmaniasis* ADULT: 2 to 4 mg/kg I.M. daily or every other day, up to 15 doses PEDIATRIC: 4 mg/kg I.M. daily or every other day, up to 15 doses	• Pentamidine is contraindicated in a patient with a history of hypersensitivity. • This drug requires cautious use in a patient with hypotension, hypertension, hypoglycemia, hyperglycemia, hypocalcemia, leukopenia, thrombocytopenia, anemia, or hepatic or renal dysfunction.
eflornithine	*Treatment of meningoencephalitic stage of* Trypanosoma brucei gambiense *infections* ADULT: 100 mg/kg/dose I.V. every 6 hours for 14 days; adjust dose for patients with renal dysfunction	• Eflornithine use requires caution in a patient with renal dysfunction. • Use in pregnancy only if the benefit to mother justifies the risk to the fetus. Women should not breast-feed during therapy. • Safety and efficacy in children have not been established.
trimetrexate	*Treatment of moderate to severe* P. carinii *pneumonia* ADULT: 45 mg/m^2 I.V. daily for 21 days with folinic acid	• Trimetrexate is contraindicated in a patient who is hypersensitive to trimetrexate, leucovorin, or methotrexate, and in pregnant or breast-feeding women. • Cautious use in patients with impaired hematologic, renal, or hepatic function. • Safety and efficacy in children have not been established.

For treatment of malaria caused by chloroquine-resistant or multidrug-resistant strains of *P. falciparum,* quinine is the drug of choice and is given with slower-acting antimalarial agents.

Primaquine is the drug of choice to prevent *Plasmodium vivax* or *P. ovale* malaria relapse.

Mefloquine is used for treatment of malaria caused by susceptible strains of *P. falciparum, P. vivax, P. ovale,* and *P.*

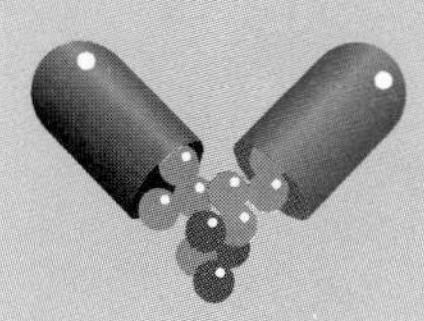

DRUG INTERACTIONS

Antimalarial agents

Antimalarial agents can produce a variety of interactions. The most serious are additive, occurring with concomitant therapy with other drugs that produce similar adverse reactions.

DRUG	INTERACTING DRUGS	POSSIBLE EFFECTS	NURSING IMPLICATIONS
chloroquine	oral antacids that contain magnesium trisilicate	Decreased chloroquine absorption	• Administer antacid doses as far apart as possible from chloroquine doses if these drugs must be used concomitantly.
hydroxychloroquine	digoxin	Increased digoxin levels	• Monitor the patient's serum digoxin level when hydroxycholoroquine therapy begins or ends.
mefloquine	beta-adrenergic blockers, quinine, quinidine, other drugs that may prolong cardiac conduction	Electrocardiogram abnormalities or cardiac arrest	• Avoid concomitant administration.
	chloroquine	Increased risk of seizures	• Monitor the patient closely if concomitant administration occurs.
	valproic acid	Decreased valproic acid blood levels, increased risk of seizures	• Monitor serum valproic acid levels; adjust the dosage as necessary.
primaquine	quinacrine	Increased risk of primaquine toxicity	• Monitor the patient for adverse reactions. • Avoid administration to patients who have recently received quinacrine.
pyrimethamine	folic acid	Inhibited antimicrobial effect	• Monitor the patient for a decreased therapeutic effect.
quinine	antacids that contain aluminum	Delayed or decreased quinine absorption	• Administer antacid doses as far apart as possible from quinine doses if these drugs must be used concomitantly.
	neuromuscular blockers (pancuronium, tubocurarine, succinylcholine)	Neuromuscular blockade, which may lead to respiratory difficulties	• Monitor the patient's respirations. • Have emergency resuscitation equipment nearby. • Monitor the patient's arterial blood gas values, as needed. • Adjust dose of neuromuscular agent as necessary.
	oral anticoagulants (warfarin type)	Increased hypoprothrombinemia	• Monitor the patient receiving an oral anticoagulant for altered anticoagulant effect when quinine therapy begins or ends.
	cardiac glycosides (digoxin, digitoxin)	Increased plasma levels of the cardiac glycoside	• Monitor the patient's serum cardiac glycoside level, and adjust the dosage as prescribed.

malariae. It also is indicated to prevent malaria infections, including chloroquine-resistant strains of *P. falciparum.*

Pyrimethamine, in combination with sulfadoxine, is used with other antimalarial agents to treat chloroquine-resistant malaria and with chloroquine **prophylaxis** for self-treatment of febrile illness when medical care is not immediately available in areas where chloroquine-resistant *P. falciparum* is found.

Quinidine is the parenteral drug of choice for the treatment of malaria in patients who cannot tolerate oral therapy.

Drug interactions

Various interactions can occur between antimalarial agents and other drugs. (See Drug Interactions: *Antimalarial agents.*)

Adverse reactions of antimalarial agents

This chart summarizes the adverse reactions to antimalarial agents, grouping them by frequency. Most of the adverse reactions result from high dosages.

DRUG	COMMON	OCCASIONAL	RARE
chloroquine, hydroxychloroquine	Epigastric discomfort, anorexia, nausea, vomiting, abdominal cramps, diarrhea	Blurred vision, difficulty in focusing, corneal inclusions, corneal changes, rash, pruritus, changes in skin and mucosal pigment, hair bleaching, headache, fatigue, nervousness, anxiety, irritability, personality changes	Retinal changes, exfoliative dermatitis, psychotic episodes, seizures, hypotension, electrocardiogram changes, ototoxicity, tinnitus, neutropenia, granulocytopenia, aplastic anemia, thrombocytopenia, hemolytic anemia, neuropathy, neuromyopathy, hypersensitivity reaction
mefloquine	Vomiting, dizziness, myalgia, nausea, fever, headache, chills, diarrhea, skin rash, abdominal pain, fatigue, loss of appetite, tinnitus	Bradycardia, hair loss, emotional problems, pruritus, asthenia, transient emotional disturbances, seizures	Encephalopathy
primaquine	Nausea, vomiting, epigastric discomfort, abdominal cramps	Headache, difficulty in focusing, pruritus, hemolytic anemia, methemoglobinemia, mild anemia, leukocytosis, leukopenia	Hypertension, arrhythmias, granulocytopenia, extreme mental confusion, hypersensitivity reaction
pyrimethamine	Anorexia, vomiting, abdominal cramps	Megaloblastic anemia, leukopenia, thrombocytopenia, ataxia, tremor, hypersensitivity reaction	Granulocytopenia, hemolytic anemia, seizures, respiratory failure, photosensitivity, malaise, fatigue, irritability, hypersensitivity reaction
quinine	Mild cinchonism	Moderate cinchonism, thrombocytopenic purpura, hypoprothrombinemia, hemolytic anemia, hearing disturbances, ventricular tachycardia, angina, fever, hypothermia, apprehensiveness, restlessness, confusion, syncope, excitement, delirium	Severe cinchonism, granulocytopenia, optic atrophy, hepatitis, hypoglycemia, deafness, hypersensitivity reaction

ADVERSE DRUG REACTIONS

In the low dosages used to prevent or treat malaria, these agents usually produce few serious adverse reactions. (See *Adverse reactions of antimalarial agents.*)

NURSING PROCESS APPLICATION

The following information assists the nurse in caring for a patient who is receiving an antimalarial agent. It includes an overview of assessment activities as well as examples of appropriate nursing diagnoses and related interventions. It also highlights the importance of evaluation.

Assessment

Before drug therapy begins, review the patient's history for conditions that contraindicate or require cautious use of the prescribed antimalarial agent. Also review the patient's medication history to identify use of drugs that may interact with it. During therapy, assess the patient for adverse drug reactions and signs of drug interactions. Also, periodically assess the effectiveness of antimalarial therapy. Finally, evaluate the patient's and family's knowledge of the prescribed drug.

Nursing diagnoses

- Risk for injury related to adverse drug reactions or drug interactions
- Altered protection related to the adverse hematologic effects of the prescribed antimalarial agent
- Knowledge deficit related to the prescribed antimalarial agent regimen

Planning and implementation

- Do not administer an antimalarial agent to a patient with a condition that contraindicates its use.
- Administer an antimalarial agent cautiously to a patient with a preexisting condition.
- Monitor the patient periodically for adverse reactions and drug interactions during antimalarial therapy.

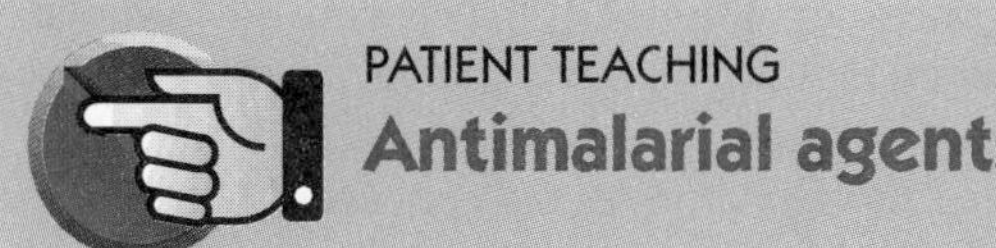

PATIENT TEACHING
Antimalarial agents

- Teach the patient and family the name, dose, frequency, action, and adverse effects of the prescribed antimalarial agent.
- Instruct the patient receiving primaquine or quinine to take the drug with food to minimize adverse gastrointestinal reactions.
- Advise the patient that these medications should not be taken with antacids.
- Instruct the patient to exercise caution while driving or operating hazardous machinery during antimalarial therapy.
- Inform the patient and family that the antimalarial agent may affect the patient's behavior and emotional state. Instruct them to report personality changes, confusion, or other such alterations to the physician.
- Advise the patient to report any visual or auditory changes immediately to the physician and to have regular ophthalmic and auditory examinations.
- Teach the patient receiving quinine to recognize and report the signs and symptoms of hypoglycemia and cinchonism.
- Warn a female patient of childbearing age who is traveling to an area where malaria is endemic against becoming pregnant. Instruct her to continue contraceptive precautions for 2 months after the last dose of medication.
- Explain to the patient that children are extremely sensitive to chloroquine and hydroxychloroquine and that accidental ingestion can cause death. Instruct the patient to keep these and all other medications out of the reach of children.
- Stress the importance of having a complete blood count and liver and renal function studies done. If thrombocytopenia occurs, teach the patient to take bleeding precautions.
- Instruct the patient to report adverse reactions.

• Administer chloroquine, primaquine, or quinine with food to minimize adverse gastrointestinal (GI) reactions. (See Patient Teaching: *Antimalarial agents.*)
• Do not administer medications concurrently with antacids.
***** *Monitor the patient's vital signs for abnormalities, such as fever, hypothermia, increased or decreased heart rate or blood pressure, or decreased respiratory rate. Also monitor the electrocardiogram (ECG) to detect arrhythmias or other ECG changes.***
• Observe the patient's behavior and emotional state for irritability, personality changes, excitability, or other such changes during antimalarial therapy. If changes are observed, notify the primary health care provider to discuss changing the patient to a different antimalarial.
***** *Monitor the patient for visual or auditory changes when administering chloroquine, hydroxychloroquine, primaquine, or quinine.***
• Regularly monitor the patient's blood glucose level and observe for signs and symptoms of hypoglycemia (profuse sweating, nervousness, and headache) when administering quinine.

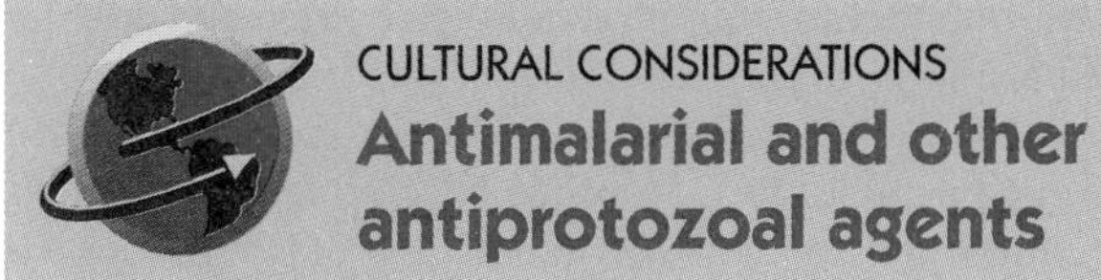

CULTURAL CONSIDERATIONS
Antimalarial and other antiprotozoal agents

Glucose-6-phosphate dehydrogenase (G6PD) determinations should be made before treatment with primaquine, especially in Blacks, Asians, and Whites of Mediterranean origin. If a deficiency is found, administer primaquine with caution because it may cause hemolytic anemia in these individuals.

***** *Initiate seizure precautions when administering chloroquine, hydroxychloroquine, mefloquine, or pyrimethamine.***
• Notify the primary health care provider if adverse reactions or drug interactions occur.
• Monitor the patient's complete blood count (CBC) and liver and renal function studies for abnormalities. Notify the primary health care provider if any abnormalities occur.
• Initiate bleeding precautions if thrombocytopenia occurs and observe the patient for signs of bleeding, such as spontaneous epistaxis, bruises, hematuria, and occult blood in the urine or feces, until the patient's platelet count returns to normal.
• Stagger the patient's activities and promote frequent rest periods if anemia occurs.
• Notify the primary health care provider of hematologic changes. (See Cultural Considerations: *Antimalarial and other antiprotozoal agents.*)

Evaluation

For each nursing diagnosis, prepare an evaluation statement that describes the patient's or family's response to nursing interventions.

Other antiprotozoal agents

Although many agents are used to treat protozoal infections, this section focuses on the following readily obtainable antiprotozoal agents: atovaquone, eflornithine, furazolidone, iodoquinol, metronidazole, pentamidine isethionate, and trimetrexate. Other antiprotozoal agents include investigational new drugs that can be obtained only from the Centers for Disease Control and Prevention, such as dehydroemetine, diloxanide furoate, melarsoprol, nifurtimox, and suramin sodium. Amphotericin B, paromomycin, and co-trimoxazole are also used sometimes as antiprotozoals.

PHARMACOKINETICS

After oral administration, atovaquone absorption varies. The bioavailability increases approximately threefold when administered with meals. It is approximately 99.9% plasma protein-bound. Atovaquone is not metabolized and is excreted primarily in the feces. The pharmacokinetics of iodoquinol and pentamidine are unclear. After oral administration, furazolidone is absorbed poorly and is inactivated in the intestine. About 5% of an oral dose of furazolidone is excreted in the urine as unchanged drug and metabolites. From 80% to 90% of a metronidazole dose is absorbed after oral administration. It is distributed widely, metabolized partially in the liver, and excreted in the urine and, to a lesser degree, in the feces.

Atovaquone shows double-peak concentrations, with the first peak occurring between 1 and 8 hours after administration and the second 24 to 96 hours after administration. This double peak suggests that the drug is excreted into the bile from the systemic circulation and then reabsorbed.

Little or no information exists about the onsets of action, peak concentration levels, or durations of action of furazolidone, iodoquinol, and pentamidine. Information about trimetrexate pharmacokinetics is limited due to the small number of patients studied. Pharmacokinetic parameters appear to differ in patients with *P. carinii* pneumonia and those with cancer. Concurrent administration with folinic acid also appears to alter these pharmacokinetic parameters.

Route	Onset	Peak	Duration
P.O.	Unknown	Double peak: 1-8 hr; 24 to 96 hr	2-3 days, unknown
Inhalation	Unknown	Unknown	Unknown
I.M.	Unknown	30-60 min	Unknown
I.V.	Variable	Variable	Unknown

PHARMACODYNAMICS

Atovaquone is thought to inhibit electron transport, causing decreased activity of several mitochondrial enzymes and thereby inhibiting nucleic acid and adenosine triphosphate synthesis.

Furazolidone may kill **bacteria** by interfering with their enzyme systems and by inhibiting monoamine oxidase.

Iodoquinol is a contact or luminal amebicide that acts directly on **protozoa** in the GI tract.

The **bactericidal, amebicidal,** and trichomonacidal properties of metronidazole may result from disruption of protozoal DNA and inhibition of nucleic acid synthesis, eventually causing cellular death.

Pentamidine may work by several mechanisms that may vary with the protozoan involved. These mechanisms include inhibition of dihydrofolate reductase, interference with aerobic glycolysis, and inhibition of oxidative phosphorylation and nucleic acid synthesis.

Eflornithine inhibits the enzyme ornithine decarboxylase, resulting in a disruption of cell division and differentiation.

Trimetrexate is an inhibitor of the enzyme dihydrofolate reductase. This results in disruption of DNA, ribonucleic acid, and protein synthesis, and, ultimately, cell death. Trimetrexate must be administered concurrently with folinic acid to protect the patient's normal cells.

PHARMACOTHERAPEUTICS

Atovaquone is only indicated for patients with mild to moderate *Pneumocystis carinii* pneumonia who cannot tolerate co-trimoxazole therapy. Eflornithine is indicated for treatment of the meningoencephalitic stage of *Trypanosoma brucei gambiense* infections. Trimetrexate with concurrent folinic acid is indicated as an alternate for the treatment of moderate to severe *P. carinii* pneumonia in patients who are intolerant of, or are refractory to, co-trimoxazole or for whom co-trimoxazole therapy is contraindicated. The other antiprotozoal agents are used for a wide range of disorders, including *P. carinii* infections, amebiasis, giardiasis, trichomoniasis, toxoplasmosis, African trypanosomiasis, and leishmaniasis.

Drug interactions

No significant drug interactions occur with the administration of atovaquone. However, many interactions occur between the other antiprotozoal agents and other drugs. (See Drug Interactions: *Other antiprotozoal agents.*)

ADVERSE DRUG REACTIONS

Adverse reactions to atovaquone reported by 10% or more of patients in clinical trials include rash, nausea, diarrhea, headache, vomiting, fever, and cough. Several other antiprotozoal agents can produce severe, even life-threatening, adverse reactions. The recommended dosages and duration of therapy for these agents must not be exceeded. (See *Adverse reactions of other antiprotozoal agents,* page 466.)

NURSING PROCESS APPLICATION

The following information assists the nurse in caring for a patient who is receiving an antiprotozoal agent. It includes an overview of assessment activities as well as examples of appropriate nursing diagnoses and related interventions. It also highlights the importance of evaluation.

Assessment

Before drug therapy begins, review the patient's history for conditions that contraindicate or require cautious use of the prescribed antiprotozoal agent. Also review the patient's medication history to identify use of drugs that may interact with it. During therapy, assess the patient for adverse drug reactions and signs of drug interactions. Also, periodically assess the effectiveness of antiprotozoal therapy. Finally, evaluate the patient's and family's knowledge of the prescribed drug.

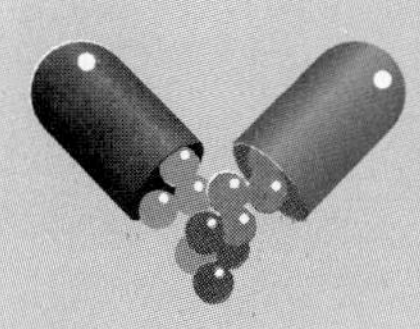

DRUG INTERACTIONS

Other antiprotozoal agents

Many interactions can occur between antiprotozoal agents and other drugs. Because most interactions are unpredictable, the nurse should monitor the patient closely.

DRUG	INTERACTING DRUGS	POSSIBLE EFFECTS	NURSING IMPLICATIONS
furazolidone	alcohol	A disulfiram-like reaction (flushing, weakness, lightheadedness, and lacrimation) may occur	• Instruct the patient to avoid alcohol use during furazolidone therapy. • Take a detailed social history.
	meperidine	Increased mepridine levels; may lead to seizures, agitation, diaphoresis, fever, coma, and apnea	• Avoid concomitant therapy.
	tricyclic antidepressants (TCAs)	Increased TCA blood levels leading to hypertension, hypyrexia, seizures, tachycardia, and psychosis	• Avoid concomitant therapy. • Take a detailed drug history.
	anorexiant sympathomimetics	Increased pressor effects caused by monamine oxidase inhibition	• Avoid concomitant therapy. • Take a detailed drug history.
iodoquinol	preparations that contain iodine	Increased binding of iodine to protein, thus causing interference with thyroid function tests	• Explain to the patient that thyroid function tests may be abnormal for up to 6 months after iodoquinol therapy is discontinued.
metronidazole	anticoagulants (warfarin type)	Increased hypoprothrombinemia	• Monitor the patient receiving an oral anticoagulant for altered anticoagulant effect when metronidazole therapy begins or ends.
	disulfiram	Acute psychotic reaction, confusion	• Monitor the patient's psychological status for changes.
	alcohol	Disulfiram-like reaction, including flushing, headache, nausea, vomiting, abdominal cramps, and sweating	• Instruct the patient to avoid alcohol use during metronidazole therapy.
	barbiturates	Increased metronidazole metabolism and possible therapeutic failure	• Adjust metronidazole dosage as prescribed.
pentamidine	aminoglycosides, cisplatin, amphotericin B	Increased nephrotoxic effects	• Observe for therapeutic failure. • Reduce the doses or adjust the dose intervals, as prescribed, when these medications are used concomitantly.
eflornithine	erythromycin, rifampin, rifabutin, ketoconazole, fluconazole, cimetidine or other drugs known to induce P-450 liver enzyme system	Altered trimetrexate metabolism	• Monitor the patient's renal failure by measuring fluid intake and output and assessing the serum creatinine and blood urea nitrogen levels.
trimetrexate	zidovudine	Additive toxicity	• Avoid concomitant therapy.

Adverse reactions of other antiprotozoal agents

This chart summarizes the adverse reactions to antiprotozoal agents, grouping them by frequency.

DRUG	COMMON	OCCASIONAL	RARE
furazolidone	Nausea, vomiting	Abdominal pain, diarrhea, headache, malaise	Hypersensitivity reaction, hypoglycemia, granulocytopenia, hemolytic anemia, disulfiram-like reaction
iodoquinol	Anorexia, vomiting, diarrhea, abdominal cramps, constipation, pruritus ani	Neurotoxicity, optic neuritis, optic atrophy, peripheral neuropathy, iodism, subacute myelo-opticoneuropathy (with muscle pain, weakness, optic atrophy, and ataxia), urticaria, pruritus, thyroid enlargement, fever, chills, headache, vertigo, malaise, discoloration of hair and nails	Agitation, amnesia, hair loss, granulocytopenia, hypersensitivity reaction
metronidazole	Nausea, headache, anorexia, dry mouth, metallic taste	Vomiting, diarrhea, epigastric distress, abdominal discomfort, constipation, dizziness, vertigo, lack of coordination, ataxia, confusion, irritability, depression, weakness, insomnia, urethral burning, dysuria, vaginal dryness, dyspareunia, decreased libido	Pseudomembranous colitis, peripheral neuropathy, transient leukopenia, hypersensitivity reaction, furry tongue, glossitis, stomatitis, disulfiram-like reaction, flattening of T wave on electrocardiogram
pentamidine	Nephrotoxicity, pain or induration at the injection site, elevated liver function tests, leukopenia, nausea, anorexia, bronchospasm, cough with inhalation therapy	Hypotension, arrhythmias, phlebitis, pruritus, urticaria, hypoglycemia, hyperglycemia, thrombocytopenia, hypocalcemia, vomiting, sterile abscess	Stevens-Johnson syndrome, pancreatitis, anemia, neutropenia, thrombocytopenic purpura, toxic epidermal necrolysis
eflornithine	anemia, leukopenia	Diarrhea, thrombocytopenia, seizures	Hearing loss, vomiting, alopecia, abdominal pain, anorexia, headache, asthenia, facial edema, eosinophilia
trimetrexate	bone marrow depression	Rash, peripheral neuropathy, elevated liver function test results, fever, electrolyte imbalance	Nausea, vomiting, confusion, fatigue, increased kidney function test values

Nursing diagnoses

- Risk for injury related to adverse drug reactions or drug interactions
- Risk for fluid volume deficit related to the adverse GI effects of the prescribed antiprotozoal agent
- Knowledge deficit related to the prescribed antiprotozoal agent regimen

Planning and implementation

- Do not administer an antiprotozoal agent to a patient with a condition that contraindicates its use.
- Administer an antiprotozoal agent cautiously to a patient with a preexisting condition.
- Monitor the patient periodically for adverse reactions and drug interactions during antiprotozoal therapy.

Monitor the patient's blood pressure and ECG before, during, and after pentamidine administration. Infuse intravenous (I.V.) pentamidine over 1 hour with the patient supine to minimize severe hypotension and arrhythmias. Have emergency resuscitation equipment nearby.

- Monitor the patient's blood glucose level during pentamidine therapy and several weeks after it is discontinued.
- Dissolve nebulized pentamidine in sterile water and administer it via a Respirgard II nebulizer.
- Perform a respiratory assessment after administering nebulized pentamidine, particularly watching for bronchospasm and cough. (See Patient Teaching: *Other antiprotozoal agents.*)
- Inspect the infusion site for evidence of phlebitis when administering I.V. pentamidine.
- Be aware that atovaquone is only indicated for patients with mild to moderate *P. carinii* pneumonia.
- Administer atovaquone with food for maximum absorption and therapeutic value. Patients with GI disorders may not be candidates for therapy.

• Dilute eflornithine with sterile water for injection prior to use; administer infusion over a *minimum* of 45 minutes; do not administer concomitantly with other I.V. drugs.
• Monitor patients receiving eflornithine for seizure activity.
• Monitor patients receiving eflornithine for hearing loss.
• Administer trimetrexate concomitantly with folinic acid.
• Reconstitute trimetrexate with dextrose 5% or sterile water; further dilute with dextrose 5% prior to administration.
• Expect that trimetrexate dosages will be lower in patients with hematologic, renal, or hepatic impairment.
• Monitor CBCs and renal and hepatic function tests in patients receiving trimetrexate.
• Notify the primary health care provider if adverse reactions or drug interactions occur.
• Monitor hydration if the patient experiences anorexia, nausea, vomiting, or diarrhea. Obtain a prescription for an antiemetic or antidiarrheal agent as needed.
• Notify the primary health care provider if adverse GI reactions persist or worsen.

Evaluation

For each nursing diagnosis, prepare an evaluation statement that describes the patient's or family's response to nursing interventions.

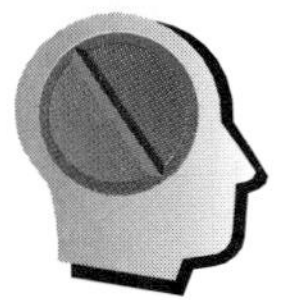

CRITICAL THINKING. To enhance your critical thinking about antiprotozoal agents, consider the following situation and its analysis.
Situation: Buddy Hansen is a 27-year-old male who is HIV-positive. He is admitted to the hospital with suspected *P. carinii* pneumonia. His past medical history is significant for a similar admission 5 months ago when treated with co-trimoxazole for 21 days. After discharge, he was placed on pentamidine 300 mg for inhalation once every 4 weeks for *P. carinii* prophylaxis. He complained of severe bronchospasm and shortness of breath because he thinks he is allergic to the medication. What are your thoughts about whether his therapy has failed or succeeded?
Analysis: Co-trimoxazole therapy is the drug of choice for treatment of *P. carinii* pneumonia. Mr. Hansen appears to have been successfully treated in the past. It has been 5 months since the last episode, so a second course of co-trimoxazole would be warranted. Chances are that this is not a failure of the first therapy. In addition to the general monitoring for a patient on co-trimoxazole, the patient should be closely monitored for worsening of his condition as a result of treatment failure. If his condition worsens, an alternate treatment regimen may be initiated. Co-trimoxazole may be given orally or intravenously (I.V.); if Mr. Hansen does well on this regimen, he may be discharged on oral therapy. Trimetrexate plus folinic acid could also be used as an alternative therapy. This regimen is more toxic and requires more frequent and intense monitoring. Additionally, trimetrexate is only available as an I.V. medication. It would be the regimen of choice if co-trimoxazole failure is suspected; however, he did have a documented adverse event to pentamidine (bronchospasm and shortness of breath). In either case, baseline laboratory values including complete blood counts and renal function tests must be taken prior to initiation of either regimen.

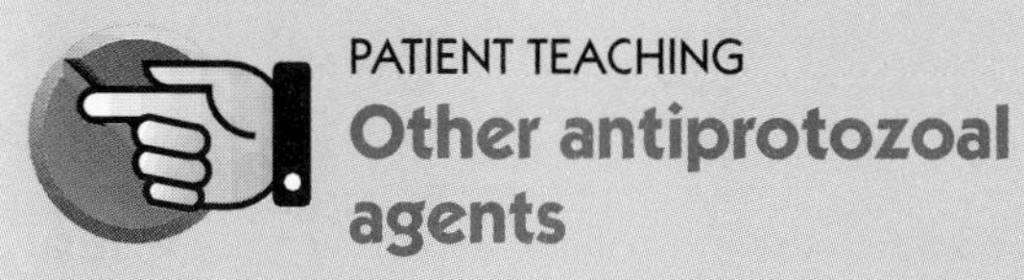

PATIENT TEACHING
Other antiprotozoal agents

- Teach the patient and family the name, dose, frequency, action, and adverse effects of the prescribed antiprotozoal agent.
- Inform the patient that pain may occur at the injection site with intramuscular (I.M.) administration of pentamidine.
- Advise the patient to alert the nurse or physician if a cough or shortness of breath occurs after pentamidine inhalation therapy or if pruritus or skin changes occur during I.M. or intravenous pentamidine therapy. Review the signs and symptoms of hyperglycemia or hypoglycemia with the patient.
- Advise the patient that metronidazole may darken the urine and cause dysuria and a lingering metallic taste in the mouth.
- Caution the patient to avoid activities that require mental alertness or physical coordination if adverse central nervous system reactions occur.
- Advise the patient to take a laxative if constipation occurs. Also, teach the patient how to prevent constipation.
- Inform the patient receiving metronidazole that decreased libido may occur. Inform the female patient that she may experience vaginal dryness and dyspareunia.
- Teach the patient how to manage metronidazole-induced insomnia through relaxation techniques and other nonpharmacologic measures.
- Advise the patient to take metronidazole with food to minimize the risk of adverse gastrointestinal reactions. Also instruct the patient to avoid alcoholic beverages during therapy and for 48 hours after it is discontinued.
- Advise the patient to refrain from sexual intercourse during treatment for trichomoniasis or to have her partner use a condom to avoid reinfection. Recommend that all sexual partners be evaluated for infection.
- Instruct the patient to avoid drinking alcohol during furazolidone therapy because it can cause serious systemic adverse reactions.
- Teach the patient mouth care techniques if metronidazole causes glossitis or stomatitis.
- Inform the patient that iodoquinol can interfere with thyroid function tests.
- Inform the patient receiving iodoquinol that hair loss or nail and hair discoloration can occur.
- Instruct the patient to take atovaquone with food.
- Advise the patient on long-term antiprotozoal therapy to have periodic ophthalmologic examinations and to report any vision disturbances to the physician.
- Teach the patient about drug interactions that can occur with furazolidone. Advise the patient to avoid tyramine-rich foods, such as cheese, chocolate, and sausage, and over-the-counter medications containing sympathomimetics, such as cold capsules and anorexiants.
- Instruct the patient to report adverse reactions to the physician.

CHAPTER SUMMARY

Chapter 35 discussed antimalarial and other antiprotozoal agents as they are used to prevent or treat malaria and other protozoal infections. Here are the chapter highlights.

The major agents used to prevent and treat malaria include the 4-aminoquinolines (chloroquine hydrochloride, chloroquine phosphate, and hydroxychloroquine sulfate), mefloquine hydrochloride, the 8-aminoquinoline primaquine phosphate, pyrimethamine, quinine sulfate, and quinidine gluconate.

Antimalarial agents can produce a wide variety of adverse reactions. Quinine commonly produces cinchonism; the others typically produce adverse GI reactions. Less common adverse reactions range from blood disorders to deafness to psychotic episodes.

Different antiprotozoal agents are used to manage amebiasis, giardiasis, leishmaniasis, *P. carinii* infections, toxoplasmosis, trichomoniasis, and African trypanosomiasis. These agents include atovaquone, furazolidone, iodoquinol, metronidazole, pentamidine isoethionate, eflornithine, and trimetrexate .

The other antiprotozoal drugs produce a range of adverse reactions, which include GI distress, central nervous system disturbances, and nephrotoxicity. More severe, but less common, adverse reactions affecting most body systems also may occur.

The nurse should instruct the patient and family about the administration, therapeutic effects, and possible adverse effects of antimalarial and other antiprotozoal agents, monitor the patient throughout therapy, and notify the primary health care provider if adverse reactions occur.

Questions to consider

See Appendix 1 for answers.

1. James Ti-Ku Lee has a history of seizures, controlled by phenobarbital. He is diagnosed with acute intestinal amebiasis and will be treated with metronidazole. Which of the following dosage adjustments would the nurse expect?
   (a) The dose of metronidazole will be increased.
   (b) The dose of metronidazole will be decreased.
   (c) The dose of phenobarbital will be decreased.
   (d) The dose of phenobarbital will be increased.

2. Mary Hellitus will be discharged today. She is scheduled to receive an I.V. pentamidine infusion. Which of the following nursing actions should be taken to prepare for the infusion?
   (a) Prepare a chair so that the I.V. can be administered while Mrs. Hellitus is sitting.
   (b) Prepare a quiet room with a flat bed for use during I.V. administration.
   (c) Prepare the resuscitation equipment and a well lit room for use during I.V. administration.
   (d) Order a home infusion to administer the drug after discharge.

3. Felix Berallini develops epigastric discomfort while taking chloroquine. To minimize this adverse reaction, the nurse should give him which of the following instructions?
   (a) Take the medication with antacids.
   (b) Take the medication with meals.
   (c) Take the medication at bedtime.
   (d) Take the medication before meals.

4. Sylvia Brown, age 42, is diagnosed with giardiasis caused by *Giardia lamblia.* Which of the following drugs is her physician most likely to prescribe?
   (a) quinine sulfate
   (b) atovaquone
   (c) pyrimethamine
   (d) furazolidone

37 Urinary antiseptic agents

OBJECTIVES

After reading and studying this chapter, the student should be able to:

1. describe the actions of the fluoroquinolones, sulfonamides, and nitrofurantoin.
2. discuss drug interactions associated with urinary antiseptic agents.
3. describe adverse reactions associated with the fluoroquinolones, sulfonamides, and nitrofurantoin.
4. describe how to apply the nursing process when caring for a patient who is receiving a urinary antiseptic agent.

INTRODUCTION

This chapter discusses the urinary antiseptic agents. The most commonly used urinary antiseptics are the fluoroquinolones (ciprofloxacin, norfloxacin, levofloxacin, lomefloxacin, ofloxacin), sulfonamides (co-trimoxazole, sulfadiazine, sulfamethoxazole, and sulfisoxazole), and nitrofurantoin. These agents are used in patients with **bacteriuria** because they inhibit the growth of many species of **bacteria** in the urine and greatly diminish the symptoms of lower urinary tract **infections** (UTIs). Less commonly used urinary antiseptic agents include cinoxacin, methenamine, nalidixic acid, and trimethoprim. (See *Selected major urinary antiseptic agents,* page 470.)

Drugs covered in this chapter include:

- cinoxacin
- ciprofloxacin
- co-trimoxazole
- levofloxacin
- lomefloxacin
- methenamine
- nalidixic acid
- nitrofurantoin
- norfloxacin
- ofloxacin
- sulfadiazine
- sulfamethoxazole
- sulfisoxazole
- trimethoprim.

Fluoroquinolones

Ciprofloxacin, norfloxacin, levofloxacin, lomefloxacin, and ofloxacin are structurally similar synthetic antibiotics. They primarily are administered orally to treat UTIs.

PHARMACOKINETICS

After oral administration, the fluoroquinolones are absorbed well. The onset of action of norfloxacin occurs within 30 minutes. These drugs are not highly protein-bound, minimally metabolized in the liver, and excreted primarily by the kidneys in the urine.

Route	Onset	Peak	Duration
P.O.	Unknown	0.5-2.3 hr	3-8 hr, then 20-25 hr (biphasic pattern)
I.V.	Immediate	Immediate	4-5 hr, then 20-25 hr

PHARMACODYNAMICS

The effectiveness of fluoroquinolones in treating UTIs relates to an affinity for enzymes within the bacterial cell. These drugs interrupt deoxyribonucleic acid synthesis during bacterial replication.

PHARMACOTHERAPEUTICS

The fluoroquinolones can be used to treat a wide variety of UTIs. In addition, ciprofloxacin is used to treat lower respiratory tract infections; skin, bone, or joint infections; and infectious diarrhea. Lomefloxacin also is used to treat lower respiratory tract infections and to prevent UTIs in patients who are undergoing transurethral procedures. Ofloxacin also is used to treat selected sexually transmitted diseases, lower respiratory infections, skin and skin-structure infections, and prostatitis. All fluoroquinolones require dosage reductions when they are used to treat patients with renal dysfunction. Levofloxacin is also indicated for treatment of lower respiratory infections.

Drug interactions

Several drug interactions are associated with the fluoroquinolones. These agents interact with antacids that contain magnesium or aluminum hydroxide, resulting in decreased absorption of the fluoroquinolone. With the exception of lomefloxacin and levofloxacin, the fluoroquinolones also interact with xanthine derivatives, such as aminophylline or

Selected major urinary antiseptic agents

This chart lists the major antiseptic agents currently in clinical use.

DRUG	MAJOR INDICATIONS AND USUAL DOSAGES	CONTRAINDICATIONS AND PRECAUTIONS
Fluoroquinolones		
ciprofloxacin (Cipro)	*Urinary tract infection (UTI)* ADULT: 250 to 500 mg P.O. every 12 hours *Respiratory tract, skin, bone, or joint infections* ADULT: 500 to 750 mg P.O. every 12 hours *Infectious diarrhea* ADULT: 500 mg P.O. every 12 hours	• Ciprofloxacin is contraindicated in a pediatric, pregnant, or breast-feeding patient or one with known hypersensitivity to the drug or other fluoroquinolones. • This drug requires cautious use in a patient with known or suspected central nervous system disorders.
norfloxacin (Noroxin)	*Uncomplicated UTI* ADULT: 400 mg P.O. b.i.d. for 7 to 10 days *Complicated UTI* ADULT: 400 mg P.O. b.i.d. for 10 to 21 days	• Norfloxacin is contraindicated in a pediatric, pregnant, or breast-feeding patient or one with known hypersensitivity to the drug or other fluoroquinolones. • This drug requires cautious use in a patient with a condition that predisposes the patient to seizures.
lomefloxacin (Maxaquin)	*Treatment of UTI and lower respiratory tract infections caused by susceptible organisms; prevention of UTI in patients undergoing transurethral procedures* ADULT: 400 mg P.O. daily for 10 to 14 days	• Lomefloxacin is contraindicated in a patient with known hypersensitivity to the drug or other fluoroquinolones. • This drug requires cautious use in a patient with impaired renal function. • Safety and efficacy in pregnant patients, breast-feeding patients, and children have not been established.
ofloxacin (Floxin)	*Uncomplicated and complicated UTI* ADULT: 200 mg P.O. every 12 hours for 10 days *Prostatitis* ADULT: 300 mg P.O. every 12 hours for 6 weeks	• Ofloxacin is contraindicated in children and in pregnant or breast-feeding patients. • This drug is contraindicated in a patient with hypersensitivity to fluoroquinolones. • Use with caution in a geriatric patient because adverse effects can be more pronounced due to decreased renal function. • The patient should avoid excessive exposure to sunlight while receiving this drug.
levofloxacin (Levaquin)	*Acute pylonephritis and complicated UTI* ADULT: 250 mg P.O. every 24 hours for 10 days	• Levofloxacin is contraindicated in a patient with hypersensitivity to fluoroquinolones. • This drug is not indicated for use in children or in pregnant or breast-feeding patients. • Use with caution in elderly patients or those with impaired renal function or seizure disorders. • The patient should avoid excessive exposure to sunlight.
Sulfonamides		
sulfamethoxazole (Gantanol)	*UTI* ADULT: for severe infections, 2 g P.O. initially, then 1 g P.O. b.i.d. to t.i.d. PEDIATRIC: for children over age 2 months, initially, 50 to 60 mg/kg P.O. every 12 hours, then 25 to 30 mg/kg P.O. every 12 hours *Lymphogranuloma venereum (genital, inguinal, or anorectal infections)* ADULT: 1 g P.O. b.i.d. for at least 21 days	• Sulfamethoxazole is contraindicated in a pregnant patient who is at term, a breast-feeding patient, or one with known hypersensitivity. • This drug requires cautious use in a patient with impaired renal or hepatic function, severe allergy to sulfa drugs, bronchial asthma, or glucose-6-phosphate dehydrogenase deficiency.

Selected major urinary antiseptic agents *(continued)*

DRUG	MAJOR INDICATIONS AND USUAL DOSAGES	CONTRAINDICATIONS AND PRECAUTIONS
Nitrofurantoin		
nitrofurantoin (Furadantin, Macrodantin)	*Uncomplicated UTI* ADULT: 50 to 100 mg P.O. q.i.d. for 7 to 14 days PEDIATRIC: for children over age 1 month, 5 to 7 mg/kg P.O. daily in four divided doses for at least 7 days and for at least 3 days after sterility of urine is ascertained *Suppression of recurrent UTI* ADULT: 50 to 100 mg P.O. daily h.s. PEDIATRIC: for children over age 1 month, 1 mg/kg P.O. daily as a single dose or in two divided doses	• Nitrofurantoin is contraindicated in an infant under age 1 month, a pregnant patient who is at term, or one with anuria, oliguria, significant renal impairment, or known hypersensitivity. • This drug requires cautious use in a breast-feeding patient.

theophylline, increasing the plasma theophylline concentration and the risk of theophylline **toxicity.** Ciprofloxacin, norfloxacin, and lomefloxacin interact with probenecid, resulting in decreased renal elimination of these fluoroquinolones—thus increasing their serum concentrations and half-lives.

ADVERSE DRUG REACTIONS

Well tolerated by most patients, the fluoroquinolones produce few adverse reactions. The most common reactions affect the gastrointestinal (GI) tract and include nausea, vomiting, diarrhea, and abdominal pain. About 1% of patients have developed adverse central nervous system (CNS) reactions, such as headache, drowsiness, seizures, vision disturbances, hallucinations, depression, and agitation. Photosensitivity has been reported in 2.4% of patients receiving lomefloxacin during clinical trials. Lomefloxacin also may cause dizziness. Ofloxacin and levofloxacin may cause insomnia and dizziness.

Less common adverse reactions affect the integumentary system. In 1% of patients or fewer, the fluoroquinolones produce hypersensitivity reactions that include urticaria, nonspecific rashes, pruritus, and edema. Some patients experience transient arthralgia or myalgia.

Other rare reactions include hematologic problems, such as hemolytic anemia, that are associated with glucose-6-phosphate dehydrogenase (G6PD) deficiency and disturbances of blood glucose, including symptomatic hyperglycemia and hypoglycemia.

NURSING PROCESS APPLICATION

The following information assists the nurse in caring for a patient who is receiving a fluoroquinolone. It includes an overview of assessment activities as well as examples of appropriate nursing diagnoses and related interventions. It also highlights the importance of evaluation.

Assessment

Before drug therapy begins, review the patient's history for conditions that contraindicate or require cautious use of the prescribed fluoroquinolone. Also review the patient's medication history to identify use of drugs that may interact with it. During therapy, assess the patient for adverse drug reactions and signs of drug interactions. Also, periodically assess the effectiveness of fluoroquinolone therapy. Finally, evaluate the patient's and family's knowledge about the prescribed drug.

Nursing diagnoses

- Risk for injury related to adverse drug reactions or drug interactions
- Risk for trauma related to fluoroquinolone-induced seizures
- Knowledge deficit related to the prescribed fluoroquinolone regimen

Planning and implementation

- Do not administer a fluoroquinolone to a patient with a condition that contraindicates its use.
- Administer a fluoroquinolone cautiously to a patient at risk because of a preexisting condition.
- Monitor the patient for adverse reactions and drug interactions during fluoroquinolone therapy.
- Take safety precautions if the patient experiences adverse CNS reactions, such as drowsiness, vision disturbances, or dizziness. For example, place the bed in the lowest position, keep the bed rails raised, and supervise the patient's ambulation.

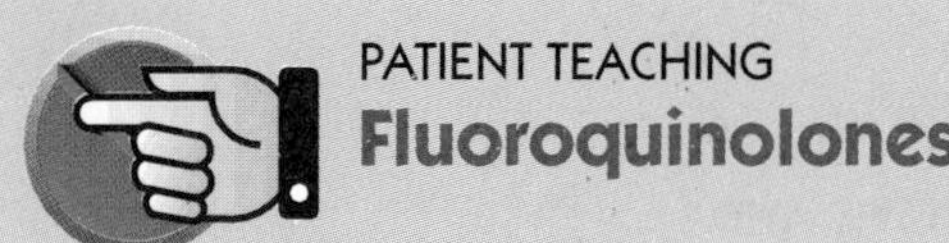

- Teach the patient and family the name, dose, frequency, action, and adverse effects of the prescribed fluoroquinolone.
- Advise the patient taking a fluoroquinolone to use extreme caution when driving or operating machinery because these drugs may cause dizziness, drowsiness, or other adverse central nervous system reactions.
- Advise the patient to take a mild analgesic if headache occurs.
- Teach the patient nonpharmacologic measures to use if ofloxacin causes insomnia. If these measures are ineffective, instruct the patient to request a prescription for a sedative from the physician.
- Instruct the patient to report rash, urticaria, ankle swelling, or pruritus because these signs may indicate a fluoroquinolone hypersensitivity reaction.
- Inform the patient when to take antacids if they also are part of the patient's treatment regimen.
- Instruct the patient to notify the physician if adverse reactions occur.

- Adjust the dosage as prescribed for a patient with impaired renal function because the elimination rate will decrease and the serum half-life will increase.
- Administer antacids, as prescribed, at least 2 hours after administering a fluoroquinolone.
- Question the patient about any history of head trauma, seizures, or use of drugs known to cause seizures before administering a fluoroquinolone. (See Patient Teaching: *Fluoroquinolones*.)
- Monitor the patient for seizures during fluoroquinolone therapy.
- Take seizure precautions such as padding the bed rails, if needed.
- Notify the physician immediately if seizures occur.
- Notify the physician if other adverse reactions or drug interactions occur.

Evaluation

For each nursing diagnosis, prepare an evaluation statement that describes the patient's or family's response to nursing interventions.

Sulfonamides

The sulfonamides were the first effective systemic **antibacterial** agents. Today, they are less useful because strains of bacteria that resist sulfonamides have emerged. The sulfonamides discussed in this chapter include co-trimoxazole, sulfadiazine, sulfamethoxazole, and sulfisoxazole.

PHARMACOKINETICS

Most sulfonamides are absorbed well and distributed widely in the body. They are metabolized in the liver to inactive metabolites and excreted by the kidneys. Sulfonamides are classified as short-acting, intermediate-acting, and long-acting, depending on their absorption and excretion rates. Sulfadoxine (in combination with pyrimethamine as Fansidar) is the only long-acting sulfonamide available in the United States. It is used to treat and prevent malaria caused by chloroquine-resistant *Plasmodium falciparum.*

Route	Onset	Peak	Duration
P.O.	Unknown	2-17 hr	4 hr-days
I.V.	Immediate	3-17 hr	7-17 hr

PHARMACODYNAMICS

Sulfonamides are **bacteriostatic** agents that prevent the growth of **microorganisms** by inhibiting folic acid production. The decreased folic acid synthesis decreases the number of bacterial nucleotides and inhibits bacterial growth.

PHARMACOTHERAPEUTICS

Sulfonamides are used primarily to treat acute UTIs. With recurrent or chronic UTIs, the infecting organism may or may not be susceptible to sulfonamides; therefore, the choice of therapy should be based on bacteria susceptibility tests. Sulfonamides also are used to treat infections caused by *Nocardia asteroides, Toxoplasma gondii,* and *Chlamydia trachomatis.* Sulfonamides exhibit a wide **spectrum** of activity against gram-positive and gram-negative bacteria. However, the increasing **resistance** of formerly susceptible bacteria has decreased the clinical usefulness of these drugs. Sulfonamide **prophylaxis** against *Neisseria meningitidis* is variably effective.

Drug interactions

All sulfonamides interact with para-aminobenzoic acid, sulfonylureas (hypoglycemic agents), and methenamine. Co-trimoxazole also interacts with coumarin anticoagulants and cyclosporine. (See Drug Interactions: *Sulfonamides.*)

ADVERSE DRUG REACTIONS

The sulfonamides cause numerous adverse reactions. Excessively high doses of less water-soluble sulfonamides can produce crystalluria and tubular deposits of sulfonamide crystals. These complications can be minimized by maintaining a high urine flow rate and alkalinized urine. With the newer water-soluble sulfonamides, these complications usually do not occur. Nausea, vomiting, and diarrhea are common.

The incidence of hypersensitivity reactions appears to increase as the dosage increases. Various dermatologic reac-

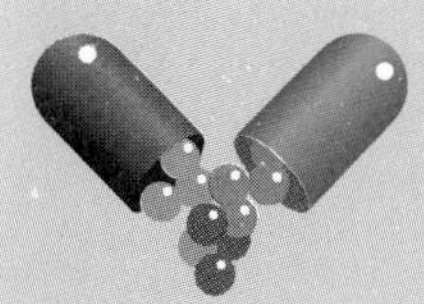

DRUG INTERACTIONS

Sulfonamides

The following chart summarizes the significant interactions between sulfonamides and other drugs.

DRUG	INTERACTING DRUGS	POSSIBLE EFFECTS	NURSING IMPLICATIONS
co-trimoxazole, sulfadiazine, sulfamethoxazole, sulfisoxazole	para-aminobenzoic acid	Decreased antibacterial activity	• Avoid concurrent use.
	sulfonylureas (hypoglycemic agents)	Increased hypoglycemic effect	• Monitor the patient's blood glucose level frequently. • Decrease the sulfonylurea dosage, as prescribed.
	methenamine	Crystalluria	• Avoid concomitant use.
co-trimoxazole	coumarin anticoagulants	Increased anticoagulant effect	• Monitor the patient's prothrombin time frequently. • Decrease the anticoagulant dosage, as prescribed.
	cyclosporine	Increased nephrotoxicity	• Closely monitor the patient's renal function.

tions, including rash, pruritus, erythema nodosum, erythema multiforme of the Stevens-Johnson type, and exfoliative dermatitis, can occur. Sulfonamides also can produce photosensitivity.

Fever may develop 7 to 10 days after the initial sulfonamide dose. A reaction that resembles **serum sickness** may occur, producing fever, joint pain, urticarial eruptions, bronchospasm, and leukopenia. Extremely rare reactions, such as granulocytopenia, aplastic anemia, and hemolytic anemia, have been reported.

NURSING PROCESS APPLICATION

The following information assists the nurse in caring for a patient who is receiving a sulfonamide. It includes an overview of assessment activities as well as examples of appropriate nursing diagnoses and related interventions. It also highlights the importance of evaluation.

Assessment

Before drug therapy begins, review the patient's history for conditions that contraindicate or require cautious use of the prescribed sulfonamide. Also review the patient's medication history to identify use of drugs that may interact with it. During therapy, assess the patient for adverse drug reactions and signs of drug interactions. Also, periodically assess the effectiveness of sulfonamide therapy. Finally, evaluate the patient's and family's knowledge about the prescribed drug.

Nursing diagnoses

- Risk for injury related to adverse drug reactions or drug interactions
- Altered urinary elimination related to sulfonamide-induced crystalluria and tubular deposits of sulfonamide crystals
- Knowledge deficit related to the prescribed sulfonamide regime

Planning and implementation

- Do not administer a sulfonamide to a patient with a condition that contraindicates its use.
- Administer a sulfonamide cautiously to a patient at risk because of a preexisting condition.
- Monitor the patient for adverse reactions and drug interactions during sulfonamide therapy.
- Withhold the sulfonamide dose and notify the physician if dermatologic reactions occur. Expect to provide dermatologic care to relieve discomfort caused by the reaction.
- Administer oral preparations of sulfonamides with ample amounts of fluids. (See Patient Teaching: *Sulfonamides,* page 474.)
- Notify the physician if adverse reactions or drug interactions occur.
- Monitor the patient's urine elimination pattern for such changes as an increase or decrease in the amount voided, urinary frequency, or dysuria.

***** ***Monitor the patient's fluid intake and output. The urine output should be at least 1,500 ml per day to ensure proper hydration. Inadequate urine output can lead to crystalluria or tubular deposits of the sulfonamide.***

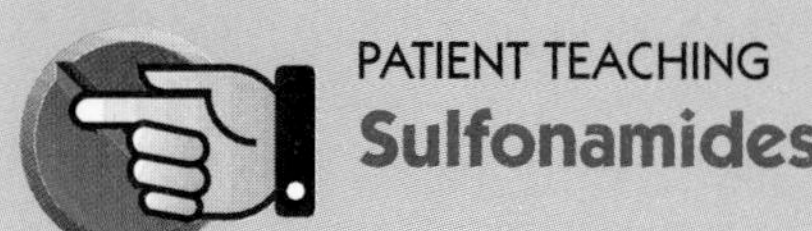

PATIENT TEACHING
Sulfonamides

- Teach the patient and family the name, dose, frequency, action, and adverse effects of the prescribed sulfonamide.
- Advise the patient to avoid direct sunlight to help prevent a photosensitivity reaction.
- Instruct the patient to notify the physician if signs and symptoms of a hematologic reaction (such as sore throat, pallor, purpura, jaundice, or weakness) or a dermatologic reaction (such as rash or pruritus) occur.
- Stress the importance of completing the course of sulfonamide therapy.
- Instruct the patient to consume at least eight 8-oz (240-ml) glasses of fluid daily while taking a sulfonamide.
- Instruct the patient to notify the physician if adverse reactions occur.

• Notify the primary health care provider if the patient cannot consume adequate amounts of fluid or if the patient's urine elimination pattern changes for no apparent reason.

Evaluation

For each nursing diagnosis, prepare an evaluation statement that describes the patient's or family's response to nursing interventions.

Nitrofurantoin

Nitrofurantoin is used primarily to treat acute and chronic UTIs.

PHARMACOKINETICS

After oral administration, nitrofurantoin is absorbed rapidly and well from the GI tract. Concomitant ingestion of food enhances the bioavailability of nitrofurantoin. The drug is 20% to 60% protein-bound. Nitrofurantoin crosses the placental barrier and is secreted in breast milk; it also is distributed in bile. Two-thirds of a nitrofurantoin dose is metabolized by the liver and one-third is excreted unchanged in the urine.

Route	Onset	Peak	Duration
P.O.	Unknown	20 min	<1 hr

PHARMACODYNAMICS

Usually bacteriostatic, nitrofurantoin may become **bactericidal** depending on its urinary concentration and the susceptibility of the infecting organisms. Although the exact mechanism of action has not been described, the drug appears to inhibit formation of acetyl coenzyme A from pyruvic acid, thereby inhibiting the energy production of the infecting organism. Nitrofurantoin also may disrupt bacterial cell wall formation.

PHARMACOTHERAPEUTICS

Nitrofurantoin is used to treat UTIs; its antibacterial activity is higher in acid urine. It is not effective against systemic bacterial infections.

Drug interactions

Probenecid and sulfinpyrazone inhibit the renal excretion of nitrofurantoin, reduce its efficacy, and increase its toxic potential. Antacids can decrease the extent and rate of nitrofurantoin absorption. Nitrofurantoin may decrease the antibacterial activity of norfloxacin and nalidixic acid. It may produce false-positive results for urine glucose determinations when Benedict's reagent (Clinitest) is used, but does not affect results when glucose oxidase methods (Clinistix, Tes-Tape) are used.

ADVERSE DRUG REACTIONS

GI irritation is the most common adverse reaction to nitrofurantoin. Anorexia, nausea, and vomiting occur more commonly than diarrhea and abdominal pain. Some patients have experienced peripheral neuropathy, which usually begins with paresthesia and dysesthesia of the legs and can progress to a debilitating state.

Hypersensitivity reactions may occur and involve the skin, lungs, blood, and liver. Chills, fever, arthralgia (a characteristic of systemic lupus erythematosus), and anaphylaxis also may occur. Dermatologic hypersensitivity reactions include maculopapular, erythematous, or eczematous rashes; urticaria; angioneurotic edema; and pruritus. Pulmonary reactions include asthmatic attacks in patients with a history of asthma and acute pneumonitis. Acute pneumonitis is manifested by sudden fever, chills, cough, dyspnea, chest pain, eosinophilia, and pulmonary infiltration that may appear as consolidation or pleural effusion on X-rays. It is most common in geriatric patients, with symptoms appearing within the 1st week of treatment.

Hematologic reactions are rare but may include leukopenia, granulocytopenia, and megaloblastic anemia. In patients with G6PD deficiency, nitrofurantoin can precipitate an acute episode of hemolytic anemia, although this is rare. Non-dose-related hepatotoxicity occurs rarely as well as chronic active hepatitis, cholestatic jaundice, and cholestatic hepatitis. Nitrofurantoin may color the urine dark yellow or brown.

NURSING PROCESS APPLICATION

The following information assists the nurse in caring for a patient who is receiving nitrofurantoin. It includes an overview of assessment activities as well as examples of appropriate nursing diagnoses and related interventions. It also highlights the importance of evaluation.

Assessment

Before drug therapy begins, review the patient's history for conditions that contraindicate or require cautious use of nitrofurantoin. Also review the patient's medication history to identify use of drugs that may interact with it. During therapy, assess the patient for adverse drug reactions and signs of drug interactions. Also, periodically assess the effectiveness of nitrofurantoin therapy. Finally, evaluate the patient's and family's knowledge about the prescribed drug.

Nursing diagnoses

• Risk for injury related to adverse drug reactions or drug interactions
• Risk for injury related to hypersensitivity reactions to the prescribed nitrofurantoin
• Knowledge deficit related to the prescribed nitrofurantoin regime

Planning and implementation

• Do not administer nitrofurantoin to a patient with a condition that contraindicates its use.
• Administer nitrofurantoin cautiously to a patient at risk because of a preexisting condition.
• Avoid concomitant administration of nitrofurantoin with probenecid, sulfinpyrazone, antacids, nalidixic acid, and norfloxacin.
• Monitor the patient for adverse reactions and drug interactions during nitrofurantoin therapy.
• Monitor the patient for hypersensitivity reactions that may involve the skin, lungs, blood, and liver. Keep standard emergency equipment nearby because anaphylaxis may occur.
• Withhold the drug and notify the physician if a hypersensitivity reaction occurs during nitrofurantoin therapy. Provide symptomatic relief as prescribed. (See Patient Teaching: *Nitrofurantoin.*)
• Administer nitrofurantoin with food or milk to minimize adverse GI reactions.
∗ Obtain a urine culture and sensitivity test before beginning and during therapy, as prescribed, to determine drug effectiveness. Nitrofurantoin therapy should be continued for 3 days after sterility of urine is ascertained.
• Notify the physician if adverse reactions or drug interactions occur.

Evaluation

For each nursing diagnosis, prepare an evaluation statement that describes the patient's or family's response to nursing interventions.

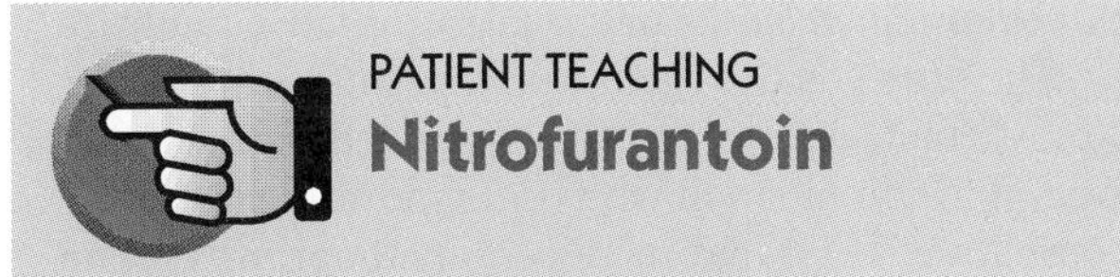

PATIENT TEACHING
Nitrofurantoin

- Teach the patient and family the name, dose, frequency, action, and adverse effects of nitrofurantoin.
- Stress the importance of taking the drug for the prescribed length of time.
- Inform the patient that nitrofurantoin may turn urine brown or dark yellow.
- Instruct the patient to take nitrofurantoin with food or milk.
- Advise the patient that gastrointestinal upset is a common adverse reaction.
- Instruct the patient to stop taking nitrofurantoin and notify the physician if paresthesia, dysesthesia, or hypersensitivity reaction occurs.
- Caution the patient against performing activities that require alertness, such as operating a motor vehicle or machinery, if paresthesia or dysesthesia occur.
- Teach the patient the proper procedure for collecting a urine sample for culture and sensitivity testing.
- Instruct the diabetic patient not to perform urine glucose determinations using Clinitest, because false-positive results may occur during nitrofurantoin therapy.
- Instruct the patient to notify the physician if adverse reactions occur.

Other urinary antiseptic agents

Less commonly used urinary antiseptic agents include cinoxacin, methenamine, nalidixic acid, and trimethoprim.

Cinoxacin is a quinolone derivative indicated for acute and chronic uncomplicated UTIs. Its antibacterial spectrum is somewhat greater than that of nalidixic acid. It is effective against all *Proteus, Escherichia coli,* and most strains of *Klebsiella, Enterobacter, Citrobacter, Providencia,* and *Serratia.* It is ineffective against *Pseudomonas, Staphylococcus aureus,* and enterococci.

Methenamine is prescribed to prevent recurrent UTIs, especially for long-term suppressive therapy. It is active against all gram-positive and gram-negative bacteria. However, UTIs caused by urea-splitting organisms such as *Proteus* may not respond, because acidifying the urine is difficult in the presence of these bacteria that increase urinary pH.

Nalidixic acid is a quinolone derivative used to treat acute and chronic UTIs. It has a limited antibacterial spectrum. Although the development of resistance may limit the usefulness of this drug against *E. coli, Proteus mirabilis,* other *Proteus, Klebsiella,* and *Enterobacter,* it is bactericidal at easily achieved concentrations in the urine of 16 mcg/ml or less. *Pseudomonas* is resistant to nalidixic acid.

Trimethoprim is used to treat initial episodes of acute uncomplicated UTIs caused by *E. coli, P. mirabilis, Klebsiella pneumoniae, Enterobacter,* or coagulase-negative staphylococci. The drug is active against most gram-positive **cocci** and most gram-negative rods. Using trimethoprim alone instead of in combination with co- trimoxazole for acute uncomplicated UTIs may increase trimethoprim-resistant organisms.

CHAPTER SUMMARY

Chapter 37 presented the urinary antiseptic agents that can be used against UTIs. Here are the chapter highlights.

The fluoroquinolones, a major class of urinary antiseptic agents, include ciprofloxacin, norfloxacin, levofloxacin, lomefloxacin, and ofloxacin.

Ciprofloxacin also is used to treat lower respiratory tract infections; skin, bone, or joint infections; and infectious diarrhea. Ofloxacin also is indicated to treat lower respiratory infections, some sexually transmitted diseases, skin and skin-structure infections, and prostatitis.

The sulfonamides include co-trimoxazole, sulfadiazine, sulfamethoxazole, and sulfisoxazole. They are used primarily to treat acute UTIs. With recurrent or chronic UTIs, the infecting organism may or may not be susceptible to sulfonamides.

Nitrofurantoin, another urinary antiseptic agent, is effective in acute UTIs and recurrent bacteriuria.

Other, less commonly used urinary antiseptic agents include cinoxacin and nalidixic acid, which are quinolone derivatives, and the anti-infective agents methenamine and trimethoprim.

The nurse should administer urinary antiseptic agents cautiously because various adverse reactions can occur. The nurse also must teach the patient and family about the importance of compliance with therapy to prevent recurrent UTIs.

Questions to consider

See Appendix 1 for answers.

1. Tammy Winslow, age 24, is an adult asthmatic who takes theophylline in conjunction with her treatment regimen for asthma. She comes to you complaining of signs of a UTI, which is soon confirmed by testing. Which of the following drugs would be the best choice for Ms. Winslow?
   (a) ofloxacin
   (b) lomefloxacin
   (c) ciprofloxacin
   (d) norfloxacin

2. Mohammud El-Al, age 38, tells the nurse that he takes an antacid whenever he experiences heartburn. What should the nurse tell him about taking the antacid in relationship to the ciprofloxacin dose?
   (a) Take the antacid whenever it is needed.
   (b) Take the antacid 15 minutes before the ciprofloxacin dose.
   (c) Take the antacid 2 hours after the ciprofloxacin dose.
   (d) Take the antacid immediately after the ciprofloxacin dose.

3. Amos Nutley, age 47, develops an acute lower UTI. He tells the nurse he has never had a UTI before. The physician prescribes the sulfonamide co-trimoxazole for 10 days. Which of the following instructions should the nurse give Mr. Nutley about co-trimoxazole?
   (a) Continue to take his oral hypoglycemic agent as usual.
   (b) Take the medication with an antacid.
   (c) Limit the fluid intake to 32 oz (1 L) daily.
   (d) Drink at least eight 8-oz (240-ml) glasses of fluid daily.

4. Lurethra Walker, age 38, has developed a recurrent UTI. You, as her nurse practitioner, prescribe nitrofurantoin. Which of the following instructions should *not* be included in her instructions?
   (a) Nitrofurantoin may turn her urine bright red.
   (b) Nitrofurantoin should be taken with food or milk.
   (c) Nitrofurantoin should be discontinued and the nurse notified if paresthesia or dysesthesia occur.
   (d) Nitrofurantoin should be taken for the full course of treatment.

UNIT

XI

Drugs to control inflammation, allergy, and organ rejection

Certain agents used to control **inflammation,** allergic reactions, and organ rejection are used for more than one purpose. Glucocorticoids, for example, exert anti-inflammatory and immunosuppressant effects, the antiallergy drugs block inflammation caused by **antigen-antibody** reactions, and immunosuppressant drugs are used to prevent organ rejection. To understand the mechanisms of action of these drugs, the nurse needs an overview of immune and inflammatory responses.

IMMUNE AND INFLAMMATORY RESPONSES

Immune and inflammatory responses protect the body from foreign substances and insults. (See *Immune responses,* page 478.) These responses usually help maintain homeostasis, but sometimes are inappropriate, as in a patient undergoing organ transplantation or experiencing an **autoimmune** disease. In such instances, drugs are used to suppress these responses.

The immune system is a highly complicated and regulated system. It's categorized into two major components, the cellular and humoral immune systems.

Cell-mediated response depends on the T **lymphocyte (T cell)** system. Stem cells in the bone marrow give rise to T cell precursors, which later are released from the thymus as mature T cells. (They are called T cells because they come from the thymus.) T cells may be helper or suppressor cells. **Helper T cells** enhance the body's immune response; **suppressor T cells** inhibit it. Helper T cells usually outnumber suppressor T cells by two to one. In a disease such as acquired immunodeficiency syndrome (AIDS), however, the number of helper T cells drops to almost zero.

In an autoimmune disease, such as systemic lupus erythematosus or rheumatoid arthritis, the cell-mediated response is activated by the individual's cells, which the immune system treats as foreign substances. (See Cultural Considerations: *Systemic lupus erythematosus.*)

The humoral response depends on B lymphocyte **(B cell)** activity. B cells (lymphocytes that originate as stem cell precursors in the bone marrow) respond to an antigen by differentiating into plasma cells that secrete antigen-specific antibodies. This antigen-antibody reaction activates the **complement** system, which causes lysis of antigenic cells.

Immune responses commonly result in inflammation, the local reaction of vascularized tissue to injury. When injury occurs, chemical reactions involving bradykinins, prostaglandins, and histamines ensue. These reactions cause vasodilation at the injury site, which increases blood flow, redness, and warmth. Capillary permeability also increases, causing edema (swelling). Pain results from the edema and the effects of **histamine** and bradykinin on nerve endings. Leukocyte migration to the area to remove cellular debris contributes to the edema and pain.

An exaggerated immune response, or **hypersensitivity** reaction, can occur in a sensitized individual. Reexposure to an **allergen** can cause such symptoms as **rhinitis,** wheezing, and red, tearing eyes.

DRUG THERAPY

Unit XI presents drugs that modify immune or inflammatory responses. These drugs are used in such diverse disorders as allergic rhinitis, hypersensitivity reactions, and organ transplant rejection.

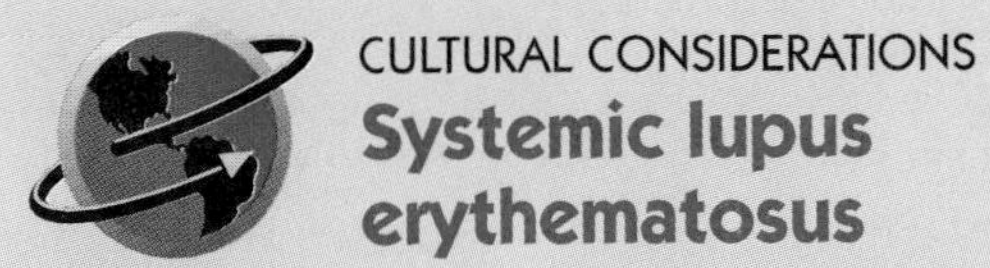

CULTURAL CONSIDERATIONS

Systemic lupus erythematosus

Systemic lupus erythematosus (SLE) is most prevalent among Asians and Blacks. The prognosis improves with early detection and treatment, so make sure you include related questions as part of your health history and observe for signs of SLE during physical assessment. Be aware that corticosteriods are often used in the treatment of the disorder.

Immune responses

When an antigen stimulates the bone marrow stem cells, the immune system produces one of two responses, shown below.

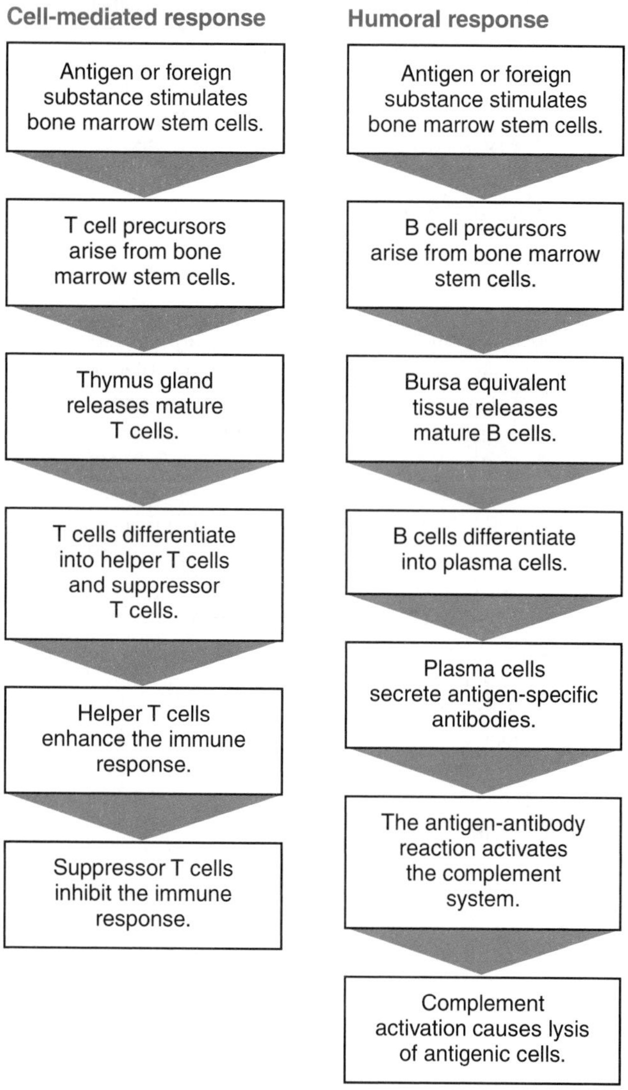

Cell-mediated response

Antigen or foreign substance stimulates bone marrow stem cells.

T cell precursors arise from bone marrow stem cells.

Thymus gland releases mature T cells.

T cells differentiate into helper T cells and suppressor T cells.

Helper T cells enhance the immune response.

Suppressor T cells inhibit the immune response.

Humoral response

Antigen or foreign substance stimulates bone marrow stem cells.

B cell precursors arise from bone marrow stem cells.

Bursa equivalent tissue releases mature B cells.

B cells differentiate into plasma cells.

Plasma cells secrete antigen-specific antibodies.

The antigen-antibody reaction activates the complement system.

Complement activation causes lysis of antigenic cells.

For example, antihistaminic agents block the effects of histamine on target tissues, which makes them useful in treating allergies and some hypersensitivity reactions. Corticosteroids are used to suppress immune responses and reduce inflammation. Noncorticosteroid immunosuppressants most commonly are prescribed to prevent rejection of transplanted organs, but can be used to treat autoimmune disease, such as **rheumatoid arthritis.** Gold salts reduce joint inflammation caused by rheumatoid arthritis, possibly by altering the body's immune response.

38 Antihistaminic agents

OBJECTIVES

After reading and studying this chapter, the student should be able to:

1. explain the action of histamine$_1$ (H_1)- receptor antagonists and explain how they relieve allergy symptoms.
2. identify drugs in the six major antihistamine drug classes.
3. describe the interactions between H_1-receptor antagonists and other drugs.
4. discuss the major adverse reactions to the H_1-receptor antagonists.
5. describe how to apply the nursing process when caring for a patient who is receiving an antihistaminic agent.

INTRODUCTION

Antihistamines primarily act to block **histamine** effects that occur in an immediate (type I) **hypersensitivity** reaction, commonly called an allergic reaction. By doing this, antihistamines diminish most histamine effects and relieve the symptoms of a type I hypersensitivity reaction. They are available alone or in combination products, by prescription, or over-the-counter (OTC). (See *Selected major antihistaminic agents,* pages 480 to 482.)

Drugs covered in this chapter include:

- astemizole
- azatadine maleate
- brompheniramine maleate
- chlorpheniramine maleate
- clemastine fumarate
- cyclizine lactate
- cyproheptadine hydrochloride
- dexchlorpheniramine maleate
- dimenhydrinate
- diphenhydramine hydrochloride
- hydroxyzine hydrochloride
- hydroxyzine maleate
- loratadine
- meclizine hydrochloride
- methdilazine hydrochloride
- phenindamine tartrate
- phenyltoloxamine citrate
- promethazine hydrochloride
- pyrilamine maleate
- trimeprazine tartrate
- tripelennamine citrate
- tripelennamine hydrochloride
- triprolidine hydrochloride.

Histamine$_1$-receptor antagonists

The term *antihistamine* refers to drugs that act as H_1-receptor antagonists. Drugs that antagonize histamine-$_2$ (H_2) receptors are not considered antihistamines and are discussed separately. Based on chemical structure, antihistamines are categorized into six major classes: ethanolamines, ethylenediamines, alkylamines, phenothiazines, piperidines, and miscellaneous agents.

The ethanolamines include clemastine fumarate, dimenhydrinate, diphenhydramine hydrochloride, and phenyltoloxamine citrate. The ethylenediamines are pyrilamine maleate, tripelennamine citrate, and tripelennamine hydrochloride. The alkylamines include brompheniramine maleate, chlorpheniramine maleate, dexchlorpheniramine maleate, and triprolidine hydrochloride. The phenothiazines include methdilazine hydrochloride, promethazine hydrochloride, and trimeprazine tartrate. The piperidine class consists of azatadine maleate, cyclizine lactate, cyproheptadine hydrochloride, meclizine hydrochloride, and phenindamine tartrate. Astemizole, loratadine, hydroxyzine hydrochloride, and hydroxyzine maleate are miscellaneous antihistamines; astemizole and loratadine are longer-acting and produce fewer central nervous system (CNS) effects than the other antihistamines.

PHARMACOKINETICS

H_1-receptor antagonists are absorbed well after oral or parenteral administration. Some may also be given rectally. They are distributed widely throughout the body and CNS, with the exceptions of astemizole and loratadine. The "nonsedating" antihistamines penetrate the blood-brain barrier so poorly that very little drug is distributed in the CNS. Antihistamines are metabolized by hepatic enzymes and excreted in the urine. Small amounts are secreted in breast milk.

(Text continues on page 482.)

Selected major antihistaminic agents

This chart summarizes the major antihistaminic agents currently in clinical use.

DRUG	MAJOR INDICATIONS AND USUAL DOSAGES	CONTRAINDICATIONS AND PRECAUTIONS
Ethanolamines		
dimenhydrinate (Dimetabs, Dramamine, Marmine)	*Nausea, vomiting, and vertigo associated with motion sickness* ADULT: 50 to 100 mg P.O. every 4 to 6 hours, as needed, not to exceed 400 mg daily PEDIATRIC: for children over age 12, 50 to 100 mg P.O. every 4 to 6 hours, as needed, not to exceed 400 mg daily; for children ages 6 to 12, 25 to 50 mg P.O. every 6 to 8 hours, as needed, not to exceed 150 mg daily; for children ages 2 to 5, 12.5 to 25 mg P.O. every 6 to 8 hours, as needed, not to exceed 75 mg daily; alternatively, for all children, 1.25 mg/kg or 37.5 mg/m^2 P.O. q.i.d., as needed, up to a maximum of 300 mg daily *Vestibular system disease* ADULT: 50 to 100 mg P.O. every 4 to 6 hours, as needed, not to exceed 400 mg daily	• Dimenhydrinate is contraindicated in a breast-feeding patient, a patient who is receiving monoamine oxidase (MAO) inhibitor therapy, or one with known hypersensitivity. • This drug requires cautious use in a patient with acute angle-closure glaucoma, stenosed peptic ulcer, pyloroduodenal obstruction, symptomatic prostatic hyperplasia, bladder neck obstruction, bronchial asthma, increased intraocular pressure (IOP), hyperthyroidism, cardiovascular (CV) disease, or hypertension.
diphenhydramine (Benadryl, Benylin, Compoz, Nytol, Sominex)	*Motion sickness, rhinitis, and other allergy symptoms* ADULT: 25 to 50 mg P.O. t.i.d. or q.i.d. (do not exceed 300 mg daily), or 10 to 50 mg I.V. or deep I.M. injection PEDIATRIC: for children over age 12, 25 to 50 mg P.O. every 4 to 6 hours, as needed, not to exceed 300 mg daily; for children ages 6 to 12, 12.5 to 25 mg P.O. every 4 to 6 hours, as needed, not to exceed 150 mg daily; for children ages 2 to 5, 6.25 mg P.O. every 4 to 6 hours, as needed, not to exceed 37.5 mg daily *Dyskinesia, Parkinson's disease* ADULT: 25 to 50 mg P.O. one to four times a day, or 25 to 50 mg I.V. or deep I.M. injection *Hypnotic effects* ADULT: 25 to 50 mg P.O. h.s. PEDIATRIC: for children over age 12, 25 to 50 mg P.O. h.s.; for children ages 2 to 12, 1 mg/kg (up to a maximum of 50 mg) P.O. h.s.	• Diphenhydramine is contraindicated in a neonate, a premature neonate, a breast-feeding patient, a patient who is receiving MAO inhibitor therapy, or one with known hypersensitivity to this drug or any other antihistamine with a similar chemical structure. • This drug requires cautious use in a patient with acute angle-closure glaucoma, stenosed peptic ulcer, pyloroduodenal obstruction, symptomatic prostatic hyperplasia, bladder neck obstruction, bronchial asthma, increased IOP, hyperthyroidism, CV disease, or hypertension.
clemastine (Tavist)	*Allergic rhinitis* ADULT: 1.34 mg b.i.d. to 2.68 mg t.i.d; do not exceed 8.04 mg daily	• Clemastine is contraindicated in a breast-feeding patient, a pregnant patient in her third trimester, or a patient with acute asthma or known hypersensitivity. • Use with caution in patients with bronchial asthma, acute angle-closure glaucoma, prostatic hyperplasia, bladder neck obstruction, stenosed peptic ulcer, pyloroduodenal obstruction, or known hypersensitivity. • This drug requires cautious use in a pregnant patient in her first or second trimester or a patient with increased IOP, hyperthyroidism, CV disease, or hypertension.
Ethylenediamines		
tripelennamine hydrochloride (PBZ, PBZ-SR, Pelamine)	*Allergy symptoms* ADULT: 25 to 50 mg of tripelennamine hydrochloride P.O. every 4 to 6 hours, not to exceed 600 mg daily; or 100 mg sustained-release form of tripelennamine hydrochloride P.O. b.i.d. or t.i.d.	• Tripelennamine is contraindicated in a neonate, a premature neonate, a pregnant or breast-feeding patient, a patient who is receiving MAO inhibitor therapy, or one with prostatic hyperplasia, bladder neck ob–

(continued)

Selected major antihistaminic agents *(continued)*

DRUG	MAJOR INDICATIONS AND USUAL DOSAGES	CONTRAINDICATIONS AND PRECAUTIONS
Ethylenediamines *(continued)*		
tripelennamine hydrochloride (PBZ, PBZ-SR, Pelamine) *(continued)*	PEDIATRIC: 5 mg/kg or 150 mg/m^2 P.O. every 4 to 6 hours, not to exceed 300 mg daily; do not use sustained-released in children	struction, acute angle-closure glaucoma, bronchial asthma, stenosed peptic ulcer, pyloroduodenal obstruction, or known hypersensitivity to this drug or related compounds. Sustained-release tablets are contraindicated in children. • This drug requires cautious use in a patient with increased IOP, hyperthyroidism, CV disease, or hypertension.
Alkylamines		
brompheniramine (Bromphen, Dimetane, Dimetane Extentabs, Veltane)	*Allergy symptoms, seasonal and perennial allergic rhinitis* ADULT: 4 mg P.O. every 4 to 6 hours, not to exceed 24 mg daily; 8 to 12 mg sustained-release form P.O. every 8 to 12 hours; or 10 mg I.V., I.M., or S.C. every 6 to 12 hours, as needed, not to exceed 40 mg daily PEDIATRIC: for children over age 12, 4 mg P.O. every 4 to 6 hours, not to exceed 24 mg daily or, alternatively, 8 to 12 mg sustained-release form P.O. every 12 hours, not to exceed 24 mg daily; for children ages 6 to 12, 2 to 4 mg P.O. t.i.d. or q.i.d. or, alternatively, 8 to 12 mg sustained-release form P.O. every 12 hours, not to exceed 24 mg daily; for children ages 2 to 5, 1 mg P.O. every 4 to 6 hours, not to exceed 6 mg daily or, alternatively, 0.5 mg/kg or 15 mg/m^2 daily in three or four divided doses	• Brompheniramine is contraindicated in a neonate, a premature infant, a pregnant or breast-feeding patient, a patient who is receiving MAO inhibitor therapy, or one with prostatic hyperplasia, bladder neck obstruction, acute angle-closure glaucoma, bronchial asthma, stenosed peptic ulcer, pyloroduodenal obstruction, or known hypersensitivity to this drug or related compounds. Sustained release tablets are contraindicated in children under age 6. • This drug requires cautious use in a patient with increased IOP, hyperthyroidism, CV disease, or hypertension.
chlorpheniramine (Chlor-Trimeton, Chlor-Trimeton Repetabs, Teldrin)	*Allergy symptoms* ADULT: 4 mg P.O. every 4 to 6 hours, not to exceed 24 mg daily; or 8 to 12 mg sustained-release form P.O. b.i.d. PEDIATRIC: for children over age 12, 4 mg P.O. every 4 to 6 hours, not to exceed 24 mg daily or, alternatively, 8 to 12 mg sustained-release form P.O. b.i.d.; for children ages 6 to 12, 2 mg P.O. every 4 to 6 hours, not to exceed 12 mg daily or, alternatively, 8 mg sustained-release form P.O. once daily; for children ages 2 to 5, 1 mg P.O. every 4 to 6 hours. Do not exceed 4 mg/24 hours. *Uncomplicated allergic reactions* ADULT: 5 to 20 mg I.V. or I.M. PEDIATRIC: for children age 12 and over, 5 to 20 mg I.V. *Anaphylactic reactions* ADULT: 10 to 20 mg I.V. or I.M. PEDIATRIC: for children age 12 and over, 10 to 20 mg I.V.	• Chlorpheniramine is contraindicated in a neonate, a premature infant, a breast-feeding patient, a pregnant patient in her third trimester, a patient receiving MAO inhibitor therapy, or one with bronchial asthma, acute angle-closure glaucoma, prostatic hyperplasia, bladder neck obstruction, stenosed peptic ulcer, pyloroduodenal obstruction, or known hypersensitivity. • This drug requires cautious use in a pregnant patient in her first or second trimester or a patient with increased IOP, hyperthyroidism, CV disease, or hypertension.
Miscellaneous antihistaminic agents		
astemizole (Hismanal)	*Chronic allergic rhinitis* ADULT: 10 mg P.O. daily on empty stomach PEDIATRIC: for children age 12 and over, 10 mg P.O. daily on empty stomach	• Astemizole is strongly contraindicated in patients receiving erythromycin (macrolide antibiotic), itraconazole, fluconazole, ketoconazole, or miconazole due to risk of serious CV events.

(continued)

Selected major antihistaminic agents *(continued)*

DRUG	MAJOR INDICATIONS AND USUAL DOSAGES	CONTRAINDICATIONS AND PRECAUTIONS
Miscellaneous antihistaminic agents *(continued)*		
astemizole (Hismanal) *(continued)*		• Astemizole is contraindicated in a patient with known hypersensitivity to the drug or any of its active ingredients. • This drug requires cautious use in a pregnant or breast-feeding patient or one with asthma or other lower airway disease, cirrhosis or other liver disease, or renal impairment. • Safety and efficacy in children under age 12 have not been established. • Drug should be taken on a empty stomach.
loratadine (Claritin)	*Allergic rhinitis* ADULT: 10 mg P.O. q.d. on an empty stomach	• Loratadine is contraindicated in patient with known hypersensitivity to the drug or any of its ingredients. • This drug requires cautious use in a pregnant or breast-feeding patient. • Patients with hepatic failure and renal impairment may require a lower initial dose.

The onset of action, peak concentration level, and duration of action vary among the antihistamines.

Route	Onset	Peak	Duration
P.O.	15-60 min	1-2 hr	4-8 hr
P.O. (delayed onset)	1-4 hr	3-4 hr	12-24 hr
I.M., I.V.	20-30 min	1-2 hr	4-8 hr
P.R.	30-40 min	1-2 hr	4-8 hr

PHARMACODYNAMICS

H_1-receptor antagonists compete with histamine for H_1-receptor sites on effector cells in the small blood vessels, smooth muscles, peripheral nerves, adrenal medulla, **exocrine glands,** and brain. Through this antagonism, histamine binding on these target tissues is blocked, but the overall release of histamine continues. This action prevents further responses to histamine but does not reverse the present effects of histamine, which means that continued exposure to the **allergen** will cause continued histamine release. If the amount of histamine increases rapidly, antihistamines may not be able to block the numerous histamine molecules from the receptors. When that happens, epinephrine or another physiologic histamine antagonist must be administered to produce the opposite effects of histamine: constricting small blood vessels and relaxing bronchial smooth muscles.

H_1-receptor antagonists effectively block the action of histamine on the small blood vessels. (See *How antihistamines block allergic response.*) They can decrease small arteriole dilation and engorgement of related tissues. They significantly reduce capillary permeability, thereby decreasing interstitial leakage of plasma proteins and fluids and lessening edema.

H_1-receptor antagonists inhibit most smooth-muscle responses to histamine. In particular, they block the constriction of bronchial, gastrointestinal (GI), and vascular smooth muscle. They are less effective on histamine-induced vasodilation. However, administration of an H_2-receptor antagonist may correct this problem.

H_1-receptor antagonists also relieve symptoms by acting on the terminal nerve endings in the skin. Nerve endings stimulated by histamine produce a flare (redness around an urticarial lesion) and itching. H_1-receptor antagonists suppress both symptoms, possibly by blocking histamine receptors that occupy nerve endings.

The drugs also selectively suppress adrenal medulla stimulation, autonomic ganglia stimulation, and exocrine gland secretion, such as lacrimal and salivary secretion. The drugs, however, do not affect parietal cell secretion, which is suppressed more effectively by H_2-receptor antagonists.

Several antihistaminic agents have a high affinity for H_1-receptors in the brain and are used for their CNS effects. These agents include diphenhydramine, dimenhydrinate, promethazine, and various piperidine derivatives.

How antihistamines block allergic response

Although an antihistamine can't reverse symptoms of an allergic response, it can stop the progression of the response. Here's what happens.

When a mast cell becomes sensitized to an antigen (below, top illustration), it reacts to repeated exposure by releasing chemical mediators. One of them, histamine, binds to histamine$_1$ (H_1) receptors found on effector cells, responsible for allergic symptoms (below, middle illustration). This initiates the allergic response that affects the major systems, including the respiratory (bronchial constriction and bronchospasm, shown in bottom illustration), cardiovascular (elevated heart rate), gastrointestinal (smooth-muscle contraction), endocrine (increased release of epinephrine), and integumentary (hives, flushing) systems.

The same process happens before a person takes an antihistamine. The mast cell is sensitized to an antigen (below, top illustration). The mast cell releases chemical mediators, including histamine. An antihistamine such as chlorpheniramine competes with histamine for H_1-receptor sites on the effector cells (below, middle illustration). By binding to these sites first, the drug prevents more histamine from binding to effector cells, stopping the allergic response and preventing allergic symptoms from becoming worse (below, bottom illustration).

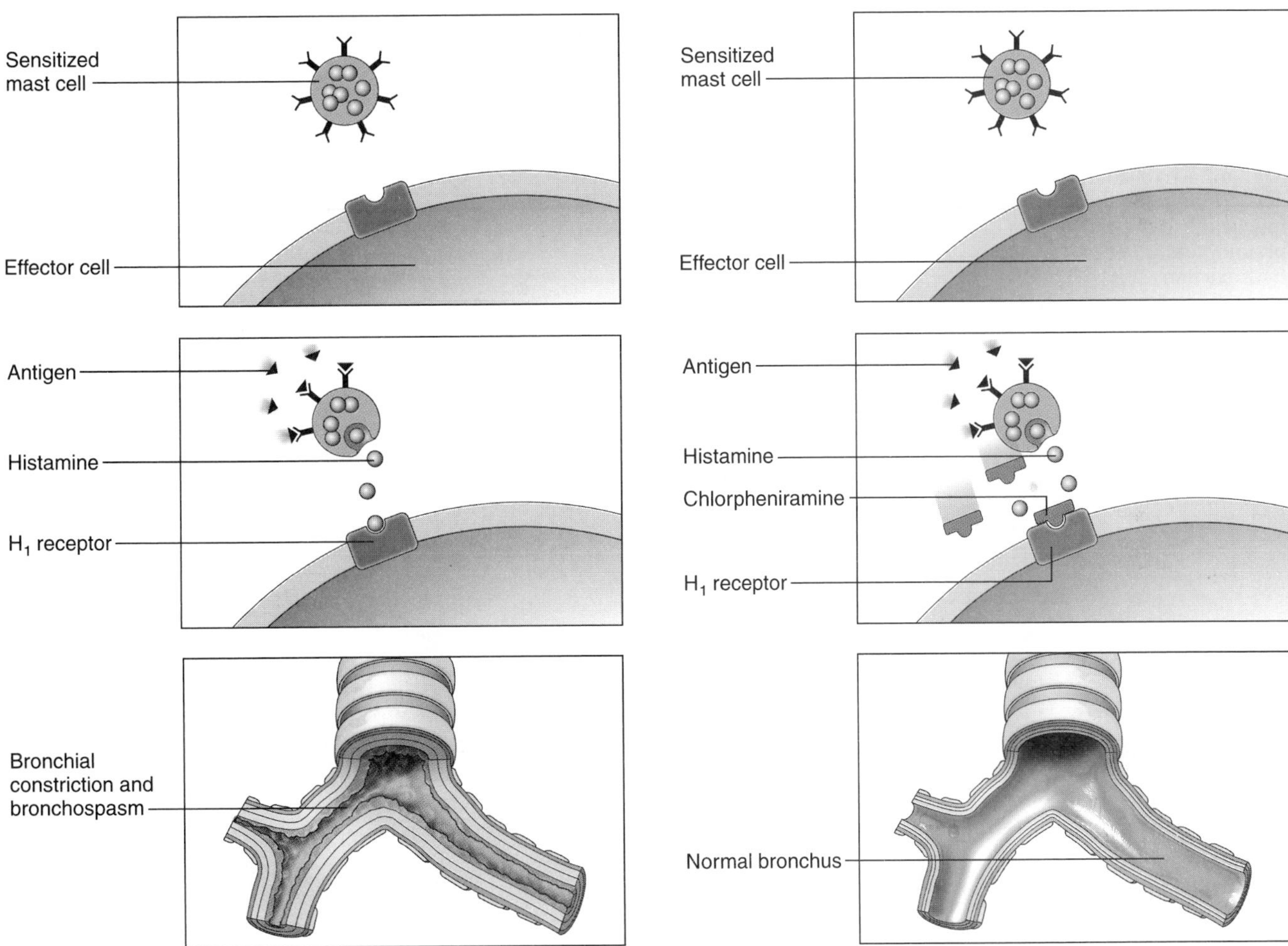

PHARMACOTHERAPEUTICS

Antihistaminic agents are used to treat the symptoms of type I hypersensitivity reactions, such as allergic **rhinitis,** vasomotor rhinitis, allergic **conjunctivitis, urticaria** (hives), and angioedema (submucosal swelling in the hands, face, and feet). They also are used as adjunctive therapy to treat an anaphylactic reaction after its acute manifestations are controlled. Additional clinical indications include nausea, vomiting, motion sickness, vertigo, and preoperative sedation. In fact, some of these drugs are used primarily as antiemetics. Diphenhydramine can help treat Parkinson's disease (parkinsonism) and drug-induced extrapyramidal reactions. Because of its antiserotonin qualities, cyprohepta-

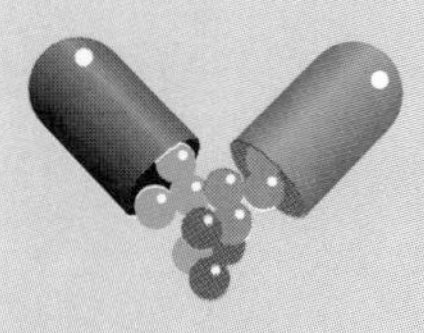

DRUG INTERACTIONS

Antihistaminic agents

Antihistamines can increase the anticholinergic effects of anticholinergic drugs and the sedative effects of central nervous system (CNS) depressants, such as tricyclic antidepressants, tranquilizers, barbiturates, and alcohol. The combination of these drugs with antihistamines can cause life-threatening consequences.

DRUG	INTERACTING DRUGS	POSSIBLE EFFECTS	NURSING IMPLICATIONS
clemastine, dimenhydrinate, diphenhydramine, phenyltoloxamine, pyrilamine, tripelennamine, brompheniramine, chlorpheniramine, dexchlorpheniramine, triprolidine, methdilazine, promethazine, trimeprazine, azatadine, cyclizine, cyproheptadine, meclizine, phenindamine, hydroxyzine	CNS depressants, including barbiturates, tranquilizers, alcohol, and opiates	CNS depression	• Use caution when administering these drugs concurrently to avoid excessive CNS depression or sedation. • Inform an ambulatory patient of possible additive effects.
	anticholinergic drugs, including tricyclic antidepressants, phenothiazines, and antiparkinsonian agents; monoamine oxidase inhibitors	Additive anticholinergic effects	• Assess for signs of increased anticholinergic activity, such as constipation, dry mouth, vision disturbances, and urine retention. • Notify the physician if anticholinergic effects occur.
	ototoxic drugs, including aminoglycosides and salicylates	Masked signs and symptoms of ototoxicity	• Monitor the patient for signs of hearing loss and conduct an audiometric test weekly or biweekly. • Notify the physician of changes in the patient's hearing.
	epinephrine	Vasodilation, increased heart rate, decreased blood pressure	• Monitor the patient's heart rate and blood pressure. • Notify the physician if the patient displays abnormal vital signs.
astemizole, loratadine	macrolide antibiotics (such as erythromycin), fluconazole, ketoconazole, itraconazole, miconazole, cimetidine, ciprofloxacin, clarithromycin	Serious adverse cardiac effects	• Do not administer concurrently.

dine may be used to treat Cushing's disease, serotonin-associated diarrhea, vascular cluster headaches, and anorexia nervosa.

Drug interactions

When given with other drugs, antihistamines may cause three types of interactions. (See Drug Interactions: *Antihistaminic agents.*) The first type may occur when a patient simultaneously receives two or more drugs that have similar effects. The patient will display additive or cumulative drug effects characteristic of drug overdose. Drugs that are likely to cause this interaction with antihistamines include CNS depressants, antimuscarinics, tricyclic antidepressants, and monoamine oxidase inhibitors.

The second type of interaction may occur when an antihistamine blocks or reverses the effects of another drug. For instance, if epinephrine is administered to a patient receiving one of the phenothiazines, the antihistamine may block — or reverse — the intended vasopressor effect. If a vasopressor is required for a patient receiving phenothiazines, norepinephrine or phenylephrine should be used. Similarly, antihistamines may block H_1 receptors in the skin, suppressing the flare reaction to antigen skin testing. Therefore, antihistamines should be discontinued for 4 days before skin testing, whenever possible.

The third type of interaction occurs when antihistamine use masks the toxic signs and symptoms of another drug. For example, an antihistamine used to depress vestibular stimulation and labyrinthine function in motion sickness and vertigo can mask the signs of ototoxicity associated with aminoglycosides or large dosages of salicylates. If antihistamines must be given with an aminoglycoside, the patient must be monitored closely for signs of ototoxicity.

ADVERSE DRUG REACTIONS

The most common adverse reaction that antihistamines produce is CNS depression, which can produce sedation and other symptoms. Occurring with usual dosages, sedation can range from mild drowsiness to deep sleep. Other

CNS reactions may include dizziness, lassitude, disturbed coordination, and muscle weakness. After 2 to 3 days of antihistamine therapy, these adverse reactions may disappear spontaneously. Less common reactions include CNS excitation, restlessness, insomnia, palpitations, and seizures.

The next most common adverse reactions are GI symptoms, including epigastric distress, loss of appetite, nausea, vomiting, constipation, and diarrhea. Taking the drug with meals or with milk may reduce these symptoms.

The third most common reactions are anticholinergic ones, which occur especially with the ethanolamines. Dryness of the mouth, nose, and throat and thickening of bronchial secretions commonly occur. Other anticholinergic effects include urine retention and dysuria; vertigo, tinnitus, and **labyrinthitis;** and vision disturbances, such as diplopia and blurred vision. Cardiovascular effects, such as hypotension, hypertension, tachycardia, and arrhythmias, also may occur.

Sensitivity reactions to antihistamines are not as common but may include hypersensitivity, drug fever, hematologic complications, and teratogenic effects (effects that interfere with fetal development). Hypersensitivity manifested by urticaria, drug rash, and photosensitivity may occur with oral drug administration, but usually results from topical application. Once a local hypersensitivity reaction has occurred, topical or systemic reuse of the drug or any drug in the same chemical class will produce a similar reaction.

Although rare, hematologic complications include leukopenia, granulocytopenia, hemolytic anemia, thrombocytopenia, and pancytopenia.

Drug fever is a sign of a toxic reaction or overdose. Because of the wide use and ready availability of OTC antihistamines, acute poisoning commonly occurs, especially in children. The CNS effects of the drugs pose the greatest threat and account for most of the signs and symptoms of poisoning: hallucinations, excitement, ataxia, athetosis, involuntary movements, and seizures. Fever is more common in children than in adults. Fixed, dilated pupils accompany other anticholinergic effects and may be followed by coma and death.

NURSING PROCESS APPLICATION

The following information assists the nurse in caring for a patient receiving an antihistamine. It includes an overview of assessment activities as well as examples of appropriate nursing diagnoses and related interventions (see "Planning and implementation"). It also highlights the importance of evaluation.

Assessment

Before drug therapy begins, review the patient's history for conditions that contraindicate or require cautious use of the prescribed antihistamine. Also review the patient's medication history to identify use of drugs that may interact with it. During therapy, assess the patient for adverse drug reactions and signs of drug interactions. Also, periodically assess the effectiveness of antihistamine therapy. Finally, evaluate the patient's and family's knowledge about the prescribed drug.

Nursing diagnoses

- Risk for injury related to a preexisting condition that contraindicates or requires cautious use of an antihistamine
- Risk for injury related to adverse drug reactions or drug interactions
- Risk for trauma related to the sedative effects of an antihistamine
- Knowledge deficit related to the prescribed antihistamine

Planning and implementation

- Do not administer an antihistamine to a patient with a condition that contraindicates its use.
- Administer an antihistamine cautiously to a patient at risk because of a preexisting condition.
- Monitor the patient for adverse reactions and drug interactions during antihistamine therapy.
- Expect to decrease the dosage or use a different antihistamine, as prescribed, if a mild adverse reaction occurs.

* ***Monitor the patient — especially a pediatric patient — for signs of acute poisoning. Keep standard emergency equipment nearby. If acute poisoning occurs, discontinue the antihistamine and prepare to give symptomatic and supportive treatment such as mechanical ventilation. If acute poisoning is not recognized early, coma and death may occur.***

- Observe the patient for signs of a hypersensitivity reaction, such as urticaria, drug rash, and photosensitivity, especially when administering a topical antihistamine.
- Administer the prescribed antihistamine with meals or milk to decrease adverse GI reactions (except for the longer-acting preparations that should be taken on an empty stomach or 2 hours after a meal).
- Monitor the patient's complete blood count for adverse hematologic reactions to the prescribed antihistamine.
- Consult the physician about discontinuing the antihistamine for 4 days before the patient receives an allergy skin test to avoid masking abnormal results.
- Administer a parenteral antihistamine by deep intramuscular injection, using the Z-track method to prevent subcutaneous irritation.
- Notify the physician if adverse reactions or drug interactions occur or if the prescribed antihistamine is ineffective.
- Monitor the patient for sedation, the most common adverse reaction to antihistamines, especially during concomitant therapy with other CNS depressants. (See Patient Teaching: *Antihistamines,* page 486.)

* ***Take safety precautions if sedation occurs. For example, keep the bed rails up and supervise the patient's ambula-***

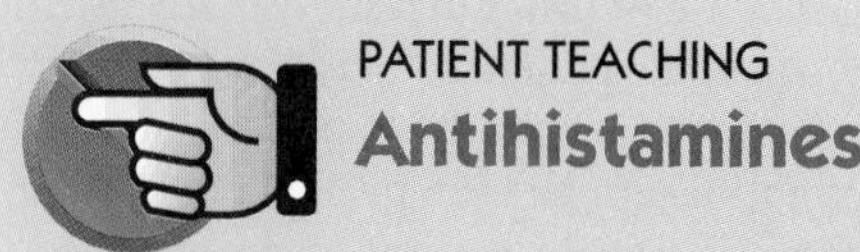

PATIENT TEACHING
Antihistamines

- Teach the patient and family the name, dose, frequency, action, and adverse effects of the prescribed antihistamine.
- Review all contraindications with the patient to help prevent misuse of an over-the-counter (OTC) antihistamine. Advise against using an antihistamine during pregnancy, while breast-feeding, or if the patient has a history of asthma, enlarged prostate, cardiovascular disease, hypertension, intestinal blockage, renal disease, overactive thyroid, stomach ulcer, or urinary tract blockage. Caution the patient against taking an antihistamine concurrently with an antimuscarinic (muscle relaxant and antispasmodic), monoamine oxidase inhibitor, or a drug that can produce tinnitus or balance problems, such as aspirin, other salicylates, or aminoglycosides.
- Advise a patient with a severe allergy to carry identification or wear an identification band that lists the type of allergy, the usual treatment, and the physician's name.
- Review adverse central nervous system (CNS), anticholinergic, and gastrointestinal (GI) reactions with the patient.
- Explain that the antihistamine can produce drowsiness and reduce alertness. Tell the patient that taking the drug at bedtime can minimize these symptoms (but may cause continued drowsiness in the morning) and that these effects may lessen after 2 to 3 days of use. Advise the patient not to drive or engage in activities that require mental alertness until the reaction to the drug is known.
- Inform the patient that combining an antihistamine with alcohol or another CNS depressant adds to the sedative effects of these drugs. Advise the patient taking an antihistamine to consult the physician before taking any CNS depressants, such as narcotics, sedatives, barbiturates, OTC sleep aids, tranquilizers, tricyclic antidepressants, muscle relaxants, anesthetics, and alcohol.
- Remind the patient to keep this and other drugs out of the reach of children. Instruct the patient to be alert for signs of an overdose, such as clumsiness, unsteadiness, seizures, severe drowsiness, and hallucinations. Advise the patient to seek help immediately if an overdose is suspected.
- Instruct the patient to drink fluids, chew sugarless gum, or suck on sugarless candy if the antihistamine produces mouth dryness.
- Advise the patient to avoid exposure to the sun or to wear sunscreen, sunglasses, and a hat when in the sun.
- Suggest that the patient take an oral antihistamine with food or milk to avoid adverse GI reactions.
- Instruct the patient to take an antihistamine prescribed for motion sickness at least 30 minutes — preferably 1 to 2 hours — before traveling.
- Advise the patient to take a sustained-release capsule or long-acting tablet in whole form. Remind the patient not to break, cut, crush, or chew the medication.
- Instruct the patient to report adverse reactions to the physician because a change in dosage may be indicated.

tion. Keep in mind that these effects may disappear spontaneously 2 to 3 days after antihistamine therapy begins.

• Notify the physician if sedation is pronounced or does not disappear 2 to 3 days after antihistamine therapy begins.

Evaluation

For each nursing diagnosis, prepare an evaluation statement that describes the patient's or family's response to nursing interventions.

CHAPTER SUMMARY

Chapter 38 discussed the antihistaminic agents, specifically the H_1-receptor antagonists. Here are the chapter highlights.

The classes of antihistamines include ethanolamines, ethylenediamines, alkylamines, phenothiazines, piperidines, and miscellaneous agents. Ethanolamines are potent and effective H_1-receptor antagonists that can produce extreme CNS depression and sedation. This class includes clemastine fumarate, dimenhydrinate, diphenhydramine hydrochloride, and phenyltoloxamine citrate.

Ethylenediamines include pyrilamine maleate, tripelennamine citrate, and tripelennamine hydrochloride. In most cases, these drugs produce low to moderate sedative effects and low anticholinergic and antiemetic effects.

Because alkylamines produce few CNS effects, they are more suitable for daytime use. Alkylamines include brompheniramine maleate, chlorpheniramine maleate, dexchlorpheniramine maleate, and triprolidine hydrochloride.

Phenothiazines are used primarily for their antiemetic effects. The phenothiazines are methdilazine hydrochloride, promethazine hydrochloride, and trimeprazine tartrate.

The piperidines are used to manage allergic pruritus and to prevent or treat motion sickness. This class consists of azatadine maleate, cyclizine lactate, cyproheptadine hydrochloride, meclizine hydrochloride, and phenindamine tartrate.

The miscellaneous antihistaminic agents astemizole and loratadine offer the benefits of a longer duration of action and significantly less sedation. Hydroxyzine hydrochloride and hydroxyzine maleate are two other miscellaneous antihistamines.

When caring for a patient who is taking an antihistamine, the nurse should monitor closely for signs of acute poisoning — especially in a pediatric patient — because coma and death can result.

Questions to consider

See Appendix 1 for answers.

1. Jeffrey Arnold, age 24, is stung by a bee while taking a walk in the park. He informs the physician in the emergency department that he came immediately after being stung because he is allergic to bees. The physician holds Mr. Arnold for observation and prescribes diphenhydramine 50 mg P.O. For Mr. Arnold, how does diphenhydramine exert its therapeutic effects?

(a) It acts as a competitive H_1-receptor antagonist to reverse histamine effects.
(b) It acts as a competitive H_1-receptor antagonist to prevent further response to histamine.
(c) It acts as a competitive H_2-receptor antagonist to reverse histamine effects.
(d) It acts as a competitive H_2-receptor antagonist to prevent further response to histamine.

2. The nurse should monitor Mr. Arnold for adverse reactions to diphenhydramine. What is the most common adverse reaction to antihistamines?
(a) Drug fever
(b) GI distress
(c) Sedation
(d) Urine retention

3. Twenty minutes after receiving diphenhydramine, Mr. Arnold suddenly remembers that he took a tranquilizer 1 hour before he was stung. Although he had denied any recent drug use when asked earlier, he told the nurse he forgot in the excitement because he doesn't take the tranquilizer often. Which of the following drug interactions is this CNS depressant likely to cause when given with an antihistamine?
(a) Additive anticholinergic effects
(b) Profound CNS depression
(c) Hyperexcitability
(d) Paradoxical allergic response

4. When administering antihistaminic agents, such as astemizole or loratadine, which of the following should the nurse caution the patient not to do?
(a) Use sugarless candy or gum to alleviate thirst.
(b) Take the tablet without chewing it.
(c) Take the drug on an empty stomach.
(d) Restrict fluid intake.

5. Adam Wingate, age 6, has seasonal allergies and is given dimenhydrinate 25 mg P.O. for motion sickness. His parents should monitor Adam carefully for all but which of the following signs and symptoms?
(a) Wheezing
(b) Drowsiness
(c) Increased urine output
(d) Increased thirst

39 Corticosteroid and other immunosuppressant agents

OBJECTIVES

After reading and studying this chapter, the student should be able to:

1. discuss the mechanisms of action of the systemic corticosteroids (glucocorticoids and mineralocorticoids) and immunosuppressants.
2. identify the common clinical uses of the systemic corticosteroids and immunosuppressants.
3. describe the most common adverse reactions to systemic corticosteroids and immunosuppressants.
4. describe how to apply the nursing process when caring for a patient who is receiving a systemic corticosteroid or immunosuppressant.

Drugs covered in this chapter include:

- azathioprine
- beclomethasone dipropionate
- betamethasone
- cortisone acetate
- cyclophosphamide
- cyclosporine
- dexamethasone
- dexamethasone acetate
- dexamethasone sodium phosphate
- fludrocortisone acetate
- hydrocortisone
- hydrocortisone acetate
- hydrocortisone sodium phosphate
- hydrocortisone sodium succinate
- lymphocyte immune globulin
- methylpredisolone
- methylprednisolone acetate
- methylprednisolone sodium succinate
- muromonab CD3
- paramethasone acetate
- prednisolone
- prednisolone acetate
- prednisolone sodium phosphate
- prednisolone tebutate
- prednisone
- tacrolimus
- triamcinolone.

INTRODUCTION

Corticosteroid drugs, which are available as natural or synthetic steroids, are used to suppress immune responses and to reduce **inflammation.** Natural corticosteroids are hormones produced by the adrenal cortex; most corticosteroid drugs are synthetic forms of these hormones. Natural and synthetic corticosteroids are classified according to their biological activities. The **glucocorticoids,** such as cortisone acetate and dexamethasone, affect carbohydrate and protein metabolism; the **mineralocorticoids,** such as aldosterone and fludrocortisone acetate, regulate electrolyte and water balance.

Besides their primary uses as anti-inflammatory and immunosuppressant agents, glucocorticoids and mineralocorticoids are used for replacement therapy in patients with adrenocortical insufficiency (decreased secretion of endogenous corticosteroids) and for suppression of adrenocortical hyperfunction in patients with adrenogenital syndrome.

The noncorticosteroid immunosuppressant agents include azathioprine, cyclophosphamide, cyclosporine, lymphocyte immune **globulin** (better known as antithymocyte globulin [ATG]), and muromonab-CD3. Except for cyclophosphamide, they are used to prevent rejection of transplanted organs and experimentally to treat various autoimmune disorders. Cyclophosphamide is used primarily to treat cancer. (See *Selected major corticosteroid and other immunosuppressant agents.*)

Systemic glucocorticoids

Most glucocorticoids are synthetic analogues of hormones secreted by the zona fasciculata of the adrenal cortex. They exert anti-inflammatory, metabolic, and immunosuppressant effects. Drugs in this class include beclomethasone dipropionate, betamethasone (also available in topical form, betamethasone valerate), cortisone acetate, dexamethasone, dexamethasone acetate, dexamethasone sodium phosphate, hydrocortisone, hydrocortisone acetate, hydrocortisone sodium phosphate, hydrocortisone sodium succinate, methylprednisolone, methylprednisolone acetate, methylprednisolone sodium succinate, paramethasone acetate, prednisolone, prednisolone acetate, prednisolone sodium phosphate, prednisolone tebutate, prednisone, and triamcinolone.

PHARMACOKINETICS

The glucocorticoids are absorbed well when administered orally. After intramuscular (I.M.) administration, they are absorbed completely, but their onset and duration of action may vary. Duration of action also varies for glucocorticoids

Selected major corticosteroid and other immunosuppressant agents

This chart summarizes the major corticosteroid and other immunosuppressant agents currently in clinical use.

DRUG	MAJOR INDICATIONS AND USUAL DOSAGES	CONTRAINDICATIONS AND PRECAUTIONS
Systemic glucocorticoids		
cortisone (Cortone)	*Replacement therapy for adrenocortical insufficiency, anti-inflammatory conditions* ADULT: 25 to 300 mg P.O. daily or 20 to 300 mg I.M. q 12 hours PEDIATRIC: 0.7 to 10 mg/kg P.O. daily or 20 to 300 mg/m² P.O. daily in four divided doses; or 0.2 to 1.25 mg/kg I.M. or 7 to 37.5 mg/m² I.M. once daily or b.i.d.	• Cortisone is contraindicated in a patient with a systemic fungal infection or known hypersensitivity to any component of the drug. • This drug requires cautious use in a patient with gastrointestinal (GI) ulceration, renal disease, hypertension, osteoporosis, varicella infection, vaccinia, exanthema, diabetes mellitus, hypothyroidism, thromboembolic disorder, seizures, myasthenia gravis, heart failure, tuberculosis (TB), ocular herpes simplex, or hypoalbuminemia. It also requires cautious use in a patient who is emotionally unstable or psychotic. • Use with caution in a pregnant or breast-feeding woman.
dexamethasone sodium phosphate (Decadron Phosphate, Hexadrol Phosphate)	*Cerebral edema* ADULT: initially, 10 mg I.V., followed by 4 to 6 mg I.M. every 6 hours for 2 to 4 days, then taper over 5 to 7 days *Asthma* ADULT: 3 inhalations t.i.d. or q.i.d. up to 12 inhalations daily PEDIATRIC: 2 inhalations three to four times daily, maximum 8 inhalations daily *Inflammatory conditions* ADULT: 2 to 4 mg injected into large joints, 0.8 to 1 mg injected into small joints	• Dexamethasone sodium phosphate is contraindicated in a patient with a systemic fungal infection or known hypersensitivity to any component of the drug. • This drug requires cautious use in a patient with GI ulceration, renal disease, hypertension, osteoporosis, varicella infection, vaccinia, exanthema, diabetes mellitus, hypothyroidism, thromboembolic disorders, seizures, myasthenia gravis, heart failure, TB, tuberculosis, ocular herpes simplex, or hypoalbuminemia. It also requires cautious use in a patient who is emotionally unstable or psychotic. • Use with caution in a pregnant or breast-feeding woman.
methylprednisolone (Medrol, Solu-Medrol, A-Methapred, Depo-Medrol)	*Inflammatory conditions and those requiring immunosuppression* ADULT: initially, 4 to 48 mg P.O. daily; further therapy must be individualized PEDIATRIC: initially, 0.117 to 1.66 mg/kg or 3.3 to 50 mg/m² P.O. daily in three to four divided doses; further therapy must be individualized	• Methylprednisolone is contraindicated in a patient with a systemic fungal infection or known hypersensitivity to any component of the drug. • This drug requires cautious use in a patient with GI ulceration, renal disease, hypertension, osteoporosis, varicella infection, vaccinia, exanthema, diabetes mellitus, hypothyroidism, thromboembolic disorder, seizures, myasthenia gravis, heart failure, TB, ocular herpes simplex, or hypoalbuminemia. It also requires cautious use in a patient who is emotionally unstable or psychotic. • Use with caution in a pregnant or breast-feeding woman.
prednisone (Deltasone, Orasone)	*Inflammatory conditions and those requiring immunosuppression* ADULT: initially, 5 to 60 mg P.O. daily; further therapy must be individualized PEDIATRIC: initially, 0.14 to 2 mg/kg or 4 to 60 mg/m² P.O. daily in four divided doses; further therapy must be individualized	• Prednisone is contraindicated in a patient with a systemic fungal infection or known hypersensitivity to any component of the drug. • This drug requires cautious use in a patient with GI ulceration, renal disease, hypertension, osteoporosis, varicella infection, vaccinia, exanthema, diabetes mellitus, hypothyroidism, thromboembolic disorder, seizures, myasthenia gravis, heart failure, TB, ocular herpes simplex, or hypoalbuminemia. It also requires cautious use in a patient who is emotionally unstable or psychotic. • Use with caution in a pregnant or breast-feeding woman.
Mineralocorticoids		
fludrocortisone (Florinef)	*Adrenocortical insufficiency, salt-losing adrenogenital syndrome* ADULT: 0.1 to 0.2 mg P.O. daily with 10 to 37.5 mg cortisone P.O. daily or with 10 to 30 mg hydrocortisone P.O. daily in three or four divided doses	• Fludrocortisone is contraindicated in a patient with a systemic fungal infection or known hypersensitivity to any component of the drug.

(continued)

Selected major corticosteroid and other immunosuppressant agents

(continued)

DRUG	MAJOR INDICATIONS AND USUAL DOSAGES	CONTRAINDICATIONS AND PRECAUTIONS
Mineralocorticoids		
fludrocortisone (Florinef) *(continued)*		• This drug requires cautious use in a pregnant or breast-feeding woman, a patient with GI ulceration, renal disease, hypertension, osteoporosis, varicella infection, vaccinia, exanthema, diabetes mellitus, cushingoid symptoms, thromboembolic disorder, myasthenia gravis, metastatic cancer, heart failure, TB, ocular herpes simplex, or hypoalbuminemia. It also requires cautious use in a patient who is emotionally unstable or psychotic. • Monitor electrolytes carefully; may need to supplement potassium.
Immunosuppressants		
azathioprine (Imuran)	*Prevention of allograft rejection* ADULT: 3 to 5 mg/kg P.O. daily, starting on the day of transplantation or 1 to 3 days before; after transplantation, the same dosage I.V. until the patient can tolerate the oral form; can reduce maintenance dose to 1 to 3 mg/kg/day PEDIATRIC: same as adult dosage above	• Azathioprine is contraindicated in a pregnant or breast-feeding patient, one with known hypersensitivity, or one who has received previous treatment with an alkylating agent. • Notify physician if infection, bleeding, or bruising occurs; monitor blood counts.
cyclosporine (Sandimmune, Neoral)	*Prevention of allograft rejection* ADULT: 15 mg/kg P.O. 4 to 12 hours before transplantation, followed by 15 mg/kg P.O. daily for 1 to 2 weeks after transplantation, and then a decrease of 5% per week to a maintenance dosage of 5 to 10 mg/kg daily PEDIATRIC: same as adult dosage above	• Cyclosporine is contraindicated in a breast-feeding patient or one with known hypersensitivity. • This drug requires cautious use in a pregnant patient. • Neoral must be given in two equal doses daily.
lymphocyte immune globulin [antithymocyte globulin, ATG] (Atgam)	*Prevention or delay of allograft rejection* ADULT: 15 mg/kg I.V. daily for 14 days, followed by alternate-day therapy with the same dosage for 14 more days *Prevention of graft-versus-host disease after bone marrow allograft transplantation* ADULT: 7 to 10 mg/kg I.V. every other day for six doses *Management of acute allograft rejection* ADULT: 10 to 15 mg/kg I.V. daily for 14 days, followed by alternate-day therapy with the same dosage for up to 14 more days *Treatment of graft-versus-host disease after bone marrow allograft transplantation* ADULT: 7 mg/kg I.V. every other day for six doses	• ATG is contraindicated in a pregnant patient or one who has had a severe systemic hypersensitivity reaction to the drug or other equine immunoglobulin G preparation. • This drug requires cautious use in a patient with a systemic hypersensitivity reaction to the skin test.

Selected major corticosteroid and other immunosuppressant agents

(continued)

DRUG	MAJOR INDICATIONS AND USUAL DOSAGES	CONTRAINDICATIONS AND PRECAUTIONS
Immunosuppressants *(continued)*		
lymphocyte immune globulin [antithymocyte globulin, ATG] (Atgam) *(continued)*	*Treatment of aplastic anemia* ADULT: 10 to 20 mg/kg daily for 8 to 14 days followed by alternate-day therapy with the same dose for up to 14 additional days	
muromonab-CD3 (Orthoclone OKT3)	*Treatment or "rescue" of allograft rejection unresponsive to other therapies; prevention of allograft rejection* ADULT: 5 mg I.V. as a bolus given over less than 1 minute, daily for 10 to 14 days	• Muromonab-CD3 is contraindicated in a patient with fluid overload or known hypersensitivity to the drug or any other product of murine origin. • This drug requires cautious use in a pregnant patient or one who has previously received the drug.
tacrolimus (Prograf)	*Organ rejection prophalaxis* ADULT: 0.05 to 1 mg/kg/day as a continous I.V. infusion, start no sooner than 6 hours after transplantation; convert to P.O. form as soon as possible, 0.15 to 0.3 mg/kg/day in two divided doses 8 to 12 hours after discontinuing I.V. dosing PEDIATRIC: 0.1 mg/kg/day I.V. and 0.3 mg/kg/day P.O.; doses are individualized	• Tracrolimus is contraindicated in patients with known hypersensitivity reaction. • Use with caution in a pregnant or breast-feeding patient or one with renal impairment. • Monitor blood pressure, hypertension is a common adverse effect.

given intravenously. Glucocorticoids are bound to plasma proteins and distributed via the blood. They are metabolized in the liver and excreted by the kidneys. Many of the glucocorticoids peak quickly. For instance, prednisone reaches its peak within 1 hour.

No positive correlation exists between the half-lives of these drugs and their biological effects. Glucocorticoid preparations may be short-acting (half-life of 8 to 18 hours), intermediate-acting (half-life of 18 to 36 hours), or long-acting (half-life of 36.1 to 54 hours), but their pharmacologic effects can last days, weeks, or longer. In fact, after prolonged therapy with high doses of these drugs, adrenal suppression of the corticotropin response may persist for up to 12 months.

Route	Onset	Peak	Duration
P.O.	Rapid	1 hr	Variable
I.M. (sodium phosphate and sodium succinate combinations)	Variable	1 hr	Variable
I.M., I.V. (acetate combinations)	Variable	24-48 hr	Variable

PHARMACODYNAMICS

Glucocorticoids suppress **hypersensitivity** and immune responses through a process not entirely understood. Researchers believe that glucocorticoids inhibit these responses by suppressing or preventing cell-mediated immune reactions; reducing the concentration of thymus-dependent leukocytes, monocytes, and eosinophils; decreasing the binding of immunoglobulins to cell surface receptors; and inhibiting interleukin synthesis. Unfortunately, this clinically useful process also may mask the signs and symptoms of serious concomitant infections.

Glucocorticoids suppress the redness, edema, heat, and tenderness associated with the inflammatory response. On the cellular level, the glucocorticoids stabilize the lysosomal membranes so that they do not release their store of hydrolytic enzymes into the cells. The drugs also prevent plasma exudation, suppress the migration of **polymorphonuclear leukocytes,** inhibit **phagocytosis,** decrease **antibody** formation in injured or infected tissues, and disrupt **histamine** synthesis, **fibroblast** development, collagen deposition, microvasculature dilation, and capillary permeability.

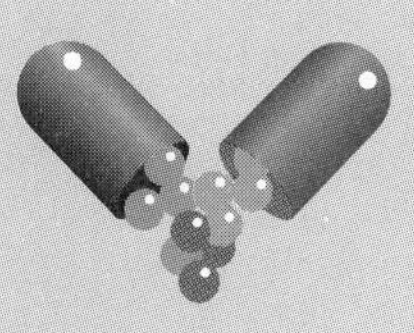

DRUG INTERACTIONS

Systemic glucocorticoids and mineralocorticoids

Corticosteroids interact with many other drugs. The nurse must be aware that these interactions affect electrolytes as well as medication dosages.

DRUG	INTERACTING DRUGS	POSSIBLE EFFECTS	NURSING IMPLICATIONS
systemic glucocorticoids, mineralocorticoids	barbiturates, phenytoin, rifampin, aminoglutethimide	Decreased corticosteroid effect	• Increase the corticosteroid dosage, as prescribed.
	amphotericin B, chlorthalidone, ethacrynic acid, furosemide, thiazide diuretics	Increased risk or severity of hypokalemia	• Monitor the patient's serum potassium level, and observe for signs of hypokalemia. • Administer potassium supplements, as prescribed, and recommend high-potassium foods, such as bananas and grapes.
	erythromycin, troleandomycin	Decreased corticosteroid metabolism	• Observe for signs of increased corticosteroid effect. • Decrease the corticosteroid dosage, as prescribed.
	salicylates	Increased risk of gastrointestinal (GI) ulceration; decreased plasma concentration and effects of salicylates	• Watch for signs of GI irritation (heartburn) and ulceration (melena). • Increase the salicylate dosage, as prescribed, when administered concomitantly with a corticosteroid. • Observe the patient for signs of salicylate intoxication, such as tinnitus or hyperventilation, when the corticosteroid dosage is decreased.
	nonsteroidal anti-inflammatory drugs	Increased risk of peptic ulcer	• Watch for signs of GI irritation. • Administer these drugs at least 2 hours apart or with food or milk.
	vaccines, toxoids	Decreased response to vaccines and toxoids; increased replication of attenuated viruses	• Administer with extreme caution and only as prescribed. • Observe for signs of specific viral infection after vaccine or toxoid administration.
	estrogen, oral contraceptives that contain estrogen	Increased corticosteroid effect	• Observe for signs of increased corticosteroid effects. • Decrease the corticosteroid dosage, as prescribed.
	hypoglycemic agents	Increased blood glucose level in patients with diabetes mellitus	• Monitor the patient's blood glucose level. • Monitor the patient for signs of hyperglycemia, such as polyuria, polydipsia, polyphagia, and weight loss.
	cholestyramine	Decreased corticosteroid absorption	• Observe the patient for signs of reduced response to corticosteroid therapy. • Administer colestyramine at least 2 hours before or after the corticosteroid.
	isoniazid	Reduced effect of isoniazid; reduced metabolism and increased effect of corticosteroid	• Monitor the patient for signs of reduced response to isoniazid, such as exacerbation of tuberculosis, or increased corticosteroid effect. • Increase the isoniazid dosage, as prescribed.
	antihypertensive agents	Decreased antihypertensive effect	• Monitor the patient for increased blood pressure and edema. • Limit the patient's sodium and fluid intake. • Increase the antihypertensive dosage, as prescribed.

Adverse reactions to systemic corticosteroids

Systemic corticosteroids — both glucocorticoids and mineralocorticoids — affect almost all body systems, so they can cause widespread adverse reactions. The list below groups the most common reactions by body system.

Central nervous system
- Behavioral changes ranging from mood alterations to psychosis and suicidal behavior
- Insomnia
- Increased intracranial pressure
- Seizures
- Cerebral edema
- Blunted sensorium

Endocrine system (and metabolic functions)
- Diabetes mellitus
- Hyperlipidemia
- Adrenal atrophy
- Hypothalamic-pituitary axis suppression
- Dysmenorrhea
- Altered protein, fat, and carbohydrate metabolism and protein catabolism
- Cushingoid signs and symptoms
- Increased serum cholesterol levels
- Inhibited protein synthesis

Urinary system
- Increased sodium and water retention
- Increased potassium excretion

Immune system
- Suppressed immune response
- Suppressed inflammation
- Increased susceptibility to infection
- Suppressed signs and symptoms of infection

Ophthalmic system
- Glaucoma
- Posterior subcapsular cataracts

Musculoskeletal system
- Osteoporosis
- Aseptic necrosis of bone
- Increased susceptibility to fractures
- Muscle wasting
- Myopathy
- Arthralgia

Gastrointestinal system
- Intestinal perforation
- Peptic ulcer
- Pancreatitis

Cardiovascular system
- Hypertension
- Edema
- Hypercoagulability
- Thrombophlebitis
- Embolism
- Atherosclerosis
- Polycythemia

Integumentary system
- Impaired wound healing
- Hirsutism
- Ecchymoses
- Acne
- Striae
- Thin, fragile skin

PHARMACOTHERAPEUTICS

Besides their use as replacement therapy for patients with adrenocortical insufficiency, the glucocorticoids are prescribed for **immunosuppression** and reduction of inflammation and for their effects on the blood and lymphatic systems. Specific indications include suppression of adrenocortical hyperfunction in patients with adrenogenital syndrome and treatment of hypercalcemia in patients with cancer with bone metastasis such as breast cancer (glucocorticoids increase calcium excretion), multiple myeloma, and vitamin D intoxication. (See *Adverse reactions to systemic corticosteroids.*) In patients with rheumatoid arthritis, osteoarthritis, rheumatic fever, nephrotic syndrome, inflammatory bowel disease, or collagen disease, glucocorticoids are used for their anti-inflammatory effects. They may cause a rapid and marked reduction in symptoms but do not affect disease progression. The glucocorticoids also are used to relieve hypersensitivity reactions by suppressing the inflammatory response in patients with asthma, food and drug hypersensitivities, bee stings, hay fever, contact or exfoliative dermatitis, ulcerative colitis, or vasculitis. These drugs also contribute antilymphocytic effects in treating leukemias, lymphomas, and myelomas; reduce or prevent cerebral edema associated with neoplasms, neurosurgery, and trauma; are used in chronic obstructive pulmonary disease; and are combined with other immunosuppressants to prevent or treat transplant rejection. Finally, glucocorticoids commonly are used to decrease ocular inflammatory processes.

Drug interactions

Many drugs interact with the systemic glucocorticoids. (See Drug Interactions: *Systemic glucocorticoids and mineralocorticoids.*)

ADVERSE DRUG REACTIONS

Because systemic glucocorticoids affect nearly every body system, they can cause widespread adverse reactions. Such reactions are unlikely to occur with short-term therapy, even at high dosages. However, when glucocorticoids are given for more than a brief period, devastating reactions can occur. If long-term therapy with these drugs is necessary, alternate-day therapy (a single dose administered every other morning) may decrease the severity of adverse reactions.

Glucocorticoids also can retard normal growth in children by their effects on the epiphyseal cartilage. Even small doses of glucocorticoids can inhibit or even arrest growth by interfering with deoxyribonucleic acid (DNA) synthesis and cell division.

Reported anaphylactic reactions in patients who have received parenteral glucocorticoids may have resulted from hypersensitivity to the preservative used in some parenteral formulations.

NURSING PROCESS APPLICATION

The following information assists the nurse in caring for a patient who is receiving a systemic glucocorticoid. It includes an overview of assessment activities as well as examples of appropriate nursing diagnoses and related interventions (see "Planning and implementation"). It also highlights the importance of evaluation.

Assessment

Before drug therapy begins, review the patient's history for conditions that contraindicate or require cautious use of the prescribed systemic glucocorticoid. Also review the patient's medication history to identify use of drugs that may interact with it. During therapy, assess the patient for adverse drug reactions and signs of drug interactions. Also, periodically assess the effectiveness of systemic glucocorticoid therapy. Finally, evaluate the patient's and family's knowledge about the prescribed drug.

Nursing diagnoses

- Risk for injury related to a preexisting condition that contraindicates or requires cautious use of a systemic glucocorticoid
- Risk for injury related to adverse drug reactions or drug interactions
- Altered protection related to immunosuppression caused by long-term systemic glucocorticoid therapy
- Knowledge deficit related to the prescribed systemic glucocorticoid

Planning and implementation

- Do not administer a systemic glucocorticoid to a patient with a condition that contraindicates its use.
- Administer a systemic glucocorticoid cautiously to a patient at risk because of a preexisting condition.
- Monitor the patient frequently for adverse reactions and drug interactions during systemic glucocorticoid therapy.

*** *Observe the patient closely for an anaphylactic reaction after drug administration. Keep standard emergency equipment nearby.***

- Monitor the following during systemic glucocorticoid therapy: the patient's serum glucose level, body weight, blood pressure, complete blood count (CBC), blood chemistries (particularly electrolytes), and intraocular pressure. Also obtain chest and spinal X-rays regularly.
- Monitor the patient for signs of adrenocortical insufficiency, such as hypotension, dehydration, fatigue, hyponatremia, diarrhea, and anorexia, during glucocorticoid therapy and after it is discontinued.
- Monitor the patient for potential stressors, such as surgery, trauma, and infections, and adjust the dosage accordingly, as prescribed.
- Monitor the patient for signs of Cushing's syndrome. (See *Cushingoid signs and symptoms.*)
- Prevent severe gastrointestinal (GI) complications by assessing the patient for epigastric pain 1 to 3 hours after meals and for nausea, vomiting, bloody stools, hematemesis, coffee-ground vomitus, decreased hemoglobin and hematocrit level, and a positive guaiac stool test.
- Observe for and report any emotional changes. Suicide precautions may be needed for a severely depressed patient.
- Administer the daily dosage in four equally divided doses or in one single dose in the early morning for a patient who needs short-term oral therapy. Keep in mind that early-morning administration simulates the natural circadian rhythm of corticosteroid secretion — higher in the morning, lower in the evening.
- Expect to administer alternate-day therapy for a patient who needs long-term therapy (longer than a month). This minimizes the risk or severity of adverse reactions.

Cushingoid signs and symptoms

Prolonged corticosteroid therapy may result in the signs and symptoms associated with Cushing's syndrome — a condition marked by widespread abnormalities, including obvious fat deposits in the face, between the shoulders, and around the waist.

During corticosteroid therapy, the nurse should assess the patient for the following cushingoid signs and symptoms:

- acne
- moon face
- hirsutism and masculinization
- cervicodorsal fat (buffalo hump)
- protruding abdomen
- girdle obesity
- amenorrhea
- purplish abdominal striae
- edema
- thinning and atrophy of extremities
- muscle weakness or atrophy
- hypertension
- hyperglycemia
- glycosuria
- renal disorder
- mental changes, ranging from euphoria to depression
- lowered resistance to infection.

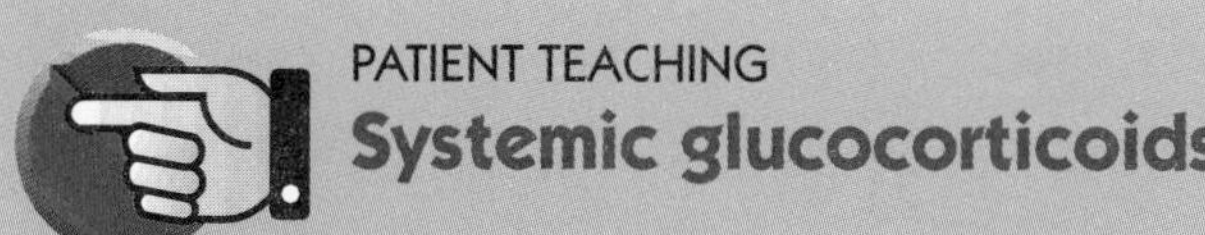

PATIENT TEACHING

Systemic glucocorticoids

- Teach the patient and family the name, dose, frequency, action, and adverse effects of the prescribed systemic glucocorticoid.

Dosage and storage guidelines

- Ensure that the patient and family clearly understand why the systemic glucocorticoid has been prescribed and know the risks associated with it. Advise the patient who is taking the drug for more than 1 week not to stop taking it abruptly. Explain that the dosage must be decreased gradually before the drug can be discontinued.
- Emphasize the importance of taking the drug exactly as prescribed.
- Review guidelines for missed doses with the patient. In general, a missed daily dose should be taken as soon as the patient remembers it (but not the next day — doses should never be doubled). The patient who misses one portion of a divided daily dose should take the next dose on schedule. A patient on alternate-day therapy, however, should not take a missed dose, even if it is remembered that same morning. Instead, the patient should take the missed dose the next morning, skip a day, then resume alternate-day therapy on the following day.
- Advise the patient to take extra medication along when traveling in case the trip lasts longer than expected. Also advise the patient not to pack the medication in a suitcase, but to carry it at all times.
- Instruct the patient about storage requirements.

Adverse drug reactions and drug interactions

- Review the signs and symptoms of adrenocortical insufficiency with the patient. Instruct the patient to notify the physician if they occur.
- Advise the patient to avoid the use of alcohol, cigarettes, caffeine, aspirin, or aspirin-containing compounds without first consulting the physician.
- Teach the patient to recognize the signs and symptoms of gastrointestinal disorders and to notify the physician immediately if they appear.
- Inform the patient that the systemic glucocorticoid may cause emotional changes that should be reported to the physician.
- Instruct the patient about therapy-related dietary precautions, including adequate intake of proteins, vitamins, and calcium. Foods high in potassium and low in sodium also may be prescribed. Have the patient keep a weekly weight record and report any gain over 5 lb (2.2 kg).
- Explain the need for the patient to keep active to prevent osteoporosis. (Periodic X-rays also may be required to monitor bone status.)
- Instruct the patient to take an oral glucocorticoid with food or milk to decrease the risk of gastric irritation.
- Instruct the patient to wear a medical identification tag or to carry an identification card at all times. The patient also should notify any health care professionals (dentists or oral surgeons, for example) about the glucocorticoid therapy before undergoing any other kind of treatment.
- Help the patient reduce the risk of infection by teaching self-care practices to prevent skin injury and proper care of minor injuries.
- Instruct the patient to call the physician if signs or symptoms of infection such as fever develop.
- Advise the patient to avoid people with infections, especially respiratory infections.
- Stress the importance of scrupulous oral hygiene during oral inhalation therapy, especially immediately after treatment.
- Inform the patient receiving long-term therapy about the possibility of changes in appearance, such as fat deposits in the face, acne, hirsutism, and truncal obesity. Reassure the patient that these changes are therapy-related.
- Instruct the patient to notify the physician if adverse reactions occur.

Inhaler use

- Teach the patient the correct way to use a beclomethasone oral inhaler: shake the inhaler well immediately before use; invert the inhaler; exhale completely; place the mouthpiece of the inhaler in the mouth and close the lips around it; while pressing the metal canister down with a finger, inhale slowly and deeply through the mouth; after holding the breath as long as possible, remove the mouthpiece and exhale as slowly as possible. Wait 1 minute (breathing normally) before inhaling again.

• Inject an I.M. glucocorticoid preparation deeply into gluteal muscle, and avoid using the same site for repeated injections to help prevent atrophy at injection sites. Know that subcutaneous injection usually is contraindicated.

*** *Do not administer beclomethasone via oral inhalation to a patient experiencing an acute asthmatic attack because the drug cannot stop bronchospasm.***

• Notify the physician if adverse reactions or drug interactions occur.

• Closely monitor the patient for signs of infection, such as delayed wound healing and an increased white blood cell (WBC) count, because systemic glucocorticoids increase susceptibility to infection. (See Patient Teaching: *Systemic glucocorticoids.*)

• Handle or dress all wounds, surgical sites, tubes, and catheters with meticulous care to help prevent contamination and reduce the risk of infection.

• Notify the physician if an infection is suspected.

• Apply a topical glucocorticoid in the smallest amount and lowest concentration possible.

Evaluation

For each nursing diagnosis, prepare an evaluation statement that describes the patient's or family's response to nursing interventions.

Mineralocorticoids

The mineralocorticoid fludrocortisone acetate is a synthetic analogue of hormones secreted by the zona glomerulosa layer of the adrenal cortex. This drug affects electrolyte and water balance. Aldosterone, a natural mineralocorticoid, is the prototype drug in this class, but its use has been limited by its high cost, limited availability, and requirement of parenteral administration.

PHARMACOKINETICS

Fludrocortisone acetate is absorbed well and distributed to all parts of the body. This drug is metabolized to its inactive forms, in part, by the body tissues, but the liver is the major metabolic site. The drug is excreted by the kidneys, primarily as inactive metabolites.

Route	Onset	Peak	Duration
P.O.	30 min	Unknown	1-2 days

PHARMACODYNAMICS

Fludrocortisone acetate affects fluid and electrolyte balance by acting on the distal renal tubule to enhance sodium resorption and potassium and hydrogen secretion. The glomerular filtration rate is increased, favoring sodium excretion. However, the net effect of the mineralocorticoid usually is sodium retention.

PHARMACOTHERAPEUTICS

Fludrocortisone acetate is used as part of replacement therapy for patients with adrenocortical insufficiency. It also is used to treat salt-losing congenital adrenogenital syndrome after the patient's electrolyte balance has been restored.

Drug interactions

The drug interactions associated with the mineralocorticoids are similar to those associated with the systemic glucocorticoids.

ADVERSE DRUG REACTIONS

The mineralocorticoids cause the same adverse reactions that are associated with systemic glucocorticoids. Although fludrocortisone itself does not cause hypersensitivity reactions, chemicals used in formulating the preparation may do so.

NURSING PROCESS APPLICATION

The following information assists the nurse in caring for a patient receiving a mineralocorticoid. It includes an overview of assessment activities as well as examples of appropriate nursing diagnoses and related interventions (see "Planning and implementation"). It also highlights the importance of evaluation.

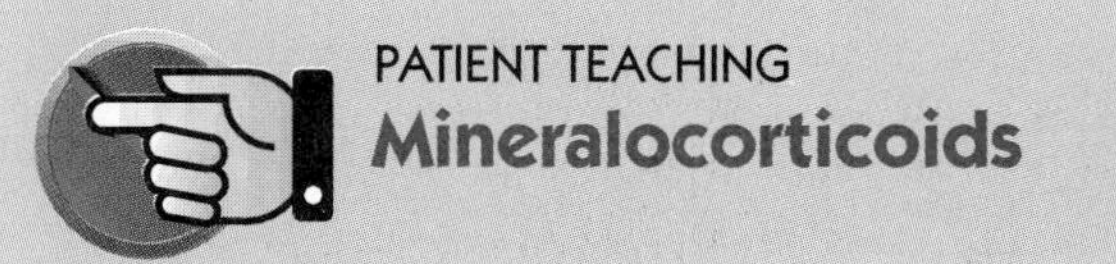

PATIENT TEACHING
Mineralocorticoids

- Teach the patient and family the name, dose, frequency, action, and adverse effects of the prescribed mineralocorticoid.
- Inform the patient of the importance of periodic evaluations of serum electrolyte levels and blood pressure.
- Advise the patient to control salt intake and to monitor weight daily. Teach the patient to recognize and report signs of edema, such as swollen ankles and feet.
- Instruct the patient to consume high-potassium foods and to avoid high-sodium foods.
- Teach the patient to note and report adverse reactions associated with systemic glucocorticoids.
- Instruct the patient to notify the physician if adverse reactions occur.

Assessment

Before drug therapy begins, review the patient's history for conditions that contraindicate or require cautious use of the prescribed mineralocorticoid. Also review the patient's medication history to identify use of drugs that may interact with it. During therapy, assess the patient for adverse drug reactions and signs of drug interactions. Also, periodically assess the effectiveness of mineralocorticoid therapy. Finally, evaluate the patient's and family's knowledge about the prescribed drug.

Nursing diagnoses

- Risk for injury related to a preexisting condition that contraindicates or requires cautious use of a mineralocorticoid
- Risk for injury related to adverse drug reactions or drug interactions
- Fluid volume excess related to sodium and water retention caused by a mineralocorticoid
- Knowledge deficit related to the prescribed mineralocorticoid

Planning and implementation

- Do not administer a mineralocorticoid to a patient with a condition that contraindicates its use.
- Administer a mineralocorticoid cautiously to a patient at risk because of a preexisting condition.
- Monitor the patient regularly for fluid and electrolyte imbalances during mineralocorticoid therapy.
- Periodically monitor plasma sodium, potassium, and calcium levels.
- Monitor the patient for additional adverse reactions, which usually are associated with mineralocorticoids. Also monitor for drug interactions.

• Notify the physician if adverse reactions or drug interactions occur.
• Monitor the patient for signs of fluid retention by measuring blood pressure and body weight daily, inspecting for edema, and auscultating lung fields. (See Patient Teaching: *Mineralocorticoids.*)
• Do not allow the patient to consume more than eight 8-oz (240-ml) glasses of fluid daily, unless prescribed.
• Provide a low-sodium, high-potassium diet for the patient, as prescribed.
• Notify the physician if fluid retention occurs.

Evaluation

For each nursing diagnosis, prepare an evaluation statement that describes the patient's or family's response to nursing interventions.

Immunosuppressants

Several drugs used for their immunosuppressant effects in patients undergoing **allograft** transplantation also are used experimentally to treat **autoimmune** diseases. Drugs in this immunosuppressant class include azathioprine, cyclosporine, lymphocyte immune globulin (ATG [equine]), muromonab-CD3, and tacrolimus. Cyclophosphamide, classified as an alkylating agent, also is used as an immunosuppressant, but it is used primarily to treat cancer.

PHARMACOKINETICS

When administered orally, azathioprine is absorbed readily from the GI tract, whereas absorption of cyclosporine is varied and incomplete. ATG and muromonab-CD3 are administered only by I.V injection.

The distribution of azathioprine is not understood fully. Cyclosporine and muromonab-CD3 are distributed widely throughout the body. Azathioprine and cyclosporine cross the placental barrier. The distribution of ATG is not defined clearly, but it may be distributed to breast milk.

Azathioprine and cyclosporine are metabolized in the liver. Muromonab-CD3 is consumed by **T cells** circulating in the blood. The metabolism of ATG is unknown.

Azathioprine and ATG are excreted in the urine; cyclosporine is excreted principally in the bile. The excretion of muromonab-CD3 is unknown.

Route	Onset	Peak	Duration
P.O.	Variable	2-3.5 hr	12-24 days
I.V.	Minutes	3 hr	1 wk

PHARMACODYNAMICS

The action of azathioprine has not been determined precisely. It antagonizes metabolism of the amino acid purine and therefore may inhibit ribonucleic acid and DNA structure and synthesis. It also may inhibit coenzyme formation and function. In patients receiving kidney allografts, the drug suppresses cell-mediated hypersensitivities and produces various alterations in antibody production.

The precise mechanism of action of cyclosporine also is unknown, but experimental data suggest that the drug inhibits **helper T cells** and **suppressor T cells.**

ATG has an unknown mechanism of action, but it may eliminate **antigen**-reactive T cells in peripheral blood, alter T-cell function, or both.

Muromonab-CD3 is a monoclonal antibody that blocks the function of T cells.

PHARMACOTHERAPEUTICS

The immunosuppressant drugs are used mainly to prevent rejection in patients who undergo organ transplantation.

Drug interactions

Most drug interactions with this class of drugs involve other immunosuppressant and anti-inflammatory agents and various antibiotic and antimicrobial drugs. (See Drug Interactions: *Immunosuppressants,* page 498.)

ADVERSE DRUG REACTIONS

The primary adverse reaction to azathioprine is bone marrow suppression, evidenced by leukopenia, macrocytic anemia, pancytopenia, and thrombocytopenia. This may alter clotting mechanisms and cause hemorrhaging. Nausea, vomiting, anorexia, and diarrhea can occur with high dosages; mouth ulcerations, esophagitis, and steatorrhea also can occur. In a small number of patients, hepatic dysfunction has been reported. Other adverse reactions to azathioprine include alopecia, arthralgia, retinopathy, Raynaud's disease, and pulmonary edema.

The most severe adverse reaction to cyclosporine is nephrotoxicity, usually characterized by increased blood urea nitrogen (BUN) and serum creatinine levels. More common adverse reactions include hyperkalemia, hyperuricemia, decreased serum bicarbonate level, hypertension, tremor, gingival hyperplasia, hirsutism, diarrhea, nausea, vomiting, generalized abdominal discomfort, and infection. Less common reactions are gastritis, hiccups, and peptic ulcers. Occasional complaints include central nervous system effects (flushing, paresthesia, headache) and hepatotoxicity (usually occurring during the first month of therapy and with high dosages). Leukopenia, thrombocytopenia, and anemia are uncommon, and hematuria and psychiatric disorders are rare. In 3% of patients undergoing cyclosporine therapy, sinusitis and gynecomastia have been reported; conjunctivitis, hearing loss, tinnitus, hyperglycemia, edema, fever, and muscle pain have been reported in 2% or less.

With ATG therapy, the most common adverse reaction is fever accompanied by chills. Up to 20% of patients receiving kidney allografts experience leukopenia, thrombocytopenia, or both while receiving this drug. Early **myelosup-**

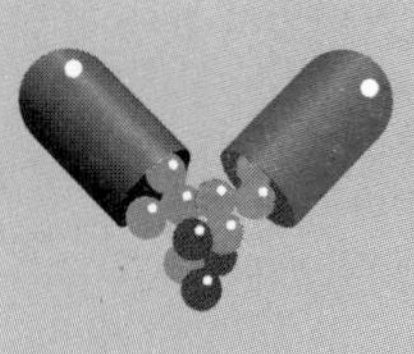

DRUG INTERACTIONS

Immunosuppressants

Interactions involving the immunosuppressants and other drugs can increase the patient's risk of infection greatly. The nurse should assess the patient continually for fever, malaise, and other signs and symptoms of infection.

DRUG	INTERACTING DRUGS	POSSIBLE EFFECTS	NURSING IMPLICATIONS
azathioprine	allopurinol	Increased blood level of azathioprine	• Decrease the azathioprine dosage, as prescribed, during concomitant use of these drugs.
cyclosporine	acyclovir, aminoglycosides, amphotericin B	Increased risk for nephrotoxicity	• Monitor the patient's blood urea nitrogen (BUN) and serum creatinine levels. • Monitor the patient's fluid intake and output. • Decrease the dosage of both nephrotoxic drugs, as prescribed.
	other immunosuppressant agents (except corticosteroids)	Increased risk of infection and lymphoma	• Monitor the patient for signs and symptoms of infection.
	ketoconazole	Increased serum cyclosporine level	• Monitor the patient for excessive cyclosporine effect (neurotoxicity). • Monitor the patient's BUN and serum creatinine levels. • Monitor the patient's fluid intake and output. • Decrease the cyclosporine dosage, as prescribed.
	barbiturates, rifampin, phenytoin, sulfonamides, trimethoprim	Decreased plasma cyclosporine level	• Increase the cyclosporine dosage, as prescribed.
	calcium channel blockers, cimetidine	Increased plasma cyclosporine level	• Decrease the cyclosporine dosage, as prescribed.
	anabolic steroids, oral contraceptives	Increased serum cyclosporine level	• Monitor the patient's serum cyclosporine concentration. • Decrease the cyclosporine dosage, as prescribed. • Monitor the patient's BUN and serum creatinine levels. • Advise the patient to avoid concomitant use with oral contraceptives or anabolic steroids.
	cardiac glycosides	Increased serum digoxin level	• Monitor for signs and symptoms of digitalis toxicity, such as cardiac, gastrointestinal, and neurologic dysfunction. • Monitor the patient's serum digoxin concentration. • Decrease the glycoside dosage, as prescribed.
	erythromycin, metoclopramide	Increased serum cyclosporine level	• Monitor the patient's BUN and serum creatinine levels. • Monitor the serum cyclosporine concentration.
lymphocyte immune globulin (antithymocyte globulin, ATG)	other immunosuppressant agents	Increased risk of infection and lymphoma	• Monitor the patient's white blood cell count for leukocytosis.
muromonab-CD3	other immunosuppressant agents	Increased immunosuppressant effect	• Monitor the patient for signs and symptoms of infection.

pression also may occur and force discontinuation of ATG. The immunosuppressant effects of ATG may lead to local and systemic infections. Nausea, vomiting, diarrhea, stomatitis, hiccups, epigastric pain, and abdominal distention also may occur. Rash, pruritus, urticaria, and erythema have been reported in 10% to 15% of patients. Adverse cardiovascular reactions to ATG, such as hypotension, hypertension, tachycardia, edema, pulmonary edema, iliac vein obstruction, and renal artery stenosis, are uncommon.

Most adverse reactions to muromonab-CD3 occur during the first 2 days of therapy. The most common reactions are fever and chills. Others include dyspnea, chest pain, vomiting, wheezing, nausea, diarrhea, and tremor. Severe — potentially fatal — pulmonary edema has been reported in 2% or less of patients receiving this drug. The incidence of infection associated with muromonab-CD3 therapy is comparable to that associated with high dosages of corticosteroids. The most common infections, which involve cytomegalovirus and herpes simplex virus, occur during the first 45 days of therapy.

All drugs in this class can cause hypersensitivity reactions, which range from rash and serum sickness to anaphylaxis. Azathioprine may cause hypersensitivity-induced pancreatitis.

NURSING PROCESS APPLICATION

The following information assists the nurse in caring for a patient receiving an immunosuppressant. It includes an overview of assessment activities as well as examples of appropriate nursing diagnoses and related interventions (see "Planning and implementation"). It also highlights the importance of evaluation.

Assessment

Before drug therapy begins, review the patient's history for conditions that contraindicate or require cautious use of the prescribed immunosuppressant. Also review the patient's medication history to identify use of drugs that may interact with it. During therapy, assess the patient for adverse drug reactions and signs of drug interactions. Also, periodically assess the effectiveness of immunosuppressant therapy. Finally, evaluate the patient's and family's knowledge about the prescribed drug. (See Patient Teaching: *Immunosuppressants.*)

Nursing diagnoses

- Risk for injury related to a preexisting condition that contraindicates or requires cautious use of an immunosuppressant
- Risk for injury related to adverse drug reactions or drug interactions
- Altered protection related to immunosuppression caused by long-term immunosuppressant therapy
- Knowledge deficit related to the prescribed immunosuppressant

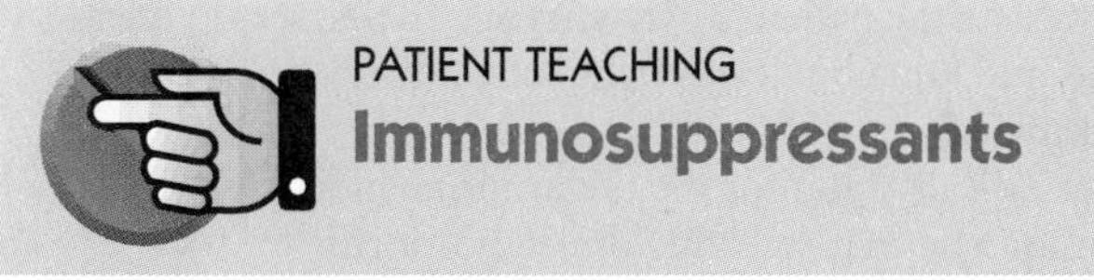

- Teach the patient and family the name, dose, frequency, action, and adverse effects of the prescribed immunosuppressant.
- Thoroughly explain the therapeutic purpose of the immunosuppressant.
- Inform the patient that infection, which can be life-threatening, is the most common hazard associated with immunosuppressant therapy.
- Emphasize that preventing infection requires scrupulous oral and personal hygiene during immunosuppressant therapy.
- Advise the patient to avoid crowds and people who have infections while taking the immunosuppressant.
- Urge the patient to postpone immunizations until after immunosuppressant therapy is discontinued.
- Urge a female patient to avoid conception during immunosuppressant therapy and for up to 4 months after it is stopped.
- Emphasize the importance of having laboratory tests and periodic monitoring by the physician.
- Teach the patient to take bleeding precautions if the platelet count falls below normal.
- Instruct the patient receiving cyclosporine to notify the physician if paresthesia, tinnitus, or hearing loss occurs.
- Inform the diabetic patient that hyperglycemia may occur during cyclosporine therapy. Instruct such a patient to monitor the blood glucose level closely and strictly adhere to the prescribed treatment regimen strictly.
- Prepare the patient for immunosuppressant-induced changes in appearance, such as alopecia, hirsutism, gynecomastia, or rashes.
- Instruct the patient to notify the physician if adverse reactions occur.

Planning and implementation

- Do not administer an immunosuppressant to a patient with a condition that contraindicates its use.
- Administer an immunosuppressant cautiously to a patient at risk because of a preexisting condition.
- Monitor the patient frequently for adverse reactions or drug interactions during immunosuppressant therapy.

*** *Monitor the patient closely for hypersensitivity reactions. Keep standard emergency equipment nearby.***

- Give the patient 1 mg/kg of methylprednisolone sodium succinate I.V., as prescribed, before administering muromonab-CD3 I.V. to reduce the risk of a first-dose reaction.
- Administer 100 mg of hydrocortisone sodium succinate I.V., as prescribed, 30 minutes after muromonab-CD3 I.V. administration to reduce the risk of a first-dose reaction.

*** *Perform an intradermal skin test, as prescribed, before administering the first dose of ATG to assess the patient's risk for severe systemic adverse reactions.***

- Monitor the patient's CBC (including platelets) and liver function tests frequently during azathioprine therapy.

• Evaluate the patient's liver enzymes, BUN, serum creatinine, and bilirubin levels frequently during cyclosporine therapy.
• Periodically monitor the cyclosporine blood concentration for a patient receiving oral cyclosporine.
• Document that the patient starting muromonab-CD3 therapy has had a chest X-ray 24 hours before receiving the first dose; the chest must be clear of fluid.
• Regularly monitor the patient's T-cell assays during muromonab-CD3 therapy.
• Administer azathioprine in divided doses after meals, as prescribed, to reduce the risk or severity of adverse GI reactions.
• Administer azathioprine I.V., as prescribed, if the patient cannot tolerate the oral drug, but resume oral therapy as soon as possible.
• Give I.V. azathioprine as a bolus or diluted in normal saline solution or dextrose 5% in water (D_5W) and infuse over 30 to 60 minutes.
• Mix oral cyclosporine in a glass container with milk or orange juice at room temperature to increase its palatability. Stir it well with a metal spoon and administer the drink immediately. Then put a little more milk or orange juice in the container and have the patient drink it to receive the entire dose.
• Dilute each milliliter of cyclosporine for I.V. infusion in 20 to 100 ml of normal saline solution or D_5W immediately before administration and infuse over 2 to 6 hours. Ensure that the solution is free from particulate matter and discoloration. If it is not, discard it and start over.
• Administer I.V. ATG as an infusion, diluted in 250 to 1,000 ml of normal or half-normal saline solution over 4 to 8 hours.
• Refrigerate the ATG solution if it will not be given immediately. If refrigeration time plus infusion time exceeds 12 hours, do not use the solution.
• Administer the ATG solution into high-flow veins to decrease the risk of phlebitis and thrombosis. Always use an in-line filter and make sure the solution is free from particulate matter and discoloration.
• Administer a muromonab-CD3 I.V. bolus in less than 1 minute. Do not administer it as an infusion or with other solutions.
• Notify the physician if adverse reactions, drug interactions, or signs of organ or graft rejection occur.
*** *Monitor the patient for signs and symptoms of infection during immunosuppressant therapy. Keep in mind that classic signs of infection may be suppressed. However, the WBC count remains a reliable indicator.***
• Regularly monitor the patient's WBC and differential counts during immunosuppressant therapy.
*** *Take infection control measures such as maintaining reverse isolation.***
• Notify the physician immediately if the patient displays signs of infection. Prepare to begin appropriate treatment, such as antibiotic therapy, as prescribed.

Evaluation

For each nursing diagnosis, prepare an evaluation statement that describes the patient's or family's response to nursing interventions.

CHAPTER SUMMARY

Chapter 39 discussed the systemic corticosteroids and other immunosuppressant agents. Here are the chapter highlights.

Systemic corticosteroids affect nearly every body system and have the potential to cause severe adverse reactions. They are synthetic analogues of natural corticosteroids secreted by the adrenal cortex. When caring for a patient receiving a systemic glucocorticoid, the nurse should monitor closely for adverse reactions and teach the patient about the correct timing and self-administration of doses as well as the signs and symptoms of adverse reactions.

Fludrocortisone is a mineralocorticoid that also is a synthetic analogue of natural corticosteroids excreted by the adrenal cortex. It exerts its principal effect on the body's fluid and electrolyte balance and extracellular fluid volume. The drug is used chiefly for replacement therapy in patients with adrenocortical insufficiency. Aldosterone is a natural mineralocorticoid that is not commonly used because of its cost, availability, and administration route. Nursing care related to mineralocorticoid therapy includes preparing the patient for long-term use of the drug.

The major immunosuppressant agents, used to prevent or treat allograft rejection, are highly potent and can cause severe — even life-threatening — adverse reactions. Nursing care for a patient receiving an immunosuppressant includes taking all possible measures to prevent infection, teaching the patient the importance of preventing infection, and stressing the need for the patient to report any change in health status because it may signal infection.

Questions to consider

See Appendix 1 for answers.

1. Mark Edge, age 29, has ulcerative colitis and takes prednisone 10 mg P.O. daily. Mr. Edge should take prednisone at what time?
   (a) At bedtime to minimize adverse reactions
   (b) In the morning to mimic normal hormone secretion
   (c) On an empty stomach to enhance absorption
   (d) In the evening when normal hormone secretion is low

2. Because long-term use of a corticosteroid can produce cushingoid signs and symptoms, the nurse assesses a patient regularly for these effects during prednisone therapy. Which of the following signs and symptoms suggest this adverse reaction?
   (a) Alopecia and dysmenorrhea
   (b) Hypoglycemia and thrombocytopenia
   (c) Hypotension, tachycardia, and dyspnea
   (d) Girdle obesity, glycosuria, and moon face

3. Beth Walker, 52, is diagnosed with psoriasis. Her physician prescribes betamethasone valerate cream to be applied three times a day. How should the nurse teach Ms. Walker to apply this glucocorticoid cream?
   (a) Apply the smallest amount possible in a thin coat over the affected area.
   (b) Apply a thick coat to ensure maximum therapeutic effects.
   (c) Apply to nearby unaffected areas to prevent the spread of psoriasis.
   (d) Apply an occlusive dressing after putting a thick coat on the affected area.

4. Jeff White, age 57, has just received a heart transplant. To prevent transplant rejection, his physician prescribes cyclosporine 1 g P.O. daily, azathioprine 100 mg P.O. daily, and prednisone 30 mg P.O. daily. When caring for Mr. White, the nurse should assess for which of the following primary adverse reactions to azathioprine?
   (a) Renal failure
   (b) Peptic ulcer
   (c) Severe pulmonary edema
   (d) Bone marrow suppression

40 Uricosurics, other antigout agents, and gold salts

OBJECTIVES

After reading and studying this chapter, the student should be able to:
1. identify the specific clinical indications for the following drugs: probenecid, sulfinpyrazone, allopurinol, colchicine, auranofin, aurothioglucose, and gold sodium thiomalate.
2. describe the action of the uricosurics probenecid and sulfinpyrazone and the antigout agents allopurinol and colchicine.
3. describe the adverse reactions to the major drugs used to treat acute gouty attacks and rheumatoid arthritis.
4. differentiate between the pharmacokinetic properties of parenteral and oral gold salt preparations.
5. describe how to apply the nursing process when caring for a patient who is receiving a uricosuric, other antigout agents, or gold salt.

INTRODUCTION

Joint **inflammation** can be treated with many drugs, depending on its etiology. For example, **gout** and **rheumatoid arthritis** produce joint inflammation that responds to different drug interventions. Gout is best treated with **uricosurics,** such as probenecid and sulfinpyrazone, or other antigout medications, such as allopurinol and colchicine. Indomethacin, naproxen, and phenylbutazone also are used to treat gout. The drugs of choice for rheumatoid arthritis include auranofin (an oral gold salt) and aurothioglucose or gold sodium thiomalate (two parenteral forms of gold salt therapy). These three drugs are used only after other agents, such as nonsteroidal anti-inflammatory drugs (NSAIDs), have failed to work effectively. All the drugs discussed in this chapter exert their effects through their anti-inflammatory actions — they are not analgesics. (See *Selected major uricosurics, other antigout agents, and gold salts.*)

Drugs covered in this chapter include:

- allopurinol
- auranofin
- aurothioglucose
- ColBenemid
- colchicine
- gold sodium thiomalate
- probenecid
- sulfinpyrazone.

Uricosurics

The two major uricosurics, probenecid and sulfinpyrazone, act by increasing uric acid excretion in the urine. The primary goal in using uricosurics is to prevent or control the frequency of gouty arthritis attacks.

PHARMACOKINETICS

Uricosurics are absorbed from the gastrointestinal (GI) tract. Distribution of the two drugs also is similar, with 75% to 95% of probenecid and 98% of sulfinpyrazone being protein-bound. Metabolism of the drugs occurs in the liver, and excretion is primarily by the renal system. Only small amounts of these two drugs are excreted in the feces. Probenecid reaches peak plasma concentrations in 2 to 4 hours; sulfinpyrazone, in 1 to 2 hours.

Route	Onset	Peak	Duration
P.O.	30 min	1-4 hr	4-10 hr

PHARMACODYNAMICS

Probenecid and sulfinpyrazone competitively inhibit the active resorption of uric acid at the proximal convoluted tubules. This leads to urine excretion of uric acid and a subsequent reduction of the serum urate level.

PHARMACOTHERAPEUTICS

Probenecid and sulfinpyrazone, which lower the serum urate level, are indicated for patients with chronic gouty arthritis and tophaceous gout. Uricosuric drugs also are used in patients with visible **tophi,** with a serum urate level above 8.5 to 9 mg/dl, and with a family history of tophi or decreased uric acid excretion. Probenecid and sulfinpyrazone are not indicated during an acute gouty attack. If taken at that time, the drugs only prolong inflammation. Probenecid is also used to promote uric acid excretion in patients experiencing **hyperuricemia.**

Recently colchicine and probenecid have been combined to form the drug ColBenemid. This new formulated drug's purpose is to facilitate the administration of these two products. Therapy with ColBenemid should not be started until an acute gouty attack has subsided.

Selected major uricosurics, other antigout agents, and gold salts

This table summarizes the major uricosurics, other antigout agents, and gold salts currently in clinical use.

DRUG	MAJOR INDICATIONS AND USUAL DOSAGES	CONTRAINDICATIONS AND PRECAUTIONS
Uricosurics		
probenecid (Benemid)	*Chronic gouty arthritis, tophaceous gout* ADULT: 250 mg P.O. b.i.d. during the 1st week, then 500 mg b.i.d.; can be increased by 500 mg every 4 weeks until a maximum of 2 g daily is achieved	• Probenecid is contraindicated in a patient who is taking penicillin and has impaired renal function or one with known hypersensitivity, blood dyscrasias, or uric acid renal calculi. • This drug requires cautious use in a patient with a history of peptic ulcer disease.
Other antigout agents		
allopurinol (Zyloprim)	*Gout, hyperuricemia* ADULT: 100 mg P.O. daily, then increased at weekly intervals by 100 mg, up to a maximum of 800 mg daily	• Allopurinol is contraindicated in a patient with known hypersensitivity. • This drug requires cautious use in a pregnant or breast-feeding patient, a patient with impaired renal function, or one who is taking a thiazide diuretic and has impaired renal function.
colchicine	*Acute gouty arthritis* ADULT: initial dose of 0.5 to 1.3 mg P.O., then 0.5 to 0.6 mg every hour or 1 to 1.2 mg P.O. every 2 hours, up to a maximum of 8 mg, until pain relief occurs or until patient suffers nausea, vomiting, or diarrhea; course of oral therapy should not be repeated for at least 3 days; or initial dose of 2 mg I.V. followed by 0.5 mg P.O. every 6 hours until a satisfactory response occurs, with a maximum daily dosage of 4 mg; course of I.V. therapy should not be repeated for several weeks	• Colchicine is contraindicated in a pregnant patient or a patient with a serious gastrointestinal (GI), renal, hepatic, or cardiac disease. • This drug requires cautious use in a geriatric, debilitated, or breast-feeding patient.
Gold salts		
auranofin (Ridaura)	*Rheumatoid arthritis* ADULT: 6 mg P.O. daily in a single dose or divided doses	• Auranofin is contraindicated in a pregnant or breast-feeding patient or a patient with a history of a gold-induced disorder, such as anaphylactic reaction, necrotizing enterocolitis, pulmonary fibrosis, exfoliative dermatitis, bone marrow aplasia, or other severe hematologic disorder. • This drug requires cautious use in a patient with GI distress, such as nausea, vomiting, diarrhea, constipation, or abdominal pain. • Safety and efficacy in children have not been established.
aurothioglucose (Solganal)	*Rheumatoid arthritis* ADULT: 10 mg I.M during the first week, 25 mg I.M. during the 2nd and 3rd weeks, then 50 mg I.M. weekly until 0.8 to 1 g I.M. has been administered; for maintenance, 25 to 50 mg I.M. every 3 to 4 weeks PEDIATRIC: for children ages 6 to 12, 1 mg/kg I.M. weekly for 20 weeks; for children over age 12, same as adult dosage above	• Aurothioglucose is contraindicated in a pregnant or breast-feeding patient, a severely debilitated patient, one who has recently undergone radiation therapy, or one with known hypersensitivity, uncontrolled diabetes mellitus, systemic lupus erythematosus, renal disease, hepatic dysfunction, uncontrolled heart failure, marked hypertension, granulocytopenia, other blood dyscrasias, hemorrhagic diathesis, history of infectious hepatitis, urticaria, eczema, or colitis. • This drug requires cautious use in a patient with compromised cardiovascular or cerebral circulation. • Safety and efficacy in children under age 6 have not been established.

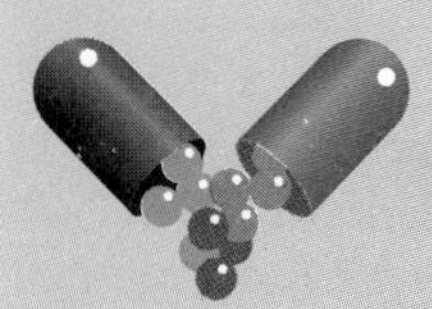

DRUG INTERACTIONS
Uricosurics

Some drug interactions involving the uricosurics represent potentially serious complications for the patient.

DRUG	INTERACTING DRUGS	POSSIBLE EFFECTS	NURSING IMPLICATIONS
probenecid	weakly acidic organic antibiotics	Increased plasma level of the antibiotic	• Monitor the patient's serum antibiotic level as prescribed.
	salicylates	Inhibited action of probenecid, which decreases the drug's effects	• Explain to the patient that prolonged use of salicylates is contraindicated. • Administer acetaminophen as prescribed if an analgesic or antipyretic is needed.
	antineoplastic drugs	Increased serum urate level	• Do not administer these drugs together.
	dapsone	Increased serum dapsone level	• Monitor the patient's hemoglobin level and hematocrit. • Observe for signs of methemoglobinemia, such as cyanosis and shortness of breath. • Monitor the patient for peripheral neuropathy (pain or change in sensation in extremities). • Reduce the dapsone dosage, as prescribed.
	dyphylline	Increased serum dyphylline level	• Monitor the signs and symptoms of theophylline toxicity, such as nausea, tachycardia, and nervousness. • Monitor the patient's serum theophylline level. • Administer theophylline instead of dyphylline, as prescribed.
	ketoprofen	Increased serum ketoprofen level	• Monitor the signs and symptoms of excessive ketoprofen effect, such as nausea, abdominal pain, dizziness, drowsiness, headache, tinnitus, and impaired renal function. • Decrease the ketoprofen dosage, as prescribed.
	methotrexate	Increased serum methotrexate level	• Monitor for signs and symptoms of methotrexate toxicity, such as stomatitis, bone marrow suppression, and fatigue. • Decrease the methotrexate dosage, as prescribed.
sulfinpyrazone	warfarin	Increased hypoprothrombinemic response to warfarin as exhibited by increased prothrombin time (PT); increased risk of bleeding	• Monitor the patient's PT when beginning or discontinuing therapy with either drug. • Teach the patient the signs and symptoms of bleeding, such as epistaxis, hematuria, and easy bruising. • Monitor for changes in the patient's red blood cells, hemoglobin level, and hematocrit. • Monitor the patient's urine, feces, and vomitus for blood.
	salicylates	Inhibited uricosuric effect of sulfinpyrazone	• Avoid the concomitant use of salicylates during uricosuric therapy.
	theophylline	Increased clearance of theophylline	• Monitor theophylline levels.
	tobutamide	Increased half-life of tolbutamide	• Monitor patient's blood glucose level for hypoglycemia.

Because these agents may increase the chance of an acute gouty attack when therapy begins and whenever the serum urate level changes rapidly, colchicine is administered in prophylactic dosages during the first 3 to 6 months of probenecid or sulfinpyrazone therapy.

Drug interactions

Numerous drugs interact with uricosurics. (See Drug Interactions: *Uricosurics.*)

Uricosurics also may interact with Clinitest, a reactive agent used to test for urine glucose. This interaction produces a false-positive test result.

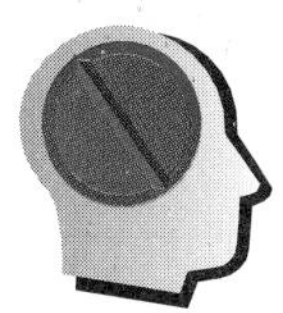

CRITICAL THINKING. To enhance your critical thinking about probenecid, consider the following situation and its analysis.

Situation: Mr. Allen is a 51-year-old patient who calls the telephone advice program that you staff. He tells you he is taking probenecid for his gout but forgot that he was not supposed to take aspirin. He relates taking aspirin for the past week, and he wants to know what he should do.

Analysis: First find out why he is taking aspirin and how many he took, and then determine if he needs more definitive medical care. If there are no contraindications to Mr. Allen taking acetaminophen, suggest that he stop taking aspirin and switch to acetaminophen. Because aspirin inhibits the action of probenecid, you want to ask him if he is experiencing signs or symptoms, such as pain, warmth, or swelling, indicating that his gout is flaring up, so other medical consultations can be arranged.

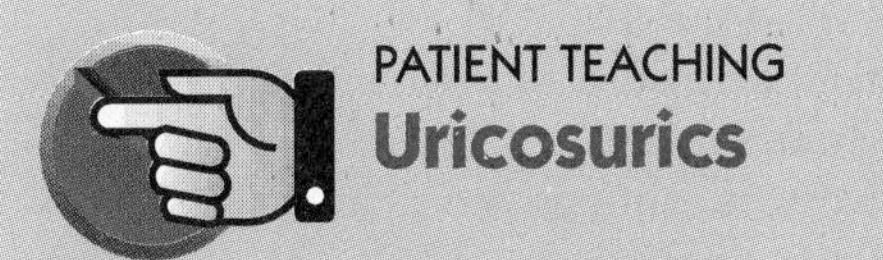

PATIENT TEACHING

Uricosurics

- Teach the patient and family the name, dose, frequency, action, and adverse effects of the prescribed uricosuric.
- Instruct the patient to take the drug exactly as prescribed and not to stop the drug without consulting the physician because gout symptoms may reappear.
- Advise the patient to notify the physician if gastrointestinal distress persists.
- Instruct the patient not to take aspirin during uricosuric therapy. If an analgesic or antipyretic is needed, the patient should take acetaminophen.
- Ensure that the patient understands that the uricosuric should not be taken during an acute attack of gout. Explain that taking the drug at that time will prolong the inflammation and will not relieve the acute symptoms. Inform the patient that the drug usually is not started until 2 to 3 weeks after an acute attack.
- Alert the diabetic patient who tests the urine glucose level with Clinitest of the possibility of false-positive test results. Recommend that the patient use Clinistix or another urine glucose testing product.
- Advise the patient not to perform activities that require mental alertness if dizziness or vertigo occurs.
- Emphasize the importance of having laboratory studies performed regularly as ordered.
- Instruct the patient to notify the physician if adverse reactions occur.

ADVERSE DRUG REACTIONS

When given in therapeutic dosages, probenecid usually is tolerated well by patients. Its most common adverse effects are headache and GI distress, including anorexia, nausea, and vomiting. Other adverse reactions include flushing, dizziness, urinary frequency, sore gums, and anemia.

When given in therapeutic dosages, sulfinpyrazone usually is tolerated well. Nausea, dyspepsia, GI pain, and GI blood loss are the most commonly reported adverse reactions to sulfinpyrazone. Reactivation or aggravation of peptic ulcer disease also can occur. Other adverse reactions include dizziness, rash, vertigo, tinnitus, and edema. Blood dyscrasias, such as anemia, leukopenia, granulocytopenia, and thrombocytopenia, are rare.

Some patients taking probenecid or sulfinpyrazone may form uric acid calculi. This usually occurs upon initiation of therapy. Acute gouty attacks also can occur in some patients during the first 6 to 12 months of therapy.

Hypersensitivity reactions can occur in some patients taking probenecid. Signs and symptoms of such reactions may include dermatitis, pruritus, fever, sweating, or hypotension. Rarely, a patient may experience an anaphylactic reaction, nephrotic syndrome, hepatic necrosis, or aplastic anemia. In some patients, discontinuation of sulfinpyrazone therapy has reversed renal dysfunction.

NURSING PROCESS APPLICATION

The following information assists the nurse in caring for a patient receiving a uricosuric. It includes an overview of assessment activities as well as examples of appropriate nursing diagnoses and related interventions (see "Planning and implementation"). It also highlights the importance of evaluation.

Assessment

Before drug therapy begins, review the patient's history for conditions that contraindicate or require cautious use of the prescribed uricosuric. Also review the patient's medication history to identify use of drugs that may interact with it. (See Patient Teaching: *Uricosurics.*) During therapy, assess the patient for adverse drug reactions and signs of drug interactions. Also, periodically assess the effectiveness of uricosuric therapy. Finally, evaluate the patient's and family's knowledge about the prescribed drug.

Nursing diagnoses

- Risk for injury related to a preexisting condition that contraindicates or requires cautious use of a uricosuric
- Risk for injury related to adverse drug reactions or drug interactions
- Risk for fluid volume deficit related to the adverse GI effects of the prescribed uricosuric
- Knowledge deficit related to the prescribed uricosuric

Planning and implementation

- Do not administer a uricosuric to a patient with a condition that contraindicates its use.
- Administer a uricosuric cautiously to a patient at risk because of a preexisting condition.
- Monitor the patient frequently for adverse reactions and drug interactions during uricosuric therapy.

*** *Observe the patient closely for hypersensitivity reactions to probenecid. Have standard emergency equipment nearby because anaphylaxis can occur.***

- Monitor appropriate laboratory values, including a complete blood count (CBC), urinalysis, and serum uric acid level. Regularly monitor renal function tests and the blood urea nitrogen level.
- Notify the physician if the patient has an acute gouty attack. Discuss temporary discontinuation of the uricosuric, because it may prolong inflammation in an acute gouty attack.
- Administer colchicine, as prescribed, with the uricosuric to help prevent an acute attack of gouty arthritis, which can occur at the start of uricosuric therapy.
- Encourage the patient to drink ten to twelve 8-oz (240-ml) glasses of water daily, unless contraindicated. Maintaining a high fluid intake minimizes calculi formation.
- Encourage the patient to ingest a high-vegetable diet to alkalinize the urine. Maintaining alkaline urine decreases the formation of uric acid calculi.
- Notify the physician if adverse reactions or drug interactions occur.
- Monitor hydration if the patient experiences adverse GI reactions, such as anorexia, nausea, or vomiting. Obtain a prescription for an antiemetic agent, as needed.
- Notify the physician if the patient cannot tolerate oral therapy.
- Administer the drug with food, milk, or an antacid to prevent GI distress, which is the most common adverse reaction to uricosurics.

Evaluation

For each nursing diagnosis, prepare an evaluation statement that describes the patient's or family's response to nursing interventions.

Other antigout agents

Two other drugs, allopurinol and colchicine, commonly are prescribed to treat gout. Allopurinol is used to inhibit uric acid synthesis, thereby reducing the metabolic pool of uric acid in the body and preventing gouty attacks. Colchicine has a relatively specific use: to treat acute gouty attacks.

PHARMACOKINETICS

After oral administration, allopurinol and colchicine are absorbed from the GI tract. Allopurinol and its inactive metabolite oxypurinol are distributed throughout the tissue fluid, metabolized by the liver, and excreted in the urine.

Allopurinol

Route	Onset	Peak	Duration
P.O.	30-60 min	2-6 hr	2-3 days

Colchicine is partially metabolized in the liver. The drug and its metabolites then reenter the intestinal tract via biliary secretions. After reabsorption from the intestines, colchicine is distributed to various tissues. The drug is excreted primarily in the feces and to a lesser degree in the urine.

Colchicine

Route	Onset	Peak	Duration
P.O.	≤12 hr	0.5-2 hr	12-48 hr
I.V.	6-12 hr	Unknown	4-12 hr

PHARMACODYNAMICS

Allopurinol and its primary metabolite oxypurinol inhibit uric acid synthesis, which contributes to the pharmacologic effectiveness of allopurinol. The long half-life of oxypurinol contributes significantly to the inhibition of xanthine oxidase, the enzyme responsible for converting hypoxanthine to xanthine as well as xanthine to uric acid.

Colchicine appears to reduce the inflammatory response to monosodium urate crystals deposited in joint tissues. Colchicine may produce its effects by interfering with the activity of **polymorphonuclear leukocytes** that results when metabolism, mobility, **chemotaxis,** or other leukocyte functions become inhibited.

PHARMACOTHERAPEUTICS

Allopurinol is used to treat primary gout and gout associated with blood dyscrasias and related therapy. This drug is recommended for primary or secondary uric acid nephropathy, with or without the accompanying symptoms of gout, and for patients with recurrent uric acid calculi formation. Allopurinol also proves effective in patients who respond poorly to maximum dosages of uricosurics or who have allergic reactions or intolerance to uricosuric drugs. Allopurinol is useful in preventing hyperuricemia in patients who also are receiving cancer chemotherapy for myeloproliferative disorders. It also is effective when given with uricosurics, where smaller dosages of each drug are used. Allopurinol is the drug of choice for patients at risk for renal calculi, such as those who have renal disease or who excrete excessive amounts of uric acid in the urine. By reducing uric acid formation, allopurinol eliminates the hazards of hyperuricuria.

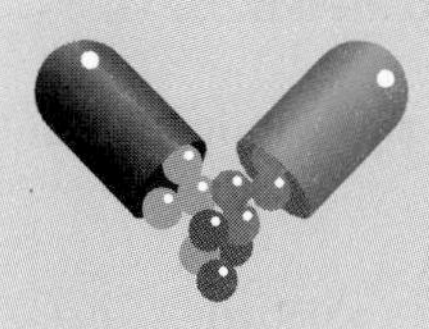

DRUG INTERACTIONS
Allopurinol

When given with other drugs, allopurinol may cause interactions that adversely affect the patient. The nurse should exercise caution and closely monitor the patient.

DRUG	INTERACTING DRUGS	POSSIBLE EFFECTS	NURSING IMPLICATIONS
allopurinol	oral anticoagulants	Inhibited anticoagulant metabolism, leading to a prolonged half-life	• Monitor the patient's prothrombin time. • Teach the patient the signs and symptoms of bleeding, such as spontaneous epistaxis, hematuria, and easy bruising. • Monitor the patient's urine, feces, and vomitus for blood.
	mercaptopurine, azathioprine	Increased antimetabolite effect of these drugs	• Expect to reduce the drug dosages as prescribed. • Monitor the patient for signs and symptoms of toxicity, such as additive bone marrow suppression and fatigue.
	angiotensin-converting enzyme inhibitors	Increased risk of hypersensitivity reactions to allopurinol	• Monitor the patient for rash, fever, and arthralgia. • Avoid concomitant use of these drugs.
	theophylline	Increased serum theophylline level	• Monitor the patient for signs and symptoms of theophylline toxicity, such as nervousness, nausea, and tachycardia. • Monitor the patient's serum theophylline level.
	cyclophosphamide	Increased myelosuppression	• Monitor infection and bleeding risks.

Colchicine is used to relieve acute attacks of gouty arthritis. When initiated early enough and in adequate amounts, the drug proves especially effective in relieving pain. Colchicine also is recommended for prevention of recurrent gouty arthritis. Also, concomitant use of colchicine during the first several months of allopurinol, probenecid, or sulfinpyrazone therapy may prevent the acute gouty attacks that sometimes accompany the use of these drugs. Colchicine can be especially valuable in diagnosing gouty arthritis.

Drug interactions

When allopurinol is used concomitantly with other drugs, the resulting interactions can affect the patient seriously. (For more information, see Drug Interactions: *Allopurinol.*) Colchicine does not interact significantly with other drugs.

ADVERSE DRUG REACTIONS

The most common reaction to allopurinol is a rash, which usually is maculopapular. Adverse GI reactions include nausea, vomiting, diarrhea, and intermittent abdominal pain. Less common reactions include those that cause hematopoietic changes, such as granulocytopenia, anemia, aplastic anemia, and bone marrow suppression. However, these reactions usually result from concomitant use of allopurinol and any drug known to cause such reactions. Peripheral neuritis and drowsiness also may occur. Rare instances of sensitivity reactions, such as alopecia and altered liver function test results, have occurred during allopurinol therapy.

The most common adverse reactions to orally administered colchicine include nausea, vomiting, abdominal discomfort, and diarrhea. These reactions usually occur with dosages used to achieve a therapeutic level of colchicine. However, they also indicate drug toxicity, and the colchicine should be discontinued. Therapy should not be resumed for 3 days; by waiting this period, the possibility of cumulative toxicity is minimized. GI symptoms also can occur when colchicine is administered intravenously (I.V.), but these adverse reactions usually occur only when the recommended dosage is exceeded.

Other adverse reactions involving colchicine primarily affect the skin, vascular system, and central nervous system (CNS). The most common skin problems include dermatitis, urticaria, and alopecia. Prolonged administration may cause bone marrow suppression and related hematologic problems, such as aplastic anemia, granulocytopenia, leukopenia, and thrombocytopenia. The only adverse CNS reaction is peripheral neuritis. Rare adverse reactions in-

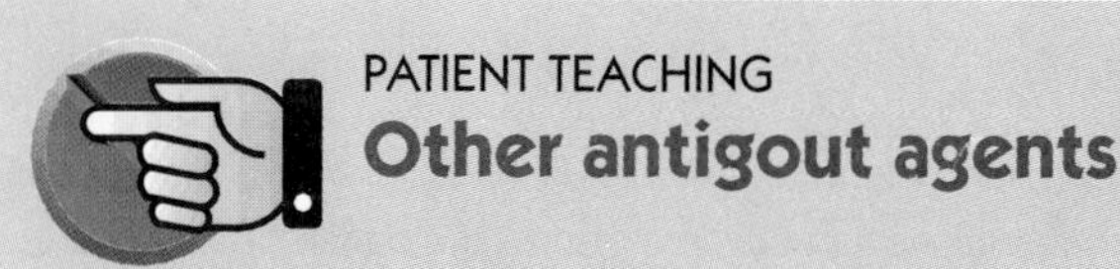

PATIENT TEACHING
Other antigout agents

- Teach the patient and family the name, dose, frequency, action, and adverse effects of the prescribed antigout agent.
- Instruct the patient to keep colchicine readily available so that it can be taken as soon as symptoms of an acute gouty attack occur. Explain that a delay in taking the drug can impair its effectiveness.
- Advise the patient to discontinue colchicine if nausea, vomiting, or diarrhea occurs and to notify the physician.
- Instruct the patient to discontinue allopurinol and to notify the physician at the first sign of a rash because this reaction may precede a severe hypersensitivity reaction.
- Instruct the patient to store allopurinol or colchicine in a tightly closed, light-resistant container.
- Advise the patient to exercise caution when engaging in activities that require alertness because allopurinol may cause drowsiness.
- Instruct the patient to notify the physician if adverse reactions occur.

clude renal damage, muscle weakness, reversible azoospermia, and an increased serum alkaline phosphatase level.

Colchicine produces few hypersensitivity reactions. These include bladder spasms, paralytic ileus, stomatitis, hypothyroidism, and nonthrombocytopenic purpura. Fever, chills, leukopenia, eosinophilia, arthralgia, rash, and pruritus also may be present.

NURSING PROCESS APPLICATION

The following information assists the nurse in caring for a patient receiving an antigout agent. It includes an overview of assessment activities as well as examples of appropriate nursing diagnoses and related interventions (see "Planning and implementation"). It also highlights the importance of evaluation.

Assessment

Before drug therapy begins, review the patient's history for conditions that contraindicate or require cautious use of the prescribed antigout drug. If the patient must receive allopurinol, also review the patient's medication history to identify use of drugs that may interact with it. During therapy, assess the patient for adverse drug reactions and signs of drug interactions. Also, periodically assess the effectiveness of therapy with the antigout agent. Finally, evaluate the patient's and family's knowledge about the prescribed drug.

Nursing diagnoses

- Risk for injury related to a preexisting condition that contraindicates or requires cautious use of an antigout agent
- Risk for injury related to adverse drug reactions or drug interactions
- Risk for fluid volume deficit related to the adverse GI effects of the prescribed antigout agent
- Knowledge deficit related to the prescribed antigout agent

Planning and implementation

- Do not administer an antigout agent to a patient with a condition that contraindicates its use.
- Administer an antigout agent cautiously to a patient at risk because of a preexisting condition.
- Monitor the patient closely for adverse reactions and drug interactions during antigout therapy.
- Monitor CBC, urinalysis, serum uric acid level, and liver and kidney function test results before beginning and periodically during antigout therapy as instructed.
- Auscultate the patient's bowel sounds regularly during colchicine therapy to detect paralytic ileus.
- Administer allopurinol in divided doses, as prescribed, if the dosage exceeds 300 mg daily.
- Expect to adjust the allopurinol dosage, as prescribed, based on the serum creatinine level and a 12- or 24-hour urine creatinine level for a patient with renal failure.

∗ ***Do not give more than 4 mg/ml of colchicine I.V. during a 24-hour period.*** Parenteral colchicine is available in a strength of 0.5 mg/ml; if a lower concentration is needed for I.V. injection, dilute the drug with normal saline solution or sterile water. If the diluted solution is not clear, do not use.

- Prevent extravasation of colchicine into surrounding tissues. During I.V. administration, properly position the needle in the vein and check for good blood return before injecting the drug. If extravasation occurs, apply heat or cold to relieve the discomfort and notify the physician. Analgesics also may be given.

∗ ***Do not give more than 12 tablets of oral colchicine for any single acute gouty attack in a 24-hour period.***

- Notify the physician if adverse reactions or drug interactions occur.
- Monitor hydration if the patient experiences adverse GI reactions, such as nausea, vomiting, or diarrhea. Notify the physician and obtain a prescription for an antiemetic or antidiarrheal agent as needed. Expect to discontinue colchicine until GI distress has subsided. (See Patient Teaching: *Other antigout agents.*
- Administer allopurinol after meals and administer oral colchicine with food or milk to decrease GI distress.
- Inform the physician of the GI effects of the prescribed antigout agent on the patient.

Evaluation

For each nursing diagnosis, prepare an evaluation statement that describes the patient's or family's response to nursing interventions.

Gold salts

Gold salts are administered primarily to treat rheumatoid arthritis. The oral gold salt is auranofin, and the parenteral forms are aurothioglucose and gold sodium thiomalate.

PHARMACOKINETICS

Auranofin is absorbed from the GI tract. Distribution of auranofin is related primarily to its binding with erythrocytes. Within an erythrocyte, 90% of auranofin is distributed intracellularly; the remaining 10% is membrane-bound. The metabolic fate of auranofin is not understood completely. About 60% of the absorbed auranofin is excreted in the urine, with the remainder excreted in the feces. The unabsorbed auranofin is excreted primarily in the feces.

Gold sodium thiomalate is absorbed rapidly after intramuscular (I.M.) administration; aurothioglucose is absorbed more slowly and irregularly. The parenteral gold salts are distributed throughout the body. The metabolic fate of the parenteral gold salts remains obscure. They are excreted slowly from the body, with about 70% excreted in the urine and the remainder in the feces.

Route	Onset	Peak	Duration
P.O.	Unknown	1-2 hr	Unknown
I.M.	Unknown	Few hr	Variable

PHARMACODYNAMICS

The complexity of rheumatoid arthritis and the pharmacologic effects of gold salts makes understanding the mechanism of action of these drugs difficult. They may act by decreasing liposomal enzyme release and altering the immune response.

PHARMACOTHERAPEUTICS

Gold salts are prescribed only for patients who have an established diagnosis of rheumatoid arthritis and display an insufficient therapeutic response to an adequate trial of one or more NSAIDs. Because of the slow therapeutic response to gold salts, concomitant use of an NSAID or salicylate usually is prescribed until the patient begins to experience symptomatic relief. If cartilage and bone destruction also have occurred, gold salts cannot reverse the structural damage to the joints.

Drug interactions

Gold salts do not interact significantly with other drugs.

ADVERSE DRUG REACTIONS

The numerous adverse reactions to gold salts explain why these drugs are not the first choice for treating rheumatoid arthritis.

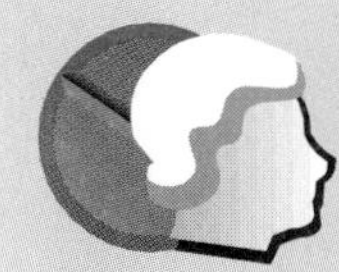

GERIATRIC CONSIDERATIONS

Gold salts

A major adverse effect with gold salts is dose-related loose stools and diarrhea. Geriatric patients receiving gold salts must be carefully monitored for signs of dehydration (dry skin and mouth, central nervous system changes, tachycardia) if reports of diarrhea ensue. The geriatric population tends to be at a higher risk for dehydration.

The most common adverse reactions to auranofin involve the GI system. Patients taking auranofin may experience dose-related diarrhea or loose stools. Nausea, vomiting, anorexia, abdominal cramps, and flatulence are less common. Ulcerative enterocolitis is a rare but serious adverse reaction. (See Geriatric Considerations: *Gold salts* for more information.)

Patients on oral gold therapy also experience mucocutaneous reactions. A rash, commonly preceded by pruritus, has occurred in about 25% of patients taking auranofin. Other mucocutaneous reactions include conjunctivitis, glossitis, and stomatitis. Stomatitis has occurred in about 13% of patients and produces shallow ulcers on the buccal membranes, palate, pharynx, and borders of the tongue. Alopecia, a dermatologic reaction, also may occur.

Other less common adverse reactions to auranofin involve the renal and hematologic systems. Renal effects include nephrotic syndrome and glomerulonephritis with proteinuria and hematuria. Blood dyscrasias, including leukopenia, thrombocytopenia, and anemia, have occurred.

The most common adverse reactions to parenteral gold salts involve mucocutaneous conditions, including stomatitis, gingivitis, glossitis, pharyngitis, tracheitis, and vaginitis. Parenteral gold salts also can produce severe blood dyscrasias as well as renal and hepatic damage, which warrant immediate attention. Adverse GI reactions rarely develop.

Most hypersensitivity reactions seem to occur with the parenteral gold salts. Up to 5% of patients receiving gold sodium thiomalate have experienced a vasomotor reaction, commonly called the nitritoid reaction. This reaction is characterized by flushing, dizziness, nausea, weakness, tachycardia, and syncope. Having the patient lie down can alleviate the nitritoid reaction; then the patient should be switched to aurothioglucose.

Rare incidents of anaphylactic shock, syncope, bradycardia, difficulty swallowing, and angioedema have occurred with injectable gold salt. These reactions usually occur immediately or within 10 minutes of injection.

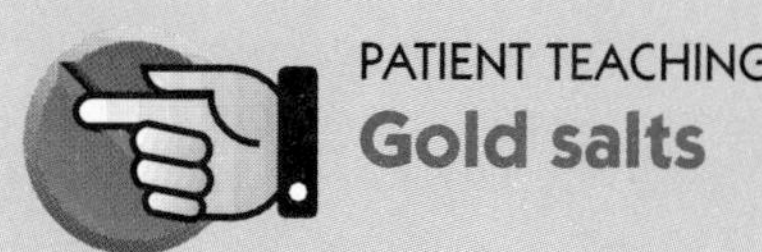

PATIENT TEACHING

Gold salts

- Teach the patient and family the name, dose, frequency, action, and adverse effects of the prescribed gold salt.
- Instruct the patient to report diarrhea that persists for more than 3 to 4 days or that interferes with daily activities.
- Stress the importance of compliance with gold therapy. Explain to the patient that the therapeutic effects of the gold salt usually occur 8 to 12 weeks after treatment begins or may not occur for 6 months or longer.
- Counsel the patient to keep follow-up appointments with the physician.
- Explain that monthly platelet counts are needed, and teach the patient the signs and symptoms of a decreased platelet count, such as purpura, ecchymoses, petechiae, and bleeding gums. If the platelet count drops below 100,000/mm^3, the drug may need to be discontinued.
- Explain to the patient that rinsing the mouth with 1 tsp of salt in 8 oz (240 ml) of water can help treat symptomatic, mild mouth ulcers.
- Instruct the patient to store oral gold in a tightly closed, light-resistant container and to use capsules before their expiration date, 4 years after the date of manufacture.
- Instruct the patient to notify the physician if adverse reactions occur.

NURSING PROCESS APPLICATION

The following information assists the nurse in caring for a patient receiving a gold salt. It includes an overview of assessment activities as well as examples of appropriate nursing diagnoses and related interventions (see "Planning and implementation"). It also highlights the importance of evaluation.

Assessment

Before drug therapy begins, review the patient's history for conditions that contraindicate or require cautious use of the prescribed gold salt. During therapy, assess the patient for adverse drug reactions and periodically assess the effectiveness of therapy with the gold salt. Finally, evaluate the patient's and family's knowledge about the prescribed drug. (See Patient Teaching: *Gold salts.*)

Nursing diagnoses

- Risk for injury related to a preexisting condition that contraindicates or requires cautious use of a gold salt
- Risk for injury related to adverse drug reactions
- Noncompliance related to long-term use and adverse effects of auranofin
- Knowledge deficit related to the prescribed gold salt

Planning and implementation

- Do not administer a gold salt to a patient with a condition that contraindicates its use.
- Administer a gold salt cautiously to a patient at risk because of a preexisting condition.
- Monitor the patient closely for adverse reactions, especially during the first 6 months of therapy.
- Obtain a baseline urinalysis, CBC, and platelet count as instructed for later comparison with subsequent monthly laboratory values to assess the patient's response to therapy.

*** *Assess the patient for anaphylactic shock, syncope, bradycardia, difficulty swallowing, and angioedema, which can occur up to 10 minutes after injection of a gold salt. Keep standard emergency equipment nearby.***

*** *Monitor the patient for flushing, dizziness, nausea, weakness, tachycardia, and syncope during administration of gold sodium thiomalate. If such a vasomotor response occurs, have the patient lie down during and for 10 minutes after administration. Continue to observe the patient for adverse reactions for another 15 minutes. Expect to switch the patient to aurothioglucose as prescribed if this response occurs.***

- Ensure that physical therapy accompanies gold salt therapy as prescribed to maximize the drug's beneficial effects. Schedule patient activities around the physical therapy sessions.
- Administer auranofin orally; give aurothioglucose and gold sodium thiomalate I.M., preferably in the gluteal muscle.
- Take special care to withdraw a uniform suspension of aurothioglucose from the vial because it is an oil-based suspension. To do this, immerse the vial in warm water and then remove the medication with a dry needle and syringe.
- Monitor for gold salt toxicity by asking the patient at each visit about any signs and symptoms that indicate an adverse reaction.
- Ensure that the patient is reevaluated after receiving 1 g of a parenteral gold salt.
- Notify the physician if adverse reactions occur.
- Question the patient regularly about compliance with auranofin therapy.
- Notify the physician if noncompliance occurs.

Evaluation

For each nursing diagnosis, prepare an evaluation statement that describes the patient's or family's response to nursing interventions.

CHAPTER SUMMARY

Chapter 40 presented the uricosurics, other antigout agents, and gold salts. Here are the chapter highlights.

The uricosurics, antigout agents, and gold salts exert their effects through their anti-inflammatory actions; they are not analgesics.

The drug administered to treat gout depends on the acuity of the disease. During an acute gout attack, colchicine is prescribed. The uricosurics and allopurinol are used only when a patient has chronic gouty arthritis or hyperuricemia, which places the patient at risk for an acute attack of gout.

The use of gold salts can help a patient with rheumatoid arthritis achieve a remission. The effects of gold salts can be dramatic, but the drugs can be toxic.

When caring for a patient receiving a uricosuric, antigout agent, or gold salt, the nurse should teach the patient about the risks and benefits of the prescribed treatment. The nurse also should monitor the patient closely for adverse reactions. Monitoring involves comparing periodic laboratory test results and discussing with the patient the response to drug therapy.

Questions to consider

See Appendix 1 for answers.

1. Wayne Locks, age 68, takes probenecid as maintenance therapy for chronic gouty arthritis. What is the most common adverse reaction to probenecid?
   (a) Edema
   (b) Vertigo
   (c) Tinnitus
   (d) GI distress

2. Mr. Locks becomes noncompliant with his uricosuric therapy and develops an acute attack of gouty arthritis. What is the drug of choice for treating this problem?
   (a) auranofin
   (b) colchicine
   (c) allopurinol
   (d) aurothioglucose

3. The nurse assesses Mr. Locks for adverse reactions to his antigout therapy. Which body system is most likely to be affected adversely?
   (a) GI
   (b) Renal
   (c) Cardiac
   (d) Respiratory

4. Mr. Locks' adverse reactions quickly disappear. How long should the nurse tell Mr. Locks to wait before restarting his oral colchicine?
   (a) 24 hours
   (b) 48 hours
   (c) 3 days
   (d) Never

5. Robin Lawson, age 38, takes aurothioglucose for chronic rheumatoid arthritis. How may a gold salt like aurothioglucose relieve the signs and symptoms of rheumatoid arthritis?
   (a) It may act primarily as an analgesic.
   (b) It may provide skeletal muscle relaxant effects.
   (c) It may decrease liposomal enzyme release.
   (d) It may reverse rheumatoid arthritis deformation.

6. When should Ms. Lawson expect to see the benefits of gold salt therapy?
   (a) 10 to 24 hours after administration
   (b) 7 to 10 days after administration
   (c) 3 to 4 weeks after administration
   (d) 8 to 12 weeks after administration

7. Sue Smith, age 33, has just been prescribed auranofin for the treatment of her rheumatoid arthritis. Which of the following medications should she discontinue?
   (a) Nonsteroidal anti-inflammatory drugs
   (b) Thyroid medications
   (c) Birth control pills
   (d) None of the above

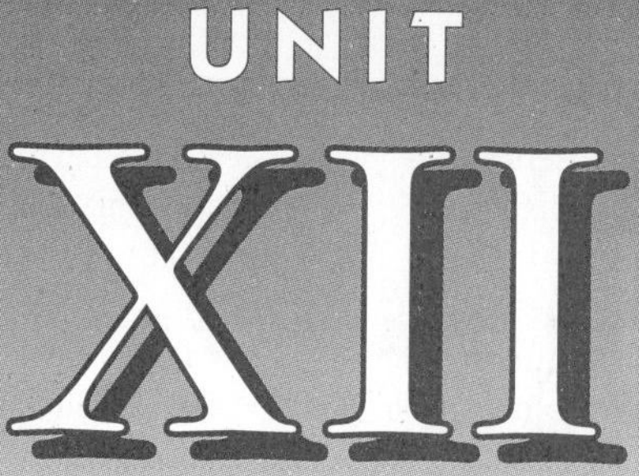

UNIT XII

Drugs to alter psychogenic behavior and promote sleep

Pharmacologic treatment of psychiatric disorders is relatively new. In the past 35 years, many drugs have become available for various psychiatric disorders. For example, phenothiazines were found to help patients with **schizophrenia,** changing the nurse's relationship with the patient from a custodial one to a therapeutic one. Also, antianxiety agents, such as lorazepam and buspirone, and **antidepressant** agents, such as fluoxetine and paroxetine, became commonly prescribed drugs. Although these medications sometimes are used alone, psychiatric drugs usually are intended to be used with other therapeutic modalities such as psychotherapy.

Unit 12 presents the drugs that are used to treat various sleep and psychogenic disorders, such as **insomnia,** agitation, **depression, mania, bipolar disorders, anxiety,** and schizophrenia.

When caring for a patient who is receiving a drug to alter psychogenic behavior or promote sleep, the nurse should keep in mind that such a drug is likely to be prescribed for long-term therapy. Because of this and because the drug may cause intolerable adverse reactions, the nurse should monitor the patient closely for adverse reactions, check the blood level of the drug as instructed, and watch for signs of noncompliance, such as a return of the original symptoms. Because some of these drugs are addictive, the nurse also should be alert for signs of dependence and, when the drug is discontinued, withdrawal symptoms.

SLEEP DISORDERS

Although researchers know that lack of sleep causes physical and psychological symptoms and generally believe that the body requires sleep for restoration, they have not yet identified the precise relationship between sleep and cellular renewal. The four major categories of sleep disorders are insomnias, **hypersomnias, parasomnias,** and disorders of the sleep-awake schedule.

PSYCHOGENIC DISORDERS

Depression and mania are the most common **affective disorders** producing mood disturbances not related to any other physical or psychiatric conditions. These disorders affect twice as many women as men, with unipolar depressions accounting for 90% of the cases.

A diagnosis of depression requires a prominent and persistent mood disturbance and the presence of several of the following signs and symptoms for at least 2 weeks: poor appetite, weight loss, sleep disturbances, agitation, loss of interest in activities, fatigue, feelings of worthlessness, slowed thinking or the inability to concentrate, and thoughts of death. For 30% to 50% of these patients, depression occurs as a single episode; for the remainder, depression recurs.

Unlike depression, mania produces periods of **euphoria,** rapid speech, flight of ideas, lack of need for sleep, and overactivity. Mania may occur alone or it may alternate with depression, resulting in **manic-depressive disorder,** a bipolar disorder that is much less common than depression.

Anxiety disorders are classified as nonphobic or phobic. Nonphobic anxieties can be subdivided into generalized anxiety disorders (the most common), **obsessive-compulsive disorders,** and panic disorders. Phobic anxieties can take many forms, such as **phobias** of crowds or heights. An anxiety disorder may be a primary medical condition or may occur secondary to another medical or social problem.

Psychoses, such as paranoia and schizophrenia, result in inappropriate or abnormal behavior or thinking. One theory suggests that schizophrenia results from excess dopamine in the limbic system. This theory is based on evidence that dissociated thought patterns and drives, hallucinations, and delusions tend to disappear when psychotic patients receive **antipsychotic** drugs that inhibit dopamine action.

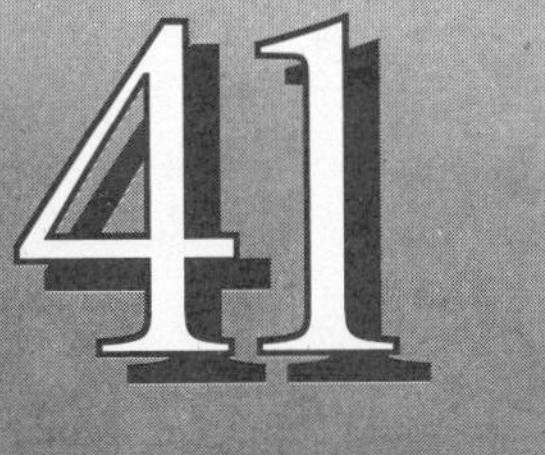

Sedative and hypnotic agents

OBJECTIVES

After reading and studying this chapter, the student should be able to:

1. differentiate between a sedative and a hypnotic agent.
2. describe the pharmacokinetic properties of the benzodiazepines, barbiturates, and the nonbenzodiazepine-nonbarbiturate drugs.
3. identify the clinical indications for each of the three major groups of sedative and hypnotic agents.
4. describe significant adverse reactions associated with each of the three major classes of sedative and hypnotic agents.
5. describe how alcohol and over-the-counter (OTC) products function as sleep aids.
6. describe how to apply the nursing process when caring for a patient receiving a sedative or hypnotic agent.

INTRODUCTION

Sedatives are drugs that act to reduce activity or excitement, thereby calming a patient. Some degree of drowsiness commonly accompanies sedative use. When administered in large doses, sedatives are considered **hypnotics,** which induce a state resembling natural sleep. Chapter 41 discusses three main classes of synthetic drugs used as sedatives and hypnotics: the benzodiazepines, the barbiturates, and the nonbenzodiazepine-nonbarbiturate drugs. The chapter also discusses other sedatives, including alcohol and OTC sleep aids. (See *Selected major sedative and hypnotic agents,* pages 514 to 516.)

Drugs covered in this chapter include:

- alcohol
- amobarbital
- aprobarbital
- butabarbital sodium
- chloral hydrate
- diphenhydramine
- doxylamine
- estazolam
- ethchlorvynol
- flurazepam hydrochloride
- glutethimide
- lorazepam
- mephobarbital
- methylprylon
- paraldehyde
- pentobarbital sodium
- phenobarbital
- pyrilamine maleate
- quazepam
- secobarbital sodium
- temazepam
- triazolam
- zolpidem tartrate.

Benzodiazepines

Benzodiazepines produce many effects, including daytime and preanesthetic sedation, sleep inducement, relief of anxiety and tension, skeletal muscle relaxation, and anticonvulsant activity. The benzodiazepines discussed here are used primarily for their sedative or hypnotic effects. Such benzodiazepines include estazolam, flurazepam hydrochloride, lorazepam, quazepam, temazepam, and triazolam. When the other benzodiazepines are used in other clinical situations, they secondarily exert a sedative or hypnotic effect.

PHARMACOKINETICS

Benzodiazepines are absorbed well from the gastrointestinal (GI) tract and distributed widely in the body. They may be given parenterally. All benzodiazepines are metabolized in the liver and excreted primarily in the urine.

Route	Onset	Peak	Duration
P.O.	15 min-2 hr	Unknown	3-8 hr
I.V.	1-5 min	1 hr-90 min	Variable
I.M.	15-30 min	1-1.5 hr	Variable

PHARMACODYNAMICS

Researchers believe that the principal sites of action for the benzodiazepines are the cerebral cortex and the limbic, thalamic, and hypothalamic levels of the central nervous system (CNS). They probably indirectly stimulate gamma aminobutyric acid receptors in the ascending reticular system. (See *How benzodiazepines work,* page 517.)

When administered at low therapeutic dosages, benzodiazepines decrease anxiety by acting on the limbic system and related brain areas that help regulate emotional activity. The drugs usually can calm or sedate the patient without causing drowsiness. At higher dosages, benzodiazepines exhibit sleep-producing properties, probably because the drugs depress the activating system located in the reticular formation of the midbrain.

The clinical use of benzodiazepines results in a net increase in total sleep time and produces a deep, refreshing sleep. Many experts hypothesize that the benzodiazepines improve the quality of sleep because of their effect on **rapid**

(Text continues on page 516.)

Selected major sedative and hypnotic agents

This chart summarizes some of the major sedative and hypnotic agents currently in clinical use.

DRUG	MAJOR INDICATIONS AND USUAL DOSAGES	CONTRAINDICATIONS AND PRECAUTIONS
Benzodiazepines		
estazolam (ProSom)	*Hypnotic for insomnia* ADULT: 1 to 2 mg P.O. h.s.	• Estazolam is contraindicated in a pregnant or breast-feeding patient or a patient with known hypersensitivity. • This drug requires cautious use in a geriatric or debilitated patient, a depressed patient, or one with impaired renal or hepatic function or compromised respiratory function. • Safety and efficacy in children have not been established.
flurazepam (Dalmane)	*Hypnotic for insomnia* ADULT: 15 to 30 mg P.O. h.s.	• Flurazepam is contraindicated in a pregnant patient or a patient with known hypersensitivity. • This drug requires cautious use in a patient with severe or latent depression, impaired renal or hepatic function, or chronic pulmonary insufficiency. • Safety and efficacy in children under age 15 have not been established.
lorazepam (Ativan)	*Sedative before surgery* ADULT: 0.05 mg/kg (up to a maximum of 4 mg) I.M. 2 hours before operative procedure	• Lorazepam is contraindicated in a pregnant or breast-feeding patient, a psychotic patient, or one with known hypersensitivity, acute angle-closure glaucoma, or a primary depressive disorder. • This drug requires cautious use in a geriatric patient, a patient with impaired renal or hepatic function, or any patient over a prolonged time. • Safety and efficacy of lorazepam in children under age 12 and of lorazepam injection in children under age 18 have not been established.
triazolam (Halcion)	*Hypnotic for insomnia resulting from anxiety or transient situational stress; anxiety disorders* ADULT: 0.125 to 0.25 mg P.O. h.s.	• Triazolam is contraindicated in a pregnant or breast-feeding patient or a patient with known hypersensitivity. • This drug requires cautious use in a depressed patient or one with impaired renal or hepatic function or chronic pulmonary insufficiency. • Safety and efficacy in children have not been established.
Barbiturates		
amobarbital (Amytal)	*Sedative for anxiety and tension* ADULT: 30 to 50 mg P.O. or I.M. b.i.d. or t.i.d. *Hypnotic for insomnia* ADULT: 65 to 200 mg P.O. or I.M. h.s., for a maximum of 2 weeks	• Amobarbital is contraindicated in a pregnant patient or a patient with porphyria, bronchopneumonia, or other severe pulmonary insufficiency or known hypersensitivity. • This drug requires cautious use in a depressed or suicidal patient or one with acute or chronic pain, a history of drug abuse, or hepatic disease. The parenteral form of the drug requires cautious use in a patient who recently has received another respiratory depressant, a patient who is in shock, or one with hypertension, hypotension, pulmonary or cardiovascular disease, or uremia. • Safety and efficacy in children have not been established.
pentobarbital (Nembutal)	*Daytime sedative* ADULT: 20 to 40 mg P.O. b.i.d. to q.i.d. PEDIATRIC: 2 to 6 mg/kg I.M. daily (up to a maximum of 100 mg daily) in three divided doses *Sedative before surgery* ADULT: 150 to 200 mg I.M. for maximum of 2 weeks PEDIATRIC: 5 mg/kg P.O., I.M., or P.R.	• Pentobarbital is contraindicated in a pregnant patient or one with porphyria or known hypersensitivity. • This drug requires cautious use in a breast-feeding patient, a patient with acute or chronic pain, a depressed or suicidal patient, or one with hepatic damage or a history of drug abuse. The parenteral form of the drug requires cautious use in a patient who has recently received another respiratory depressant, a patient who is in shock, or one with hypertension, hypotension, pulmonary or cardiovascular disease, or uremia.

Selected major sedative and hypnotic agents *(continued)*

DRUG	MAJOR INDICATIONS AND USUAL DOSAGES	CONTRAINDICATIONS AND PRECAUTIONS
Barbiturates *(continued)*		
pentobarbital (Nembutal) *(continued)*	*Hypnotic for insomnia* ADULT: 100 mg P.O., 120 to 200 mg P.R., or 150 to 200 mg I.M. for a maximum of 2 weeks PEDIATRIC: for children ages 2 months to 1 year, 30 mg P.R.; for children ages 1 to 4, 30 or 60 mg P.R.; for children ages 12 to 14, 60 or 120 mg P.R.; alternatively for all children, 2 to 6 mg/kg or 125 mg/m^2 I.M., to a maximum dose of 100 mg	• Do not give I.V. more than 50 mg/minute.
phenobarbital (Luminal, Solfoton)	*Daytime sedative* ADULT: 15 to 30 mg P.O. b.i.d. to q.i.d. PEDIATRIC: 6 mg/kg or 180 mg/m^2 P.O. in three equally divided doses *Sedative before surgery* ADULT: 100 to 200 mg I.M. 60 to 90 minutes before surgery PEDIATRIC: 16 to 100 mg I.M. 60 to 90 minutes before surgery *Hypnotic for insomnia* ADULT: 100 to 320 mg P.O. or I.M. h.s. for maximum of 2 weeks	• Phenobarbital is contraindicated in a pregnant patient or a patient with porphyria, nephritis, renal insufficiency, or known hypersensitivity. • This drug requires cautious use in a breast-feeding patient, a depressed or suicidal patient, or one with hepatic damage or a history of drug abuse. The parenteral form of the drug requires cautious use in a patient who recently has received another respiratory depressant, a patient who is in shock, or one with hypertension, hypotension, pulmonary or cardiovascular disorders, or uremia. • Do not give I.V. more than 60 mg/minute.
secobarbital (Seconal)	*Daytime sedative* ADULT: 100 to 300 mg P.O. or P.R. in three divided doses PEDIATRIC: 6 mg/kg P.O. or P.R. in three divided doses *Sedative before surgery* ADULT: 200 to 300 mg P.O. 1 to 2 hours before surgery PEDIATRIC: 50 to 100 mg P.O. 1 to 2 hours before surgery; alternatively, 4 to 5 mg/kg I.M. or P.R. 1 to 2 hours before surgery *Hypnotic for insomnia* ADULT: 100 to 200 mg P.O., 100 to 200 mg P.R., or 100 to 200 mg I.M. h.s. for a maximum of 2 weeks PEDIATRIC: 3 to 5 mg/kg or 125 mg/m^2 I.M. h.s. to a maximum dose of 100 mg	• Secobarbital is contraindicated in a pregnant patient or one with porphyria or known hypersensitivity. • This drug requires cautious use in a breast-feeding patient, a depressed or suicidal patient, or one with hepatic damage or a history of drug abuse. The parenteral form of the drug requires cautious use in a patient who has recently received another respiratory depressant, a patient who is in shock, or one with hypertension, hypotension, pulmonary or cardiovascular disorders, or uremia. • Do not exceed doses of 250 mg I.M.
Nonbenzodiazepines-nonbarbiturates		
chloral hydrate (Aquachloral, Noctec)	*Daytime sedative* ADULT: 250 mg P.O. or 325 mg P.R. t.i.d. after meals PEDIATRIC: 8.3 mg/kg or 250 mg/m^2 t.i.d., up to a maximum dose of 500 mg t.i.d. *Hypnotic for insomnia* ADULT: 0.5 to 1 g P.O. or P.R. 15 to 30 minutes before bedtime PEDIATRIC: 50 mg/kg or 1.5 g/m^2 up to a maximum single dose of 1 g	• Chloral hydrate is contraindicated in a patient with known hypersensitivity, gastroenteritis, or esophageal ulcers. • This drug requires cautious use in a pregnant or breast-feeding patient, a depressed or suicidal patient, or one with severe hepatic, renal, or cardiac disease.

(continued)

Selected major sedative and hypnotic agents *(continued)*

DRUG	MAJOR INDICATIONS AND USUAL DOSAGES	CONTRAINDICATIONS AND PRECAUTIONS
Nonbenzodiazepines-nonbarbiturates *(continued)*		
ethchlorvynol (Placidyl)	*Hypnotic for insomnia* ADULT: 0.5 to 1 g P.O. h.s.	• Ethchlorvynol is contraindicated in a pregnant patient during her first and second trimester and in a patient with porphyria or known hypersensitivity. • This drug requires cautious use in a breast-feeding patient, a pregnant patient in her third trimester, a depressed or suicidal patient, or one with impaired renal or hepatic function or a history of drug abuse. • Safety and efficacy in children have not been established.
glutethimide (Doriden)	*Hypnotic for insomnia* ADULT: 250 to 500 mg P.O. h.s.	• Glutethimide is contraindicated in a breast-feeding patient or a patient with porphyria, severe renal impairment, uncontrolled pain, or known hypersensitivity. • This drug requires cautious use in a pregnant patient, a depressed or suicidal patient, or one with a history of drug abuse, prostatic hyperplasia, stenosed peptic ulcer, pyloroduodenal obstruction, bladder neck obstruction, angle-closure glaucoma, or cardiac arrhythmias. • Safety and efficacy in children have not been established. • Use cautiously in patients with conditions that effect hemodynamic states and those with respiratory compromise.
zolpidem (Ambien)	*Hypnotic for insomnia* ADULT: 10 mg h.s.	• Safety and efficacy in children have not been established. • This drug requires cautious use in a pregnant patient, a depressed or suicidal patient, or one with a history of drug abuse.

eye movement (REM) sleep. In most cases, benzodiazepines decrease the frequency of eyeball movement and the time spent in REM sleep. Flurazepam (in low dosages) and temazepam, however, do not diminish REM sleep significantly. Benzodiazepines that do decrease total REM sleep time also allow for more frequent REM cycles later in the sleep period.

PHARMACOTHERAPEUTICS

Clinical indications for the benzodiazepines include relaxing and calming the patient during the day or before surgery and treating **insomnia** characterized by difficulty falling or staying asleep or early morning awakenings. Other clinical indications include producing intravenous (I.V.) anesthesia, treating alcohol withdrawal symptoms, treating anxiety and seizure disorders, and producing skeletal muscle relaxation.

In most cases, benzodiazepines are preferred over barbiturates because of their effectiveness and safety. Benzodiazepines offer many advantages, including fewer adverse reactions, decreased potential for abuse, fewer drug interactions, a wide margin of safety between therapeutic and toxic dosages that makes overdose less likely, and a reduced risk of physical and psychological dependence with therapeutic dosages.

Drug interactions

Except for other CNS depressants, few drugs interact with benzodiazepines. (See Drug Interactions: *Benzodiazepines,* page 518.) No interactions involving benzodiazepines and food have been documented.

ADVERSE DRUG REACTIONS

Benzodiazepines cause few adverse reactions. The most common adverse reactions are daytime sedation and hangover effect. Rebound insomnia may occur, especially with short-acting drugs such as triazolam. Some benzodiazepines may cause amnesia. Dose-related dizziness and **ataxia** also may occur. Geriatric patients, debilitated patients, and patients with liver disease are more likely to experience dose-related adverse reactions to benzodiazepines (See Geriatric Considerations: *Benzodiazepines and barbiturates,* page 519.)

Fatigue, muscle weakness, mouth dryness, nausea, and vomiting occasionally result from benzodiazepine use. Respiratory depression is more common in geriatric or de-

How benzodiazepines work

This illustration shows how benzodiazepines work at the cellular level.

The speed of impulses from a presynaptic neuron across a synapse is influenced by the presence or absence of chloride ions in a postsynaptic neuron. The passage of the chloride ions into the postsynaptic neuron depends on the release from the brain of an inhibitory neurotransmitter called gamma-aminobutyric acid, or GABA.

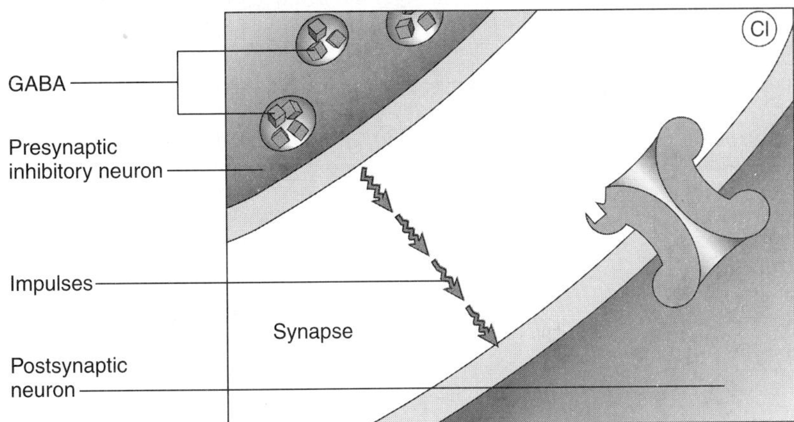

GABA, when released, opens the chloride channel of a supramolecular unit known as the benzodiazepine-GABA receptor-chloride ionophore complex. This mechanism controls the flow of chloride ions into the postsynaptic neuron.
As chloride ions flow into the neuron, the cell becomes hyperpolarized, which reduces neuronal activity and leads to slowed nerve impulses.

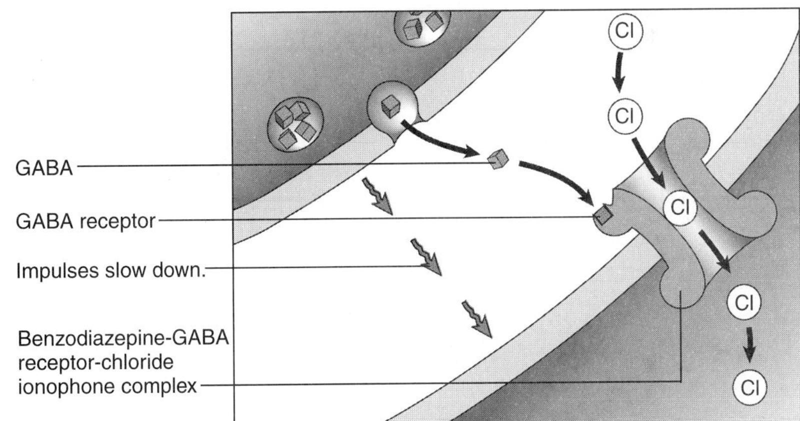

The benzodiazepine-GABA receptor-chloride ionophore complex houses a benzodiazepine receptor on or near the GABA receptor. When a benzodiazepine molecule attaches to a benzodiazepine receptor, GABA's effect on its own receptor is enhanced. This enhanced effect allows more chloride ions to flow into the postsynaptic neuron, which causes nerve impulses to slow or stop.

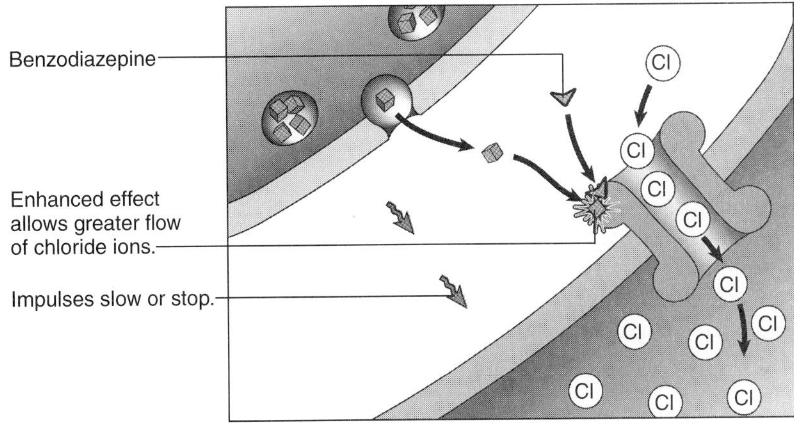

bilitated patients, patients with limited ventilatory reserve, and patients receiving other CNS depressants. Signs and symptoms of psychological and physical dependence occur with prolonged use and high dosages, but rarely with usual dosages. If a patient becomes physically dependent, sudden withdrawal of the benzodiazepine may cause weakness, delirium, and tonic-clonic seizures.

Rare and usually mild allergic reactions include rash, pruritus, urticaria, burning eyes, and photosensitivity.

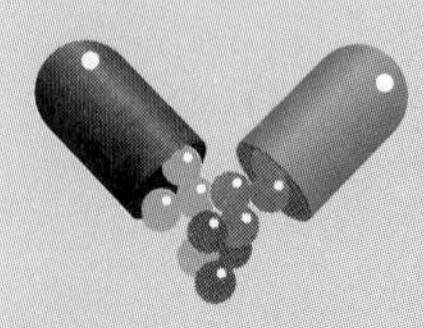

DRUG INTERACTIONS
Benzodiazepines

Few drug interactions involving the benzodiazepines discussed in this chapter occur. However, when interactions do occur, they are seen more commonly with the concurrent use of other central nervous system (CNS) depressants, including alcohol. The additive effects of CNS depressants and benzodiazepines can be lethal.

DRUG	INTERACTING DRUGS	POSSIBLE EFFECTS	NURSING IMPLICATIONS
estazolam, flurazepam, lorazepam, quazepam, temazepam, triazolam	CNS depressants (including anticonvulsants) theophylline	Enhanced sedative and other CNS depressant effects (may become supra-additive, causing motor skill impairment and respiratory depression); lethal effect, especially with high dosages; changes in seizure activity, especially in frequency or severity (with anticonvulsants) Antagonism of benzodiazepine effects	• Monitor the changes in level of consciousness and muscle coordination. • Monitor for signs of respiratory depression. • Advise the patient about possible additive effects of other CNS depressants. • Warn the patient that alcohol increases the effect of the drug and also can cause serious CNS depression. • Supervise ambulation; raise bed rails, especially with geriatric patients. • Advise against operating a motor vehicle or heavy machinery because of possible motor skill impairment. • Observe for changes in frequency and severity of seizures when these drugs are used with anticonvulsants. • Monitor response to benzodiazepines.
flurazepam, quazepam	cimetidine	Inhibited hepatic metabolism, causing increased sedative effects and increased CNS depressant effects	• Monitor for signs of increased CNS depressant effects; notify the physician of any changes. • Advise against operating a motor vehicle or heavy machinery because increased sedation is possible. • Supervise ambulation; raise bed rails, especially with geriatric patients.
flurazepam	oral contraceptives	Decreased oxidative metabolism	• Monitor the patient for excessive sedation. • Expect to decrease the benzodiazepine dosage.
lorazepam, temazepam	oral contraceptives	Increased glucuronide conjugation	• Expect to increase the benzodiazepine dosage to produce the desired effect.

NURSING PROCESS APPLICATION

The following information assists the nurse in caring for a patient who is receiving a benzodiazepine as a sedative or hypnotic agent. It includes an overview of assessment activities as well as examples of appropriate nursing diagnoses and related interventions (see "Planning and implementation"). It also highlights the importance of evaluation.

Assessment

Before drug therapy begins, review the patient's history for conditions that contraindicate or require cautious use of the prescribed benzodiazepine. Also review the patient's medication history to identify use of drugs that may interact with it. During therapy, assess the patient for adverse drug reactions and signs of drug interactions. Also, periodically assess the effectiveness of benzodiazepine therapy. Finally, evaluate the patient's and family's knowledge about the prescribed drug. Careful use of these medications is important, as patients may develop both psychologic and physical dependence.

Nursing diagnoses

- Risk for injury related to a preexisting condition that contraindicates or requires cautious use of a benzodiazepine
- Risk for injury related to adverse drug reactions or drug interactions
- Ineffective breathing pattern related to the respiratory depression caused by a benzodiazepine
- Knowledge deficit related to the prescribed benzodiazepine

Planning and implementation

- Do not administer a benzodiazepine to a patient with a condition that contraindicates its use.

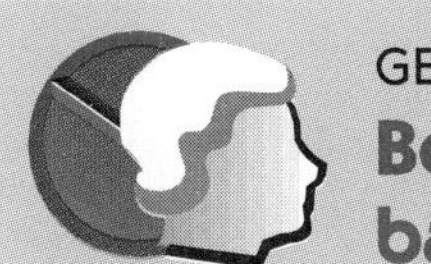

GERIATRIC CONSIDERATIONS
Benzodiazepines and barbiturates

Benzodiazepines: Geriatric patients are a population at risk for the many dose-related effects of benzodiazepines. Rare idiosyncratic reactions that primarily occur in the geriatric population include nervousness, restlessness, talkativeness, apprehension, euphoria, and excitement.
Barbiturates: Use of barbiturates for their hypnotic effects may be dangerous for the elderly. After hypnotic dosages, the hangover effect commonly occurs, accompanied by impairment of judgment and motor skills that can last for many hours and may lead to falls in geriatric patients. When hypnotic dosages are discontinued, the patient may experience a change in sleep pattern. Patients, especially geriatric ones, may exhibit excitement and confusion, particularly when taking short-acting compounds such as secobarbital.

- Administer a benzodiazepine cautiously to a patient at risk because of a preexisting condition.
- Monitor the patient regularly for adverse reactions to the prescribed benzodiazepine, especially in a geriatric or debilitated patient or one with liver disease. Also monitor for drug interactions.

*** *Consult with the physician if other CNS depressants also are prescribed during benzodiazepine therapy; this combination may cause lethal depressant effects.***

- Expect to discontinue benzodiazepine therapy in a patient who hallucinates or behaves violently.
- Assist with gastric lavage, respiratory support, and other support measures, such as I.V. fluid or drug administration, if overdose occurs. Frequently monitor vital signs and fluid intake and output. Flumazenil is an antidote for a benzodiazepine overdose.

*** *Keep epinephrine and corticosteroids readily available for emergency care of a patient who experiences a hypersensitivity reaction to the prescribed benzodiazepine.***

- Plan care and administer drugs based on the hospitalized patient's daily routines and bedtime rituals. Do not awaken a patient to administer a benzodiazepine. (See Patient Teaching: *Benzodiazepines.*)
- Watch the patient take the benzodiazepine to prevent drug hoarding for later use.
- Use nursing judgment when considering administration of a second dose of a benzodiazepine during the night. Try to find out why the patient cannot sleep. For example, if pain is causing insomnia, use comfort-inducing measures, such as back rubs, and administer analgesics. Remember, the hangover effect can result from injudicious use of a benzodiazepine during the night.
- Notify the physician if adverse reactions or drug interactions occur.

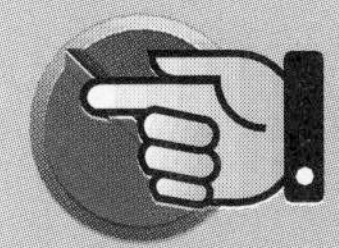

PATIENT TEACHING
Benzodiazepines

- Teach the patient and family the name, dose, frequency, action, and adverse effects of the prescribed benzodiazepine.
- Instruct the patient with insomnia or a similar sleep disorder to try other measures before taking the prescribed benzodiazepine. Suggest a warm bath or shower or a glass of warm milk before the patient retires; encourage moderate daily exercise several hours before sleeping; advise the patient to eliminate daytime naps; and encourage reading and the use of other relaxation techniques.
- Instruct the family to take safety measures, such as assisting with the patient's ambulation, during benzodiazepine therapy.
- Teach the family what to do if the patient awakens confused and excited after taking a benzodiazepine. Tell them not to awaken the patient during the night unless necessary.
- Instruct the patient and family to alert the physician if adverse reactions occur.
- Instruct the patient not to drink alcoholic beverages while taking a benzodiazepine.
- Instruct the patient not to abruptly stop drug therapy because of adverse effects.

- Monitor the patient's vital signs frequently, particularly noting signs of respiratory depression, such as decreased number of respirations or respiratory pattern changes.
- Perform a respiratory assessment before and after giving each dose of the prescribed benzodiazepine.

*** *Withhold the benzodiazepine dose and notify the physician if respiratory depression occurs.***

- Expect to reduce the benzodiazepine dosage for a patient who is receiving another CNS depressant because of the risk of increased respiratory depression.
- Position the debilitated patient to maximize respiratory function. For example, help the patient into a semi-Fowler's or high Fowler's position.

Evaluation

For each nursing diagnosis, prepare an evaluation statement that describes the patient's or family's response to nursing interventions.

Barbiturates

The major pharmacologic action of the barbiturates reduces overall CNS alertness. The uses of barbiturates include daytime and preoperative sedation, hypnotic effects for patients with insomnia, anesthesia, relief of anxiety, and anticonvulsant activity. This section discusses the barbiturates used primarily as sedatives and hypnotics, including amobarbital, aprobarbital, butabarbital sodium, mephobarbital, pentobarbital sodium, phenobarbital, and secobarbital sodium.

PHARMACOKINETICS

Barbiturates are absorbed well from the GI tract, distributed rapidly, metabolized by the liver, and excreted via the metabolic processes as well as in the urine.

The duration of action represents the main difference among barbiturates. The duration may be ultrashort-acting, short-acting, intermediate-acting, or long-acting. Peak concentration levels also vary, depending on the onset of action.

A barbiturate's duration of action depends in part on the rate of drug metabolism and the rate of drug redistribution throughout the body. The duration of action varies among patients and even in the same patient from time to time.

The half-lives of barbiturates vary from drug to drug. For example, secobarbital has a half-life of 15 to 40 hours, mephobarbital 11 to 67 hours, and phenobarbital 50 to 170 hours. Note, however, that because of the rapid distribution of some barbiturates, no correlation exists between duration and half-life. When used over an extended period, all barbiturates will accumulate.

Route	Onset	Peak	Duration
P.O., I.M., I.V.	Variable	Variable	Variable

PHARMACODYNAMICS

Barbiturates are considered to be nonspecific CNS depressants. The sites of barbiturate action appear to be less selective than the sites of benzodiazepine action. As sedative-hypnotics, barbiturates depress the sensory cortex, decrease motor activity, alter cerebral function, and produce drowsiness, sedation, and hypnosis. These drugs appear to act at the level of the thalamus, where they inhibit the ascending conduction in the reticular formation, thus interfering with impulse transmission to the cortex.

PHARMACOTHERAPEUTICS

Barbiturates have many clinical indications, including daytime sedation, hypnotic effects, anesthesia, and anticonvulsant effects. Barbiturates usually are not used for daytime sedation; when used for this indication, they are given for short periods, typically less than 2 weeks. The use of barbiturates as sedatives and hypnotics is declining because benzodiazepines now are regarded as the sedatives and hypnotics of choice.

Drug interactions

Barbiturates interact with many other drugs. (See Drug Interactions: *Barbiturates.*)

ADVERSE DRUG REACTIONS

The most commonly reported adverse reactions to barbiturates relate to the CNS and include drowsiness, lethargy, headache, depression, and vertigo.

The patient can experience serious adverse respiratory reactions, including hypoventilation, laryngospasm, bronchospasm, and severe respiratory depression, especially when large dosages are administered I.V. and too rapidly. Large dosages of barbiturates suppress the hypoxic and chemoreceptor drive of the respiratory system, resulting in decreased respiratory rate and rhythm.

The patient also can sustain adverse cardiovascular reactions, such as mild bradycardia and hypotension. Less common adverse reactions to barbiturates affect the GI tract, resulting in nausea, vomiting, diarrhea, and epigastric pain.

Acute barbiturate toxicity causes overdose symptoms, which can be severe. The symptoms are characterized by CNS and respiratory depression, and death can result from respiratory failure followed by cardiac arrest.

With prolonged use, the patient can develop drug tolerance as well as psychological and physical dependence on the barbiturate. Withdrawal symptoms resemble those associated with chronic alcoholism and occur with sudden discontinuation after long-term use.

Allergic reactions mainly involve the skin and mucous membranes and occur more commonly in patients with past allergies or asthma. Allergic reactions include various rashes, urticaria, angioedema, and fever. Rare occurrences of photosensitivity also have been reported. Other allergic reactions include rare blood dyscrasias, such as pancytopenia, leukopenia, granulocytopenia, thrombocytopenia, and megaloblastic anemia secondary to folic acid depletion.

Idiosyncratic reactions include paradoxical anxiety, agitation, restlessness, and rage or paradoxical excitement (delirium rather than sedation). The idiosyncratic reactions occur most commonly among geriatric patients and those with severe uncontrolled pain.

NURSING PROCESS APPLICATION

The following information assists the nurse in caring for a patient who is receiving a barbiturate as a sedative or hypnotic agent. It includes an overview of assessment activities as well as examples of appropriate nursing diagnoses and related interventions (see "Planning and implementation"). It also highlights the importance of evaluation.

Assessment

Before drug therapy begins, review the patient's history for conditions that contraindicate or require cautious use of the prescribed barbiturate. Also review the patient's medication history to identify use of drugs that may interact with it. During therapy, assess the patient for adverse drug reactions and signs of drug interactions. Also, periodically assess the effectiveness of barbiturate therapy. Finally, evaluate the patient's and family's knowledge about the prescribed drug.

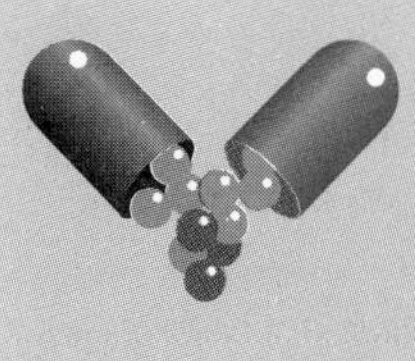

DRUG INTERACTIONS

Barbiturates

Drug interactions involving barbiturates are common and can be serious. Interactions typically occur with concurrent use of other central nervous system (CNS) depressants, including alcohol. The additive effects can be lethal. Most of the clinically significant interactions from barbiturates occur with phenobarbital, and some of the barbiturates are converted to phenobarbital in the body.

DRUG	INTERACTING DRUGS	POSSIBLE EFFECTS	NURSING IMPLICATIONS
amobarbital, aprobarbital, butabarbital, mephobarbital, pentobarbital, phenobarbital, secobarbital	hydantoins	Decreased phenobarbital metabolism, resulting in increased toxic effects	• Monitor serum concentration levels; phenobarbital dosage may need to be decreased. • Advise the patient to report adverse reactions. • Assess for change in level of consciousness (LOC). • Alert the patient not to operate a motor vehicle or heavy machinery until the effect of the drug combination is known. • Advise the patient to avoid alcohol consumption.
	beta blockers (metoprolol, propranolol)	Increased beta blocker metabolism, resulting in decreased effectiveness of beta blockers	• Monitor desired effect in the patient (antianginal, antihypertensive, or antiarrhythmic); beta blocker dosage may need to be increased. • Instruct the patient to report changes in desired effect during drug therapy. • Advise the patient to report periodically for blood pressure and pulse check.
	chloramphenicol	Increased chloramphenicol metabolism, resulting in decreased effectiveness of chloramphenicol; decreased phenobarbital metabolism	• Monitor desired effect in the patient (anti-infective); chloramphenicol dosage may need to be increased. • Monitor serum chloramphenicol and phenobarbital levels.
	corticosteroids	Increased corticosteroid metabolism, resulting in decreased effectiveness of corticosteroids	• Expect to increase the corticosteroid dosage because of the drug's decreased effectiveness. • Monitor the patient's weight and blood pressure. • Monitor serum electrolyte levels.
	doxycycline	Increased doxycycline metabolism, resulting in decreased effectiveness of doxycycline	• Expect to substitute tetracycline for doxycycline or increase the doxycycline dosage because of the drug's decreased effectiveness.
	oral anticoagulants	Increased oral anticoagulant metabolism, resulting in decreased effectiveness of oral anticoagulants	• Monitor prothrombin levels; oral anticoagulant dosage may need to be increased. • Advise the patient to be alert for signs and symptoms of thrombus formation: pain, tenderness, and edema in the calf.
	oral contraceptives	Increased oral contraceptive metabolism, resulting in decreased effectiveness of oral contraceptives	• Alert the patient that contraceptive effect may be impaired; breakthrough bleeding may occur. • Suggest use of an alternative or additional contraceptive method during barbiturate therapy.
	quinidine	Increased quinidine metabolism, resulting in decreased effectiveness of quinidine	• Expect to increase the quinidine dosage, as prescribed. • Advise the patient to see the physician frequently for monitoring of cardiac status. • Alert the patient to report signs and symptoms of arrhythmias, such as palpitations and irregular pulse.
	methoxyflurane	Increased activity of hepatic microsomal enzymes that may stimulate metabolism of methoxyflurane to nephrotoxic metabolites	• Avoid concurrent use of phenobarbital and methoxyflurane.

(continued)

Barbiturates *(continued)*

DRUG	INTERACTING DRUGS	POSSIBLE EFFECTS	NURSING IMPLICATIONS
amobarbital, aprobarbital, butabarbital, mephobarbital, pentobarbital, phenobarbital, secobarbital *(continued)*	tricyclic antidepressants	Increased tricyclic antidepressant metabolism, resulting in decreased effectiveness of tricyclic antidepressants	• Expect to increase the tricyclic antidepressant dosage, as prescribed. • Monitor serum tricyclic antidepressant level. • Advise the patient to report any change in therapeutic effect such as lack of mood elevation.
	CNS depressants (antianxiety agents, sedatives, hypnotics, most narcotic analgesics, and alcohol)	Increased CNS effects, resulting in toxicity	• Assess frequently for changes in LOC and respirations. • Supervise ambulation; raise bed rails, especially for geriatric patients. • Advise the patient not to operate a motor vehicle or heavy machinery until the effect of the drug combination is known. • Advise the patient to avoid alcohol consumption while taking these medications.
	valproic acid	Decreased hepatic metabolism of phenobarbital	• Monitor for excessive phenobarbital effect such as drowsiness. • Expect to reduce the phenobarbital dosage because of increased serum phenobarbital levels.
	metronidazole	Increased metronidazole metabolism	• Expect to increase the metronidazole dosage, as prescribed.
	digitoxin	Decreased digitoxin effect	• Monitor for the desired effect of digitoxin related to arrhythmias and cardiac function. • Expect to increase the digitoxin dosage, as prescribed.
	theophylline	Increased rate of theophylline metabolism, causing decreased serum theophylline concentration level	• Monitor serum theophylline level. • Adjust the theophylline dosage, as prescribed.
	cyclosporine	Decreased plasma cyclosporine level	• Monitor plasma cyclosporine level. • Expect to increase the cyclosporine dosage, as prescribed.
	monoamine oxidase inhibitors	Increased sedative effect	• Use cautiously together.
	acetaminophen	Increased risk of hepatotoxicity	• Use cautiously together.
	rifampin	Decreased barbiturate effectiveness	• Adjust doses as needed.

Nursing diagnoses

- Risk for injury related to a preexisting condition that contraindicates or requires cautious use of a barbiturate
- Risk for injury related to adverse drug reactions or drug interactions
- Altered role performance related to barbiturate dependence
- Knowledge deficit related to the prescribed barbiturate

Planning and implementation

- Do not administer a barbiturate to a patient with a condition that contraindicates its use.
- Administer a barbiturate cautiously to a patient at risk because of a preexisting condition.
- Monitor the patient periodically for adverse reactions to the prescribed barbiturate. Be alert for idiosyncratic reactions, such as paradoxical anxiety or excitement, in a geriatric patient or one with severe uncontrolled pain. Also monitor for drug interactions.

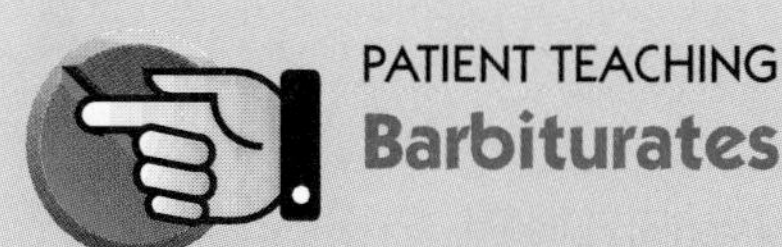

PATIENT TEACHING
Barbiturates

- Teach the patient and family the name, dose, frequency, action, and adverse effects of the prescribed barbiturate.
- Advise the patient not to discontinue the drug suddenly without consulting the physician because withdrawal symptoms may occur.
- Instruct the patient not to operate a motor vehicle or heavy machinery, at least until the patient knows how the drug affects his or her mental alertness.
- Instruct the patient not to drink alcohol during drug therapy because respiratory depression can occur.
- Advise the patient to consult the physician before taking any tranquilizers, narcotics, or other prescription pain relievers.
- Counsel the patient not to give any of the prescribed drug to family members or friends.
- Advise the patient to keep the drug and all other medications out of the reach of children.
- Tell the patient to notify the physician if adverse reactions occur.

• Expect to administer a reduced dosage, as prescribed, to a geriatric or debilitated patient.
• Discontinue the drug slowly after long-term therapy, as prescribed, to prevent rebound REM sleep.
• Monitor prothrombin time, as instructed, for a patient who also is receiving an anticoagulant. Keep in mind that abrupt withdrawal of a barbiturate may cause serious bleeding. Adjust the anticoagulant dosage as prescribed.
• Rotate the amobarbital ampule (do not shake), mix the solution with sterile water only, discard solutions that do not become clear in 5 minutes, use the solution within 30 minutes after opening to minimize deterioration, and inject the solution slowly and deeply into a large muscle mass when using the intramuscular (I.M.) route of administration.
• Do not use a cloudy pentobarbital, phenobarbital, or secobarbital solution or mix the solution with other medications; use the solution within 30 minutes after opening to minimize deterioration; and inject the solution into a large muscle mass when using the I.M. route of administration.
• Remember that the I.M. route is a poor route for administering barbiturates.
• Notify the physician if adverse reactions or drug interactions occur.
• Encourage the patient to be honest about barbiturate use because dependence can occur with long-term use.
∗ ***Do not discontinue barbiturate therapy abruptly.*** Otherwise, the patient receiving long-term therapy may develop withdrawal symptoms similar to those associated with alcohol abuse. (See Patient Teaching: *Barbiturates.*)
• Alert the physician if barbiturate dependence is suspected.

Evaluation

For each nursing diagnosis, prepare an evaluation statement that describes the patient's or family's response to nursing interventions.

Nonbenzodiazepines-nonbarbiturates

The nonbenzodiazepine-nonbarbiturate drugs act as hypnotics for short-term treatment of simple insomnia, but lose their effectiveness by the end of the second week. These drugs offer no special advantages over other sedatives and hypnotics. They include chloral hydrate, ethchlorvynol, glutethimide, methyprylon, and zolpidem as well as paraldehyde, which rarely is used.

PHARMACOKINETICS

Nonbenzodiazepine-nonbarbiturate drugs are absorbed rapidly from the GI tract, metabolized in the liver, and excreted in the urine.

Route	Onset	Peak	Duration
P.O.	15-45 min	1-6 hr	4-25 hr

PHARMACODYNAMICS

The mechanisms of action for the nonbenzodiazepine-nonbarbiturate drugs are not fully known, but the drugs produce depressant effects similar to the barbiturates. At high dosages, the drugs can produce CNS depression of the respiratory center, causing respiratory failure and death.

PHARMACOTHERAPEUTICS

Nonbenzodiazepine-nonbarbiturate drugs typically are used for short-term treatment of simple insomnia and for sedation before surgery. These drugs also provide sedation before electroencephalogram studies.

Drug interactions

The main interaction between nonbenzodiazepines-nonbarbiturates occurs when they are used with other CNS depressants, causing additive CNS depression. (For details, see Drug Interactions: *Nonbenzodiazepines-nonbarbiturates,* page 524.) These drugs do not interact with food.

ADVERSE DRUG REACTIONS

The most common dose-related adverse reactions involving nonbenzodiazepines-nonbarbiturates include GI symptoms and some hangover effects. Adverse GI reactions include nausea, vomiting, and some gastric irritation. Adverse CNS reactions, which occur especially with hypnotic dosages, can

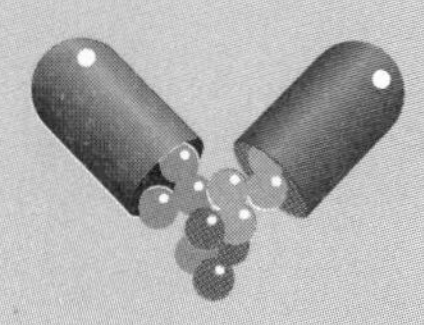

DRUG INTERACTIONS

Nonbenzodiazepines-nonbarbiturates

Drug interactions that occur with this drug class are mainly from nonbenzodiazepines-nonbarbiturates used with other central nervous system (CNS) depressants.

DRUG	INTERACTING DRUGS	POSSIBLE EFFECTS	NURSING IMPLICATIONS
chloral hydrate, ethchlorvynol, glutethimide, methyprylon, paraldehyde, zolpidem	CNS depressants	Drowsiness, respiratory depression, stupor, coma, death	• Assess for CNS and respiratory changes. • Advise the patient to prohibit or sharply curtail alcohol use during therapy. (Combination of alcohol with chloral hydrate is called a "Mickey Finn.") • Supervise ambulation; use bed rails, especially with geriatric patients. • Caution the patient not to operate a motor vehicle or heavy machinery until the effect of the drug combination is known.
paraldehyde	disulfiram	Increased paraldehyde blood levels, causing increased CNS depression; possibly toxic disulfiram reaction (respiratory depression, cardiac arrhythmias, seizures, unconsciousness)	• Monitor for increased signs of CNS and respiratory depression. • Warn the patient not to consume alcohol because doing so can be lethal.
chloral hydrate	oral anticoagulants	Increased bleeding	• Monitor the patient's prothrombin time (PT); adjust the anticoagulant dosage, as prescribed. • Assess the patient for signs of bleeding, such as epistaxis, bleeding gums, hematuria, and bruising.
	furosemide	Blood pressure changes, flushing	• Do not use concurrently.
glutethimide, ethchlorvynol	oral anticoagulants	Increased risk of clotting	• Monitor the patient's PT carefully; anticoagulant dosage may need to be adjusted. • Assess the patient for signs and symptoms of thromboembolism, such as pain, swelling, and redness in calf, and for signs of pulmonary embolism, such as shortness of breath, chest pain, and fever.

include the hangover effect. Compared with the hangover produced by barbiturates and benzodiazepines, the nonbenzodiazepine-nonbarbiturate hangover occurs less commonly, especially in geriatric patients.

At high dosages, the drugs can produce CNS depression of the respiratory center, thereby causing respiratory depression, respiratory failure, and death — especially in geriatric patients. Habitual use can cause tolerance and dependence. Chronic and acute toxicity can occur, and abrupt withdrawal from large dosages may cause dangerous withdrawal symptoms similar to those seen in barbiturate withdrawal.

Rare and mild hypersensitivity reactions include rashes and urticaria. Also rare, idiosyncratic reactions can include marked excitement, hysteria, prolonged hypnosis, profound muscle weakness, and syncope without marked hypotension.

NURSING PROCESS APPLICATION

The following information assists the nurse in caring for a patient who is receiving a nonbenzodiazepine-nonbarbiturate. It includes an overview of assessment activities as well as examples of appropriate nursing diagnoses and related interventions (see "Planning and implementation"). It also highlights the importance of evaluation.

Assessment

Before drug therapy begins, review the patient's history for conditions that contraindicate or require cautious use of the prescribed nonbenzodiazepine-nonbarbiturate. Also review

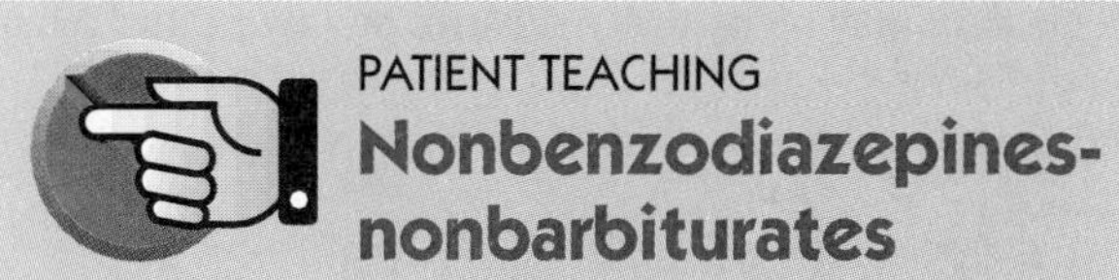

PATIENT TEACHING
Nonbenzodiazepines-nonbarbiturates

- Teach the patient and family the name, dose, frequency, action, and adverse effects of the prescribed nonbenzodiazepine-nonbarbiturate.
- Advise the patient and family to take safety precautions during nonbenzodiazepine-nonbarbiturate therapy.
- Clearly describe the risk of drug dependence.
- Teach the patient how to self-administer and store chloral hydrate.
- Teach the patient how to dilute and self-administer oral paraldehyde.
- Instruct the patient to inform the physician if any adverse reactions occur.

the patient's medication history to identify use of drugs that may interact with it. During therapy, assess the patient for adverse drug reactions and signs of drug interactions. Also, periodically assess the effectiveness of therapy with the nonbenzodiazepine-nonbarbiturate. Finally, evaluate the patient's and family's knowledge about the prescribed drug.

Nursing diagnoses

- Risk for injury related to a preexisting condition that contraindicates or requires cautious use of a nonbenzodiazepine-nonbarbiturate
- Risk for injury related to adverse drug reactions or drug interactions
- Ineffective breathing pattern related to the respiratory depression caused by the prescribed nonbenzodiazepine-nonbarbiturate
- Knowledge deficit related to the prescribed nonbenzodiazepine-nonbarbiturate agent

Planning and implementation

- Do not administer a nonbenzodiazepine-nonbarbiturate to a patient with a condition that contraindicates its use.
- Administer a nonbenzodiazepine-nonbarbiturate cautiously to a patient at risk because of a preexisting condition.
- Monitor the patient regularly for adverse reactions and drug interactions during therapy. (See Patient Teaching: *Nonbenzodiazepines-nonbarbiturates.*)
- Expect to administer a lower dosage to a geriatric or debilitated patient.
- Minimize gastric irritation from the liquid or capsule form of chloral hydrate by giving the drug after meals. Dilute liquid chloral hydrate with a fluid that minimizes its unpleasant taste, such as juice or soda. Store chloral hydrate in a light-resistant container, and refrigerate suppositories.
- Store ethchlorvynol and glutethimide in tightly closed, light-resistant containers to avoid possible deterioration; a slight darkening of the liquid from exposure to light and air will not affect its safety or potency.
- Use paraldehyde from containers that have been opened for less than 24 hours because the drug decomposes on exposure to light; do not give the drug if it is brown or has a vinegary odor. Dilute the oral liquid form in iced milk, syrup, or fruit juice to disguise the taste and odor and to reduce gastric distress.
- Use glass syringes and metal needles with paraldehyde because the drug reacts with some plastics. When administering I.M., inject deeply into a large muscle mass and massage the site. For rectal administration, minimize irritation by diluting the drug with vegetable oil (one part drug to two parts diluent); then administer as a retention enema.
- Notify the physician if adverse reactions or drug interactions occur.

* ***Frequently monitor the patient's vital signs, particularly noting such signs of respiratory depression as decreased number of respirations or respiratory pattern changes.***

- Perform a respiratory assessment before and after giving each dose of the prescribed nonbenzodiazepine-nonbarbiturate.

* ***Withhold the prescribed dose and notify the physician if respiratory depression occurs.***

- Position the debilitated patient to maximize respiratory function. For example, help the patient into a semi-Fowler's or high Fowler's position.

Evaluation

For each nursing diagnosis, prepare an evaluation statement that describes the patient's or family's response to nursing interventions.

Other sedatives

Alcohol and many OTC products, especially those containing antihistamines, are commonly used as sedatives.

Alcohol is the most widely used and abused drug in the United States. Alcohol is a CNS depressant and can be considered a sleep aid, a purpose it has served since ancient times. Small amounts of alcohol have been used to improve appetite and digestion and, in geriatric patients, to promote sleep. Alcohol causes many adverse reactions in the body, and continual consumption of large amounts can have serious effects on gastric and hepatic function. Alcohol use with other CNS depressants can be lethal. The nurse needs to be prepared to teach patients about alcohol and its effects on the body.

OTC sleep aids are readily available for purchase in the United States. These drugs usually contain an antihistamine (primarily diphenhydramine, doxylamine, or pyrilamine maleate), which has some sedative properties. Because the antihistamines are CNS depressants, they affect sleep; however, researchers have not studied this effect extensively. Minor atropine-like adverse reactions such as dry mouth can result from use of OTC sleep aids. Confusion and disorientation also can occur, especially in geriatric patients.

CHAPTER SUMMARY

Chapter 41 presented sedatives, which act to reduce activity or excitement and calm a patient, and hypnotics, which are sedatives given in large doses to induce a state resembling natural sleep. Here are the chapter highlights.

The three main classes of sedative and hypnotic agents are benzodiazepines, barbiturates, and nonbenzodiazepines-nonbarbiturates. Alcohol and OTC drugs also are used to promote sleep.

The benzodiazepines include these primary sedative and hypnotic drugs: estazolam, flurazepam, lorazepam, quazepam, temazepam, and triazolam. Benzodiazepines usually are preferred because of their effectiveness and safety; they produce few adverse reactions.

Barbiturates include amobarbital, aprobarbital, butabarbital, mephobarbital, pentobarbital, phenobarbital, and secobarbital. Like benzodiazepines, barbiturates are CNS depressants capable of producing a wide range of effects, from sedation to hypnosis and anesthesia to coma. Barbiturates exhibit a high potential for physical and psychological dependence, high potential for abuse, and life-threatening toxicity with overdose (causing severe CNS and respiratory depression).

Nonbenzodiazepines-nonbarbiturates include chloral hydrate, ethchlorvynol, glutethimide, methylprylon, paraldehyde, and zolpidem. The most common adverse reactions to these drugs are GI distress and some hangover effects. Respiratory depression also can occur. Hypersensitivity and idiosyncratic reactions to these drugs are rare.

Other sources of sedative and hypnotic effects include alcohol and OTC drugs. OTC sleep aids contain antihistamines, such as diphenhydramine, doxylamine, and pyrilamine.

When caring for a patient who is receiving a sedative or hypnotic agent, the nurse applies the nursing process, paying particular attention to prevention of respiratory depression, detection of drug dependence, and safety measures.

Questions to consider

See Appendix 1 for answers.

1. Jill Neilson, age 48, sees her physician because of a recent onset of insomnia. Her physician prescribes the benzodiazepine triazolam 0.125 mg P.O. h.s. Which condition in Ms. Neilson's health history would require cautious use of this benzodiazepine?
   (a) Diabetes mellitus
   (b) Depression
   (c) Seizure disorder
   (d) Peptic ulcer disease

2. Triazolam may be used as a sedative or a hypnotic. What is the difference?
   (a) Sedatives produce more adverse reactions than hypnotics.
   (b) Sedatives are Schedule II drugs; hypnotics are Schedule IV drugs.
   (c) Sedatives reduce activity or excitement; hypnotics induce sleep.
   (d) Sedatives require larger doses than hypnotics to produce desired effects.

3. Louise Eagan, age 49, is scheduled for an abdominal hysterectomy. The physician prescribes butabarbital 50 mg P.O. h.s. as a hypnotic the night before surgery. When Ms. Eagan awakens in the morning, she says she feels like she has a hangover. What is the probable cause of this effect?
   (a) Anxiety related to impending surgery
   (b) Unusually large dose of barbiturate
   (c) Hypersensitivity to the barbiturate
   (d) Adverse reaction to the barbiturate

4. Barbiturates are not used for sedative or hypnotic purposes as commonly as benzodiazepines. Which characteristic of barbiturates may account for this?
   (a) High incidence of hepatotoxicity
   (b) Unpredictable therapeutic effects
   (c) High potential for drug dependence
   (d) Paradoxical effects with prolonged use

5. Henry Garfield, age 62, has been having difficulty sleeping. His physician prescribes the nonbenzodiazepine-nonbarbiturate chloral hydrate 0.5 g P.O. h.s. Mr. Garfield is *most* likely to experience which adverse reactions?
   (a) Severe CNS and respiratory depression
   (b) Severe withdrawal symptoms
   (c) Hypersensitivity reactions
   (d) GI symptoms and hangover effects

6. Which of the following drug interactions cause the most problems for a patient taking phenobarbital?
   (a) Rapid drug absorption
   (b) Decrease in drug elimination
   (c) Enhancement of drug metabolism
   (d) Impaired drug distribution

7. Which of the following patients are more likely to experience dose-related adverse effects of benzodiazepines?
   (a) Active 70-year-old golfer
   (b) Anorexic college student
   (c) High school football player
   (d) Perimenopausal woman

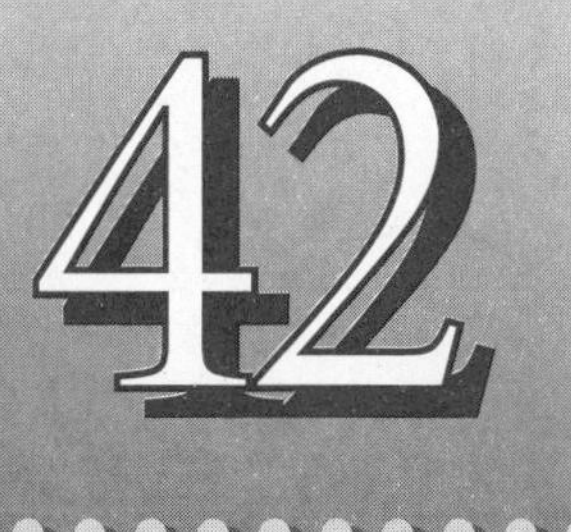

Antidepressant and antimanic agents

OBJECTIVES

After reading and studying this chapter, the student should be able to:
1. identify the clinical indications for antidepressant and antimanic agents.
2. explain the mechanisms of action of antidepressant and antimanic agents.
3. describe the major adverse effects of monoamine oxidase (MAO) inhibitors, tricyclic and second-generation antidepressants, and lithium.
4. describe how to apply the nursing process when caring for a patient who is receiving an antidepressant or antimanic agent.

INTRODUCTION

Antidepressant and **antimanic** agents are used to treat **affective disorders.** MAO inhibitors, tricyclic antidepressants, and second-generation antidepressants are used to treat unipolar disorders, which are characterized by periods of clinical **depression.** Lithium is used to treat **bipolar disorders,** which are characterized by alternating periods of manic behavior and clinical depression. (See *Selected major antidepressant and antimanic agents,* pages 528 and 529.)

Drugs covered in this chapter include:

- amitriptyline hydrochloride
- amoxapine
- bupropion hydrochloride
- clomipramine hydrochloride
- desipramine hydrochloride
- doxepine hydrochloride
- fluoxetine hydrochloride
- fluvoxamine maleate
- imipramine hydrochloride
- lithium carbonate
- lithium citrate
- maprotiline hydrochloride
- nefazodone
- nortriptyline hydrochloride
- paroxetine hydrochloride
- phenelzine sulfate
- protriptyline hydrochloride
- sertraline hydrochloride
- tranylcypromine sulfate
- trazodone hydrochloride
- trimipramine maleate
- venlafaxine.

MAO inhibitors

MAO inhibitors are divided into two classifications based on chemical structure: the hydrazines, which include phenelzine sulfate, and the single nonhydrazine tranylcypromine sulfate. All of these drugs nonselectively inhibit the enzyme MAO, which metabolizes neurotransmitters at receptor sites. Researchers have subdivided this enzyme into type A, which can produce hypertensive crisis in a patient who eats food containing tyramine, and type B, which is sensitive to different amines and is not associated with hypertensive reactions.

PHARMACOKINETICS

MAO inhibitors are absorbed rapidly and completely from the gastrointestinal (GI) tract and are metabolized in the liver to inactive metabolites. These metabolites are excreted mainly by the GI tract and to a lesser degree by the kidneys.

Route	Onset	Peak	Duration
P.O.	1-2 wk	Unknown	1-2 wk after discontinuing

PHARMACODYNAMICS

Although their exact mechanism of action is unclear, MAO inhibitors appear to work by inhibiting monoamine oxidase (the enzyme that normally metabolizes the neurotransmitters norepinephrine and **serotonin**) because they inhibit neurotransmitter intracellular metabolism. This action makes more norepinephrine and serotonin available to the receptors, thereby relieving the symptoms of depression.

PHARMACOTHERAPEUTICS

MAO inhibitors are used to treat psychiatric conditions, especially atypical depression. This disorder produces the signs opposite to those of typical depression. For example, the patient gains weight, lacks suicidal tendencies, and has an increased libido. MAO inhibitors may be used to treat typical depression when it is resistant to other therapies or when other therapies are contraindicated. Other clinical uses include depression accompanied by anxiety, phobic

Selected major antidepressant and antimanic agents

This chart summarizes the major antidepressant and antimanic agents currently in clinical use.

DRUG	MAJOR INDICATIONS AND USUAL DOSAGES	CONTRAINDICATIONS AND PRECAUTIONS
Monoamine oxidase (MAO) inhibitors		
phenelzine (Nardil)	*Atypical depression* ADULT: Initial dose is 15 mg P.O. t.i.d.; dosages up to 90 mg daily may be needed in some patients; maintenance dose is reduced to as low as 15 mg every other day when condition improves	• Phenelzine is contraindicated in a geriatric or debilitated patient; one with known hypersensitivity, severe hepatic or renal impairment, heart failure, pheochromocytoma, severe or frequent headaches, or hypertensive, cardiovascular, or cerebrovascular disease; one receiving another MAO inhibitor, a tricyclic antidepressant, psychotropic agent, meperidine, buspirone, clomipramine, central nervous system (CNS) depressant, or sympathomimetic; one who has been ingesting foods that have a high tryptophan or tyramine content or excessive amounts of caffeine; or within 10 days before and after a patient undergoes elective surgery involving general anesthesia, cocaine, or a local anesthetic containing a sympathomimetic vasoconstrictor. • This drug requires cautious use in a pregnant or breast-feeding patient; a hyperactive, agitated, schizophrenic, or suicidal patient; one receiving an antihypertensive drug (including thiazide diuretics); or one with diabetes or epilepsy. • Safety and efficacy in children under age 16 have not been established.
tranylcypromine (Parnate)	*Atypical depression* ADULT: 10 mg P.O. b.i.d., increased after 2 to 3 weeks, as needed, up to a maximum dose of 30 mg daily	• Tranylcypromine is contraindicated in a patient with a cerebrovascular defect, cardiovascular disorder, pheochromocytoma, liver disease, or known hypersensitivity; one receiving another MAO inhibitor, dibenzazepine, fluoxetine, buspirone, meperidine, dextromethorphan, or a sympathomimetic or hypotensive agent; one undergoing elective surgery; or one who has been ingesting narcotics, alcohol, excessive amounts of caffeine, or foods that have a high tyramine content. • This drug requires cautious use in a pregnant or breast-feeding patient; a patient with impaired renal function, epilepsy, diabetes, or hyperthyroidism; or one receiving an antiparkinsonian agent or disulfiram. • Safety and efficacy in children under age 16 have not been established.
Tricyclic antidepressants		
amitriptyline (Elavil, Emitrip, Endep)	*Depression* ADULT: 50 to 75 mg P.O. daily, increased to 200 mg daily, then to a maximum dose of 300 mg daily, as needed; or 20 to 30 mg I.M. q.i.d. or as a single dose h.s.	• Amitriptyline is contraindicated in a patient with known hypersensitivity or one who is in the acute recovery phase of myocardial infarction. • This drug requires cautious use in a pregnant or breast-feeding patient, a patient receiving electroconvulsive therapy or undergoing elective surgery, a suicidal patient, or one with seizures, urine retention, acute angle-closure glaucoma, increased intraocular pressure, cardiovascular disease, hyperthyroidism, or impaired hepatic function. • Safety and efficacy in children under age 12 have not been established.
doxepin (Adapin, Sinequan)	*Depression* ADULT: Initially, 25 to 50 mg P.O. daily, increased to a maximum dose of 300 mg daily, as needed	• Doxepin is contraindicated in a patient with urine retention, acute angle-closure glaucoma, or known hypersensitivity. • This drug requires cautious use in a pregnant, breast-feeding, or suicidal patient. • Safety and efficacy in children under age 12 have not been established.

Selected major antidepressant and antimanic agents *(continued)*

DRUG	MAJOR INDICATIONS AND USUAL DOSAGES	CONTRAINDICATIONS AND PRECAUTIONS
Second-generation antidepressants		
sertraline (Zoloft)	*Depression* ADULT: 50 mg P.O. daily, increased as needed, up to a maximum dose of 200 mg daily	• Sertraline is contraindicated in a patient with known hypersensitivity or one who has received an MAO inhibitor within the past 14 days. • This drug requires cautious use in a pregnant patient or one with severe hepatic or renal impairment, seizure disorder, or a history of mania or hypomania. • Safety and efficacy in children have not been established.
trazodone (Desyrel)	*Depression* ADULT: 150 P.O. daily in divided doses, increased by 50 mg daily every 3 to 4 days up to a maximum dose of 400 mg daily; for severely ill patients, 600 mg daily	• Trazodone is contraindicated in a patient with known hypersensitivity. • This drug requires cautious use in a pregnant or breast-feeding patient or one with cardiac disease. • Safety and efficacy in children have not been established.
fluoxetine (Prozac)	*Major depression, obsessive-compulsive disorders* ADULT: Initially, 20 mg P.O. daily in a.m.; if response not adequate, may increase according to patient response; may be given b.i.d. in the morning and at noon; maximum dosage is 80 mg/day	• Fluoxetine is contraindicated in a breast-feeding patient, a patient with known hypersensitivity, or one who has received an MAO inhibitor within the past 14 days. • This drug requires cautious use in a pregnant patient or one with severe hepatic or renal impairment, diabetes, or seizure disorder.
Lithium		
lithium carbonate (Eskalith, Lithane, Lithobid)	*Mania and bipolar disorder relapse* ADULT: 300 to 600 mg P.O. up to q.i.d., adjusted to achieve lithium blood level of 1 to 1.5 mEq/L for acute mania; 0.6 to 1.2 mEq/L to prevent bipolar disorder relapses, adjusted to achieve a maximum dosage of 2 mEq/L	• Lithium is contraindicated in a pregnant, breast-feeding, geriatric, or debilitated patient; a patient who cannot be monitored closely; or one with epilepsy, renal or cardiovascular disease, brain damage, severe dehydration, or sodium depletion. • This drug requires cautious use in a patient with a thyroid disorder. • Safety and efficacy in children under age 12 have not been established.

anxieties, neurodermatitis, hypochondriasis, and refractory narcoleptic states.

Drug interactions

Certain foods and drugs can interact with MAO inhibitors and may produce severe reactions. The most serious reactions involve tyramine-rich foods and sympathomimetic agents. (See *Foods that may interact with MAO inhibitors,* page 530, and Drug Interactions: *MAO inhibitors,* page 531.)

ADVERSE DRUG REACTIONS

The most serious adverse reaction to MAO inhibitors is hypertensive crisis, which can lead to death. Hypertensive crisis is characterized by increased blood pressure, severe headache, palpitations, nausea, vomiting, neck stiffness or soreness, fever, clammy skin, mydriasis, or photophobia or other vision disturbances. It also may be associated with tachycardia or bradycardia, constricting chest pain, or intracranial hemorrhage.

The most common adverse reactions are restlessness, drowsiness, dizziness, headache, insomnia, constipation, anorexia, nausea, vomiting, weakness, arthralgia, dry mouth, blurred vision, peripheral edema, urine retention, transient impotence, rash, and purpura. Orthostatic hypotension is also common, especially in geriatric patients, and may lead to syncope with high dosages. Orthostatic hypotension usually occurs in patients with preexisting hypertension, although it also may occur in patients with normal blood pressure.

Other adverse reactions to MAO inhibitors include urinary frequency, increased appetite, weight gain, increased perspiration, flushing, numbness, paresthesia, muscle spasms, tremor, myoclonic jerks, and hyperreflexia. With high dosages, these drugs may cause hyperexcitability, agita-

Foods that may interact with MAO inhibitors

Foods that contain tyramine (listed below) can produce a hypertensive crisis in a patient receiving a monoamine oxidase (MAO) inhibitor. Hypertensive crisis is signaled by a sudden severe increase in blood pressure, severe headache, sudden visual changes, and dizziness. To avoid this severe drug-food interaction, teach the patient which foods to avoid during treatment. Foods with a high tyramine content should be avoided completely, those with a moderate content may be eaten occasionally, and those with low tyramine levels are allowable in limited quantities.

Foods with a high tyramine content

- Red wines, such as chianti and burgundy
- Beer
- Aged cheese, such as blue, Swiss, and cheddar
- Aged or smoked meats, such as herring, sausage, and corned beef
- Liver, such as chicken or beef liver
- Yeast extracts such as brewer's yeast
- Fava or broad beans such as Italian green beans

Foods with a moderate tyramine content

- Sour cream
- Ripe avocados
- Yogurt
- Ripe bananas
- Meat extracts such as bouillon

Foods with a low tyramine content

- Chocolate
- Figs
- American, mozzarella, cottage, and cream cheese
- Distilled spirits, such as gin, vodka, and scotch
- White wines

tion, activation of latent schizophrenic disorder, mania, and hypomania. Such reactions require a dosage reduction or concomitant use of a phenothiazine.

Rare reactions include amblyopia, aggravation of glaucoma, other vision disturbances, impaired water excretion, leukopenia, granulocytopenia, thrombocytopenia, and normocytic or normochromic anemia.

With high dosages of tranylcypromine, dependence and addiction may occur. When this drug is discontinued, the patient may display anxiety, depression, confusion, hallucinations, diarrhea, and other withdrawal symptoms.

NURSING PROCESS APPLICATION

The following information assists the nurse in caring for a patient who is receiving an MAO inhibitor. It includes an overview of assessment activities as well as examples of appropriate nursing diagnoses and related interventions (see "Planning and implementation"). It also highlights the importance of evaluation.

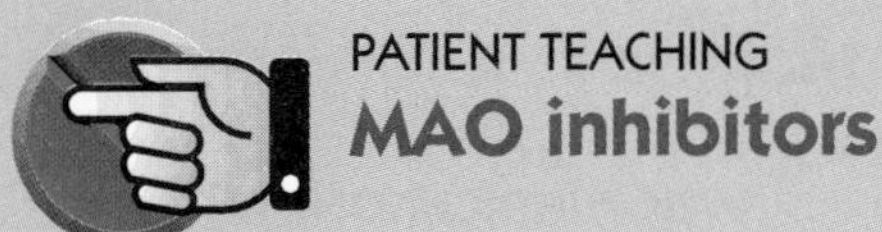

PATIENT TEACHING
MAO inhibitors

- Teach the patient and family the name, dose, frequency, action, and adverse effects of the prescribed monoamine oxidase (MAO) inhibitor.
- Teach the patient which drugs and foods to avoid during MAO inhibitor therapy and provide the patient with a written list.
- Teach the patient and family to recognize the symptoms of a hypertensive crisis, such as severe headache, sudden vision changes, and dizziness.
- Instruct the patient to inform other physicians about the MAO inhibitor therapy. For example, the drug should be discontinued 10 to 14 days before surgery.
- Caution the patient not to stop taking the MAO inhibitor abruptly, and explain that the drug should be tapered off as prescribed by the physician.
- Instruct the patient to take the drug at bedtime if it produces drowsiness or to take the last daily dose in the afternoon if it causes insomnia.
- Inform the male patient that impotence may occur during MAO inhibitor therapy but should subside when the drug is discontinued.
- Teach the patient to recognize and report to the physician signs of urine retention.
- Instruct the patient to notify the physician if adverse reactions occur.

Assessment

Before drug therapy begins, review the patient's history for conditions that contraindicate or require cautious use of the prescribed MAO inhibitor. Also review the patient's medication history to identify use of drugs that may interact with it. During therapy, assess the patient for adverse drug reactions and signs of drug interactions. Also, periodically assess the effectiveness of therapy with the MAO inhibitor. Finally, evaluate the patient's and family's knowledge about the prescribed drug. (See Patient Teaching: *MAO inhibitors.*)

Nursing diagnoses

- Risk for injury related to a preexisting condition that contraindicates or requires cautious use of an MAO inhibitor
- Risk for injury related to adverse drug reactions or drug interactions
- Urinary retention related to the adverse genitourinary (GU) effects of the prescribed MAO inhibitor
- Knowledge deficit related to the prescribed MAO inhibitor

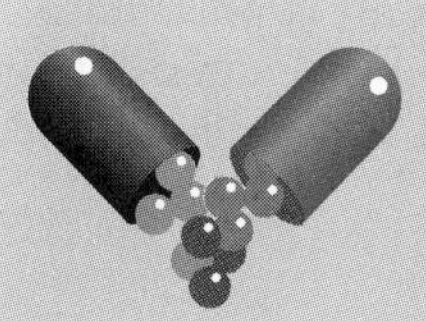

DRUG INTERACTIONS
MAO inhibitors

Monoamine oxidase (MAO) inhibitors can interact with several commonly used drugs, causing potentially severe effects.

DRUG	INTERACTING DRUGS	POSSIBLE EFFECTS	NURSING IMPLICATIONS
phenelzine, tranylcypromine	amphetamines, methylpheidate, fenfluramine	Increased catecholamine release, hypertension	• Do not use amphetamines with an MAO inhibitor.
	fluoxetine, tricyclic antidepressants, clomipramine, trazodone, sertraline, paroxetine, flovoxamine	Hyperpyrexia, excitation, seizures	• Monitor the patient's temperature and level of consciousness.
	doxapram	Hypertension and arrhythmias; increased risk of an adverse reaction to doxapram	• Monitor the patient's vital signs frequently.
	sympathomimetics, nonamphetamine anorexigenics	Increased catecholamine release, hypertension	• Avoid giving sympathomimetics or nonamphetamine anorexigenics to a patient receiving an MAO inhibitor.
	levodopa	Hypertension	• Avoid giving levodopa to a patient receiving an MAO inhibitor.
	hypoglycemic agents	Hypoglycemia	• Monitor the patient for signs and symptoms of hypoglycemia, such as hunger, diaphoresis, weakness, tremor, dizziness, and tachycardia.
	meperidine	Excitation, hypertension or hypotension, hyperpyrexia, coma	• Avoid concurrent use of meperidine as well as use within 10 days of last MAO inhibitor dose.

Planning and implementation

• Do not administer an MAO inhibitor to a patient with a condition that contraindicates its use.

• Administer an MAO inhibitor cautiously to a patient at risk because of a preexisting condition.

• Monitor the patient regularly for adverse reactions to the prescribed MAO inhibitor. Also monitor for drug interactions.

*✱ **Monitor the patient for signs and symptoms of hypertensive crisis, such as increased blood pressure, severe headache, palpitations, neck stiffness or soreness, nausea, or vomiting.***

*✱ **Prepare for emergency interventions if hypertensive crisis occurs. For example, expect to discontinue the MAO inhibitor immediately and administer 5 to 10 mg of phentolamine by intravenous injection to reduce the blood pressure, as prescribed.***

• Expect to change the patient to a different MAO inhibitor if adverse reactions do not diminish with time or make a dosage adjustment.

• Expect to change the administration time to the early evening or the morning if drowsiness or insomnia occurs.

*✱ **Do not discontinue tranylcypromine therapy abruptly. If discontinuation is necessary, expect to taper off the dosage over 2 weeks to prevent withdrawal reactions, such as anxiety, depression, confusion, and hallucinations.***

• Continue to monitor the patient for 7 to 10 days after discontinuation of the prescribed MAO inhibitor because of its long-lasting effects.

• Notify the physician if adverse reactions or drug interactions occur.

• Record the patient's fluid intake and output to help detect urine retention. Also, palpate and percuss the bladder after the patient voids.

• Ask the patient to report symptoms of urine retention, such as urinary hesitancy, frequent voiding of small amounts, and a sensation of fullness in the lower abdomen.

• Notify the physician if urine retention occurs and prepare to catheterize the patient, as directed.

Evaluation

For each nursing diagnosis, prepare an evaluation statement that describes the patient's or family's response to nursing interventions.

Tricyclic antidepressants

Most tricyclic antidepressants produce similar effects in treating depression, but differ in their abilities to increase neurotransmitter concentration levels. This section discusses the following tricyclic antidepressants: amitriptyline hydrochloride, desipramine hydrochloride, doxepin hydrochloride, imipramine hydrochloride, nortriptyline hydrochloride, protriptyline hydrochloride, and trimipramine maleate. It also discusses the tricyclic antidepressant clomipramine hydrochloride, which is the first agent approved by the Food and Drug Administration to treat **obsessive-compulsive disorder.**

PHARMACOKINETICS

Tricyclic antidepressants are absorbed completely after oral administration, but their bioavailability ranges from 30% to 70% because of the first-pass effect. The extreme fat solubility of these drugs accounts for their wide distribution throughout the body, slow excretion, and long half-lives. The tricyclic antidepressants are metabolized extensively in the liver. All of the tricyclic antidepressants are active pharmacologically, and some of their metabolites also are active. Eventually, the metabolites are hydroxylated and then conjugated to form inactive compounds that are excreted in the urine. Only small amounts of active drug are excreted.

Route	Onset	Peak	Duration
P.O.	Unknown	7-30 hr	Unknown

PHARMACODYNAMICS

Researchers hypothesize that tricyclic antidepressants increase the amount of norepinephrine, serotonin, or both, through reuptake inhibition. This normalizes the hyposensitive receptor site associated with depression. Normalization takes up to several weeks, thus slowing the onset of antidepressant action.

PHARMACOTHERAPEUTICS

Tricyclic antidepressants are the drugs of choice for episodes of major depression. They are especially effective in treating depression of insidious onset accompanied by weight loss, anorexia, or insomnia. Physical signs and symptoms may respond after 1 to 2 weeks of therapy; psychological symptoms, after 2 to 4 weeks. Tricyclic antidepressants are much less effective in patients with hypochondriasis, atypical depression, or depression accompanied by delusions. However, they may be helpful in treating acute episodes of depression, having produced a response in about two-thirds of these patients.

Clomipramine is a tricyclic antidepressant used to treat obsessive-compulsive disorder. However, tricyclic antidepressants also are being investigated for use in preventing migraine headaches and in treating phobias, enuresis, attention deficit disorders, duodenal or peptic ulcer disease, and diabetic neuropathies.

Drug interactions

Tricyclic antidepressants interact with many drugs, especially MAO inhibitors and sympathomimetics. (See Drug Interactions: *Tricyclic antidepressants.*)

ADVERSE DRUG REACTIONS

Orthostatic hypotension commonly occurs with tricyclic antidepressant therapy. In these cases, the dosage may be reduced or nortriptyline may be prescribed — especially for geriatric patients — because it is less likely to cause this adverse reaction.

A conduction delay, demonstrated by a widening QT interval, also may occur with tricyclic antidepressant therapy. This adverse reaction can exacerbate heart failure or an existing bundle-branch block. A patient taking a tricyclic antidepressant will need to be monitored for palpitations, tachycardia, and electrocardiogram (ECG) changes.

Adverse anticholinergic reactions commonly occur with tricyclic antidepressant therapy, but they may diminish or disappear as treatment continues. Reactions include blurred vision, urine retention, dry mouth, and constipation.

At high dosages, tricyclic antidepressants can cause seizures. Other adverse reactions include sedation, jaundice, a fine resting tremor, decreased libido, inhibited ejaculation, transient eosinophilia and leukopenia and, rarely, granulocytopenia.

Rashes may occur during the first 2 months of therapy, particularly with amitriptyline and imipramine. They usually are mild and do not require discontinuation of therapy. Photosensitivity reactions also may occur. Inappropriate use may trigger manic episodes in patients with bipolar disorders.

NURSING PROCESS APPLICATION

The following information assists the nurse in caring for a patient who is receiving a tricyclic antidepressant. It includes an overview of assessment activities as well as examples of appropriate nursing diagnoses and related interventions (see "Planning and implementation"). It also highlights the importance of evaluation.

Assessment

Before drug therapy begins, review the patient's history for conditions that contraindicate or require cautious use of the prescribed tricyclic antidepressant. Also review the patient's medication history to identify use of drugs that may interact with it. During therapy, assess the patient for adverse drug reactions and signs of drug interactions. Also, periodically assess the effectiveness of therapy with the tricyclic an-

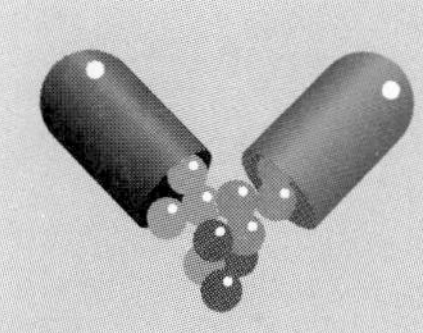

DRUG INTERACTIONS

Tricyclic antidepressants

Tricyclic antidepressants can interact with several commonly used drugs, causing potentially severe effects.

DRUG	INTERACTING DRUGS	POSSIBLE EFFECTS	NURSING IMPLICATIONS
amitriptyline, clomipramine, desipramine, doxepin, imipramine, nortriptyline, protriptyline, trimipramine	amphetamines	Increased catecholamine effects, leading to hypertension	• Administer amphetamines cautiously to a patient receiving a tricyclic antidepressant. • Monitor the patient's blood pressure frequently.
	barbiturates	Increased metabolism and decreased blood level of tricyclic antidepressant	• Monitor the patient for decreased therapeutic effect.
	cimetidine	Impaired hepatic metabolism of tricyclic antidepressant, leading to toxicity	• Monitor the patient for signs and symptoms of toxicity, such as dry mouth, blurred vision, orthostatic hypotension, urine retention, and tachycardia, if these drugs must be given together.
	monoamine oxidase inhibitors	Hyperpyrexia, excitation, seizures	• Monitor the patient's body temperature and level of consciousness.
	sympathomimetics	Increased catecholamine effects, leading to hypertension	• Monitor the patient's blood pressure and heart rate frequently if these drugs must be given together.
	anticholinergic drugs	Increased anticholinergic effects	• Monitor the patient for signs and symptoms of anticholinergic effects, such as dry mouth, urine retention, and constipation.
	clonidine, guanethidine	Decreased antihypertensive effects	• Avoid concomitant use, if possible. • Monitor the patient's blood pressure frequently.

tidepressant. Finally, evaluate the patient's and family's knowledge about the prescribed drug.

Nursing diagnoses

- Risk for injury related to a preexisting condition that contraindicates or requires cautious use of a tricyclic antidepressant
- Risk for injury related to adverse drug reactions or drug interactions
- Sexual dysfunction related to the adverse GU effects of the tricyclic antidepressant
- Knowledge deficit related to the prescribed tricyclic antidepressant

Planning and implementation

- Do not administer a tricyclic antidepressant to a patient with a condition that contraindicates its use.
- Administer a tricyclic antidepressant cautiously to a patient at risk because of a preexisting condition.
- Monitor the patient frequently for adverse reactions during tricyclic antidepressant therapy. Closely observe any patient who receives more than 200 mg of trimipramine maleate daily because of the increased incidence of adverse reactions with high dosages. Also monitor the patient for drug interactions.
- Expect to change the patient to a different tricyclic antidepressant if intolerable adverse reactions occur because adverse reactions can differ markedly among these agents.
- Consult with the physician about dividing a once-daily dosage if adverse reactions occur because smaller doses that are given more frequently decrease the risk of adverse reactions.
- Be aware that a geriatric patient should have an ECG before beginning tricyclic antidepressant therapy.

✱ ***Notify the physician if the QT interval widens on the ECG.***

✱ ***Monitor a suicidal patient closely until the drug takes full effect.***

- Reassure the patient that adverse anticholinergic reactions may diminish or disappear as therapy continues.
- Notify the physician if adverse reactions or drug interactions occur.
- Reassure the patient that drug-induced decreased libido and inhibited ejaculation should resolve when the tricyclic antidepressant is discontinued. (See Patient Teaching: *Tricyclic antidepressants,* page 534.)

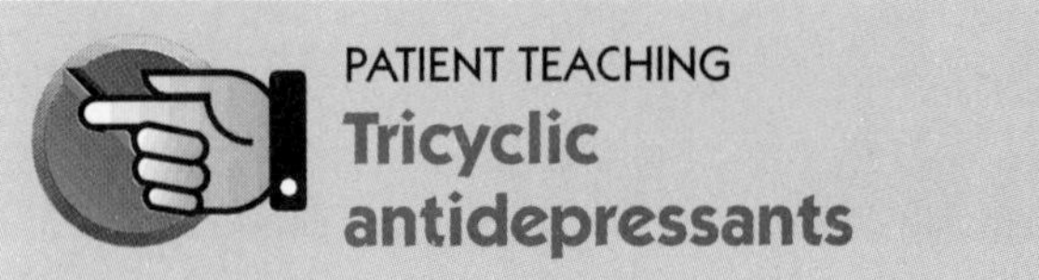

PATIENT TEACHING
Tricyclic antidepressants

- Teach the patient and family the name, dose, frequency, action, and adverse effects of the prescribed tricyclic antidepressant.
- Caution the patient not to stop taking a tricyclic antidepressant abruptly after long-term use; abrupt withdrawal can produce nausea, headache, and malaise.
- Advise the patient not to operate a motor vehicle or dangerous machinery if blurred vision or sedation occurs.
- Inform the patient that urine retention may occur.
- Teach the patient to identify high-fiber foods and include them in the diet to prevent constipation.
- Teach the patient how to manage orthostatic hypotension.
- Inform the patient that decreased libido may occur. Tell the male patient that inhibited ejaculation also may occur.
- Alert the patient that a full therapeutic response may take up to 30 days. The patient taking amitriptyline should notice an antidepressant response in 10 to 14 days.
- Instruct the patient to take the entire daily dosage at bedtime to avoid sedation and anticholinergic effects, unless otherwise prescribed.
- Warn the patient that the use of alcohol or other central nervous system depressants may increase sedation.
- Warn the patient to keep tricyclic antidepressants out of the reach of children.
- Instruct the patient to notify the physician if adverse reactions occur.

Evaluation

For each nursing diagnosis, prepare an evaluation statement that describes the patient's or family's response to nursing interventions.

Second-generation antidepressants

Developed to treat depression with fewer adverse reactions, these antidepressants are chemically different from each other and from tricyclic antidepressants and MAO inhibitors. Some of the second-generation antidepressants currently are available: amoxapine, bupropion hydrochloride, fluoxetine hydrochloride, fluvoxamine, maprotiline hydrochloride, nefazodone, paroxetine hydrochloride, sertraline hydrochloride, trazodone hydrochloride and venlafaxine.

PHARMACOKINETICS

The second-generation antidepressants are absorbed completely after oral administration and distributed widely throughout the body, except for cardiac tissue. Their peak times vary. For instance, sertraline peaks in 4.5 to 8.4 hours.

Route	Onset	Peak	Duration
P.O.	1-2 hr	1-24 hr	2-30 days

PHARMACODYNAMICS

Second-generation antidepressants inhibit reuptake of the neurotransmitters norepinephrine, serotonin, or both, thus restoring hyposensitive receptor sites to normal so that increased neurotransmitter concentrations can exert a therapeutic effect. Amoxapine and maprotiline primarily inhibit the reuptake of norepinephrine, inhibiting serotonin reuptake to a lesser extent. Sertraline, fluvoxamine, nefazodone, and trazodone inhibit reuptake of serotonin only. Paroxetine is a potent inhibitor of serotonin reuptake and a weak inhibitor of norepinephrine uptake. Bupropion weakly blocks reuptake of serotonin and norepinephrine. Fluoxetine strongly inhibits serotonin reuptake and has some inhibiting effect on norepinephrine reuptake. Venlafaxine is a potent inhibitor of both norepinephrine and serotonin reuptake.

PHARMACOTHERAPEUTICS

Second-generation antidepressants are used to treat the same major depressive episodes as the tricyclic antidepressants and have the same degree of effectiveness.

Drug interactions

Few interactions have been documented between amoxapine or maprotiline and other drugs. Patients receiving drugs that interact with tricyclic antidepressants, however, should be observed for similar interactions with the second-generation antidepressants.

Bupropion may stimulate hepatic enzymes needed for drug metabolism. It should be used cautiously in therapy with other drugs that may affect drug metabolism, such as carbamazepine, cimetidine, phenobarbital, and phenytoin. Bupropion may increase levodopa's adverse effects when used concurrently. Therefore, bupropion therapy should begin with small doses and be increased gradually in a patient receiving levodopa.

Fluoxetine increases the half-life of diazepam and displaces highly protein-bound drugs, which can lead to drug toxicity. It also may produce a potentially fatal interaction when used with an MAO inhibitor; this drug combination should be avoided. This second-generation antidepressant also may increase serum levels of other antidepressants during concomitant therapy.

Paroxetine should not be used with tryptophan because this combination can cause headache, nausea, sweating, and dizziness. (See Patient Teaching: *Second-generation antidepressants.*) Concomitant use with an MAO inhibitor can cause a serious, potentially fatal reaction; therefore, MAO inhibitor use contraindicates paroxetine therapy. Paroxetine may interact with warfarin, causing increased bleeding; with procyclidine, causing anticholinergic effects; and with other highly protein-bound drugs, causing adverse reactions to either drug. Cimetidine, phenobarbital, and phenytoin may alter the hepatic metabolism of paroxetine.

Concomitant use of sertraline with a highly protein-bound drug, such as warfarin and digitoxin, may increase the plasma concentration of either drug. Administration of sertraline with an MAO inhibitor may cause elevated sertraline levels, resulting in serious and sometimes fatal reactions; they should not be used together. Sertraline may decrease diazepam and tolbutamide clearance.

Trazodone may produce additive effects when combined with other drugs. For instance, it can increase sedation when combined with a central nervous system (CNS) depressant and may produce an additive hypotensive effect when used with a hypotensive agent. It also can increase phenytoin levels during concomitant therapy.

ADVERSE DRUG REACTIONS

Seizures may occur with all second generation antidepressants except sertraline. Amoxapine and maprotiline also may cause anticholinergic effects, orthostatic hypotension, and tachycardia.

Bupropion causes dose-related CNS stimulation, including restlessness, hallucinations, seizures, insomnia, and psychotic episodes. This distinguishes bupropion from the other tricyclic antidepressants, which commonly produce sedation. Bupropion produces fewer cardiovascular and anticholinergic symptoms than other antidepressants.

The most common adverse reactions to fluoxetine are headache, nervousness, anxiety, insomnia, nausea, anorexia, diarrhea, and diaphoresis. Rash also may occur.

In clinical trials, paroxetine has produced CNS, GI, and other adverse reactions. Adverse CNS reactions include somnolence, dizziness, and insomnia. Adverse GI reactions include nausea, dry mouth, constipation, and diarrhea. Other reactions were headache, asthenia, sweating, and ejaculatory and other disturbances of the male genitals.

During clinical trials, at least 10% of patients reported these adverse reactions to sertraline: dry mouth, headache, dizziness, tremor, diarrhea, nausea, insomnia or somnolence, sexual dysfunction in males, and fatigue.

Trazodone sometimes produces sedation, dizziness, and priapism, but rarely produces anticholinergic effects.

NURSING PROCESS APPLICATION

The following information assists the nurse in caring for a patient who is receiving a second-generation antidepressant. It includes an overview of assessment activities as well as examples of appropriate nursing diagnoses and related interventions (see "Planning and implementation"). It also highlights the importance of evaluation.

Assessment

Before drug therapy begins, review the patient's history for conditions that contraindicate or require cautious use of the prescribed second-generation antidepressant. Also review the patient's medication history to identify use of drugs that may interact with it. During therapy, assess the patient for adverse drug reactions and signs of drug interactions. Also, periodically assess the effectiveness of therapy with the second-generation antidepressant. Finally, evaluate the patient's and family's knowledge about the prescribed drug.

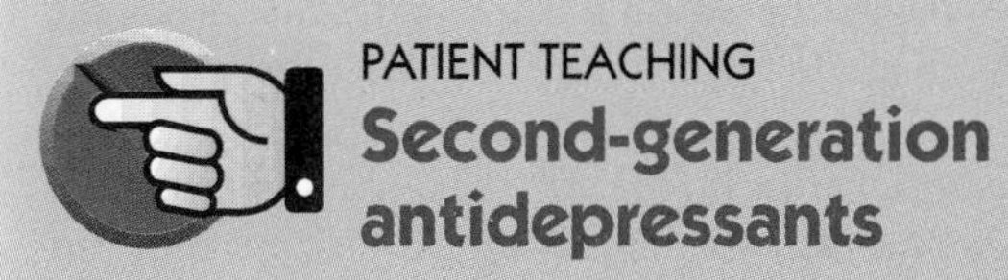

PATIENT TEACHING

Second-generation antidepressants

- Teach the patient and family the name, dose, frequency, action, and adverse effects of the prescribed second-generation antidepressant.
- Advise the patient to avoid operating a motor vehicle or dangerous machinery because sedation may occur.
- Teach the patient to take most of the daily dosage at bedtime if sedation is a problem.
- Instruct the patient to take the drug with meals or a snack to enhance absorption and to decrease dizziness.
- Instruct the female patient to notify her physician if she becomes pregnant or intends to become pregnant.
- Advise the patient to notify the physician if adverse reactions occur.

Nursing diagnoses

- Risk for injury related to a preexisting condition that contraindicates or requires cautious use of a second-generation antidepressant
- Risk for injury related to adverse drug reactions or drug interactions
- Knowledge deficit related to the prescribed second-generation antidepressant

Planning and implementation

- Do not administer a second-generation antidepressant to a patient with a condition that contraindicates its use.
- Administer a second-generation antidepressant cautiously to a patient at risk because of a preexisting condition.
- Monitor the patient periodically for adverse reactions and drug interactions during therapy.

∗ ***Take seizure precautions such as padding the bed rails during therapy with these agents (except for sertraline).*** Also, expect to administer less-than-maximum dosages of maprotiline and bupropion to prevent seizures.

- Give the drug before bedtime or with food to minimize anticholinergic effects.
- Expect to administer a reduced paroxetine dosage to a patient with a renal or hepatic impairment.
- Expect to administer a fluoxetine dosage that exceeds 20 mg daily in two divided doses — in the morning and at noon.

• Expect to begin bupropion therapy with small doses and increase them gradually in a patient who also is receiving levodopa.

* ***Withhold fluoxetine and notify the physician if the patient develops a rash.*** Also notify the physician if other adverse reactions or drug interactions occur.

Evaluation
For each nursing diagnosis, prepare an evaluation statement that describes the patient's or family's response to nursing interventions.

Lithium

Lithium carbonate and lithium citrate are the drugs of choice to prevent or treat **mania.** The discovery of lithium was a milestone in treating mania and bipolar disorders.

PHARMACOKINETICS
After oral administration, lithium is absorbed rapidly and completely and is distributed to body tissues. An active drug, lithium is not metabolized and is excreted from the body unchanged. Steady-state concentration is reached in 6 days with fixed-dosage administration.

Route	Onset	Peak	Duration
P.O.	1-3 wk	0.5-2 hr	Unknown

PHARMACODYNAMICS
In mania, the patient experiences excessive catecholamine stimulation. In a bipolar disorder, the patient is affected by swings between the excessive catecholamine stimulation of mania and the diminished catecholamine stimulation of depression. Lithium may normalize the catecholamine receptors by increasing norepinephrine and serotonin uptake, reducing the release of norepinephrine from the synaptic vesicles, and inhibiting norepinephrine's postsynaptic action. Researchers are also examining its effects on electrolyte and ion transport. It may also modify actions of second messengers such as cyclic adenosine monophosphate.

PHARMACOTHERAPEUTICS
Lithium is used primarily to treat acute episodes of mania and to prevent relapses of bipolar disorders. Other uses of lithium under investigation include preventing unipolar depression and migraine headaches and treating depression that has not responded to other therapies, alcohol dependence, anorexia nervosa, syndrome of inappropriate antidiuretic hormone, and neutropenia.

Drug interactions
Serious interactions with other drugs can occur because of lithium's narrow therapeutic range. (See Drug Interactions: *Lithium.*)

ADVERSE DRUG REACTIONS
Adverse reactions to lithium affect various body systems and may occur in any phase of therapy; most are dose-related. Because GI complaints are associated with increasing blood levels of lithium, they are most common during the initial phase of therapy and after dosage adjustments. About 50% of patients experience a fine tremor that may diminish with dosage reduction and worsen with dosage increase. Polyuria of 2 to 3 L/day may appear, accompanied by polydipsia. When blood levels exceed 1.5 mEq/L, toxicity may occur, producing confusion, lethargy, slurred speech, hyperreflexia, and seizures. Long-term lithium therapy may result in distal tubule atrophy and decreased glomerular filtration rate. Diabetes insipidus syndrome may occur, producing a daily urine output exceeding 3 L and having a low specific gravity. Hypothyroidism and nontoxic goiters may affect about 4% of patients. Other adverse reactions include weight gain, skin eruptions, alopecia, and leukocytosis.

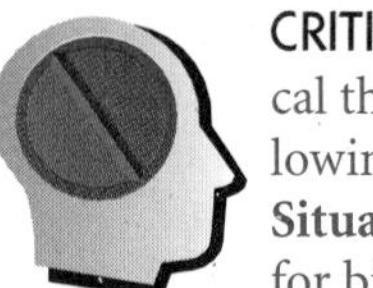

CRITICAL THINKING: To enhance your critical thinking about lithium, consider the following situation and its analysis.

Situation: Beth Jones has been taking lithium for bipolar disease for the past 10 years. She has been diagnosed with mild heart failure and started on a diuretic. Since taking the diuretic, she has become confused and lethargic with slurred speech. Her son has brought her to the emergency department for evaluation, because he is afraid she is having a cerebrovascular accident. What other potential problem could Ms. Jones be experiencing?

Analysis: Ms. Jones should be evaluated for lithium toxicity because sodium depletion from the diuretic will increase lithium levels. Both Ms. Jones and her son should be reminded to tell all health care providers that she is taking lithium before taking any other medications. Should she continue to need a diuretic, her lithium dosage may need to be reduced. Her lithium levels need to be carefully monitored.

NURSING PROCESS APPLICATION
The following information assists the nurse in caring for a patient who is receiving lithium. It includes an overview of assessment activities as well as examples of appropriate nursing diagnoses and related interventions (see "Planning and implementation"). It also highlights the importance of evaluation.

Assessment
Before drug therapy begins, review the patient's history for conditions that contraindicate or require cautious use of

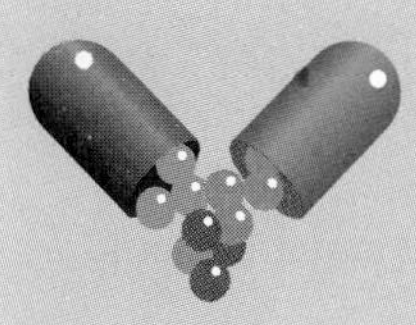

DRUG INTERACTIONS
Lithium

Lithium can interact with several drugs; most interactions affect lithium excretion and require a dosage adjustment.

DRUG	INTERACTING DRUGS	POSSIBLE EFFECTS	NURSING IMPLICATIONS
lithium	thiazide diuretics, loop diuretics	Increased lithium reabsorption in the kidneys	• Monitor the patient's serum lithium level and renal function.
	nonsteroidal anti-inflammatory drugs (NSAIDs)	Inhibited lithium excretion	• Monitor the patient's serum lithium level. • Expect to substitute sulindac for the interacting NSAID.
	potassium iodide	Increased hypothyroid activity	• Avoid concomitant use. If these drugs must be given together, observe the patient for signs and symptoms of hypothyroidism, such as fatigue, cold sensitivity, and a decreased pulse rate.
	sodium bicarbonate	Increased lithium excretion	• Monitor the patient's serum lithium level.
	sodium chloride	Altered lithium excretion (in proportion to sodium chloride intake)	• Be aware that a patient on a severe salt-restricted diet is susceptible to lithium toxicity. • Advise the patient that increased salt intake will decrease lithium's therapeutic effects.
	carbamazepine	Neurotoxicity	• Assess the patient's level of consciousness (LOC). • Instruct the patient to report dizziness, headache, fatigue, or slurred speech.
	phenothiazines, haloperidol	Neurotoxicity, seizures	• Assess the patient's LOC. • Instruct the patient to report dizziness, headache, fatigue, or slurred speech. • Take seizure precautions, such as padding the patient's bed rails.
	theophylline	Increased renal clearance of lithium	• Monitor the patient's serum lithium level.

lithium. Also review the patient's medication history to identify use of drugs that may interact with it. During therapy, assess the patient for adverse drug reactions and signs of drug interactions. Also, periodically assess the effectiveness of lithium therapy. Finally, evaluate the patient's and family's knowledge about lithium.

Nursing diagnoses

- Risk for injury related to a preexisting condition that contraindicates or requires cautious use of lithium
- Risk for injury related to adverse drug reactions or drug interactions
- Risk for fluid volume deficit related to possible lithium-induced diabetes insipidus syndrome
- Knowledge deficit related to lithium

Planning and implementation

- Do not administer lithium to a patient with a condition that contraindicates its use.
- Administer lithium cautiously to a patient at risk because of a preexisting condition.
- Observe the patient frequently for adverse reactions during lithium therapy. (See Patient Teaching: *Lithium*, page 538.)
- Obtain baseline tests of the patient's thyroid and renal functions and an ECG reading, as prescribed.
- Monitor the patient's lithium concentration periodically during therapy and after dosage adjustments. Expect to draw blood and evaluate the lithium concentration 12 hours after the last daily dose. Particularly note a concentration that exceeds 1.5 mEq/L, which may be toxic.
- Monitor the patient's white blood cell count.
- Monitor the patient for drug interactions.

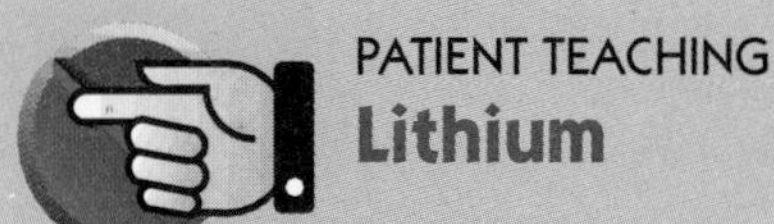

PATIENT TEACHING
Lithium

- Teach the patient and family the name, dose, frequency, action, and adverse effects of lithium.
- Advise the patient that lithium may take 1 to 3 weeks to produce a therapeutic response.
- Instruct the patient to take lithium with food to reduce gastrointestinal distress.
- Stress the importance of having blood drawn for lithium level and white blood cell counts.
- Teach the patient and family to recognize signs and symptoms of toxicity (confusion, lethargy, slurred speech, hyperreflexia, and seizures) and to notify the physician if toxicity occurs before administering the next dose.
- Instruct the patient to notify other physicians about lithium therapy to avoid serious drug interactions.
- Advise the patient to measure fluid intake and output and to notify the physician if output exceeds 3 qt (2.8 L) daily.
- Advise the patient who develops a fine tremor that it may diminish with a dosage reduction and worsen with a dosage increase. Reassure the patient that the tremor will cease when lithium is discontinued.
- Reassure the patient that weight gain, skin eruptions, and alopecia will cease when lithium is discontinued.
- Instruct the female patient to notify the physician if she becomes pregnant or intends to become pregnant.
- Instruct the patient to notify the physician if adverse reactions occur.

• Monitor the patient for GI complaints, especially during the initial phase of lithium therapy.
• Administer lithium with food to reduce GI distress.
• Notify the physician if adverse reactions or drug interactions occur.
• Record the patient's fluid intake and output; polyuria of 2 to 3 L/day may occur in a patient with diabetes insipidus syndrome.
• Monitor the patient with polyuria for signs of dehydration, such as dry mucous membranes, polydipsia, and poor skin turgor.
• Note the specific gravity and color of the patient's urine. With diabetes insipidus syndrome, the specific gravity is low and the urine is light yellow (diluted) rather than dark yellow (concentrated), which usually occurs in dehydration.
*** *Notify the physician if the urine output significantly exceeds fluid intake.***
• Administer fluids to replace fluid loss, as needed.

Evaluation

For each nursing diagnosis, prepare an evaluation statement that describes the patient's or family's response to nursing interventions.

CHAPTER SUMMARY

Chapter 42 discussed the antidepressant and antimanic agents. Here are the chapter highlights.

Although MAO inhibitors can interact with many drugs and foods, they remain the treatment of choice for atypical depression. They also may be used to treat other types of depression when it is resistant to other therapies or when other therapies are contraindicated.

The tricyclic antidepressants are preferred for treating major depressive episodes; however, they can interact with numerous drugs.

The second-generation antidepressants are used to treat depression. They have fewer adverse effects than tricyclic antidepressants and MAO inhibitors.

Lithium effectively treats acute manic episodes and prevents relapses of bipolar disorders. Because this drug has a narrow therapeutic range and a high incidence of adverse effects, a patient receiving lithium requires close monitoring.

For a patient who is receiving an antidepressant or antimanic agent, the nurse applies the nursing process. Nursing care focuses on monitoring for CNS effects, taking safety precautions, and ensuring compliance with the drug regimen.

Questions to consider

See Appendix 1 for answers.

1. Glen Bateman age 25, is diagnosed as having atypical depression. Which of the following antidepressants is the physician most likely to prescribe for Mr. Bateman?
   (a) lithium
   (b) An MAO inhibitor
   (c) A tricyclic antidepressant
   (d) A second-generation antidepressant

2. Veronica Zantz, age 52, has typical depression that has not responded to conventional therapy. Her physician prescribes the MAO inhibitor tranylcypromine. The nurse cautions Ms. Zantz to avoid high-tyramine foods. Which of the following adverse reactions is most likely to occur if Ms. Zantz eats this type of food?
   (a) MAO inhibitor inactivation
   (b) MAO inhibitor-induced hypersensitivity
   (c) Paradoxical drug effects
   (d) Hypertensive crisis

3. Mary Haines, age 55, is about to begin therapy with the tricyclic antidepressant amitriptyline. Before teaching Ms. Haines about this drug, the nurse reviews her medication history. Which of the following drugs could interact with amitriptyline?
   (a) Nonsteroidal anti-inflammatory drugs (NSAIDs)
   (b) Hypoglycemic agents
   (c) cimetidine
   (d) erythromycin

4. Bill Deglin, age 38, takes the second-generation antidepressant sertraline, as prescribed, for episodes of major depression. This drug acts by inhibiting the reuptake of which of the following neurotransmitter?
   (a) acetylcholine
   (b) epinephrine
   (c) norepinephrine
   (d) serotonin

5. Jeffrey Hallman, age 41, takes lithium citrate 300 mg P.O. t.i.d. for bipolar disorder. Which of the following actions should the nurse take to help prevent lithium toxicity?
   (a) Assess for decreased urine output.
   (b) Administer an NSAID for mild pain.
   (c) Regularly monitor his lithium concentration.
   (d) Maintain his lithium concentration between 1.5 and 2 mEq/L.

6. Mary Smith, age 21, was started on lithium 600 mg daily for a bipolar disorder. Which of the following medications should she avoid?
   (a) Oral contraceptives
   (b) Tetracycline products
   (c) Loop diuretics
   (d) Oral hypoglycemics

7. Bill Jones, age 42, was started on fluoxetine for an obsessive-compulsive disorder. On administering the first dose, Bill wants some information on possible adverse effects. Which of the following is *not* an adverse effect of fluoxetine?
   (a) Headache
   (b) Nausea
   (c) Dry mouth
   (d) Thyroid disorders

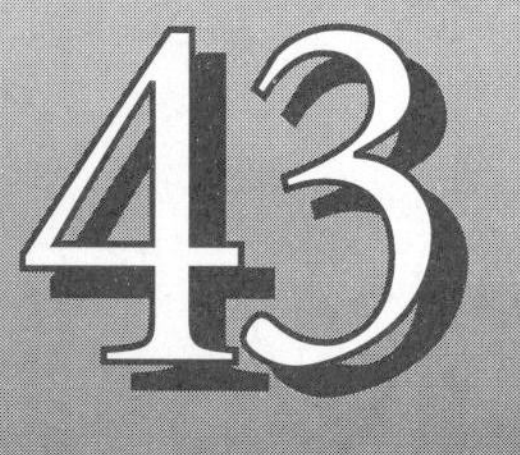

Antianxiety agents

OBJECTIVES

After reading and studying this chapter, the student should be able to:

1. describe the three major types of antianxiety agents.
2. explain why the benzodiazepines are the drugs of choice for treating anxiety.
3. compare the mechanism of action of the benzodiazepines with that of the barbiturates, and describe how each type of drug produces different adverse reactions.
4. describe the pharmacokinetic, pharmacodynamic, and pharmacotherapeutic properties of buspirone.
5. describe how to apply the nursing process when caring for a patient receiving an antianxiety agent.

INTRODUCTION

Antianxiety agents, also called **anxiolytics,** include some of the most commonly prescribed drugs in the United States. They are used primarily to treat **anxiety disorders,** which affect 7% to 18% of Americans.

This chapter presents the three main types of drugs used to treat anxiety disorders: the commonly prescribed benzodiazepines, buspirone, and the former drugs of choice, the barbiturates. It also briefly discusses meprobamate and several other drugs that are used (rarely) to treat **anxiety.** (See *Selected major antianxiety agents.*)

Drugs covered in this chapter include:

- alprazolam
- buspirone hydrochloride
- chlordiazepoxide hydrochloride
- clorazepate dipotassium
- diazepam
- diphenhydramine hydrochloride
- halazeprem
- hydroxyzine hydrochloride
- lorazepam
- meprobamate
- oxazepam
- pentobarbital sodium
- phenobarbital sodium
- prazepam.

Benzodiazepines

Currently, the benzodiazepines are the drugs of choice in treating anxiety disorders. They include alprazolam, chlordiazepoxide hydrochloride, clorazepate dipotassium, diazepam, halazepam, lorazepam, oxazepam, and prazepam. Diazepam also is used as a muscle relaxant.

PHARMACOKINETICS

Benzodiazepines may be given orally or parenterally. They are absorbed well and distributed widely in the body. In the liver, long-acting agents are broken down into active metabolites. Short-acting agents are metabolized to inactive metabolites. (However, alprazolam is a short- to intermediate-acting agent metabolized to an active compound.) All benzodiazepines are excreted primarily in the urine.

Prolonged half-lives of the long-acting agents, such as diazepam, may occur in geriatric patients because they have an increased percentage of fatty tissue in their bodies. Prolonged half-lives also may occur in patients with liver disease because they have decreased clearance of these drugs. Short-acting benzodiazepines with no active metabolites will accumulate more rapidly and reach steady-state concentrations in 2 to 4 days. These agents require multiple doses every day. If the patient misses 1 day of therapy, the blood level — and the therapeutic response — will decline rapidly.

Route	Onset	Peak	Duration
P.O.	0.5-2 hr	Unknown	3-8 hr
I.V.	1-5 min	1-1.5 hr	Variable
I.M.	15-30 min	1-1.5 hr	Variable

PHARMACODYNAMICS

Current theories suggest that the benzodiazepines enhance the effects of **gamma-aminobutyric acid (GABA).** A natural inhibitor of excitatory stimulation, GABA affects the limbic system and helps control emotions. Unlike barbiturates, which can depress the central nervous system (CNS) directly, benzodiazepines work indirectly by enhancing GABA activity. This synergistic action may explain the safer adverse

Selected major antianxiety agents

This chart summarizes the major antianxiety agents currently in clinical use.

DRUG	MAJOR INDICATIONS AND USUAL DOSAGES	CONTRAINDICATIONS AND PRECAUTIONS
Benzodiazepines		
alprazolam (Xanax)	*Anxiety associated with depression* ADULT: 0.25 to 0.5 mg P.O. t.i.d., increased as tolerated, up to a maximum dose of 4 mg daily in divided doses	• Alprazolam is contraindicated in a pregnant or breast-feeding patient or one with acute angle-closure glaucoma or known hypersensitivity. • This drug requires cautious use in a geriatric or debilitated patient, a patient receiving another psychotropic agent, or one with impaired renal or hepatic function or a history of drug dependence. • Safety and efficacy in children have not been established.
diazepam (Valium)	*Anxiety* ADULT: 2 to 10 mg P.O. b.i.d. to q.i.d. PEDIATRIC: 1 to 2.5 mg P.O. t.i.d. or q.i.d. *Alcohol withdrawal* ADULT: 10 mg P.O. t.i.d. or q.i.d. for 24 hours, then decreased to 5 mg t.i.d. or q.i.d. *Skeletal muscle spasms* ADULT: 2 to 10 mg P.O. t.i.d. or q.i.d. PEDIATRIC: 1 to 2.5 mg P.O. t.i.d. or q.i.d. *Status epilepticus* ADULT: 5 to 10 mg slow I.V. push repeated every 10 to 15 minutes, up to a maximum dose of 30 mg PEDIATRIC: For children ages 31 days to 5 years, 0.2 to 0.5 mg slow I.V. push, repeated every 2 to 5 minutes, up to a maximum dose of 5 mg; for children age 5 and over, 1 mg slow I.V. push, repeated every 2 to 5 minutes, up to a maximum dose of 10 mg	• Diazepam is contraindicated in a pregnant patient or one with acute angle-closure glaucoma or known hypersensitivity. • This drug requires cautious use in a patient with severe or latent depression, impaired renal or hepatic function, or a history of drug dependence. • Safety and efficacy of oral diazepam in children under age 6 months have not been established. Safety and efficacy of parenteral diazepam in infants age 30 days or under have not been established.
Buspirone		
buspirone hydrochloride (BuSpar)	*Anxiety* ADULT: 5 mg P.O. t.i.d., increased by 5 mg every 2 to 3 days, as needed, up to a maximum of 60 mg daily	• Buspirone is contraindicated in a breast-feeding patient, one receiving a monoamine oxidase inhibitor, or one with impaired renal or hepatic function or known hypersensitivity. • This drug requires cautious use in a pregnant patient. • Safety and efficacy in children have not been established.
Barbiturates		
pentobarbital sodium (Nembutal Sodium)	*Anxiety, sedation* ADULT: 20 mg P.O. t.i.d. or q.i.d.	• Pentobarbital is contraindicated in a pregnant patient or one with porphyria, bronchopneumonia or other severe pulmonary insufficiency, or known hypersensitivity. • This drug requires cautious use in a breast-feeding patient, a depressed or suicidal patient, or one with hepatic damage, a history of drug abuse, or acute or chronic pain.
phenobarbital sodium	*Anxiety* ADULT: 30 to 120 mg P.O. daily in two or three divided doses	• Phenobarbital is contraindicated in a pregnant patient or one with porphyria, nephritis, renal insufficiency, bronchopneumonia or other severe pulmonary insufficiency, or known hypersensitivity. • This drug requires cautious use in a breast-feeding patient, a depressed or suicidal patient, or one with hepatic damage, a history of drug abuse, or acute or chronic pain.

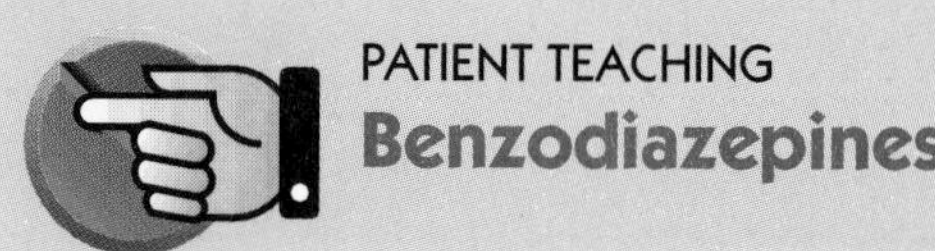

PATIENT TEACHING
Benzodiazepines

- Teach the patient and family the name, dose, frequency, action, and adverse effects of the prescribed benzodiazepine.
- Instruct the female patient to notify her physician if she becomes pregnant or intends to become pregnant.
- Advise the family to provide close supervision and take safety measures, such as assisting with ambulation, if the patient experiences adverse central nervous system reactions.
- Instruct the patient and family to notify the physician if adverse reactions occur.
- Advise the patient to avoid alcohol, driving, and operating machinery.

reaction profile of the benzodiazepines, especially in overdoses.

PHARMACOTHERAPEUTICS

Benzodiazepines are used for short-term treatment of generalized anxiety. Other clinical uses include producing sedative and hypnotic effects, treating seizure disorders, producing skeletal muscle relaxation, treating insomnia, providing light anesthesia, and managing alcohol withdrawal symptoms. Alprazolam also is used to treat **panic** attacks.

Currently, the benzodiazepines are the drugs of choice for treating anxiety. They have replaced the barbiturates because they produce fewer adverse reactions, less respiratory depression, fewer drug interactions, and milder withdrawal symptoms and because they have a relatively low abuse potential. They are, however, more expensive than barbiturates.

Drug interactions

The major interactions relate to the use of benzodiazepines with other CNS depressants, thereby producing additive effects.

ADVERSE DRUG REACTIONS

Most adverse reactions to the benzodiazepines affect the CNS; less than 1% affect other body systems. Sedation is the most common adverse reaction, affecting 4% to 12% of all patients taking chlordiazepoxide or diazepam. Benzodiazepines also can impair motor coordination, reaction time, and cognitive reasoning, especially in geriatric patients. Benzodiazepines — particularly alprazolam, diazepam, and lorazepam — also can cause dosage-related amnesia.

The benzodiazepines have a potential for abuse, tolerance, and physical dependence. As a result, abrupt discontinuation of long-term, high-dosage therapy can cause a withdrawal reaction with such signs and symptoms as weakness, delirium, and tonic-clonic seizures. Because some benzodiazepines have long half-lives, withdrawal symptoms may take a week to appear. Alprazolam is most likely to cause withdrawal symptoms because it is used in high dosages, usually for long periods, to treat panic attacks. Rarely, benzodiazepines may cause mild allergic reactions, such as rash, pruritus, and urticaria. They also may cause paradoxical excitation in geriatric patients.

Overdose of benzodiazepines is treated with flumazenil, which blocks the action of benzodiazepines. Repeated dosing with flumazenil may be necessary to block the effects of the drug, due to longer bioactive metabolites of benzodiazepines.

NURSING PROCESS APPLICATION

The following information assists the nurse in caring for a patient who is receiving a benzodiazepine as an antianxiety agent. It includes an overview of assessment activities as well as examples of appropriate nursing diagnoses and related interventions (see "Planning and implementation"). It also highlights the importance of evaluation.

Assessment

Before drug therapy begins, review the patient's history for conditions that contraindicate or require cautious use of the prescribed benzodiazepine. Also review the patient's medication history to identify use of drugs that may interact with it. During therapy, assess the patient for adverse drug reactions and signs of drug interactions. Also, periodically assess the effectiveness of benzodiazepine therapy. Finally, evaluate the patient's and family's knowledge about the prescribed drug. (See Patient Teaching: *Benzodiazepines.*)

Nursing diagnoses

- Risk for injury related to a preexisting condition that contraindicates or requires cautious use of a benzodiazepine
- Risk for injury related to adverse drug reactions or drug interactions
- Altered thought processes related to the adverse CNS effects of the prescribed benzodiazepine
- Knowledge deficit related to the prescribed benzodiazepine

Planning and implementation

- Do not administer a benzodiazepine to a patient with a condition that contraindicates its use.
- Administer a benzodiazepine cautiously to a patient at risk because of a preexisting condition.
- Monitor the patient periodically for adverse reactions or drug interactions during benzodiazepine therapy.
- Monitor the patient for a therapeutic response to a long-acting benzodiazepine. Keep in mind that, after steady-state levels are reached, the therapeutic response may persist for days after discontinuation.

• Avoid intramuscular (I.M.) administration, if possible, because absorption after I.M. injection is slow and erratic.
• Prepare I.M. chlordiazepoxide with the diluent provided and administer it deeply into a muscle.
* ***Administer intravenous (I.V.) preparations slowly to reduce the risk of phlebitis and cardiovascular collapse.*** Administer I.V. diazepam at no more than 5 mg/minute and repeat, as needed, every 10 to 15 minutes, up to a maximum of 30 mg.
* ***Do not discontinue benzodiazepine therapy abruptly.*** Otherwise, the patient may develop withdrawal symptoms, such as weakness, delirium, and tonic-clonic seizures.
• Notify the physician if adverse reactions or drug interactions occur.
* ***Take safety precautions if the patient develops adverse CNS reactions, such as sedation or amnesia. For example, place the patient's bed in a low position, keep the bed rails up, and supervise the patient's ambulation.***
• Expect to decrease the benzodiazepine dosage, as prescribed, if CNS reactions occur.

Evaluation

For each nursing diagnosis, prepare an evaluation statement that describes the patient's or family's response to nursing interventions.

Buspirone

The first anxiolytic in a new class of agents, buspirone hydrochloride's structure and mechanism of action differ from those of other antianxiety agents. It is less sedating, it does not increase the CNS depressant effects of alcohol or sedative hypnotics, and it has less chance of being abused.

PHARMACOKINETICS

Buspirone is absorbed rapidly. Although buspirone's distribution has not been explained fully, researchers have found that some of its metabolites accumulate in the brain at higher levels than the parent compound. Buspirone's metabolism also remains largely unknown. After administration, 29% to 63% of a dose appears in the urine as metabolites, less than 1% is excreted unchanged, and nearly 18% to 38% is excreted in the feces.

Route	Onset	Peak	Duration
P.O.	1-2 wk	1 hr	Unknown

PHARMACODYNAMICS

Researchers theorize buspirone's mechanism of action as a partial agonist of serotonin receptors, but they know that, in contrast to theories about the benzodiazepines, buspirone does not affect GABA receptors. Rather, it seems to produce various effects in the midbrain and acts as a midbrain modulator possibly due to its high affinity for serotonin receptors.

PHARMACOTHERAPEUTICS

Currently, buspirone is indicated to treat generalized anxiety states. Few clinical trials have compared buspirone to other agents, but patients who have not been exposed previously to benzodiazepines seem to respond better to buspirone. This drug's slow onset of action, however, makes it ineffective for quick results.

Drug interactions

When buspirone is given concomitantly with monoamine oxidase (MAO) inhibitors, hypertensive reactions may occur. Therefore, these drugs should not be used together. Unlike other antianxiety agents, buspirone does not interact with alcohol or other CNS depressants.

ADVERSE DRUG REACTIONS

The most common reactions to buspirone include dizziness, light-headedness, insomnia, tachycardia, palpitations, and headache. At this time, no data exist regarding buspirone overdose, and the drug does not appear to have an abuse potential.

NURSING PROCESS APPLICATION

The following information assists the nurse in caring for a patient who is receiving buspirone. It includes an overview of assessment activities as well as examples of appropriate nursing diagnoses and related interventions (see "Planning and implementation"). It also highlights the importance of evaluation.

Assessment

Before drug therapy begins, review the patient's history for conditions that contraindicate or require cautious use of buspirone. Also review the patient's medication history to identify use of drugs that may interact with it. During therapy, assess the patient for adverse drug reactions and signs of drug interactions. Also, periodically assess the effectiveness of buspirone therapy. Finally, evaluate the patient's and family's knowledge about the prescribed drug.

Nursing diagnoses

• Risk for injury related to a preexisting condition that contraindicates or requires cautious use of buspirone
• Risk for injury related to adverse drug reactions or drug interactions
• Sleep pattern disturbance related to buspirone-induced insomnia
• Knowledge deficit related to buspirone

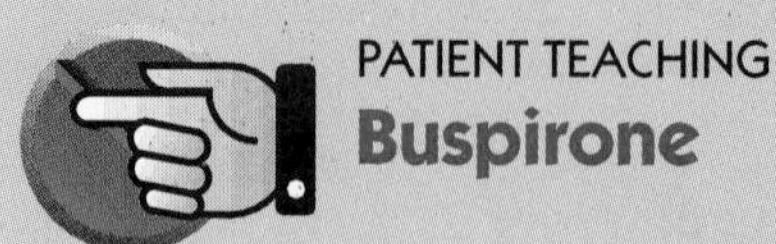

PATIENT TEACHING
Buspirone

- ➤ Teach the patient and family the name, dose, frequency, action, and adverse effects of buspirone.
- ➤ Instruct the patient to use safety precautions at home and tell family members to supervise the patient's ambulation if dizziness or light-headedness occurs.
- ➤ Instruct the patient to take the last daily dose of buspirone several hours before bedtime to prevent insomnia. Also suggest alternative methods for inducing sleep if insomnia occurs.
- ➤ Advise the patient to ask the physician to recommend an analgesic if headaches occur.
- ➤ Instruct the female patient to notify her physician if she becomes pregnant or plans to breast-feed her infant.
- ➤ Instruct the patient to notify the physician if adverse reactions occur.

Planning and implementation

- Do not administer buspirone to a patient with a condition that contraindicates its use.
- Administer buspirone cautiously to a patient at risk because of a preexisting condition.
- Monitor the patient for adverse reactions and drug interactions during buspirone therapy.
- Expect to change a patient from long-term benzodiazepine therapy to buspirone therapy by tapering off the benzodiazepine dosage as prescribed to avoid a benzodiazepine withdrawal reaction.
- Notify the physician if adverse reactions or drug interactions occur.
- Prevent insomnia by administering the last daily dose of buspirone several hours before bedtime, if possible. (See Patient Teaching: *Buspirone.*)
- Help the patient explore alternative methods for inducing sleep if insomnia occurs, such as a warm bath or quiet meditation. Request a prescription for a hypnotic agent, as needed.

Evaluation

For each nursing diagnosis, prepare an evaluation statement that describes the patient's or family's response to nursing interventions.

Barbiturates

Until benzodiazepines were introduced about 30 years ago, barbiturates were the most commonly prescribed antianxiety agents. This section presents two representative barbiturates: pentobarbital sodium and phenobarbital sodium.

PHARMACOKINETICS

Barbiturates are absorbed well, distributed rapidly, metabolized in the liver, and excreted in the urine. They fall into four classifications based on their duration of action: long-acting, intermediate-acting, short-acting, and ultrashort-acting.

These medications induce their own metabolism. This may account for the tolerance that develops to them. However, they also increase the rate of metabolism of other medications.

Route	Onset	Peak	Duration
P.O.	15-60 min	30-60 min	1-12 hr
I.V.	Immediate	Immediate	Variable
I.M.	10-25 min	Unknown	Variable
P.R.	15 min	Unknown	1-4 hr

PHARMACODYNAMICS

The mechanism of action of the barbiturates in treating anxiety is not understood completely. However, these agents may cause an imbalance in the central inhibitory and facilitatory mechanisms, which affects the cerebral cortex and reticular formation. They also increase the action of GABA at high concentrations, mimicking its activity.

PHARMACOTHERAPEUTICS

In treating anxiety, barbiturates are more effective than meprobamate and equally as effective as the benzodiazepines. Because barbiturates cause many adverse reactions, including severe respiratory depression, they largely have been replaced by the benzodiazepines as antianxiety agents. Phenobarbital also is used to manage barbiturate or nonbarbiturate withdrawal in dependent patients and is under investigation for use in treating congenital biliary defects and hyperbilirubinemia in neonates.

Drug interactions

When administered with other CNS depressants, the barbiturates can produce additive depressant effects. Other drug interactions also are likely to occur because barbiturates can stimulate the enzymes that degrade other drugs, thereby decreasing their duration of action.

ADVERSE DRUG REACTIONS

The most common dose-related adverse reactions involve the CNS and include sedation, lethargy, ataxia, headache, depression, and impaired motor coordination and reaction time. When used as hypnotics, barbiturates can produce a hangover effect or confused state the next day, especially in elderly patients. (See Patient Teaching: *Barbiturates.*)

In an otherwise healthy person, barbiturates produce respiratory depression equal to that produced by sleep. In a patient with a pulmonary disease, respiratory depressant effects are more pronounced. Even low dosages of phenobarbital can produce severe changes in the blood oxygen saturation and blood pH levels. Respiratory effects are more drastic in a patient who has taken an overdose.

Long-term use can lead to tolerance and physical or psychological dependence on the barbiturate. If therapy is discontinued abruptly, a withdrawal reaction may occur 8 to 12 hours later. Withdrawal signs and symptoms include anxiety, insomnia, nausea, vomiting, hallucinations, muscle twitches, and seizures.

Other reactions include dermatologic and allergic manifestations, paradoxical excitation, and blood dyscrasias.

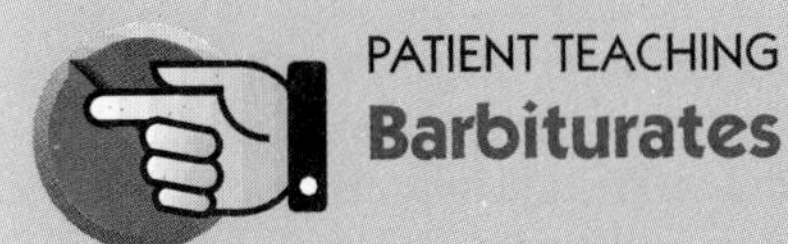

PATIENT TEACHING
Barbiturates

- Teach the patient and family the name, dose, frequency, action, and adverse effects of the prescribed barbiturate.
- Teach the patient to take the drug exactly as prescribed and not to change the dosage without consulting the physician.
- Advise the patient not to discontinue the drug suddenly without consulting the physician because withdrawal symptoms may occur.
- Instruct the patient not to operate a motor vehicle or heavy machinery, at least until the patient knows the drug's effects on mental alertness.
- Instruct the patient not to drink alcohol during drug therapy because respiratory depression can occur.
- Instruct the patient to read drug labels and avoid over-the-counter drugs that contain central nervous system depressants, such as alcohol or antihistamines.
- Advise the patient to consult the physician before taking any tranquilizers, narcotics, or other prescription pain relievers.
- Counsel the patient not to give any prescribed drugs to family members or friends.

NURSING PROCESS APPLICATION

The following information assists the nurse in caring for a patient who is receiving a barbiturate as an antianxiety agent. It includes an overview of assessment activities as well as examples of appropriate nursing diagnoses and related interventions (see "Planning and implementation"). It also highlights the importance of evaluation.

Assessment

Before drug therapy begins, review the patient's history for conditions that contraindicate or require cautious use of the prescribed barbiturate. Also review the patient's medication history to identify use of drugs that may interact with it. During therapy, assess the patient for adverse drug reactions and signs of drug interactions. Also, periodically assess the effectiveness of barbiturate therapy. Finally, evaluate the patient's and family's knowledge about the prescribed drug.

Nursing diagnoses

- Risk for injury related to a preexisting condition that contraindicates or requires cautious use of a barbiturate
- Risk for injury related to adverse drug reactions or drug interactions
- Ineffective breathing pattern related to the adverse respiratory effects of the prescribed barbiturate
- Knowledge deficit related to the prescribed barbiturate

Planning and implementation

- Do not administer a barbiturate to a patient with a condition that contraindicates its use.
- Administer a barbiturate cautiously to a patient at risk because of a preexisting condition.
- Monitor the patient for adverse reactions and drug interactions during barbiturate therapy.
- Monitor prothrombin time if the patient also is receiving an anticoagulant. Adjust the anticoagulant dosage, as prescribed. Remember that abrupt withdrawal of barbiturates may cause bleeding.

∗ ***Take safety measures when administering a barbiturate.***

∗ ***Do not discontinue a barbiturate abruptly.*** Otherwise, the patient may develop withdrawal signs and symptoms, such as anxiety, insomnia, nausea, vomiting, hallucinations, muscle twitches, and seizures.

- Notify the physician if adverse reactions or drug interactions occur.
- Monitor the patient's vital signs frequently, particularly noting such signs of respiratory depression as decreased respirations or respiratory pattern changes.

∗ ***Perform a respiratory assessment before and after giving each dose of the prescribed barbiturate.***

∗ ***Delay the prescribed barbiturate dose until the physician is notified, if respiratory depression occurs.***

Evaluation

For each nursing diagnosis, prepare an evaluation statement that describes the patient's or family's response to nursing interventions.

Other antianxiety agents

Although benzodiazepines, buspirone, and barbiturates commonly are used to treat anxiety disorders, meprobamate, beta blockers, and antihistamines also may be used as antianxiety agents.

Meprobamate was used widely in the past to treat anxiety. It rarely is used today, however, because of its low degree of effectiveness, the severity of its adverse effects, and the existence of safer, more effective agents. Although meprobamate is a CNS depressant, its exact site and mechanism of action in anxiety relief is unknown. When administered with other CNS depressants, meprobamate usually causes additive depressant effects. Meprobamate's CNS depressant action accounts for its adverse effects, which commonly include sedation, ataxia, and hypotension. Dependence can develop, and severe withdrawal reactions have occurred after abrupt discontinuation of high dosage, long-term therapy.

Beta blockers can relieve the somatic symptoms associated with anxiety. Although most studies show that benzodiazepines are more effective in treating anxiety disorders, beta blockers are useful in treating acute situational anxiety that causes somatic symptoms.

Antihistamines, particularly hydroxyzine hydrochloride and diphenhydramine hydrochloride, may be used to treat anxiety. This use of antihistamines is rare, however, and most studies indicate that they are not effective antianxiety agents.

CHAPTER SUMMARY

Chapter 43 explored drugs used to treat anxiety disorders. Here are the chapter highlights.

Benzodiazepines have replaced barbiturates as the drugs of choice to treat anxiety. They interact with fewer drugs and offer a safer adverse reaction profile.

Buspirone is the newest antianxiety agent. Preliminary data indicate it interacts only with MAO inhibitors. Buspirone appears to have no abuse potential, causes almost no sedation, and produces only minor adverse reactions.

Although barbiturates are effective in treating anxiety, they largely have been replaced by the benzodiazepines because benzodiazepines interact with fewer drugs and cause fewer adverse reactions.

Other drugs that are used rarely to treat anxiety include meprobamate, beta blockers, and antihistamines.

When caring for a patient receiving an antianxiety agent, the nurse uses the nursing process. Key aspects of nursing care include monitoring the drug's effectiveness, observing for signs of drug tolerance, assessing for adverse reactions, and ensuring patient safety.

Questions to consider

See Appendix 1 for answers.

1. Bruce Plaid, age 62, sees his doctor because of symptoms caused by the death of his wife. His physician prescribes the benzodiazepine diazepam. Mr. Plaid is *most* likely to experience which of the following adverse reactions to diazepam?
   (a) Tachycardia
   (b) Rash
   (c) Hypertension
   (d) Sedation

2. Diazepam is able to relieve anxiety because of which of the following properties?
   (a) Inhibited neurotransmitter release
   (b) Enhanced GABA activity
   (c) Direct CNS depression
   (d) Midbrain modulation

3. Kim Wall, age 37, takes buspirone 5 mg P.O. t.i.d. for generalized anxiety. Which of the following statements accurately characterizes buspirone?
   (a) Buspirone has a rapid onset of action.
   (b) Buspirone has a high potential for abuse.
   (c) Buspirone does not interact with alcohol or other CNS depressants.
   (d) Buspirone produces more adverse reactions than the benzodiazepines.

4. Jason Ralph, age 29, sees his physician because of increased anxiety caused by financial problems. Because he is allergic to benzodiazepines, the physician prescribes the barbiturate phenobarbital 20 mg P.O. t.i.d. Which of the following disorders would require cautious use of phenobarbital in Mr. Ralph?
   (a) Epilepsy
   (b) Acute angle-closure glaucoma
   (c) Anorexia nervosa
   (d) Hepatic damage

44 Antipsychotic agents

OBJECTIVES

After reading and studying this chapter, the student should be able to:

1. identify the clinical indications for the antipsychotic agents.
2. describe the mechanisms of action of the antipsychotic agents.
3. identify common adverse reactions to the antipsychotic agents.
4. explain the drug regimen and adverse effects of an antipsychotic agent to the patient.
5. describe how to apply the nursing process when caring for a patient receiving an antipsychotic agent.

INTRODUCTION

Antipsychotic agents can control psychotic symptoms, such as delusions, hallucinations, and thought disorders, that can occur with **schizophrenia, mania,** and other **psychoses.** They can help treat organic psychiatric disorders, such as **dementia,** delirium, and stimulant-induced psychoses, and can sedate agitated patients. They also are used to treat the movement disorders of **Gilles de la Tourette syndrome** and **Huntington's disease,** to augment the effects of preoperative analgesics and anesthetics to control pain, and to treat nausea, vomiting, intractable hiccups, and pruritus.

Antipsychotic agents also are called major tranquilizers or **neuroleptics:** *antipsychotic* because they can eliminate signs and symptoms of psychoses, *major tranquilizer* because they can calm an agitated patient, and *neuroleptic* because they have an adverse neurobiological effect that causes abnormal body movements.

Regardless of what they are called, all antipsychotic agents belong to one of two major groups: phenothiazines or nonphenothiazines. This chapter discusses both groups. (See *Selected major antipsychotic agents,* page 548.)

Drugs covered in this chapter include:

- acetophenazine maleate
- chlorpromazine hydrochloride
- chlorprothixene
- clozapine
- fluphenazine decanoate
- fluphenazine enanthate
- fluphenazine hydrochloride
- haloperidol
- haloperidol decanoate
- loxapine succinate
- mesoridazine besylate
- molindone hydrochloride
- perphenazine
- pimozide
- prochlorperazine maleate
- prochlorperazine maleate
- promazine hydrochloride
- thioridazine hydrochloride
- thiothixene
- thiothixene hydrochloride
- trifluoperazine hydrochloride.

Phenothiazines

Antipsychotics can be classified on the basis of chemical structure. Many clinicians believe that one of these groups, the phenothiazines, should be treated as three distinct drug classes because of the differences in their adverse effects. The three classes include aliphatics (which primarily cause sedation and anticholinergic effects), piperazines (which primarily cause extrapyramidal reactions), and piperidines (which primarily cause sedation). Aliphatics are considered moderately potent.

The phenothiazines include chlorpromazine hydrochloride and promazine hydrochloride of the aliphatic subgroup; acetophenazine maleate, fluphenazine decanoate, fluphenazine enanthate, fluphenazine hydrochloride, perphenazine, and trifluoperazine hydrochloride of the piperazine subgroup; and mesoridazine besylate and thioridazine hydrochloride of the piperidine subgroup. Prochlorperazine maleate, also a phenothiazine, is used almost exclusively for controlling nausea and vomiting.

PHARMACOKINETICS

Although the phenothiazines are absorbed erratically, they are very lipid soluble and highly protein-bound. Therefore, they are distributed to many tissues and are highly concentrated in the brain. All phenothiazines are metabolized in the liver and excreted in urine and bile. Because fatty tissues slowly release accumulated phenothiazine metabolites into the plasma, the phenothiazines may produce effects up to 3 months after their discontinuation.

Selected major antipsychotic agents

This chart summarizes the major antipsychotic agents currently in clinical use.

DRUG	MAJOR INDICATIONS AND USUAL DOSAGES	CONTRAINDICATIONS AND PRECAUTIONS
Phenothiazines		
chlorpromazine (Thorazine)	*Symptomatic relief of psychoses* ADULT: initially, 200 to 600 mg P.O. daily in divided doses; for maintenance dosage, 500 to 1,000 mg P.O. daily in divided doses PEDIATRIC: for children age 6 months and over, 0.55 mg/kg P.O. or I.M. every 4 to 6 hours or 1.1 mg/kg P.R. every 6 to 8 hours	• Chlorpromazine is contraindicated in a pregnant or breast-feeding patient, a patient with bone marrow depression or known hypersensitivity, a comatose patient, a patient receiving a high dosage of a central nervous system (CNS) depressant, or a pediatric patient with signs and symptoms of Reye's syndrome. • This drug requires cautious use in a geriatric or debilitated patient, one receiving atropine or a related drug, one who has been exposed to extreme heat or organophosphate insecticides, or one with cardiovascular or liver disease, a history of seizures, chronic respiratory disorder (such as severe asthma or emphysema), acute respiratory infections (especially a pediatric patient), or glaucoma.
fluphenazine decanoate (Prolixin Decanoate)	*Symptomatic relief of psychoses* ADULT: initially, 12.5 to 25 mg I.M. or S.C. every 3 to 4 weeks	• Fluphenazine decanoate is contraindicated in a comatose or severely depressed patient or one with known hypersensitivity to the drug, suspected or proven subcortical brain damage, blood dyscrasias, or liver damage. • This drug requires cautious use in a geriatric, debilitated, or pregnant patient; one who has been exposed to extreme heat or organophosphate insecticides; one undergoing surgery who is taking large doses of fluphenazine; or one with cholestatic jaundice, dermatoses, or other allergic reactions to phenothiazine derivatives, seizure disorder, cardiovascular disease (such as mitral insufficiency), or pheochromocytoma. • Safety and efficacy in children under age 12 have not been established.
Nonphenothiazines		
haloperidol (Haldol), haloperidol decanoate (Haldol Decanoate)	*Symptomatic relief of psychoses* ADULT: 0.5 to 2 mg P.O. b.i.d. or t.i.d., increased as needed, up to a maximum of 100 mg daily PEDIATRIC: for children ages 3 to 12, 0.05 to 0.15 mg/kg P.O. daily given in two or three divided doses *Relief of dyskinesia in Gilles de la Tourette syndrome* ADULT: 0.5 to 2 mg P.O. b.i.d. or t.i.d., increased as needed, up to a maximum of 100 mg daily PEDIATRIC: for children ages 3 to 12, 0.05 to 0.075 mg/kg P.O. daily given in two or three divided doses	• Haloperidol and haloperidol decanoate are contraindicated in a pregnant or breast-feeding patient, a comatose patient, or one with toxic CNS depression, Parkinson's disease, or known hypersensitivity. • These drugs require cautious use in a patient who is receiving an anticonvulsant or anticoagulant or one with severe cardiovascular disease, thyrotoxicosis, or known allergies. • Safety and efficacy of haloperidol in children under age 3 have not been established. Safety and efficacy of haloperidol decanoate in children have not been established.
clozapine (clozaril)	*Management of severely ill schizophrenic patients* ADULT: 12.5 mg qd or b.i.d. P.O., then increase in 25-to 50-mg increments until a target dose of 300 to 450 mg/day is reached	• Clozapine is contraindicated in patients with uncontrolled epilepsy, a previous hypersensitivity reaction, a white blood cell count below 3,500/mm^3, severe CNS depression, and myelosuppression disorders. • Use cautiously in patients with prostatic hyperplasia; angle-closure glaucoma; hepatic, renal, or cardiac disease; and those receiving general anesthesia.

Route	Onset	Peak	Duration
P.O.	Variable	30 min	6-8 hr
I.M.	15-30 min	1.5-2 hr	6-8 hr

PHARMACODYNAMICS

Although the mechanism of action of phenothiazines is not understood fully, researchers believe that these drugs work through strong postsynaptic blockade of dopaminergic receptors. They depress the reticular activating system, the hypothalamus, the chemoreceptor trigger zone and, to some extent, the vomiting center. Phenothiazines also stimulate the extrapyramidal system.

PHARMACOTHERAPEUTICS

Phenothiazines are used primarily to treat schizophrenia, to calm anxious or agitated patients, to improve a patient's thought processes, and to alleviate delusions and hallucinations. These agents may be used to treat other psychiatric disorders, such as brief reactive psychosis, atypical psychosis, schizoaffective psychosis, pervasive development disorder (autism), bipolar affective disorder (**manic-depressive disorder**), and major **depression** with psychosis. In manic-depressive patients, the phenothiazines are administered with lithium until the slower-acting lithium produces its therapeutic effect. They can be used to quiet mentally retarded children and agitated geriatric patients, particularly those with dementia.

The phenothiazines also are used to augment the preoperative effects of analgesics and to manage pain, anxiety, and nausea in patients with cancer. Additional indications vary with the specific phenothiazine.

Initial dosing with phenothiazines can be rapid or slow, depending on the severity of symptoms and the patient's age and physical condition. In acute psychosis, the patient receives a loading dose; a patient receiving a high dosage must be hospitalized so that the drug's effectiveness and adverse reactions can be monitored. When the symptoms are under control, the patient receives a low maintenance dosage. Because phenothiazines have long half-lives, the maintenance dosage may consist of a single bedtime dose. If severe orthostatic hypotension occurs in the morning, the patient may require divided doses.

Unlike other adults, a geriatric or debilitated patient will receive a small initial dosage that is increased gradually until a favorable response is achieved. After the patient has taken that dosage for about 2 weeks, it is reduced gradually to the lowest effective maintenance dosage.

Drug interactions

Phenothiazines interact with many different types of drugs. (See Drug Interactions: *Phenothiazines,* page 550.)

ADVERSE DRUG REACTIONS

Neurologic reactions are the most common and serious adverse reactions associated with phenothiazines. They include extrapyramidal effects, which may appear any time after the first few days of therapy, and **tardive dyskinesia,** which usually occurs after several years of treatment. Phenothiazines also may lower the seizure threshold. (See *Common neurologic effects of antipsychotic agents,* page 551.)

Phenothiazines can cause severe and possibly irreversible tardive dyskinesia, especially in geriatric and debilitated patients. However, their actions sometimes mask tardive dyskinesia. A **drug holiday** may be prescribed for a patient on long-term phenothiazine therapy to unmask this adverse reaction. The patient receives no antipsychotic drugs for 4 or more weeks and is observed for adverse reactions. A drug holiday also is used to delay the appearance of tardive dyskinesia, which is related to the total accumulated phenothiazine dosage.

Phenothiazines are not associated with psychological dependence, tolerance, or addiction. On abrupt withdrawal, however, they produce signs and symptoms that resemble physical dependence, such as nausea, vomiting, gastritis, dizziness, tremors, sweating, tachycardia, headache, and insomnia.

Phenothiazines also may produce adverse reactions in the autonomic nervous and endocrine systems, including sedation, hypotension, orthostatic hypotension, and anticholinergic effects.

Hypersensitivity to phenothiazines can cause additional effects such as photosensitive skin reactions. Other skin reactions, such as urticaria and dermatitis, are less common.

Although they are rare, more serious adverse reactions can occur, including blood dyscrasias and jaundice. Neuroleptic malignant syndrome is a serious condition that produces muscle rigidity, hyperpyrexia, autonomic instability, and cardiovascular collapse. Dantrolene and bromocriptine are used to treat this life-threatening syndrome.

NURSING PROCESS APPLICATION

The following information assists the nurse in caring for a patient who is receiving a phenothiazine. It includes an overview of assessment activities as well as examples of appropriate nursing diagnoses and related interventions (see "Planning and implementation"). It also highlights the importance of evaluation.

Assessment

Before drug therapy begins, review the patient's history for conditions that contraindicate or require cautious use of the prescribed phenothiazine. Also review the patient's medication history to identify use of drugs that may interact with it. During therapy, assess the patient for adverse drug reactions and signs of drug interactions. Also, periodically assess the effectiveness of phenothiazine therapy. Finally, evaluate

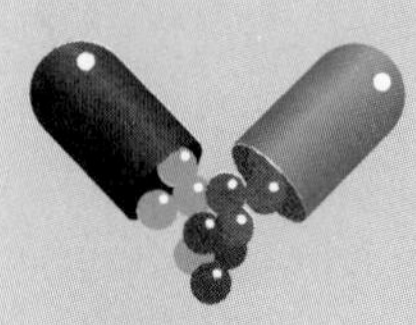

DRUG INTERACTIONS

Phenothiazines

Drug interactions involving phenothiazines can be serious. Interactions occur commonly with concurrent use of alcohol or other central nervous system (CNS) depressants.

DRUG	INTERACTING DRUGS	POSSIBLE EFFECTS	NURSING IMPLICATIONS
chlorpromazine, fluphenazine, mesoridazine, perphenazine, promazine, thioridazine, trifluoperazine	guanethidine	Inhibited uptake of guanethidine	• Monitor the patient's blood pressure frequently. • Expect to increase the guanethidine dosage or replace guanethidine with another antihypertensive agent, as prescribed.
	amphetamines, nonamphetamine anorexigenic agents	Decreased effects of both drugs	• Do not administer these drugs concurrently.
	anticholinergic agents	Increased anticholinergic effects, decreased antipsychotic effects	• Do not administer together routinely. If the drugs must be given concurrently, assess the patient for signs of reduced phenothiazine effects such as increased psychotic behavior. • Perform abdominal assessments to monitor the patient for diminished or absent bowel sounds, abdominal pain, constipation, and other abdominal problems.
	CNS depressants (barbiturates, narcotic analgesics, general anesthetics, alcohol)	Increased CNS depressant effects; increased phenothiazine metabolism	• Observe the patient for erratic therapeutic effects by behavior changes such as increased psychotic behavior or agitation, for hypotension and CNS and respiratory depression, and for increased CNS depressant effects such as stupor.
	levodopa	Decreased antiparkinsonian effects of levodopa	• Avoid concurrent administration, if possible.
	lithium	Increased risk of neurotoxicity, seizures, delirium, and encephalopathy in manic patients; respiratory depression and hypotension	• Monitor the patient for an increase in parkinsonian symptoms. • Monitor the patient for reduced phenothiazine response and changes in neurologic status. • Monitor the patient's vital signs frequently.
	droperidol	Increased risk of extrapyramidal effects	• Monitor the patient for tremors. • Monitor the patient's vital signs frequently.
	anticonvulsants	Lowered seizure threshold	• Monitor the patient for seizures. • Expect to increase the anticonvulsant dosage, as prescribed.
	tricyclic antidepressants, beta blockers	Increased serum levels of either agent	• Monitor the patient for adverse reactions to either agent.

the patient's and family's knowledge about the prescribed drug.

Nursing diagnoses

- Risk for injury related to a preexisting condition that contraindicates or requires cautious use of a phenothiazine
- Risk for injury related to adverse drug reactions or drug interactions
- Altered cerebral tissue perfusion related to the hypotensive effects of the prescribed phenothiazine
- Knowledge deficit related to the prescribed phenothiazine

Planning and implementation

- Do not administer a phenothiazine to a patient with a condition that contraindicates its use.
- Administer a phenothiazine cautiously to a patient at risk because of a preexisting condition.
- Monitor the patient for adverse reactions and drug interactions during phenothiazine therapy.

Common neurologic effects of antipsychotic agents

Phenothiazines and other antipsychotic drugs commonly produce adverse neurologic reactions ranging from extrapyramidal effects to tardive dyskinesia. These effects are illustrated below.

Dystonia

In the 1st week of antipsychotic therapy, the patient may exhibit an acute dystonic reaction — an extrapyramidal effect manifested by spasms in the tongue, face, neck, back, and sometimes legs that may resemble a seizure. Spasms sometimes affect certain groups of muscles only. Contracted cervical muscles can result in torticollis, an unnatural or twisted position of the neck. Opisthotonos, grimacing, perioral spasms, or pharyngeal or laryngeal spasms with dysphagia or dyspnea also can occur. Eye muscle spasms can cause oculogyrations — abnormal eye movements. Commonly accompanied by excessive salivation, these dystonic spasms typically occur when a patient receives large doses of an antipsychotic agent that is likely to produce extrapyramidal symptoms. They usually disappear with a dosage reduction or administration of 25 to 50 mg intramuscular (I.M.) diphenhydramine or 1 to 2 mg I.M. or intravenous benztropine.

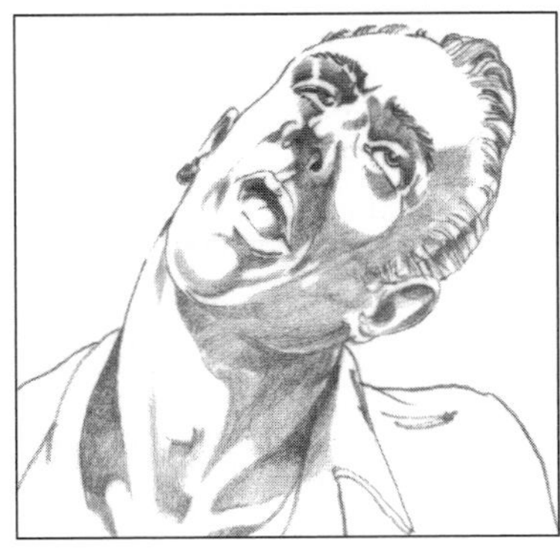

Akathisia

Another extrapyramidal effect, akathisia (a continuous restlessness or inability to sit or stand still) may occur in the first 90 days of therapy. The patient attempts to relieve the discomfort of remaining quiet by tapping a foot, moving about in a chair, or pacing constantly. This symptom can easily be mistaken for agitation, which requires treatment with a higher dosage of an antipsychotic agent. However, akathisia should be managed by decreasing the antipsychotic dosage or by giving an antiparkinsonian agent such as benztropine.

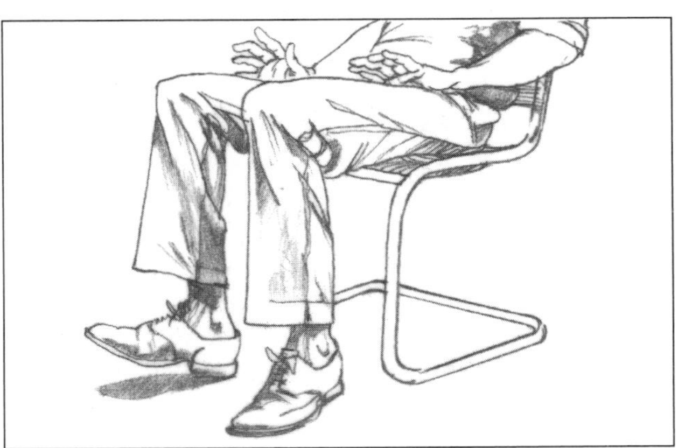

Pseudoparkinsonism

Later in the course of treatment, pseudoparkinsonism may occur. This extrapyramidal effect produces muscle tremors, cogwheel rigidity (muscle rigidity that gives way in little jerks when the muscle is stretched passively), shuffling gait, drooling, and a decrease in arm swing and associative movements when walking. Bradykinesia (slow movement) and akinesia (immobility) also may occur. Pseudoparkinsonism results from a direct blockade of dopamine receptors by antipsychotic agents. This reaction may be controlled with the use of antiparkinsonian agents, such as amantadine or cogentin.

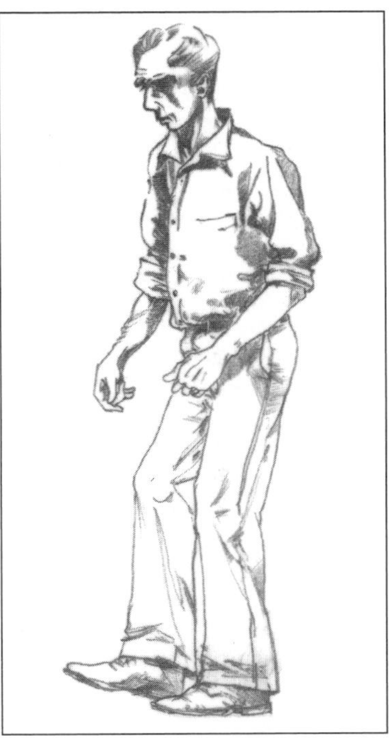

Tardive dyskinesia

Tardive dyskinesia may appear after several months or years of treatment with antipsychotic drugs. It is characterized by abnormal muscle movements, primarily around the mouth, such as lip smacking, rhythmic darting of the tongue, and constant chewing movements. Slow, aimless, involuntary movements of the arms or legs also may occur. Although the exact mechanism of tardive dyskinesia is not clear, researchers believe that it may differ from that of the other extrapyramidal symptoms. Tardive dyskinesia usually affects geriatric female patients, but can occur in younger patients as well, even after short-term antipsychotic therapy. If the medication is discontinued when the first signs such as fine wormlike tongue movements are detected, tardive dyskinesia sometimes can be prevented.

Prevention of this adverse reaction is vital because no effective treatment is available and the reaction usually is irreversible.

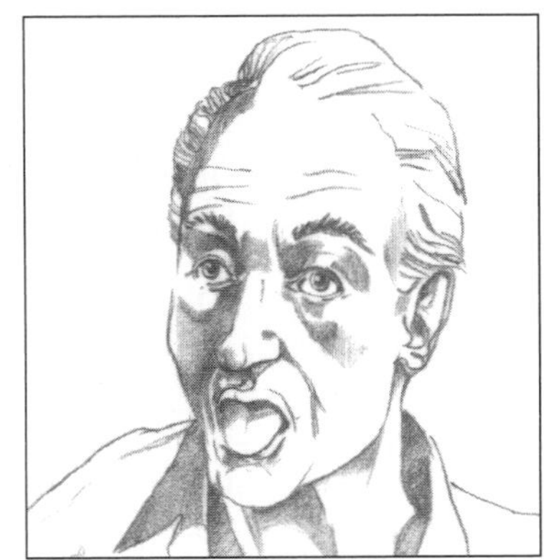

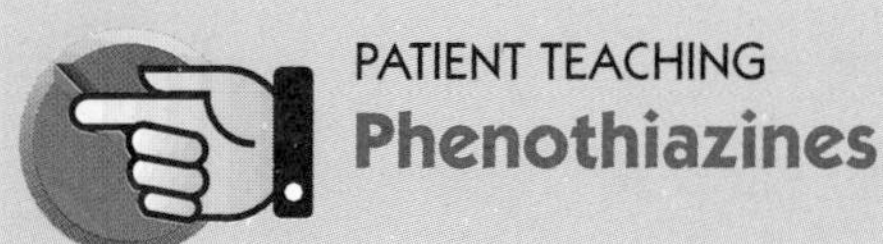

PATIENT TEACHING
Phenothiazines

- Teach the patient (if appropriate) and family the name, dose, frequency, action, and adverse effects of the prescribed phenothiazine.
- Alert the family that psychological dependence can occur with phenothiazine use.
- Inform the family that they can expect to see normalization of thoughts, moods, and actions in the patient after several weeks or months of phenothiazine therapy.
- Stress the importance of taking the phenothiazine exactly as prescribed and not discontinuing it without the physician's approval because psychotic symptoms may return.
- Ask the family to tell the physician if the patient does not comply with the drug regimen. The physician may change the drug to fluphenazine decanoate or fluphenazine enanthate because their effects last for up to 6 weeks.
- Advise the patient to obtain the physician's approval before ingesting other central nervous system depressants.
- Teach the patient how to manage troublesome anticholinergic effects.
- Instruct the patient to return regularly for follow-up care, which includes periodic dosage adjustments.
- Instruct the family to notify the physician at the first sign of tardive dyskinesia to prevent permanent damage.
- Prepare the patient receiving long-term phenothiazine therapy for a drug holiday, as instructed. During the 4 or more weeks of the drug holiday, the patient and family should watch for — and report to the physician — signs of tardive dyskinesia.
- Advise the patient not to discontinue the drug abruptly.
- Teach the patient how to manage orthostatic hypotension.
- Instruct the family to use safety precautions such as supervising the patient's ambulation if mild sedation occurs and to alert the physician if sedation worsens or seizures occur.
- Teach the patient to recognize and report the signs of urine retention.
- Instruct the patient and family to notify the physician of other adverse reactions or changes in psychotic symptoms.

*** *Observe for extrapyramidal symptoms. Notify the physician immediately if the patient exhibits acute dystonic reactions, particularly if face or neck spasms interfere with swallowing or breathing.***

• Assess the patient for early signs of tardive dyskinesia such as wormlike movements of the tongue. If these signs appear, suggest a change in the drug regimen.

• Expect a drug holiday to be prescribed to check for tardive dyskinesia in a patient receiving long-term phenothiazine therapy. When beginning the drug holiday, remember not to discontinue the drug abruptly to prevent withdrawal symptoms. During the 4 or more weeks of the drug holiday, observe the patient closely for tardive dyskinesia, which is exhibited by abnormal muscle movement primarily around the mouth (such as lip smacking, rhythmic darting of the tongue, and constant chewing movements) and by slow, aimless, involuntary movements of the arms and legs.

• Do not give intramuscular (I.M.) trifluoperazine injections more frequently than every 4 hours if the dosage exceeds 10 mg daily because of the drug's cumulative effects.

• Do not administer more than 800 mg of thioridazine daily because retinal pigmentation may occur.

• Relieve anticholinergic effects, for example, by offering the patient sugarless gum or chipped ice to relieve dry mouth and increasing the patient's fluid and fiber intake to prevent constipation. (See Patient Teaching: *Phenothiazines.*)

• Observe and report patient behavior carefully because the response to treatment can vary widely among individuals.

• Document the effects of therapy so that the patient may receive the lowest effective dosage. Note, in particular, whether the patient is sedated, stimulated, agitated, or overactive, and describe any changes in thought patterns and speech that might indicate hallucinations or delusions.

• Notify the physician if adverse reactions or drug interactions occur.

• Monitor the patient's blood pressure regularly to detect hypotension.

*** *Use caution when administering phenothiazines with narcotics or other central nervous system (CNS) depressants because they can induce hypotension.***

• Expect to administer the prescribed phenothiazine in divided doses if severe orthostatic hypotension occurs in the morning.

• Have the patient sit up for 1 to 2 minutes before standing to minimize the effects of orthostatic hypotension.

*** *Monitor the patient for signs of altered cerebral perfusion, such as decreased blood pressure or changes in level of consciousness or behavior. If these signs occur, take safety precautions and notify the physician.***

Evaluation

For each nursing diagnosis, prepare an evaluation statement that describes the patient's or family's response to nursing interventions.

Nonphenothiazines

Based on their chemical structure, nonphenothiazine antipsychotics can be divided into several drug classes, including the butyrophenones, such as haloperidol and haloperidol decanoate; dibenzodiazepines such as clozapine; dibenzoxazepines such as loxapine succinate; dihydroindolones such as molindone hydrochloride; diphenylbutylpiperidines such as pimozide; and thioxanthenes, such as chlorprothixene, thiothixene, and thiothixene hydrochloride. Clozapine is the newest nonphenothiazine.

PHARMACOKINETICS

Nonphenothiazines are absorbed, distributed, metabolized, and excreted in the same manner as the phenothiazines.

Route	Onset	Peak	Duration
P.O.	Unknown	3-6 hr	Variable
I.M.	Unknown	10-20 min	Unknown

PHARMACODYNAMICS

Except for clozapine, the mechanism of action of the nonphenothiazines resembles that of the phenothiazines. Clozapine's structure differs from that of the other nonphenothiazines. Unlike the other drugs in this category, which block dopamine receptors, clozapine is a weak blocker of dopamine receptors but a potent blocker of **serotonin** activity.

PHARMACOTHERAPEUTICS

As a group, nonphenothiazines are used to treat psychotic disorders. Specific drugs in this group may serve additional functions. For example, thiothixene also is used to control acute agitation. Haloperidol and pimozide may be used to treat Gilles de la Tourette syndrome. Because of its adverse effects, clozapine is reserved for patients who have not responded to therapy with other antipsychotic agents or who have developed tardive dyskinesia. It is beneficial in the treatment of negative symptoms, such as emotional blunting and poor socialization.

Drug interactions

Nonphenothiazines interact with fewer drugs than the phenothiazines. However, their dopamine-blocking activity can inhibit levodopa and may cause disorientation in patients receiving both medications. Haloperidol also may augment the effects of lithium, producing encephalopathy. Concomitant administration of clozapine with anticholinergic agents may result in additive anticholinergic effects. The hypotensive effects of antihypertensive agents may be potentiated by clozapine use. Additive CNS effects may result when clozapine is administered with other agents that affect the CNS. Clozapine may cause granulocytopenia and should not be administered with other agents known to suppress the bone marrow. Because clozapine is highly protein-bound, it may cause protein-binding displacement when administered with such other highly bound drugs as warfarin or phenytoin and may lead to drug toxicity.

ADVERSE DRUG REACTIONS

Most nonphenothiazines cause the same adverse reactions as the phenothiazines. Compared with the other nonphenothiazines, clozapine produces fewer extrapyramidal reactions and no tardive dyskinesia. Divided doses and cautious titration of clozapine help minimize the risk of hypotension, sedation, and seizures. Its major adverse reaction is the development of life-threatening neutropenia or granulocytopenia, which typically occur within the first 6 months of therapy. Weekly blood counts should be done on all patients receiving clozapine.

NURSING PROCESS APPLICATION

The following information assists the nurse in caring for a patient who is receiving a nonphenothiazine. It includes an overview of assessment activities as well as examples of appropriate nursing diagnoses and related interventions (see "Planning and implementation"). It also highlights the importance of evaluation.

Assessment

Before drug therapy begins, review the patient's history for conditions that contraindicate or require cautious use of the prescribed nonphenothiazine. Also review the patient's medication history to identify use of drugs that may interact with it. During therapy, assess the patient for adverse drug reactions and signs of drug interactions. Also, periodically assess the effectiveness of nonphenothiazine therapy. Finally, evaluate the patient's and family's knowledge about the prescribed drug. (See Patient Teaching: *Nonphenothiazines,* page 554.)

Nursing diagnoses

- Risk for injury related to a preexisting condition that contraindicates or requires cautious use of a nonphenothiazine
- Risk for injury related to adverse drug reactions or drug interactions
- Urinary retention related to the anticholinergic effects of the prescribed nonphenothiazine
- Knowledge deficit related to the prescribed nonphenothiazine

Planning and implementation

- Do not administer a nonphenothiazine to a patient with a condition that contraindicates its use.
- Administer a nonphenothiazine cautiously to a patient at risk because of a preexisting condition.
- Monitor the patient for adverse reactions and drug interactions during nonphenothiazine therapy.

*✱ **Observe for extrapyramidal symptoms. Notify the physician immediately if the patient exhibits acute dystonic reactions, particularly if face or neck spasms interfere with swallowing or breathing.***

- Assess the patient for early signs of tardive dyskinesia such as wormlike movements of the tongue. If these signs appear, suggest a change in the drug regimen.
- Expect a drug holiday to be prescribed to check for tardive dyskinesia in a patient receiving long-term nonphenothiazine therapy. During the 4 or more weeks of the drug holiday, observe the patient for tardive dyskinesia, exhibited by abnormal muscle movements primarily around the

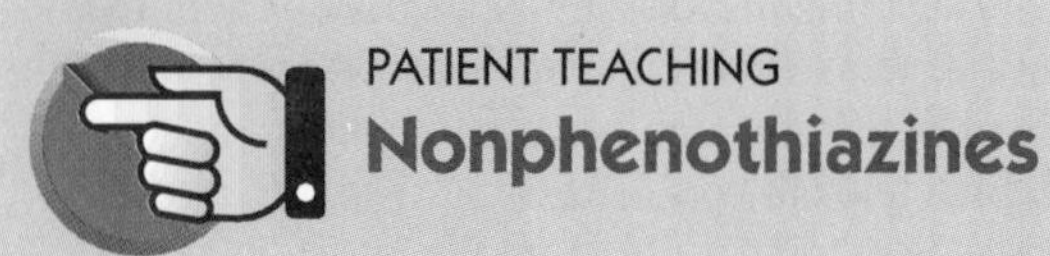

PATIENT TEACHING
Nonphenothiazines

- ➤ Teach the patient (if appropriate) and family the name, dose, frequency, action, and adverse effects of the prescribed nonphenothiazine.
- ➤ Inform the family that they can expect to see normalization of thoughts, moods, and actions in the patient after several weeks or months of nonphenothiazine therapy.
- ➤ Stress the importance of taking the nonphenothiazine exactly as prescribed and not discontinuing it without physician approval because psychotic symptoms may return.
- ➤ Teach the patient how to manage troublesome anticholinergic effects.
- ➤ Encourage the patient to return regularly for follow-up care, which includes periodic dosage adjustments and laboratory studies.
- ➤ Instruct the family to notify the physician at the first sign of tardive dyskinesia to prevent permanent damage.
- ➤ Prepare the patient receiving long-term nonphenothiazine therapy for a drug holiday, as instructed. During the 4 or more weeks of the drug holiday, the patient and family should watch for — and report to the physician — signs of tardive dyskinesia.
- ➤ Advise the patient to use a sunscreen and wear protective clothing outdoors to prevent a photosensitivity reaction.
- ➤ Teach the patient how to manage orthostatic hypotension.
- ➤ Teach the patient to recognize and report the signs of urine retention.
- ➤ Teach the patient to recognize and report the signs of agranulocytosis if the patient is taking clozapine.
- ➤ Instruct the patient and family to notify the physician of other adverse reactions or changes in psychotic symptoms.

mouth (such as lip smacking, rhythmic darting of the tongue, and constant chewing movements) and by slow, aimless, involuntary movements of the arms or legs.

- Expect the patient to be changed to clozapine if tardive dyskinesia occurs or if the patient does not respond to standard drug therapy.
- Administer clozapine in divided doses, as prescribed, and titrate it cautiously to minimize the risk of hypotension, sedation, and seizures, as prescribed.
- Monitor the patient taking chlorprothixene for an allergic reaction because it contains tartrazine.
- Expect to administer a small initial dosage of the prescribed nonphenothiazine and gradually increase it until a favorable response is achieved in a geriatric or debilitated patient. With thiothixene, a geriatric patient should receive only one-half to one-third of the normal I.M. or oral dosage.
- Protect haloperidol from exposure to light. Haloperidol may be administered if it becomes slightly yellow, but it must be discarded if the solution is markedly discolored because its potency will have decreased.

∗ Avoid abrupt discontinuation of the prescribed nonphenothiazine unless severe adverse reactions make this necessary.

- Relieve anticholinergic effects, for example, by offering the patient sugarless gum or chipped ice to relieve dry mouth and increasing the patient's fluid and fiber intake to prevent constipation, unless otherwise contraindicated.
- Observe and report patient behavior carefully because the response to treatment can vary widely among individuals.
- Document the effects of therapy so that the patient may receive the lowest effective dosage. Note, in particular, whether the patient is stimulated, agitated, or overactive, and describe any changes in thought patterns and speech that might indicate hallucinations or delusions.
- Notify the physician if adverse reactions or drug interactions occur.
- Monitor the patient for signs of urine retention, such as frequent trips to the bathroom, complaints of a sense of fullness in the lower abdomen, dullness on percussion of the lower abdomen, and palpation of a distended bladder.
- Notify the physician and prepare to catheterize the patient if assessment findings suggest urine retention. Expect to decrease the nonphenothiazine dosage or change the patient to another drug.

Evaluation

For each nursing diagnosis, prepare an evaluation statement that describes the patient's or family's response to nursing interventions.

CHAPTER SUMMARY

Chapter 44 presented antipsychotic agents used to control the symptoms of psychoses. Here are the chapter highlights.

All antipsychotic agents belong to one of two major groups: phenothiazines or nonphenothiazines. Phenothiazines include chlorpromazine, promazine, acetophenazine, fluphenazine, perphenazine, trifluoperazine, mesoridazine, and thioridazine. Nonphenothiazines include haloperidol, clozapine, loxapine, molindone, pimozide, chlorprothixene, and thiothixene.

Antipsychotic agents also are used to calm or sedate agitated or disturbed patients with psychotic symptoms, to alleviate nausea and vomiting, and to enhance the effects of preoperative analgesics and anesthetics to control pain.

The newest nonphenothiazine, clozapine can cause severe neutropenia and granulocytopenia. Because of these adverse reactions, clozapine is reserved for patients who do not respond to therapy with standard antipsychotic agents or who have tardive dyskinesia.

During antipsychotic therapy, the nurse uses the nursing process to guide patient care. Nursing activities typically include monitoring the patient and promoting compliance. The nurse also should teach the patient about the drug, its regimen, its therapeutic and adverse effects, and other considerations.

Questions to consider

See Appendix 1 for answers.

1. Amy Halstead, age 32, requires emergency hospitalization for an acute psychiatric disorder. As part of her admission orders, the physician prescribes the phenothiazine chlorpromazine 125 mg P.O. q.i.d. After receiving the drug for a week, Ms. Halstead develops constipation. Which of the following drug effects is responsible for this adverse reaction?
   (a) Antiadrenergic
   (b) Anticholinergic
   (c) Extrapyramidal
   (d) Adrenergic

2. Which of the following instructions should the nurse provide for a patient about to be discharged with a prescription for the drug chlorpromazine?
   (a) Stop taking the drug as soon as you begin to feel better.
   (b) Take the drug exactly as prescribed, even if symptoms disappear.
   (c) Take the drug with an antacid if gastric distress occurs.
   (d) Increase or decrease the dosage, depending on how you feel.

3. Jonathan Batts, age 80, has dementia and becomes agitated while in the hospital for treatment of a fractured hip. The physician prescribes haloperidol 0.5 mg I.M. b.i.d until symptoms are controlled. When preparing a haloperidol injection for Mr. Batts, the nurse notices that the medication is slightly yellow. What should the nurse do?
   (a) Administer the medication; a slightly yellow color is acceptable.
   (b) Administer the medication; the normal color is light yellow.
   (c) Discard the medication; its potency will have decreased.
   (d) Double the dosage to offset the deterioration of the drug.

4. Neuroleptic malignant syndrome is associated with the use of which of the following medications?
   (a) clonazepam
   (b) phenytoin
   (c) promazine
   (d) sertraline

5. James Compher is prescribed clozapine. Which of the following adverse reactions should the nurse be concerned about?
   (a) Hypertension
   (b) Dyspnea
   (c) Tardive dyskinesia
   (d) Blood dyscrasias

UNIT XIII

Drugs to treat endocrine system disorders

This unit presents agents used to treat endocrine system disorders. Endocrine pharmacology encompasses a wide range of agents, including natural hormones and their synthetic analogues, hormonelike substances, and drugs that stimulate or suppress hormone secretion. To understand endocrine pharmacology, the nurse needs to know about the endocrine system and its hormones. (See *Endocrine hormones.*)

PANCREATIC HORMONES

The pancreas performs endocrine and exocrine functions. The exocrine functions include the production of enzymes necessary for the digestion of proteins, carbohydrates, and fats. The endocrine functions arise from the islets of Langerhans in the pancreas. The islet cells of Langerhans consist of three specialized cell types: alpha, beta, and delta. The alpha cells produce glucagon. The beta cells produce insulin. The delta cells produce somatostatin.

Insulin promotes glucose uptake, storage, and use; glucagon increases **glycogenolysis** and **gluconeogenesis.** Insulin also inhibits **lipolysis** and promotes cellular uptake of amino acids and protein synthesis. The blood glucose level primarily controls insulin and glucagon secretion. At a normal fasting blood glucose level, (70 to 110 mg/dl), little insulin is secreted. When the blood glucose level rises above 110 mg/dl, insulin secretion rapidly increases. When it falls below 70 mg/dl, glucagon secretion increases, rapidly increasing hepatic glucose production. Thus, glucagon prevents **hypoglycemia** and insulin prevents **hyperglycemia.**

Somatostatin inhibits the release of glucagon and insulin and prolongs the absorption of nutrients into the bloodstream. There is a continual feedback and interaction between somatostatin, insulin, and glucagon that maintains normal blood sugar values.

THYROID HORMONES

The thyroid gland secretes triiodothyronine (T_3) and thyroxine (T_4), which influence the body's metabolic rate, and **calcitonin,** which helps regulate calcium metabolism. Secretion of these thyroid hormones is controlled primarily by thyroid-stimulating hormone (TSH), which is secreted by the anterior pituitary gland.

The thyroid gland secretes more T_4 than T_3. Although the hormones function the same physiologically, they differ in onset and intensity of action. T_3 is about four times as potent as T_4 and produces effects much more rapidly. Yet both hormones increase protein synthesis, stimulate cellular enzyme activity, promote growth, and enhance carbohydrate and fat metabolism. They also increase cardiac output and heart rate, respiratory rate and depth, and gastrointestinal (GI) motility.

Calcitonin is secreted primarily by the thyroid gland. When the serum calcium level is high, calcitonin secretion increases. Calcitonin reduces the serum calcium level by inhibiting bone resorption, reducing osteoclast activity (bone absorption and removal), and increasing renal excretion of calcium.

PARATHYROID HORMONE

Secretion of parathyroid hormone by the parathyroid glands is regulated primarily by the plasma calcium concentration. Any physiologic or pathologic alteration that increases the serum calcium level will suppress parathyroid gland secretion. Any decrease in serum calcium level will increase parathyroid gland secretion.

Parathyroid hormone stimulates the absorption of calcium and phosphate from bone. It also increases GI absorption and decreases renal excretion of calcium.

ANTERIOR PITUITARY HORMONES

The anterior pituitary gland secretes a variety of hormones that help control metabolic processes throughout the body: growth hormone (GH), corticotropin, TSH, prolactin, follicle-stimulating hormone (FSH), and luteinizing hormone (LH).

Endocrine hormones

In the endocrine system, various glands secrete different endocrine hormones, listed below. These hormones either stimulate or inhibit the activity of target glands or cells to maintain homeostasis.

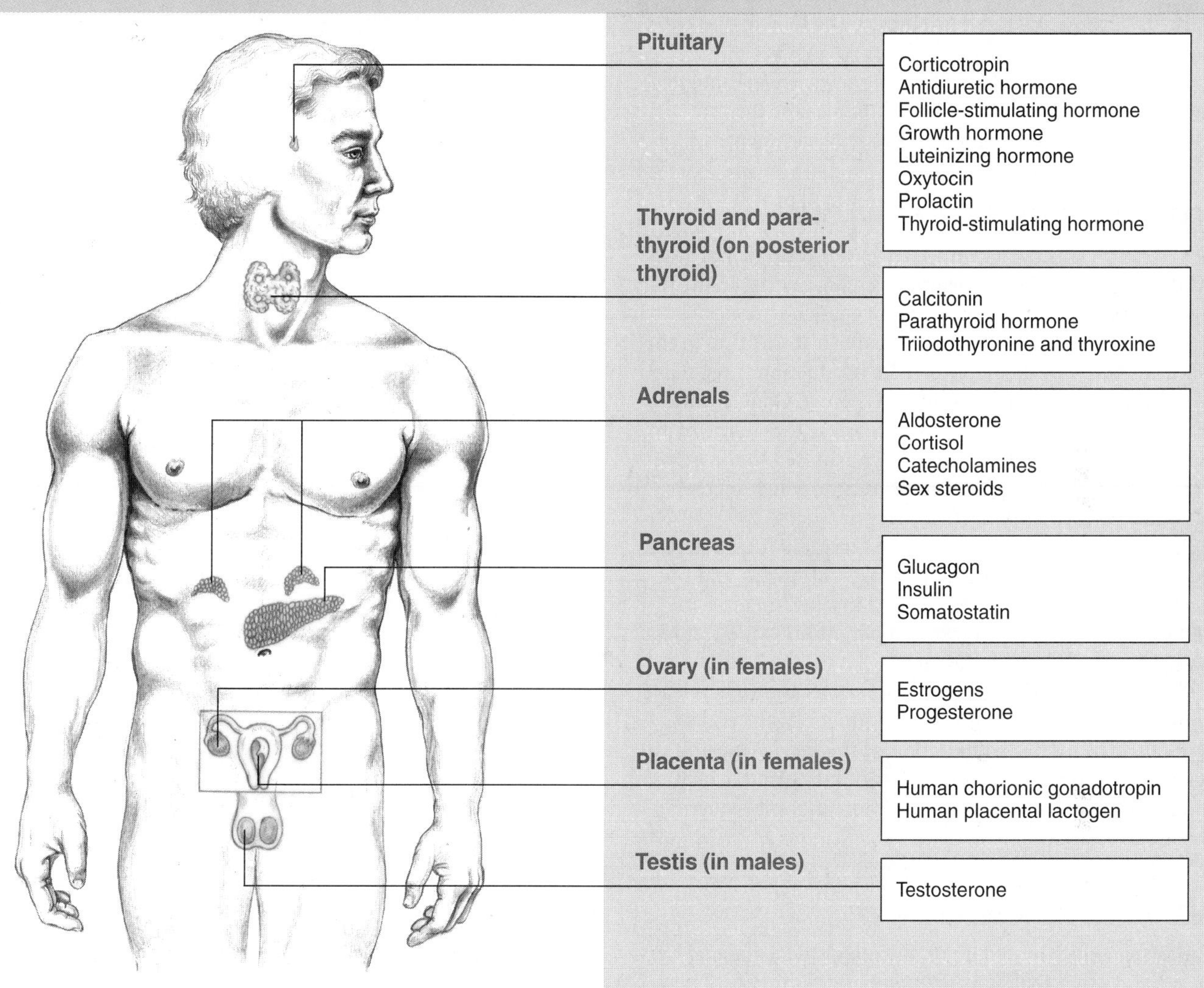

Also called somatotropic hormone or somatotropin, GH promotes growth by increasing protein synthesis, decreasing carbohydrate use, and increasing fat mobilization and use for energy.

Corticotropin, also called **adrenocorticotropin**, controls cortisol secretion and enhances androgen production by the adrenal gland. It also influences aldosterone secretion.

TSH, or **thyrotropin,** stimulates the thyroid gland to increase T_3 and T_4 production and secretion. Normally, the thyroid hormone level remains fairly constant because of an effective feedback mechanism. Increased levels of thyroid hormone inhibit TSH secretion from the pituitary gland; decreased levels stimulate TSH secretion. A hypothalamic hormone, thyrotropin-releasing hormone, regulates the increase in TSH secretion.

Prolactin promotes mammary gland development and milk production. Prolactin secretion predominantly is under the negative control of the hypothalamus, which synthesizes a hormone that suppresses its secretion from the pituitary gland. During lactation, however, formation of this prolactin inhibitory hormone is suppressed, and sucking or breast manipulation stimulates prolactin secretion.

FSH and LH are **gonadotropic** hormones secreted in response to a hypothalamic-releasing hormone and regulated by plasma estrogen and progesterone levels. During each female reproductive cycle, FSH and LH plasma levels increase and decrease. During the first phase of the cycle, increased hormone secretion stimulates new follicle growth in the ovaries. Eventually, one follicle becomes more highly developed than the others and begins to secrete large amounts of estrogen, which triggers a feedback mechanism that inhibits

FSH secretion by the anterior pituitary gland. This makes the other follicles stop growing and involute. The one large follicle continues to grow through the self-stimulating effect of the secreted estrogen. Shortly before ovulation, LH and FSH secretion by the anterior pituitary gland increases markedly, producing rapid swelling of the follicle that culminates in ovulation.

LH and FSH also has an effect on males. FSH stimulates the testes to produce sperm. LH stimulates the interstitial cells in the testes to develop and produce testosterone.

POSTERIOR PITUITARY HORMONES

The posterior pituitary gland secretes antidiuretic hormone (ADH) and oxytocin. Nerve impulses originating in the hypothalamus regulate the secretion of these hormones.

ADH, or vasopressin, increases water reabsorption in the collecting ducts of the nephrons. Its production is regulated by osmotic receptors and volume receptors. Concentration of body fluids stimulates the osmotic receptors in the hypothalamus, increasing the impulses transmitted to the posterior pituitary to stimulate ADH secretion, which increases the water permeability of the collecting ducts.

Blood loss stimulates the volume receptors (atrial stretch receptors and baroreceptors in the carotid, aortic, and pulmonary arteries). This precipitates a marked increase in ADH secretion. ADH also exerts a potent pressor effect to maintain arterial blood pressure.

Oxytocin produces uterine contractions and milk release from the breast alveoli into the milk ducts. At the end of pregnancy, stretching or irritation of the cervix transmits a neurogenic reflex to the posterior pituitary gland, which stimulates increased oxytocin secretion and, subsequently, uterine contraction.

GONADAL HORMONES

The testes secrete testosterone, the major male gonadal hormone, and other male sex hormones, or androgens. These hormones produce **androgenic** (masculinizing) effects but also exert some **anabolic** effects. The adrenal gland also secretes androgens, but they are much less potent and do not produce significant androgenic effects.

The ovaries secrete estrogens and progesterone in response to FSH and LH. Estrogens stimulate the cellular proliferation and growth of female sex organs and related reproductive tissues. They also affect skeletal growth, fat deposition, skin vascularity, and various intracellular functions. Progesterone promotes secretory changes in the endometrium to prepare the uterus for implantation of the fertilized ovum. It also evokes secretory changes in the fallopian tubes and breasts.

Estrogen or progesterone can inhibit ovulation by a negative feedback effect on the hypothalamus and subsequent suppression of FSH and LH release.

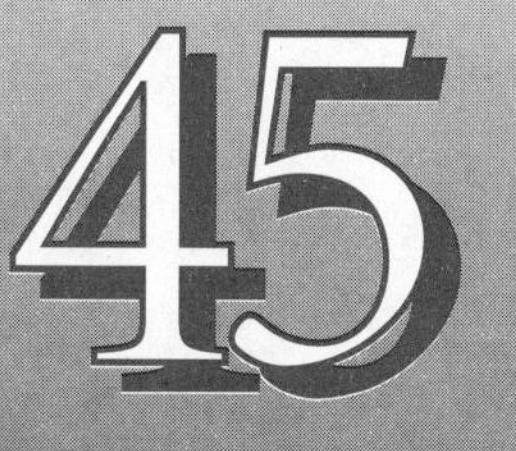

Antidiabetic agents and glucagon

OBJECTIVES

After reading and studying this chapter, the student should be able to:

1. Identify the different sources of insulins and describe how they are classified.
2. Describe the action by which insulin decreases the blood glucose level.
3. Identify the important points the nurse should teach a diabetic patient about taking insulin.
4. Discuss the pharmacokinetics of oral antidiabetic agents.
5. Identify the clinical uses of oral antidiabetic agents.
6. Explain how glucagon increases the blood glucose level.
7. Describe how to apply the nursing process when caring for a patient who is receiving an antidiabetic agent or glucagon.

INTRODUCTION

Scattered throughout the pancreas are cell clusters known as the islets of Langerhans. Beta cells in the islets of Langerhans produce insulin; alpha cells there produce glucagon. Insulin decreases the blood glucose level, whereas glucagon increases it.

During normal carbohydrate metabolism, insulin facilitates glucose uptake, storage, and metabolism. It also increases protein synthesis, inhibits protein breakdown, stimulates triglyceride synthesis, and inhibits fat breakdown. Without insulin, the body cannot metabolize glucose and must break down protein and fat for fuel.

Glucagon opposes the actions of insulin. It stimulates **glycogenolysis** (conversion of glycogen to glycose) and **gluconeogenesis** (glucose production from protein breakdown), increases **lipolysis** (fat breakdown), and inhibits triglyceride storage.

Insulin and oral hypoglycemic preparations are classified as antidiabetic or hypoglycemic agents because they lower blood glucose levels. Glucagon is classified as a hyperglycemic agent because it raises blood glucose levels. (See *Selected major antidiabetic agents and glucagon,* page 560.)

Drugs covered in this chapter include:

- acarbose
- acetohexamide
- chlorpropamide
- glipizide
- glucagon
- glyburide
- insulin
- metformin
- tolazamide
- tolbutamide
- troglitazone

Insulin

Patients with type 1 **diabetes mellitus** require exogenous insulin to control the blood glucose level. Insulin also may be given to patients with type 2 diabetes mellitus.

Four sources of insulin are available:

- beef insulin, from the bovine pancreas
- pork insulin, from the porcine pancreas
- "human" insulin, from a recombinant deoxyribonucleic acid (DNA) process in which insulin is synthesized from *Escherichia coli* bacteria that have been altered genetically
- "human" insulin, from an enzymatic conversion of pork insulin through which the pork insulin molecule becomes identical to the insulin produced by the human pancreas.

Three concentrations of insulin are available: U-40, or 40 units of insulin per milliliter; U-100, or 100 units of insulin per milliliter; and U-500, or 500 units of insulin per milliliter.

PHARMACOKINETICS

Insulin is *not* effective when taken orally because the gastrointestinal (GI) tract breaks down the protein molecule before it reaches the bloodstream. All insulins, however, may be given by subcutaneous (S.C.) injection. Absorption of S.C. insulin varies according to the injection site and the vascular supply and degree of tissue hypertrophy at the injection site. Also, regular (unmodified) insulin may be given intravenously (I.V.) or intramuscularly (I.M.) as well as in dialysate fluid infused into the peritoneal cavity for patients on peritoneal dialysis therapy.

After absorption into the bloodstream, insulin is distributed throughout the body. Insulin-responsive tissues are located in the liver, adipose tissue, and muscle. Insulin is metabolized primarily in the liver, to a lesser extent in the kidneys, and in the muscle tissue and is excreted in the feces and in urine.

Selected major antidiabetic agents and glucagon

This chart summarizes the major antidiabetic agents currently in clinical use. It also lists glucagon.

DRUG	MAJOR INDICATIONS AND USUAL DOSAGES	CONTRAINDICATIONS AND PRECAUTIONS
Insulin		
insulin	*Hyperglycemia* ADULT: individualized according to the patient's blood glucose level PEDIATRIC: individualized according to the patient's blood glucose level	• Insulin is contraindicated in a patient with hypoglycemia or known hypersensitivity. • This drug requires cautious use in a patient with impaired renal or hepatic function.
Oral antidiabetic agents		
acarbose (Precose)	*Hyperglycemia* ADULT: initially, 25 mg P.O. t.i.d. given with first bite of morning meal. Maintenance should not exceed 100 mg P.O. t.i.d. with meals. If patient weighs 60 kg or less, 50 mg t.i.d. is maximum dosage	• Acarbose is contraindicated in a pregnant or breast-feeding patient, one with chronic intestinal disease, or one with known hypersensitivity. • Use cautiously in patients with mild to moderate renal impairment and in those receiving insulin or a sulfonylurea. • Safety and efficacy in children have not been established.
chlorpropamide (Diabinese, Glucamide)	*Hyperglycemia* ADULT: 100 to 750 mg P.O. daily	• Chlorpropamide is contraindicated in a pregnant or breast-feeding patient or one with diabetic ketoacidosis (DKA) or known hypersensitivity. • This drug requires cautious use in a patient with impaired renal or hepatic function. • Safety and efficacy in children have not been established.
glipizide (Glucotrol)	*Hyperglycemia* ADULT: 2.5 to 40 mg P.O. daily	• Glipizide is contraindicated in a pregnant or breast-feeding patient or one with DKA or known hypersensitivity. • This drug requires cautious use in a patient with impaired renal or hepatic function. • Safety and efficacy in children have not been established.
glyburide (DiaBeta, Micronase)	*Hyperglycemia* ADULT: 1.25 to 20 mg P.O. daily	• Glyburide is contraindicated in a pregnant or breast-feeding patient or one with DKA or known hypersensitivity. • This drug requires cautious use in a patient with impaired renal or hepatic function. • Safety and efficacy in children have not been established.
metformin (Glucophage)	*Hyperglycemia* ADULT: initially, 500 mg P.O. b.i.d. with morning and evening meals. Maintenance: 500 or 850 mg P.O. b.i.d. or t.i.d. with meals	• Metformin is contraindicated in a patient needing close glucose control, a patient with history of active lactic acidosis, or one with renal or hepatic disease or known hypersensitivity to the drug. • Use cautiously in a pregnant or breast-feeding patient. • Safety and efficacy in children have not been established.
troglitazone (Rezulin)	*Hyperglycemia, adjunctive treatment* ADULTS: Continue with present insulin dose and initiate with 200 mg P.O. q.d. Increase as needed after 2 to 4 weeks. Decrease insulin dose 10% to 25% once fasting gluose levels are below 120 mg/dl	• Troglitazone is contraindicated in a breast-feeding patient or one with known hypersensitivity to the drug. • This drug requires cautious use in a patient with hepatic disease or one with class III or IV status heart failure. • Insulin is the preferred agent in pregnancy. Troglitazone should be used only when the benefits outweigh the risks to the fetus. • Safety and efficacy in children have not been established.
Glucagon		
glucagon	*Emergency treatment of hypoglycemia* ADULT: 0.5 to 1 mg S.C., I.M., or I.V., repeated in 20 minutes once or twice if no response after the first injection. PEDIATRIC: 0.025 mg/kg S.C., I.M., or I.V., repeated once or twice if no response after the first injection	• Glucagon is contraindicated in a patient with pheochromocytoma or known hypersensitivity. • This drug requires cautious use in a pregnant or breast-feeding patient or one with a history that suggests insulinoma or pheochromocytoma.

How insulin aids glucose uptake

These illustrations show how insulin allows a cell to use glucose for energy.

1. Glucose cannot enter the cell without the aid of insulin.

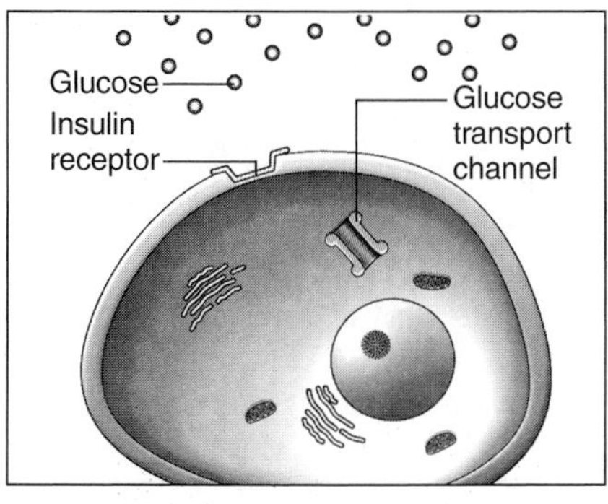

2. Normally produced by the beta cells of the pancreas, insulin binds to the receptors on the surface of the target cell. Insulin and its receptor first move to the inside of the cell, which activates glucose transporter channels to move to the surface of the cell.

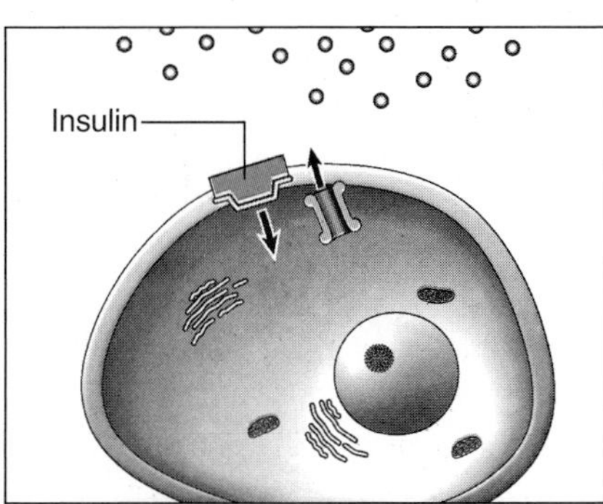

3. These channels allow glucose to enter the cell. The cell can then utilize the glucose for metabolism.

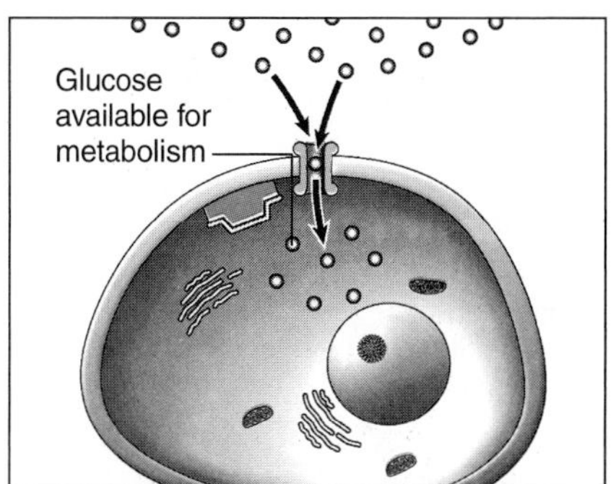

The exact times for onset, peak, and duration, however, are not absolute.

They vary not only from patient to patient, but also from injection to injection in the same patient. If insulin absorption is altered, the insulin onset of action, peak concentration level, and duration of action also are altered. If insulin absorption occurs more rapidly, the onset of action and peak concentration times occur more rapidly. Conversely, if insulin absorption is prolonged, onset of action and peak concentration are delayed, and duration of action is prolonged.

Route	Onset	Peak	Duration
S.C. (Rapid-acting)	30 min-1 hr	2-10 hr	5-16 hr
S.C. (Intermediate-acting)	1-2 hr	4-15 hr	22-28 hr
S.C. (Long-acting)	4-8 hr	10-30 hr	36 hr

PHARMACODYNAMICS

Insulin is an **anabolic,** or building, hormone. It promotes the storage of glucose as glycogen, increases protein and fat synthesis, and inhibits the breakdown of glycogen, protein, and fat. Although it has no antidiuretic effect, insulin can correct the polyuria and polydipsia associated with the osmotic diuresis of **hyperglycemia** by decreasing the blood glucose level. (See *How insulin aids glucose uptake.*)

Insulin also facilitates the movement of potassium from the extracellular fluid into the cell.

PHARMACOTHERAPEUTICS

Insulin is indicated for type 1 diabetes mellitus. It also is administered to patients with type 2 diabetes mellitus when other methods of maintaining a normal blood glucose level are ineffective or contraindicated. Patients with type 2 diabetes mellitus may find the usual methods of maintaining a normal blood glucose level ineffective during periods of emotional or physical stress (such as infection and surgery) or contraindicated because of pregnancy or hypersensitivity. These patients may need insulin to control blood glucose more stringently. Insulin also is indicated for two of the comas that are complications of diabetes: diabetic ketoacidosis, more common with type 1 diabetes mellitus, and hyperosmolar hyperglycemic nonketotic syndrome, which is more common with type 2 diabetes mellitus.

Sometimes, insulin is prescribed for patients who do not have diabetes mellitus. Because insulin stimulates cellular uptake of potassium, it may be administered with hypertonic glucose to patients with severe hyperkalemia. This insulin and glucose mixture produces a shift of serum potassium into cells and lowers the serum potassium level for a short time.

All insulins have the same effect in the body. The advantages or disadvantages of a particular kind of insulin reflect the differences in onset of action, peak concentration, and duration of action as well as in concentration, source, and purity. Many different insulin preparations are available on the U.S. market. Several of these are available in more than one concentration. (See *Available insulins,* page 562.)

Available insulins

The insulins currently available are divided into standard and purified categories and into rapid-acting, intermediate-acting, and long-acting subcategories.

TRADE NAME	MANUFACTURER	SPECIES
Standard		
Rapid-acting		
Humalog	Lilly	Human
Regular Iletin I	Lilly	Beef or pork
Regular Insulin	Novo Nordisk	Pork
Intermediate-acting		
NPH Iletin I	Lilly	Beef and pork
Lente Iletin I	Lilly	Beef and pork
NPH Insulin	Novo Nordisk	Beef
Lente Insulin	Novo Nordisk	Beef
Long-acting		
Ultralente U	Novo Nordisk	Beef
Purified		
Rapid-acting		
Regular Purified Pork Insulin Injection	Novo Nordisk	Pork Human
Velosulin Human	Novo Nordisk	Pork
Humulin R	Lilly	Human*
Novolin R	Novo Nordisk	Human**
Intermediate-acting		
NPH-N	Novo Nordisk	Pork
Lente L	Novo Nordisk	Pork
Humulin 70/30	Lilly	Human
Humulin L	Lilly	Human*
Humulin N	Lilly	Human*
Novolin L	Novo Nordisk	Human**
Novolin 70/30	Novo Nordisk	Human
Novolin N	Novo Nordisk	Human**
Long-acting		
Humulin U, Ultralente	Lilly	Human

*Recombinant deoxyribonucleic acid alteration of *Escherichia coli*
**Enzymatic conversion of porcine insulin

Adult and pediatric dosages of insulin, which vary widely, represent the amount needed to keep the blood glucose at a normal or near-normal level. The dosage varies from person to person as well as at different times for the same person. Insulin requirements are increased by growth, pregnancy, increased food intake, stress, surgery, infection, illness, increased insulin antibodies, and some medications. Insulin requirements are decreased by hypothyroidism, decreased food intake, exercise, and some medications.

Drug interactions

Some drugs interact with insulin to alter its ability to decrease the blood glucose level; other drugs directly alter these levels. (See Drug Interactions: *Insulin.*)

ADVERSE DRUG REACTIONS

Hypoglycemia (below-normal blood glucose levels) is a relatively common adverse reaction to insulin. Specific signs and symptoms may vary and include nervousness or shakiness, diaphoresis, weakness, light-headedness, confusion, paresthesia, irritability, headache, hunger, tachycardia, and changes in speech, hearing, or vision. If untreated, signs and symptoms may progress to unconsciousness, seizures, coma, and death.

The Somogyi phenomenon occurs when hypoglycemia is followed by a compensatory period of rebound hyperglycemia as the body increases glucose production to correct the problem. Typically, it occurs during the late night or early morning when the patient is asleep. During this time, insulin continues to be absorbed from the S.C. injection site, although insufficient glucose may be present for insulin to act. As a result, the blood glucose level drops rapidly. In response, the body secretes glucagon, norepinephrine, and corticosteroids to correct the hypoglycemia. An overshoot phenomenon occurs, resulting in hyperglycemia. Although the patient awakens with symptoms of hyperglycemia, hypoglycemia is the condition that must be corrected.

The dawn phenomenon (an early morning rise in blood glucose level) may result from uneven therapy. Unlike the Somogyi phenomenon, the dawn phenomenon is not preceded by hypoglycemia. It may result from nocturnal secretion of growth hormone, which causes insulin resistance.

A patient can develop local or systemic hypersensitivity reactions to any type of insulin, but such reactions to purified and human insulin are unlikely. Local reactions are characterized by redness, itching, or burning at the injection site. Local hypersensitivity usually disappears after 1 or 2 months of continued insulin use. A systemic hypersensitivity reaction to insulin is characterized by generalized urticaria (hives), angioedema (swelling of submucosa), dyspnea, tachycardia and, possibly, anaphylactic shock. Systemic hypersensitivity reactions rarely occur.

Two kinds of **lipodystrophy** (disturbance in fat metabolism) can occur with insulin injections. **Lipoatrophy** (loss of fat tissue at the injection site) and **lipohypertrophy** (thickening of subcutaneous fat tissue) can be prevented by rotating insulin injection sites.

Patients can develop a resistance to insulin. Although anti-insulin antibodies may play a role, insulin resistance usually results from a decreased number of insulin receptors, a postreceptor defect in insulin action, or an excess of hormones antagonistic to insulin. Insulin antibodies seem more likely to develop during episodic insulin therapy with type 2 diabetes mellitus. Therefore, human insulin is preferred for episodic insulin therapy because it is the least antigenic.

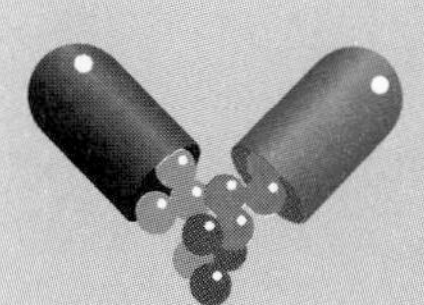

DRUG INTERACTIONS
Insulin

Interactions with other drugs can increase insulin's effect, resulting in an inappropriately altered blood glucose level for the patient. The nurse must be aware of these interactions.

DRUG	INTERACTING DRUGS	POSSIBLE EFFECTS	NURSING IMPLICATIONS
insulin	alcohol	Hypoglycemia	• Discourage alcohol consumption. • Monitor the patient for signs and symptoms of hypoglycemia, such as hunger, diaphoresis, weakness, tremor, dizziness, and tachycardia. • Decrease the insulin dosage, as prescribed.
	anabolic steroids, salicylates, monoamine oxidase inhibitors	Hypoglycemia	• Monitor the patient for signs and symptoms of hypoglycemia, such as hunger, diaphoresis, weakness, tremor, dizziness, and tachycardia. • Decrease the insulin dosage, as prescribed.
	corticosteroids, sympathomimetic agents, thiazide diuretics, dextrothyroxine sodium	Hyperglycemia	• Monitor the patient for signs and symptoms of hyperglycemia, such as thirst, polyuria, stupor, and a rapid, weak pulse. • Increase the insulin dosage, as prescribed.
	beta blockers	Masked symptoms of and delayed recovery from hypoglycemia	• Teach the patient that concomitant use of these drugs may mask the signs and symptoms of hypoglycemia, except for diaphoresis, which may become more profuse. • Monitor the patient for prolonged hypoglycemia.

NURSING PROCESS APPLICATION

The following information assists the nurse in caring for a patient receiving insulin. It includes assessment activities, examples of appropriate nursing diagnoses, and related interventions. It also highlights the importance of evaluation.

Assessment

Before drug therapy begins, review the patient's history for conditions that contraindicate or require cautious use of the prescribed insulin. Also review the patient's medication history to identify use of drugs that may interact with it.
During therapy, assess the patient for adverse drug reactions and signs of drug interactions. Also, periodically assess the effectiveness of insulin therapy. Finally, evaluate the patient's and family's knowledge about the prescribed drug.

Nursing diagnoses

• Risk for injury related to a preexisting condition that contraindicates or requires cautious use of insulin
• Risk for injury related to adverse drug reactions or drug interactions
• Noncompliance related to long-term use of insulin
• Knowledge deficit related to the prescribed insulin

Planning and implementation

• Do not administer insulin to a patient with a condition that contraindicates its use.
• Administer insulin cautiously to a patient at risk because of a preexisting condition.
• Frequently monitor the patient for adverse reactions, especially hypoglycemia, during insulin therapy. Also monitor for drug interactions.
***** ***Monitor the patient's blood glucose level regularly and more frequently after the insulin dosage is increased. Expect to check the blood glucose level during the night and in the early morning if the Somogyi or dawn phenomenon is suspected.***
• Avoid delays in the patient's mealtimes to prevent hypoglycemia.
• Monitor the patient's intake to ensure that daily caloric requirements are met. Be sure to count the calories in I.V. solutions in the patient's daily caloric intake.
***** ***Keep a source of glucose or glucagon readily available to treat a hypoglycemic reaction. After such a reaction, provide a complex carbohydrate snack.***
• Notify the physician if the patient experiences hypoglycemia frequently and expect a dosage adjustment or dietary increase in calories.
• Avoid dosage errors by measuring U-100 insulin in U-100 insulin syringes and U-40 insulin in U-40 insulin syringes.
• Prepare a U-500 dose with extreme caution. A small, inadvertent overdose of U-500 insulin could cause death.
• Do not shake insulin because the resulting froth prevents withdrawal of an accurate dose and may damage protein molecules.

Mixing insulin

The patient may withdraw two different types of insulin into the same syringe. In this series of diagrams, a rapid-acting insulin (R vial) is combined with an intermediate-acting insulin (N vial).

1. After cleaning the rubber stopper on both vials with an alcohol wipe, inject an amount of air equal to the dose of the intermediate-acting insulin into the N vial.

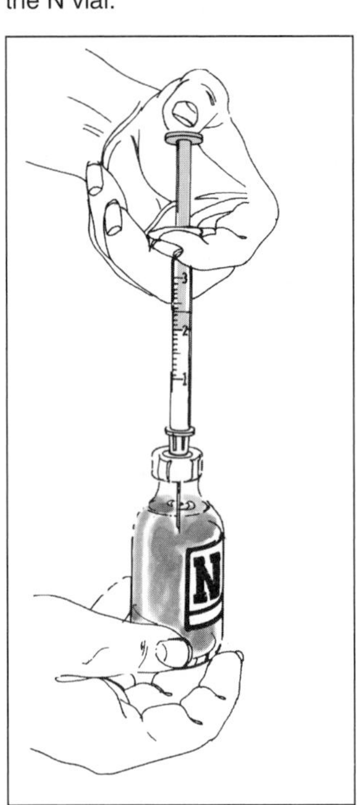

2. Inject an amount of air equal to the dose of the rapid-acting insulin into the R vial.

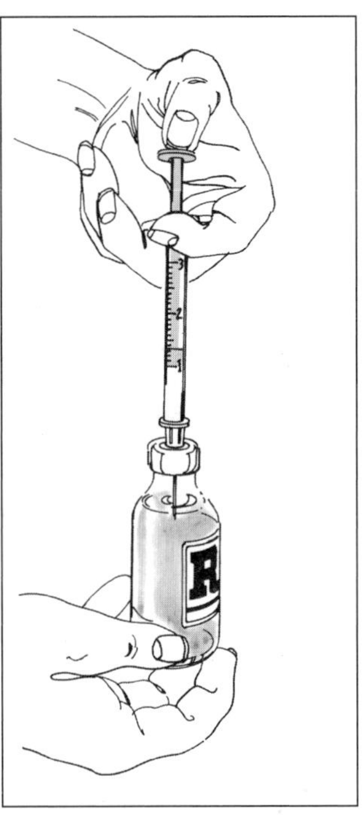

3. Withdraw the correct amount of rapid-acting insulin.

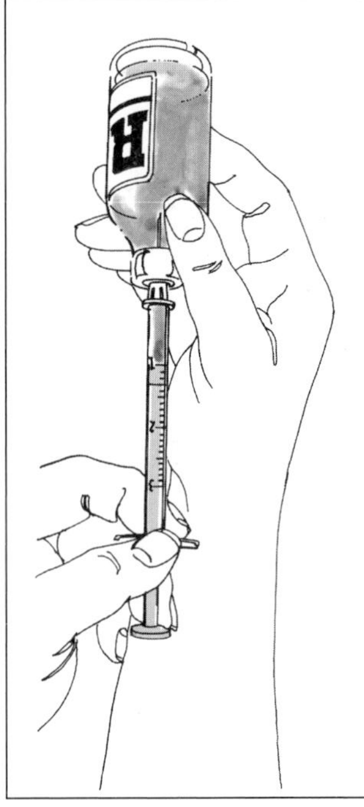

4. Withdraw the correct amount of intermediate-acting insulin. (Note: Pull the plunger down to the unit mark that equals the dose of rapid-acting insulin *plus* the dose of intermediate-acting insulin. The insulins will mix immediately in the syringe. If too large an amount of intermediate-acting insulin is withdrawn, the entire contents of the syringe must be discarded.)

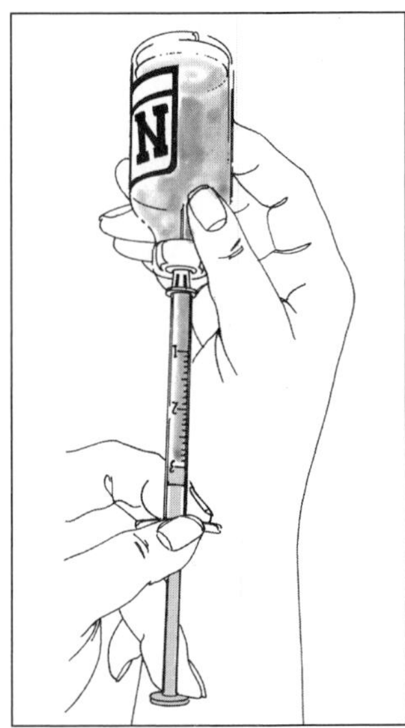

- Mix insulins in the same order every time. (See *Mixing insulin.*)
- Administer mixed insulins within 5 minutes after mixing.
- Do not administer regular insulin that appears cloudy or any insulin solution that contains particles.
- Expect to administer insulin S.C. If prescribed, however, administer regular insulin I.V. or I.M., or mix it with dialysate fluid and infuse it into the peritoneal cavity during peritoneal dialysis.
- Administer a once-daily morning dosage of insulin 30 minutes before breakfast or a split morning and evening dosage 30 minutes before breakfast and 30 minutes before dinner, unless otherwise prescribed.
- Rotate and document insulin injection sites.

∗ ***Observe the S.C. or I.M. injection site for signs and symptoms of a local hypersensitivity reaction, such as redness, itching, or burning at the site.*** If the reaction persists for more than 2 months or becomes worse in a patient who is taking a standard insulin, expect to switch the patient to a human or purified insulin.

∗ ***Observe the patient during initial or episodic insulin therapy, particularly noting systemic hypersensitivity reactions. Have standard emergency equipment nearby. If such a reaction occurs, expect to switch the patient to an insulin from another source. If prescribed, begin desensitization therapy.***

∗ ***Observe the patient for signs and symptoms of hyperglycemia, such as polyuria, polydipsia, polyphagia, weight loss, and fatigue. These suggest a need to change the insulin regimen.***

- Administer only human insulin as prescribed for episodic insulin therapy.
- Notify the physician if hyperglycemia, other adverse reactions, or drug interactions occur.
- Question the patient with uncontrolled diabetes mellitus about compliance with the prescribed insulin regimen. (See Patient Teaching: *Insulin.*)
- Notify the physician if the patient is not complying with the prescribed therapy, and try to determine the patient's reasons for doing so.

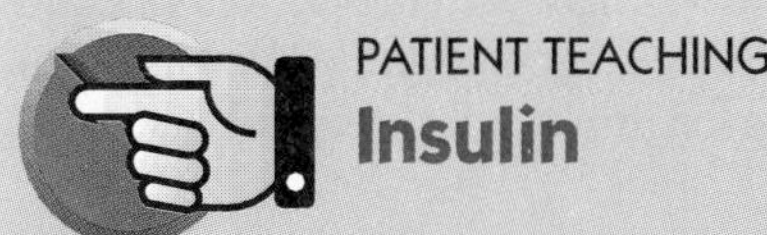

PATIENT TEACHING
Insulin

- Teach the patient and family the name, dose, frequency, action, and adverse effects of the prescribed insulin.
- Teach the patient and family how to draw up and administer the prescribed insulin.
- Instruct the patient to rotate vials of intermediate- and long-acting insulin gently before withdrawing the dose. This ensures proper dispersion of the suspension.
- Advise the patient to use a U-40 insulin syringe with U-40 insulin and a U-100 syringe with U-100 insulin.
- Inform the patient with impaired vision of the numerous aids available to help withdraw the correct amount of insulin into a syringe.
- Instruct the patient who must mix insulins always to follow the same order when drawing the insulins into the syringe.
- Instruct the patient using mixtures to withdraw and administer the mixture within 5 minutes or to store the mixture in the refrigerator and administer after the binding period (15 minutes for regular insulin with NPH insulin; 24 hours for regular insulin with lente insulin).
- Teach the patient that proper rotation of subcutaneous injection sites helps prevent lipodystrophy.
- Instruct the patient to let insulin reach room temperature before injection to minimize pain on administration.
- Instruct the patient to store insulin at a temperature less than 80° F (27° C) and greater than 36° F (2° C). Unopened vials can be stored in the refrigerator, but insulin should never be frozen or left in direct sunlight.
- Instruct the patient using an insulin pump how to care for the device.
- Instruct the patient not to change the manufacturer, type, purity, species, or dosage of insulin unless instructed to do so by the physician.
- Teach the patient the signs and symptoms of hypoglycemia and hyperglycemia and what to do if they occur.
- Teach the patient how to monitor the blood glucose level. Monitoring blood glucose is especially important for a patient who needs rigid control of the blood glucose level or requires sliding-scale insulin coverage (dose varies according to the body's need). Instruct the patient to monitor the blood glucose level during times of stress or infection because the insulin requirement may increase. Some patients may monitor the urine glucose level rather than the blood glucose level, though this method typically provides less accurate and less reliable information.
- Teach the patient how to monitor urine acetone levels to detect ketosis, especially during illness or stress.
- Review all aspects of diabetic care that may affect insulin therapy and predispose the patient to hypoglycemia or hyperglycemia, such as diet, exercise, and stress.
- Review sick-day rules to follow during insulin therapy. For example, instruct the patient to contact the physician for insulin dosage adjustments and to test blood glucose more frequently when illness occurs.
- Instruct the patient receiving insulin to wear medical identification and to have ready access to a source of glucose such as hard candy.
- Advise the patient to notify the physician if hyperglycemia or other adverse reactions occur.

Evaluation

For each nursing diagnosis, prepare an evaluation statement that describes the patient's or family's response to nursing interventions.

Oral antidiabetic agents

Most oral antidiabetic agents approved for use in the United States are sulfonylureas. The initially developed drugs, known as first-generation sulfonylureas, include acetohexamide, chlorpropamide, tolazamide, and tolbutamide. Developed more recently, the second-generation sulfonylureas include glipizide and glyburide. Troglitazone is one of the newest nonsulfonylureas available. It is a thiazolidinedione antidiabetic agent. Metformin is a biguanide. Acarbose is an alpha-glucosidase inhibitor.

PHARMACOKINETICS

Available only in oral form, oral antidiabetic agents are absorbed well from the GI tract. Their onsets of action vary. For example, glipizide acts within 1 to 1.5 hours. Oral antidiabetic agents are distributed via the bloodstream throughout the body. Oral antidiabetic agents are metabolized primarily in the liver and are excreted primarily in the urine, with some excreted in the bile. Glyburide is excreted equally in the urine and feces.

Route	Onset	Peak	Duration
P.O.	0.5-6 hr	2-6 hr	Variable

PHARMACODYNAMICS

Generally accepted theory suggests that oral hypoglycemic agents produce pancreatic and extrapancreatic actions to regulate blood glucose. These drugs probably stimulate pancreatic beta cells to release insulin. The pancreas already must be functioning at a minimal level. Within a few weeks to a few months of the initial response to the sulfonylureas, pancreatic insulin secretion drops to pretreatment levels. However, blood glucose levels remain normal or near-normal. Extrapancreatic actions of oral hypoglycemic agents probably maintain this continued control of blood glucose.

Oral antidiabetic agents may provide several extrapancreatic actions to decrease and control blood glucose. They probably decrease glucose production by the liver and also may increase the number of cellular insulin receptors. With more available receptors, the cells can bind with insulin sufficiently to initiate the process of glucose metabolism. Oral antidiabetic agents also may partially reverse the postreceptor deficit in insulin action, enabling the completion of intracellular glucose metabolism. The ability to restore tissue sensitivity to insulin at the receptor and postreceptor level is not restricted to sulfonylureas; weight reduction and exercise probably provide similar effects.

Troglitazone inhibits glucose production and enhances the effects of circulating insulin. Metformin decreases hepatic glucose production and intestinal absorption of glucose and improves insulin sensitivity. Acarbose inhibits an enzyme, delaying glucose absorption.

PHARMACOTHERAPEUTICS

Oral antidiabetic agents are indicated for patients with type 2 diabetes mellitus if diet and exercise do not maintain blood glucose at normal or near-normal levels. These agents are not indicated for patients with type 1 diabetes mellitus because pancreatic beta cells are not functioning at a sufficient level. Combination oral antidiabetic agent and insulin therapy may be indicated for some patients who do not respond to either drug alone.

Drug interactions

Some drugs interact with the oral antidiabetic agents and alter their ability to decrease the blood glucose level, but other drugs directly alter the patient's blood glucose level. (See Drug Interactions: *Oral antidiabetic agents.*)

ADVERSE DRUG REACTIONS

Hypoglycemia, the major adverse reaction to oral antidiabetic agents, typically results from too little food or too much medication. Hypoglycemia also can occur after an incorrect dose or, more likely, from drug or metabolite accumulation in the body. Patients with decreased liver or kidney function and those taking chlorpropamide must be especially careful to note signs of hypoglycemia.

Other relatively uncommon reactions to oral antidiabetic agents include GI effects (nausea, vomiting, cholestasis), skin reactions (rash, pruritus, photosensitivity), a diffuse pulmonary reaction, hematologic reactions (leukopenia, thrombocytopenia, hemolytic anemia), hepatic effects (abnormal liver function tests), and renal effects (severe diuretic or antidiuretic effect). Oral antidiabetic agents also may cause an allergic reaction.

When a patient does not respond initially to sulfonylurea therapy, the patient is said to exhibit primary failure. Primary failure occurs in about 20% of patients receiving oral hypoglycemic agents; the mechanism of drug failure is unknown. In secondary failure, the sulfonylurea maintains a normal or near-normal blood glucose level for a time, but then, for unknown reasons, no longer can do so. Each year, secondary failure occurs in 5% to 10% of patients receiving oral antidiabetic agents. However, 25% to 60% of patients with secondary failure to one oral antidiabetic agent will respond to another agent. Therefore, trial with a different agent may be warranted.

NURSING PROCESS APPLICATION

The following information assists the nurse in caring for a patient who is receiving an oral antidiabetic agent. It includes an overview of assessment activities as well as examples of appropriate nursing diagnoses and related interventions. It also highlights the importance of evaluation.

Assessment

Before drug therapy begins, review the patient's history for conditions that contraindicate or require cautious use of the prescribed oral antidiabetic agent. Also review the patient's medication history to identify use of drugs that may interact with it. During therapy, assess the patient for adverse drug reactions and signs of drug interactions. Also, periodically assess the effectiveness of therapy with the oral antidiabetic agent. Finally, evaluate the patient's and family's knowledge about the prescribed drug.

Nursing diagnoses

- Risk for injury related to a preexisting condition that contraindicates or requires cautious use of an oral antidiabetic agent
- Risk for injury related to adverse drug reactions or drug interactions
- Noncompliance related to long-term use of the oral antidiabetic agent
- Knowledge deficit related to the prescribed oral antidiabetic agent

Planning and implementation

- Do not administer an oral antidiabetic agent to a patient with a condition that contraindicates its use.
- Administer an oral antidiabetic agent cautiously to a patient at risk because of a preexisting condition.
- Monitor the patient for adverse reactions, especially hypoglycemia, during therapy with an oral antidiabetic agent. Also monitor for drug interactions.
- Monitor the patient's blood glucose level regularly and more frequently after the dosage is increased.
- Avoid delays in mealtimes to prevent glucose alterations.
- Monitor the patient's intake to ensure that daily caloric requirements are met. Be sure to include the calories in I.V. solutions in the patient's daily caloric intake.

* ***Keep a source of glucose or glucagon readily available to treat a hypoglycemic reaction. After such a reaction, provide a complex carbohydrate snack.***

- Notify the physician if the patient experiences hypoglycemia frequently, and expect a dosage adjustment.
- Give most oral antidiabetic agents 30 minutes before breakfast; if the daily drug dosage is divided, give the second dose 30 minutes before dinner (some are given with meals). Oral antidiabetic agents should be taken on a regular schedule to minimize wide fluctuations in the blood glucose level.
- Notify the physician if adverse reactions or drug interations occur.
- Question the patient about compliance with the prescribed drug regimen. If the patient is not complying with therapy, try to determine the patient's reasons for doing so. (See Patient Teaching: *Oral antidiabetic agents,* page 568.)
- Notify the physician if noncompliance occurs or is suspected.

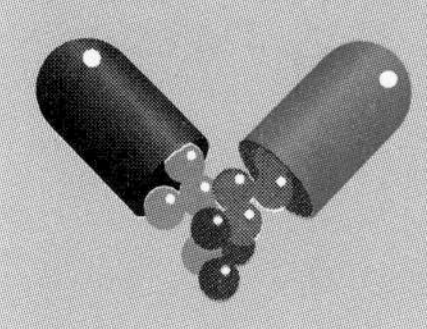

DRUG INTERACTIONS

Oral antidiabetic agents

Numerous drugs can interact with the oral antidiabetic agents to produce hypoglycemia or hyperglycemia.

DRUG	INTERACTING DRUGS	POSSIBLE EFFECTS	NURSING IMPLICATIONS
acetohexamide, chlorpropamide, tolazamide, tolbutamide, glipizide, glyburide	alcohol	Hypoglycemia or hyperglycemia	• Monitor the patient for signs and symptoms of hyperglycemia (thirst, polyuria, stupor, and a rapid, weak pulse) and hypoglycemia (hunger, diaphoresis, weakness, tremor, dizziness, and tachycardia). • Discourage alcohol consumption. • Teach the patient about the possibility of a disulfiram-like reaction with chlorpropamide.
	coumarin	Hypoglycemia, increased anticoagulant effect	• Monitor the patient for signs and symptoms of hypoglycemia. • Monitor the patient for increased anticoagulant effect, such as epistaxis, bruises, and hematuria. • Change the patient to another medication for anticoagulant therapy, as prescribed.
	anabolic steroids, chloramphenicol, clofibrate, gemfibrozil, monoamine oxidase inhibitors, phenylbutazone, salicylates, sulfonamides, fluconazole, cimetidine, ranitidine	Hypoglycemia	• Monitor the patient for signs and symptoms of hypoglycemia.
	corticosteroids, dextrothyroxine, rifampin, sympathomimetic agents, thiazide diuretics	Hyperglycemia	• Monitor the patient for signs and symptoms of hyperglycemia. • Increase the dosage of the oral hypoglycemic agent, as prescribed.
	beta blockers, clonidine	Masked signs of hypoglycemia	• Be aware that beta blockers will block the epinephrine-induced symptoms of hypoglycemia but not alter the hypoglycemia itself. • Monitor the patient for hypoglycemia by testing the blood glucose level. • Teach the patient that most typical signs and symptoms of hypoglycemia, such as tachycardia and tremor, may be masked, but that diaphoresis will be detectable and may become more profuse.
acarbose	digestive enzymes and charcoal	Effect of acarbose is reduced	• Do not use together.
metformin	cimetidine, nifedipine, procainamide, ranitidine, vancomycin	Inhibits metformin excretion	• Monitor the patient by testing the blood glucose level.
troglitazone	cholestyramine	Reduced absorption of troglitazone	• Do not use cholestyramine while taking troglitazone.
	oral contraceptives	Loss of contraceptive properties	• Use additional forms of contraception.
	terfenadine	Decrease terfenadine effectiveness	• Monitor the patient.

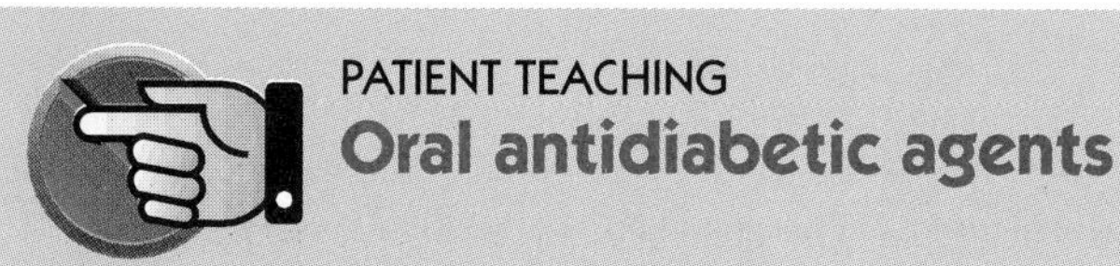

PATIENT TEACHING
Oral antidiabetic agents

- Teach the patient and family the name, dose, frequency, action, and adverse effects of the prescribed oral antidiabetc agent.
- Teach the patient the signs and symptoms of hypoglycemia and hyperglycemia and what to do if they occur.
- Instruct the patient to eat meals on a regular schedule; skipping a meal increases the risk of hypoglycemia.
- Advise the patient to adjust the drug dosage *only* under medical supervision. A change in body weight, diet, or amount of exercise may require a change in the drug dosage. Severe stress also may require a dosage change or the addition of insulin to the treatment regimen.
- Teach the patient how to monitor the blood glucose level. Blood glucose testing is a better indicator for management of diabetes than urine glucose measurement because of individual variations in the renal threshold for glucose.
- Instruct the patient to carry or wear medical identification and to have ready access to a source of glucose such as hard candy.
- Advise the patient to notify the physician if increased diuresis or signs of fluid retention (ankle swelling and weight gain unrelated to caloric intake) occur.
- Inform the patient that the oral antidiabetic agent may cause photosensitivity and to avoid exposure to the sun. When this is not possible, the patient should use protective measures, such as wearing sunglasses, sunscreen lotion, and a hat when outdoors.
- Advise the patient to obtain alcohol-use guidelines from the physician.
- Advise the patient to notify the physician if adverse reactions occur.

Evaluation
For each nursing diagnosis, prepare an evaluation statement that describes the patient's or family's response to nursing interventions.

Glucagon

Unlike insulin and the oral antidiabetic agents, which decrease the blood glucose level, glucagon increases it. This hyperglycemic agent is a hormone normally produced by the alpha cells of the islets of Langerhans in the pancreas.

PHARMACOKINETICS
After S.C., I.M., or I.V. injection, glucagon is absorbed rapidly. It cannot be taken orally because it is a protein, and it would be destroyed in the GI tract. Glucagon is distributed throughout the body, although its effect occurs primarily in the liver. The exact metabolic fate of glucagon is unknown, although it is degraded extensively in the liver. Glucagon is removed from the body by the liver and the kidneys.

Route	Onset	Peak	Duration
S.C., I.M., I.V.	5-20 min	30 min	1-2 hr

PHARMACODYNAMICS
Glucagon regulates the rate of glucose production through glycogenolysis, gluconeogenesis, and lipolysis. A glucagon deficiency results in hypoglycemia. Although glucagon stimulates insulin secretion, insulin antagonizes glucagon's actions through a negative feedback system.

PHARMACOTHERAPEUTICS
Glucagon is used for emergency treatment of severe hypoglycemia. It also is used during radiologic examination of the GI tract to produce a hypokinetic state.

Drug interactions
Glucagon interacts adversely only with oral anticoagulants, thereby increasing the anticoagulant effects. Although glucagon does not interact adversely with food, it is ineffective in poorly nourished or starving patients. If the patient has no glycogen stored in the liver, glycogenolysis cannot occur even with glucagon.

ADVERSE DRUG REACTIONS
Adverse reactions to glucagon are rare. Nausea and vomiting may occur occasionally. Because of the short half-life of glucagon, overdose is unlikely. No evidence of glucagon toxicity exists. With large dosages or prolonged treatment, hypokalemia can result. Because glucagon is a protein, a patient can develop an allergy to it, but this reaction is rare. A patient can also develop antibodies to glucagon, though the effect of such antibodies remains unknown.

NURSING PROCESS APPLICATION
The following information assists the nurse in caring for a patient receiving glucagon. It includes assessment activities, examples of nursing diagnoses, and related interventions. It also highlights the importance of evaluation.

Assessment
Before drug therapy begins, review the patient's history for conditions that contraindicate or require cautious use of glucagon. Also review the patient's medication history to identify use of drugs that may interact with it. During therapy, assess the patient for adverse drug reactions and signs of drug interactions. Also, periodically assess the effectiveness of glucagon therapy. Finally, evaluate the patient's and family's knowledge about the prescribed drug.

Nursing diagnoses
- Risk for injury related to a preexisting condition that contraindicates or requires cautious use of glucagon

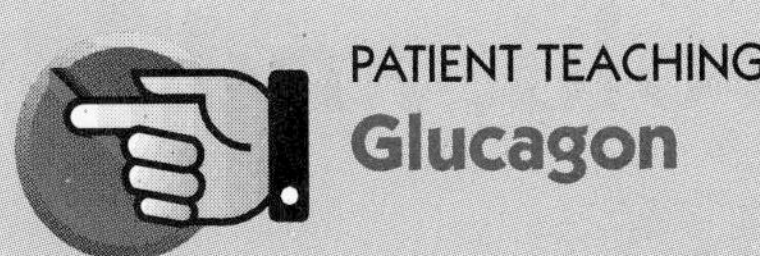

PATIENT TEACHING
Glucagon

- ➤ Teach the patient and family the name, dose, conditions that require administration, action, and adverse effects of glucagon.
- ➤ Teach the family to recognize the signs and symptoms of hypoglycemia. Also show them how to prepare and administer glucagon in an emergency. Instruct the family to use only the diluent provided for glucagon preparation.
- ➤ Instruct the family to provide a complex carbohydrate snack after the patient awakens from the coma. Also advise them to notify the physician because the patient's medication may need to be changed.
- ➤ Advise the family to seek emergency help immediately if the patient does not respond to glucagon therapy.

- Risk for injury related to adverse drug reactions or drug interactions
- Knowledge deficit related to glucagon

Planning and implementation

- Do not administer glucagon to a patient with a condition that contraindicates its use. Administer glucagon cautiously to a patient at risk because of a preexisting condition.
- Observe the patient receiving high-dosage or long-term glucagon therapy for signs of hypokalemia.

***** ***Monitor the patient for signs of bleeding in concomitant therapy with an oral anticoagulant. Notify the physician if bleeding occurs and expect to decrease the oral anticoagulant dosage, as prescribed.***

- Give the patient with type 1 diabetes mellitus who requires glucagon a complex carbohydrate snack as soon as possible to restore the liver glycogen level and prevent secondary hypoglycemia. (See Patient Teaching: *Glucagon.*)

***** ***Contact the physician immediately to obtain a prescription for I.V. glucose if the patient does not respond to glucagon.***

***** ***Administer I.V. glucose with glucagon, as prescribed, if the patient is in a deep coma or does not awaken from the coma after glucagon administration.***

- Mix glucagon powder only with the diluent provided.
- Do not administer I.V. glucagon in a solution that contains calcium, potassium, or sodium chloride because precipitation can occur.

***** ***Notify the physician if adverse reactions or drug interactions occur.***

Evaluation

For each nursing diagnosis, prepare an evaluation statement that describes the patient's or family's response to nursing interventions.

CHAPTER SUMMARY

Chapter 45 discussed insulin, oral antidiabetic agents, and glucagon. Here are the chapter highlights.

Hypoglycemia is the most common adverse reaction to insulin therapy. When caring for a patient receiving insulin, the nurse should help the patient balance diet, exercise, and insulin requirements and prevent complications of therapy.

Most oral antidiabetic agents currently on the market in the United States are sulfonylureas. They are used to treat hyperglycemia in patients with type 2 diabetes mellitus. Hypoglycemia and drug failure are the most common adverse reactions. For a patient receiving an oral antidiabetic agent, the nurse should teach about diet, exercise, and prevention of adverse reactions to the prescribed agent. Glucagon is used in the emergency treatment of severe hypoglycemia. It regulates the rate of glucose production through glycogenolysis, gluconeogenesis, and lipolysis. Glucagon produces few adverse reactions. Nursing care for a diabetic patient receiving glucagon should include teaching the patient and family how and when to administer the drug.

Questions to consider

See Appendix 1 for answers.

1. How does insulin lower the blood glucose level?
   (a) It prevents glucose absorption from the GI tract.
   (b) It increases glucose excretion from the GI tract.
   (c) It promotes glucose storage as glycogen and inhibits glycogen breakdown.
   (d) It promotes gluconeogenesis.

2. Which of the following are signs of hypoglycemia?
   (a) Polyuria, headache, and fatigue.
   (b) Polyphagia and flushed, dry skin.
   (c) Polydipsia, pallor, and irritability.
   (d) Nervousness, diaphoresis, and confusion.

3. When should a patient with type 2 diabetes mellitus take the oral antidiabetic agent glipizide?
   (a) With meals.
   (b) After meals.
   (c) 30 minutes before bedtime.
   (d) 30 minutes before breakfast.

4. A patient takes a double dose of insulin and is semiconscious when he arrives at the hospital. His blood glucose level is 40 mg/dl. The physician prescribes glucagon I.V. Why is this drug not administered orally?
   (a) It would irritate the GI tract too much.
   (b) It would have a delayed onset of action.
   (c) It would be destroyed by the GI tract.
   (d) It would be absorbed unpredictably.

Thyroid, antithyroid, and parathyroid agents

OBJECTIVES

After reading and studying this chapter, the student should be able to:

1. describe the pharmacokinetics, pharmacodynamics, and pharmacotherapeutics of individual thyroid and antithyroid agents.
2. identify the major drug interactions and adverse reactions for the major thyroid and antithyroid agents.
3. describe the pharmacokinetics and mechanisms of action of parathyroid agents.
4. identify adverse reactions associated with the calcium-regulating drugs.
5. describe how to apply the nursing process when caring for a patient who is receiving a thyroid, antithyroid, or parathyroid agent.

INTRODUCTION

Thyroid and antithyroid agents are drugs that function to correct thyroid hormone imbalances—hypothyroidism and hyperthyroidism. This chapter discusses the use of thyroid agents as replacement therapy in patients with hypothyroidism (thyroid hormone deficiency). It also describes antithyroid agents and their ability to interfere with thyroid hormone synthesis in patients with hyperthyroidism (thyroid hormone excess). (See *Selected major thyroid, antithyroid, and parathyroid agents.*)

Parathyroid agents, also known as calcium-regulating drugs, are drugs that function to maintain calcium homeostasis. This chapter discusses the following calcium-regulating drugs: parathyroid hormone (PTH), **calcitonin,** alendronate, etidronate disodium, and the vitamin D analogues calcifediol, calcitriol, and dihydrotachysterol.

Although no therapeutic use of exogenous PTH currently exists, the drug formerly was used to increase serum calcium concentrations. Today, PTH is available for diagnostic and research purposes only. The effects of vitamin D analogues on serum calcium concentrations resemble the effects of endogenous and exogenous PTH; however, other drugs discussed in this chapter—calcitonin and etidronate disodium—produce effects opposite to those of PTH.

Drugs covered in this chapter include:

- alendronate
- calcifediol
- calcitonin
- calcitriol
- dihydrotachysterol
- etidronate disodium
- iodine
- levothyroxine sodium
- liotrix
- methimazole
- parathyroid hormone
- propylthiouracil
- protirelin
- radioactive iodine
- thyroid USP
- thyrotropin.

Thyroid agents

Thyroid agents can be natural or synthetic hormones and may contain triiodothyronine (T_3), thyroxine (T_4), or both. Natural thyroid agents, which are derived from animal thyroid, include thyroid USP (desiccated) and **thyroglobulin.** Both contain T_3 and T_4. Synthetic thyroid agents actually are the sodium salts of the L-isomers of the hormones. These synthetic hormones include levothyroxine sodium, which contains T_4, liothyronine sodium, which contains T_3, and liotrix, which contains T_3 and T_4. All of these agents are used for exogenous replacement of thyroid hormone.

PHARMACOKINETICS

Thyroid hormones are absorbed variably from the gastrointestinal (GI) tract, distributed in plasma, and bound to serum proteins. They are metabolized through deiodination, primarily in the liver, and excreted unchanged in the feces.

Route	Onset	Peak	Duration
P.O.	24-72 hr	2 days-4 wk	3 days-3 wk
I.V.	6-8 hr	3-4 wk	1-3 wk

PHARMACODYNAMICS

In an adult, thyroid hormones act on tissues through various mechanisms, including intracellular transport of amino acids and electrolytes, synthesis of specific intracellular enzymes, and enhancement of intracellular processes that lead to changes in cell size and number.

The principal pharmacologic effect of exogenous thyroid hormones is an increased metabolic rate in body tissues.

Selected major thyroid, antithyroid, and parathyroid agents

This chart summarizes the drugs most commonly used in treating hypothyroidism, hyperthyroidism, and calcium imbalances.

DRUG	MAJOR INDICATIONS AND USUAL DOSAGES	CONTRAINDICATIONS AND PRECAUTIONS
Thyroid agents		
thyroid USP (S-P-T, Thyrar)	*Mild hypothyroidism* ADULT: initially, 60 mg P.O. daily, increased until desired response is achieved *Adult myxedema* ADULT: 16 mg P.O. daily; may double dosage every 2 weeks, up to a maximum of 120 mg daily *Congenital hypothyroidism, severe hypothyroidism in children* PEDIATRIC: initially, 15 mg P.O. daily; increased at 2-week intervals, as needed	• Thyroid USP is contraindicated in a patient with thyrotoxicosis, acute myocardial infarction (MI) uncomplicated by hypothyroidism, uncorrected adrenal insufficiency, or known hypersensitivity. • This drug requires cautious use in a geriatric or breast-feeding patient or one with angina pectoris, hypertension, or other cardiovascular disease.
levothyroxine (T_4), L-thyroxine sodium, Synthroid)	*Mild hypothyroidism* ADULT: initially, 50 mcg P.O. daily, increased by 25 to 50 mcg every 2 to 4 weeks; for maintenance, 100 to 400 mcg P.O. daily PEDIATRIC: for children under age 1, 6 to 15 mcg P.O. daily; for children age 1 and over, 3 to 5 mcg/kg P.O. daily *Myxedema coma* ADULT: initially, 400 mcg I.V. in a concentration of 100 mcg/ml; increased, as needed, by 100 to 300 mcg or more	• Levothyroxine is contraindicated in a patient with thyrotoxicosis, acute MI uncomplicated by hypothyroidism, uncorrected adrenal insufficiency, or known hypersensitivity. • This drug requires cautious use in a geriatric or breast-feeding patient or one with a history of lactose intolerance or angina pectoris, hypertension, or other cardiovascular disease.
Antithyroid agents		
propylthiouracil (Propyl-Thyracil)	*Hyperthyroidism, adjunct preparation before thyroid surgery or radioactive iodine therapy* ADULT: initially, 100 to 200 mg P.O. t.i.d.; for maintenance, 100 to 150 mg P.O. daily PEDIATRIC: for children ages 6 to 10, 50 to 150 mg P.O. daily; for children over age 10, 150 to 300 mg P.O. daily *Thyroid crisis* ADULT: 100 to 200 mg P.O. t.i.d., increased as needed up to a maximum of 1,200 mg daily	• Propylthiouracil is contraindicated in a breast-feeding patient or one with known hypersensitivity. • This drug requires cautious use in a pregnant patient, one who is receiving another drug known to cause granulocytopenia, or one older than age 40 because of the risk of heart disease.
iodine (potassium iodide solution, USP [SSKI]; sodium iodide, USP; strong iodine solution, USP [Lugol's solution])	*Adjunct preparation before thyroid surgery* ADULT: 3 to 5 drops of Lugol's solution P.O. t.i.d. or 1 to 5 drops of SSKI P.O. t.i.d. for 10 to 14 days before surgery PEDIATRIC: 3 to 5 drops of strong iodine solution P.O. t.i.d. *Thyroid crisis* ADULT: 1 g I.V. of sodium iodide or 10 drops of SSKI every 8 hours, or 30 drops of Lugol's solution P.O. or by nasogastric tube daily *Hyperthyroidism* ADULT: 3 to 5 drops of Lugol's solution P.O. t.i.d. or 1 drop of SSKI P.O. t.i.d.	• Iodine is contraindicated in a pregnant patient or one with acute bronchitis or known hypersensitivity. • This drug requires cautious use in a patient with tuberculosis.

(continued)

Selected major thyroid, antithyroid, and parathyroid agents *(continued)*

DRUG	MAJOR INDICATIONS AND USUAL DOSAGES	CONTRAINDICATIONS AND PRECAUTIONS
Parathyroid agents		
calcitonin (salmon) (Calcimar, Miacalcin, Osteocalcin)	*Paget's disease* ADULT: 100 IU S.C. or I.M. daily for first few months; for maintenance, 50 to 100 IU daily or every other day *Osteoporosis* ADULT: 100 IU daily, S.C. or I.M.; or 200 IU nasally daily	• Calcitonin (salmon) is contraindicated in a pregnant or breast-feeding patient or one with hypersensitivity to fish or to the gelatin in the diluent. • This drug has no known precautions. • Safety and efficacy in children have not been established.
etidronate disodium (Didronel)	*Paget's disease* ADULT: 5 to 10 mg/kg P.O. daily for no more than 6 months, or 11 to 20 mg/kg P.O. daily for no more than 3 months	• Etidronate disodium has no known contraindications. • This drug requires cautious use in a pregnant or breast-feeding patient or one with renal dysfunction. • Safety and efficacy in children have not been established.
calcitriol (Rocaltrol)	*Hypoparathyroidism and pseudohypoparathyroidism* ADULT: 0.25 mcg P.O. daily, with dosages possibly increased at 2- to 4-week intervals PEDIATRIC: 0.25 mcg (ages 1 to 5); 0.5-2 mcg (age 6) P.O. daily, with dosages possibly increased at 2- to 4-week intervals	• Calcitriol is contraindicated in a breast-feeding patient or one with hypercalcemia or vitamin D toxicity. • This drug requires cautious use in a pregnant patient or one receiving a digitalis glycoside.
alendronate (Fosamax)	*Paget's disease* ADULT: 40 mg P.O. daily for 6 months *Osteoporosis* ADULT: 10 mg P.O. daily	• Alendronate is contraindicated in a patient with known hypersensitivity, hypocalcemia, or severe renal insufficiency. • Use with caution in patients with moderate renal insufficiency or one with an upper gastrointestinal disorder.

These hormones affect protein and carbohydrate metabolism and stimulate protein synthesis. They promote **gluconeogenesis** (carbohydrate formation from noncarbohydrate molecules) and increase the use of glycogen stores. By decreasing hepatic and serum cholesterol concentrations, thyroid hormones affect lipid metabolism. They stimulate the heart and increase cardiac output. They may even increase the heart's sensitivity to catecholamines and increase the number of myocardial beta-adrenergic receptors. Thyroid hormones may increase renal blood flow and the glomerular filtration rate in hypothyroid patients, producing diuresis within 24 hours after administration.

PHARMACOTHERAPEUTICS

Thyroid agents act as replacement or substitute hormones when the body's hormone level cannot meet its needs. Therefore, they are used to treat the many forms of hypothyroidism.

Thyroid agents also may be used with antithyroid agents to prevent goitrogenesis (goiter formation) and hypothyroidism. In diagnostic tests, these agents help differentiate between primary and secondary hypothyroidism.

Levothyroxine is the drug of choice for thyroid hormone replacement and thyroid-stimulating hormone (TSH) suppression therapy. Treating papillary or follicular thyroid carcinoma also may require the use of thyroid agents.

Drug interactions

Thyroid agents interact with several common medications. (See Drug Interactions: *Thyroid agents.*)

ADVERSE DRUG REACTIONS

Most adverse reactions to thyroid agents result from toxicity. Discontinuation of the drugs will reverse the signs and symptoms.

Common GI signs and symptoms of thyroid toxicity include diarrhea, abdominal cramps, weight loss, and increased appetite. Cardiovascular signs and symptoms, including palpitations, diaphoresis, tachycardia, increased blood pressure, angina pectoris, and arrhythmias, also may occur. Other manifestations of toxicity may include headache, tremor, insomnia, nervousness, fever, heat intolerance, and menstrual irregularities.

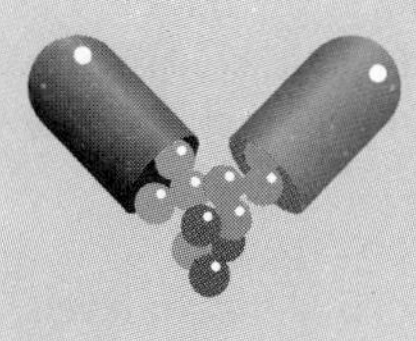

DRUG INTERACTIONS

Thyroid agents

Thyroid agents interact with several common drugs, including oral anticoagulants, cholestyramine, and phenytoin. The nurse should monitor for the effects of drug interactions in any patient who is receiving one of these drugs and a thyroid agent.

DRUG	INTERACTING DRUGS	POSSIBLE EFFECTS	NURSING IMPLICATIONS
levothyroxine, liothyronine, liotrix, thyroglobulin, thyroid USP	oral anticoagulants	Increased risk of bleeding	• Monitor the patient for signs of bleeding, such as epistaxis, bleeding gums, hematuria, or easy bruising. • Monitor the patient's prothrombin time (PT) when thyroid therapy begins. • Reduce the anticoagulant dosage as prescribed when thyroid therapy begins. Readjust it as prescribed according to the PT results.
	cholestyramine, colestipol	Decreased absorption and recirculation of thyroid hormones	• Administer these medications at least 4 to 6 hours apart. • Monitor the results of the patient's thyroid function tests.
	phenytoin	Increased metabolism of thyroid hormones; increased thyroxine levels	• Monitor the results of the patient's thyroid function tests. • Adjust the thyroid dosage, as prescribed.
	cardiac glycosides	Decreased serum digitoxin or digoxin levels; increased risk of arrhythmias	• Monitor the patient's serum digitoxin or digoxin level. • Monitor the patient's pulse and electrocardiogram.
	carbamazepine	Increased metabolism of thyroid hormones	• Assess the patient for signs of ineffectiveness of thyroid therapy. • Monitor the results of the patient's thyroid function tests when beginning or ending carbamazepine therapy.
	theophylline	Increased serum theophylline level	• Monitor the patient's theophylline level closely when starting thyroid agent therapy. • Monitor the patient's respiratory status during concomitant therapy.

Geriatric patients beginning thyroid therapy require close monitoring because the cardiostimulatory effect of the thyroid agent may produce angina pectoris or a myocardial infarction (MI) if coronary artery disease is present.

A patient with adrenal insufficiency should receive corticosteroids to correct the insufficiency before thyroid therapy begins. Because thyroid agents increase tissue demand for adrenal hormones, thyroid therapy could precipitate an acute adrenal crisis in a patient with adrenal insufficiency.

Euthroid and synthroid tablets contain tartrazine yellow dye, which may produce bronchial asthma and other hypersensitivity reactions in a susceptible individual. Although rare, these reactions are more likely to occur in an aspirin-sensitive patient. A lactose-sensitive patient may need to avoid levothyroxine because it contains lactose. A patient who is sensitive to pork may experience GI distress when taking thyroid USP or thyroglobulin.

NURSING PROCESS APPLICATION

The following information assists the nurse in caring for a patient who is receiving a thyroid agent. It includes an overview of assessment activities as well as examples of appropriate nursing diagnoses and related interventions. It also highlights the importance of evaluation.

Assessment

Before drug therapy begins, review the patient's history for conditions that contraindicate or require cautious use of the prescribed thyroid agent. Review the patient's medication history to identify use of drugs that may interact with it. During therapy, assess the patient for adverse drug reactions and signs of drug interactions. Periodically assess the effectiveness of therapy with the thyroid agent. Finally, evaluate

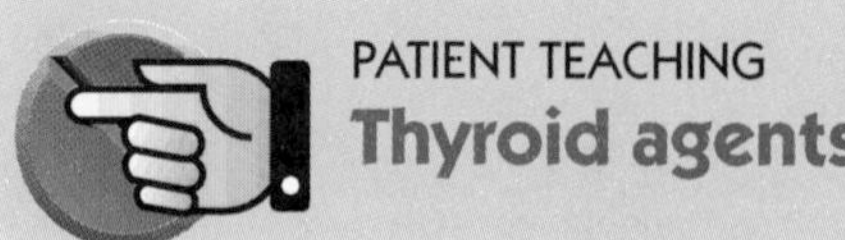

PATIENT TEACHING

Thyroid agents

- Teach the patient and family the name, dose, frequency, action, and adverse effects of the prescribed thyroid agent.
- Teach the patient to recognize and report the signs and symptoms of hyperthyroidism, such as fatigue, breathlessness, and heat intolerance. Also instruct the patient to report headaches, palpitations, or nervousness, which are symptoms of thyroid hormone overdose.
- Discuss the prescribed medication regimen with the patient. A prescription for triiodothyronine (T_3) may require the patient to take it two to three times per day because of its rapid plasma half-life. A thyroxine (T_4) prescription usually specifies that it be taken once a day. Remind the patient to take levothyroxine on an empty stomach to promote regular absorption and to take it in the morning to help prevent insomnia and to mimic normal hormone release.
- Remind the patient to store the thyroid agent in a tightly capped, light-resistant container at 59° to 86° F (15° to 30° C) to prevent deterioration.
- Teach the patient that different brands of thyroid agents may vary slightly in concentration. Instruct the patient to check that the physician orders the drug by brand name and that the pharmacist does not substitute a different brand.
- Stress the importance of returning for routine thyroid studies to assess the drug's effectiveness and to detect drug toxicity.
- Instruct the patient to notify the physician if adverse reactions occur.

the patient's and family's knowledge about the prescribed drug.

Nursing diagnoses

- Risk for injury related to a preexisting condition that contraindicates or requires cautious use of a thyroid agent
- Risk for injury related to adverse drug reactions or drug interactions
- Pain related to thyroid agent-induced angina pectoris or acute MI
- Knowledge deficit related to the prescribed thyroid agent

Planning and implementation

- Do not administer a thyroid agent to a patient with a condition that contraindicates its use.
- Administer a thyroid agent cautiously to a patient at risk because of a preexisting condition.

* ***Monitor the patient for toxicity and other adverse reactions during therapy with a thyroid agent.*** If toxicity occurs, notify the physician. Also, expect to discontinue the drug temporarily and to decrease the dosage as prescribed when therapy begins again.

- Monitor the patient for drug interactions.
- Assess for any history of pork sensitivity before administering thyroid USP or thyroglobulin, lactose sensitivity before administering levothyroxine, and aspirin sensitivity before administering euthroid or synthroid. If the patient has a history of hypersensitivity to a thyroid agent, consult the physician about using a different thyroid preparation. (See Patient Teaching: *Thyroid agents.*)
- Evaluate the patient's response to therapy regularly. Appropriate treatment should restore normal serum levels of T_3 and T_4. With thyroid USP or levothyroxine, expect to see a change in the patient's physical appearance and well-being in 1 to 3 weeks. With liothyronine, expect a change in 1 to 3 days.
- Reconstitute levothyroxine for injection immediately before administration. Do not add it to other I.V. fluids. Discard any unused portions.
- Ensure that a patient with adrenal insufficiency receives corticosteroid therapy as prescribed before beginning thyroid therapy.

* ***Do not withdraw a thyroid agent abruptly in a patient with myxedema because it may precipitate myxedema coma.***

- Notify the physician if adverse reactions or drug interactions occur.
- Monitor for cardiac problems if the patient is elderly or has a history of cardiac disease because T_4 may aggravate angina pectoris and lead to MI.

* ***Notify the physician immediately if the patient experiences chest pain during therapy with a thyroid agent. Obtain a prescription for a drug such as nitroglycerin to relieve pain. Also obtain an electrocardiogram, if prescribed.***

- Hypocalcemia and other mineral disorders should be corrected before alendronate therapy begins.

Evaluation

For each nursing diagnosis, prepare an evaluation statement that describes the patient's or family's response to nursing interventions.

Other thyroid agents

Several thyroid agents are used in diagnostic tests. The most common ones—**thyrotropin** and protirelin—help differentiate between the various forms of hypothyroidism. Made from bovine pituitary glands, thyrotropin aids in the differential diagnosis of primary and secondary hypothyroidism. Parenteral administration of 10 IU of thyrotropin for 1 to 3 days precedes serum T_3 and T_4 measurements.

A synthetic version of the natural hypothalamic tripeptide hormone, protirelin assists in the differential diagnosis of secondary and tertiary hypothyroidism. After blood is drawn to obtain a baseline TSH level, the patient receives 400 to 500 mcg of protirelin I.V. A second blood sample is drawn for a TSH level 30 minutes after administration, and a third is drawn 30 minutes later. The patient requires careful monitoring for 1 hour after injection because complications can occur, including transient hypotension or hypertension.

Antithyroid agents

A number of agents act as antithyroid agents or thyroid antagonists. Used for patients with hyperthyroidism (**thyrotoxicosis**), these agents include the thionamides (propylthiouracil and methimazole) and the iodides (stable iodine and radioactive iodine).

PHARMACOKINETICS

The thionamides and the iodides are absorbed through the GI tract, concentrated in the thyroid, metabolized by conjugation, and excreted in the urine. The thionamides inhibit the synthesis, rather than the release, of hormones, so their onset of action may occur 3 to 4 weeks after therapy begins.

Route	Onset	Peak	Duration
P.O.	2 days-weeks	1 hr-15 days	Variable

PHARMACODYNAMICS

The thionamides prevent thyroid hormone synthesis by blocking the combination of iodide and tyrosine. Stable iodine inhibits hormone synthesis through the Wolff-Chaikoff effect, in which above-critical concentrations of intracellular iodide seem to deter hormone synthesis. Radioactive iodine limits hormone secretion by destroying thyroid tissue. Radioactive iodine works in two ways: by inducing acute radiation **thyroiditis** and chronic gradual thyroid atrophy. These mechanisms destroy thyroid tissue. Acute radiation thyroiditis usually occurs 3 to 10 days after administering radioactive iodine. Chronic thyroid atrophy may take several years to appear.

PHARMACOTHERAPEUTICS

Antithyroid agents commonly are used to treat hyperthyroidism, especially in the form of Graves' disease, which accounts for 85% of all hyperthyroidism. (Other causes of hyperthyroidism that require therapy include toxic multinodular goiter, thyroiditis, excessive intake of thyroid hormones, and neoplasms.)

Propylthiouracil, which lowers serum T_3 levels faster than methimazole, usually is used for rapid improvement of severe hyperthyroidism. It also is the thionamide of choice to treat pregnant patients because its rapid action lessens placental transfer and because it does not cause aplasia cutis (a severe dermatologic disorder) in the fetus. Because methimazole blocks thyroid hormone formation for a longer time, it is better suited for administration once a day to patients with mild to moderate hyperthyroidism. Therapy may continue for 12 to 24 months before remission occurs.

To help treat hyperthyroidism, the thyroid gland may be removed by surgery or destroyed by radiation. Preoperatively, stable iodine is used to prepare the gland for surgical removal by firming it and decreasing its vascularity. Stable iodine also is used after radioactive iodine therapy to control symptoms of hyperthyroidism while the radiation takes effect.

Drug interactions

Iodide preparations may react synergistically with lithium, causing hypothyroidism. Other interactions have not proven clinically significant.

ADVERSE DRUG REACTIONS

The most serious adverse reaction to thionamide therapy is potentially fatal granulocytopenia. It typically appears 4 to 8 weeks after treatment begins and usually produces a precipitous drop in white blood cell count. The patient may develop a sore throat or fever.

Hypersensitivity reactions to the thionamides commonly produce pruritus, rash, or fever in the first 3 weeks of treatment.

The iodides can cause **iodism** (chronic toxicity related to iodine therapy), which is dosage-dependent. Iodism can produce an unpleasant brassy taste and burning sensation in the mouth and increased salivation and swelling of the parotid and submaxillary glands. Other signs and symptoms may include headache, rhinitis, conjunctivitis, gastric irritation, bloody diarrhea, anorexia, and depression. These reactions should disappear a few days after iodine therapy is discontinued.

Potassium iodide can cause tooth discoloration. Radioactive iodine can produce a feeling of fullness in the neck and a metallic taste and can increase the risk of birth defects and leukemia.

Rarely, I.V. iodine administration can cause an acute hypersensitivity reaction characterized by angioedema, hemorrhagic skin lesions, and serum sickness. Radioactive iodine also can cause a rare—but acute—reaction 3 to 14 days after administration. During this time, thyroglobulin pours out of damaged follicles and can lead to acute exacerbation of hyperthyroidism and thyroid crisis. Thyroid crisis also may occur after propylthiouracil withdrawal or after administering iodine or iodinated contrast dye.

NURSING PROCESS APPLICATION

The following information assists the nurse in caring for a patient who is receiving an antithyroid agent. It includes an overview of assessment activities as well as examples of appropriate nursing diagnoses and related interventions. It also highlights the importance of evaluation.

Assessment

Before drug therapy begins, review the patient's history for conditions that contraindicate or require cautious use of the prescribed antithyroid agent. Review the patient's medication history to identify use of lithium, which may interact with it. During therapy, assess the patient for adverse drug reactions and signs of drug interactions. Also, periodically

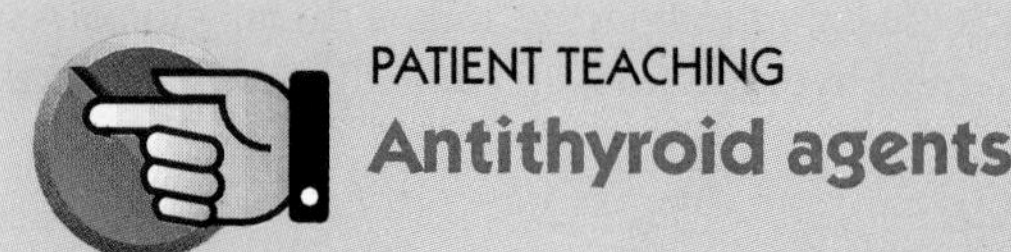

PATIENT TEACHING
Antithyroid agents

- Teach the patient and family the name, dose, frequency, action, and adverse effects of the prescribed antithyroid agent.
- Instruct the patient receiving a thionamide agent to call the physician immediately if a sore throat and fever develop. Explain that the patient may need blood tests and a throat culture if these symptoms appear. Inform the patient that these symptoms are most likely to occur 4 to 8 weeks after drug therapy begins.
- Teach the patient to recognize and report the signs and symptoms of iodism during iodide therapy.
- Advise the patient discharged fewer than 7 days after receiving radioactive iodine for thyroid cancer to avoid close prolonged contact with small children. Also, instruct the patient not to sleep in the same room with anyone else for 7 days after treatment because of the risk of thyroid cancer for people exposed to radioactive iodine. Inform the patient that using the same bathroom as the rest of the family is safe.
- Review radiation precautions with the patient receiving radioactive iodine for hyperthyroidism.
- Teach the patient to recognize the signs and symptoms of a hypersensitivity reaction, such as pruritus and rash. Explain that these symptoms may occur during the first 3 weeks of therapy, and if they do, the physician may prescribe a different medication or treat the reaction with an antihistamine.
- Teach the patient to recognize the signs and symptoms of hypothyroidism, which may occur after radioactive iodine therapy.
- Advise a pregnant patient that she should not receive radiation therapy. Counsel a female patient to wait several months after therapy before becoming pregnant. Advise a male patient not to father a child for several months after therapy.
- Teach the patient to keep the antithyroid agent in a light-resistant container.
- Advise the patient to take the antithyroid agent with meals to prevent adverse gastrointestinal reactions. Radioactive iodine, however, requires overnight fasting before administration.
- Instruct the patient to dilute potassium iodide with water, milk, or fruit juice to mask the salty taste and to drink it through a straw to avoid tooth discoloration.
- Advise the patient to consult the physician before eating iodized salt and iodine-rich foods, such as shellfish, during treatment with an antithyroid agent. The patient also should consult the physician before using any over-the-counter cough medicines because they may contain iodine.
- Instruct the patient to notify the physician if adverse reactions occur.

assess the effectiveness of therapy with the antithyroid agent. Finally, evaluate the patient's and family's knowledge about the prescribed drug.

Nursing diagnoses

- Risk for injury related to a preexisting condition that contraindicates or requires cautious use of an antithyroid agent
- Risk for injury related to adverse drug reactions or drug interactions
- Noncompliance related to long-term use of the antithyroid agent
- Knowledge deficit related to the prescribed antithyroid agent

Planning and implementation

- Do not administer an antithyroid agent to a patient with a condition that contraindicates its use.
- Administer an antithyroid agent cautiously to a patient at risk because of a preexisting condition.
- Watch for effects of propylthiouracil in 3 to 4 weeks.
- Monitor the patient for adverse reactions and drug interactions during therapy with the antithyroid agent.

* ***Monitor the patient's complete blood count periodically to detect impending granulocytopenia, leukopenia, and thrombocytopenia.*** Notify the physician if any of these conditions exist. If laboratory results reveal fewer than 1,500 granulocytes/mm^3, expect to discontinue the drug and administer antibiotics as prescribed.

- Monitor the patient receiving an iodide for signs and symptoms of iodism, such as increased salivation and swelling of the parotid and submaxillary glands, rhinitis, GI distress, and depression. Expect to discontinue iodide therapy if iodism occurs.
- Observe the patient for hypersensitivity reactions to the antithyroid agent.

* ***Monitor the patient for signs and symptoms of thyroid crisis after administering iodine, iodinated contrast dye, or radioactive iodine or after discontinuing propylthiouracil. Be prepared to begin emergency treatment as needed.***

- Evaluate the patient's response to treatment. With propylthiouracil, expect the serum T_4 level to return to normal 14 to 60 days after therapy begins. The average time to reach a **euthyroid** state is 42 to 49 days, but this can vary with drug dosage.

* ***Monitor the patient for signs of toxicity such as thyroid gland enlargement. Also monitor for signs and symptoms of hypothyroidism, such as depression, cold intolerance, and nonpitting edema.***

* ***Take full radiation precautions for 24 hours after a patient receives a dose of radioactive iodine for hyperthyroidism.*** The patient will have slightly radioactive urine and saliva for 24 hours, and highly radioactive vomitus for 6 to 8 hours after taking the dose.

* ***Isolate a patient who receives a dose of radioactive iodine for thyroid cancer because the patient will have radioactive urine, saliva, and perspiration for 3 days.*** Observe the following precautions: Ensure that pregnant personnel do not take care of the patient, use disposable eating utensils and linens, and have the patient save all urine for 24 to 48 hours in a lead container so that the laboratory can measure the amount of radioactive material excreted. Have the patient drink as much fluid as possible for 48 hours after drug administration to facilitate excretion. Limit contact with the patient to 30 minutes per person per shift on the 1st day and 1 hour on the 2nd day. (See Patient Teaching: *Antithyroid agents.*)

• Notify the physician if adverse reactions or drug interactions occur.
• Question the patient about compliance with the prescribed antithyroid regimen. Notify the physician if noncompliance occurs.

Evaluation

For each nursing diagnosis, prepare an evaluation statement that describes the patient's or family's response to nursing interventions.

Other antithyroid agents

Other agents may be used as thyroid antagonists, although they currently are not used as first-line drug therapy for hyperthyroidism. These agents include ionic inhibitors, primarily potassium perchlorate; adrenergic blockers, primarily propranolol; and ipodate, a cholecystographic agent used experimentally to decrease serum T_3 levels.

Ionic inhibitors interfere with the ability of the thyroid gland to concentrate iodide ions. One of the ionic inhibitors, perchlorate, is concentrated in the thyroid gland and excreted unchanged by the kidneys. However, the occasional incidence of granulocytopenia has limited its use.

Researchers recently have recognized lithium as a cation-exchange agent that induces hypothyroidism. But they have not established indications yet for lithium therapy in hyperthyroidism.

Adrenergic blockers deplete catecholamines or prevent their release. These agents, which include propranolol, guanethidine, and reserpine, have been used to reduce the signs and symptoms of hyperthyroidism, such as nervousness, tremor, palpitations, tachycardia, and diaphoresis. Currently, propranolol is used as a short-term adjunct treatment in hyperthyroidism when tachycardia is a problem. Although propranolol reduces conversion of T_4 to T_3, it is not effective when used alone.

Ipodate is an oral cholecystographic agent that has decreased serum T_3 levels in experiments. When given to a hyperthyroid patient, it can reduce serum T_3 levels by almost 70% in 48 hours. Ipodate shows promise for use in the short-term management of hyperthyroidism, as an adjunct therapy after radioactive iodine administration, for more rapid control of hyperthyroidism when given with thionamides, and in preparation for thyroid surgery.

Parathyroid agents

The parathyroid agents, also referred to as calcium regulators, include calcitonin (human), calcitonin (salmon), etidronate disodium, alendronate, and vitamin D analogues, such as calcifediol, calcitriol, and dihydrotachysterol.

PHARMACOKINETICS

After parenteral administration, calcitonin is absorbed directly into the circulation. It is metabolized rapidly by conversion to smaller inactive fragments, primarily in the kidneys, but also in the blood and peripheral tissues. A small amount of unchanged hormone and its inactive metabolites are excreted in the urine.

Route	Onset	Peak	Duration
P.O.	2 hr	Variable	Variable
S.C., I.M.	15 min	4 hr	8-24 hr

PHARMACODYNAMICS

A potent hypocalcemic agent, calcitonin reduces bone resorption and increases renal calcium clearance. Etidronate disodium and alendronate decrease serum calcium primarily by reducing bone resorption. The vitamin D analogues produce their effects by promoting bone resorption, increasing GI absorption of calcium, and decreasing renal calcium clearance. (See *Serum calcium regulation by parathyroid hormone,* page 578.)

PHARMACOTHERAPEUTICS

Calcitonin, alendronate, and etidronate disodium are the drugs of choice for treating **Paget's disease.** Vitamin D analogues are the drugs of choice for increasing the serum calcium concentration.

Drug interactions

Several types of drugs and some foods can interact with the calcium regulators to alter their therapeutic effects. (See Drug Interactions: *Parathyroid agents,* page 579.)

ADVERSE DRUG REACTIONS

The use of these agents to regulate calcium and bone metabolism may produce hypercalcemia. However, because some of these drugs work in opposition to each other, hypocalcemia also may result. With the use of vitamin D analogues, vitamin D intoxication associated with hypercalcemia may occur.

Clinical use of calcitonin can cause flushing, nausea, vomiting, and urticaria. Because calcitonin also is a protein, a severe systemic reaction may occur. In many cases, long-term calcitonin therapy produces swelling and tenderness of the hands. Diarrhea and neurologic symptoms, such as headache, also may occur. Calcitonin antibody formation may result from the activation of the body's antigen-antibody complex. A local inflammatory reaction at the injection site has been documented after long-term use. Rarely, hypocalcemic **tetany** may occur.

Serum calcium regulation by parathyroid hormone

Homeostatic serum calcium concentration levels are maintained by an elaborate feedback system that begins with the stimulation or inhibition of parathyroid hormone (PTH) secretion. The increase or decrease of the PTH level elicits concurrent responses in the renal, gastrointestinal (GI), and skeletal systems. These responses return the serum calcium concentration to normal, as shown.

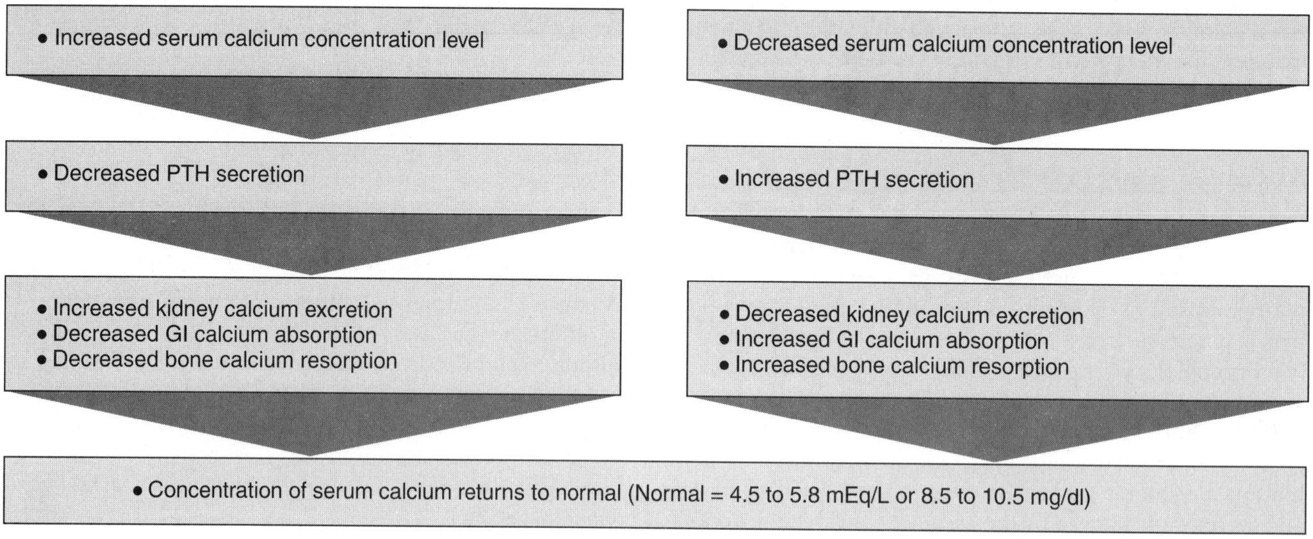

- Increased serum calcium concentration level
- Decreased PTH secretion
- Increased kidney calcium excretion
- Decreased GI calcium absorption
- Decreased bone calcium resorption

- Decreased serum calcium concentration level
- Increased PTH secretion
- Decreased kidney calcium excretion
- Increased GI calcium absorption
- Increased bone calcium resorption

- Concentration of serum calcium returns to normal (Normal = 4.5 to 5.8 mEq/L or 8.5 to 10.5 mg/dl)

Adverse reactions to etidronate disodium are dose-related and uncommon. Usually affecting the GI tract, adverse reactions include nausea, vomiting, abdominal cramps, and diarrhea. Alendronate may cause the same adverse effects. Also, an increased serum phosphate concentration may occur. Etidronate disodium may cause hypocalcemic crisis in which the threshold potential of the neuron is lowered, enabling the neurons to fire more easily. This enhanced motor nerve activity is accompanied by sensory symptoms, including numbness, tingling, muscle twitches, and cramps. Finally, suppressed bone mineralization in the uninvolved skeleton increases the risk of bone fractures in patients with Paget's disease. These patients also experience increased bone pain at the affected sites as well as at previously uninvolved sites.

Normal dosages of vitamin D analogues produce no significant dose-related adverse reactions. Adverse reactions associated with excessive amounts of vitamin D analogues and an increased responsiveness to normal amounts of vitamin D represent a clinical syndrome that probably results from deranged calcium metabolism. The syndrome involves vitamin D intoxication associated with hypercalcemia. Initial signs and symptoms include weakness, fatigue, lassitude, headache, nausea, vomiting, and diarrhea. Signs and symptoms of impaired renal function caused by hypercalcemia include polyuria, polydipsia, nocturia, hyposthenuria (excretion of urine with a low specific gravity), and proteinuria. During chronic hypercalcemia, calcium deposits occur in soft tissue, especially the kidneys, which can lead to nephrolithiasis (kidney stones) and nephrocalcinosis (calcium deposits in the kidneys, leading to infection, hematuria, renal colic, and decreased renal function). Osteoporosis may occur during vitamin D intoxication from the mobilization of calcium from bone. Some infants may exhibit hyperactivity even when small amounts of vitamin D are administered.

NURSING PROCESS APPLICATION

The following information assists the nurse in caring for a patient who is receiving a parathyroid agent. It includes an overview of assessment activities as well as examples of appropriate nursing diagnoses and related interventions. It also highlights the importance of evaluation.

Assessment

Before drug therapy begins, review the patient's history for conditions that contraindicate or require cautious use of the prescribed parathyroid agent. Review the patient's medication history to identify use of drugs that may interact with it. During therapy, assess the patient for adverse drug reactions and signs of drug interactions. Periodically assess the effectiveness of therapy with the parathyroid agent. Finally, evaluate the patient's and family's knowledge about the prescribed drug.

Nursing diagnoses

- Risk for injury related to a preexisting condition that contraindicates or requires cautious use of a parathyroid agent
- Risk for injury related to adverse drug reactions or drug interactions

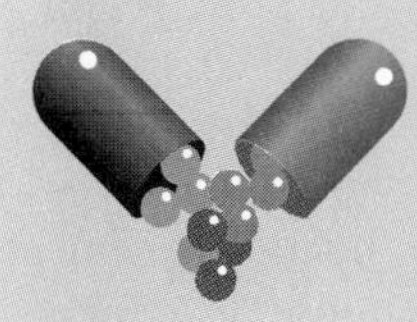

DRUG INTERACTIONS

Parathyroid agents

Drug interactions involving parathyroid agents can increase or decrease bone resorption, kidney reabsorption, and intestinal absorption of calcium. These interactions can produce hypercalcemia or hypocalcemia.

DRUG	INTERACTING DRUGS	POSSIBLE EFFECTS	NURSING IMPLICATIONS
alendronate	aspirin	Adverse gastrointestinal (GI) effects in doses more than 10 mg	• Monitor for GI bleeding, gastritis, or esophagitis.
	calcium supplements and antacids	Decreased alendronate absorption	• Administer at least 2 hours apart.
calcitonin	theophylline, isoproterenol	Increased bone resorption, intestinal absorption, and kidney reabsorption of calcium	• Monitor the patient's calcium and phosphate levels. • Observe for signs and symptoms of calcium imbalance.
etidronate disodium	foods and drugs that contain calcium, iron, magnesium, or aluminum	Decreased absorption of etidronate disodium	• Administer etidronate disodium between meals. • Instruct the patient not to ingest interacting substances within 2 hours after administration of this drug. • Monitor for signs and symptoms of calcium imbalance.
vitamin D analogue (calcifediol)	cholestyramine, colestipol	Decreased calcifediol absorption	• Observe the patient closely for desired therapeutic effect of calcifediol if given with cholestyramine or colestipol.
	thiazide diuretics	Hypercalcemia in patients with hypoparathyroidism	• Observe for signs and symptoms of calcium imbalance. • Discontinue the vitamin D analogue, as instructed.

- Risk for fluid volume deficit related to the adverse GI effects of the prescribed parathyroid agent
- Knowledge deficit related to the prescribed parathyroid agent

Planning and implementation

- Do not administer a parathyroid agent to a patient with a condition that contraindicates its use.
- Administer a parathyroid agent cautiously to a patient at risk because of a preexisting condition.
- Monitor the patient for adverse reactions and drug interactions during therapy with a parathyroid agent.
- Monitor the serum calcium level frequently, assess for signs of hypocalcemic tetany, report the earliest signs of tetany, and ascertain drug compliance if a relapse occurs.

∗ *Monitor for signs of hypocalcemic tetany, such as a positive Chvostek's or Trousseau's sign and a serum calcium concentration of 7 to 8 mg/dl (latent tetany) or less than 7 mg/dl (manifest tetany).*

∗ *Take seizure precautions until the calcium level is restored in a hypocalcemic patient.*

- Prevent vitamin D intoxication by administering the drug exactly as prescribed and by monitoring the serum calcium level. (Serum calcium level multiplied by serum phosphate level should not exceed 70 mg/dl.) Ensure that the patient's daily calcium intake is adequate. (See Patient Teaching: *Parathyroid agents,* page 580).
- Expect to perform or assist with a skin test before administering calcitonin because this drug can cause a systemic allergic reaction. The appearance of more than mild erythema 15 minutes after injection constitutes an abnormal test, indicating that the drug should not be administered.

∗ *Have emergency equipment and medications, such as oxygen, epinephrine, and steroids, nearby during calcitonin therapy to manage a systemic allergic reaction. Also, have calcium readily available for the emergency treatment of hypocalcemic tetany, which also may result from calcitonin therapy.*

- Refrigerate reconstituted calcitonin to maintain its potency.
- Administer oral etidronate disodium with 8 oz (240 ml) of water or juice to reduce GI distress. To enhance etidronate disodium absorption, administer the drug 2 hours before or after the patient consumes food, especially milk, or an antacid high in metals (calcium, iron, magnesium, or aluminum).

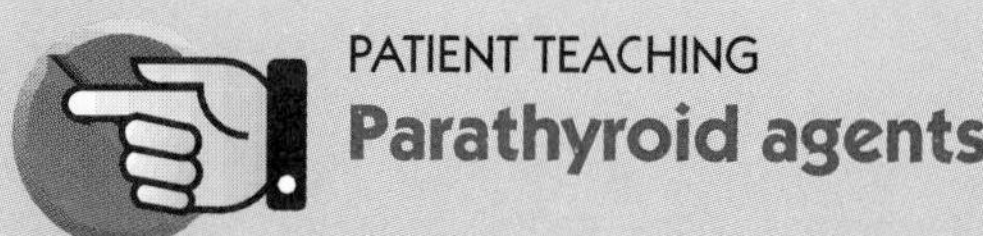

PATIENT TEACHING
Parathyroid agents

- Teach the patient and family the name, dose, frequency, action, and adverse effects of the prescribed parathyroid agent.
- Teach the patient to self-administer calcitonin subcutaneously, the preferred route of administration. If the calcitonin dose exceeds 2 ml, however, instruct the patient to use the intramuscular route and to rotate the injection sites.
- Teach the patient how to use aseptic technique when reconstituting calcitonin and when administering the injection. Teach the patient to recognize and seek advice about local inflammation at injection sites.
- Teach the patient receiving calcitonin to recognize the signs and symptoms of hypocalcemia. Explain to the patient that the initial nausea and vomiting tend to disappear with continued therapy. Inform the patient that facial flushing and warmth occur in some patients within minutes of a calcitonin injection, and assure the patient that these effects usually last no longer than 1 hour. Stress the importance of having periodic laboratory tests to assess renal function.
- Advise the patient taking calcitonin to consult the physician before using over-the-counter (OTC) preparations during treatment because some combination vitamins, hematinic agents, and antacids contain calcium. The patient using calcitonin may have to reduce dietary calcium intake. High-calcium foods include green, leafy vegetables and milk and other dairy products.
- Teach the patient receiving etidronate disodium to maintain a well-balanced diet with an adequate intake of calcium and vitamin D. Advise the patient to include milk and other dairy products as well as green, leafy vegetables in the diet. However, advise the patient not to eat such foods within 2 hours of taking the drug.
- Instruct the patient to report promptly the sudden onset of unexplained bone pain. Urge the patient to keep follow-up appointments for periodic testing.
- Advise the patient receiving a vitamin D analogue to maintain the prescribed diet and calcium supplementation and to avoid OTC drugs. Teach the patient to report signs and symptoms of hypercalcemia and to store the drugs properly. Also, explain that although these drugs are vitamins, they are potent and must not be taken by anyone for whom they were not prescribed because serious toxicity may result.
- Instruct the patient to notify the physician if adverse reactions occur.

• Alendronate must be taken 30 minutes before the first food, beverage, or medication of the day. It should be taken with 6 to 8 oz water only, and the patient should then stay upright for 30 minutes.
• Protect calcitriol and dihydrotachysterol from heat and light to prevent loss of potency. Do not refrigerate dihydrotachysterol.
• Notify the physician if adverse reactions or drug interactions occur.
• Monitor for signs and symptoms of dehydration in a patient with nausea, vomiting, or diarrhea caused by calcitonin, alendronate, or etidronate sodium. If the patient is dehydrated, notify the physician and obtain a prescription for an antiemetic or antidiarrheal, as needed.

Evaluation

For each nursing diagnosis, prepare an evaluation statement that describes the patient's or family's response to nursing interventions.

CHAPTER SUMMARY

Chapter 46 discussed the thyroid agents used to treat hypothyroidism, the antithyroid agents used to treat hyperthyroidism, and the parathyroid agents used to regulate calcium. Here are the chapter highlights.

Thyroid agents are used as replacements when the body's thyroid hormone production cannot meet its needs. These agents include levothyroxine, liothyronine, liotrix, thyroglobulin, and thyroid USP. Thyroid agents are natural or synthetic preparations that contain T_3, T_4, or both. Although the onset of action varies widely among thyroid agents, their principal pharmacologic effect is the same: an increase in the metabolic rate of body tissues.

Antithyroid agents are used to treat hyperthyroidism. Major drugs in this class include the thionamides (propylthiouracil and methimazole) and the iodides (stable iodine and radioactive iodine). Antithyroid agents function by interfering with hormone synthesis, modifying the tissue response to hormones, or destroying the thyroid gland.

When caring for a patient receiving a thyroid or antithyroid agent, the nurse should teach the patient about the signs and symptoms of hypothyroidism and hyperthyroidism, the importance of compliance with the drug regimen, the need for follow-up care, and the signs and symptoms of adverse reactions.

The major parathyroid agents include calcitonin, etidronate disodium, alendronate, and the vitamin D analogues. Calcitonin, alendronate, and etidronate disodium decrease the serum calcium concentration; vitamin D analogues increase this concentration. Calcitonin, alendronate, and etidronate disodium are the drugs of choice for treating Paget's disease. Most adverse reactions to parathyroid agents are dosage-dependent. Because some parathyroid agents increase the serum calcium concentration and others decrease it, toxicity can result in hypercalcemia or hypocalcemia. A systemic allergic reaction may occur with calcitonin administration.

When caring for a patient receiving a parathyroid agent, the nurse should monitor the patient for allergic reactions, signs and symptoms of hypercalcemia or hypocalcemia, and kidney dysfunction. The nurse also should teach the patient about administering the specific drug, following the prescribed diet, and avoiding over-the-counter products, especially those containing calcium.

Questions to consider

See Appendix 1 for answers.

1. Which of the following are signs and symptoms of thyroid toxicity?
   (a) Diarrhea and weight loss
   (b) Weight gain and constipation
   (c) Bradycardia and hypotension
   (d) Lethargy and cold intolerance

2. Joel Grey, age 35, has Graves' disease and takes methimazole 5 mg P.O. t.i.d. How does this drug correct hyperthyroidism?
   (a) It inhibits thyroid hormone synthesis.
   (b) It inhibits thyroid hormone release.
   (c) It destroys excess thyroid tissue.
   (d) It inactivates thyroid hormones.

3. Sally Kennedy, age 45, is diagnosed with hypoparathyroidism. Her physician prescribes the vitamin D analogue calcitriol 0.25 mcg P.O. daily. How does calcitriol increase the calcium concentration?
   (a) It reduces bone resorption.
   (b) It increases GI absorption and bone resorption of calcium.
   (c) It stimulates the parathyroid gland to secrete PTH.
   (d) It decreases osteoclastic activity.

47 Pituitary agents

OBJECTIVES

After reading and studying this chapter, the student should be able to:

1. compare the pharmacokinetic properties of the anterior pituitary agents.
2. describe several diagnostic and therapeutic uses of the anterior pituitary agents corticotropin, cosyntropin, and somatrem.
3. explain why the patient must be monitored carefully for adverse reactions during corticotropin therapy.
4. identify the uses of the posterior pituitary agents.
5. describe the interactions between posterior pituitary agents and other drugs.
6. identify common adverse reactions to posterior pituitary agents.
7. describe how to apply the nursing process when caring for a patient who is receiving a pituitary agent.

INTRODUCTION

Pituitary agents are natural or synthetic hormones that mimic the hormones produced by the pituitary gland. The pituitary agents consist of two groups: anterior pituitary agents and posterior pituitary agents. The anterior pituitary hormone drugs may be used diagnostically or therapeutically to control the function of other endocrine glands, such as the thyroid gland, adrenals, and gonads. Posterior pituitary hormone drugs may be used to regulate fluid volume and stimulate smooth-muscle contraction in selected clinical situations. (See *Selected major pituitary agents.*)

Drugs covered in this chapter include:

- chorionic gonadotropin
- corticotropin
- corticotropin repository
- corticotropin zinc hydroxide
- cosyntropin
- desmopressin acetate
- lypressin
- menotropins
- oxytocin
- oxytocin citrate
- protirelin
- somatrem
- thyroid-stimulating hormone
- thyrotropin
- vasopressin.

Anterior pituitary agents

The protein hormones produced in the anterior pituitary gland regulate growth, development, and sexual characteristics by stimulating the actions of other endocrine glands. Anterior pituitary hormone drugs include the adrenocorticotropics (corticotropin, corticotropin repository, corticotropin zinc hydroxide, and cosyntropin), growth hormone (somatrem), the gonadotropics (chorionic gonadotropin and menotropins), and the thyrotropics (thyroid-stimulating hormone or thyrotropin and protirelin).

PHARMACOKINETICS

The anterior pituitary agents have peptide links, which enable peptidases in the gastrointestinal (GI) tract to destroy the hormones. Therefore, oral administration proves ineffective. Some of these hormones can be administered topically, but most require injection. The pharmacokinetic fate of some anterior pituitary hormone drugs remains unknown. Usually, natural hormones are absorbed, distributed, and metabolized rapidly. Some analogues, however, are absorbed and metabolized more slowly. Anterior pituitary hormone drugs are metabolized at the receptor site and in the liver and kidneys. The hormones are excreted primarily in the urine.

Route	Onset	Peak	Duration
I.V.	5 min	1 hr	2-4 hr
I.M., S.C.	6 hr	Unknown	18-72 hr

PHARMACODYNAMICS

The anterior pituitary agents exert a profound effect on the body's growth and development. Under the control of neurohormonal-stimulating and neurohormonal-inhibiting release factors from the hypothalamus, these hormone drugs alter the functions of their target tissues. The concentration of hormones in the circulating blood helps determine hormone production rate. Increased hormone levels inhibit hormone production; decreased levels raise production and secretion. The relationship between hormone concentration and hormone production critically affects the regulation of

Selected major pituitary agents

The following chart summarizes the major pituitary agents currently in clinical use.

DRUG	MAJOR INDICATIONS AND USUAL DOSAGES	CONTRAINDICATIONS AND PRECAUTIONS
Anterior pituitary agents		
corticotropin (Acthar), corticotropin repository (ACTH Gel, Cortigel, Cortrophin Gel, H.P. Acthar Gel), corticotropin zinc hydroxide (Cortrophin-Zinc)	*Diagnostic testing of adrenal function* ADULT: up to 80 units in a single I.M. or S.C. injection; 10 to 25 units I.V. (aqueous form) in 500 ml dextrose 5% in water (D_5W) infused over 8 hours *Adrenal insufficiency* ADULT: 20 units I.M. or S.C. q.i.d.; 40 to 80 units repository preparation I.M. or S.C. every 24 to 72 hours; or 40 to 80 units zinc hydroxide preparation I.M. every 12 to 24 hours	• Corticotropin is contraindicated in a patient who recently has undergone surgery or one with adrenocortical hyperfunction, primary adrenal insufficiency, systemic fungal infection, peptic ulcer disease, ocular herpes simplex, heart failure, scleroderma, osteoporosis, uncontrolled hypertension, or known hypersensitivity to the drug or to porcine proteins. • This drug requires cautious use in a woman of childbearing age, a pregnant or breast-feeding patient, a patient being immunized, a psychotic patient, or one with myasthenia gravis, latent tuberculosis, hypothyroidism, impaired hepatic function, diabetes mellitus, diverticulitis, abscess or other pyogenic infection, thromboembolic disorder, seizures, or renal insufficiency.
cosyntropin (Cortrosyn)	*Diagnostic testing of adrenal function* ADULT: 0.25 to 0.75 mg I.M. or 0.25 mg I.V. infused over 4 to 8 hours	• Cosyntropin is contraindicated in a patient with known hypersensitivity to the drug or to corticotropin. • This drug has no known precautions.
Posterior pituitary agents		
vasopressin (Pitressin)	*Diabetes insipidus* ADULT: 5 to 10 units S.C. or I.M., 2 to 4 times daily PEDIATRIC: 2.5 to 10 units I.M. or S.C. b.i.d. to q.i.d. *Abdominal distention* ADULT: initially, 5 units I.M., followed by 10 units every 3 to 4 hours PEDIATRIC: highly individualized *GI hemorrhage* ADULT: dilute with normal saline solution or D_5W and infused at 0.2 to 0.4 units/minute up to 0.9 units/minute	• Vasopressin is contraindicated in a patient who is experiencing or recovering from anaphylaxis or one with known hypersensitivity or chronic nephritis with nitrogen retention. • This drug requires cautious use in a pediatric, geriatric, pregnant, or breast-feeding patient or one with epilepsy, migraine headaches, asthma, cardiovascular disease, or fluid overload.
oxytocin (Pitocin, Syntocinon)	*Induction of labor* ADULT: initially, 1 to 2 mU/minute I.V., increased gradually as needed, up to a maximum of 20 mU/minute	• Oxytocin is contraindicated in significant cephalopelvic disproportion, unfavorable fetal position, fetal distress when delivery is not imminent, cord prolapse, placenta previa, fetal prematurity, uterine overdistention, grand multiparity, traumatic delivery, or in a patient with invasive cervical carcinoma, known hypersensitivity, or a history of cesarean delivery or uterine sepsis. • This drug has no known precautions.

hormone levels. (See *Control and effects of anterior and posterior pituitary hormones,* page 584.)

PHARMACOTHERAPEUTICS

The clinical indications for anterior pituitary hormone drugs are diagnostic and therapeutic. Corticotropin and cosyntropin are used diagnostically to differentiate between primary and secondary failure of the adrenal cortex. Corticotropin also is used to treat certain progressive diseases. Somatrem is used to treat pituitary dwarfism.

Because the physiologic need for hormones fluctuates greatly with the patient's age, state of health, stress level, and other variables, dosages must vary. Continual assessment of the patient's response to hormone therapy helps determine the drug regimen.

Control and effects of anterior and posterior pituitary hormones

The hypothalamus and stress stimulate the anterior pituitary gland to secrete hormones that act on various target organs in the endocrine system. The hypothalamus also stimulates the posterior pituitary gland to secrete hormones that act on specific target organs. This chart summarizes the specific action of each hormone and the target organs involved.

STIMULUS	HORMONE	TARGET ORGAN	ACTION
Anterior pituitary			
Hypothalamic neurohormonal releasing factors and stress	thyroid-stimulating hormone	• Thyroid gland	• Synthesis and secretion of thyroid hormone • Metabolic rate control
	growth hormone	• Body muscles • Adipose tissue	• Growth stimulation • Increased protein synthesis
	prolactin	• Mammary glands	• Lactation
	corticotropin	• Adrenal cortex	• Growth stimulation • Cortisol (hydrocortisone) secretion • Increased protein, fat, and carbohydrate metabolism
	follicle-stimulating hormone	• Ovaries • Testes	• Ovulation • Spermatogenesis
	luteinizing hormone	• Testes • Ovaries	• Testosterone production • Progesterone and estrogen production
Posterior pituitary			
Hypothalamic neurocontrol (direct)	oxytocin	• Mammary glands • Kidneys • Uterus	• Lactation • Water reabsorption • Uterine contractions

Drug interactions

Anterior pituitary agents interact with several different types of drugs. (See Drug Interactions: *Anterior pituitary agents.*)

ADVERSE DRUG REACTIONS

Because of the polypeptide nature of all pituitary agents, the major adverse drug reactions are hypersensitivity reactions. Short-term, intensive hormone drug therapy with preparations derived from animal sources increases the possibility of a hypersensitivity reaction. However, these reactions occur less commonly when the therapy involves synthetic hormones.

Because the dosage must vary, the number and types of adverse reactions also vary. The most common dose-related reactions from corticotropin include sodium and water retention, impaired wound healing, dizziness, seizures, and euphoria. Less common dose-related reactions include hypokalemia, hypertension, ketosis, immunosuppression, skin hyperpigmentation, and mood elevation. Long-term use of corticotropin can cause iatrogenic Cushing's syndrome that is indistinguishable from the naturally occurring condition.

Cosyntropin administration may cause pruritus and flushing.

Somatrem may cause glucose intolerance and hypothyroidism. A large percentage of patients treated with somatrem develop antibodies to the hormone. However, the antibodies usually do not interfere with the effectiveness of the therapy.

NURSING PROCESS APPLICATION

The following information assists the nurse in caring for a patient who is receiving an anterior pituitary agent. It includes an overview of assessment activities as well as examples of appropriate nursing diagnoses and related interventions. It also highlights the importance of evaluation.

Assessment

Before drug therapy begins, review the patient's history for conditions that contraindicate or require cautious use of the prescribed anterior pituitary agent. Also review the patient's medication history to identify use of drugs that may interact with it. During therapy, assess the patient for adverse drug reactions and signs of drug interactions. Also, periodi-

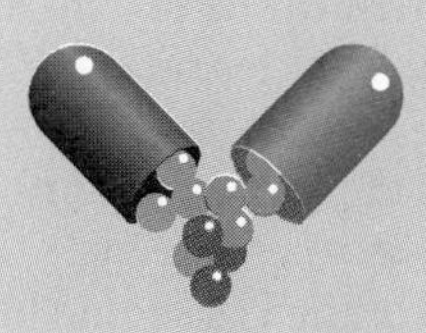

DRUG INTERACTIONS

Anterior pituitary agents

Drug interactions with anterior pituitary agents may reduce the effectiveness of therapy or create additional abnormalities.

DRUG	INTERACTING DRUGS	POSSIBLE EFFECTS	NURSING IMPLICATIONS
corticotropin	immunizations	Neurologic complications, lack of antibody response	• Assess the patient's neurologic status.
	aspirin	Decreased salicylate levels	• Assess for decreased therapeutic effects of aspirin.
	diuretics	Enhanced potassium losses	• Monitor the patient's electrolyte levels, particularly the potassium level.
	barbiturates, phenytoin, rifampin	Decreased corticotropin effect	• Expect to increase the corticotropin dosage, as prescribed.
	estrogens	Increased corticotropin effect	• Adjust the corticotropin dosage as prescribed if estrogens are added to or withdrawn from the patient's drug regimen.
cosyntropin	amphetamines, estrogens, lithium	Altered test results	• Obtain a complete and current drug history. • Consult with the physician to reschedule the test.
somatrem	thyroid hormone and androgens (concurrently)	Epiphyseal closure	• Assess the patient annually for bone age.
	corticosteroids	Diminished growth response, decreased hyperglycemia, decreased sensitivity to insulin	• Document the patient's growth rate carefully for 6 to 12 months before treatment begins. • Instruct a family member to record the pediatric patient's height accurately at regular intervals. • Monitor the patient continually for glycosuria or an increased blood glucose level.

cally assess the effectiveness of therapy with the anterior pituitary agent. Finally, evaluate the patient's and family's knowledge about the prescribed drug. (See Patient Teaching: *Anterior pituitary agents,* page 586.)

Nursing diagnoses

- Risk for injury related to a preexisting condition that contraindicates or requires cautious use of an anterior pituitary agent
- Risk for injury related to adverse drug reactions or drug interactions
- Fluid volume excess related to sodium and water retention caused by corticotropin
- Knowledge deficit related to the prescribed anterior pituitary agent

Planning and implementation

- Do not administer an anterior pituitary agent to a patient with a condition that contraindicates its use.
- Administer corticotropin cautiously to a patient at risk because of a preexisting condition.
- Monitor the patient for hypersensitivity reactions, electrolyte imbalances, and other adverse reactions during therapy with the anterior pituitary agent. Also monitor for drug interactions.
- Perform a hypersensitivity skin test before administering any anterior pituitary agent. After the test, document the result. If it is normal, therapy can begin as prescribed. If it is abnormal, notify the physician.

*∗ **Have epinephrine 1:1,000 readily available for emergency treatment of an allergic reaction.***

*∗ **Observe the patient for hypersensitivity reactions during the first 15 minutes of intravenous (I.V.) administration or immediately after intramuscular (I.M.) or subcutaneous (S.C.) injection.***

*∗ **Observe the patient for signs of hypersensitivity, such as urticaria, tachycardia, and pruritus, after the cosyntropin test (rapid adrenocorticotropic hormone test).***

- Monitor the patient's thyroid function and blood glucose, blood urea nitrogen, and electrolyte levels during somatrem therapy.
- Check the urine and plasma corticosteroid values, as prescribed, to measure the adrenal response before and after administering corticotropin to test adrenocortical function.
- Place the patient on a high-potassium diet, as prescribed, to offset corticotropin-induced loss of potassium.

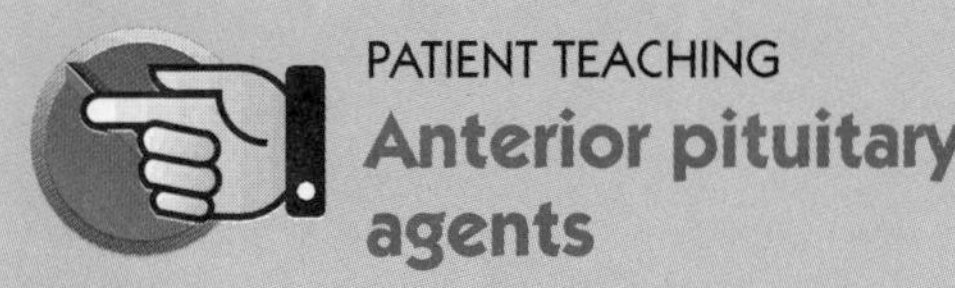

PATIENT TEACHING

Anterior pituitary agents

- Teach the patient and family the name, dose, frequency, action, and adverse effects of the prescribed anterior pituitary agent.
- Inform the patient that a skin test must be performed before drug administration to assess for hypersensitivity reactions.
- Instruct the patient to report promptly any signs of hypersensitivity, such as hives or pruritus, during therapy with an anterior pituitary agent.
- Review the signs and symptoms of infection, peptic ulcer disease, Cushing's syndrome, hypothyroidism, hyperglycemia, and electrolyte imbalances with the patient, and discuss what to do if they occur. Stress the importance of returning for regular laboratory tests to detect these abnormalities.
- Encourage the patient to consume a low-sodium, high-protein, and high-potassium diet during the therapy.
- Warn the patient that corticotropin injections are painful.
- Caution the patient to avoid activities that require mental alertness if dizziness occurs.
- Inform the patient with a wound that healing may be delayed during corticotropin therapy.
- Instruct the patient to record body weight daily and report a sudden weight gain of 2 lb (1 kg) or more. Also teach the patient to recognize and report other signs of fluid retention. If appropriate, advise the patient not to drink more than eight 8-oz (240-ml) glasses of fluid daily.
- Explain the purpose of the cosyntropin test (rapid corticotropin test) before administering it. Advise the patient to fast for 12 hours, rest for 30 minutes, and take no corticotropin or steroids before the test.
- Advise the patient to notify the physician as soon as an adverse reaction occurs.

• Use caution when matching the type of preparation to the administration method. I.V. infusions of corticotropin require aqueous solutions; I.M. and S.C. injections require suspension and gelatin solutions.
• Be aware that corticotropin repository preparation is viscid at room temperature. Corticotropin repository and corticotropin zinc preparations are not suitable for I.V. use and should be shaken before they're injected into the gluteal muscle.
*** *Taper off doses of corticotropin during high-dosage therapy, as prescribed, rather than suddenly withdrawing the drug because withdrawal usually causes 2 to 5 days of hypofunction.***
• Protect corticotropin solutions from heat, temperatures below freezing, and agitation to avoid denaturing the protein molecules in the drug.
• Reconstitute cosyntropin (a synthetic peptide powder) by adding 1 ml of normal saline solution to a 0.25-mg vial to provide 0.25 mg/ml. Reconstituted solutions have a pH of 5.5 to 7.5 and remain stable for 12 hours at room temperature or for 21 days if refrigerated.
• Reconstitute each 5-mg vial of somatrem with 1 to 5 ml of bacteriostatic water for injection. Use only bacteriostatic water preserved with benzyl alcohol. To prepare the solution, inject the bacteriostatic water into the 5-mg vial, aiming the stream against the glass wall. Then rotate the vial gently without shaking it. The contents of the vial should be clear after reconstitution. Discard any drug that appears cloudy or contains particulate material. Use small syringes to validate the accuracy of the dose and a needle of adequate length (1" [2.5 cm] or greater) to ensure muscle insertion.
• Refrigerate the anterior pituitary agent for storage but avoid freezing. Use the contents of reconstituted vials within 1 week.
• Notify the physician if adverse reactions or drug interactions occur.
• Monitor the patient for signs of fluid retention (such as ankle swelling, jugular vein distention, and crackles in the lungs upon auscultation) during corticotropin therapy.
• Provide a low-sodium diet and restrict fluids throughout corticotropin therapy, if appropriate.
• Weigh the patient daily, particularly noting any sudden increase of 2 lb (1 kg) or more.
• Monitor the patient's blood pressure regularly to detect any increase. Also monitor the patient's fluid intake and output to identify any imbalance.
• Notify the physician if fluid retention occurs.

Evaluation

For each nursing diagnosis, prepare an evaluation statement that describes the patient's or family's response to nursing interventions.

Posterior pituitary agents

Protein hormones synthesized by the nerve bodies of the hypothalamus and stored in the posterior pituitary are secreted into the blood by the pituitary gland. Posterior pituitary hormone drugs include all forms of antidiuretic hormone (ADH), such as desmopressin acetate, lypressin, and vasopressin, and the oxytocic agents oxytocin and oxytocin citrate.

PHARMACOKINETICS

Because enzymes in the GI tract can destroy all protein hormones, oral administration of these drugs proves ineffective. Preparations of posterior pituitary agents may be given by injection or intranasal spray.

The precise pharmacokinetics of the oxytocic drugs remains unclear. Like other natural hormones, however, oxytocic drugs usually are absorbed, distributed, and metabolized rapidly. Parenterally administered oxytocin is absorbed rapidly, but when it is administered intranasally, absorption is erratic.

Type	Onset	Peak	Duration
Intranasal	5 min-1 hr	30 min-4 hr	20 min-20 hr
I.V.	1 min	Unknown	Unknown
I.M	3-7 min	Unknown	2-12 hr

PHARMACODYNAMICS

Under neural control, the posterior pituitary hormones affect smooth-muscle contraction in the uterus, bladder, and GI tract; fluid balance via renal reabsorption of water; and blood pressure via stimulation of the arterial wall muscles.

As with other protein hormones, an increase in cyclic adenosine monophosphate in the target cells mediates the effects of ADH. In the kidneys, ADH is bound by receptors on the surfaces of collecting duct cells, thereby regulating the threshold for water reabsorption by the distal tubules, collecting tubules, and collecting ducts. High dosages of ADH stimulate vessel contraction, producing pressor effects and increasing blood pressure. Desmopressin, which has an antidiuretic action, also increases the plasma level of factor VIII (antihemophilic factor). Oxytocin may stimulate uterine contractions by increasing the permeability of uterine cell membranes to sodium ions. It also can stimulate lactation through its effect on mammary glands.

PHARMACOTHERAPEUTICS

ADH is prescribed for hormone replacement therapy in patients affected by neurogenic **diabetes insipidus.** However, it does not treat nephrogenic diabetes insipidus effectively. Short-term ADH treatment is indicated for patients with transient diabetes insipidus after head injury or surgery, but may be lifelong for patients with idiopathic hormone deficiencies. The drugs of choice for chronic deficiency, the synthetic extracts desmopressin and lypressin, are administered intranasally two to four times a day based on the degree of polyuria. These drugs prove particularly useful for patients allergic or refractory to a vasopressin of animal origin. When given in large dosages by the I.V. route, desmopressin is used to increase factor VIII in patients with mild to moderate hemophilia A or B or type I von Willebrand's disease. Used for short-term therapy, vasopressin elevates blood pressure in patients with hypotension caused by lack of vascular tone. It also relieves postoperative gaseous distention.

The oxytocics are used to induce labor and complete incomplete abortions. They also may be used to stimulate lactation; treat **preeclampsia, eclampsia,** and premature rupture of membranes; control postpartal hemorrhage and uterine atony; and hasten uterine involution.

Drug interactions

Drug interactions with posterior pituitary agents can occur with various drugs. (See Drug Interactions: *Posterior pituitary agents,* page 588.)

ADVERSE DRUG REACTIONS

Hypersensitivity reactions are the most common adverse reactions to ADH drugs and oxytocics. These reactions occur more commonly with natural hormone extracts than with synthetic drug preparations. Large dosages of ADH can cause GI distress and cardiovascular problems.

Common dose-related reactions to natural ADHs include circumoral and facial pallor, increased GI motility, and abdominal and uterine cramps. Other adverse reactions can include tinnitus, anxiety, hyponatremia, albuminuria, eclamptic attacks, mydriasis, and transient edema. Nasal preparations can cause irritation, rhinorrhea, and nasal passage ulceration. Accidental deep inhalation of the powder preparation into the bronchial passages may cause substernal tightness, coughing, and transient dyspnea. Large dosages may increase blood pressure. Anaphylaxis may occur after injection.

Adverse reactions to synthetic ADH drugs are rare, although high dosages can cause transient headaches, nausea, nasal congestion, rhinitis, flushing, mild abdominal cramps, and vulvar pain. Decreasing the dosage usually reduces these reactions.

Synthetic extracts have replaced natural oxytocics. Synthetic oxytocin, however, can cause adverse reactions for the pregnant patient, such as postpartum hemorrhage, GI disturbances, diaphoresis, headache, dizziness, and tinnitus. Severe water intoxication has been associated with slow oxytocin infusion over 24 hours. Excessive dosages as well as hypersensitivity to the drug may result in uterine hypertonicity, tetany, or uterine rupture. Uterine hypertonicity can produce fetal asphyxia, which may lead to fetal bradycardia, neonatal jaundice, cardiac arrhythmias, or death.

NURSING PROCESS APPLICATION

The following information assists the nurse in caring for a patient who is receiving a posterior pituitary agent. It includes an overview of assessment activities as well as examples of appropriate nursing diagnoses and related interventions. It also highlights the importance of evaluation.

Assessment

Before drug therapy begins, review the patient's history for conditions that contraindicate or require cautious use of the prescribed posterior pituitary agent. Also review the patient's medication history to identify use of drugs that may interact with it. During therapy, assess the patient for adverse drug reactions and signs of drug interactions. Also, periodically assess the effectiveness of therapy with the posterior pituitary agent. Finally, evaluate the patient's and family's knowledge about the prescribed drug. (See Patient Teaching: *Posterior pituitary agents,* page 589.)

Nursing diagnoses

- Risk for injury related to a preexisting condition that contraindicates the use of a posterior pituitary agent

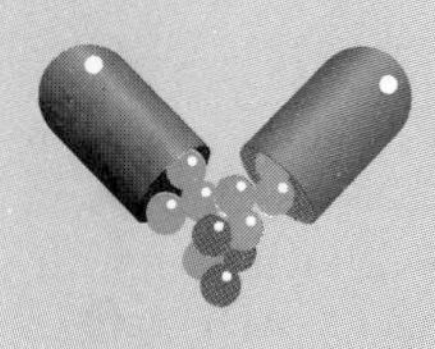

DRUG INTERACTIONS

Posterior pituitary agents

Drug interactions with posterior pituitary agents can be antagonistic, synergistic, or potentiating. Patients receiving hormone therapy should be monitored continually for drug interactions that can alter the desired therapeutic effect.

DRUG	INTERACTING DRUGS	POSSIBLE EFFECTS	NURSING IMPLICATIONS
desmopressin, lypressin, vasopressin	alcohol, demeclocycline, lithium	Decreased antidiuretic hormone (ADH) activity	• Monitor for signs of dehydration, such as acute weight loss, increased pulse rate, dry skin and mucous membranes, decreased orthostatic systolic blood pressure, decreased skin turgor, thirst, and fatigue. • Monitor urine output, specific gravity of urine, and serum osmolality. • Monitor vital signs and weight. • Monitor laboratory values for hematocrit, hemoglobin, red blood cell (RBC) count, and blood urea nitrogen.
	chlorpropamide, clofibrate, carbamazepine, cyclophosphamide	Increased ADH activity	• Monitor for signs and symptoms of water intoxication, such as drowsiness, increased blood pressure, dyspnea, headache, confusion, and weight gain. • Monitor urine output, specific gravity of urine, and serum osmolality. • Monitor vital signs and weight. • Monitor laboratory values for hematocrit, hemoglobin, and RBC counts.
	barbiturate or cyclopropane anesthetics	Synergistic effects, leading to coronary insufficiencies or cardiac arrhythmias	• Monitor vital signs.
oxytocin	cyclophosphamide	Increased oxytocic effect	• Monitor uterine contractions. • Monitor for signs and symptoms of water intoxication.
	vasopressors (anesthetics, ephedrine, methoxamine)	Increased risk of hypertensive crisis and postpartum rupture of cerebral blood vessels	• Monitor vital signs. • Monitor the patient for neurologic changes such as decreased level of consciousness.

- Risk for injury related to a preexisting condition that requires cautious use of vasopressin
- Risk for injury related to adverse drug reactions or drug interactions
- Fluid volume excess related to water intoxication caused by a posterior pituitary agent
- Knowledge deficit related to the prescribed posterior pituitary agent

Planning and implementation

- Do not administer a posterior pituitary agent to a patient with a condition that contraindicates its use.
- Administer vasopressin cautiously to a patient at risk because of a preexisting condition.
- Monitor the patient for adverse reactions and drug interactions during therapy with a posterior pituitary agent.

∗ ***Monitor the patient for hypersensitivity reactions to the posterior pituitary agent, and be prepared to deliver emergency treatment, as prescribed.***

- Monitor hydration if the patient experiences GI distress. Obtain a prescription for an antiemetic or antidiarrheal agent as needed.
- Assess the patient's cardiovascular function frequently. Particularly note vital sign abnormalities, such as irregular heartbeat or increased blood pressure, as well as such signs and symptoms as chest discomfort, shortness of breath, or skin color changes. Notify the physician if abnormalities occur.
- Monitor the patient's urine output to assess the effectiveness of antidiuretic therapy used to treat diabetes insipidus.
- Inspect the nasal passages frequently when natural ADH is given nasally. Be alert for nasal irritation, nasal ulcerations, or rhinorrhea.

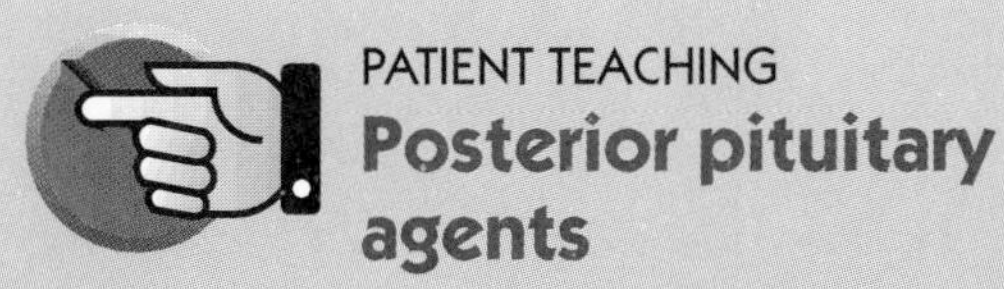

PATIENT TEACHING
Posterior pituitary agents

- Teach the patient and family the name, dose, frequency, action, and adverse effects of the prescribed posterior pituitary agent.
- Teach the patient how to administer the agent, as needed.
- Instruct the patient to clear the nasal passages before administering a nasal preparation, to hold the squeeze bottle upright, and to spray into the nostril while sitting with the head vertical. A nasal preparation should not be administered with the patient lying down or with the head tilted back.
- Teach the patient how to measure fluid intake and output and how to interpret 24-hour fluid measurement during antidiuretic hormone therapy.
- Instruct the patient to never increase the number of vasopressin sprays without speaking to the physician.
- Explain the purpose of intravenous (I.V.) oxytocin administration to the patient and describe the expected outcome. Advise the patient that I.V. oxytocin always is administered under a physician's supervision.
- Advise the patient to notify the physician as soon as an adverse reaction occurs.

• Assess the patient for bowel sounds, flatus passage, and resumption of bowel movements during ADH therapy used to improve peristalsis in the GI tract.
• Check the expiration date on the desmopressin label before administering the drug. Nasal solutions expire 1 year after the date of manufacture.
• Store parenteral and nasal desmopressin in a refrigerator at 39° F (4° C). Discard any cloudy or discolored solution.
Ensure that a physician is present during I.V. or I.M. administration of oxytocin.
Keep magnesium sulfate available during I.M. administration of oxytocin to produce endometrial relaxation, if needed.
Rotate the oxytocin solution container gently to distribute the drug throughout the solution during I.V. administration. Add a Y-connector to the infusion tubing; this provides an alternate route for another solution and ensures patency of the vein if the oxytocin must be discontinued. Always control oxytocin administration with an infusion pump and never administer it by more than one route at a time.
• Use one of the following solutions when infusing oxytocin, as prescribed: dextrose 5% in water (D_5W), D_5W and Ringer's solution, D_5W and lactated Ringer's solution, or D_5W and normal saline solution.
• Reconstitute oxytocin by adding 1 ml (10 units) to 1,000 ml of normal saline solution or other I.V. fluid to provide a solution containing 10 mU/ml (0.01 units/ml).
Assess uterine contractions and the fetal heart rate during oxytocin administration. Discontinue the I.V. infusion immediately, administer oxygen, and notify the physician if contractions become more frequent than every 2 minutes and last longer than 60 seconds without uterine relaxation, if contractions become excessively strong or exceed 50 mm Hg as measured on a monitor, or if the fetal heart rate indicates bradycardia, tachycardia, or irregular rhythm as measured on a monitor.
• Keep the plastic nasal tube for oxytocin administration clean and dry. Measure the nasal oxytocin dosage exactly because the drug is potent.
• Notify the physician if adverse reactions or drug interactions occur or if the drug is ineffective.
• Monitor the patient for early signs of water intoxication when administering a posterior pituitary agent. Document the patient's fluid intake and output.
• Notify the physician if the patient displays signs of water intoxication.

Evaluation
For each nursing diagnosis, prepare an evaluation statement that describes the patient's or family's response to nursing interventions.

CHAPTER SUMMARY

Chapter 47 discussed the anterior and posterior pituitary agents. Here are the chapter highlights.

Anterior pituitary agents act on other endocrine glands, such as the thyroid gland, adrenals, and gonads, to control their function. The three major anterior pituitary agents are corticotropin, cosyntropin, and somatrem.

Posterior pituitary agents regulate fluid volume, stimulate smooth-muscle contraction, and affect blood pressure by stimulating the arterial wall muscles. They include desmopressin acetate, lypressin, vasopressin, oxytocin, and oxytocin citrate.

Pituitary agents are administered parenterally or, for some drugs, intranasally.

Interactions between anterior pituitary agents and other drugs can produce a wide variety of reactions. Interactions between posterior pituitary agents and other drugs can alter ADH activity and can produce cardiovascular dysfunction and water intoxication.

The most significant adverse reaction to these agents is hypersensitivity to the natural hormone drugs. Administering synthetic ones decreases the risk of hypersensitivity.

Nursing care for a patient receiving a pituitary agent typically includes assessing for hypersensitivity reactions and providing emergency treatment, and monitoring for signs and symptoms of other adverse reactions. It also includes patient teaching that explains hormone therapy, stresses the importance of taking accurate dosages, demonstrates correct administration, and emphasizes compliance with the prescribed drug regimen.

Questions to consider

See Appendix 1 for answers.

1. Gail Deana, age 32, is suspected of having adrenal insufficiency. As part of the diagnostic workup, she is given an I.V. infusion of corticotropin 25 units in 500 ml of D_5W over 8 hours. The nurse should observe Ms. Deana for which of the following major adverse reactions?
(a) Sodium and water retention
(b) Orthostatic hypotension
(c) Paroxysmal supraventricular tachycardia
(d) Confusion

2. Keith Deleon, age 22, develops neurogenic diabetes insipidus after sustaining a head injury from a rock climbing fall. The physician prescribes vasopressin 5 units stat. Which of the following administration routes would render vasopressin ineffective?
(a) Intranasal
(b) I.M.
(c) S.C.
(d) P.O.

3. Kristin Applegate, age 26 and 8 months pregnant, experiences premature rupture of membranes and is brought to the hospital by her husband. After an evaluation, her physician decides to induce labor with oxytocin. During labor induction, the nurse determines that Ms. Applegate's contractions occur every 90 seconds and last 70 seconds. How should the nurse intervene?
(a) Continue the medication and notify the physician.
(b) Increase the dosage until the cervix is fully dilated.
(c) Decrease the dosage and continue to monitor the patient.
(d) Stop the medication immediately and notify the physician.

4. Nancy Smith, age 20, is suspected of having hypopituitarism. In order to test her adrenal function, the physician decides to use corticotropin. Why should this drug be used cautiously?
(a) The patient is of childbearing age.
(b) The response to the hormone is unknown.
(c) The drug is used only for hypothyroidism.
(d) Corticotropin can cause ventricular tachycardia.

48 Estrogens, progestins, and oral contraceptive agents

OBJECTIVES

After reading and studying this chapter, the student should be able to:

1. identify the therapeutic uses of estrogens, progestins, and oral contraceptives.
2. identify the major adverse reactions to estrogens, progestins, and oral contraceptives.
3. describe how oral contraceptives prevent pregnancy.
4. compare the monophasic, biphasic, and triphasic oral contraceptives and the progestin implant.
5. describe how to apply the nursing process when caring for a patient who is receiving an estrogen, progestin, or oral contraceptive agent.

INTRODUCTION

Estrogens, progestins, and oral contraceptives mimic the physiologic effects of the naturally occurring female sex hormones, the estrogens and progesterone. The naturally occurring estrogens and progesterone serve a vital function in the development of the female reproductive tract and secondary sex characteristics. Also, estrogens and progesterone are responsible for the maturation of the ovum and its development after fertilization. Therapy with estrogens and progestins includes their use as contraceptives and as replacement therapy after menopause.

This chapter details the natural and synthetic estrogens, used to correct estrogen-deficient states and to prevent pregnancy; the natural and synthetic progestins, used to restore or regulate the menstrual cycle and to treat premenstrual syndrome (PMS) as well as the progestin implant to prevent pregnancy; and the oral contraceptives, used to prevent pregnancy. (See *Selected major estrogens, progestins, and oral contraceptive agents,* page 592.)

Drugs in this chapter include:

- chlorotrianisene
- dienestrol
- diethylstilbestrol
- diethylstilbestrol disphosphate
- estradiol
- estradiol cypionate
- estradiol valerate
- estrone
- ethynodiol diacetate
- ethinyl estradiol
- hydroxyprogesterone caproate
- levonogestrel
- medroxyprogesterone acetate
- norethindrone
- norethindrone acetate
- norgestrel
- quinestrol.

Estrogens

The estrogens discussed in this section include the natural products (conjugated estrogenic substances, estradiol, and estrone) as well as the synthetic estrogens (chlorotrianisene, dienestrol, diethylstilbestrol, diethylstilbestrol diphosphate, esterified estrogens, estradiol cypionate, estradiol valerate, ethinyl estradiol, and quinestrol).

PHARMACOKINETICS

Estrogens are absorbed well and distributed throughout the body. Metabolism occurs in the liver, and the metabolites are excreted primarily by the kidneys.

Estrogens exert their pharmacologic effects via protein synthesis at the cellular level. The time required for this process varies greatly among the preparations.

Route	Onset	Peak	Duration
P.O.	Days to months	Within hours	Variable

PHARMACODYNAMICS

The exact mechanism of action of estrogen is not clearly understood but is believed to involve cytoplasmic receptor proteins found in estrogen-responsive tissues in the female breast and genitourinary (GU) tract. After estrogen binds to these cytoplasmic receptors, the resulting estrogen-receptor complex is transported into the nucleus. This action stimulates the synthesis of messenger ribonucleic acid (mRNA) and deoxyribonucleic acid, which in turn promotes the synthesis of specific proteins responsible for the actions of the estrogens.

PHARMACOTHERAPEUTICS

Estrogens are prescribed primarily for hormonal replacement therapy in postmenopausal women to relieve symp-

Selected major estrogens, progestins, and oral contraceptive agents

This table summarizes the major estrogens, progestins, and oral contraceptives currently in clinical use.

DRUG	MAJOR INDICATIONS AND USUAL DOSAGES	CONTRAINDICATIONS AND PRECAUTIONS
Estrogens		
conjugated estrogenic substances, estradiol (Climara, Vivelle, Estraderm)	*Atrophic vaginitis, kraurosis vulvae* ADULT: 0.3 to 1.25 mg P.O. daily or 2 to 4 g cream administered vaginally daily in 21-day cycle *Female hypogonadism* ADULT: 2.5 mg P.O. daily to t.i.d. for 20 consecutive days each month *Surgical castration, primary ovarian failure* ADULT: 1.25 mg P.O. daily in 21-day cycle *Menopausal symptoms* ADULT: 0.3 to 1.25 mg P.O. daily in 21-day cycle *Osteoporosis* ADULT: 0.625 mg P.O. daily in 21-day cycle *Abnormal uterine bleeding caused by hormonal imbalance* ADULT: 25 mg I.V. or I.M., repeated in 6 to 12 hours, as prescribed *Atrophic vaginitis, female hypogonadism, menopausal symptoms, prophylaxis of osteoporosis, postmenopausal; ovariectomy, primary ovarian failure or vulvar squamous hyperplasia* ADULT: patch replaced twice weekly (Vivelle, Estraderm) or weekly (Climara)	• Conjugated estrogenic substances and estradiol are contraindicated in a patient with known or suspected pregnancy, thrombophlebitis or a thromboembolic disorder, estrogen-dependent cancer of the breast or reproductive organs (except when used as palliative therapy for inoperable cancer in a postmenopausal woman), or undiagnosed abnormal uterine bleeding. • These drugs require cautious use in a depressed patient or one with a condition that may be aggravated by fluid retention, metabolic bone disease, blood dyscrasias, gallbladder disease, seizure disorder, diabetes mellitus, amenorrhea, or a family history of breast or genital cancer.
Progestins		
medroxyprogesterone acetate (Amen, Curretab, Depo-Provera, Provera)	*Amenorrhea or abnormal uterine bleeding caused by hormonal imbalance* ADULT: 5 to 10 mg P.O. daily for 5 to 10 days beginning on day 16 of the menstrual cycle; if the patient has previously received estrogen, 10 mg P.O. daily for 10 days beginning on day 16 of the menstrual cycle	• Medroxyprogesterone acetate is contraindicated in a patient with thrombophlebitis or a thromboembolic disorder, known or suspected pregnancy, cancer of the breast or reproductive organs (except when used as palliative therapy for inoperable cancer in a postmenopausal woman), hepatic disease or dysfunction, undiagnosed abnormal uterine bleeding, or missed abortion. It also is contraindicated as a test for pregnancy. • This drug has no known precautions.
levonorgestrel (Norplant System)	*Long-term prevention of pregnancy* ADULT: six 36-mg capsules of levonorgestrel implanted subdermally in the upper arm during the first 7 days of menses; 150 mg Depo-Provera I.M. every 13 weeks	• Levonorgestrel is contraindicated in a patient with thrombophlebitis or thromboembolic disorders, undiagnosed abnormal genital bleeding, known or suspected pregnancy, acute liver disease, benign or malignant liver tumors, or known or suspected breast cancer. • This drug requires cautious use in a patient who has a strong family history of breast cancer or hyperlipidemia, develops breast nodules during implant use, or has a condition that might be aggravated by fluid retention.
Oral contraceptives		
estrogen-progestin combination products	*Contraception* ADULT: 21-tablet therapy: one tablet P.O. at the same time each day for 21 days beginning on day 5 of the menstrual cycle. 28-tablet therapy: one active tablet P.O. at	• Estrogen-progestin combination products are contraindicated in a patient with known or suspected pregnancy, thrombophlebitis or a thromboembolic disorder, estrogen-dependent cancer (except when used as palliative therapy for inoperable cancer in a postmenopausal woman), or undiagnosed abnormal bleeding.

Selected major estrogens, progestins, and oral contraceptive agents *(continued)*

DRUG	MAJOR INDICATIONS AND USUAL DOSAGES	CONTRAINDICATIONS AND PRECAUTIONS
Oral contraceptives *(continued)*		
estrogen-progestin combination products *(continued)*	the same time each day for 21 days beginning on day 5 of the menstrual cycle, then one inactive tablet P.O. daily for 7 days; when all 28 tablets have been taken, the patient should start a new pill pack. Alternate 28-tablet therapy: one active or inactive tablet P.O. daily based on manufacturer's instructions	• These drugs require cautious use in a depressed patient or one with a condition that may be aggravated by fluid retention, metabolic bone disease, blood dyscrasias, gallbladder disease, seizure disorder, diabetes mellitus, amenorrhea, or a family history of breast or genital cancer.

toms caused by loss of ovarian function. Specific postmenopausal indications include the relief of vasomotor symptoms (hot flashes) and urogenital atrophy as well as the prevention of osteoporosis. Less commonly, estrogens are used for hormonal replacement therapy in patients with primary ovarian failure or female **hypogonadism** and in patients who have undergone surgical castration. Estrogens also are used to prevent postpartal breast engorgement in women who are not breast-feeding and palliatively to treat advanced, inoperable breast cancer in postmenopausal women and prostate cancer in men.

Estrogens most commonly are administered in a cyclic manner during 3 out of 4 weeks of a calendar month. However, this method can cause confusion because therapy may start or end on a different day each month. As an alternative, the patient may take the drug for the first 25 days of the month, not take the drug for the remaining 5 to 6 days, then resume the therapy. This regimen may prove easier to follow because it starts on the first day of the calendar month and always ends on day 25. If a progestin is added, it is administered during the last 10 days of each 25-day cycle.

Drug interactions

Relatively few drugs interact with estrogens. Those that do, such as rifampin, barbiturates, carbamazepine, phenytoin, and primidone, typically result in decreased estrogenic activity, which may not be significant. Estrogens may decrease the anticoagulant effects of anticoagulants. They potentiate the anticonvulsant effects of anticonvulsants. Antibiotics decrease the effects of estrogens. Estrogens interfere with the absorption of dietary folic acid, which may result in a folic acid deficiency.

ADVERSE DRUG REACTIONS

Most adverse reactions to estrogens are mild and do not have serious or long-term consequences. However, endometrial and breast cancer may be more likely to occur in women taking estrogens. The risk of endometrial cancer increases fourfold to eightfold in women taking estrogens. Most of the risk appears to be dose-related—higher dosages over longer periods increase the risk. An increased risk of breast cancer associated with low-dosage estrogen replacement therapy has not been determined definitely.

Thromboembolic disorders have not been linked clearly to estrogen replacement therapy in postmenopausal women.

The incidence of gallbladder disease increases with estrogen use. Increased blood pressure also may occur. Although such increases usually are minor and reversible, some women may develop hypertension.

Adverse metabolic reactions may include decreased glucose tolerance, altered thyroid and liver function test results, increased serum lipoprotein levels, fluid retention, decreased absorption of dietary folic acid, and cholestatic jaundice.

Adverse GU reactions may include breakthrough bleeding, spotting, altered menstrual flow, dysmenorrhea, amenorrhea, and increased risk of vaginal candidiasis. Breast tenderness, enlargement, and secretions also can occur. Adverse central nervous system (CNS) reactions may include depression, migraine headaches, dizziness, and altered libido. Changed corneal curvature may cause vision disturbances or intolerance to hard or rigid gas-permeable contact lenses. Adverse reactions involving the skin include melasma and acne. Urticaria, skin rashes and, rarely, hypersensitivity reactions may occur.

NURSING PROCESS APPLICATION

The following information assists the nurse in caring for a patient who is receiving an estrogen. It includes an overview of assessment activities as well as examples of appropriate nursing diagnoses and related interventions. It also highlights the importance of evaluation.

Assessment

Before drug therapy begins, review the patient's history for conditions that contraindicate or require cautious use of the

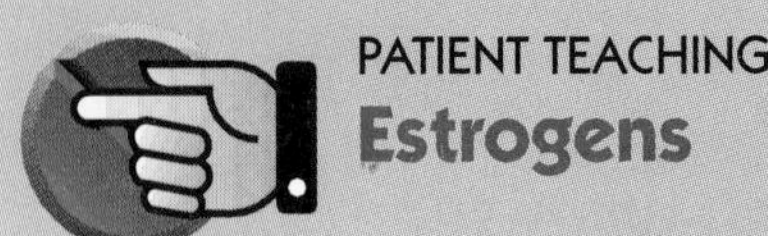

PATIENT TEACHING
Estrogens

- Teach the patient and family the name, dose, frequency, action, and adverse effects of the prescribed estrogen.
- Advise the patient to read the estrogen package insert. Explain and reinforce this information, as needed.
- Instruct the patient to report signs and symptoms of disorders associated with estrogen use, such as abdominal pain, abdominal mass, severe headache, slurred speech, vomiting, dizziness, faintness, weakness, numbness, heaviness in the chest, shortness of breath, blurred vision, blind spots, breast lumps, yellow skin or sclera, dark urine, or light-colored stools.
- Counsel a sexually active patient of childbearing age to use an effective contraceptive method because estrogens (especially diethylstilbestrol) can cause congenital fetal defects.
- Inform the patient that corneal curvature may change, causing vision disturbances or intolerance to hard or rigid gas-permeable contact lenses.
- Explain to the patient on cyclic therapy for postmenopausal symptoms that withdrawal bleeding may occur but does not indicate fertility restoration.
- Instruct the diabetic patient to monitor the blood glucose level regularly and adjust the insulin or oral hyperglycemic agent dosage as prescribed if estrogen causes hyperglycemia.
- Instruct the patient to avoid activities that require mental alertness if dizziness occurs.
- Stress the importance of returning for follow-up examinations and laboratory tests to detect adverse reactions.
- Teach the patient how to perform breast self-examination.
- Instruct the patient to notify the physician if adverse reactions occur.

prescribed estrogen. Also review the patient's medication history to identify use of drugs that may interact with it. During therapy, assess the patient for adverse drug reactions and signs of drug interactions. Also, periodically assess the effectiveness of estrogen therapy. Finally, evaluate the patient's and family's knowledge about the prescribed drug.

Nursing diagnoses

- Risk for injury related to a preexisting condition that contraindicates or requires cautious use of an estrogen
- Risk for injury related to adverse drug reactions and drug interactions.
- Fluid volume excess related to fluid retention caused by the prescribed estrogen
- Knowledge deficit related to the prescribed estrogen

Planning and implementation

- Do not administer an estrogen to a patient with a condition that contraindicates its use.
- Administer an estrogen cautiously to a patient at risk because of a preexisting condition. (See Patient Teaching: *Estrogens.*)
- Monitor the patient for adverse reactions and drug interactions during estrogen therapy.
- Obtain a complete health history and perform a physical examination before estrogen therapy begins and every 6 to 12 months thereafter.
- Determine if the patient is hypersensitive to natural oils (sesame, peanut, or castor oil) before estrogen administration because some intramuscular (I.M.) injections are dispersed in such oils.

∗ ***Observe the patient for signs of a thromboembolic disorder, such as deep vein thrombosis (calf tenderness, redness, and warmth) or pulmonary embolism (sudden onset of shortness of breath, chest pain, and anxiety). Notify the physician immediately if they occur. Be prepared to administer treatment as prescribed.***

- Monitor the patient's blood pressure frequently to detect estrogen-induced hypertension.
- Monitor the patient's blood glucose level regularly. For a diabetic patient, adjust the insulin or antidiabetic agent dosage as prescribed.
- Observe the patient for signs of folic acid deficiency, such as progressive fatigue, shortness of breath, weakness, irritability, and pallor.
- Monitor the results of the following tests to detect estrogen-induced abnormalities: metyrapone test, platelet count, thyroid and liver function tests, prothrombin time, and serum folate, serum triglyceride, and phospholipid level determinations. When any relevant specimen is submitted, inform the laboratory that the patient is receiving estrogen. Notify the physician of any abnormal test results.
- Roll the vial for I.M. administration between the palms to mix the contents completely.
- Administer an I.M. injection deeply into a large muscle.
- Notify the physician if adverse reactions or drug interactions occur.
- Monitor the patient for signs of fluid retention.
- Place the patient on a low-sodium diet and restrict fluid intake to no more than 64 oz (2 L) daily, as prescribed, if fluid retention occurs.
- Notify the physician if fluid retention increases.

Evaluation

For each nursing diagnosis, prepare an evaluation statement that describes the patient's or family's response to nursing interventions.

Progestins

Progesterone is the major natural hormone in this drug class, but it has limited usefulness. It has a short duration of action because it undergoes rapid and extensive first-pass metabolism in the liver. To overcome this disadvantage, researchers have developed several synthetic progestins that remain active when administered orally. Of these, medroxyprogesterone acetate, norethindrone, and norethindrone acetate are used most commonly. Hydroxyprogesterone caproate is a synthetic agent that is administered I.M. Levonorgestrel is the only progestin contraceptive agent currently available as a subdermal implant.

PHARMACOKINETICS

Progestins that are micronized are absorbed well when administered orally and distributed throughout the body. Metabolism occurs in the liver, and the metabolites are excreted primarily by the kidneys.

Route	Onset	Peak	Duration
P.O.	Unknown	Within hours	9-17 days
S.C. (implant)	Up to 24 hr	Up to 24 hr	5 yr

PHARMACODYNAMICS

At the cellular level, progestins act on receptor proteins in cellular cytoplasm. The resulting progesterone-receptor complex is transported into the cell nucleus, where the synthesis of mRNA is stimulated. Under the direction of mRNA, the cell produces various proteins that are responsible for the pharmacologic effects of the progestins.

PHARMACOTHERAPEUTICS

Natural progesterone and its synthetic derivatives are used to treat ovarian disorders. The primary clinical indications for progestin therapy are amenorrhea and abnormal uterine bleeding caused by hormonal imbalance. These conditions are characterized by an absent or abnormal menstrual flow, so the goal of therapy is to restore a regular menstrual cycle. This goal is accomplished by administering estrogens and progestins in a cyclic pattern that resembles the natural secretion pattern of estrogen and progesterone.

Continuous progestin therapy is used to treat endometriosis by preventing menstruation for several months, thereby relieving the symptoms and promoting the regression of the ectopic endometrial growths.

Used singly and in combination with estrogens, progestins also are used commonly as oral contraceptives. Levonorgestrel is a nonoral form of progestin used as a subdermal implant to prevent pregnancy. Progestasert is a plastic intrauterine device embedded with 38 mg of progesterone that prevents pregnancy in two ways. The device prevents implantation and the progesterone thickens cervical mucus to obstruct sperm passage.

Progestins are used less commonly to treat PMS and to provide palliative therapy for advanced metastatic endometrial and renal cancer.

Drug interactions

Rifampin and other drugs that enhance hepatic drug metabolism may increase the clearance of progestins, reducing their effectiveness. For example, concomitant use with carbamazepine or phenytoin may decrease levonorgestrel's efficacy as a contraceptive by increasing its metabolism.

ADVERSE DRUG REACTIONS

Breakthrough bleeding, spotting, changes in menstrual flow, and amenorrhea are the most common adverse reactions to the progestins. In addition, difficult implant removal may occur with levonorgestrel. Progestasert is an intrauterine device that increases the risk of pelvic infection.

Other adverse reactions associated with progestins include cervical erosions or abnormal secretions, uterine fibromas, vaginal candidiasis, edema, weight gain or loss, depression, cholestatic jaundice, thromboembolic disorders, and melasma. Occasional adverse CNS reactions include migraine headaches, dizziness, nervousness, insomnia, and fatigue. Rare reactions include breast tenderness and galactorrhea.

Progestins and estrogens used in combination as oral contraceptives have been associated with an increased risk of thrombophlebitis, pulmonary embolism, and cerebral embolism.

Hypersensitivity reactions, including urticaria, pruritus, angioedema, and generalized skin rashes (with or without pruritus), have occurred. Anaphylaxis is rare.

NURSING PROCESS APPLICATION

The following information assists the nurse in caring for a patient who is receiving a progestin. It includes an overview of assessment activities as well as examples of appropriate nursing diagnoses and related interventions. It also highlights the importance of evaluation.

Assessment

Before drug therapy begins, review the patient's history for conditions that contraindicate or require cautious use of the prescribed progestin. Also review the patient's medication history to identify use of drugs that may interact with it. During therapy, assess the patient for adverse drug reactions and signs of drug interactions. Also, periodically assess the effectiveness of progestin therapy. Finally, evaluate the patient's and family's knowledge about the prescribed drug.

Nursing diagnoses

- Risk for injury related to a preexisting condition that contraindicates or requires cautious use of a progestin
- Risk for injury related to adverse reactions and drug interactions
- Risk for infection with intrauterine device utilization
- Fluid volume excess related to fluid retention caused by the prescribed progestin
- Alteration in comfort related to adverse reactions, such as headache, breast tenderness, and cramping
- Knowledge deficit related to the prescribed progestin

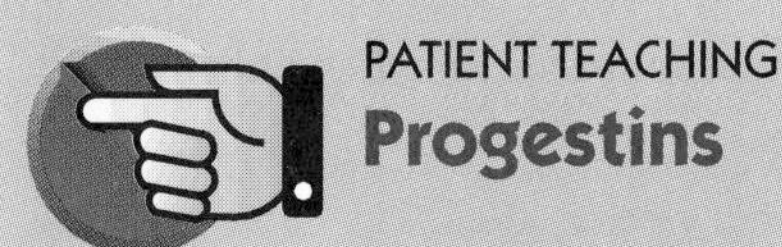

PATIENT TEACHING
Progestins

- ➤ Teach the patient and family the name, dose, frequency, action, and adverse effects of the prescribed progestin.
- ➤ Advise the patient to read the progestin package insert. Explain and reinforce this information, as needed.
- ➤ Explain to the patient that routine follow-up examinations should be performed every 6 to 12 months, with special attention given to the breasts and pelvic organs, the Papanicolaou test, and liver function tests.
- ➤ Teach the patient how to perform breast self-examination.
- ➤ Advise the patient to avoid activities that require mental alertness if dizziness occurs.
- ➤ Teach the patient to report any signs of thromboembolic disorders, including pain in the chest, groin, or calf; headache or changes in vision; shortness of breath; or slurred speech.
- ➤ Counsel a sexually active patient of childbearing age to use an effective contraceptive method because progestins can cause congenital fetal defects.
- ➤ Teach the patient with insomnia to use relaxation techniques, such as reading or taking a warm bath before bedtime, to promote sleep. If insomnia persists, advise the patient to ask the physician to prescribe a hypnotic agent.
- ➤ Teach patient about pelvic inflammatory disease. Instruct the patient to notify the physician of vaginal discharge.
- ➤ Instruct the patient to notify the physician if adverse reactions occur or if concerns arise regarding progestin therapy.

Planning and implementation

- Do not administer a progestin to a patient with a condition that contraindicates its use.
- Administer a progestin cautiously to a patient at risk because of a preexisting condition.
- Monitor the patient for adverse reactions and drug interactions during progestin therapy. (See Patient Teaching: *Progestins.*)

*** Observe the patient for signs and symptoms of thromboembolic disorders, such as thrombophlebitis (calf tenderness, redness, and warmth), pulmonary embolism (sudden onset of shortness of breath, chest pain, and anxiety), or cerebral embolism (abrupt change in consciousness). Notify the physician immediately if any of these signs or symptoms occur and prepare to administer treatment as prescribed.***

- Determine if the patient is hypersensitive to natural oils (sesame, castor, or peanut oil) before progestin administration because I.M. solutions are dispersed in such oils.

*** Have standard emergency equipment nearby because anaphylaxis may occur. Observe the patient for signs of hypersensitivity reactions when beginning progestin therapy. If these signs occur, consult with the physician about discontinuing therapy.***

- Monitor the results of these tests, as prescribed, to detect progestin-induced abnormalities: urine pregnanediol determination and serum alkaline phosphatase, plasma amino acid, and urine nitrogen levels. When any specimen is submitted for testing, inform the laboratory that the patient is receiving progestin.
- Roll the vial for I.M. administration between the palms to mix the contents completely.
- Administer an I.M. injection deeply into a large muscle.
- Be aware that levonorgestrel implants must be removed if a patient becomes pregnant. Also, a patient who develops active thrombophlebitis or thromboembolic disease or who will be immobile for a prolonged period should have the implants removed. Prepare the patient for the possibility of implant removal if jaundice or significant depression occurs.
- Obtain immediate evaluation and medical attention for patients with levonorgestrel implants who develop unexplained partial or complete loss of vision, exophthalmos, diplopia, papilledema, or vascular retinal lesions—these indicate thromboembolism.
- Notify the physician if adverse reactions or drug interactions occur.
- Monitor the patient for signs of fluid retention.
- Place the patient on a low-sodium diet and restrict fluid intake to no more than 64 oz (2 L) daily, as prescribed, if fluid retention occurs.
- Notify the physician if fluid retention increases.

Evaluation

For each nursing diagnosis, prepare an evaluation statement that describes the patient's or family's response to nursing interventions.

Oral contraceptives

The oral contraceptives were the first drugs developed for use in healthy individuals. (See Cultural Considerations: *Oral contraceptives.*) They are used not to cure disease, but to prevent a condition that arises from normal physiologic events. Currently available contraceptive agents are combination products containing 50 mcg or less of estrogen and 1 mg or less of progestin. The few progestin-only oral preparations are known as minipills.

This section discusses the following oral contraceptives: ethinyl estradiol and ethynodiol diacetate, ethinyl estradiol and levonorgestrel, ethinyl estradiol and norethindrone, ethinyl estradiol and norethindrone acetate, ethinyl estradiol and norgestrel, mestranol and norethindrone, norethindrone, and norgestrel.

PHARMACOKINETICS

Oral contraceptives are absorbed well and are distributed throughout the body. Metabolism occurs in the liver, and the metabolites are excreted primarily by the kidneys.

The onset of action of the oral contraceptives is delayed somewhat because of their mechanisms of action. Full contraceptive benefits are not experienced until the contraceptive agents have been taken for at least 10 days.

Oral contraceptives remain effective throughout the 21-day cycle. When the woman has taken all of the tablets properly, the contraceptive efficacy extends through the 7-day contraceptive-free period each month. If doses are missed immediately before or after the contraceptive-free period, however, the likelihood of breakthrough ovulation and contraceptive failure is high. This is especially true for low-dosage products containing estrogen and progestin.

Route	Onset	Peak	Duration
P.O.	Unknown	Unknown	Variable

PHARMACODYNAMICS

Estrogens act as contraceptives by suppressing ovulation and inhibiting implantation of the fertilized ovum. Oral contraceptives create negative feedback to the hypothalamus and pituitary gland, reducing follicle-stimulating hormone (FSH) and luteinizing hormone (LH) concentrations. The diminished FSH concentration prevents follicle development, and the absence of the midcycle surge of LH prevents ovulation.

Estrogens can interfere with implantation of the fertilized ovum by altering ovum transport and by inhibiting the normal secretory development of the endometrium. Alteration of ovum transport can cause the fertilized ovum to be delivered to the uterus at a time improper for implantation. Inhibited secretory development of the endometrium can result in unfavorable conditions for implantation. Interference with ovum implantation is the main mechanism of action of the estrogen-only postcoital contraceptives.

Progestins also inhibit ovulation via the negative feedback mechanism, making combinations of estrogen and progestin nearly 100% effective.

Besides inhibiting ovulation, pharmacologically increased concentrations of progestin occurring during the first half of the female reproductive cycle promote changes in the endometrium that make it unsuitable for ovum implantation. Progestins also thicken cervical mucus, blocking sperm migration toward the ovum. Finally, progestins can slow ovum transport through the fallopian tubes. This may be why women taking the minipill have a higher incidence of tubal and ectopic pregnancies.

PHARMACOTHERAPEUTICS

Oral contraceptives are used primarily to prevent pregnancy and are the most effective form of reversible contraception available.

Oral contraceptives containing high dosages of estrogen and progestin may be used to treat hypermenorrhea and endometriosis and to promote cyclic withdrawal bleeding.

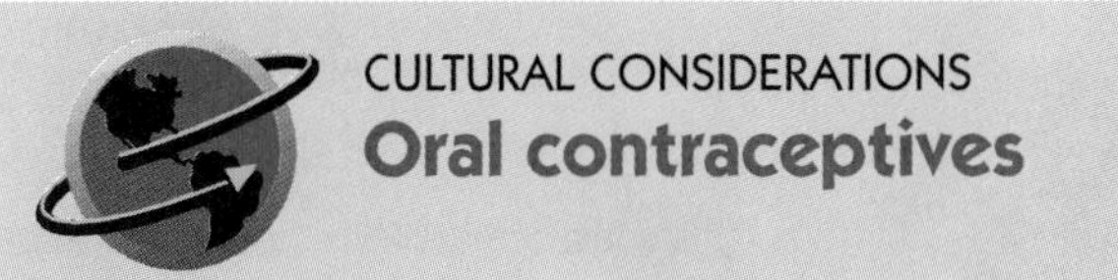

CULTURAL CONSIDERATIONS

Oral contraceptives

Certain religions teach against the use of contraceptives. The Catholic religion specifically disallows the use of unnatural means of interference in the natural act of intercourse. Any use of contraception other than "natural family planning" is unacceptable in the eyes of the Catholic Church. When counseling women and men about contraception, it is important to be aware of their cultural and religious values.

Progestin-dominant oral contraceptives (those providing mainly progestin effects) sometimes are used to treat dysmenorrhea.

Several types of combination oral contraceptives are available. Most are monophasic, providing fixed doses of estrogen and progestin throughout the 21-day cycle. One biphasic product delivers a constant amount of estrogen throughout the 21-day cycle but an increased amount of progestin for the last 11 days. The newest oral contraceptives are triphasic formulations. Two of these provide fixed doses of estrogen throughout the 21-day cycle, with progestin doses varying every 7 days. The others are tablets that vary the estrogen and progestin doses every 7 days throughout the 21-day cycle.

Drug interactions

Relatively few interactions occur between oral contraceptives and other drugs. However, these few interactions are clinically significant. (See Drug Interactions: *Oral contraceptives,* page 598.)

ADVERSE DRUG REACTIONS

The oral contraceptives can produce adverse reactions that range from mild to severe. The most common adverse reaction is nausea. Other gastrointestinal reactions can include vomiting, abdominal cramping, diarrhea, and constipation.

Melasma is the most common adverse dermatologic reaction. Facial hyperpigmentation may develop 1 month to 2 years after the initiation of oral contraceptive therapy and may fade slowly or be permanent. Acne may improve or develop; estrogen-dominant products tend to improve it, progestin-dominant products tend to cause or worsen it.

Serious cardiovascular reactions can result from oral contraceptive use. The incidence of hypertension in women using oral contraceptives is about two to three times that of nonusers. Women taking oral contraceptives also are at greater risk for developing myocardial infarction. This risk increases with age, duration of oral contraceptive use and, especially, cigarette smoking.

Oral contraceptives also are associated with an increased risk of thromboembolic disorders because of their estrogen

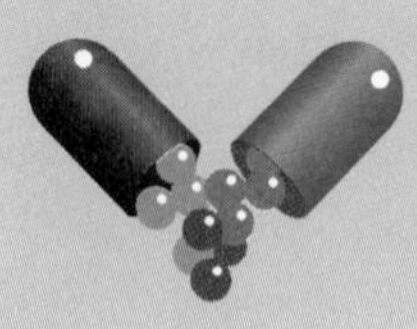

DRUG INTERACTIONS

Oral contraceptives

This chart summarizes the major interactions that can occur between oral contraceptives and other drugs.

DRUG	INTERACTING DRUGS	POSSIBLE EFFECTS	NURSING IMPLICATIONS
all combination oral contraceptives, especially the low-dosage monophasic and the biphasic and triphasic products	barbiturates, carbamazepine, phenylbutazone, phenytoin, primidone, rifampin	Rapid metabolism of oral contraceptives, leading to breakthrough bleeding and decreased contraceptive efficacy	• Advise the patient to use an alternative contraceptive method if therapy with known enzyme-inducers is necessary. A higher dose pill may be prescribed.
	ampicillin, penicillin V, tetracycline	Altered gastrointestinal bacterial flora, leading to decreased contraceptive efficacy and breakthrough bleeding	• Advise the patient to use an alternative contraceptive method during anti-infective therapy and for 1 week after its discontinuation.
	benzodiazepines	Decreased metabolism of oxidatively metabolized benzodiazepines and increased elimination of benzodiazepines that undergo glucuronide conjugation	• Monitor the patient for enhanced therapeutic effects of oxidatively metabolized benzodiazepines (alprazolam, chlordiazepoxide, clorazepate, diazepam, flurazepam, halazepam, and prazepam). • Expect to administer a higher dosage of a benzodiazepine eliminated via glucuronide conjugation (lorazepam, oxazepam, and temazepam), as prescribed.
	corticosteroids	Increased effects of corticosteroids	• Observe the patient for signs of excessive corticosteroid effects. • Adjust the corticosteroid dosage, as prescribed, when oral contraceptive therapy is started or discontinued.
	cyclosporine	Increased plasma concentration of cyclosporine	• Monitor the patient's plasma cyclosporine concentration. • Reduce the cyclosporine dosage, as prescribed.
	anticoagulants	Increase or decrease of anticoagulant effects	• Monitor patient's prothrombin time or partial thromboplastin time, and adjust dose accordingly.

and progestin content. (The current lower-dosage formulations, however, are less likely to cause thromboembolic disorders than the original formulations.) The risk of developing cerebrovascular accidents and subarachnoid hemorrhage, which is already high in patients taking oral contraceptives, is increased further if the patient smokes or has hypertension.

Adverse endocrine and metabolic reactions may occur. Decreased glucose tolerance appears to be related primarily to estrogen, but progestin also may be involved. Estrogens can increase the concentration of high-density lipoproteins; progestins can decrease it. Thus, the overall effect of an oral contraceptive on cholesterol level depends on whether it is estrogen- or progestin-dominant. Oral contraceptive use also may lead to folate deficiency.

Oral contraceptives can affect several serum proteins produced by the liver, elevate the thyroxine-binding globulin concentration, and alter the albumin and immunoglobulin concentrations. Oral contraceptive users also have an increased incidence of liver tumors (primarily benign hepatic adenomas) and gallbladder disease.

Recent epidemiologic studies indicate that oral contraceptives may not be as carcinogenic as was believed previously. For example, none of the currently available oral contraceptives increases the risk of endometrial cancer. However, they may increase the risk of cervical cancer. Recent studies have found no association between oral contraceptive use and breast cancer.

Adverse GU reactions may occur, depending on the estrogen or progestin dominance of the oral contraceptive. Dizziness, headache, depression, lethargy, decreased libido, fluid retention, and edema are associated with oral contraceptive use. Oral contraceptives may worsen myopia or astigmatism and alter the fit of rigid contact lenses. (See Patient Teaching: *Oral contraceptives.*)

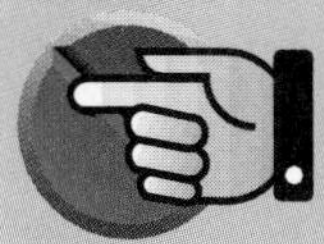

PATIENT TEACHING

Oral contraceptives

- Teach the patient the name, dose, frequency, action, and adverse effects of the prescribed oral contraceptive.
- Advise the patient to read the oral contraceptive package insert. Explain and reinforce this information, as needed.
- Ensure that the patient understands the sequence to follow in taking the pills.
- Instruct the patient to start the first cycle by taking the first pill on day 5 of menstrual bleeding or on the first Sunday after bleeding begins, as directed.
- Teach the patient to swallow the pills whole and to take them at the same time every day (for example, at bedtime or with breakfast) to ensure effectiveness.
- Counsel the patient to use an alternate contraceptive method, such as condoms, spermicides, or a diaphragm, for the first cycle to ensure full protection.
- Advise the patient to expect her period to begin while taking the last seven pills of a 28-pill pack or a few days after taking the last pill in a 21-pill pack.
- Teach the patient to stop taking the pills and contact the physician if pregnancy is suspected or confirmed.
- Reassure the patient that mild nausea, weight gain, breast tenderness, and skin blotching are not unusual and that spotting or bleeding may occur during the first two cycles of oral contraceptives. Instruct the patient to report spotting or bleeding that persists after the second cycle.
- Instruct the patient to take the pill at bedtime if nausea occurs.
- Teach the patient to contact the physician immediately if she experiences any of these signs of blood clots: pain in the chest, arms, or legs; numbness; dizziness; headaches; or vision changes.
- Instruct the patient to store the oral contraceptives in their original container and to keep them out of the reach of children.
- Provide these instructions for missed doses: If the patient misses one pill, she should take it as soon as she remembers. (If she does not remember it until the next day, she should take two pills — the one she forgot and the one scheduled for that day.) If the patient misses two pills in a row, she should take two pills daily for the next 2 days and use an alternative contraceptive method during the rest of the cycle. If the patient misses three or more pills in a row, she should not take any more pills from that cycle and should discard the pack. She should use an alternate contraceptive method until her period begins and then start a new pack on the regular schedule.
- Stress the importance of a semiannual Papanicolaou test and blood pressure check and an annual gynecologic examination.
- Teach the patient how to perform breast self-examination.
- Advise the patient who smokes to stop. Explain the increased risks of cardiovascular dysfunction and thromboembolic events associated with smoking while using an oral contraceptive.
- Instruct the patient to weigh herself at least twice a week and to report any sudden weight gain or swelling to her physician.
- Counsel the patient to use an alternate contraceptive method before surgery to decrease the risk of thromboembolism.
- Explain to the patient that if she misses one menstrual period after having taken all the pills on time, she should start her next cycle of pills at the regularly scheduled time. However, if she misses one menstrual period and has not taken all the pills on time, or if she misses two consecutive menstrual periods even though she has taken all the pills on time, she should stop taking the pills and have a pregnancy test. Explain to the patient that progestins and estrogens can cause birth defects if taken early in pregnancy.
- Explain to the patient that achieving pregnancy may be difficult for a short time after the oral contraceptive is discontinued. Advise her to wait 3 months before trying to become pregnant and to use an alternative contraceptive method in the interim because the endometrium may take up to 3 months to return to normal.
- Advise the patient that oral contraceptive use may alter the fit of rigid contact lenses.
- Instruct the patient to notify the physician if adverse reactions occur or if other concerns arise.
- Instruct the patient that oral contraceptives do not prevent the spread of sexually transmitted diseases such as human immunodeficiency virus. Instruct the patient to use latex condoms during sex with a partner of unknown history.

Some oral contraceptive users have experienced hypersensitivity reactions, such as skin rashes, urticaria, and pruritus.

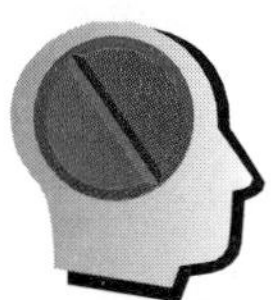

CRITICAL THINKING: To enhance your critical thinking about oral contraceptives, consider the following situation and its analysis.

Situation: Elaine Murray is a 20-year-old obese female who presents to the emergency department complaining of shortness of breath. She denies allergies. She is taking birth control pills. She complains of sharp, right-sided chest pain and has an oxygen saturation of 89% on room air. Her initial chest X-ray is normal, and she has no fever or cough. She denies trauma, and the pain is not reproducible with palpation. What is your impression?

Analysis: Elaine could be suffering from a pulmonary embolism. Classic symptoms include chest pain, shortness of breath, and hypoxia. The use of estrogen and progesterone coupled with obesity would increase her risk for a pulmonary embolus. The physician will want to rule it out by a ventilation perfusion scan or arteriogram.

NURSING PROCESS APPLICATION

The following information assists the nurse in caring for a patient who is receiving an oral contraceptive. It includes an overview of assessment activities as well as examples of appropriate nursing diagnoses and related interventions. It also highlights the importance of evaluation.

Assessment

Before drug therapy begins, review the patient's history for conditions that contraindicate or require cautious use of the prescribed oral contraceptive. Also review the patient's medication history to identify use of drugs that may interact with it. During therapy, assess the patient for adverse drug reactions and signs of drug interactions. Also, periodically assess the effectiveness of oral contraceptive therapy. Finally, evaluate the patient's and family's knowledge about the prescribed drug.

Nursing diagnoses

- Risk for injury related to a preexisting condition that contraindicates or requires cautious use of an oral contraceptive
- Risk for injury related to adverse drug reactions or drug interactions
- Knowledge deficit related to the prescribed oral contraceptive

Planning and implementation

- Do not administer an oral contraceptive to a patient with a condition that contraindicates its use.
- Administer an oral contraceptive cautiously to a patient at risk because of a preexisting condition.
- Monitor the patient for adverse reactions and drug interactions during oral contraceptive therapy.
- Notify the physician if the patient reports or exhibits adverse reactions or drug interactions. Be prepared to implement treatment, as prescribed.

Evaluation

For each nursing diagnosis, prepare an evaluation statement that describes the patient's or family's response to nursing interventions.

CHAPTER SUMMARY

Chapter 48 presented the estrogens, progestins, and oral contraceptives. Here are the chapter highlights.

Estrogens are prescribed primarily for hormonal replacement therapy in postmenopausal women. They also are used as contraceptives, either alone or in combination with progestins.

Progestins are used to treat ovarian disorders (such as abnormal menstrual flow), endometriosis, PMS, and advanced metastatic endometrial or renal cancer. They also are used as contraceptives, either alone or in combination with estrogens. Levonorgestrel is an implantable progestin available for use as a contraceptive.

Oral contraceptives are used to prevent pregnancy and to treat hypermenorrhea, endometriosis, and dysmenorrhea and to promote cyclic withdrawal bleeding. They act primarily by inhibiting ovulation. Most oral contraceptives contain estrogen and progestin. The monophasic preparations provide fixed doses of both hormones throughout the 21-day cycle. The biphasic preparations deliver a constant amount of estrogen throughout the 21-day cycle but an increased amount of progestin during the last 11 days. The progestin dose in triphasic preparations varies every 7 days; the estrogen dose may remain fixed throughout the 21-day cycle or may vary every 7 days.

When caring for a patient who is taking an estrogen, progestin, or oral contraceptive, the nurse should monitor for adverse reactions and teach the patient how to take the drug safely and effectively.

Questions to consider

See Appendix 1 for answers.

1. Joan Tarr, age 42, develops abnormal uterine bleeding caused by a hormonal imbalance. Her physician prescribes conjugated estrogenic substances 25 mg I.M. Before administering the drug, the nurse obtains a thorough medical history. Which of the following conditions would contraindicate estrogen therapy for Ms. Tarr?
   (a) Epilepsy
   (b) Thromboembolic disorder
   (c) Diabetes insipidus
   (d) Gallbladder disease

2. What should a nurse tell a patient about conception during progestin therapy?
   (a) Conception should be avoided because progestin may cause congenital defects.
   (b) Conception is safe during progestin therapy because progestin is a natural hormone.
   (c) Conception is unlikely because progestin acts as a safe and effective contraceptive.
   (d) Conception is common during therapy with progestin, the "pregnancy hormone."

3. Eileen Erskine, age 25, sees her gynecologist for information about birth control methods. After considering her options, she requests an oral contraceptive. The physician prescribes the triphasic oral contraceptive Ortho-Novum 7/7/7. Which of the following drugs may decrease the effectiveness of an oral contraceptive if taken concomitantly?
   (a) diazepam
   (b) aspirin
   (c) cyclosporine
   (d) ampicillin

4. The nurse teaches Margaret McConnahy about oral contraceptives. If Ms. McConnahy misses a dose, what should she do?
   (a) Double the prescribed dosage for the next 7 days.
   (b) Abstain from sexual intercourse, and call her physician immediately.
   (c) Take the missed dose as soon as she remembers or take two pills the next day.
   (d) Wait until the next scheduled dose and use an additional contraceptive method until then.

5. Jane Heme presents to her physician's office and tells the nurse she has not had her period in 9 months, since her levonorgestrel implant was inserted. What should the nurse tell Jane?
   (a) Don't worry; it is normal.
   (b) Inform the physician later.
   (c) Provide urine for a pregnancy test.
   (d) Douche with vinegar and water for 4 days.

6. Jane finds out she is pregnant. She asks if the implants will remain in place. Which of the following is the best answer?
   (a) Yes, there is no sense in removing them now.
   (b) No, they must be removed.
   (c) The decision is up to Jane.
   (d) Yes, but only for 6 more months.

Androgenic and anabolic steroid agents

OBJECTIVES

After reading and studying this chapter, the student should be able to:

1. differentiate between the effects of the androgenic and anabolic steroid agents.
2. describe the mechanisms of action of these agents.
3. describe the major drug interactions that occur with androgenic and anabolic steroid agents.
4. identify the common adverse reactions to these agents and explain how to manage them.
5. describe how to apply the nursing process when caring for a patient receiving an androgenic or anabolic steroid agent.

INTRODUCTION

Androgenic steroids stimulate the growth of male accessory sex organs and produce masculinizing effects, such as facial hair growth and voice deepening. **Anabolic** steroids promote a positive nitrogen balance in the body, which stimulates tissue building and reverses tissue depletion.

In reality, these sharp distinctions are blurred. No purely androgenic or anabolic steroids exist. All androgenic steroids provide some anabolic effects, and all anabolic steroids provide some androgenic effects. However, the distinction between androgenic and anabolic remains useful because one effect always predominates. Predominantly androgenic steroid agents include danazol, fluoxymesterone, methyltestosterone, testolactone, and all forms of testosterone. Predominantly anabolic steroid agents include ethylestrenol, nandrolone decanoate, nandrolone phenpropionate, oxandrolone, oxymetholone, and stanozolol. (See *Selected major androgenic and anabolic steroid agents.*)

Drugs covered in this chapter include:

- danazol
- ethylestrenol
- fluoxymesterone
- methyltestosterone
- nandrolone decanoate
- nandrolone phenpropionate
- oxandrolone
- oxymetholone
- stanozolol
- testolactone
- testosterone.

Androgenic and anabolic steroid agents

These steroid agents have many clinical uses and produce predominantly androgenic or anabolic effects, depending upon the agent used. In androgen-deficient males, androgenic agents can correct **hypogonadism** and related disorders. In females, they may be used to treat certain types of breast cancer and related disorders. Anabolic agents can promote weight gain in underweight patients affected by a catabolic disorder or drug. They also may be used to treat certain types of osteoporosis and anemia.

PHARMACOKINETICS

Anabolic and androgenic steroids are absorbed rapidly and highly bound to plasma proteins. These lipid-soluble agents are distributed widely throughout the body, metabolized in the liver, and excreted mainly by the kidneys. Their onsets of action, peak concentration levels, and durations of action are largely unknown.

PHARMACODYNAMICS

Steroids such as testosterone produce androgenic and anabolic effects by binding to androgen receptors in target organs, such as skeletal muscle, the prostate gland, and bone marrow. Receptor binding not only stimulates development in these organs, but also increases protein synthesis. These actions produce dramatic effects in androgen-deficient patients (such as castrated men, men with pituitary hormone deficiencies, and normal women).

Steroids may promote anabolic effects by blocking cortisol uptake in muscle and liver cells. Secreted by the adrenal gland, cortisol normally acts as a catabolic agent, increasing muscle breakdown and activating the body's stress mechanisms. By blocking cortisol uptake in muscle cells, steroids reduce muscle breakdown and increase muscle mass. By blocking cortisol uptake in liver cells, they maximize its effect on the body's reactions to stress. Steroids also decrease plasma protein synthesis in the liver, which enhances their effects by increasing the amount of free, or unbound, drug in the plasma.

The anabolic steroid agents reduce urine excretion of nitrogen and electrolytes, causing water retention and weight

Selected major androgenic and anabolic steroid agents

The following chart summarizes the major androgenic and anabolic steroids currently in clinical use.

DRUG	MAJOR INDICATIONS AND USUAL DOSAGES	CONTRAINDICATIONS AND PRECAUTIONS
fluoxymesterone (Halotestin, Android-F)	*Hypogonadism and impotence caused by testicular deficiency* ADULT: 5 to 20 mg P.O. daily *Breast cancer in women* ADULT: 10 to 40 mg P.O. daily in divided doses, adjusted to individual's needs and reduced to a minimum dosage when therapeutic effects are noted	• Fluoxymesterone is contraindicated in suspected pregnancy, a pregnant or breast-feeding patient, a male patient with breast or prostate cancer, or a patient with serious cardiac, hepatic, or renal disease or known hypersensitivity. • This drug requires cautious use in a male patient who has experienced delayed onset of puberty.
stanozolol (Winstrol)	*Treatment and prophylaxis of hereditary angioedema* ADULT: Initially, 2 mg P.O. t.i.d.; then decreased at 1- to 3-month intervals to a maintenance dosage of 2 mg daily or every other day	• Stanozolol is contraindicated in suspected pregnancy, a pregnant or breast-feeding patient, a male patient with breast or prostate cancer, or a patient with serious cardiac, hepatic, or renal disease or known hypersensitivity. • This drug requires cautious use in a prepubertal male patient, a patient with diabetes or coronary disease, or a patient receiving corticotropin, a corticosteroid, or an anticoagulant. • Safety and efficacy in children have not been established because this drug may cause serious disturbances in linear growth, thereby affecting adult height.
testosterone cypionate (Andro-Cyp, Depo-Testosterone); Testosterone Transdermal Systems (Androderm, Testoderm)	*Impotence, hypogonadism, male hormone deficiency after castration, male climacteric symptoms* ADULT: 50 to 400 mg I.M. every 2 to 4 weeks ADULT: (Androderm) 2 systems applied nightly for 24 hours. A nonvirilized patient may begin with 1 system applied nightly to back, upper abdomen or thighs. ADULT: (Testoderm) 6 mg/24-hr system applied nightly to the scrotal skin. If scrotal skin is inadequate, a 4 mg/24-hr patch should be applied to scrotal skin. *Metastatic breast cancer in women* ADULT: 200 to 400 mg I.M. every 2 to 4 weeks	• Testosterone cypionate is contraindicated in a pregnant or breast-feeding patient, a male patient with breast or prostate cancer, a patient who is easily sexually stimulated, or a patient with serious cardiac, hepatic, or renal disease; hypercalcemia; or known hypersensitivity. • This drug requires cautious use in a male patient who has experienced delayed onset of puberty. • This drug requires cautious use in a premenopausal patient.
testolactone (Teslac)	*Adjunct therapy in treating advanced or disseminated postmenopausal breast cancer or premenopausal women with terminated ovarian function* ADULT: 250 mg P.O. q.i.d.	• Testolactone is contraindicated in a male patient with breast cancer or a patient with known hypersensitivity. • This drug requires cautious use in a premenopausal patient.

gain. (See Patient Teaching: *Androgenic and anabolic steroids,* page 604.)

PHARMACOTHERAPEUTICS

Although each agent produces androgenic and anabolic effects, one effect always predominates and helps determine the agent's clinical indications.

Androgenic steroids, such as testosterone cypionate and testosterone enanthate, best serve as androgen replacements for castrated males and males with hypogonadism. They produce pronounced effects in prepubertal males. Danazol and other agents can be used to treat hereditary angioedema (an immune disorder that causes transient attacks of subcutaneous, submucosal, or visceral edema) because they can stabilize the immunologic defect by increasing or restoring components in the complement system. Testosterone propionate and related agents can provide palliative treatment for some hormonally responsive breast cancers.

Some predominantly anabolic steroids, such as oxymetholone, can stimulate erythropoiesis (red blood cell

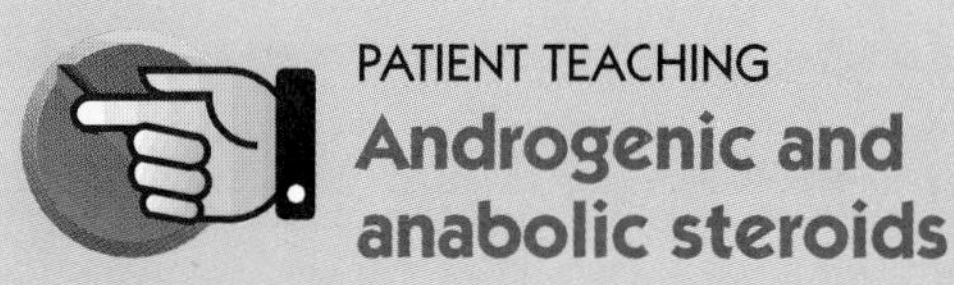

PATIENT TEACHING

Androgenic and anabolic steroids

- Teach the patient and family the name, dose, frequency, action, and adverse effects of the prescribed androgenic or anabolic steroid.
- Teach the patient to take the drug exactly as prescribed for the specified duration of time. Advise the patient not to eliminate any doses or discontinue the drug without consulting the physician.
- Advise the patient receiving a parenterally administered steroid to report irritation at the injection site.
- Teach the patient to store an oral steroid in a dry, light-resistant, and tightly closed container.
- Instruct the patient to carry medical identification or another source of drug information.
- Advise the patient to return as directed for follow-up laboratory tests and physician consultations.
- Help the patient maximize tissue growth by establishing a diet that includes calcium, protein, vitamins, adequate calories, and ample fluids.
- Warn the patient not to take an androgenic or anabolic steroid for body-building or aphrodisiac effects. The risks outweigh the benefits.
- Prepare the patient for changes in appearance, and encourage expression of concerns or fears about these changes.
- Advise the female patient to report to the physician any masculinizing effects, such as hoarseness or voice changes, facial hair growth, clitoral enlargement, acne, increased libido, and menstrual irregularities. Tell her to be particularly alert for increased libido, which may be an early indication of toxicity.
- Reassure the female patient that such effects as facial hair growth and acne should disappear when the drug is discontinued. Other effects, such as voice changes caused by structural alterations in the larynx, may be irreversible.
- Advise the male patient to report to the physician increased libido, priapism, or urinary hesitancy. These reactions may require a dosage reduction or discontinuation of the drug.
- Advise the prepubertal boy and his family that steroid therapy may cause premature development of secondary sex characteristics, such as facial hair and phallic enlargement. The patient or family should report any of these changes to the physician.
- Instruct the patient to notify the physician if adverse reactions occur or other concerns about therapy arise.

production) in the bone marrow, which makes them effective against aplastic and other types of anemia in 25% of patients. Other anabolic steroids, such as oxandrolone, sometimes are used to treat malnourished patients. For some, they can promote a positive nitrogen balance, enhance the appetite, and increase the sense of well-being.

Drug interactions

Although testosterone and its salts do not interact significantly with other drugs, some other androgenic and anabolic steroid agents do. Oral methyltestosterone or oral oxymetholone may increase the effects of oral anticoagulants when used together. Androgenic and anabolic steroids also may interact with high-sodium foods, causing sodium and fluid retention.

ADVERSE DRUG REACTIONS

Androgenic and anabolic steroids can cause many adverse reactions, ranging from changes in sexual characteristics to life-threatening liver failure.

In females, long-term or high-dosage therapy may cause masculinizing reactions, including hoarseness or voice deepening, male pattern hair distribution, menstrual irregularities, acne, increased libido, and clitoral enlargement. Many of these reactions are reversible upon discontinuation of the drug.

In males, adverse reactions result from the conversion of steroids to female sex hormone metabolites in the body. This commonly causes **gynecomastia** — especially in adolescent males — and also may produce testicular atrophy, decreased levels of pituitary reproductive hormones, and prostatic hypertrophy. Other adverse reactions may include priapism (persistent erection), increased libido, and oligospermia.

In children, androgenic and anabolic steroids may cause premature epiphyseal closure (closure of the growth plate in the long bones), thus retarding growth. Prepubertal boys may develop secondary sex characteristics prematurely.

These agents can produce serious toxic effects. In many patients, they elevate liver enzyme levels, resulting in jaundice. In some patients, peliosis hepatis (blood-filled liver cysts) may occur, leading to liver failure. In others, long-term oral therapy may cause liver cancer.

Androgenic and anabolic steroids can affect metabolism in several ways. They commonly increase the serum cholesterol level and decrease the high-density lipoprotein level, predisposing the patient to atherosclerotic heart disease. These agents may increase serum calcium to a dangerous level in a patient with metastatic bone disease or parathyroid hormone hypersecretion. They also may cause sodium and water retention, leading to edema.

Chronic use of anabolic steroids can result in abuse or physical dependence. Physical, psychological, and behavioral changes can ensue, including aggressive behavior. These changes can be seen upon drug withdrawal or when drug levels fluctuate. Collegiate and olympic athletic organizations regularly test athletes for the use of these drugs. The Drug Enforcement Agency now considers androgenic and anabolic steroids schedule III controlled substances.

Androgenic and anabolic steroids do not appear to precipitate allergic or other hypersensitivity reactions.

NURSING PROCESS APPLICATION

The following information assists the nurse in caring for a patient who is receiving an androgenic or anabolic steroid. It includes an overview of assessment activities as well as examples of appropriate nursing diagnoses and related interventions (see "Planning and implementation"). It also highlights the importance of evaluation.

Assessment

Before drug therapy begins, review the patient's history for conditions that contraindicate or require cautious use of the prescribed androgenic or anabolic steroid. Also review the patient's medication history to identify use of drugs that may interact with it. During therapy, assess the patient for adverse drug reactions and signs of drug interactions. Also, periodically assess the effectiveness of therapy with the androgenic or anabolic steroid. Finally, evaluate the patient's and family's knowledge about the prescribed drug.

Nursing diagnoses

- Risk for injury related to a preexisting condition that contraindicates or requires cautious use of an androgenic or anabolic steroid
- Risk for injury related to adverse drug reactions or drug interactions
- Fluid volume excess related to sodium and water retention caused by the androgenic or anabolic steroid
- Knowledge deficit related to the prescribed androgenic or anabolic steroid

Planning and implementation

- Do not administer an androgenic or anabolic steroid to a patient with a condition that contraindicates its use.
- Administer an androgenic or anabolic steroid cautiously to a patient at risk because of a preexisting condition.
- Monitor the patient for adverse reactions and drug interactions during therapy with an androgenic or anabolic steroid.
- Perform a complete physical and nutritional assessment before therapy begins to develop a baseline against which the drug's effects can be measured. Include the patient's blood pressure, pulse rate, and respirations in the physical assessment. Monitor serum protein determinations, which indicate nitrogen and protein balance, as part of the nutritional assessment. Also monitor baseline values for the patient's complete blood count, serum cholesterol and serum calcium levels, and hepatic and cardiac function.

∗ ***Inspect the patient's sclera and skin for jaundice in natural — not fluorescent or incandescent — light.*** If jaundice occurs, notify the physician.

∗ ***Monitor the patient for and report other signs and symptoms of hepatotoxicity.***

∗ ***Monitor for signs and symptoms of hypercalcemia in a patient with metastatic bone disease or parathyroid hormone hypersecretion.*** Monitor the patient's serum calcium level and administer fluids to decrease the risk of renal calculi, which may develop with hypercalcemia and result in flank pain, fever, and hematuria.

- Notify the physician if adverse reactions or drug interactions occur.

∗ ***Monitor the patient's fluid intake and output and weigh the patient daily during dosage determination.*** Report to the physician any weight gain of more than 2 lb (1 kg) in 1 week or any signs of edema, such as swelling in the feet or ankles. Expect to administer a diuretic and a low-sodium diet, as prescribed, to relieve water retention.

Evaluation

For each nursing diagnosis, prepare an evaluation statement that describes the patient's or family's response to nursing interventions.

CHAPTER SUMMARY

Chapter 49 discussed steroid agents, which produce a predominantly androgenic, or masculinizing, effect or a predominantly anabolic, or protein-sparing, effect. Here are the chapter highlights.

Predominantly androgenic steroids include danazol, fluoxymesterone, methyltestosterone, testolactone, and all forms of testosterone. Predominantly anabolic steroids include ethylestrenol, nandrolone decanoate, nandrolone phenpropionate, oxandrolone, oxymetholone, and stanozolol.

Steroids are used in males to treat hypogonadism and related disorders, in females to treat breast cancer and related disorders, and in both sexes to stimulate weight gain.

When caring for a patient receiving an androgenic or anabolic steroid, the nurse should obtain baseline data, monitor the patient for adverse reactions, teach the patient how to store and use the prescribed agent, and help the patient cope with drug-induced changes in the body or in sexuality patterns.

Questions to consider

See Appendix 1 for answers.

1. Sarah Kiley, age 56, has metastatic breast cancer. Her physician prescribes testosterone, an androgenic steroid. Although androgenic and anabolic steroids produce similar effects, generally how do they differ?
   (a) Androgenic steroids produce masculinizing effects; anabolic steroids build muscle mass.
   (b) Androgenic steroids promote development of female sex characteristics; anabolic steroids suppress their development.
   (c) Androgenic steroids promote a positive nitrogen balance; anabolic steroids stimulate cellular protein synthesis.
   (d) Androgenic steroids promote tissue development; anabolic steroids stimulate development of male accessory sex characteristics.

2. During androgenic steroid therapy, the nurse should monitor the patient for which of the following serious toxic effects?
   (a) Anaphylaxis
   (b) Liver failure
   (c) Blood dyscrasias
   (d) Cardiac arrhythmias

3. The nurse should assess a patient receiving an androgenic steroid for which of the following adverse reactions?
   (a) Gynecomastia
   (b) Decreased libido
   (c) Voice deepening
   (d) Growth retardation

4. John Jones, age 12 , is being evaluated for poor growth. His past medical history is significant for hypogonadism and he has been taking androgenic steroids for the past year. John's mother appears worried and asks the nurse, "What do you think?" Which of the following responses best suits the situation?
   (a) I have no idea; you had better ask the physician.
   (b) Tell me what you know about John's medicines.
   (c) It is not the size of the child but the quality that matters.
   (d) This is a common adverse effect of steroids.

UNIT XIV

Drugs for fluid, electrolyte, and nutritional balance

Illness can easily disturb the homeostatic mechanisms that help maintain normal fluid, **electrolyte,** and nutritional balance. Such occurrences as loss of appetite, medication administration, vomiting, and diagnostic tests can also alter this delicate balance. Fortunately, numerous drugs can be used to correct fluid, electrolyte, acid-base, or nutritional imbalances. Unit 14 provides a full range of information about these drugs.

FLUID AND ELECTROLYTE BALANCE

About 60% of an adult's body is made up of water: 60% of this body water is intracellular, 40% is extracellular. The ingestion of food and fluids and the metabolism of nutrients add water to the body — 1,500 to 3,000 ml/day for an average adult. Ordinarily, the fluid intake equals the fluid output, but an illness can upset this delicate balance.

Intracellular and **extracellular fluid** compartments have specific chemical compositions of electrolytes. This unit addresses the major electrolytes: sodium, potassium, chloride, calcium, phosphorus, magnesium, and bicarbonate. (See *Normal electrolyte concentrations in intracellular and extracellular fluid,* page 608.)

Many disorders and diseases can alter electrolyte levels in the fluid compartments, profoundly affecting the body's water distribution, cell function, neuromuscular activity, and acid-base balance. When such imbalances occur, the agents discussed in this unit are used to reestablish homeostasis.

NUTRITIONAL BALANCE

Unit 14 also includes agents used to maintain nutritional balance or to correct a nutritional imbalance. Maintaining nutrition is important because the body relies on exogenous sources of carbohydrate, fat, and protein to sustain life. Nutritional requirements within the body can vary according to a person's weight, age and activity level. Malnutrition must be corrected because it can decrease the ability of organ systems to function, thereby complicating a patient's treatment.

Nutritional assessment

Assessing the type and degree of malnutrition will help determine necessary nutritional support and the goals of therapy. To assess malnutrition, the nurse can use laboratory tests and daily clinical evaluations, including the patient's daily weight and other anthropometric measurements to help determine the status of protein and fat reserves. A triceps skinfold measurement estimates the body's fat reserve. Midarm muscle circumference indicates the protein deficit. The creatinine-height index helps evaluate muscle status. When assessing a patient, the nurse should compare the value of each measurement to the standard value to estimate the degree of depletion.

Certain laboratory tests can help assess visceral protein depletion. For example, a low serum albumin, serum transferrin, and total lymphocyte count may indicate this type of nutritional deficiency.

Nutritional supplements

A complete nutritional supplement will supply carbohydrates, proteins, lipids, electrolytes, **vitamins,** and trace elements. Patients need adequate nonprotein calories to allow optimal protein use, and carbohydrate calories should be given in amounts approximating the basal energy expenditure. Of the daily caloric requirements, 4% to 10% should include essential fatty acids. Daily protein requirements depend on the stress level because stress increases protein use. Maintenance therapy usually requires 0.5 to 1 g of protein/kg/day; high-stress states or moderate protein repletion, 1.5 to 2 g of protein/kg/day; extensive repletion, 2 to 4 g of protein/kg/day. Two types of nutritional supplements may be prescribed: enteral agents, administered through the alimentary canal, and parenteral agents, administered through other routes.

Enteral nutrition

Many physicians prefer enteral nutrition to parenteral nutrition for patients with functional gastrointestinal tracts because it uses the normal metabolic pathways and processes. It allows the body to use nutrients more efficiently and

Normal electrolyte concentrations in intracellular and extracellular fluid

Blood contains intracellular fluid (fluid in red blood cells) and extracellular fluid (plasma fluid). Because their cells allow different substances to permeate, intracellular and extracellular fluids contain different electrolyte concentration levels. For example, intracellular fluid contains about 30 times more potassium than extracellular fluid, whereas extracellular fluid contains about 14 times more sodium than intracellular fluid.

Alterations in electrolyte balance will affect a patient's total physiologic functioning. Some drugs will alter that balance. Various electrolytes are prescribed to treat electrolyte imbalance.

In the clinical setting, the nurse will see values reflecting the components of extracellular fluid only because intracellular fluids are not measured routinely.

Be aware that standards for these values vary among health care facilities.

ELECTROLYTE	INTRACELLULAR CONCENTRATION	EXTRACELLULAR CONCENTRATION
Sodium	10 mEq/L	135 to 145 mEq/L
Potassium	140 mEq/L	3.5 to 5 mEq/L
Calcium	10 mEq/L	4.5 to 5.8 mEq/L
Magnesium	40 mEq/L	1.5 to 2.5 mEq/L
Chloride	4 mEq/L	100 to 108 mEq/L
Bicarbonate	10 mEq/L	24 to 28 mEq/L
Phosphate	100 mEq/L	1.8 to 2.6 mEq/L

tends to cause fewer metabolic problems. Enteral nutrition also is much less expensive, averaging approximately one-tenth the cost of parenteral nutrition. And because there is also little chance of sepsis with tube or oral formulas, they are safer than parenteral forms.

The nurse can administer enteral nutrition by the bolus, gravity drip, or continuous drip method. The bolus method delivers 240 to 400 ml of feeding solution by gravity over several minutes and is repeated every 4 to 6 hours. Because most patients tolerate this method poorly, its use is limited. The gravity drip method infuses 240 to 400 ml of feeding solution over 30 to 60 minutes and is repeated every 4 to 6 hours. Patients usually tolerate this method better than the bolus method. The continuous drip method delivers the feeding solution continuously over 24 hours, usually at a rate of 50 to 125 ml/hour. Ideally, an infusion pump is used to control the infusion rate. Studies show that this method is the most reliable and best tolerated of the three enteral nutrition methods.

Parenteral nutrition

Patients who cannot tolerate oral feeding or enteral nutrition may need parenteral nutrition. Total parenteral nutrition (TPN) or intravenous (I.V.) hyperalimentation, as it is sometimes called, provides carbohydrates, proteins, lipids, electrolytes, vitamins, and trace elements I.V. It supplies carbohydrates as a dextrose solution that provides 3.4 kcal/gram of dextrose. Concentrations of dextrose 5% to 10% may be given via a peripheral vein, but hypertonic solutions greater than 12.5% must be given via a central catheter. Parenteral nutrition supplies proteins in amino acid solutions that provide 4 kcal/gram, and lipids in 10% or 20% fat emulsions that provide 1.1 kcal/ml or 2 kcal/ml, respectively.

The nurse typically initiates central TPN solutions slowly at about 40 to 50 ml/hour, increasing the rate over 24 to 48 hours to the maximum desired rate to avoid severe hyperglycemia. If a low dextrose concentration is used, the nurse may use a rate of 100 to 125 ml/hour. When discontinuing central TPN, the nurse must taper the rate gradually over 24 hours to avoid hypoglycemia.

Because some people are allergic to the egg protein in fat emulsions, therapy should begin with a test dose of 1 ml/minute for 30 minutes. If no adverse reactions occur, the rate may be advanced to the desired rate. The nurse may give fat emulsions through a central or peripheral catheter but should not use an in-line filter because the fat particles are too large to pass through the pores. (See *Comparing types of parenteral nutrition.*)

DRUG THERAPY FOR FLUID, ELECTROLYTE, AND NUTRITIONAL IMBALANCES

Various substances may be used to treat fluid, electrolyte, and nutritional imbalances. For example, a fat-soluble vitamin, water-soluble vitamin, or trace **mineral** may be prescribed, depending on the patient's specific deficiency.

The patient may receive the primary intracellular electrolyte, potassium; a major extracellular electrolyte, calcium; or another electrolyte replacement agent, such as magnesium or sodium, based on the specific electrolyte imbalance.

The patient may require an alkalinizing or acidifying agent to correct abnormal **pH** in the blood or urine. A systemic agent, such as sodium bicarbonate or ammonium chloride, may be used to treat **metabolic acidosis** or **alkalosis;** a **urinary alkalinizer,** such as sodium bicarbonate or acetazolamide, or a **urinary acidifier,** such as ascorbic acid or ammonium chloride, may be needed to treat other disorders.

Comparing types of parenteral nutrition

This chart summarizes the uses and special considerations of the various forms of parenteral nutrition, that can be used for a patient who needs nutritional supplements.

SOLUTION COMPONENTS PER LITER	USES	SPECIAL CONSIDERATIONS
Total parenteral nutrition (TPN) via central venous line		
• Dextrose 15% to 35% (1 L dextrose 25% = 850 nonprotein calories) • Crystalline amino acids 2.5% to 5% • Electrolytes, vitamins, trace elements, insulin, and heparin as prescribed • Fat emulsion 10% to 20% (may be infused as a separate solution; can be given peripherally or centrally)	• Is used for 1 week or more (long-term therapy) • Is used for patients with large caloric and nutrient needs • Provides needed calories, essential vitamins, electrolytes, minerals, and trace elements; restores nitrogen balance • Promotes tissue synthesis, wound healing, and normal metabolic function • Allows bowel rest and healing; reduces activity in the gallbladder, pancreas, and small intestine	**Basic solution** • Is nutritionally complete except for essential fatty acids • Requires minor surgical procedure for central line insertion • Delivers hypertonic solutions • May cause metabolic complications (glucose intolerance, electrolyte imbalances, essential fatty acid deficiency) **I.V. fat emulsion** • May not be used effectively in severely stressed patients (especially burn patients) • May interfere with immune mechanisms
Peripheral parenteral nutrition		
• Dextrose 5% to 10% • Crystalline amino acids 2.75% to 4.25% • Electrolytes, trace elements, vitamins, and heparin as prescribed • Fat emulsion 10% or 20% (1 L dextrose 10% and amino acids 3.5% infused at same time with 1 L 10% fat emulsion = 1,440 nonprotein calories: 340 from dextrose and 1,100 from fat emulsion)	• Is used for 1 week or less • Maintains nutritional status in patients who can tolerate relatively high fluid volume, those who usually resume bowel function and oral feedings in a few days, and those who are susceptible to catheter-related infections of central venous TPN	**Basic solution** • Is appropriate for short-term use only; cannot be used in nutritionally depleted patients • Cannot be used in volume-restricted patients because higher volumes of solution are needed than with central venous TPN • Avoids insertion and maintenance of central catheter, but patient must have good veins; I.V. site should be changed every 48 hours • Requires no surgery for peripheral line insertion • Delivers less hypertonic solutions than central venous TPN • May cause phlebitis **I.V. fat emulsion** • Is as effective as dextrose for caloric source • Irritates vein in long-term use • Diminishes phlebitis if infused at same time as basic nutrient solution
Protein-sparing therapy		
• Crystalline amino acids in same amounts as TPN • Electrolytes, vitamins, and minerals as prescribed	• Is used for 2 weeks or less • May preserve body protein in a stable patient • Augments oral or tube feedings	• Is nutritionally incomplete; may be initiated or stopped at any point in a patient's hospital stay • Allows administration of other I.V. fluids, some drugs, and blood by-products via same I.V. line • Is not as likely to cause phlebitis as peripheral parenteral nutrition
Standard I.V. therapy		
• Dextrose, water, electrolytes, and vitamins in varying amounts *Frequently used parenteral fluids include:* dextrose 5% = 170 cal/L dextrose 10% = 340 cal/L normal saline solution = 0 calories	• Is used for less than 1 week as nutrition source • Maintains hydration (main function) • Facilitates and maintains normal metabolic function	• Is nutritionally incomplete; does not provide sufficient calories to maintain adequate nutritional status

50 Vitamin and mineral agents

OBJECTIVES

After reading and studying this chapter, the student should be able to:

1. explain the pharmacokinetics of the four fat-soluble vitamins (A, D, E, and K), including their routes of absorption, distribution, metabolism, and excretion.
2. identify the signs of vitamin A and D toxicity.
3. discuss the pharmacokinetics of the water-soluble vitamins (B and C), and explain why these preparations are less toxic than the fat-soluble vitamins.
4. identify the clinical uses of water-soluble vitamins.
5. compare the pharmacokinetics, pharmacodynamics, pharmacotherapeutics, and adverse effects of the various minerals.
6. describe how to apply the nursing process when caring for a patient receiving a vitamin or mineral agent.

INTRODUCTION

Vitamins are organic chemicals that do not fit into the categories of protein, fat, or carbohydrate. Vitamins act mainly as coenzymes to help convert carbohydrates and fat into energy and form bones and tissues. Although the human body requires only small amounts of these chemicals, they are essential for the normal operation of various metabolic functions. Vitamins and **minerals** are naturally occurring substances. However, many vitamins can be synthesized, and natural and synthetic forms are commercially available. Both forms function identically.

Vitamins are divided into two categories based on their solubility: fat-soluble and water-soluble. Fat-soluble vitamins include A, D, E, and K. Water-soluble vitamins include B-complex vitamins and vitamin C.

Minerals are inorganic chemicals that are components of all living tissues. Like vitamins, they play a role in various metabolic functions. Because the body cannot manufacture minerals, they must be obtained from some exogenous source, usually food. This chapter discusses the trace mineral (or trace element) agents chromium, copper, fluoride, iodine, manganese, molybdenum, selenium, and zinc. (See *Selected major vitamin and mineral agents.*)

Drugs in this chapter include:

- ascorbic acid
- biotin
- cholecalciferol
- choline
- chromium
- copper
- cyanocobalamin
- ergocalciferol
- fluoride
- folic acid
- inositol
- iodine
- manganese
- menadiol sodium diphosphate
- molybdenum
- niacin
- niacinamide
- panthothenic acid
- para-aminobenzoic acid
- phytonadione
- pyridoxine
- riboflavin
- selenium
- thiamine
- vitamin A
- vitamin E
- zinc.

Fat-soluble vitamins

Pharmacologic preparations of the fat-soluble vitamins A, D, E, and K are discussed in this chapter; they include beta carotene, isotretinoin, vitamin A (as retinol), cholecalciferol (vitamin D_3), ergocalciferol (vitamin D_2), vitamin E, menadiol sodium diphosphate (vitamin K_4), and phytonadione (vitamin K_1). (See *Fat-soluble vitamins: Food sources and RDAs,* page 614.)

PHARMACOKINETICS

Fat-soluble vitamins require the presence of bile salts, pancreatic lipase, and dietary fat for absorption into the body. Vitamin A exists as beta carotene (provitamin A) in plants, and as the retinyl esters in animals. All are converted to forms of retinol in the intestines, where they are absorbed. Vitamin A is distributed widely throughout the body, metabolized in the liver, and excreted in the urine and feces via bile. Its onset of action depends on body requirements. Peak plasma concentration levels of retinol esters occur 4 to 5 hours after oral administration of retinol in an oil solution; 3 to 4 hours after using a water solution preparation.

Oral vitamin D is absorbed readily from the gastrointestinal (GI) tract in the presence of bile. Traveling in the blood bound to protein, vitamin D is stored mostly in fat and muscle, metabolized in the liver and kidneys, and excreted in the feces via bile with a small amount excreted in

Selected major vitamin and mineral agents

The following chart summarizes the major vitamin and mineral agents currently in clinical use.

DRUG	MAJOR INDICATIONS AND USUAL DOSAGES	CONTRAINDICATIONS AND PRECAUTIONS
Fat-soluble vitamins		
vitamin A (Aquasol A)	*Severe vitamin A deficiency with corneal changes* ADULT: 500,000 IU P.O. for 3 days, followed by 50,000 IU P.O. daily for 2 weeks, and then a maintenance dosage of 10,000 to 20,000 IU P.O. daily for 2 months PEDIATRIC: for children age 9 and over, 500,000 IU P.O. for 3 days, followed by 50,000 IU P.O. daily for 2 weeks, and then a maintenance dosage of 10,000 to 20,000 IU P.O. daily for 2 months; for children ages 1 to 8, 5,000 to 15,000 IU I.M. daily for 10 days or 5,000 IU/kg P.O. for 5 days or until recovery occurs; for children under age 1, 7,500 to 15,000 IU I.M. daily for 10 days *Vitamin A deficiency without corneal changes* ADULT: 10,000 to 25,000 IU P.O. daily for 1 to 2 weeks PEDIATRIC: for children age 9 and over, 10,000 to 25,000 IU P.O. daily for 1 to 2 weeks *Malabsorption syndromes* ADULT: 10,000 to 50,000 IU P.O. daily	• Vitamin A is contraindicated in a patient with hypervitaminosis A or hypersensitivity to vitamin A or other ingredients in the commercial preparation • This drug requires cautious use in a pregnant or breast-feeding patient if administered in high dosages. • Excessive intake of vitamin A can occur with vitamin abuse.
ergocalciferol (vitamin D_2) (Calciferol)	*Familial hypophosphatemia* ADULT: 250 mcg to 1.5 mg P.O. daily PEDIATRIC: initially, 1 to 2 mg P.O. daily, increased in 250- to 500-mcg increments at 3- to 4-month intervals until an adequate response is achieved *Hypoparathyroidism* ADULT: 0.625 to 5 mg P.O. or I.M. daily PEDIATRIC: 1.25 to 5 mg P.O. daily *Vitamin D deficiency* ADULT: 0.25 to 7.5 mg P.O. daily PEDIATRIC: 0.25 to 0.625 mg P.O. daily	• Ergocalciferol is contraindicated in a patient with impaired renal function, hypercalcemia, or vitamin D toxicity. • This drug requires cautious use in a patient receiving cardiac glycosides or one with heart disease, renal calculi, arteriosclerosis, or increased sensitivity to vitamin D analogues.
vitamin E (Aquasol E)	*Vitamin E deficiency* ADULT: 60 to 75 IU P.O. daily *Prevention of vitamin E deficiency* ADULT: 30 IU P.O. daily with other vitamins PEDIATRIC: for premature, low-birth-weight neonates, 5 IU P.O. daily; for full-term neonates, 5 IU per liter of formula	• Vitamin E has no known contraindications. • This drug requires cautious use in low-birth-weight neonates.
phytonadione (vitamin K_1) (Aqua-MEPHYTON, Mephyton)	*Anticoagulant-induced hypoprothrombinemia* ADULT: 2.5 to 10 mg P.O., I.M., S.C., or slow I.V. *Hypoprothrombinemia resulting from causes other than anticoagulant therapy* ADULT: 2 to 25 mg P.O., I.M., or S.C., repeated once, as needed PEDIATRIC: for infants, 2 mg P.O., I.M., or S.C.; for older children, 5 to 10 mg P.O., I.M., or S.C. *Prevention of hypoprothrombinemia from vitamin K deficiency in patients on prolonged total parenteral nutrition* ADULT: 5 to 10 mg I.M. weekly PEDIATRIC: 2 to 5 mg I.M. weekly *Hemorrhagic disease in neonates* PEDIATRIC: 0.5 to 1 mg I.M. or S.C.	• Phytonadione is contraindicated in a patient with known hypersensitivity to this drug or other ingredients in the commercial preparation. • This drug requires cautious use in a pediatric patient.

(continued)

Selected major vitamin and mineral agents *(continued)*

DRUG	MAJOR INDICATIONS AND USUAL DOSAGES	CONTRAINDICATIONS AND PRECAUTIONS
Water-soluble vitamins		
thiamine (vitamin B_1) (Betalin S)	*Thiamine deficiency* ADULT: 5 to 30 mg P.O. daily for 1 month PEDIATRIC: 10 to 50 mg P.O. daily, in divided doses *Thiamine dietary supplement* ADULT: 1 to 2 mg P.O. daily PEDIATRIC: for infants, 0.3 to 0.5 mg P.O. daily; for older children, 0.5 to 1 mg P.O. daily *Wet beriberi* ADULT: 10 to 30 mg I.V. t.i.d. *Beriberi* ADULT: 10 to 20 mg I.M. t.i.d. for 2 weeks *Wernicke's encephalopathy* ADULT: 100 mg I.V. daily	• Thiamine is contraindicated in a patient with known hypersensitivity to the drug or other ingredients in the commercial preparation. • This drug has no precautions.
riboflavin (vitamin B_2)	*Riboflavin deficiency* ADULT: 5 to 30 mg P.O. daily PEDIATRIC: 3 to 10 mg P.O. daily *Riboflavin dietary supplement* ADULT: 1 to 4 mg P.O. daily	• Riboflavin has no known contraindications or precautions.
niacin (nicotinic acid, vitamin B_3) (Nicobid, Nicolar)	*Niacin deficiency* ADULT: 10 to 20 mg P.O. daily *Pellagra* ADULT: 300 to 500 mg P.O. daily in divided doses PEDIATRIC: 100 to 300 mg P.O. daily in divided doses *Hyperlipidemia* ADULT: 1.5 to 6 g P.O. daily, in two to four divided doses	• Niacine is contraindicated in a patient with hepatic dysfunction, active peptic ulcer disease, severe hypotension, arterial hemorrhage, or known hypersensitivity. • This drug requires cautious use in a patient with gallbladder disease, diabetes mellitus, gout, or coronary artery disease.
pyridoxine (vitamin B_6) (Beesix, Hexa-Betalin)	*Pyridoxine deficiency* ADULT: 2.5 to 10 mg P.O. daily for 3 weeks, followed by 2 to 5 mg P.O. daily *Prevention of pyridoxine deficiency in patients receiving isoniazid or penicillamine* ADULT: 10 to 50 mg P.O. daily *Prevention of seizures in patients receiving cycloserine* ADULT: 100 to 300 mg P.O. daily in divided doses *Treatment of seizures caused by acute isoniazid intoxication* ADULT: 1 to 4 g I.V., followed by 1 g I.M. every 30 minutes until the total dosage is given (the total pyridoxine dosage should approximate the amount of isoniazid ingested) *Treatment of seizures in pyridoxine-dependent infants* PEDIATRIC: 10 to 100 mg I.M. or I.V.; if response to pyridoxine is positive, infant may require 2 to 100 mg P.O. daily for life	• Pyridoxine is contraindicated in a patient with known hypersensitivity; the I.V. route is contraindicated in a patient with heart disease. • Use with caution in pregnancy, can cause pyridoxine-dependent seizures.
ascorbic acid (vitamin C)	*Prevention of scurvy* ADULT: 70 to 150 mg P.O. daily *Scurvy* ADULT: 100 to 500 mg P.O. daily in divided doses for 2 to 3 weeks PEDIATRIC: 100 to 300 mg P.O. parenterally daily in divided doses for several days *To acidify the urine* ADULT: 4 to 12 g P.O. daily in divided doses	• Ascorbic acid has no contraindications. • This drug requires cautious use in a patient with a history of renal calculi who is receiving long-term or high-dosage therapy. • Excessive vitamin C intake may produce excessive amounts of oxalate in the urine which can result in renal calculi formation.

Selected major vitamin and mineral agents *(continued)*

DRUG	MAJOR INDICATIONS AND USUAL DOSAGES	CONTRAINDICATIONS AND PRECAUTIONS
Trace minerals		
iodine, sodium iodide (Iodopen)	*Additive to TPN solution* ADULT: 1 to 2 mcg/kg daily	• Iodine is contraindicated in a patient with known hypersensitivity, acute bronchitis, or tuberculosis. • This drug requires cautious use when administered for the first time, especially in patients with hypocomplementemic vasculitis, goiter, or autoimmune thyroid disease.
zinc (Zinca-Pak), zinc sulfate (Orazinc)	*Zinc deficiency* ADULT: 200 to 220 mg P.O. t.i.d. *Additive to TPN solution* ADULT: 2.5 to 6 mg I.V. daily	• Zinc is contraindicated in a pregnant or breast-feeding patient.

the urine. After oral or intramuscular (I.M.) administration of natural vitamin D, its onset of action occurs in 10 to 24 hours. Peak concentration occurs about 4 weeks after daily administration of a fixed dosage, and the duration of action can be 2 months or longer.

Vitamin E is absorbed poorly, distributed widely, metabolized in the liver, and excreted in the feces via bile. Information on the onset of action, peak concentration, and duration of action is unavailable.

Vitamin K is absorbed from the GI tract and concentrates in the liver immediately after absorption. Metabolism occurs in the liver, and metabolites are excreted in the bile and urine. Blood coagulation factors may increase in 6 to 12 hours after oral administration of phytonadione and in 1 to 2 hours after parenteral administration. Bleeding may be controlled in 3 to 8 hours, and a normal prothrombin time may be obtained 12 to 14 hours after parenteral administration. The onset of action of parenteral menadiol sodium diphosphate may require 8 to 24 hours.

Route	Onset	Peak	Duration
P.O.	6-24 hr	3 hr-4 wk	12 hr-8 wk
I.M.	1-24 hr	3 hr-4 wk	12 hr-8 wk

PHARMACODYNAMICS

Vitamin A plays a role in preventing night blindness and is essential for growth and development of epithelial tissues, bone growth, human reproduction, and embryonic development. It also plays a role in many biochemical reactions, including steroid metabolism and cholesterol synthesis. Active forms of vitamin D maintain calcium and phosphorus homeostasis in humans, primarily by facilitating their absorption, enhancing their mobilization from bone, and decreasing their renal excretion. Vitamin E may act as an antioxidant and help decrease platelet aggregation. After being produced by bacteria in the intestinal tract, vitamin K is used by the body to synthesize clotting factors and maintain hemostasis.

PHARMACOTHERAPEUTICS

Vitamin A is used primarily to treat vitamin A deficiency. Conditions that may lead to this deficiency include biliary tract or pancreatic disease, extreme dietary inadequacy, or **malabsorption** syndromes. The use of water solution preparations of vitamin A may be beneficial in patients with GI disorders in which vitamin A absorption may be decreased.

Vitamin D is used most frequently as a dietary supplement in persons with malabsorption syndromes, in breastfed and premature infants, and in individuals receiving fewer than 10 mcg of vitamin D daily from food. Patients with vitamin D-dependent rickets usually respond best to calcitriol (one of the vitamin D analogues). Ergocalciferol and dihydrotachysterol have been used with oral calcium therapy to treat osteoporosis. However, further studies are needed to determine the efficacy of vitamin D therapy in osteoporosis.

Because vitamin E is abundant in normal diets, deficiency of this vitamin normally does not occur. Deficiencies may occur in persons with abetalipoproteinemia, abnormal fat absorption, or malabsorption syndromes. The only established use for vitamin E is for treating or preventing vitamin E deficiency.

Vitamin K is used to prevent or treat hypoprothrombinemia caused by vitamin K deficiency. It is also used to treat anticoagulant-induced hypoprothrombinemia. Phytonadione is the drug of choice for treating a moderate to severe hemorrhage caused by excessive dosages of coumarin anticoagulants and for treating or preventing hemorrhagic disease of the newborn. Phytonadione also is effective in preventing neonatal hemorrhage resulting from anticonvul-

Fat-soluble vitamins: Food sources and RDAs

To prevent chronic deficiencies, the nurse should teach the patient about dietary sources and recommended daily allowances (RDAs) for vitamins A, D, E, and K. The chart below provides this information, with the RDAs grouped by patient age and condition.

VITAMIN	FOOD SOURCES	RDAs
vitamin A	Dairy products, liver, egg yolks, fish, and yellow or green fruits and vegetables	*Infants up to age 1:* 375 mcg *Children ages 1 to 10:* 400 to 700 mcg *Males age 11 and older:* 1,000 mcg *Females age 11 and older:* 800 mcg *Pregnant females:* 1,300 mcg *Breast-feeding females:* 1,200 to 1,300 mcg
vitamin D	Fortified milk and margarine	*Infants up to age 1:* 7.5 to 10 mcg *Children ages 1 to 10:* 10 mcg *Males age 11 and older:* 5 to 10 mcg *Females age 11 and older:* 5 to 10 mcg *Pregnant females:* 10 mcg *Breast-feeding females:* 10 mcg
vitamin E	Vegetable oils, margarine, milk, egg yolks, meats, green leafy vegetables, whole grains, and animal fats	*Infants up to age 1:* 3 to 4 mg *Children ages 1 to 10:* 6 to 7 mg *Males age 11 and older:* 10 mg *Females age 11 and older:* 8 mg *Pregnant females:* 10 mg *Breast-feeding females:* 11 to 12 mg
vitamin K	Liver, cheese, egg yolks, green leafy vegetables, tomatoes, meats, milk, cauliflower, wheat bran, and vegetable oils	*Infants up to age 1:* 5 to 10 mcg *Children ages 1 to 10:* 15 to 30 mcg *Males age 11 and older:* 45 to 80 mcg *Females age 11 and older:* 45 to 65 mcg *Pregnant females:* 65 mcg *Breast-feeding females:* 65 mcg

sants or anticoagulants used during pregnancy. Other causes of hypoprothrombinemia, such as malabsorption syndromes and therapy with salicylates, sulfonamides, quinidine, coumarin anticoagulants, or broad-spectrum antibiotics, also are treated with phytonadione, which is more effective than synthetic vitamin K.

Drug interactions

Vitamin A interacts with mineral oil, resulting in decreased absorption of vitamin A. When vitamin D is given concomitantly with cholestyramine, colestipol hydrochloride, or mineral oil, the interaction may interfere with intestinal absorption of vitamin D. Large doses of vitamin E may increase the anticoagulant effects of warfarin by interfering with the synthesis of vitamin K-dependent clotting factors. Vitamin E also may impair the hematologic response to iron therapy in a patient with iron deficiency anemia. Vitamin K antagonizes the effect of coumarin anticoagulants by increasing the synthesis of vitamin K-dependent clotting factors.

ADVERSE DRUG REACTIONS

In most cases, the fat-soluble vitamins are relatively nontoxic when administered in the usual adult dosages. However, higher dosages may cause various adverse reactions.

Because the primary functions of vitamin A relate to vision, development of epithelial tissues, and bone growth, adverse reactions to this drug tend to alter these functions. Changes in liver metabolism also are possible because the liver is the primary site of vitamin A storage.

Most adverse reactions to vitamin A appear to be dose-related. Toxicity, known as **hypervitaminosis** A, may be acute or chronic; signs of acute toxicity have occurred after administration of very large vitamin A doses over a short time or with a single dose. In adults, this results from doses in excess of 25,000 IU per kilogram of body weight.

In adults, chronic toxicity usually results from doses of 4,000 IU per kilogram for 6 to 15 months. Possible manifestations of toxicity include fatigue, malaise, lethargy, abdominal discomfort, anorexia, nausea, vomiting, and vision disturbances. Changes in epithelial tissues, including dry itchy skin, dry nose and mouth, inflammation of oral mucous membranes, or hair loss, may appear. Skeletal changes, including thickening of long bones, slowed growth, and migratory bone pain, also have been reported. Signs of increased intracranial pressure, such as headache and irritability, papilledema, and exophthalmos, may occur. Other signs include hypoplastic anemia, a broad category of anemias characterized by a decrease in the number of red blood cells (RBCs), and leukopenia, an abnormal decrease in the number of white blood cells (WBCs). Also, because large amounts of vitamin A accumulate in the liver, an overdose may result in jaundice, hepatomegaly, and a rise in liver enzymes.

Adverse reactions to isotretinoin, a metabolite of vitamin A used to treat acne, are similar to those caused by other forms of the vitamin. Also, eye irritation, conjunctivitis, and cheilosis (scaly, cracked lips) tend to be prominent. Elevated serum triglyceride levels and photosensitivity may result from use of isotretinoin. This drug also may cause fetal abnormalities.

Anaphylactic reactions and shock have occurred after intravenous (I.V.) administration of vitamin A. Parenteral vitamin A should be administered I.M. unless it is part of a multivitamin preparation used for total parenteral nutrition (TPN).

High dosages of vitamin D increase calcium and phosphorus absorption from the GI tract and increase calcium and phosphorus mobilization from bone. If serum levels of calcium and phosphorus rise to a particularly critical level, calcium phosphate precipitates and soft tissue calcification results. The kidneys, heart, muscles, blood vessels, eyes, and lungs may be affected. This can result in renal insufficiency and polyuria, hypertension, arrhythmias, muscle pain, renal calculi, and conjunctivitis. Bone demineralization can result in bone pain and osteoporosis in adults and growth retardation in children.

Other reactions associated with vitamin D toxicity include nausea, vomiting, anorexia, headache, weakness, and diarrhea or constipation. Elevations of aspartate aminotransferase and alanine aminotransferase levels also may occur. Because some vitamin D preparations contain tartrazine, an individual susceptible to this chemical may develop an allergic response.

Vitamin E dosages above 300 IU daily tend to result in such adverse GI reactions as nausea, vomiting, diarrhea, and abdominal cramping. Fatigue, weakness, headache, blurred vision, and rash also have been reported after vitamin E administration.

Vitamin E has been linked to increases in serum cholesterol and triglyceride levels and to decreases in serum thyroxine and triiodothyronine levels. Increases in urinary estrogen and androgen levels also have been noted.

At least two nondose-related adverse reactions have been linked to vitamin E. Sterile abscesses have been documented after I.M. injection of vitamin E; for this reason, the oral route is preferred. White hair growth has been reported after oral administration of vitamin E for skin disorders accompanied by alopecia.

Adverse reactions to vitamin K primarily depend on the route of administration. Nausea, vomiting, and headache may occur with oral administration. Rapid parenteral administration may lead to transient flushing and, occasionally, dizziness, rapid and weak pulse, transient hypotension, dyspnea, cyanosis, or chest pain. Slow I.V. administration should help prevent these reactions. Infants may develop hyperbilirubinemia and jaundice with parenteral administration of phytonadione; this is particularly a problem in premature infants.

An allergic response may occur after vitamin K administration. Reactions can range from skin rashes and urticaria to severe and sometimes fatal anaphylactic reactions. Shock and cardiac or respiratory arrest have occurred with parenteral administration despite adequate dilution and slow administration.

NURSING PROCESS APPLICATION

The following information assists the nurse in caring for a patient who is receiving a fat-soluble vitamin. It includes an overview of assessment activities as well as examples of appropriate nursing diagnoses and related interventions (see "Planning and implementation"). It also highlights the importance of evaluation.

Assessment

Before drug therapy begins, review the patient's history for conditions that contraindicate or require cautious use of the prescribed fat-soluble vitamin. Also review the patient's medication history to identify use of drugs that may interact with it. During therapy, assess the patient for adverse drug reactions and signs of drug interactions. Also, periodically assess the effectiveness of therapy with the fat-soluble vitamin. Finally, evaluate the patient's and family's knowledge about the prescribed drug.

Nursing diagnoses

- Risk for injury related to a preexisting condition that contraindicates or requires cautious use of a fat-soluble vitamin
- Risk for injury related to adverse drug reactions or drug interactions
- Knowledge deficit related to the prescribed fat-soluble vitamin
- Knowledge deficit related to adverse effects of self-prescribed megadoses of vitamins

Planning and implementation

- Do not administer a fat-soluble vitamin to a patient with a condition that contraindicates its use.
- Administer a fat-soluble vitamin cautiously to a patient with a preexisting condition, especially chronic illnesses.
- Monitor the patient for adverse reactions, especially toxicity, because fat-soluble vitamins can accumulate in the body. Also monitor for drug interactions.

* ***Monitor closely for hypersensitivity reactions during parenteral vitamin therapy. Have emergency equipment nearby.***

- Monitor the patient's fat-soluble vitamin intake from foods, dietary supplements, self-administered drugs, and prescription drugs to avoid possible toxicity.
- Administer vitamin A with food to stimulate bile secretion, which aids absorption and decreases nausea.
- Avoid I.M. or subcutaneous administration of menadiol sodium diphosphate or phytonadione in a patient with hypoprothrombinemia because hemorrhage or hematoma may develop.
- Do not administer vitamin E I.V.
- Inspect the patient's injection site for sterile abscess formation after administering vitamin E.
- Monitor the patient for signs of continued bleeding, such as hematuria, oozing around I.V. catheters, petechiae, and bruising or bleeding from mucous membranes, during vitamin K therapy. Do so until prothrombin times return to normal. Apply pressure to control bleeding after I.M. administration.
- Monitor bilirubin levels in a neonate receiving vitamin K.
- Store parenteral vitamin K in a light-resistant container.

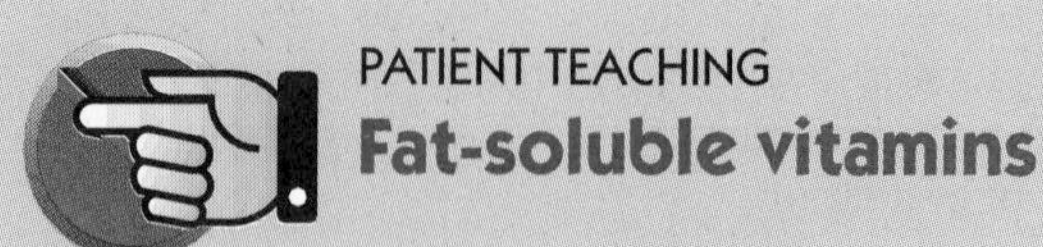

PATIENT TEACHING
Fat-soluble vitamins

- Teach the patient and family the name, dose, frequency, action, and adverse effects of the prescribed fat-soluble vitamin.
- Inform the patient of the recommended daily allowance and food sources for the prescribed fat-soluble vitamin.
- Advise the patient that fat-soluble vitamins are potent drugs that can be toxic to anyone for whom they are not prescribed.
- Instruct the patient to take vitamin A with food to aid absorption and reduce nausea.
- Instruct the patient to avoid using mineral oil during vitamin A therapy because it decreases absorption of the vitamin.
- Teach the patient to identify and report the signs and symptoms of vitamin A toxicity.
- Caution the patient receiving isotretinoin to avoid prolonged exposure to sunlight or to use a sunscreen to avoid photosensitivity reactions.
- Inform the female patient that fetal abnormalities may occur if isotretinoin is taken during pregnancy. Advise her to use an effective contraceptive method and to notify the physician if she becomes pregnant.
- Instruct the patient to protect vitamin A preparations from light and heat to prevent deterioration.
- Teach proper storage procedures to avoid loss of vitamin A in food; 5% to 10% of vitamin A activity is lost when frozen foods are stored for 12 months at –10° F (–23° C).
- Instruct the patient to take vitamin D with food to prevent adverse GI reactions and promote absorption.
- Teach the patient to identify and report the signs and symptoms of hypercalcemia.
- Caution the patient about the potential adverse effects of self-medication with high doses of vitamin E.
- Instruct the patient to store vitamin E in a cool, dark place.
- Caution the patient to take oral vitamin K with food to promote absorption and decrease nausea.
- Instruct the patient receiving oral vitamin K for vitamin K deficiency to increase the dietary intake of vitamin K in order to decrease the risk of developing an ongoing deficiency.
- Instruct the patient to notify the physician if adverse reactions occur.

• Notify the physician if adverse reactions or drug interactions occur.
• Monitor the patient receiving high-dosage vitamin A therapy for changes in epithelial tissues, such as dry nose and mouth, inflammation of oral mucous membranes, hair loss, or dry, itchy skin.
• Apply a moisturizing cream to dry skin several times a day, as prescribed, to prevent skin breakdown.
• Offer the patient frequent sips of water to relieve dry mouth and apply petroleum jelly to dry lips and nostrils to prevent further drying.
• Consult the physician regarding discontinuation of vitamin A therapy if epithelial tissue changes become severe or persist.
• Perform a baseline evaluation of the patient's usual patterns of diet and exposure to sunlight to avoid overadministration of vitamin D. Monitor diet to ensure that the patient obtains sufficient amounts of calcium to enhance the effectiveness of vitamin D. (See Patient Teaching: *Fat-soluble vitamins.*)
• Monitor serum and urine calcium levels and serum levels of phosphorus, magnesium, blood urea nitrogen, and alkaline phosphatase for a patient receiving vitamin D therapy. The product of serum calcium and serum phosphorus levels (the serum calcium level multiplied by the serum phosphorus level) should remain below 70 to avoid calcification of soft tissue. A decrease in the serum level of alkaline phosphatase usually precedes hypercalcemia. Alert the physician if abnormalities occur.
• Monitor hydration if the patient develops diarrhea during vitamin E therapy. Obtain a prescription for an antidiarrheal agent, if needed.
Monitor the patient for severe adverse reactions to I.V. phytonadione, particularly if it is given rapidly. This route is reserved for situations in which rapid correction of hypoprothrombinemia is necessary. If this drug must be given I.V., be sure to dilute it according to the manufacturer's guidelines and to administer it slowly: never faster than 1 mg/minute. Observe the patient closely for signs of allergic reaction, and notify the physician immediately if they appear. Be prepared to intervene if hypotension, bronchospasm, or cardiac or respiratory arrest occurs.

Evaluation

For each nursing diagnosis, prepare an evaluation statement that describes the patient's or family's response to nursing interventions.

Water-soluble vitamins

Water-soluble vitamins include B-complex vitamins (thiamine, riboflavin, niacin, niacinamide, pyridoxine, para-aminobenzoic acid [PABA], pantothenic acid, biotin, choline, inositol, folic acid, and cyanocobalamin) and vitamin C (ascorbic acid). Although different in structure and function, the B-complex vitamins are grouped together because they originally were derived from all liver and yeast foods that contained antiberiberi properties. This section discusses thiamine (B_1), riboflavin (B_2), niacin or nicotinic acid (B_3), niacinamide (nicotinamide), pyridoxine (B_6), and vitamin C in detail. Although PABA is not considered a true vitamin, it is a precursor to folic acid. Therefore, it is discussed briefly in a later section in this chapter along with pantothenic acid, biotin, choline, and inositol. (See *Water-soluble vitamins: Food sources and RDAs.*)

PHARMACOKINETICS

Thiamine, riboflavin, niacin, pyridoxine, and vitamin C are absorbed well after administration and are distributed widely in the body, except for pyridoxine — which is stored primarily in the liver. Thiamine and niacin are metabolized

Water-soluble vitamins: Food sources and RDAs

To prevent chronic deficiencies, the nurse should teach the patient about dietary sources of, and recommended daily allowances (RDAs) for, B-complex vitamins and vitamin C. The chart below provides this information, with the RDAs grouped by patient age and condition.

VITAMIN	FOOD SOURCES	RDAs
thiamine (B_1)	Yeast, whole grain and enriched cereals and breads, legumes, nuts, pork, egg yolks, fish, poultry, and organ meats	*Infants up to age 1:* 0.3 to 0.4 mg *Children ages 1 to 10:* 0.7 to 1.0 mg *Males age 11 and older:* 1.2 to 1.5 mg *Females age 11 and older:* 1.0 to 1.1 mg *Pregnant females:* 1.5 mg *Breast-feeding females:* 1.6 mg
riboflavin (B_2)	Milk, cheddar and cottage cheese, organ meats, eggs, whole grain and enriched cereals and breads, and green leafy vegetables	*Infants up to age 1:* 0.4 to 0.5 mg *Children ages 1 to 10:* 0.8 to 1.2 mg *Males age 11 and older:* 1.4 to 1.8 mg *Females age 11 and older:* 1.2 to 1.3 mg *Pregnant females:* 1.6 mg *Breast-feeding females:* 1.7 to 1.8 mg
niacin (B_3)	Meats, liver, poultry, fish, eggs, yeast, whole grain and enriched cereals and breads, nuts, and legumes	*Infants up to age 1:* 5 to 6 mg *Children ages 1 to 10:* 9 to 13 mg *Males age 11 and older:* 15 to 20 mg *Females age 11 and older:* 13 to 15 mg *Pregnant females:* 17 mg *Breast-feeding females:* 20 mg
pyridoxine (B_6)	Meats, eggs, liver, whole grain cereals and breads, soybeans, wheat germ, potatoes, and vegetables	*Infants up to age 1:* 0.3 to 0.6 mg *Children ages 1 to 10:* 1.0 to 1.4 mg *Males age 11 and older:* 1.7 to 2.0 mg *Females age 11 and older:* 1.5 to 1.6 mg *Pregnant females:* 2.2 mg *Breast-feeding females:* 2.1 mg
ascorbic acid (C)	Citrus fruits, tomatoes, strawberries, cabbage greens, and potatoes	*Infants up to age 1:* 30 to 35 mg *Children ages 1 to 10:* 40 to 45 mg *Males age 11 and older:* 50 to 60 mg *Females age 11 and older:* 60 mg *Pregnant females:* 70 mg *Breast-feeding females:* 90 to 95 mg

in the liver; riboflavin and pyridoxine, in RBCs and the liver. Riboflavin also undergoes metabolism in GI mucosal cells. Vitamin C is oxidized to dehydroascorbic acid. All of these water-soluble vitamins are excreted in the urine, although some riboflavin is also excreted in the feces.

For water-soluble vitamins, information about onset of action, peak concentration level, and duration of action is incomplete.

Route	Onset	Peak	Duration
P.O., I.M., I.V.	Unknown	Unknown	Unknown

PHARMACODYNAMICS

Thiamine plays an important part in carbohydrate metabolism by acting as a coenzyme. Riboflavin plays an important role in tissue respiration. Niacin is required for lipid metabolism, tissue respiration, and glycogenolysis (splitting of glycogen in the body, yielding glucose — the primary carbohydrate in the body). Pyridoxine is used in the metabolism of proteins, carbohydrates, and fats and acts as a coenzyme in many other metabolic reactions. Vitamin C functions in many important biochemical reactions in the body. It is involved in steroid synthesis, the conversion of folic acid to folinic acid, and microsomal drug metabolism. Vitamin C also plays a role in tyrosine metabolism and acts as an intracellular cement in the synthesis of many intracellular substances, such as collagen, tooth and bone matrix, and capillary endothelium.

PHARMACOTHERAPEUTICS

Thiamine is used primarily to prevent and treat thiamine deficiency syndromes, such as **beriberi,** Wernicke's encephalopathy, and peripheral neuritis associated with pellagra. Thiamine malabsorption may occur in patients with alcoholism, cirrhosis, or GI disease, requiring supplementation. Increased thiamine requirements may be associated with pregnancy, increased physical activity, hyperthyroidism, infection, and hepatic disease.

Riboflavin is used to prevent and treat riboflavin deficiency, which is rarely severe in humans and is frequently mild.

Niacin and niacinamide are used to prevent or treat niacin deficiency and pellagra. Pellagra may result from dietary deficiency, isoniazid therapy, or certain neoplasms. Niacin is also used as an adjunct to dietary therapy in patients with hyperlipidemia.

The therapeutic preparation of vitamin B_6 is pyridoxine hydrochloride. Pyridoxine is used to prevent or treat vitamin B_6 deficiency. Deficiencies may occur in a patient with uremia, alcoholism, cirrhosis, or a malabsorption syndrome or in one receiving isoniazid, cycloserine, hydralazine, ethionamide, D-penicillamine, or an oral contraceptive. An infant exposed to high amounts of pyridoxine in utero may become pyridoxine-dependent after birth. Pyridoxine is used to treat seizures that are unresponsive to standard therapy in such an infant. It is also used as an adjunct to other measures in treating toxicity resulting from isoniazid, cycloserine, or hydralazine overdose. Isoniazid-induced seizures may be treated with pyridoxine and other anticonvulsants.

Vitamin C is used primarily as a dietary supplement to prevent or treat vitamin C deficiency. It also is used to treat scurvy, the result of severe vitamin C deficiency. Vitamin C also can be used as a **urinary acidifier.**

Drug interactions

No clinically significant interactions occur with thiamine or riboflavin. Clonidine may block the flushing reaction associated with niacin. Combined therapy with niacin and lovastatin may cause rhabdomyolysis and myopathy. Pyridoxine accelerates levodopa metabolism, which decreases control of the signs and symptoms of parkinsonism. Vitamin C may increase iron absorption and decrease the effects of warfarin. Concomitant administration of large dosages of vitamin C may affect the excretion of acidic and basic drugs.

ADVERSE DRUG REACTIONS

In most cases, thiamine administration does not result in adverse reactions or toxicity. Various nonspecific reactions that have been reported include nausea, anxiety, sweating, and sensations of warmth. Allergic reactions have occurred with parenteral administration, ranging from itching and urticaria to cardiovascular failure and death.

Riboflavin is considered nontoxic, and no adverse reactions have been reported.

Although niacin and niacinamide may be used interchangeably to correct niacin deficiency, niacinamide produces fewer adverse reactions. The most common adverse reaction to niacin is vasodilation, which typically occurs with large dosages. The cutaneous blood vessels of the face, neck, and chest are affected most. Tolerance of this effect may occur within 2 weeks. Sensations of flushing and warmth, itching, tingling, and hypotension have been reported with oral and parenteral administration. GI reactions also may occur, including nausea, vomiting, diarrhea, and abdominal pain. Hyperglycemia and hyperuricemia may occur with niacin therapy. Abnormalities of liver function tests, including increased serum bilirubin, have been documented. Niacin products that contain tartrazine may cause allergic-type responses in sensitive individuals.

In therapeutic dosages, pyridoxine results in few if any adverse reactions. Very large doses, roughly 1,000 times the recommended daily allowance, have resulted in nervous system damage. Patients have developed difficulty with balance and a sensory neuropathy after ingestion of 2 to 6 g of pyridoxine. Other nervous system effects, such as drowsiness and paresthesia, have occurred with smaller doses of this vitamin.

Few adverse reactions are associated with ascorbic acid administration. Dose-related reactions include diarrhea and the precipitation of oxalate or urate renal calculi. The development of renal calculi results from urine acidification. Dental erosion has occurred with the long-term use of chewable vitamin C. Patients may complain of tenderness at the injection site after I.M. administration. Rapid I.V. administration may cause brief dizziness. Ascorbic acid products that contain tartrazine may cause allergic responses in sensitive individuals.

NURSING PROCESS APPLICATION

The following information assists the nurse in caring for a patient who is receiving a water-soluble vitamin. It includes an overview of assessment activities as well as examples of appropriate nursing diagnoses and related interventions (see "Planning and implementation"). It also highlights the importance of evaluation.

Assessment

Before drug therapy begins, review the patient's history for conditions that contraindicate or require cautious use of the prescribed water-soluble vitamin. Also review the patient's medication history to identify use of drugs that may interact with it, if appropriate. During therapy, assess the patient for adverse drug reactions and signs of drug interactions related to the prescribed water-soluble vitamin. Also, periodically assess the effectiveness of therapy. Finally, evaluate the patient's and family's knowledge about the prescribed drug.

Nursing diagnoses

- Risk for injury related to a preexisting condition that contraindicates or requires cautious use of a water-soluble vitamin
- Risk for injury related to adverse reactions or drug interactions
- Knowledge deficit related to the prescribed water-soluble vitamin

Planning and implementation

- Do not administer a water-soluble vitamin to a patient with a condition that contraindicates its use.
- Administer a water-soluble vitamin cautiously to a patient at risk because of a preexisting condition.
- Monitor the patient for adverse reactions and drug interactions during therapy with a water-soluble vitamin. (See Patient Teaching: *Water-soluble vitamins.*)
- Inquire about tartrazine or aspirin hypersensitivity before administering niacin or ascorbic acid products with tartrazine. Patients who are aspirin-sensitive commonly are sensitive to tartrazine as well. The sensitive patient should receive a test dose or another product. Monitor the patient closely for signs and symptoms of an allergic response.

✱ Monitor the patient for allergic reactions to parenteral thiamine. Have emergency equipment nearby.

- Check liver function tests, blood glucose levels, and serum uric acid levels frequently during niacin therapy to detect abnormalities.

✱ Do not test a diabetic patient's urine for glucose with a cupric sulfate tablet (Clinitest) because a false-positive reaction can occur during therapy with niacin or large doses of vitamin C. Also, do not use glucose oxidase methods (Clinistix, Diastix, or Tes-Tape) for urine glucose testing during high-dosage vitamin C therapy because a false-negative result can occur.

- Administer thiamine in divided doses with food to improve absorption. Also administer riboflavin with food.
- Begin oral niacin therapy with small doses as prescribed to avoid vasodilation.
- Notify the physician if adverse reactions or drug interactions occur.

Evaluation

For each nursing diagnosis, prepare an evaluation statement that describes the patient's or family's response to nursing interventions.

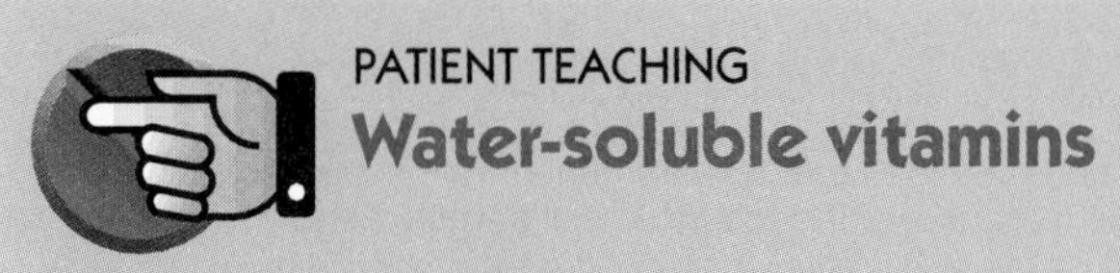

PATIENT TEACHING

Water-soluble vitamins

- ➤ Teach the patient and family the name, dose, frequency, action, and adverse effects of the prescribed water-soluble vitamin.
- ➤ Inform the patient of the recommended daily allowance and food sources for the prescribed water-soluble vitamin.
- ➤ Inform the patient that water-soluble vitamins are drugs, and stress the importance of adhering to the therapeutic regimen.
- ➤ Instruct the patient to store the water-soluble vitamin in a cool, dark place.
- ➤ Teach the patient to check expiration dates and to avoid purchasing more than a 3-month supply because potency tends to diminish rapidly.
- ➤ Teach the patient to take thiamine or riboflavin with food.
- ➤ Inform the patient that riboflavin colors the urine bright yellow. This may interfere with urinalysis based on spectrometry methods or color reactions.
- ➤ Teach the patient with diabetes mellitus or a history of renal calculi and who is receiving an oral anticoagulant to avoid large doses of ascorbic acid. Ascorbic acid can interfere with urine testing for glucose or cause precipitation of renal calculi and may interfere with the action of warfarin.
- ➤ Inform the patient that large dosages of niacin can cause vasodilation of the face, neck, and chest. Reassure the patient that tolerance usually occurs within 2 weeks, returning the color in these areas to normal.
- ➤ Inform the patient that dental erosion may occur with long-term use of chewable vitamin C.
- ➤ Advise the patient to avoid activities that require alertness if drowsiness or balance problems occur during pyridoxine therapy.
- ➤ Instruct the patient to notify the physician if adverse reactions occur.

Other water-soluble vitamins

Other water-soluble agents include the B-complex vitamins para-aminobenzoic acid (PABA), pantothenic acid, biotin, choline, and inositol. PABA has no known nutrient value. However, it is used topically as a sunscreen agent. Although pantothenic acid has no clearly defined uses, it is commonly included in multivitamin preparations. Biotin may play a role in fat and carbohydrate metabolism. Choline is not considered an essential vitamin. It plays a role in fat metabolism and is a precursor to the neurotransmitter acetylcholine. Inositol is also not an essential vitamin. However, it plays some role in fat metabolism.

Minerals (trace elements)

This section discusses minerals that are used as nutritional supplements, including chromium, copper, fluoride, iodine, manganese, molybdenum, selenium, and zinc.

These minerals are inorganic chemicals found in all living tissues. Because most are required in very small quantities in the diet, they are known as *trace elements.* Usually, minerals are widely available in foods in the normal diet. (See *Food sources of trace minerals,* page 620.) Deficiencies are unusual unless some factor inhibits absorption or a patient requires long-term TPN and does not receive adequate supplementation. Research into the effects of trace mineral

Food sources of trace minerals

To help prevent the development of nutritional deficiencies, the nurse should teach the patient about dietary sources of trace minerals. The nurse must remember, however, that the mineral content of foods depends on the mineral content of the soil, water, and grazing land.

MINERAL	SOURCES
chromium	Yeast, cereal grains, meats
copper	Meats, seafood, legumes, whole grain cereals, liver, nuts
fluoride	Fluoridated water, seafood, eggs
iodine	Iodized salt, seafood
manganese	Green leafy vegetables, whole grains, legumes
molybdenum	Liver, milk, vegetables, legumes, cereal grains
selenium	Meats, seafood, dairy products, whole grains, vegetables
zinc	Whole grains, meats, dairy products, seafood, wheat germ

deficiencies has been difficult because of the small amount of the minerals needed to maintain health and their widespread availability in the diet. For these reasons, recommended daily allowances for many minerals have not been established.

PHARMACOKINETICS

Poorly absorbed after oral administration, chromium is distributed widely to many tissues. It is excreted in the urine.

Copper is absorbed after oral administration, and is distributed mostly to the liver. It is excreted in the feces via bile.

Fluoride, as sodium fluoride, is absorbed completely from the GI tract after oral administration, but calcium fluoride and bone meal are absorbed slowly and variably. Fluoride is distributed mostly to bone and developing teeth; it is not metabolized and is excreted mainly in the urine.

Iodine is absorbed rapidly and completely from the GI tract as iodide. The highest concentration of iodine is in the thyroid gland. Iodine is not metabolized, but is incorporated into the tyrosine residues of thyroglobulin to produce thyroid hormones. When broken down, these hormones release iodine, which is reabsorbed by the thyroid. From 40% to 80% of unabsorbed iodine is excreted in the urine.

Manganese is absorbed poorly from the GI tract. It is distributed widely to bone and the pituitary gland, liver, pineal gland, and lactating mammary glands. High concentrations are found in mitochondria and cell nuclei. Manganese is not metabolized and is excreted mainly in the feces via bile.

Molybdenum is absorbed well after oral administration and is distributed mostly to the liver, kidneys, spleen, lungs, brain, and muscle. Molybdenum is not known to undergo metabolism other than its incorporation into enzymes. It is excreted primarily in the urine, with small amounts excreted in the feces via bile.

Selenium is absorbed well after oral administration and is distributed to the kidneys, liver, muscle, and skin. It is incorporated into glutathione peroxidase but otherwise is not metabolized. Selenium is excreted primarily in the urine, although significant losses occur in the feces.

Many factors influence zinc absorption. The presence of amino acids and vitamin C increases zinc absorption; calcium and phosphates decrease it. High-fiber foods, such as bran, can interfere with zinc absorption. Zinc is distributed to bone and hepatic, pancreatic, retinal, and gonadal tissues. It is not metabolized and is excreted in the urine, feces, and perspiration.

Route	Onset	Peak	Duration
P.O.	Unknown	Variable	Unknown

PHARMACODYNAMICS

Chromium potentiates the action of insulin and helps regulate lipoprotein metabolism.

Copper functions as a component of enzymes involved in RBC formation, WBC formation, cellular energy production, elastin and collagen synthesis, and glucose and catecholamine metabolism.

Fluoride is incorporated into teeth and bone. Deposited in tooth enamel, it makes teeth resistant to acid dissolution and to formation of dental caries. After tooth calcification is complete, fluoride strengthens surface enamel. Fluoride also increases skeletal mass and density.

Iodine is essential in manufacturing thyroid hormones. By itself, it has no known metabolic function.

Manganese is involved in activating many metalloenzymes, such as pyruvate carboxylase and superoxide dismutase. Manganese and other metals activate enzymes involved in the metabolism of carbohydrates, proteins, and lipids.

Molybdenum functions as a component of xanthine oxidase, sulfite oxidase, and aldehyde oxidase, all enzymes integral to a number of metabolic reactions.

Selenium functions as an antioxidant. By incorporation into glutathione peroxidase, it helps protect cell membranes and structures from destruction by oxidation.

Zinc acts as a component of many zinc metalloenzymes and metalloproteins, such as alcohol dehydrogenase and **carbonic anhydrase.** It is involved in ribonucleic acid and protein metabolism, helps stabilize cell membranes, and interacts with insulin. Physiologic functions of zinc include cell growth and proliferation, sexual maturation and reproduction, taste, wound healing, and immune defenses.

PHARMACOTHERAPEUTICS

The mineral agents chromium, copper, fluoride, iodine, manganese, molybdenum, selenium, and zinc may be used to treat specific nutritional deficiencies or to prevent deficiencies, such as in patients receiving TPN.

Drug interactions

No significant drug interactions occur with minerals.

ADVERSE DRUG REACTIONS

Concentrated amounts of minerals tend to irritate the tissues they contact. GI symptoms may occur with oral administration. Phlebitis may develop if minerals are not diluted adequately before parenteral administration. Overdose is the most common cause of adverse reactions to minerals.

Chromium therapy may produce nausea, vomiting, gastric ulceration, rash, joint swelling, bronchospasm, seizures, coma, and kidney and liver damage.

Copper therapy may produce diarrhea, lethargy, altered behavior, diminished reflexes, photophobia, and liver and kidney damage.

The patient on fluoride therapy may develop nausea, vomiting, diarrhea, abdominal pain, nervous system hyperirritability, tetany and paresthesia related to hypocalcemia, hypoglycemia, and cardiac and respiratory failure.

Iodine therapy may produce a metallic taste, skin lesions, eyelid swelling, increased saliva production, iodide goiter (thyroid gland enlargement that results from ingestion of high concentrations of iodide), bloody diarrhea, fever, depression, or mouth, gum, and salivary gland tenderness.

Manganese therapy may cause anorexia, diarrhea, headache, and Parkinson-like symptoms, such as altered gait and speech impairment.

With molybdenum, goutlike symptoms can occur.

Adverse reactions to selenium therapy may include alopecia, skin lesions, GI irritation, depression, and garlic odor of breath and sweat. Acute poisoning has led to multiple organ failure and death.

Zinc therapy can result in stomach irritation, gastric ulceration, diarrhea, vomiting, elevated serum amylase levels, hypothermia, and hypotension accompanied by signs and symptoms of shock.

Hypersensitivity reactions have occurred after iodine administration. The use of stannous fluoride solutions has led to tooth discoloration. Allergy to fluoride has resulted in rash. Some products contain tartrazine, which may cause allergic-type reactions in sensitive individuals.

NURSING PROCESS APPLICATION

The following information assists the nurse in caring for a patient who is receiving a mineral. It includes an overview of assessment activities as well as examples of appropriate nursing diagnoses and related interventions (see "Planning and implementation"). It also highlights the importance of evaluation.

Assessment

Before drug therapy begins, review the patient's history for conditions that contraindicate or require cautious use of the prescribed mineral. During therapy, assess the patient for adverse drug reactions. Also, periodically assess the effectiveness of therapy with the mineral agent. Finally, evaluate the patient's and family's knowledge about the prescribed drug.

Nursing diagnoses

- Risk for injury related to a preexisting condition that contraindicates or requires cautious use of a mineral
- Risk for injury related to adverse reactions
- Knowledge deficit related to the prescribed mineral

Planning and implementation

- Do not administer a mineral to a patient with a condition that contraindicates its use.
- Administer a mineral cautiously to a patient at risk because of a preexisting condition.
- Monitor the patient for adverse reactions to the prescribed mineral, especially during high-dose therapy.
- Monitor the patient for GI distress when administering an oral mineral preparation and for phlebitis when administering an I.V. preparation.
- Dilute liquid preparations well before administering to improve the taste and decrease GI irritation.
- Dilute a parenteral mineral solution well and administer it via a central vein as prescribed to decrease vessel irritation. Discard a solution that contains minerals within 24 hours after mixing.
- Consider the mineral content of the patient's diet in addition to the mineral supplements being taken to help prevent mineral toxicity. Watch for signs of toxicity, particularly if the patient has renal failure or hepatic disease. Monitor the patient for signs of adequate therapeutic effect so that the mineral dosage can be decreased or discontinued. (See Patient Teaching: *Minerals,* page 622.)

* ***Document patient history of allergy to iodine or shellfish before administering a preparation containing iodine. Be prepared to intervene if an allergic response occurs.***
* ***Take seizure precautions for a patient receiving large dosages of chromium or fluoride.***

- Monitor the patient's laboratory studies to detect decreased calcium or glucose levels, decreased amylase levels, or abnormal liver or renal function studies.
- Notify the physician if adverse reactions occur.

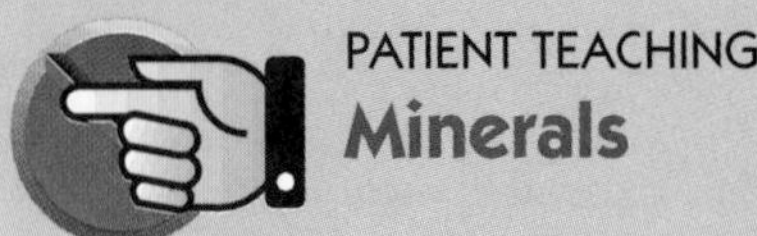

PATIENT TEACHING
Minerals

- Teach the patient and family the name, dose, frequency, action, and adverse effects of the prescribed mineral.
- Teach the patient that the best way to prevent mineral deficiencies is to eat a well-balanced diet of fresh foods, especially whole grain products, fruits, and vegetables. Deficiencies may develop if the patient usually eats large amounts of highly processed foods.
- Teach the patient to preserve minerals by cooking foods in the smallest amount of water possible.
- Teach the patient to avoid gastrointestinal irritation by taking minerals with or immediately after meals, except for fluoride and zinc. These minerals should not be taken with dairy products, and zinc should not be taken with high-fiber foods, such as bran, which interfere with its absorption.
- Teach the patient with small children to buy mineral preparations in containers with childproof caps and to store them in a safe place, out of children's reach.
- Advise the patient to take the mineral only as prescribed to prevent toxicity.
- Teach the patient how to handle bothersome adverse reactions, such as mouth or gum tenderness.
- Caution the patient not to perform an activity that requires alertness if central nervous system reactions occur.
- Instruct the patient to notify the physician if adverse reactions occur.

Evaluation

For each nursing diagnosis, prepare an evaluation statement that describes the patient's or family's response to nursing interventions.

CHAPTER SUMMARY

Chapter 50 presented vitamin and mineral agents. It focused on the three categories of drugs used as nutritional supplements: fat-soluble vitamins, water-soluble vitamins, and minerals (trace elements). Here are the chapter highlights.

Fat-soluble vitamins, which are organic chemical substances required in the diet, include vitamins A, D, E, and K. They are absorbed with dietary fats in the small intestine, so they require bile salts and pancreatic lipase for absorption. All fat-soluble vitamins are stored, but the amount stored varies with each vitamin.

The primary clinical indication for fat-soluble vitamins is dietary supplementation to compensate for low levels of the vitamin.

Because fat-soluble vitamins can accumulate in the body, the nurse must monitor patients for signs of toxicity and teach them about the potential hazards.

Water-soluble vitamins, which are organic chemical substances required in the diet, include B-complex vitamins and vitamin C. The water-soluble vitamins, except for vitamin C, all function as coenzymes in various metabolic functions. Vitamin C may function in many oxidative biochemical reactions in the body and is involved in the synthesis of intracellular substances.

Because the water-soluble vitamins are not stored to a great extent, body supplies must be replenished frequently to avoid deficiency.

Clinical indications for water-soluble vitamins include inadequate intake, impaired absorption, increased demand, or increased excretion.

Minerals are inorganic chemical substances that are components of all living tissues. They cannot be manufactured by the body and therefore must be obtained from exogenous sources, usually food. Because all minerals are stored by the body, mineral levels may become toxic.

Minerals function primarily as components of other substances, such as enzymes, hormones, bones, and teeth.

The primary clinical indications for minerals are to treat deficiencies and to function as nutritional supplements, particularly in patients receiving TPN.

The nurse should be aware of the symptoms of mineral toxicity. Toxicity usually can be prevented by limiting the patient's intake of minerals to those prescribed.

Questions to consider

See Appendix 1 for answers.

1. Frank Jones, age 57, develops hypoprothrombinemia during oral anticoagulant therapy. Which of the following vitamin agents commonly is used to treat anticoagulant-induced hypoprothrombinemia?
   (a) phytonadione
   (b) menaquinone
   (c) calcitriol
   (d) menadiol sodium diphosphate

2. Jeffrey Woods, age 67, is receiving TPN, which supplies most of his calories as dextrose. Along with TPN, which of the following vitamins should he receive because it acts as a coenzyme in carbohydrate metabolism?
   (a) niacin
   (b) pyridoxine
   (c) riboflavin
   (d) thiamine

3. Susan Hampton, age 22, has been taking large quantities of chewable vitamin C as a home remedy to treat a cold. What should the nurse teach Ms. Hammel about this vitamin?

(a) Vitamin C should be stored in a warm, well-ventilated place.
(b) Dietary sources of vitamin C include dairy products and eggs.
(c) Long-term use of chewable vitamin C may cause dental erosion.
(d) Vitamin C has a narrow margin of safety, so Ms. Hammel must be alert for signs of toxicity.

4. Michael Georges, age 48, is an alcoholic. Because his diet lacks various minerals, the physician prescribes a multimineral supplement. How should Mr. Peterson take a multimineral supplement?

(a) On an empty stomach to promote absorption
(b) With milk to minimize adverse central nervous system reactions
(c) With meals to minimize GI distress
(d) With high-fiber foods to enhance absorption

5. Joseph Davis, age 42, is ordered a fat-soluble vitamin to increase the intestinal absorption of calcium. Which of the following vitamin agents is commonly utilized for this treatment?

(a) vitamin K
(b) vitamin D
(c) vitamin E
(d) vitamin C

6. Jason Clyde, age 65, is receiving tube feedings at home. The home health nurse should include which of the following patient teaching items?

(a) Store leftover tube feeding solution at room temperature.
(b) Stop tube feedings if you have a change in bowel habits.
(c) Sit up when receiving the tube feeding.
(d) Flushing the tube after each feedings is not necessary.

51 Electrolyte replacement agents

OBJECTIVES

After reading and studying this chapter, the student should be able to:

1. describe the pharmacokinetics, pharmacodynamics, pharmacotherapeutics, and adverse effects of potassium.
2. describe the pharmacokinetics, pharmacodynamics, pharmacotherapeutics, and adverse effects of calcium.
3. explain the normal functions of magnesium and sodium, their causes of insufficiency, and replacement therapy.
4. describe how to apply the nursing process when caring for a patient who is receiving an electrolyte replacement agent.

INTRODUCTION

Electrolyte replacement agents are mineral salts that increase depleted or deficient electrolyte levels, thus helping to maintain homeostasis, or stability in body fluid composition and volume. Chapter 51 discusses the primary **intracellular fluid** (ICF) electrolyte, potassium; a major **extracellular fluid** (ECF) electrolyte, calcium; and two other electrolytes essential for homeostasis, magnesium (in ICF) and sodium (in ECF). (See *Selected major electrolyte replacement agents.*)

Drugs covered in this chapter include:

- calcium carbonate
- calcium chloride
- calcium citrate
- calcium glubionate
- calcium gluconate
- calcium lactate
- magnesium sulfate
- potassium bicarbonate
- potassium chloride
- potassium gluconate
- potassium phosphate
- sodium bicarbonate
- sodium chloride
- sodium lactate.

Potassium

Potassium is the major positively charged ion (**cation**) in ICF. Because the body cannot store potassium, adequate amounts must be ingested daily. If this is not possible, potassium replacement can be accomplished orally or intravenously (I.V.) with potassium salts, such as potassium bicarbonate, potassium chloride, potassium gluconate, or potassium phosphate.

PHARMACOKINETICS

Oral potassium is absorbed readily from the gastrointestinal (GI) tract. After absorption into ECF, 98% of the potassium passes into ICF. Normal serum levels of potassium are maintained by the kidneys, which excrete almost 90% of excessive potassium intake. The rest is excreted in feces (9%) and sweat (1%).

The onset of action of oral potassium (liquid or powder) usually is within 30 minutes. Extended-release forms have a slower onset, usually 1 to 2 hours. I.V. potassium is effective immediately.

Route	Onset	Peak	Duration
P.O.	30 min-2 hr	1-2 hr	Unknown
I.V.	Immediate	Immediate	Unknown

PHARMACODYNAMICS

Potassium moves quickly into ICF to restore depleted potassium levels and reestablish homeostasis. Potassium is an essential element in determining cell membrane potential and excitability. Therefore, it is necessary for proper functioning of all nerve and muscle cells and for nerve impulse transmission. Potassium is also essential for tissue growth and repair and for maintenance of acid-base balance.

PHARMACOTHERAPEUTICS

Potassium replacement therapy corrects **hypokalemia.** Hypokalemia is a common occurrence in conditions that increase potassium excretion. These include **malabsorption,** excessive vomiting or diarrhea, polyuria, some kidney diseases, cystic fibrosis, burns, an excess of antidiuretic hormone (ADH), or therapy with a potassium-depleting diuretic. Other causes of potassium depletion include alkalosis, insufficient potassium intake from starvation, and administration of a glucocorticoid, I.V. amphotericin B, or I.V. solutions that contain insufficient potassium.

Selected major electrolyte replacement agents

This chart summarizes the major electrolyte replacement agents currently in clinical use.

DRUG	MAJOR INDICATIONS AND USUAL DOSAGES	CONTRAINDICATIONS AND PRECAUTIONS
potassium bicarbonate (K-Lyte)	*Replacement electrolyte for symptomatic hypokalemia* ADULT: 25 to 50 mEq P.O. dissolved in 4 to 8 oz (120 to 240 ml) of cold water daily or b.i.d.	• Potassium bicarbonate is contraindicated in a breast-feeding patient or one with severe renal impairment, acute dehydration, hyperkalemia, metabolic acidosis, extensive tissue breakdown, or adrenal insufficiency. • This drug requires cautious use in a pregnant patient. • Safety and efficacy in children have not been established.
potassium chloride (Kaochlor, Slow-K, potassium chloride injection)	*Prevention of hypokalemia* ADULT: 20 to 60 mEq P.O. daily in one to three divided doses *Replacement electrolyte for symptomatic hypokalemia* ADULT: 40 to 96 mEq extended-release capsules P.O. daily in two to three divided doses; 20 mEq P.O. diluted in 4 oz (120 ml) of cold water or juice once daily to q.i.d.; or 10 mEq I.V. hourly in a concentration of 40 mEq/L or less, up to a maximum of 200 mEq daily based on patient's serum potassium level PEDIATRIC: highly individualized I.V. dosage	• Potassium chloride is contraindicated in a patient receiving a potassium-sparing diuretic or one with severe renal impairment, acute dehydration, hyperkalemia, systemic acidosis, extensive tissue breakdown, or adrenal insufficiency. The solid form is contraindicated in a patient with a condition that can arrest or delay tablet passage through the gastrointestinal tract. • This drug requires cautious use in a pregnant or breast-feeding patient. • Safety and efficacy of oral Kaochlor and Slow-K in children have not been established.
calcium carbonate (Alka-Mints, Tums)	*Dietary supplementation* ADULT: 500 mg P.O. b.i.d. to q.i.d. 1 to 2 hours after meals	• Calcium carbonate is contraindicated in a patient with hypercalcemia or ventricular fibrillation. • This drug requires cautious use in a patient with sarcoidosis or renal or cardiac disease.
calcium chloride	*Acute hypocalcemia* ADULT: 7 to 14 mEq I.V. solution infused no faster than 1 ml/minute PEDIATRIC: 0.2 ml/kg up to 10 ml/day I.V. solution administered slowly *Hypocalcemic tetany* ADULT: 4.5 to 16 mEq I.V. until response PEDIATRIC: for neonates, 2.4 mEq/kg I.V. daily in divided doses; for all other children, 0.5 to 0.7 mEq/kg I.V. t.i.d. or q.i.d. or until tetany is controlled *Cardiac arrest* ADULT: 2.7 mEq I.V., repeated as needed, or 2.7 to 5.4 mEq injected directly into ventricle as a single dose PEDIATRIC: 0.27 mEq/kg I.V., repeated in 10 minutes as needed	• Calcium chloride is contraindicated in a patient with hypercalcemia or ventricular fibrillation. • This drug requires cautious use in a patient with sarcoidosis, renal or cardiac disease, cor pulmonale, respiratory acidosis, or respiratory failure.
calcium glubionate (Neo-Calglucon syrup)	*Dietary supplementation* ADULT: 5.4 g P.O. t.i.d. or q.i.d. before meals PEDIATRIC: for children under age 1, 1.8 g P.O. five times a day before meals; for children ages 1 to 4, 3.6 g P.O. t.i.d. before meals; in children over age 4, 5.4 g P.O. t.i.d. or q.i.d. before meals	• Calcium glubionate is contraindicated in a patient with hypercalcemia or ventricular fibrillation. • This drug requires cautious use in a patient with sarcoidosis or renal or cardiac disease.
calcium gluconate	*Dietary supplementation* ADULT: 11 g P.O. daily in divided doses after meals *Replacement electrolyte for severe hypocalcemic tetany* ADULT: 4.5 to 16 mEq I.V. infused no faster than 5 ml/minute PEDIATRIC: for neonates: 2 to 4 mEq/kg I.V. in divided doses; in children 0.5 to 0.7 mEq/kg I.V. t.i.d. or q.i.d. until tetany controlled	• Calcium gluconate is contraindicated in a patient with hypercalcemia or ventricular fibrillation. • This drug requires cautious use in a patient with sarcoidosis or renal or cardiac disease.

Combination potassium replacement agents

Several potassium salts are available as combination products to be given orally as electrolyte replacements.

PRODUCT	DOSAGE	NURSING IMPLICATIONS
potassium bicarbonate and potassium chloride (Klorvess, K-Lyte/Cl)	20 to 25 mEq daily or b.i.d.	• Dissolve effervescent tablets or powder completely in 4 to 8 oz (120 to 240 ml) of cold water or juice.
potassium bicarbonate and potassium chloride (K-Lyte/Cl 50)	50 mEq daily or b.i.d.	• Be careful not to confuse these double-strength tablets with regular-strength medications.
potassium chloride, potassium bicarbonate and potassium citrate (Kaochlor-Eff)	20 mEq daily to q.i.d.	• Dissolve effervescent tablets completely in 4 to 8 oz of cold water or juice.
potassium gluconate and potassium chloride (Kolyum)	20 mEq b.i.d. to q.i.d. (for children, 20 to 40 mEq/m^2 or 2 to 3 mEq/kg daily in divided doses)	• Dissolve liquid or powder in 1 oz (30 ml) of cold water or juice.
potassium gluconate and potassium citrate (Twin-K)	20 mEq b.i.d. to q.i.d. (for children, 20 to 40 mEq/m^2 or 2 to 3 mEq/kg daily in divided doses)	• Dilute in 4 oz of cold water or juice.
potassium gluconate and potassium citrate (Twin-K)	15 mEq b.i.d. to q.i.d.	• Dilute in 4 to 8 oz of cold water or juice.
potassium acetate, potassium bicarbonate, and potassium citrate (Tri-K)	15 mEq t.i.d. or q.i.d. (for children, 15 to 30 mEq/m^2 or 2 to 3 mEq/kg daily in divided doses)	• Dilute in 4 oz of cold water or juice.
potassium and sodium phosphate tablets for oral solution (Uro-KP-Neutral)	2 tablets in 8 oz (240 ml) of water q.i.d.	• Dilute in 8 oz of water or juice. • Be aware that this agent is prescribed primarily to replace phosphorus.
potassium and sodium phosphate capsules for oral solution (Neutra-Phos)	1 to 8 capsules daily in divided doses	• Dissolve contents of capsule in 2.5 oz (75 ml) of water or juice; patient must not swallow filled capsule. • Be aware that this agent is prescribed primarily to replace phosphorus.
potassium and sodium phosphate powder for oral solution (Neutra-Phos)	2.5 to 20 oz (75 to 600 ml) of reconstituted solution daily in divided doses (for children age 4 and over, same as adult; under age 4, 2 oz reconstituted solution [60 ml] q.i.d.) Packets: 1 packet reconstituted in water q.i.d.	• Do not dilute solution. • Be aware that this agent is prescribed primarily to replace phosphorus.

Apart from its role in preventing or reversing hypokalemia, potassium is also used to decrease the toxic effects of digoxin. Because potassium inhibits the excitability of the heart, insufficient potassium enhances digitalis action, which may result in toxicity.

Potassium is available in several salts. These can be administered alone or with other potassium salts or electrolytes. (See *Combination potassium replacement agents.*)

Drug interactions

Potassium should be used cautiously in patients receiving potassium-sparing diuretics (such as amiloride, spironolactone, or triamterene) or angiotensin-converting enzyme (ACE) inhibitors (such as captopril, enalapril, or lisinopril) to avoid **hyperkalemia.**

ADVERSE DRUG REACTIONS

The use of potassium preparations may produce hyperkalemia if the patient's serum potassium level is not monitored closely. Hyperkalemia causes listlessness, confusion, flaccid paralysis, and paresthesia, weakness, and limb heaviness. Cardiovascular signs may include electrocardiogram (ECG) changes (prolonged PR interval; widened QRS complex; depressed ST segment; and tall, tented T waves), peripheral vascular collapse with a fall in blood pressure, cardiac arrhythmias, heart block, and possible cardiac arrest.

Oral potassium sometimes causes nausea, vomiting, abdominal pain, and diarrhea. Enteric-coated tablets may cause small-bowel ulceration, stenosis, hemorrhage, and obstruction. Because other formulations have largely replaced enteric-coated tablets, this adverse reaction is no longer common.

I.V. infusion of potassium preparations can cause pain at the injection site and phlebitis. Infusion of potassium in patients with decreased urine production increases the risk of hyperkalemia.

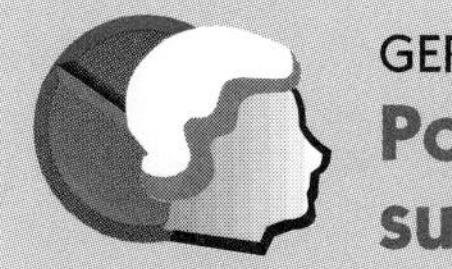

GERIATRIC CONSIDERATIONS
Potassium supplementation

Many elderly patients have some form of renal dysfunction. It is critical to be aware of the extent of dysfunction before administering potassium supplementation. If an overdose of potassium is given, the patient may exhibit cardiac arrhythmias that could become lethal. Therefore, when checking electrolyte values, also check blood urea nitrogen levels and creatinine levels to assess renal function.

Most elderly patients are taking several medications, often prescribed by different doctors. The nurse should routinely review the names, dosages, frequency and route of each. A patient could be taking two medications that do the same thing. For example, a patient may be taking K-Dur tablets and Slow-K, both of which will increase the amount of potassium in the patient's system. The situation could be deadly. Therefore, the nurse should ask the patient or a family member to bring all medications to the office or hospital so a thorough review can be performed.

NURSING PROCESS APPLICATION

The following information assists the nurse in caring for a patient who is receiving potassium. It includes an overview of assessment activities as well as examples of appropriate nursing diagnoses and related interventions (see "Planning and implementation"). It also highlights the importance of evaluation.

Assessment

Before drug therapy begins, review the patient's history for conditions that contraindicate or require cautious use of the prescribed potassium preparation. Also review the patient's medication history to identify use of drugs that may interact with it. During therapy, assess the patient for adverse drug reactions and signs of drug interactions. Also, periodically assess the effectiveness of potassium therapy. Finally, evaluate the patient's and family's knowledge about the prescribed drug. (See Geriatric Considerations: *Potassium supplementation.*)

Nursing diagnoses

- Risk for injury related to a preexisting condition that contraindicates or requires cautious use of potassium
- Risk for injury related to adverse reactions or drug interactions
- Risk for fluid volume deficit related to the adverse GI effects of the prescribed potassium preparation
- Knowledge deficit related to the prescribed potassium preparation

Planning and implementation

- Do not administer potassium to a patient with a condition that contraindicates its use.
- Administer potassium cautiously to a patient at risk because of a preexisting condition.
- Monitor the patient for adverse reactions and drug interactions during potassium therapy.
- Monitor serum potassium levels in a patient receiving potassium. Be particularly alert for hyperkalemia in a patient whose urine output decreases during potassium therapy.
- Monitor the patient regularly for signs and symptoms of hyperkalemia, such as listlessness, confusion, flaccid paralysis, paresthesia, weakness, and limb heaviness.
- Monitor the patient's ECG for changes that suggest hyperkalemia, such as prolonged PR interval, widened QRS complex, depressed ST segment, and tall, tented T waves.
- Use liquid potassium in a cardiac patient who has esophageal compression from an enlarged left atrium or one with esophageal stasis or obstruction. In such a patient, tablets in wax matrix sometimes lodge in the esophagus and cause ulceration.
- Dilute an I.V. potassium preparation as prescribed before infusion; NEVER give as a bolus or by intramuscular (I.M.) injection.
- Give diluted I.V. potassium slowly; potentially fatal hyperkalemia may result from too-rapid infusion.
- Do not mix I.V. potassium phosphate in a solution that contains calcium or magnesium because precipitates will occur.
- Inspect the patient's I.V. site regularly for signs of phlebitis. If phlebitis or pain occurs, change the I.V. site.
- Notify the physician if adverse reactions — especially hyperkalemia — or drug interactions occur.
- Administer oral potassium with or after meals to minimize GI distress. (See Patient Teaching: *Potassium*, page 628.)
- Perform an abdominal assessment if the patient reports GI distress. Notify the physician of abnormalities.

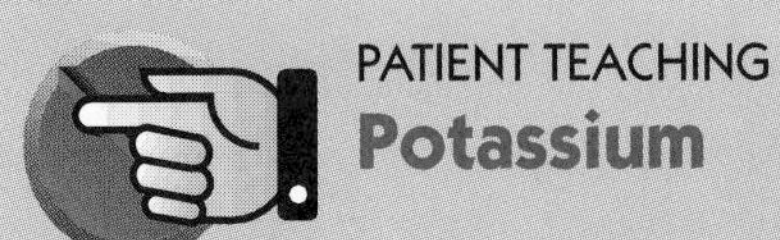

PATIENT TEACHING
Potassium

- Teach the patient and family the name, dose, frequency, action, and adverse effects of the prescribed potassium preparation.
- Instruct the patient to take oral potassium with or after meals to minimize gastrointestinal (GI) distress.
- Direct the patient to dissolve all powders and tablets in at least 4 oz (120 ml) of water or fruit juice, as directed, and to sip the solution slowly over 5 to 10 minutes. Also advise the patient to take capsules or tablets with plenty of liquid.
- Remind the patient not to crush or chew extended-release tablets, which will defeat the purpose of the special coating.
- Remind the patient that although remnants of the wax matrix may appear in the feces, the drug will be absorbed.
- Advise the patient that periodic blood tests will be needed to measure serum potassium levels.
- Teach the patient to recognize and report to the physician signs or symptoms of hyperkalemia or GI distress.

• Monitor hydration if the patient experiences nausea, vomiting, or diarrhea. Obtain a prescription for an antiemetic or antidiarrheal, as needed.

Evaluation

For each nursing diagnosis, prepare an evaluation statement that describes the patient's or family's response to nursing interventions.

CRITICAL THINKING: To enhance your critical thinking about electrolyte replacement agents, consider the following situation and its analysis.

Situation: Keith Anthony, age 63, has acute heart failure and is admitted to the intensive care unit. The goals of management of heart failure are to improve pump performance and reduce myocardial workload.

Mr. Anthony is placed in high Fowler's position to reduce pulmonary venous congestion and ease dyspnea. Oxygen is administered in high concentration by mask to relieve hypoxia and dyspnea and lessen capillary permeability. His physician has ordered a cardiac glycoside to improve cardiac output and enhance kidney perfusion, which may create a mild diuresis. When administering the cardiac glycoside, the nurse should assess for signs of digitalis toxicity, which occur in approximately one of every five clients. It may be present with systemic or cardiac manifestations.

The night nurse noted in reviewing laboratory results that Mr. Anthony's serum potassium level had dropped and he was hypokalemic. Should the nurse notify the physician regarding the laboratory results or wait until morning and relay the information through the report to the day shift?

Analysis: The night nurse should call the physician and not wait until the morning report. Hypokalemia is a particularly dangerous problem; it potentiates digitalis toxicity and can cause arrhythmias. The nurse's assessment of signs and symptoms of digitalis toxicity include the monitoring of serum potassium levels. When the client is hypokalemic, the nurse should withhold the drug and notify the physician.

Calcium

Calcium is a major cation in ECF. Almost all the calcium in the body — 99% — is stored in bone, where it can be mobilized if necessary. When dietary intake is insufficient to meet metabolic needs, calcium stores in bone are reduced. Chronic insufficient calcium intake can result in bone demineralization. Calcium is replaced orally or I.V. with calcium salts, such as calcium carbonate, calcium chloride, calcium citrate, calcium glubionate, calcium gluconate, or calcium lactate.

PHARMACOKINETICS

Oral calcium is absorbed readily from the duodenum and proximal jejunum. A pH of 5 to 7, parathyroid hormone, and vitamin D all aid calcium absorption. Absorption also depends on dietary factors, such as calcium binding to fiber, phytates, and oxalates and to fatty acids, with which calcium salts form insoluble soaps. Calcium is distributed primarily in bone. About 80% of a calcium salt is eliminated in feces; the rest is excreted in urine. An I.V. calcium infusion raises blood levels immediately; levels return to normal in 30 minutes to 2 hours.

Route	Onset	Peak	Duration
P.O.	Unknown	Unknown	Unknown
I.V.	Immediate	Immediate	30 min-2 hr

PHARMACODYNAMICS

Calcium moves quickly into ECF to restore calcium levels and reestablish homeostasis. It is the small amount of extracellular ionized calcium that plays an essential role in normal nerve and muscle excitability. Calcium is also integral to normal functioning of the heart, kidneys, and lungs, and it affects the blood coagulation rate as well as cell membrane and capillary permeability. Calcium is also a factor in neurotransmitter and hormone activity, amino acid metabolism, vitamin B_{12} absorption, and gastrin secretion. It plays a major role in normal bone and tooth formation.

PHARMACOTHERAPEUTICS

The major clinical indication for I.V. calcium is acute **hypocalcemia,** in which a rapid increase in serum calcium levels is needed. Conditions that create this need are tetany, cardiac arrest, vitamin D deficiency, parathyroid surgery, and alkalosis. I.V. calcium is also used to prevent a hypocal-

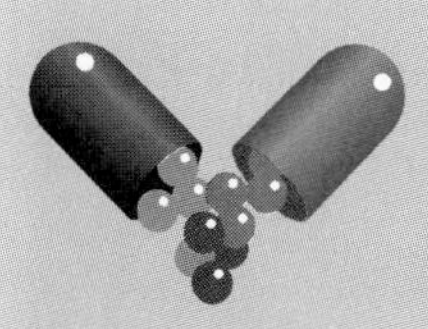

DRUG INTERACTIONS

Calcium replacement agents

Although the drug interactions involving calcium are few, they are potentially lethal and the nurse must be aware of them.

DRUG	INTERACTING DRUGS	POSSIBLE EFFECTS	NURSING IMPLICATIONS
calcium replacement agents	cardiac glycosides (digoxin, digitoxin)	Cardiac arrhythmias	• Administer calcium and cardiac glycosides simultaneously, if prescribed, by giving small amounts slowly.
	calcium channel blockers	Reduced response to calcium channel blockers	• Monitor the patient's therapeutic response to the calcium channel blocker, and expect to increase the calcium channel blocker dosage, as prescribed.
	tetracyclines	Inactivation of tetracycline through complexing	• Do not administer concurrently.

cemic reaction during exchange transfusions. Calcium is helpful in treating magnesium intoxication and in strengthening myocardial tissue after defibrillation or after a poor response to epinephrine.

Oral calcium is commonly used to supplement a calcium-deficient diet or to prevent osteoporosis. Pregnancy and lactation create a need for calcium replacement, as do periods of bone growth during childhood and adolescence. Chronic hypocalcemia from such conditions as chronic hypoparathyroidism, osteomalacia, rickets, and vitamin D deficiency is also treated with oral calcium.

Calcium is available in several salts, which can be administered alone or with other calcium salts.

Drug interactions

Calcium preparations interact with cardiac glycosides and calcium channel blockers. (See Drug Interactions: *Calcium replacement agents.*)

ADVERSE DRUG REACTIONS

Calcium preparations may produce **hypercalcemia** if the blood level is not monitored closely. Early signs of hypercalcemia include drowsiness, lethargy, muscle weakness, headache, constipation, and a metallic taste in the mouth. ECG changes include a shortened QT interval and heart block. Severe hypercalcemia can cause cardiac arrhythmias, cardiac arrest and, eventually, coma. Because calcium is excreted by the kidneys, high levels sometimes predispose patients to renal calculi.

I.V. administration of calcium may cause venous irritation; I.M. injection may cause severe local reactions, such as burning, necrosis, and tissue sloughing.

NURSING PROCESS APPLICATION

The following information assists the nurse in caring for a patient who is receiving calcium. It includes an overview of assessment activities as well as examples of appropriate nursing diagnoses and related interventions. It also highlights the importance of evaluation.

Assessment

Before drug therapy begins, review the patient's history for conditions that contraindicate or require cautious use of the prescribed calcium preparation. Also, review the patient's medication history to identify use of drugs that may interact with it. During therapy, assess the patient for adverse drug reactions and signs of drug interactions. Periodically assess the effectiveness of calcium therapy. Finally, evaluate the patient's and family's knowledge about the prescribed drug.

Nursing diagnoses

- Risk for injury related to a preexisting condition that contraindicates or requires cautious use of calcium
- Risk for injury related to adverse drug reactions or drug interactions
- Knowledge deficit related to the prescribed calcium preparation

Planning and implementation

- Do not administer calcium to a patient with a condition that contraindicates its use.
- Administer calcium cautiously to a patient at risk because of a preexisting condition.
- Monitor the patient for adverse reactions and drug interactions during calcium therapy.
- Monitor the patient's serum calcium level.

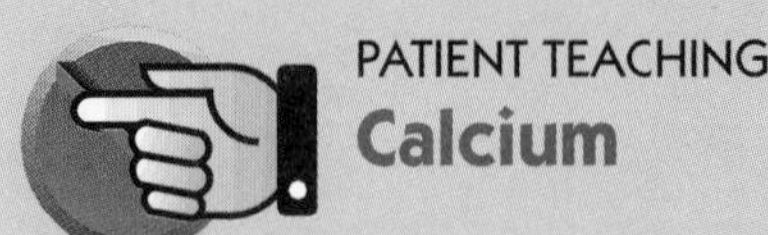

PATIENT TEACHING

Calcium

- Teach the patient and family the name, dose, frequency, action, and adverse effects of the prescribed calcium preparation.
- Advise the patient to avoid eating large amounts of spinach, rhubarb, bran, whole grain cereals and breads, and fresh fruits and vegetables when taking calcium because these foods interfere with calcium absorption. Or, unless instructed otherwise, the patient can take calcium tablets 1 to 2 hours after eating these foods.
- Suggest that the patient eat foods containing vitamin D, which enhances calcium absorption.
- Stress the importance of having blood tests to monitor calcium levels, as prescribed.
- Teach the patient to recognize and report signs of hypercalcemia to the physician.

✱ Monitor the patient regularly for early signs of hypercalcemia, such as drowsiness, lethargy, muscle weakness, headache, constipation, and a metallic taste in the mouth.

• Monitor the patient's ECG for changes that suggest hypercalcemia, such as a shortened QT interval, heart block, or arrhythmias.

• Administer I.V. calcium cautiously to prevent venous irritation. For example, warm the I.V. infusion to body temperature before administering it.

✱ Administer an I.V. infusion slowly to prevent high concentrations from reaching the heart and causing cardiac arrhythmias and arrest.

• Keep the patient recumbent for 15 minutes after injecting calcium.

• Discontinue the I.V. infusion if extravasation occurs. Also, infiltrate the area with 1% procaine and hyaluronidase to reduce vasospasm and dilute calcium, and apply warm, moist compresses to the area, as prescribed.

• Use the I.M. route in an emergency, only when the I.V. route is impossible to use. If the I.M. route is necessary, give the injection in the gluteal muscle in an adult or in the lateral thigh in an infant or small child.

• Administer an oral calcium supplement 1 to 2 hours after meals. (See Patient Teaching: *Calcium.*)

✱ Notify the physician immediately if hypercalcemia occurs. Have emergency equipment nearby.

• Administer calcium and cardiac glycosides slowly and in small amounts to avoid precipitating arrhythmias during concomitant therapy.

• Notify the physician if other adverse reactions or drug interactions occur.

Evaluation

For each nursing diagnosis, prepare an evaluation statement that describes the patient's or family's response to nursing interventions.

Other electrolytes

Besides potassium and calcium, several other electrolytes are needed in proper amounts to maintain the body's acid-base balance and to ensure proper organ functioning. Magnesium and sodium are the most important of these other electrolytes.

Magnesium is the most abundant cation in ICF after potassium. It is essential in transmitting nerve impulses to muscle and in activating enzymes necessary for carbohydrate and protein metabolism. It also stimulates parathyroid hormone secretion, thus regulating ICF calcium levels, and aids in cell metabolism and in the movement of sodium and potassium across cell membranes. Magnesium stores may be depleted by malabsorption, chronic diarrhea, prolonged treatment with diuretics, nasogastric suctioning, prolonged therapy with parenteral fluids not containing magnesium, hyperaldosteronism, hypoparathyroidism, hyperparathyroidism, and excessive release of adrenocortical hormones. Magnesium sulfate is the drug of choice for replacement therapy in magnesium deficiency. Magnesium sulfate is also used to treat seizures, severe toxemia, and acute nephritis in children.

Sodium is the major cation in ECF. It maintains the osmotic pressure and concentration of ECF, acid-base balance, and water balance; contributes to nerve conduction and neuromuscular function; and plays a role in glandular secretion. Sodium replacement is necessary in conditions that rapidly deplete it, such as excessive loss of GI fluids or excessive perspiration. Diuretics and tap water enemas can also deplete sodium, particularly when fluids are replaced by plain water. Sodium can be lost in trauma or wound drainage, adrenal gland insufficiency, cirrhosis of the liver with ascites, syndrome of inappropriate ADH, and prolonged I.V. infusion of dextrose in water without other solutes.

Severe symptomatic sodium deficiency may be treated by I.V. infusion of 3% or 5% sodium chloride (NaCl) solution. Other I.V. solutions that contain NaCl include dextrose 5% in water (D_5W) and 0.9% NaCl; D_5W and 0.45% NaCl; dextrose 2.5% in water and 0.45% NaCl; and 0.9% NaCl. Injectable sodium salts (sodium bicarbonate and sodium lactate) are also used to treat metabolic acidosis.

CHAPTER SUMMARY

Chapter 51 presented the role of electrolyte replacement agents in maintaining homeostasis, or stability in body fluid composition and volume. Here are the chapter highlights.

Potassium is the main cation in ICF; sodium is the main cation in ECF. Magnesium is the second most common cation in ICF; calcium is a major cation in ECF.

Electrolytes are primarily absorbed through the GI tract and excreted by the kidneys. Conditions that increase excretion or decrease absorption of electrolytes can lead to a deficient state that disturbs homeostasis. They can be replaced orally or parenterally.

When administering a replacement electrolyte, the nurse must monitor for elevated blood levels of the electrolyte. An excess of electrolytes can cause as serious an alteration in homeostasis as a deficit. The nurse should also monitor the patient for adverse reactions to the electrolyte, attempt to determine the cause of the electrolyte deficiency (such as inadequate dietary intake), and teach the patient about the prescribed electrolyte replacement agent.

Questions to consider

See Appendix 1 for answers.

1. William Tree, age 43, is receiving potassium chloride 40 mEq in his I.V. fluid to correct hypokalemia. The nurse assesses Mr. Tree for signs and symptoms of hyperkalemia, an adverse reaction to potassium. Which of the following assessment findings would suggest hyperkalemia?
   (a) Paresthesia, weakness, and confusion
   (b) Hyperexcitability, seizures, and confusion
   (c) Hallucinations, muscle rigidity, and clonic contractions
   (d) Drowsiness, lethargy, and muscle weakness

2. Lydia Duran, age 65, suffers cardiac arrest in the emergency department. During cardiopulmonary resuscitation, Ms. Duran received sodium bicarbonate, epinephrine, and calcium chloride. Why did Ms. Duran receive calcium chloride?
   (a) To enhance the effects of epinephrine
   (b) To treat metabolic acidosis
   (c) To strengthen myocardial tissue
   (d) To cause vasoconstriction

3. Darlene Dawson, age 28 and 9 months pregnant, develops severe toxemia. After being admitted to the maternity unit, which of the following electrolytes can the nurse expect to use to treat Ms. Dawson's toxemia?
   (a) sodium
   (b) magnesium
   (c) potassium
   (d) calcium

4. Jeffrey Davis, age 54, has been receiving furosemide therapy for several days. He begins to complain of abdominal cramping, drowsiness, muscle weakness, and nausea. What is the most likely explanation for these symptoms?
   (a) Hypomagnesemia
   (b) Hyponatremia
   (c) Hypocalcemia
   (d) Hypokalemia

5. Mariann Davis, age 65, has chronic renal failure. Her physician has ordered sodium bicarbonate 325 mg P.O. q.i.d. to maintain a normal blood pH. How should the nurse instruct Mrs. Davis to take sodium bicarbonate?
   (a) Take the pill with a small amount of water.
   (b) Combine the dose with an antacid.
   (c) Drink at least one full glass of water with each dose.
   (d) Alter the dose if GI reactions occur.

52 Alkalinizing and acidifying agents

OBJECTIVES

After reading and studying this chapter, the student should be able to:

1. identify the alkalinizing and acidifying agents.
2. discuss the pharmacokinetics of alkalinizing and acidifying agents.
3. explain how alkalinizing and acidifying agents affect blood pH.
4. discuss the adverse reactions associated with each alkalinizing and acidifying agent.
5. describe how to apply the nursing process when caring for a patient who is receiving an alkalinizing or acidifying agent.

INTRODUCTION

Alkalinizing and acidifying agents act to correct acid-base imbalances in the blood. They are commonly used to treat **metabolic acidosis** and **metabolic alkalosis,** respectively. An alkalinizing agent will increase the **pH** (hydrogen ion concentration) of the blood; an acidifying agent will decrease the pH. Some of these agents also alter urine pH, making them useful in treating some urinary tract infections and drug overdoses. This chapter covers the alkalinizing and acidifying agents as they are used to treat certain acid-base disorders. (See *Selected major alkalinizing and acidifying agents.*)

Drugs covered in this chapter include:

- acetazolamide
- ammonium chloride
- arginine hydrochloride
- ascorbic acid
- hydrochloric acid
- sodium bicarbonate
- sodium citrate
- sodium lactate
- tromethamine.

Alkalinizing agents

Four alkalinizing agents are used to increase blood pH: sodium bicarbonate, sodium citrate, sodium lactate, and tromethamine. Sodium bicarbonate also is used to increase urine pH, as is the **carbonic anhydrase** inhibitor acetazolamide (which, paradoxically, lowers the blood pH).

PHARMACOKINETICS

All of the alkalinizing agents are absorbed well when given orally. Sodium citrate and sodium lactate are metabolized to the active ingredient, bicarbonate. Sodium bicarbonate is not metabolized. Tromethamine and acetazolamide undergo little or no metabolism and are excreted unchanged in the urine. The onsets of action of the alkalinizing agents are rapid after oral administration and immediate after intravenous (I.V.) administration. Their durations of action vary widely, however, depending on use and underlying disorders.

Route	Onset	Peak	Duration
P.O.	Rapid	30 min	1-3 hr
I.V.	Rapid	Immediate	Variable

PHARMACODYNAMICS

Sodium bicarbonate dissociates in the blood to provide bicarbonate ions that are used in the blood **buffer** system to decrease the hydrogen ion concentration and raise the blood pH. As the bicarbonate ions are excreted in the urine, urine pH rises. Sodium citrate and lactate, after conversion to bicarbonate, alkalinize the blood and urine in the same way.

Tromethamine acts by combining with hydrogen ions to alkalinize the blood; the resulting tromethamine-hydrogen ion complex is excreted in the urine.

Acetazolamide promotes renal excretion of sodium, potassium, bicarbonate, and water. The bicarbonate ion excretion alkalinizes the urine and, by reducing blood bicarbonate levels, also acidifies the blood.

PHARMACOTHERAPEUTICS

Alkalinizing agents are commonly used to treat metabolic acidosis. Other uses include raising the urine pH to help remove certain substances, such as phenobarbital, after an overdose.

Drug interactions

Alkalinizing agents can interact with a wide range of drugs to increase or decrease their pharmacologic effects. (See Drug Interactions: *Alkalinizing agents,* page 634.)

Selected major alkalinizing and acidifying agents

This chart summarizes the major alkalinizing and acidifying agents currently in clinical use.

DRUG	MAJOR INDICATIONS AND USUAL DOSAGES	CONTRAINDICATIONS AND PRECAUTIONS
Alkalinizing agents		
sodium bicarbonate	*Severe metabolic acidosis in cardiac arrest* ADULT: initially, 1 mEq/kg I.V., followed by 0.5 mEq/kg every 10 minutes; or an individualized dosage PEDIATRIC: for neonates, 1 mEq/kg by slow I.V. infusion of 1 part sodium bicarbonate and 1 part dextrose 5% in water to avoid hypertonicity; for all other children, 1 mEq/kg I.V. every 10 minutes *Less severe metabolic acidosis* ADULT: 2 to 5 mEq/kg I.V. infused over 4 to 8 hours *Urine alkalinization* ADULT: initially, 48 mEq P.O., followed by 12 to 24 mEq P.O. every 4 hours	• Sodium bicarbonate is contraindicated in a patient who is predisposed to development of diuretic-induced hypochloremic acidosis, one who has ingested a strong mineral acid, or one with metabolic or respiratory alkalosis, hypocalcemia when alkalosis may induce tetany, or excessive chloride loss. • This drug requires cautious use in a patient receiving corticotropin or a corticosteroid or one with heart failure, other edematous or sodium-retaining condition, or renal insufficiency.
sodium citrate (Shohl's solution)	*Metabolic acidosis* ADULT: 10 to 30 ml of Shohl's solution P.O. after meals and at bedtime PEDIATRIC: 5 to 15 ml of Shohl's solution P.O. after meals and at bedtime	• Sodium citrate is contraindicated in a patient with severe renal impairment or one who must follow a sodium-restricted diet. • This drug requires cautious use in a patient with low urine output, heart failure, hypertension, renal dysfunction, peripheral or pulmonary edema, or toxemia of pregnancy.
Acidifying agents		
ammonium chloride	*Metabolic alkalosis related to chloride loss* ADULT: up to 5 ml/minute I.V. of diluted solution based on the patient's chloride deficit *Urine acidification* ADULT: 4 to 12 g P.O. daily in divided doses every 4 to 6 hours PEDIATRIC: 75 mg/kg daily P.O. in four divided doses	• Ammonium chloride is contraindicated in a patient with severe hepatic dysfunction, severe renal dysfunction when metabolic alkalosis is caused by vomiting and is accompanied by substantial sodium loss, primary respiratory acidosis, or high total carbon dioxide and buffer base. • This drug requires cautious use in a patient with pulmonary insufficiency or cardiac edema. • Safety and efficacy of ammonium chloride concentrate for injection in children have not been established.
ascorbic acid (Ascorbicap)	*Urine acidification* ADULT: 4 to 12 g daily P.O. in divided doses	• Ascorbic acid has no known contraindications. • This drug requires cautious use in a pregnant patient. High dosages require cautious use in a patient with a history of gouty arthritis, deep vein thrombosis, or renal calculi. • Patients should be monitored for occult blood in their stools periodically.

ADVERSE DRUG REACTIONS

The most severe adverse reaction (causing hyperirritability, tetany, or both) is metabolic alkalosis related to sodium bicarbonate overdose. In a patient with diabetic ketoacidosis, rapid administration of sodium bicarbonate that corrects acidosis too quickly may cause cerebral dysfunction, tissue hypoxia, and **lactic acidosis.** The high sodium content (12 mEq or 276 mg/gram) of this drug may cause water retention and edema in some patients, especially those with renal disease, heart failure, or other disorders that can cause fluid imbalance. Oral sodium bicarbonate may produce gastric distention and flatulence as it combines with hydrochloric acid in the stomach to release carbon dioxide. Shohl's solution, which produces less gastric upset than sodium bicarbonate, is usually preferred for this reason. I.V. administration of sodium bicarbonate can cause extravasation that may result in tissue sloughing, ulceration, and necrosis.

Sodium citrate normally produces few adverse reactions, but an overdose may cause metabolic alkalosis or tetany or

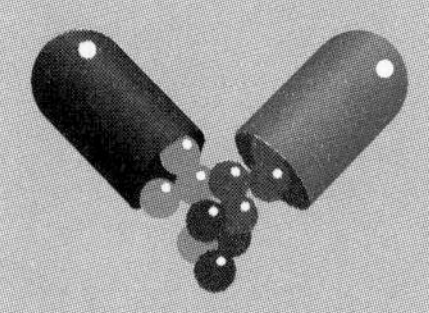

DRUG INTERACTIONS

Alkalinizing agents

Interactions involving alkalinizing agents may be severe and may alter the pharmacologic action of another drug.

DRUG	INTERACTING DRUGS	POSSIBLE EFFECTS	NURSING IMPLICATIONS
sodium bicarbonate, sodium citrate, sodium lactate	amphetamines	Decreased amphetamine excretion, resulting in increased stimulant effects	• Monitor the patient closely for signs of increased amphetamine effect, such as rapid heart rate, increased blood pressure, and restlessness.
	ketoconazole	Decreased ketoconazole absorption	• Avoid concomitant use with an oral alkalizing agent.
	lithium	Increased lithium excretion	• Monitor the patient for signs of decreased lithium effectiveness, such as increased manic-depressive behavior. • Monitor the patient's lithium blood level, as prescribed.
	methenamine	Decreased conversion of methenamine to formaldehyde, resulting in decreased antibacterial action	• Avoid concomitant use with an alkalinizing agent.
	quinidine	Decreased quinidine excretion, resulting in increased blood levels of quinidine	• Monitor the patient for signs of quinidine toxicity, such as tinnitus and a widened QT interval on electrocardiogram tracings.
	salicylates	Increased salicylate excretion if salicylate dosage exceeds 50 mg/kg daily	• Monitor the patient for signs of decreased salicylate effectiveness, such as increased pain and inflammation, at sites where relief previously had been obtained.
	pseudoephedrine	Decreased pseudoephedrine excretion	• Monitor the patient for adverse reactions to pseudoephedrine, such as increased heart rate and cardiac output.

may aggravate existing cardiac disease by decreasing serum calcium levels. Oral sodium citrate can have a laxative effect.

Sodium lactate also produces few adverse reactions except for metabolic alkalosis (from an overdose) and extravasation. Because the sodium content is high (8 to 9 mEq or 204 mg/g), this agent may cause water retention and edema in a patient whose ability to excrete sodium is impaired, particularly by renal disease or heart failure.

Adverse reactions to tromethamine may be mild, such as phlebitis or irritation at the injection site, or severe, such as hypoglycemia, respiratory depression (especially in a patient who already has depressed respirations or is receiving a drug that depresses respirations), extravasation, and hyperkalemia. In a patient with impaired renal function, this renally excreted drug may accumulate to toxic levels. In a severely ill neonate, hypertonic tromethamine given through the umbilical vein can cause hepatic necrosis. Because of these adverse reactions, tromethamine use should not exceed 24 hours for most patients.

A wide range of adverse reactions can occur with acetazolamide. Gastrointestinal (GI) signs and symptoms include nausea, vomiting, diarrhea, anorexia, and weight loss. Central nervous system reactions may include sedation, headache, confusion, and paresthesia. This drug also can elevate blood glucose levels in a diabetic patient; decrease uric acid excretion, leading to gout; cause metabolic acidosis; and precipitate hepatic coma in a patient with severe liver disease. Other adverse reactions include hypersensitivity reactions, such as cholestatic jaundice, fever, rash, skin eruptions, and bone marrow depression (which may lead to aplastic anemia).

NURSING PROCESS APPLICATION

The following information assists the nurse in caring for a patient who is receiving an alkalinizing agent. It includes an overview of assessment activities as well as examples of appropriate nursing diagnoses and related interventions (see

"Planning and implementation"). It also highlights the importance of evaluation.

Assessment

Before drug therapy begins, review the patient's history for conditions that contraindicate or require cautious use of the prescribed alkalinizing agent. Also review the patient's medication history to identify use of drugs that may interact with it. During therapy, assess the patient for adverse drug reactions and signs of drug interactions. Also, periodically assess the effectiveness of therapy with the alkalinizing agent. Finally, evaluate the patient's and family's knowledge about the prescribed drug.

Nursing diagnoses

- Risk for injury related to a preexisting condition that contraindicates or requires cautious use of an alkalinizing agent
- Risk for injury related to adverse drug reactions or drug interactions
- Fluid volume excess related to the high sodium content of sodium bicarbonate or sodium lactate
- Knowledge deficit related to the prescribed alkalinizing agent

Planning and implementation

- Do not administer an alkalinizing agent to a patient with a condition that contraindicates its use.
- Administer an alkalinizing agent cautiously to a patient at risk because of a preexisting condition. (See Patient Teaching: *Alkalinizing agents.*)
- Monitor the patient for adverse reactions and drug interactions during therapy with an alkalinizing agent.
- Monitor the patient's serum pH and serum bicarbonate levels regularly to evaluate the effectiveness of therapy and to detect problems.
- Monitor the patient's urine pH frequently when sodium bicarbonate or acetazolamide is used to alkalinize the urine.
- Inspect the I.V. site regularly for extravasation in a patient receiving sodium bicarbonate, sodium lactate, or tromethamine. Observe for phlebitis or irritation in a patient receiving tromethamine.
- Treat extravasation by elevating the affected limb, applying warm compresses, and administering lidocaine, hyaluronidase, or both, as prescribed.
- Monitor the patient for signs and symptoms of overdose with the alkalinizing agent.

*** *Administer sodium bicarbonate slowly to a patient with diabetic ketoacidosis because cerebral dysfunction, tissue hypoxia, and lactic acidosis can occur.***

- Do not administer tromethamine for more than 24 hours to help prevent severe adverse reactions.
- Monitor glucose levels regularly to detect hypoglycemia in a patient receiving acetazolamide.
- Dilute Shohl's solution with 2 to 3 oz (60 to 90 ml) of water before administration, refrigerate it to improve the taste, and administer it after meals to prevent its laxative effects.

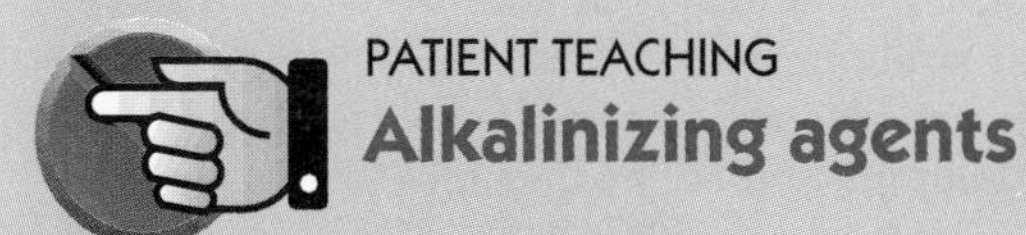

PATIENT TEACHING

Alkalinizing agents

- Teach the patient and family the name, dose, frequency, action, and adverse effects of the prescribed alkalinizing agent.
- Advise the patient receiving prolonged therapy with sodium bicarbonate tablets that gastrointestinal (GI) distress and flatulence may occur and should be reported to the physician. (Because GI distress can lead to noncompliance and subsequent acute acidosis, expect an alternate alkalinizing agent to be prescribed if the patient reports GI distress.)
- Teach the patient to recognize the signs of fluid retention, such as ankle swelling and increasing tightness of rings worn on the fingers. Emphasize the importance of immediately reporting these signs to the physician.
- Inform the diabetic patient that tromethamine can cause hypoglycemia or that acetazolamide can cause hyperglycemia. Encourage the patient to monitor blood glucose levels closely.
- Advise the patient taking acetazolamide to avoid activities that require mental alertness if sedation or mental changes occur.
- Teach the patient how to prepare and administer Shohl's solution to improve its taste and prevent its laxative effects.
- Instruct the patient to notify the physician if adverse reactions occur.
- Advise the patient to avoid milk while taking sodium bicarbonate in order to avoid milk-alkali syndrome, hypercalcemia, or renal calculi production.

- Notify the physician if adverse reactions or drug interactions occur.

*** *Monitor for signs of fluid retention, such as crackles, peripheral edema, and jugular venous distention in a patient receiving sodium bicarbonate or sodium lactate. The high sodium content of these drugs may cause fluid retention, especially in a patient with renal disease or heart failure.***

- Notify the physician if fluid retention occurs.

Evaluation

For each nursing diagnosis, prepare an evaluation statement that describes the patient's or family's response to nursing interventions.

Acidifying agents

Three acidifying agents — ammonium chloride, arginine hydrochloride, and hydrochloric acid — are used to correct metabolic alkalosis. Ammonium chloride and ascorbic acid also may serve as urinary acidifiers.

PHARMACOKINETICS

Orally administered ammonium chloride is absorbed completely in 3 to 6 hours. It is metabolized in the liver to form urea, which is excreted by the kidneys, and hydrochloric acid, the acidifying agent.

When used to treat metabolic alkalosis, arginine hydrochloride is administered intravenously. The drug is metabolized in the liver and excreted by the kidneys.

After I.V. administration, hydrochloric acid is broken down into hydrogen and chloride ions. The hydrogen ions are used as the acidifying agent.

Orally administered ascorbic acid usually is absorbed well, distributed widely in body tissues, and metabolized in the liver. Its metabolites are excreted in the urine along with excess ascorbic acid, which is excreted unchanged.

Route	Onset	Peak	Duration
P.O.	Rapid	Unknown	3-6 hr
I.V.	Rapid	Immediate	Unknown

PHARMACODYNAMICS

Ammonium chloride lowers the blood pH after being metabolized to urea and to hydrochloric acid, which provides hydrogen ions to acidify the blood or urine. Arginine hydrochloride also provides hydrogen ions via metabolism to hydrochloric acid. Hydrochloric acid lowers blood pH directly by acidifying the blood with hydrogen ions. Ascorbic acid directly acidifies the urine, providing hydrogen ions and lowering the urine pH.

PHARMACOTHERAPEUTICS

A patient with metabolic alkalosis requires therapy with an acidifying agent that provides hydrogen ions; such a patient may need chloride ion therapy as well. Although the patient can receive both in a hydrochloric acid infusion, this infusion is difficult to prepare, and an overdose can produce severe adverse reactions. That is why most patients receive both types of ions in oral or parenteral doses of ammonium chloride — a safer drug that is easy to prepare. A patient with a urinary tract infection or a drug overdose may benefit from receiving a urinary acidifier.

Drug interactions

Acidifying agents do not cause clinically significant drug interactions.

ADVERSE DRUG REACTIONS

Adverse reactions to acidifying agents are usually mild, such as GI distress. However, overdose can occur, especially with parenteral administration, and may lead to acidosis.

Oral administration of ammonium chloride may cause nausea, vomiting, anorexia, and thirst. Large dosages may cause metabolic acidosis and loss of electrolytes, especially potassium. Rapid I.V. administration may cause pain and irritation at the injection site. Ammonium toxicity may also occur, producing twitching and hyperreflexia.

Adverse reactions to arginine hydrochloride typically result from too-rapid I.V. administration and include flushing, nausea, vomiting, headache, numbness, and irritation at the infusion site. In some patients, arginine hydrochloride causes a hypersensitivity reaction that consists of a macular rash with redness and edema of the hands and face; these disappear when the drug is discontinued. This agent also may cause other hypersensitivity reactions, such as nasal obstruction and discharge, sweating, and increased pulse rate.

With hydrochloric acid administration, metabolic acidosis may occur with an overdose.

In high dosages, ascorbic acid can produce GI distress, such as nausea, vomiting, diarrhea, and abdominal cramps, and flushing, headache, and insomnia. In a patient with glucose-6-phosphate dehydrogenase (G6PD) deficiency, hemolytic anemia may develop after administration of a high dose of ascorbic acid.

CRITICAL THINKING: To enhance your critical thinking about alkalinizing and acidifying agents, consider the following situation and its analysis.

Situation: Mr. Jones is being treated for metabolic alkalosis with I.V. arginine hydrochloride. During the infusion, Mr. Jones begins to complain of blocked nasal passages and a runny nose; his heart rate is increasing on the cardiac monitor. Upon closer inspection of Mr. Jones, the nurse sees a red macular rash over his arms and face, and his hands are becoming edematous. The nurse provides Mr. Jones with an antihistamine agent (Benadryl), as ordered, and gives him a cool compress to lay over his face. Is this the correct thing to do?

Analysis: Even though arginine hydrochloride can cause minor hypersensitivity reactions such as nasal obstruction, nasal discharge, sweating, and an increased pulse rate, Mr. Jones is experiencing a more severe reaction. The red rash over his arms and face and the edematous upper extremities warrant discontinuing the infusion prior to administering antihistamine therapy and notifying the physician immediately.

NURSING PROCESS APPLICATION

The following information assists the nurse in caring for a patient who is receiving an acidifying agent. It includes an overview of assessment activities as well as examples of appropriate nursing diagnoses and related interventions (see "Planning and implementation"). It also highlights the importance of evaluation.

Assessment

Before drug therapy begins, review the patient's history for conditions that contraindicate or require cautious use of the prescribed acidifying agent. During therapy, assess the patient for adverse drug reactions. Also, periodically assess the effectiveness of therapy with the acidifying agent. Finally, evaluate the patient's and family's knowledge about the prescribed drug.

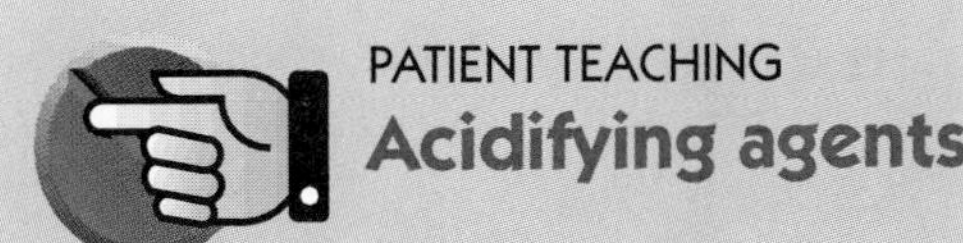

PATIENT TEACHING
Acidifying agents

- ➤ Teach the patient and family the name, dose, frequency, action, and adverse effects of the prescribed acidifying agent.
- ➤ Inform the patient receiving ascorbic acid or oral ammonium chloride to take the agent exactly as prescribed, to report severe adverse gastrointestinal reactions, and to monitor the urine pH regularly.
- ➤ Instruct the patient to withhold the next ammonium chloride dose and notify the physician if twitching occurs because twitching may indicate ammonium toxicity.
- ➤ Advise the patient to take a mild analgesic for headache as prescribed when receiving high-dosage ascorbic acid therapy. If the patient experiences insomnia, suggest relaxation techniques, such as a warm bath or reading before bedtime. If these techniques are ineffective, advise the patient to request a prescription for a hypnotic agent.
- ➤ Advise the patient to notify the physician if adverse drug reactions occur.

Nursing diagnoses

- Risk for injury related to a preexisting condition that contraindicates or requires cautious use of an acidifying agent
- Risk for injury related to adverse drug reactions
- Knowledge deficit related to the prescribed acidifying agent

Planning and implementation

- Do not administer an acidifying agent to a patient with a condition that contraindicates its use.
- Administer an acidifying agent cautiously to a patient at risk because of a preexisting condition.
- Monitor the patient for adverse reactions during therapy with an acidifying agent. (See Patient Teaching: *Acidifying agents.*)
- Monitor the patient for signs of metabolic acidosis and abnormal laboratory values of arterial blood pH, serum bicarbonate, serum chloride, and serum potassium.

***** ***Observe for signs of ammonium toxicity in a patient receiving ammonium chloride. If these signs appear, withhold the agent, notify the physician immediately, and switch the patient to a different acidifying agent as prescribed.***

***** ***Monitor the patient receiving large dosages of ammonium chloride for signs of hypokalemia. Also monitor for other electrolyte imbalances. If an electrolyte imbalance is suspected, notify the physician. Expect to draw blood to determine electrolyte levels and to start therapy to correct the imbalance, as prescribed.***

- Monitor the complete blood count, as instructed, in a patient with G6PD who is receiving high doses of ascorbic acid. Particularly note changes that suggest hemolytic anemia.
- Expect an acidifying agent to be prepared for I.V. administration under aseptic conditions, preferably in a laminar airflow hood. Expect the pharmacy to prepare a hydrochloric acid infusion, because the acid is extremely caustic.
- Administer an I.V. acidifying agent slowly to prevent pain or irritation at the infusion site as well as other adverse reactions.
- Notify the physician if adverse reactions occur.

Evaluation

For each nursing diagnosis, prepare an evaluation statement that describes the patient's or family's response to nursing interventions.

CHAPTER SUMMARY

Chapter 52 covered alkalinizing and acidifying agents as they are used to treat certain acid-base disorders and to regulate blood and urine pH. Here are the chapter highlights.

Alkalinizing agents, such as sodium bicarbonate, sodium citrate, sodium lactate, and tromethamine, are used to treat metabolic acidosis by alkalinizing the blood. They do this by decreasing the hydrogen ion concentration. Some alkalinizing agents, such as sodium bicarbonate and acetazolamide, also can alkalinize the urine. They are useful for promoting the excretion of certain weak acids, such as uric acid, or toxic drugs, such as phenobarbital.

Alkalinizing agents may cause severe adverse reactions, which are usually related to overdose. Sodium bicarbonate and sodium lactate may cause water retention and edema in patients with impaired ability to excrete sodium resulting from such disorders as heart failure or renal dysfunction.

Acidifying agents, such as ammonium chloride, arginine hydrochloride, and hydrochloric acid, are used to correct metabolic alkalosis by acidifying the blood. They do this by increasing the hydrogen ion concentration. Ammonium chloride and large dosages of ascorbic acid may be used to acidify the urine in patients with urinary tract infections.

Acidifying agents may produce adverse reactions that range from mild (GI distress) to severe (acidosis).

When administering an alkalinizing or acidifying agent, the nurse must monitor the patient's blood pH closely because overdose can occur when the pH falls outside of the narrow normal range of 7.35 to 7.45.

Questions to consider

See Appendix 1 for answers.

1. Maxwell Garfield, age 68, is given sodium bicarbonate during cardiac arrest to treat metabolic acidosis. How does sodium bicarbonate correct metabolic acidosis?

(a) By decreasing the hydrogen ion concentration
(b) By increasing the hydrogen ion concentration
(c) By combining with hydrogen ions to alkalinize the blood
(d) By promoting renal excretion of sodium, potassium bicarbonate, and water

2. A patient is receiving sodium bicarbonate. For which severe adverse reaction should he be monitored?
(a) Hepatic necrosis
(b) Metabolic alkalosis
(c) Respiratory depression
(d) Hypersensitivity reaction

3. David McKane has fluid retention, including crackles and peripheral edema. He is taking sodium bicarbonate or sodium lactate. The fluid retention may result from which of the following conditions?
(a) Insufficient renal perfusion of the sodium
(b) Low serum potassium level
(c) High sodium content of the medication
(d) Mild heart failure

4. Missy Cramer, age 42, develops metabolic alkalosis caused by the chloride-wasting diuretic furosemide. The physician prescribes 2.14% solution of ammonium chloride I.V., infused 1 ml/minute. Why is ammonium chloride used more commonly than hydrochloric acid to treat metabolic alkalosis?
(a) It is safer and easier to prepare.
(b) It provides hydrogen and chloride ions.
(c) It has a more rapid onset of action.
(d) It does not cause metabolic acidosis.

5. A patient is taking a 2.14% solution of ammonium chloride I.V. Which severe adverse reaction is associated with ammonium chloride?
(a) Renal tubular necrosis
(b) Metabolic acidosis
(c) Pain and irritation at injection site
(d) Respiratory depression

UNIT XV

Drugs to treat malignant neoplasms

In the 1940s, antineoplastic, or chemotherapeutic, drugs were used to treat **cancer** when all other therapeutic measures failed for disseminated cancers that could not be treated by surgery or radiation therapy. Then, most antineoplastic drugs commonly had serious adverse effects. Today, many of these effects can be minimized so that they are not as devastating to the patient. In fact, many childhood cancers are now considered curable because of the advent of chemotherapeutic drugs. Many of these agents are the drugs of choice for different types of cancer and are no longer considered a last resort. Also, new agents, such as interferons, are being used to treat patients with cancer.

Nurses have participated actively in administering and evaluating more than 50 drugs to treat cancer. In caring for patients receiving these drugs, nurses have helped patients and their families understand chemotherapy and cope with its adverse effects.

CLINICAL USES

Antineoplastic agents may be used to cure cancer, prevent its spread, relieve cancer symptoms or prolong survival. For patients with systemic cancer, such as **leukemia,** chemotherapy may be given as a curative treatment. In other patients, it may be given as an adjunct treatment based on the premise that micrometastases, although undetectable, exist. In patients with advanced neoplastic disorders, chemotherapy may be **palliative,** reducing **tumor** size or relieving pain and other symptoms.

Chemotherapy is commonly combined with other cancer treatments. For example, it may be given preoperatively to reduce tumor size and allow less radical surgery.

The chapters in unit 15 present **cell cycle–specific** and **cell cycle–nonspecific** agents used to treat malignant **neoplasms** or to prevent or relieve their symptoms.

CELL CYCLE

To understand the pharmacodynamics of antineoplastic agents, the nurse needs to know about the **cell cycle.** All animal cells follow a series of basic steps as they undergo division and replication. This series of steps is called the cell cycle; each step is a phase. During each phase, biochemical events that are necessary for cell division occur. (See *Cell cycle,* page 640.)

In the first phase, G_1 (G stands for gap), the cell manufactures the enzymes needed for deoxyribonucleic acid (DNA) synthesis. The time a cell spends in G_1 varies greatly but averages about 18 hours.

Next, the cell enters the S phase (S stands for synthesis). In this phase, DNA replication occurs in preparation for **mitosis** (cell division). This phase lasts from 10 to 20 hours.

Then, the cell enters the G_2 phase, when specialized DNA proteins and ribonucleic acid (RNA) are synthesized for later mitosis. This phase lasts about 3 hours.

Finally, the cell is ready to divide and enters the M phase (M stands for mitosis). During mitosis, the cell progresses through four subphases: *prophase,* when the chromosomes aggregate or clump; *metaphase,* when the chromosomes line up in the middle of the cell; *anaphase,* when the chromosomes segregate; and *telophase,* when the cell divides, producing two morphologically identical cells. The entire M phase lasts only 1 hour.

From the M phase, the cell may follow one of three paths. It may differentiate into a functional cell, enter the G_0 (resting) phase, or begin the cycle again by entering the G_1 phase. Resting cells in the G_0 phase may move on to the G_1 phase and progress through the cell cycle.

In different phases of the cycle, cells are susceptible to different drugs because the drugs interfere with specific biochemical events that occur in these phases. It should be noted that chemotherapy affects all cells that are in the cell cycle, not just cancer cells. The systems of the body with high growth rates and a large percentage of cells in the cell cycle are the hemopoietic and the epithelium systems. This explains why there is such an effect on the bone marrow of the person receiving chemotherapy.

Cell cycle

Every cell progresses through a series of phases to replicate itself. During each phase, the cell is vulnerable to certain drugs that can interfere with its replication. This susceptibility is the basis of antineoplastic therapy.

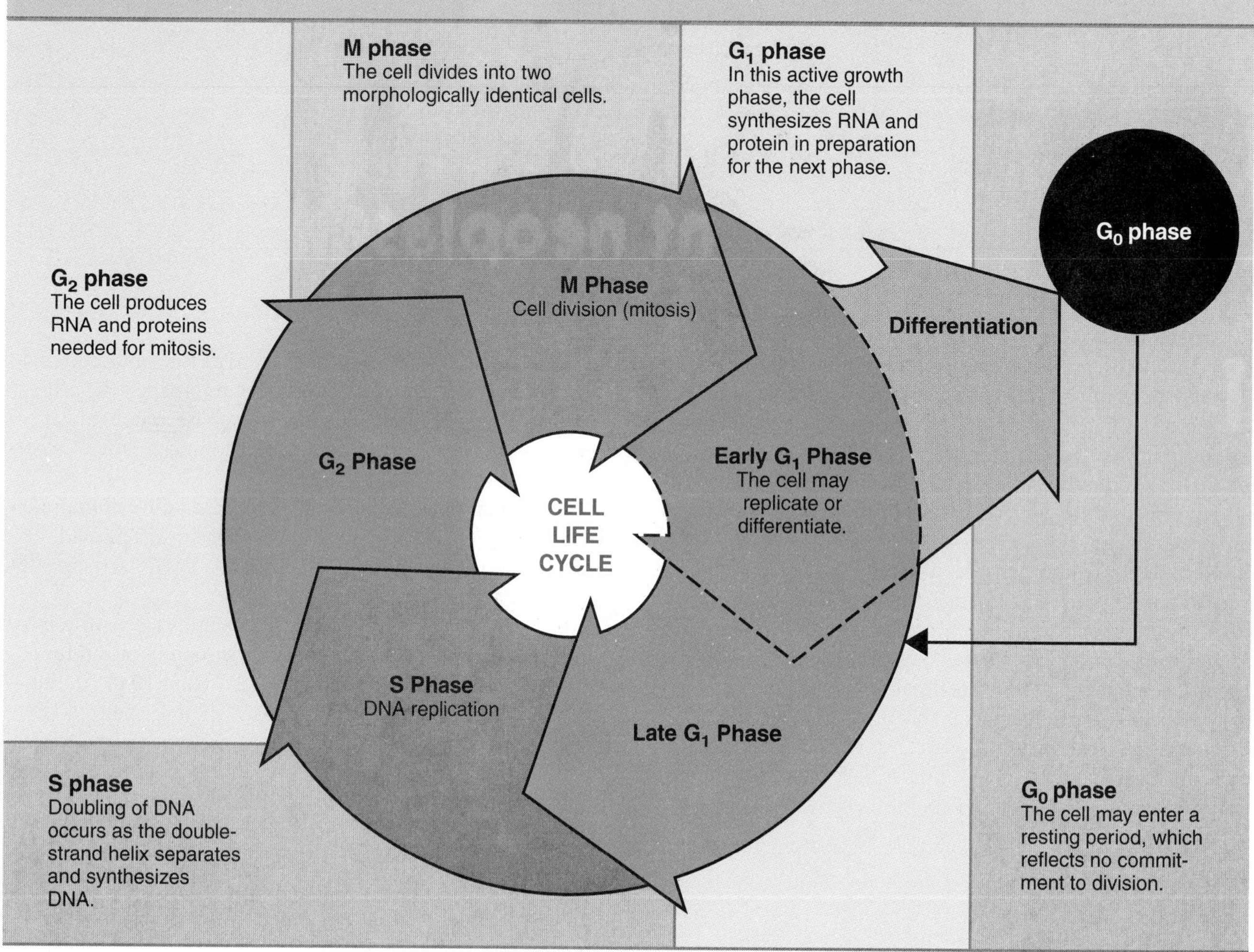

MECHANISMS OF ACTION

Although not understood completely, cancer seems to occur when one cell undergoes a malignant transformation and produces an abnormal cell. Antineoplastic agents interfere with cell reproduction, leading to tumor destruction.

During administration of an antineoplastic agent, a fixed percentage of cells die. After treatment, the remaining cells reproduce, and resting cells in the G_0 phase may return to a reproducing phase. (Cells in the G_0 phase are less sensitive to chemotherapy because they are not synthesizing DNA actively.) Total eradication of cancer cells, therefore, depends on repeated administration of the antineoplastic agent. An interval between treatments permits healthy cells to recover. The optimal interval between treatments is that which allows enough time for recovery of healthy cells, yet not enough time for the tumor to totally repopulate itself.

Because cancer cells are at various phases in the cell cycle, therapy commonly combines drugs that act on cells in different phases or that have different sites of action.

Although an antineoplastic agent kills cells as soon as they pass through a specific cell cycle, this action produces no immediate clinical response. Most patients need at least three treatments before a clinical response can be evaluated by physical examination, X-ray, computed tomography (CT) scanning, magnetic resonance imaging (MRI), or biological marker determination. (See *Common adverse reactions and associated nursing implications,* page 642.)

Tumor regression depends on several factors, such as the percentage of cells killed, the rate of regrowth, and the development of resistant cells. Evaluation of chemotherapy is difficult, however, because the cancer may be undetected clinically but still may be present. Therefore, treatments may continue for a while after the disease is no longer detectable.

TUMOR RESISTANCE

Combination drug regimens may be used for patients with tumor resistance. Tumor cell populations are heterogeneous: Some cells are sensitive to antineoplastic agents; others are not. When an antineoplastic agent is administered, it kills drug-sensitive cells initially. Repeated administration kills more drug-sensitive cells. Over time, however, tumor cells that are not drug-sensitive remain and replicate, producing a drug-resistant tumor. If these resistant cells are also resistant to other drugs, they will be even more difficult to kill. In addition, cancer cells mutate whereby drug sensitive cells become drug resistant.

Drug resistance may develop by one or more of the following mechanisms: decreased drug entry into the tumor cells, decreased drug-activating enzymes, increased drug-deactivating enzymes, increased levels of target enzymes, decreased target enzyme affinity for the drug, increased DNA repair, or development of alternate pathways that circumvent the action of the drug. In general, the greater the number of agents in a particular regimen of chemotherapy, the less likely it is that drug resistance will occur.

HANDLING ANTINEOPLASTIC AGENTS

Although the safe handling of antineoplastic agents remains controversial, most experts recommend conservative, protective methods. For maximum safety, the nurse should use the following techniques when handling antineoplastic agents:

- Mix antineoplastic agents in a Class II biological safety cabinet only.
- Wear powder-free, disposable, latex surgical gloves and a protective barrier garment with a closed front and long, cuffed sleeves to protect the body when mixing or administering antineoplastic agents. Some clinicians recommend wearing double gloves.
- Reconstitute and administer antineoplastic agents in syringes or intravenous (I.V.) sets with luer-lock syringes.
- Use a closed delivery technique when administering these agents.
- Do not prime I.V. lines and syringes into a sink or waste basket; use sterile 2"× 2" gauze pads or alcohol wipes instead.
- After mixing and administering these agents, dispose of any waste in a leakproof, punctureproof container labeled "hazardous waste." Such containers must be disposed of by incineration or burial at a hazardous chemical waste site.
- If a spill occurs, follow the health care facility's policy for cleaning up hazardous materials.

ADMINISTERING ANTINEOPLASTIC AGENTS

Before administering an antineoplastic agent, the nurse should reinforce the information about the benefits and risks of treatment that the patient received from the physician. A patient who consents to investigational chemotherapy should receive additional information. Throughout the patient's therapy, the nurse should continue to teach and reinforce this information to promote patient safety and compliance.

To administer an antineoplastic agent safely, the nurse should select an appropriate site and vein, consider drug compatibilities, determine the **vesicant** potential of the agent, consider its sequencing and delivery, and prevent or treat **extravasation** as prescribed.

For a patient who must receive several treatments with these potentially damaging agents, site and vein selection is especially important. To select an appropriate I.V. site, the nurse should begin with a distal spot, such as the hand, and proceed to proximal areas, such as up the forearm.

Before administering any antineoplastic agent, the nurse should consider drug compatibilities. As a rule, antineoplastic agents should not be mixed with any other medications. Although little research has been done to determine exact incompatibilities, the nature and toxicity of these agents usually prohibit mixing.

To choose the proper drug sequencing and delivery technique, the nurse needs to know the vesicant potential of the agent. For intermittent drug delivery, the nurse should administer a vesicant agent by direct push or delivery into the side port of an infusing I.V. line. For continuous infusion, a vesicant should be administered only via a central line or vascular access device. Nonvesicant agents (including **irritants**) may be given by direct I.V. push, through the side port of an infusing I.V. line, or as a continuous infusion. Some facilities require administration of the vesicant first because vein integrity decreases over time. Various venous access devices are available for use when vesicants are administered. These venous access devices reduce patient discomfort by removing the necessity for multiple I.V. insertions.

During the administration of any I.V. antineoplastic agent, the patient's safety depends on the nurse's assessment of the infusion site during drug delivery. To ensure patency of the vein, the nurse must elicit a blood return before, during, and after drug administration.

To prevent extravasation, the nurse should use a splint to stabilize the needle and should check frequently for blood return. Although no definitive measures exist to treat extravasation of an antineoplastic agent, conservative measures include discontinuing the infusion, aspirating any residual drug from the tubing and needle, instilling an I.V. antidote if one is available, and removing the needle. After administering an antidote as prescribed, the nurse may apply heat or cold and may elevate the affected limb.

Common adverse reactions and associated nursing implications

Antineoplastic agents share many of the same adverse reactions and require similar nursing interventions. To provide quality patient care, the nurse must be aware of the following adverse reactions and implications.

ADVERSE REACTIONS	NURSING IMPLICATIONS
Bone marrow suppression	
Bone marrow suppression. This is the most common and potentially serious adverse reaction to the antineoplastic agents.	• Watch for the blood count nadir because that is when the patient is at greatest risk for the complications of leukopenia, thrombocytopenia, and anemia (see below). • Plan a patient-teaching program about bone marrow suppression, including information about blood counts, potential sites of infection, and personal hygiene.
Leukopenia. This reaction increases the patient's risk of infection, especially if the granulocyte count is under 1,000/mm^3.	• Provide information about good hygiene and assess the patient frequently for signs and symptoms of infection. Keep in mind that a patient with leukopenia is subject to infections. • Teach the patient to recognize and report the signs and symptoms of infection, such as fever, cough, sore throat, or a burning sensation on urination. • Teach the patient how to take a temperature. • Caution the patient to avoid crowds and people with colds or the flu during the nadir. • Remember that the inflammatory response may be decreased and the complications of leukopenia more difficult to detect if the patient is receiving a corticosteroid. • Administer growth factors or colony-stimulating factors as ordered.
Thrombocytopenia. This reaction occurs with leukopenia. When the platelet count is under 50,000/mm^3, the patient is at risk for bleeding. When it is under 20,000/mm^3, the patient is at severe risk and may require a platelet transfusion.	• Assess the patient for bleeding gums, increased bruising or petechiae, hypermenorrhea, tarry stools, hematuria, and coffee-ground emesis. • Advise the patient to avoid cuts and bruises and to use a soft toothbrush and an electric razor. • Instruct the patient to report sudden headaches, which could indicate potentially fatal intracranial bleeding. • Instruct the patient to use a stool softener, as prescribed, to prevent colonic irritation and bleeding. • Instruct the patient to avoid using a rectal thermometer and receiving I.M. injections, to prevent bleeding.
Anemia. This reaction develops slowly over several courses of treatment.	• Assess the patient for dizziness, fatigue, pallor, and shortness of breath on minimal exertion. • Monitor the patient's hematocrit, hemoglobin level, and red blood cell counts. Remember that a patient dehydrated from nausea, vomiting, or anorexia may exhibit a false-normal hematocrit. Once this patient is rehydrated, the hematocrit will decrease. • Be prepared to administer a blood transfusion to a symptomatic patient, as prescribed. • Instruct the patient to rest more frequently and to increase the dietary intake of iron-rich foods. Advise the patient to take a multivitamin with iron, as prescribed. • Administer growth factors or colony-stimulating factors as ordered.
Nausea and vomiting	
Nausea and vomiting. These reactions can result from gastric mucosal irritation, chemical irritation of the central nervous system, or psychogenic factors that may be activated by sensations, suggestions, or anxiety.	• Control the chemical irritation by administering combinations of antiemetics, as prescribed. • Monitor the patient for signs and symptoms of aspiration because most antiemetics sedate. • Control psychogenic factors by helping the patient perform relaxation techniques before chemotherapy to minimize feelings of isolation and anxiety. • Encourage the patient to express feelings of anxiety. • Encourage the patient to listen to music or to engage in relaxation exercises, meditation, or hypnosis to promote feelings of control and well-being. • Adjust the drug administration time to meet the patient's needs. Some patients prefer treatments in the evening when they find sedation comfortable. Patients who are employed may prefer their treatments on their days off.

Common adverse reactions and associated nursing implications *(continued)*

ADVERSE REACTIONS	NURSING IMPLICATIONS
Stomatitis	
Stomatitis. Although epithelial tissue damage can affect any mucous membrane, the most common site is the oral mucosa. Stomatitis is temporary and can range from mild and barely noticeable to severe and debilitating. (Debilitation may result from poor nutrition during acute stomatitis.)	• Initiate preventive mouth care before chemotherapy to provide comfort and decrease the severity of the stomatitis. • Provide therapeutic mouth care, including topical antibiotics, if prescribed.
Alopecia	
Alopecia. To the patient, alopecia may be the most distressing adverse reaction. Determine whether the agent being administered does in fact cause alopecia; several agents do not have this adverse effect.	• Prepare the patient for alopecia. Inform the patient that hair loss usually is gradual and is reversible after treatment ends. • Inform the patient that alopecia may be partial or complete and that it affects men and women. • Inform the patient that alopecia may affect the scalp, eyebrows, eyelashes, and body hair.

ADVERSE REACTIONS

The adverse reactions to antineoplastic agents result from their systemic effects. Some reactions can be life-threatening, requiring modification of the drug dosage or treatment regimen. Others are less severe but may be stressful to the patient.

Nausea and vomiting are common adverse reactions. Chemotherapy can cause nausea and vomiting by three basic mechanisms. Orally administered drugs can irritate the gastric mucosa directly, causing nausea and vomiting that is less severe than that caused by the other two mechanisms.

Other antineoplastic agents can stimulate the chemoreceptor trigger zone. The incidence of nausea and vomiting from this mechanism depends on the inherent emetic potential of the drug.

Finally, chemotherapy can cause psychogenic nausea and vomiting, which originates in the cerebral cortex. Known as anticipatory emesis, this reaction can be disabling. A patient who remembers the unpleasantness of previous chemotherapy may feel nauseated or may vomit just by thinking about future treatments. This reaction may become so severe that sights, sounds, and smells associated with treatment may induce emesis, no matter how far removed the patient is from the actual treatment setting.

Chemotherapy-induced nausea and vomiting is of great concern because it can cause fluid and electrolyte imbalances, noncompliance with the treatment regimen, Mallory-Weiss syndrome (tears at the esophageal-gastric junction, leading to massive bleeding), wound dehiscence, and pathologic fractures. It also can cause distress by limiting the patient's ability and motivation to take an active role in life.

To combat the nausea and vomiting caused by chemotherapy, nurses usually administer antiemetic drugs, such as serotonin antagonists, prochlorperazine, diphenhydramine, droperidol, and dronabinol. Usually, an antiemetic drug is given with several other antiemetics that act by different mechanisms. A combination regimen is more effective than a single drug, especially for a strong emetic agent such as cisplatin. The nurse can also help control psychogenic factors related to nausea and vomiting by teaching the patient relaxation techniques that can help minimize feelings of isolation and anxiety, encouraging the patient to express anxieties, and helping the patient use relaxation techniques during chemotherapy.

53 Alkylating agents

OBJECTIVES

After reading and studying this chapter, the student should be able to:
1. explain the alkylation process and its role in the mechanisms of action of the alkylating agents: nitrogen mustards, alkyl sulfonates, nitrosoureas, triazines, ethylenimines, and alkylating-like agents.
2. identify the clinical indications for each class of alkylating agents.
3. list the common adverse reactions to the alkylating agents.
4. describe how to apply the nursing process when caring for a patient who is receiving an alkylating agent.

INTRODUCTION

Alkylating agents fall into one of six classes: nitrogen mustards, alkyl sulfonates, nitrosoureas, triazines, ethylenimines, and alkylating-like agents. Alkylating agents, given alone or with other drugs, effectively act against various malignant **neoplasms.** All of these drugs produce their antineoplastic effects through **alkylation** — linkage with deoxyribonucleic acid (DNA) that causes irreversible inhibition of the DNA molecule by enzyme modification. Bifunctional alkylation occurs when one drug molecule produces two alkylation reactions, which causes **cytotoxic** effects. Monofunctional alkylation occurs when one drug molecule is responsible for a single alkylation reaction, which eventually may lead to permanent cell damage. (See *Selected major alkylating agents.*)

Drugs covered in this chapter include:

- busulfan
- carboplatin
- carmustine
- chlorambucil
- cisplatin
- cyclophosphamide
- dacarbazine
- estramustine
- ifosfamide
- lomustine
- mechlorethamine hydrochloride
- melphalan
- semustine
- streptozocin
- thiotepa
- uracil mustard.

Nitrogen mustards

The nitrogen mustards represent the largest group of alkylating agents. Mechlorethamine hydrochloride, which was the first nitrogen mustard introduced, is also the most rapid-acting. The other nitrogen mustards include chlorambucil, cyclophosphamide, estramustine, ifosfamide, melphalan, and uracil mustard.

PHARMACOKINETICS

The absorption and distribution of nitrogen mustards, as with most alkylating agents, vary widely. The nitrogen mustards are metabolized in the liver and excreted by the kidneys.

Mechlorethamine undergoes metabolism so rapidly that no active drug remains after a few minutes. Most nitrogen mustards possess more intermediate half-lives than mechlorethamine. At 1 hour after an oral dose, the highest tissue concentration of chlorambucil occurs in the liver. Chlorambucil has a half-life of 2 hours.

Cyclophosphamide reaches a peak plasma concentration level about 1 hour after an oral dose, and has a plasma half-life of about 7 hours. However, the alkylating activity of the unbound metabolites lasts for at least 24 hours.

The plasma half-life of ifosfamide is dose-dependent. High doses have a 15-hour half-life; low doses have a 7-hour half-life.

Melphalan reaches a peak plasma concentration about 2 hours after an oral dose, and has a plasma half-life of 90 minutes.

The peak concentrations and half-lives of estramustine and uracil mustard have not been defined clearly.

Route	Onset	Peak	Duration
P.O.	Rapid	1-3 hr	3-12 hr
I.V.	Rapid	≤ 3 hr	Variable

PHARMACODYNAMICS

The nitrogen mustards form covalent bonds with DNA molecules in a chemical reaction known as alkylation. Alkylated DNA cannot replicate properly, thereby resulting

Selected major alkylating agents

This table summarizes the major alkylating agents currently in clinical use.

DRUG	MAJOR INDICATIONS AND USUAL DOSAGES	CONTRAINDICATIONS AND PRECAUTIONS
Nitrogen mustards		
mechlorethamine (Mustargen)	*Hodgkin's disease, malignant lymphoma, mycosis fungoides* ADULT: 0.4 mg/kg I.V. once every 3 to 6 weeks or 6 mg/m^2 on day 1 and 8 of a monthly regimen ADULT: 0.1 mg/ml applied topically *Malignant pleural effusions* ADULT: 0.2 to 0.4 mg/kg into the affected cavity	• Mechlorethamine is contraindicated in a pregnant or breast-feeding patient, one who has experienced an anaphylactic reaction to the drug, or one with a known infectious disease. • This drug requires cautious use in a patient with chronic lymphatic leukemia, leukopenia, thrombocytopenia, or anemia from tumor invasion of the bone marrow or in one receiving other cytotoxic agents in alternating courses or radiation therapy. • Safety and efficacy in children have not been established.
Alkyl sulfonates		
busulfan (Myleran)	*Chronic myelogenous leukemia* ADULT: 4 to 8 mg P.O. daily until the white blood cell (WBC) count falls between 10,000/mm^3 and 25,000/mm^3; resumed when the WBC count rises to 50,000/mm^3 and continued to maintain it between 10,000/mm^3 and 20,000/mm^3; maintenance, 1 to 4 mg P.O. daily PEDIATRIC: 1.8 mg/m^2 or 0.06 mg/kg to 0.12 mg/kg P.O. daily; dosage is titrated to maintain a leukocyte count of about 20,000/mm^3 *Bone marrow transplantation* ADULT: 1 mg/kg of ideal body weight q.i.d. for 4 days	• Busulfan is contraindicated in a pregnant or breast-feeding patient or one who has demonstrated resistance to the drug. • This drug requires cautious use in a patient whose bone marrow reserve may have been compromised by prior radiation therapy or chemotherapy or a patient with bone marrow suppression resulting from prior cytotoxic therapy.
Nitrosoureas		
carmustine [BCNU] (BiCNU)	*Multiple myeloma, refractory Hodgkin's disease, malignant lymphoma, brain tumors, melanoma, refractory lung cancer, colon cancer* ADULT: 75 to 100 mg/m^2 I.V. for 2 days, or up to 200 mg/m^2 in a single I.V. infusion, repeated every 6 to 8 weeks	• Carmustine is contraindicated in a pregnant or breast-feeding patient or one with known hypersensitivity. • This drug requires cautious use in a patient with a depressed platelet, leukocyte, or erythrocyte count. • Safety and efficacy in children have not been established.
Triazines		
dacarbazine (DTIC-Dome)	*Malignant melanoma, soft-tissue sarcoma* ADULT: 150 to 250 mg/m^2 I.V. daily for 5 days, repeated in 3 to 4 weeks or 375 mg/m^2 I.V. day 1 and 15 of a 28-day cycle. *Hodgkin's disease* ADULT: 2 to 4.5 mg/kg/day I.V. for 10 days or 250 mg/m^2 for 5 days.	• Dacarbazine is contraindicated in a breast-feeding patient or one with known hypersensitivity. • This drug requires cautious use in a pregnant patient.
Ethylenimines		
Thiotepa (Thiotepa)	*Bladder cancer, breast cancer* ADULT: 60 mg instilled in the bladder weekly for 4 weeks	• Thiotepa is contraindicated in a patient with hepatic, renal, or bone marrow damage or known hypersensitivity.

(continued)

Selected major alkylating agents *(continued)*

DRUG	MAJOR INDICATIONS AND USUAL DOSAGES	CONTRAINDICATIONS AND PRECAUTIONS
Ethylenimines *(continued)*		
thiotepa (Thiotepa) *(continued)*	*Palliative treatment for ovarian or breast carcinoma or lymphoma* ADULT: 0.3 to 0.4 mg/kg by rapid I.V. infusion at 1- to 4-week intervals or 0.6 to 0.8 mg/kg injected into the tumor intrapleurally or intraperitoneally; maintenance, 0.07 to 0.8 mg/kg at 1- to 4-week intervals	• This drug requires cautious use in a patient who has received treatment with other alkylating agents or radiation.
Alkylating-like agents		
cisplatin [cisplatinum] (Platinol)	*Metastatic testicular cancer; lung, head, neck, bladder, or metastatic ovarian cancer* ADULT: 20 to 40 mg/m²/day I.V. for 3 to 5 days every 3 to 4 weeks or from 20 to 120 mg/m² I.V. given as a single dose every 3 to 4 weeks	• Cisplatin is contraindicated in a patient with renal impairment, hearing impairment, myelosuppression, or known hypersensitivity to the drug or other platinum-containing compounds. • This drug requires cautious use in a pregnant patient. • Safety and efficacy in children have not been established.

in cell death. Unfortunately, **tumor** cells may develop resistance to the cytotoxic effects of nitrogen mustards. (See *How alkylating agents work.*)

PHARMACOTHERAPEUTICS

The nitrogen mustards are indicated for various malignant neoplasms. Because they produce **leukopenia,** the nitrogen mustards are effective in treating malignant neoplasms, such as **Hodgkin's disease** and **leukemia,** that have an associated elevated white blood cell (WBC) count. Also, the nitrogen mustards prove effective against many solid tumors. The sensitive malignant neoplasms include malignant **lymphoma,** multiple **myeloma, melanoma, sarcoma,** and **cancers** of the breast, ovaries, uterus, lung, brain, testes, bladder, prostate, and stomach. These drugs can be given alone or with other classes of antineoplastic agents. The activity and effectiveness of each drug depend on many factors, including the type of cancer, the extent of disease, and the patient's condition.

Drug interactions

Most drug interactions with antineoplastic agents, including the nitrogen mustards, are based theoretically on animal studies or basic chemical theory. (For more information, see the introduction to this unit.)

Human study data has revealed only two drug interactions. Cyclophosphamide interacts with succinylcholine, prolonging the neuromuscular blockade of succinylcholine. Cyclophosphamide also interacts with chloramphenicol, reducing the conversion of cyclophosphamide to active metabolites.

ADVERSE DRUG REACTIONS

Bone marrow suppression, evidenced by severe leukopenia and **thrombocytopenia,** is an anticipated adverse reaction associated with the nitrogen mustards. Nausea and vomiting from central nervous system (CNS) irritation are other common adverse reactions. Nausea and vomiting may occur 30 minutes after administration, as with mechlorethamine, or may not begin for hours, as with cyclophosphamide.

Damage to rapidly proliferating cells produces **stomatitis** and **alopecia.** The swollen, inflamed mucous membranes that characterize stomatitis can lead to a nutritional problem because of pain associated with stomatitis. Alopecia, which is caused by hair follicle damage, results in thinning hair 2 to 3 weeks after the first administration of a nitrogen mustard. However, hair loss usually is not significant for two to three courses of treatment. Once treatment ends, hair growth resumes. Many patients experience fatigue during nitrogen mustard therapy.

Because the nitrogen mustards are powerful local **vesicants** (blistering agents), direct contact with the drugs or their vapors can cause severe reactions, especially of the skin, eyes, and respiratory tract. Mechlorethamine **extravasation** may cause painful inflammation and induration.

Patients may experience alterations in fertility. After several courses of nitrogen mustard treatment, women may experience amenorrhea or irregular menses. Men may have decreased spermatogenesis. Many patients, however, experience no apparent alteration in fertility, and women treated with nitrogen mustards have conceived and given birth to normal children.

Hemorrhagic cystitis may develop within 48 hours after an intravenous (I.V.) dose of cyclophosphamide, or it may result after several months of oral low-dose therapy. Cyclophosphamide metabolites in the urine irritate the bladder lining, producing this adverse reaction. Adequate hydration usually prevents hemorrhagic cystitis, and the nurse should encourage patients receiving cyclophosphamide to consume at least eight 8-oz (240-ml) glasses of fluid daily.

Myelosuppression and hemorrhagic cystitis are dose-limiting toxicities for ifosfamide. Administration of mesna (Mesnex), a cystitis prophylactic, may alleviate the cystitis reaction. Ifosfamide may also cause adverse CNS reactions, such as somnolence, confusion, and hallucinations.

Chlorambucil may produce **hepatotoxicity,** but this reaction rarely occurs. Rarely, chlorambucil and cyclophosphamide may cause pulmonary reactions, such as interstitial pneumonitis or pulmonary fibrosis.

Like other alkylating agents, the nitrogen mustards have been implicated in producing hematologic and other malignancies, although this is rare. Anaphylaxis is another rare adverse reaction.

How alkylating agents work

Alkylating agents can attack DNA in two ways, as shown in the illustrations below.

Bifunctional alkylation

Some agents become inserted between two base pairs in the deoxyribonucleic acid (DNA) chain, forming an irreversible bond between them. This is called bifunctional alkylation.

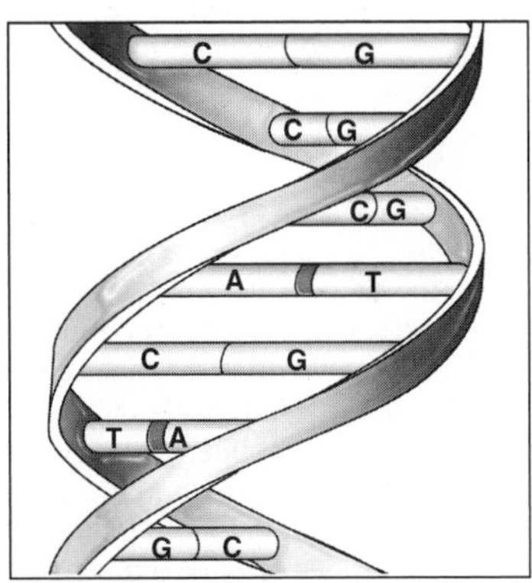

Monofunctional alkylation

Other agents react with just one part of a pair, separating it from its partner and eventually causing it and its attached sugar to break away from the DNA molecule. This is called monofunctional alkylation.

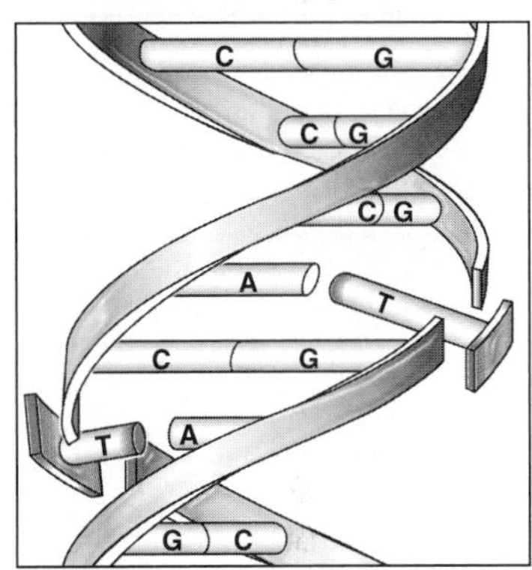

NURSING PROCESS APPLICATION

The following information assists the nurse in caring for a patient receiving a nitrogen mustard. It includes an overview of assessment activities as well as examples of appropriate nursing diagnoses and related interventions (see "Planning and implementation"). It also highlights the importance of evaluation.

Assessment

Before drug therapy begins, review the patient's history for conditions that contraindicate or require cautious use of the prescribed nitrogen mustard. Also review the patient's medication history to identify use of drugs that may interact with it. During therapy, assess the patient for adverse drug reactions and signs of drug interactions. Also, periodically assess the effectiveness of nitrogen mustard therapy. Finally, evaluate the patient's and family's knowledge about the prescribed drug.

Nursing diagnoses

- Risk for injury related to a preexisting condition that contraindicates or requires cautious use of a nitrogen mustard
- Risk for injury related to adverse drug reactions or drug interactions
- Risk for infection related to nitrogen mustard–induced leukopenia
- Knowledge deficit related to the prescribed nitrogen mustard

Planning and implementation

- Do not administer a nitrogen mustard to a patient with a condition that contraindicates its use.
- Administer a nitrogen mustard cautiously to a patient at risk because of a preexisting condition.
- Monitor the patient for adverse reactions and drug interactions during nitrogen mustard therapy.
- Administer an antiemetic concomitantly as prescribed to control or lessen nausea and vomiting. If fluid intake is inadequate despite antiemetic use, expect to replace fluids intravenously, as prescribed.
- If stomatitis occurs, monitor the patient's nutritional status. To relieve stomatitis, provide frequent oral care, apply a topical medication for pain relief as prescribed, and provide a pureed or liquid diet.
- Assist the patient with activities of daily living if fatigue occurs. Limit the patient's activities and stagger those that are necessary. Provide rest periods — especially after treatment — when the patient is most likely to feel fatigued.

*** *Monitor all infusion sites for signs of extravasation, such as pain and swelling at the insertion site. Change infusion sites according to health care facility protocol and as needed.***

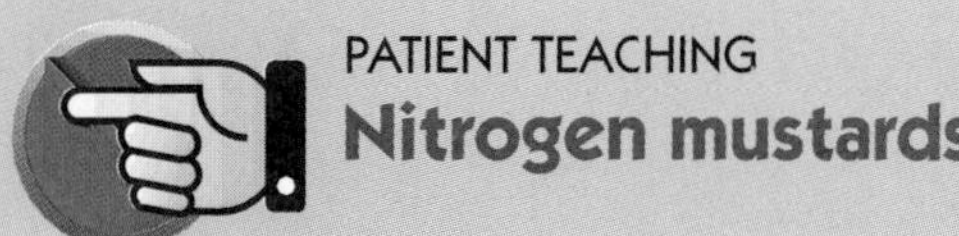

PATIENT TEACHING
Nitrogen mustards

- ➤ Teach the patient and family the name, dose, frequency, action, and adverse effects of the prescribed nitrogen mustard.
- ➤ Inform the patient that the nitrogen mustard can produce alopecia, which cannot be prevented. Explain that alopecia affects men and women and may include eyebrows, eyelashes, scalp hair, and other body hair. Reassure the patient that the hair loss is reversible when the treatment ends.
- ➤ Instruct the patient to increase oral fluid intake the day before cyclophosphamide or ifosfamide therapy to help prevent hemorrhagic cystitis. Advise the patient that fluid intake should not include beverages that contain caffeine, such as coffee or tea, because they have diuretic effects.
- ➤ Encourage the patient taking oral cyclophosphamide to take the medication earlier in the day, to maintain good fluid intake, and to void before going to bed.
- ➤ Discuss ways to relieve adverse reactions. For example, suggest dietary changes to relieve nausea, vomiting, or stomatitis; frequent oral care to help manage stomatitis; and activity restriction to help the patient manage fatigue.
- ➤ Advise the patient not to perform activities that require mental alertness until the adverse central nervous system effects of ifosfamide are known.
- ➤ Teach the patient to use infection control measures and bleeding precautions during nitrogen mustard therapy.
- ➤ Inform the patient that alterations in fertility may occur during nitrogen mustard therapy. Advise the female patient that amenorrhea or irregular menses may also occur.
- ➤ Stress the importance of returning for follow-up visits and blood tests.
- ➤ Instruct the patient to notify the physician if adverse reactions occur.
- ➤ Advise the patient to notify the physician if any other symptoms appear because the nitrogen mustard may cause a secondary hematologic or other malignancy, such as leukemia.
- ➤ Give the patient written materials about the prescribed nitrogen mustard for home reference.

*** *Monitor the patient for signs of hemorrhagic cystitis, such as hematuria and dysuria, during cyclophosphamide or ifosfamide therapy.***

• Increase the fluid intake of the patient receiving I.V. cyclophosphamide to at least 2 qt (2 L) daily. After treatment, instruct the patient to maintain increased fluids for 2 to 3 days.

• Administer cyclophosphamide or ifosfamide earlier in the day rather than at bedtime to prevent prolonged contact between the drug's metabolites and the bladder.

• Administer mesna, as prescribed, with ifosfamide and 4 and 8 hours after treatment to help prevent hemorrhagic cystitis.

*** *Wear gloves and follow the health care facility's protocol when administering the nitrogen mustard, and avoid inhaling the vapors. Direct contact with the drug or its vapors can cause severe reactions, especially of the skin, eyes, and respiratory tract.***

• Administer nitrogen mustard exactly as directed in the manufacturer's guidelines. (For more information about administration, see the introduction to this unit.)

• Administer mechlorethamine immediately after reconstitution because it is unstable in solution. Most other nitrogen mustards, which remain stable in solution, can be prepared well before administration.

• Reduce I.V. administration pain by altering the infusion rate, further diluting the drug if indicated, or warming the injection site to distend the vein and increase blood flow.

• Use other appropriate interventions for a patient with bone marrow suppression, nausea, vomiting, stomatitis, or alopecia. (For details, see the introduction to this unit.)

• Notify the physician if adverse reactions or drug interactions occur.

• Monitor the patient's blood counts frequently, especially the complete blood count (CBC).

*** *Take infection control measures and monitor the patient for signs of infection if leukopenia occurs.***

• Notify the physician if an infection is suspected. (See Patient Teaching: *Nitrogen mustards.*)

• Administer an antibiotic as prescribed if an infection occurs.

Evaluation

For each nursing diagnosis, prepare an evaluation statement that describes the patient's or family's response to nursing interventions.

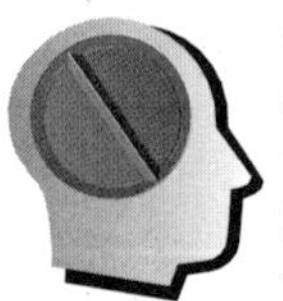

CRITICAL THINKING: To enhance your critical thinking about alkylating agents, consider the following situation and its analysis.

Situation: Mark Johnson, age 34, is diagnosed with testicular cancer and is receiving combination chemotherapy with etoposide (VP-16), ifosfamide, and cisplatin every 3 weeks. The routine laboratory tests performed prior to his scheduled third course of treatment reveal an abnormally low WBC count of 2,600 cells/mm^3. The physician orders the scheduled doses of etoposide and cisplatin, but decreases the dose of ifosfamide. Why?

Analysis: Myelosuppression is a major dose-limiting toxicity of ifosfamide. The leukopenia nadir usually occurs 7 to 14 days after treatment with recovery normally within 21 days. By decreasing the dose of Mr. Johnson's ifosfamide, his WBC count will continue to recover. This approach is preferred to withholding the next course of treatment until recovery has occurred, since it does not prolong the amount of time in which tumor cell growth can occur. Furthermore, since neither of the other two drugs in the combination have leukopenia as a major dose-limiting toxicity, administration of these two drugs is not contraindicated, and dose reduction is not necessary.

Alkyl sulfonates

The alkyl sulfonate busulfan is commonly used to treat chronic **myelogenous** leukemia and less commonly to treat **polycythemia vera** and other **myeloproliferative** disorders.

PHARMACOKINETICS

Busulfan is absorbed rapidly and well from the gastrointestinal tract. Little is known about its distribution into the brain, cerebrospinal fluid, or breast milk. Busulfan is metabolized extensively in the liver before urinary excretion. Its half-life is 2 to 3 hours. Precise data about its onset of action, peak concentration level, and duration of action are unavailable because analytical methods are insufficient.

Route	Onset	Peak	Duration
P.O., I.V.	Unknown	Unknown	Unknown

PHARMACODYNAMICS

As an alkyl sulfonate, busulfan forms covalent bonds with the DNA molecules in a chemical reaction known as alkylation.

PHARMACOTHERAPEUTICS

Busulfan primarily affects **granulocytes** and, to a lesser degree, platelets. Because of its action on granulocytes, it is the drug of choice for treating chronic myelogenous leukemia. This action also makes busulfan effective for polycythemia vera. However, other agents are usually used to treat polycythemia vera because busulfan can cause severe myelosuppression.

Drug interactions

Busulfan does not interact significantly with other drugs.

ADVERSE DRUG REACTIONS

The major adverse reaction to busulfan is bone marrow suppression, which usually is dose-related and reversible. Bone marrow suppression produces severe leukopenia, **anemia,** and thrombocytopenia. Granulocytopenia occurs rarely and can progress to **pancytopenia,** which may be fatal.

Nausea, vomiting, and diarrhea are uncommon. Hyperuricemia occurs. With long-term therapy, an addisonian-like wasting syndrome with hyperpigmentation and weight loss sometimes occurs. Busulfan may also produce irreversible interstitial pulmonary fibrosis (busulfan lung) after long-term use (1 to 3 years).

NURSING PROCESS APPLICATION

The following information assists the nurse in caring for a patient receiving busulfan. It includes an overview of assessment activities as well as examples of appropriate nursing diagnoses and related interventions (see "Planning and implementation"). It also highlights the importance of evaluation.

Assessment

Before drug therapy begins, review the patient's history for conditions that contraindicate or require cautious use of busulfan. During therapy, assess the patient for adverse drug reactions. Also, periodically assess the effectiveness of therapy with busulfan. Finally, evaluate the patient's and family's knowledge about the prescribed drug.

Nursing diagnoses

- Risk for injury related to a preexisting condition that contraindicates or requires cautious use of busulfan
- Risk for injury related to adverse drug reactions
- Risk for infection related to busulfan-induced leukopenia
- Impaired gas exchange related to busulfan-induced interstitial pulmonary fibrosis
- Knowledge deficit related to busulfan

Planning and implementation

- Do not administer busulfan to a patient with a condition that contraindicates its use.
- Administer busulfan cautiously to a patient at risk because of a preexisting condition.
- Monitor the patient for adverse reactions during busulfan therapy.
- Monitor the patient's CBC to detect such abnormalities as leukopenia, thrombocytopenia, or anemia. If abnormalities occur, notify the physician before administering the next dose of busulfan.

* ***Take infection control measures and bleeding precautions. If leukopenia occurs, monitor the patient for signs of infection. If thrombocytopenia occurs, monitor the patient for signs of bleeding. Also observe for early signs and symptoms of intracranial hemorrhage. Avoid intramuscular (I.M.) injections and venipunctures when the patient's platelet count is low. When a venipuncture must be done, apply firm pressure to the site for at least 5 minutes afterward.***
* ***Use anticoagulants cautiously and observe for signs of bleeding during concomitant administration.***

- Monitor the patient's uric acid level to detect hyperuricemia. If hyperuricemia occurs, expect to administer allopurinol as prescribed and ensure that the patient consumes at least 2 qt (2 L) of fluid daily (unless contraindicated).
- Use other appropriate interventions for a patient with bone marrow suppression, nausea, or vomiting. (For details, see the introduction to this unit.)
- Notify the physician if adverse reactions occur. (See Patient Teaching: *Alkyl sulfonates,* page 650.)

* ***Monitor pulmonary function studies for a patient receiving long-term busulfan therapy. Also monitor respiratory assessment findings regularly, particularly noting changes in the quality of respirations, such as progressive dyspnea,***

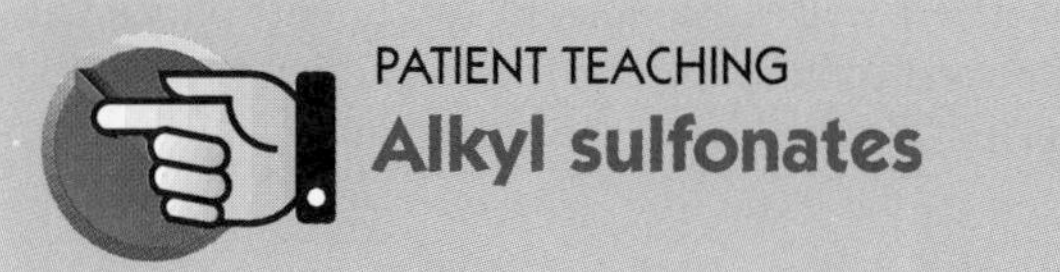

PATIENT TEACHING
Alkyl sulfonates

- Teach the patient and family the name, dose, frequency, action, and adverse effects of busulfan.
- Teach the patient to use infection control measures and bleeding precautions during busulfan therapy.
- Instruct the patient to notify the physician if fever, sore throat, unusual bleeding, bruising, or symptoms of anemia occur.
- Stress the importance of returning for follow-up visits and regular complete blood count and other blood tests.
- Advise the patient with anemia to stagger activities and rest frequently.
- Instruct the patient with hyperuricemia to drink at least eight 8-oz (240-ml) glasses of fluid a day (unless contraindicated).
- Instruct the patient to notify the physician if hyperpigmentation, weight loss, persistent cough, progressive dyspnea, or other adverse reactions occur.

or a persistent cough. Alert the physician if respiratory abnormalities occur.

Evaluation

For each nursing diagnosis, prepare an evaluation statement that describes the patient's or family's response to nursing interventions.

Nitrosoureas

The nitrosoureas include carmustine, lomustine, semustine, and streptozocin.

PHARMACOKINETICS

When administered topically to treat mycosis fungoides, carmustine is 5% to 28% systemically absorbed. After oral administration, lomustine and semustine are absorbed adequately, although incompletely. Streptozocin, which is administered intravenously, does not undergo absorption. All four nitrosoureas are lipophilic, distributing to fatty tissues and cerebrospinal fluid. They are metabolized extensively before urine excretion.

Carmustine peaks instantaneously with I.V. administration and disappears from the plasma, with a half-life of 15 to 30 minutes. The peak plasma concentration of lomustine metabolites is reached within 1 to 6 hours after oral administration. The half-life of the metabolites ranges from 24 to 48 hours. The peak plasma concentration of semustine occurs in 1 to 6 hours. Streptozocin has a plasma half-life of 35 minutes, with some streptozocin metabolites displaying a prolonged terminal half-life of more than 40 hours.

Route	Onset	Peak	Duration
P.O.	Unknown	1-6 hr	24-48 hr
I.V.	Rapid	Immediate	Unknown

PHARMACODYNAMICS

Nitrosoureas display bifunctional alkylation of DNA.

PHARMACOTHERAPEUTICS

The nitrosoureas display a high degree of lipid solubility, which allows them or their metabolites to cross the blood-brain barrier easily. Because of this ability, nitrosoureas are used to treat brain tumors and meningeal leukemias.

Drug interactions

When combined with cimetidine, carmustine seems to display an increased myelosuppressant effect, possibly because of inhibition of carmustine metabolism. Carmustine may reduce serum digoxin and phenytoin levels by altering their absorption. No significant interactions occur with lomustine, semustine, or streptozocin.

ADVERSE DRUG REACTIONS

Carmustine and lomustine produce bone marrow suppression that begins 4 to 6 weeks after treatment and lasts 1 to 2 weeks. The bone marrow suppression is cumulative — that is, it can become more severe and prolonged with repeated doses. Semustine also produces bone marrow depression, which begins 4 to 8 weeks after treatment and lasts up to 10 weeks. Severe nausea lasts 2 to 6 hours after carmustine, lomustine, or semustine administration. Lomustine and semustine may also cause anorexia for a few days after administration. The patient may also experience intense pain at the infusion site during carmustine administration. In about two-thirds of patients receiving streptozocin, renal dysfunction occurs and is dose-limiting. Severe nausea and vomiting also occur with this drug and may persist for more than 24 hours.

Nephrotoxicity and renal failure have occurred with the nitrosoureas. High-dose carmustine may produce reversible hepatotoxicity. Carmustine may also cause pulmonary toxicity characterized by pulmonary infiltrates or fibrosis. These pulmonary reactions are dose-related; their incidence is much higher in patients who receive cumulative doses of more than 1,400 mg/m^2. Hematologic toxicity and mild glucose intolerance are rare adverse reactions to streptozocin.

Streptozocin is irritating to tissues. If extravasated, it can cause necrosis. Carmustine may cause vein irritation.

NURSING PROCESS APPLICATION

The following information assists the nurse in caring for a patient receiving a nitrosourea. It includes an overview of assessment activities as well as examples of appropriate nursing diagnoses and related interventions (see "Planning and implementation"). It also highlights the importance of evaluation.

Assessment

Before drug therapy begins, review the patient's history for conditions that contraindicate or require cautious use of the prescribed nitrosourea. Also review the patient's medication history to identify use of drugs that may interact with it. During therapy, assess the patient for adverse drug reactions and signs of drug interactions. Also, periodically assess the effectiveness of nitrosourea therapy. Finally, evaluate the patient's and family's knowledge about the prescribed drug.

Nursing diagnoses

- Risk for injury related to a preexisting condition that contraindicates or requires cautious use of a nitrosourea
- Risk for injury related to adverse drug reactions or drug interactions
- Impaired tissue integrity related to the adverse effects of carmustine or streptozocin at the infusion site
- Knowledge deficit related to the prescribed nitrosourea

Planning and implementation

- Do not administer a nitrosourea to a patient with a condition that contraindicates its use.
- Administer a nitrosourea cautiously to a patient at risk because of a preexisting condition.
- Monitor the patient for adverse reactions and drug interactions during nitrosourea therapy.

✱ *Monitor the patient's CBC for abnormalities, such as delayed bone marrow suppression. Observe the patient for signs and symptoms of infection, bleeding, or anemia. Take infection control measures, bleeding precautions, or energy conservation measures as needed.*

- Monitor urinalysis, blood urea nitrogen level, and creatinine level for abnormalities that indicate nephrotoxicity and renal failure. Keep in mind that mild proteinuria may be an early sign of nephrotoxicity.
- Monitor the patient's hepatic function studies when administering high doses of carmustine. If abnormalities occur, lower the dose or change to a different agent as prescribed.
- Monitor the patient's chest X-ray results and assess the patient's respiratory status regularly during carmustine therapy to detect signs and symptoms of pulmonary toxicity, such as the appearance of pulmonary infiltrates or fibrosis on the X-ray and shortness of breath. If pulmonary toxicity occurs, decrease the dosage or change to another agent as prescribed.
- Use other appropriate nursing interventions for a patient with bone marrow suppression, nausea, or vomiting..
- Notify the physician if adverse reactions or drug interactions occur.
- Inspect the patient's I.V. site for signs of tissue damage or vein irritation, such as redness, swelling, or pain on touch, before administering each dose of carmustine or streptozocin. Change I.V. sites according to health care facility protocol and as needed. (See Patient Teaching: *Nitrosoureas.*)
- Dilute the carmustine infusion and administer it over 1 to 2 hours if vein irritation occurs. Also use warmth to dilate the veins and increase blood flow to further dilute the drug.

✱ *Stop the streptozocin infusion immediately and notify the physician if extravasation occurs. This agent is a vesicant and can cause tissue necrosis.*

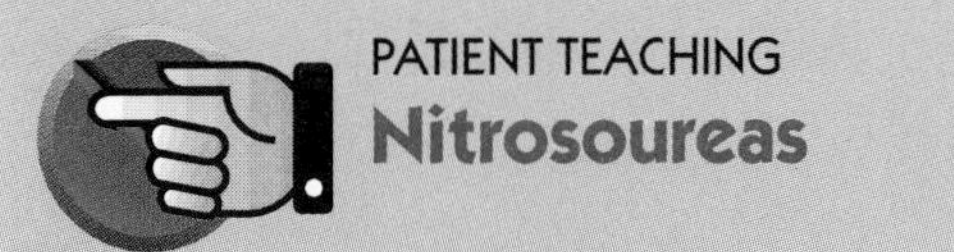

PATIENT TEACHING

Nitrosoureas

- ➤ Teach the patient and family the name, dose, frequency, action, and adverse effects of the prescribed nitrosourea.
- ➤ Alert the patient to watch for signs of infection, bleeding, and anemia. Instruct the patient to notify the physician if any occur.
- ➤ Stress the importance of returning for regular blood and urine studies.
- ➤ Teach the patient to use infection control measures, bleeding precautions, and energy conservation measures as needed.
- ➤ Inform the patient that carmustine produces pain during administration and that appropriate measures will be taken to minimize discomfort.
- ➤ Instruct the patient with adverse gastrointestinal (GI) reactions to sip fluids every hour. If nausea is severe or GI reactions persist, advise the patient to notify the physician.
- ➤ Instruct the patient to notify the physician if other adverse reactions occur.

Evaluation

For each nursing diagnosis, prepare an evaluation statement that describes the patient's or family's response to nursing interventions.

Triazines

Dacarbazine, a triazine, functions as an alkylating agent after it has been activated metabolically in the liver.

PHARMACOKINETICS

After I.V. injection, dacarbazine is distributed throughout the body and metabolized in the liver. Within 6 hours, 30% to 46% of a dose is excreted renally (50% is excreted unchanged, and 50% is excreted as one of the metabolites). Dacarbazine reaches a peak plasma concentration rapidly after I.V. administration. It has a half-life of approximately 5 hours. In patients with renal or hepatic dysfunction, the drug's half-life may increase to 7 hours.

Route	Onset	Peak	Duration
I.V.	Immediate	Immediate	5-7 hr

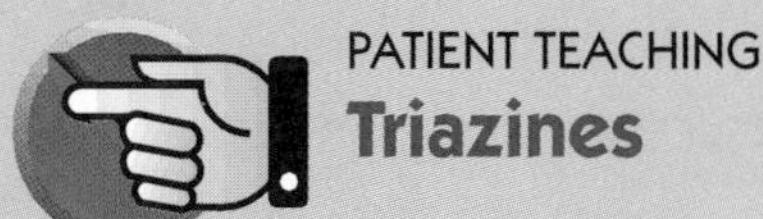

PATIENT TEACHING
Triazines

- ➤ Teach the patient and family the name, dose, frequency, action, and adverse effects of dacarbazine.
- ➤ Stress the importance of returning for complete blood counts regularly.
- ➤ Teach the patient to recognize and report signs and symptoms of infection and bleeding. Review infection control measures and bleeding precautions that the patient can use as needed.
- ➤ Advise the patient to avoid sunlight and sunlamps for the first 2 days after treatment.
- ➤ Instruct the patient to withhold food 4 to 6 hours before dacarbazine therapy to help decrease nausea.
- ➤ Reassure the patient that flulike syndrome may be treated with a mild antipyretic, such as acetaminophen.
- ➤ Inform the patient that dacarbazine may cause alopecia. Discuss ways to cope with alopecia, such as wearing a wig or an attractive scarf.
- ➤ Instruct the patient to notify the physician if adverse reactions occur.

PHARMACODYNAMICS

Dacarbazine first must be metabolized in the liver to become an alkylating agent. It seems to inhibit ribonucleic acid (RNA) and protein synthesis. Like other alkylating agents, dacarbazine is **cell cycle–nonspecific.**

PHARMACOTHERAPEUTICS

Dacarbazine is used primarily to treat patients with malignant melanoma but also is used with other drugs to treat patients with Hodgkin's disease.

Drug interactions

Dacarbazine is incompatible with hydrocortisone, sodium succinate and heparin sodium. Crystalization will develop.

ADVERSE DRUG REACTIONS

Leukopenia and thrombocytopenia occur as a result of dacarbazine use. Nausea and vomiting begin within 1 to 3 hours after administration in most patients and may last up to 12 hours. Dacarbazine infusion typically causes pain at the infusion site, which may require further dilution or a slower infusion rate. If extravasation occurs, dacarbazine may cause severe tissue damage. Phototoxicity also occurs, as does a flulike syndrome and alopecia.

NURSING PROCESS APPLICATION

The following information assists the nurse in caring for a patient receiving dacarbazine. It includes an overview of assessment activities as well as examples of appropriate nursing diagnoses and related interventions (see "Planning and implementation"). It also highlights the importance of evaluation.

Assessment

Before drug therapy begins, review the patient's history for conditions that contraindicate or require cautious use of dacarbazine. During therapy, assess the patient for adverse drug reactions. Also, periodically assess the effectiveness of dacarbazine therapy. Finally, evaluate the patient's and family's knowledge about the prescribed drug.

Nursing diagnoses

- Risk for injury related to a preexisting condition that contraindicates or requires cautious use of dacarbazine
- Risk for injury related to adverse drug reactions
- Risk for infection related to dacarbazine-induced leukopenia
- Impaired tissue integrity related to tissue damage caused by extravasation of dacarbazine
- Knowledge deficit related to the dacarbazine

Planning and implementation

- Do not administer dacarbazine to a patient with a condition that contraindicates its use.
- Administer dacarbazine cautiously to a patient at risk because of a preexisting condition.
- Monitor the patient for adverse reactions during dacarbazine therapy.

* ***Monitor the patient's CBC regularly for abnormalities that indicate leukopenia or thrombocytopenia.***

- Monitor the patient's temperature regularly, and observe for signs and symptoms of infection. Take infection control measures if leukopenia occurs.

* ***Monitor the patient for signs of bleeding. Take bleeding precautions if thrombocytopenia occurs. Avoid I.M. injections and venipunctures in a patient with a low platelet count. When venipunctures must be done, apply firm pressure to the site for at least 5 minutes afterward.***

- Withhold food for 4 to 6 hours before dacarbazine therapy, and administer an antiemetic as prescribed to decrease nausea. Nausea and vomiting usually subside after 1 to 2 days of treatment. (See Patient Teaching: *Triazines.*)
- Discard refrigerated solution after 72 hours; discard room temperature solution after 8 hours.
- Use other appropriate nursing interventions for a patient with leukopenia, thrombocytopenia, nausea, or vomiting.
- Notify the physician if adverse reactions occur.

* ***Inspect the patient's infusion site for signs of extravasation before and during dacarbazine administration. Extravasation of the drug may cause severe tissue damage.***
* ***Stop the infusion immediately if extravasation occurs and notify the physician.***

- Administer dacarbazine as an I.V. infusion in 50 to 100 ml of dextrose 5% in water or 0.9% sodium chloride (normal saline) solution over 30 minutes. If pain occurs at the infusion site, dilute the infusion up to 250 ml, slow the infusion rate, or apply warmth to the vein.

Evaluation

For each nursing diagnosis, prepare an evaluation statement that describes the patient's or family's response to nursing interventions.

Ethylenimines

The ethylenimine derivative thiotepa is a multifunctional alkylating agent.

PHARMACOKINETICS

After I.V. administration, thiotepa is 100% bioavailable. Significant systemic absorption may occur when thiotepa is administered into pleural or peritoneal spaces to treat malignant effusions or is instilled into the bladder. Thiotepa crosses the blood-brain barrier and is metabolized extensively in the liver. Thiotepa and its metabolites are excreted in the urine. The peak concentration level of thiotepa has not been quantified yet. However, the drug may have a half-life of 1 week or more.

Route	Onset	Peak	Duration
I.V.	Unknown	Unknown	2.5 hr

PHARMACODYNAMICS

Thiotepa exerts its cytotoxic activity by interfering with DNA replication and RNA transcription. Ultimately, it disrupts nucleic acid function and causes cell death.

PHARMACOTHERAPEUTICS

This alkylating agent is used to treat bladder cancer. It is also prescribed for **palliative** treatment of lymphomas and ovarian or breast **carcinomas**. The Food and Drug Administration (FDA) has approved their use for the treatment of intracavitary effusions. Thiotepa may be useful in the treatment of lung cancer.

Drug interactions

When used concomitantly with succinylcholine, thiotepa may cause prolonged respirations and apnea. Thiotepa appears to inhibit the activity of cholinesterase, the enzyme that deactivates succinylcholine.

ADVERSE DRUG REACTIONS

The major adverse reaction to thiotepa is hematologic toxicity, which is usually dose-related and cumulative. Adverse hematologic reactions include leukopenia, anemia, thrombocytopenia, and pancytopenia, which may be fatal.

Nausea, vomiting, and anorexia are uncommon after thiotepa administration. Stomatitis and ulceration of the intestinal mucosa have been reported, especially at bone marrow transplant doses.

Other adverse reactions to thiotepa include pain at the injection site, alopecia, headache, dizziness, and throat tightness as well as hyperuricemia, febrile reactions, and exudation from subcutaneous lesions.

Hypersensitivity reactions are rare, but hives, rash, and pruritus occur occasionally. In some patients, thiotepa instillation has caused lower abdominal pain, bladder irritability, hematuria and, rarely, hemorrhagic cystitis.

NURSING PROCESS APPLICATION

The following information assists the nurse in caring for a patient receiving thiotepa. It includes an overview of assessment activities as well as examples of appropriate nursing diagnoses and related interventions (see "Planning and implementation"). It also highlights the importance of evaluation.

Assessment

Before drug therapy begins, review the patient's history for conditions that contraindicate or require cautious use of thiotepa. Also review the patient's medication history to identify use of drugs that may interact with it. During therapy, assess the patient for adverse drug reactions and signs of drug interactions. Also, periodically assess the effectiveness of therapy with thiotepa. Finally, evaluate the patient's and family's knowledge about the prescribed drug.

Nursing diagnoses

- Risk for injury related to a preexisting condition that contraindicates or requires cautious use of thiotepa
- Risk for injury related to adverse drug reactions or drug interactions
- Risk for infection related to thiotepa-induced leukopenia
- Knowledge deficit related to the thiotepa

Planning and implementation

- Do not administer thiotepa to a patient with a condition that contraindicates its use.
- Administer thiotepa cautiously to a patient at risk because of a preexisting condition.
- Monitor the patient for adverse reactions and drug interactions during thiotepa therapy.
- Monitor the patient's CBC for abnormalities that indicate anemia, thrombocytopenia, or pancytopenia.
- Take bleeding precautions and monitor for signs and symptoms of bleeding.
- Stagger the patient's activities and provide frequent rest periods if the patient experiences anemia.
- Notify the physician immediately if pancytopenia occurs.
- Take safety measures if the patient experiences dizziness. For example, place the bed in the lowest position, keep the side rails up, and supervise the patient's ambulation.

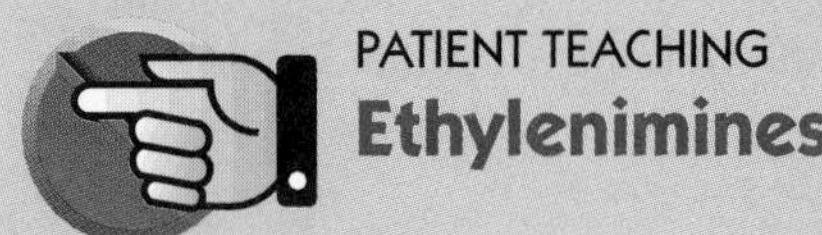

PATIENT TEACHING
Ethylenimines

- Teach the patient the name, dose, frequency, action, and adverse effects of thiotepa.
- Inform the patient that thiotepa instillation may cause lower abdominal pain, bladder irritability (with dysuria and frequent urination), and hematuria. Reassure the patient that these signs and symptoms will subside.
- Inform the patient that thiotepa may cause alopecia. Reassure the patient that hair loss is reversible when the treatment ends.
- Instruct the patient to inform the physician immediately if hives, rash, or pruritus occur. Any of these may indicate a hypersensitivity reaction.
- Caution the patient not to perform activities that require mental alertness if dizziness occurs.
- Inform the patient that pain may occur at the injection site during infusion and that appropriate measures will be taken to minimize discomfort.
- Advise the patient to notify the physician if throat tightness occurs during thiotepa therapy.
- Teach the patient to use infection control measures and bleeding precautions as needed.
- Advise the patient with anemia to stagger activities and to rest frequently.
- Teach the patient how to handle troublesome adverse reactions, such as gastrointestinal distress and stomatitis.
- Stress the importance of returning for follow-up visits and complete blood cell counts.
- Instruct the patient to notify the physician if adverse reactions occur.

• Monitor the patient's uric acid level; an elevation may indicate hyperuricemia.
• Monitor the patient for hematuria and dysuria, which indicate hemorrhagic cystitis. (See Patient Teaching: *Ethylenimines.*)
• Use other appropriate nursing interventions as needed for leukopenia, thrombocytopenia, anemia, nausea, vomiting, or stomatitis. (For more information, see the introduction to this unit.)
• Notify the physician if adverse reactions or drug interactions occur.
*** Monitor the patient's CBC for abnormalities that suggest leukopenia. If leukopenia occurs, take infection control measures and monitor the patient for signs and symptoms of infection.***
• Notify the physician if leukopenia occurs.

Evaluation
For each nursing diagnosis, prepare an evaluation statement that describes the patient's or family's response to nursing interventions.

Alkylating-like agents

Carboplatin and cisplatin are heavy metal complexes that contain platinum. Because their action resembles that of a bifunctional alkylating agent, the drugs are referred to as alkylating-like agents.

PHARMACOKINETICS
The distribution and metabolism of carboplatin are not defined clearly. After I.V. administration, carboplatin is eliminated primarily by the kidneys. The elimination of carboplatin is biphasic. It has an initial half-life of 1.1 to 2 hours and a terminal half-life of 2.5 to 6 hours.

When administered intrapleurally or intraperitoneally, cisplatin may exhibit significant systemic absorption. Highly protein-bound, cisplatin reaches high concentrations in the kidneys, liver, intestines, and testes, but displays poor CNS penetration. The drug undergoes some hepatic metabolism, followed by renal excretion. The elimination of cisplatin is also biphasic. After rapid I.V. administration, the initial half-life is 25 to 50 minutes; however, the terminal half-life may extend to 70 hours. Platinum is detectable in tissue for at least 4 months after administration.

Route	Onset	Peak	Duration
I.V.	Rapid	0.5 hr	0.5-4 hr

PHARMACODYNAMICS
Like other alkylating agents, carboplatin and cisplatin are cell cycle–nonspecific and inhibit DNA synthesis. They act like bifunctional alkylating agents by cross-linking strands of DNA and inhibiting DNA synthesis.

PHARMACOTHERAPEUTICS
Carboplatin is used primarily to treat ovarian and lung cancer. Cisplatin is prescribed to treat bladder cancer and metastatic ovarian and testicular cancers. In fact, it is the drug of choice for testicular cancer. Cisplatin may also be used to treat head, neck, and lung cancer, although these indications are not approved by the FDA.

Drug interactions
When administered concomitantly with an aminoglycoside, carboplatin or cisplatin may cause nephrotoxicity and ototoxicity.

ADVERSE DRUG REACTIONS
Carboplatin or cisplatin produce many of the same adverse reactions as the alkylating agents. Carboplatin can produce bone marrow suppression, especially platelet formation, that may require a dosage adjustment. Cisplatin usually

does not cause severe leukopenia or thrombocytopenia; however, it may cause anemia.

Nephrotoxicity occurs in 28% to 36% of patients receiving cisplatin, usually after multiple courses of therapy. With long-term cisplatin therapy, neurotoxicity can also occur, producing sensory and motor peripheral neuropathies, loss of proprioception, loss of taste, and intestinal ileus. Neurotoxicity is less common with carboplatin. Carboplatin also has a lower nephrotoxic potential.

Up to 30% of patients receiving cisplatin report tinnitus and hearing loss, which is often permanent. These adverse reactions are much less common with carboplatin. Cisplatin also produces marked nausea and vomiting in almost all patients and requires prophylactic antiemetic therapy, usually with ondansetron or granisetron hydrochloride. Carboplatin usually produces less severe nausea and vomiting that is not as prolonged.

NURSING PROCESS APPLICATION

The following information assists the nurse in caring for a patient receiving an alkylating-like agent. It includes an overview of assessment activities as well as examples of appropriate nursing diagnoses and related interventions (see "Planning and implementation"). It also highlights the importance of evaluation. (See Patient Teaching: *Alkylating-like agents.*)

Assessment

Before drug therapy begins, review the patient's history for conditions that contraindicate or require cautious use of the prescribed alkylating-like agent. Also review the patient's medication history to identify use of drugs that may interact with it. During therapy, assess the patient for adverse drug reactions and signs of drug interactions. Also, periodically assess the effectiveness of therapy with the alkylating-like agent. Finally, evaluate the patient's and family's knowledge about the prescribed drug.

Nursing diagnoses

- Risk for injury related to a preexisting condition that contraindicates or requires cautious use of an alkylating-like agent
- Risk for injury related to adverse drug reactions or drug interactions
- Altered urinary elimination related to cisplatin-induced nephrotoxicity
- Knowledge deficit related to the prescribed alkylating-like agent

Planning and implementation

- Do not administer an alkylating-like agent to a patient with a condition that contraindicates its use.
- Administer an alkylating-like agent cautiously to a patient at risk because of a preexisting condition.
- Monitor the patient for adverse reactions and drug interactions during therapy.

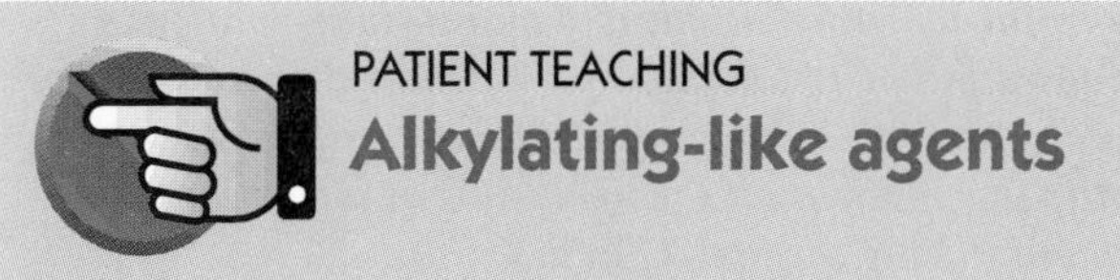

PATIENT TEACHING

Alkylating-like agents

- Teach the patient and family the name, dose, frequency, action, and adverse effects of the prescribed alkylating-like agent.
- Stress the importance of returning for routine blood and urine tests.
- Teach the patient to use infection control measures, bleeding precautions, and energy conservation measures as needed.
- Instruct the patient to report tinnitus immediately to prevent permanent hearing loss.
- Caution the patient with neurotoxicity not to perform activities that require accurate perception and coordination, such as driving.
- Instruct the patient receiving cisplatin to consume sufficient fluid to produce a urine output of 100 ml/hour for 4 consecutive hours before therapy and for 24 hours after therapy.
- Advise the patient that nausea and vomiting are possible, especially with cisplatin. Provide reassurance that an antiemetic usually is given before and after therapy to minimize these adverse reactions. Explain that intravenous therapy will be used to maintain hydration until oral fluids can be tolerated.
- Instruct the patient to report adverse reactions.

* ***Review the patient's CBC and platelet count before administering the initial dose and with each subsequent dose.***
- Monitor the patient for signs and symptoms of infection if leukopenia occurs. Take infection control measures until the patient's WBC count returns to normal.
- Monitor the patient for signs and symptoms of bleeding if thrombocytopenia occurs. Take bleeding precautions until the platelet count returns to normal. Avoid all I.M. injections and venipunctures when the platelet count is low. When a venipuncture must be done, apply firm pressure to the site for at least 5 minutes afterward.
- Reconstitute cisplatin with sterile water for injection. Cisplatin remains stable for 24 hours in 0.9% sodium chloride (normal saline) solution at room temperature; do not refrigerate solutions.

* ***Do not use an aluminum needle for reconstituting or administering carboplatin or cisplatin because the drug will interact with the aluminum, forming a black precipitate.***
- Use other appropriate nursing interventions as needed for a patient with leukopenia, thrombocytopenia, anemia, nausea, or vomiting. (For more information, see the introduction to this unit.)
- Notify the physician if adverse reactions or drug interactions occur.
- Check the results of renal function studies before administering the initial dose and with each subsequent dose. Carboplatin's dosages are based on renal function or desired platelet nadirs.

Administer sufficient fluid to maintain the patient's urine output at 100 ml/hour for 4 consecutive hours before therapy and for 24 hours after therapy with cisplatin. Notify the physician if the urine output is less than 100 ml/hour during the first 24 hours.

- Magnesium loss is common with cisplatin. Patient may require replacement therapy.
- Administer mannitol as prescribed, usually as a 12.5-g I.V. bolus, before cisplatin infusion. Also administer a mannitol infusion as prescribed, usually up to 10 g/hour, to maintain urine output during and for 6 to 24 hours after the cisplatin infusion.

Evaluation

For each nursing diagnosis, prepare an evaluation statement that describes the patient's or family's response to nursing interventions.

CHAPTER SUMMARY

Chapter 53 discussed the alkylating agents. Here are the chapter highlights.

The alkylating agents include nitrogen mustards, alkyl sulfonates, nitrosoureas, triazines, ethylenimines, and alkylating-like agents.

With the exception of the triazine dacarbazine, the alkylating agents have the same mechanisms of action in which they undergo alkylation, resulting in covalent bonds. Dacarbazine acts primarily on RNA synthesis.

Used alone or in combination with other antineoplastic drugs, alkylating agents are used to treat a wide variety of malignant neoplasms. Nitrogen mustards are indicated for Hodgkin's disease, certain leukemias, and many solid tumors. The alkyl sulfonate busulfan is used to treat chronic myelogenous leukemia and other myeloproliferative disorders. Nitrosoureas are effective against brain tumors and meningeal leukemias. The triazine dacarbazine is primarily used to treat malignant melanoma. The ethylenimine derivative thiotepa is prescribed to treat bladder cancer, ovarian or breast cancer, or lymphomas. Of the alkylating-like agents, carboplatin is used to treat ovarian cancer, and cisplatin is used primarily to treat metastatic ovarian and testicular cancers.

The most common and potentially harmful adverse reaction to the alkylating agents is bone marrow suppression, resulting in leukopenia and thrombocytopenia. Other adverse reactions include nausea, vomiting, alopecia, and fatigue. Some of these reactions may be minimized through nursing interventions.

During therapy with the alkylating agent, the nurse teaches the patient and family to minimize adverse reactions.

Questions to consider

See Appendix 1 for answers.

1. Janet Fisher, age 40, has stage III Hodgkin's disease. As part of her chemotherapy, she will receive the alkylating agent mechlorethamine (Mustargen). How does mechlorethamine exert its therapeutic effects?
   (a) It disrupts the structure of DNA.
   (b) It damages the host's immune system.
   (c) It resembles natural cell metabolites.
   (d) It destroys the cell membrane, causing lysis.

2. During mechlorethamine therapy, the nurse should assess the patient for which of the following *major* adverse reactions that is common to all alkylating agents?
   (a) Phototoxicity
   (b) Neurotoxicity
   (c) Anaphylaxis
   (d) Bone marrow suppression

3. Terry Wiggett, age 52, receives the alkyl sulfonate busulfan for chronic myelogenous leukemia. The nurse assesses him regularly for adverse drug reactions. Long-term busulfan therapy may produce which of the following adverse respiratory reactions?
   (a) Chronic obstructive pulmonary disease
   (b) Pulmonary hypertension
   (c) Pulmonary fibrosis
   (d) Asthma attacks

4. Harry Ciolla, age 55, has bladder cancer and is receiving weekly bladder instillations of thiotepa. What type of alkylating agent is thiotepa?
   (a) nitrogen mustard
   (b) nitrosourea
   (c) ethylenimine
   (d) triazine

5. Jim Collins, age 32, is receiving cisplatin for the treatment of metastatic testicular cancer. What is the organ-specific toxicity associated with cisplatin?
   (a) Cardiotoxicity
   (b) Pulmonary fibrosis
   (c) Nephrotoxicity
   (d) Photosensitivity

6. Intense pain at the infusion site during administration is associated with which of the following nitrosoureas?
   (a) carmustine
   (b) lomustine
   (c) semustine
   (d) streptozocin

54 Antimetabolite agents

OBJECTIVES

After reading and studying this chapter, the student should be able to:
1. identify the clinical uses of the antimetabolite agents.
2. differentiate among the mechanisms of action of the folic acid, pyrimidine, and purine analogues.
3. identify the common adverse reactions associated with antimetabolite agents.
4. describe how to apply the nursing process when caring for a patient who is receiving an antimetabolite agent.

INTRODUCTION

Because the antimetabolites structurally resemble natural metabolites, they can become involved in processes associated with the natural metabolites — that is, the synthesis of nucleic acids and proteins. However, the antimetabolites differ sufficiently from the natural metabolites to interfere with this synthesis. Because the antimetabolites are cell cycle–specific and primarily affect cells that actively synthesize deoxyribonucleic acid (DNA), they are referred to as S phase–specific. Normal cells that are reproducing actively as well as the cancer cells are affected by the antimetabolites. These drugs are subclassified further according to the metabolite affected and include folic acid analogues, pyrimidine analogues, and purine analogues.

Malignancies that respond to the action of antimetabolites include acute leukemia, breast cancer, adrenocarcinoma of the gastrointestinal (GI) tract, malignant lymphomas, and squamous cell carcinoma of the head, neck, and cervix. The major adverse reactions occur in the bone marrow, mucosa, skin, and hair follicles. Adverse reactions usually are dose-related and reversible, and many patients may not experience any of these reactions. (See *Selected major antimetabolite agents,* page 658.)

Drugs covered in this chapter include:
- 5-azacyitdine
- cladribine
- cytarabine
- floxuridine
- fludarabine phosphate
- fluorouracil
- gemcitabine
- mercaptopurine
- methotrexate sodium
- thioguanine

Folic acid analogues

Although researchers have developed many folic acid analogues, the early compound methotrexate sodium remains the most commonly used.

PHARMACOKINETICS

Methotrexate is absorbed well and distributed throughout the body. At usual dosages, it does not enter the central nervous system (CNS) readily. Although methotrexate is metabolized partially, it is excreted primarily unchanged in the urine. Methotrexate reaches a peak plasma concentration level 1 hour after an oral dose; this level is directly dose-related. The peak plasma concentration is achieved 30 minutes to 2 hours after parenteral administration. With **intrathecal** administration, the peak concentration is reached in 3 to 12 hours. Methotrexate exhibits a three-part disappearance from plasma; the rapid distributive phase is followed by a second phase, which reflects renal clearance. The last phase, the terminal half-life, is 3 to 10 hours for a low dose and 8 to 15 hours for a high dose.

Route	Onset	Peak	Duration
P.O.	Unknown	1 hr	Unknown
I.M.	Unknown	30-60 min	Unknown
I.V.	Unknown	30 min-2 hr	Unknown
Intrathecal	Unknown	3-12 hr	Unknown

PHARMACODYNAMICS

Methotrexate reversibly inhibits the action of dihydrofolate reductase, thereby blocking normal biochemical reactions and inhibiting DNA and ribonucleic acid (RNA) synthesis. The result is cell death.

PHARMACOTHERAPEUTICS

Methotrexate is especially useful in treating acute **lymphoblastic leukemia** in children, choriocarcinoma, osteogenic **sarcoma,** and malignant **lymphomas** as well as **carcinomas** of the head, neck, bladder, testis, and breast. The drug is also prescribed in low doses to treat severe psoriasis and rheumatoid arthritis that resist conventional therapy.

Selected major antimetabolite agents

This table summarizes the major antimetabolite agents currently in clinical use.

DRUG	MAJOR INDICATIONS AND USUAL DOSAGES	CONTRAINDICATIONS AND PRECAUTIONS
Folic acid analogues		
methotrexate (Folex, Mexate)	*Maintenance of acute lymphoblastic leukemia remission* ADULT: 20 to 30 mg/m² P.O. or I.M. twice weekly or 2.5 mg/kg I.V. every 14 days PEDIATRIC: 15 mg/m² P.O. or I.M. twice weekly or 2.5 mg/kg I.V. every 14 days *Choriocarcinoma* ADULT: 15 mg/m² P.O. or I.M. daily for 5 days at 1- to 2-week intervals *Meningeal leukemia* ADULT: 12 mg/m² intrathecally at 2- to 5-day intervals PEDIATRIC: for children under age 1, 6 mg/m² intrathecally at 2- to 5-day intervals; for children age 1, 8 mg/m² intrathecally at 2- to 5-day intervals; for children age 2, 10 mg/m² intrathecally at 2- to 5-day intervals; for children age 3 and over, 12 mg/m² intrathecally at 2- to 5-day intervals *Breast cancer* ADULT: 40 to 60 mg/m² I.V. every 21 days *Osteogenic sarcoma* ADULT: 12 to 15 g/m² I.V. with leucovorin *Malignant lymphoma* ADULT: 0.625 to 2.5 mg/kg P.O., I.M., or I.V. daily or 200 to 300 mg/m² I.V.	• Methotrexate is contraindicated in a pregnant patient or one with a blood dyscrasia. • This drug requires cautious use in a pediatric or geriatric patient or one with an infection, peptic ulcer disease, or ulcerative colitis.
Pyrimidine analogues		
cytarabine [Ara-C, cytosine arabinoside] (Cytosar-U)	*Acute myelogenous leukemia* ADULT: 100 mg/m² I.V. bolus or continuous infusion daily for 5 to 7 days PEDIATRIC: same as adult *Meningeal leukemia* ADULT: 30 mg/m² intrathecally every 4 days PEDIATRIC: same as adult	• Cytarabine is contraindicated in a pregnant or breast-feeding patient or one with known hypersensitivity. • This drug requires cautious use in a patient with drug-induced bone marrow suppression or impaired hepatic function.
fluorouracil [5 fluorouracil, 5-FU] (Adrucil, Efudex)	*Solid tumors (such as carcinomas of the gastrointestinal tract and breast* ADULT: 12 mg/kg I.V. daily, up to a maximum of 800 mg, for 4 consecutive days; if toxicity does not occur, 6 mg/kg I.V. daily on the 6th, 8th, 10th, and 12th days *Basal cell carcinomas* ADULT: Cover lesions with cream or lotion twice daily	• Fluorouracil is contraindicated in a patient with known hypersensitivity to the drug or any of its components. • This drug has no known precautions. • Safety and efficacy in children have not been established.
Purine analogues		
fludarabine (Fludara)	*B cell chronic lymphocytic leukemia for patients who have not responded to treatment with at least one standard alkylating agent* ADULT: 25 mg/m² I.V. infused over 30 minutes daily for 5 consecutive days in a 28-day cycle	• Fludarabine is contraindicated in a pregnant or breast-feeding patient or one with known hypersensitivity to the drug or any of its components. • Use cautiously in renal insufficiency. • Safety and efficacy in children have not been established.
mercaptopurine [6 MP] (Purinethol)	*Acute lymphoblastic leukemia, chronic myelocytic leukemia* ADULT: initially, 2.5 mg/kg P.O. daily (with a range of 100 to 200 mg); maintenance dosage after an adequate response is achieved, 1.5 to 2.5 mg/kg P.O. daily PEDIATRIC: same as adult	• Mercaptopurine is contraindicated in a pregnant or breast-feeding patient or one with acute lymphatic leukemia or prior resistance to the drug. • This drug requires cautious use in a patient with liver disease or one receiving another hepatotoxic drug.

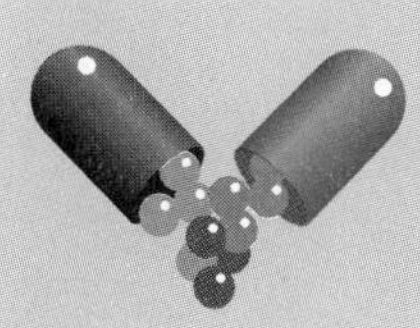

DRUG INTERACTIONS
Folic acid analogues

This chart lists drugs that interact with methotrexate, outlines possible effects for each, and presents selected nursing implications.

DRUG	INTERACTING DRUGS	POSSIBLE EFFECTS	NURSING IMPLICATIONS
methotrexate	probenecid	Decreased methotrexate excretion, which increases the risk of methotrexate toxicity	• Monitor for increased adverse reactions, such as fatigue, bone marrow suppression, and stomatitis.
	salicylates and nonsteroidal anti-inflammatory drugs, especially diclofenac, ketoprofen, indomethacin, phenylbutazone, and naproxen	Increased methotrexate toxicity	• Avoid concomitant use when possible. • Monitor for increased adverse reactions, such as fatigue, bone marrow suppression, and stomatitis.
	cholestyramine	Reduced methotrexate absorption from gastrointestinal tract	• Separate oral doses as much as possible if concomitant therapy is necessary.
	alcohol	Increased methotrexate hepatotoxicity	• Instruct the patient to avoid drinking alcohol.
	live vaccines	Increased risk of infection by organism in live vaccine	• Avoid administration of live vaccines during methotrexate therapy.
	co-trimoxazole	Megaloblastic pancytopenia	• Avoid concomitant use.
	penicillins	Decreased renal tubular secretion of methotrexate	• Monitor the patient for increased methotrexate toxicity.

Drug interactions
Various drugs can interact with methotrexate. (See Drug Interactions: *Folic acid analogues.*)

ADVERSE DRUG REACTIONS
Bone marrow suppression can occur with any methotrexate dosage schedule. It is greatest 10 to 14 days after methotrexate administration. **Stomatitis** may develop 5 to 10 days after therapy begins. Patients receiving high-dosage methotrexate therapy are susceptible to severe stomatitis, which may result in a nutritional deficit. Fatigue may also occur.

Although rare, two types of **hepatotoxicity** are associated with methotrexate: acute and chronic. Acute hepatotoxicity produces transient elevations in liver function tests 1 to 3 days after drug administration. Chronic hepatotoxicity may result in cirrhosis and, less commonly, acute liver atrophy. It is associated with high-dosage, long-term methotrexate therapy and is related to the length and frequency of dosing and to a total dose of 1.5 g or more.

Pulmonary toxicity, exhibited as pneumonitis or pulmonary fibrosis, may occur. With high doses, nephrotoxicity can also occur, raising blood urea nitrogen (BUN) and creatinine values. **Tumor** cell destruction by methotrexate may increase the uric acid concentration, which may worsen nephrotoxicity.

Photosensitivity may occur in patients despite protection from the sun. A sunburnlike rash is the primary dermatologic reaction. **Alopecia** occurs in approximately 10% of patients receiving methotrexate.

Although rare, nausea and vomiting may be the first adverse reactions to high-dose methotrexate therapy. They typically occur less than 1 hour after administration.

Intrathecal administration of methotrexate warrants special attention because severe adverse reactions have occurred, including seizures, paresis, paralysis, and death. Other less severe adverse reactions may occur, such as headaches, fever, neck stiffness, confusion, and irritability. Intrathecal administration may also produce systemic toxicity marked by tremor, ataxia, somnolence, and seizures. Rarely, systemic toxicity progresses to coma and death. Because methotrexate preparations that contain preservatives have caused more adverse reactions, only preservative-free methotrexate and diluents should be used for intrathecal drug administration.

During high-dose methotrexate therapy, leucovorin may be used to minimize adverse reactions. (See *Leucovorin rescue,* page 660.)

Leucovorin rescue

Methotrexate interferes with cell division in the S phase of the cell cycle by inhibiting dihydrofolate reductase (DHFR), an enzyme involved in deoxyribonucleic acid (DNA) synthesis. High-dose methotrexate is most effective against cells that have a high metabolic rate, such as leukemia cells. Used alone, high-dose methotrexate eventually will affect normal cells as well, producing toxicity.

To protect normal cells, methotrexate commonly is prescribed with leucovorin (folinic acid). Leucovorin rescues cells by bypassing the S phase, which methotrexate inhibits, as this diagram illustrates. It also acts by other mechanisms that are not understood completely. Leucovorin must be administered exactly on time, as prescribed, for the drug to work efficiently. When administered properly, leucovorin rescues cells before they begin active growth and division. Although leucovorin is considered a vitamin, doses must not be skipped because this drug plays an important role in preventing severe methotrexate toxicity.

Because leucovorin cannot prevent methotrexate toxicity completely, the nurse should monitor any patient on high-dose methotrexate therapy for bone marrow suppression, stomatitis, pulmonary complications, and renal damage (from drug precipitation in tubules). To prevent precipitation in tubules, the nurse also should encourage the patient to consume foods and fluids that will maintain urine alkalinity and should monitor urine output closely.

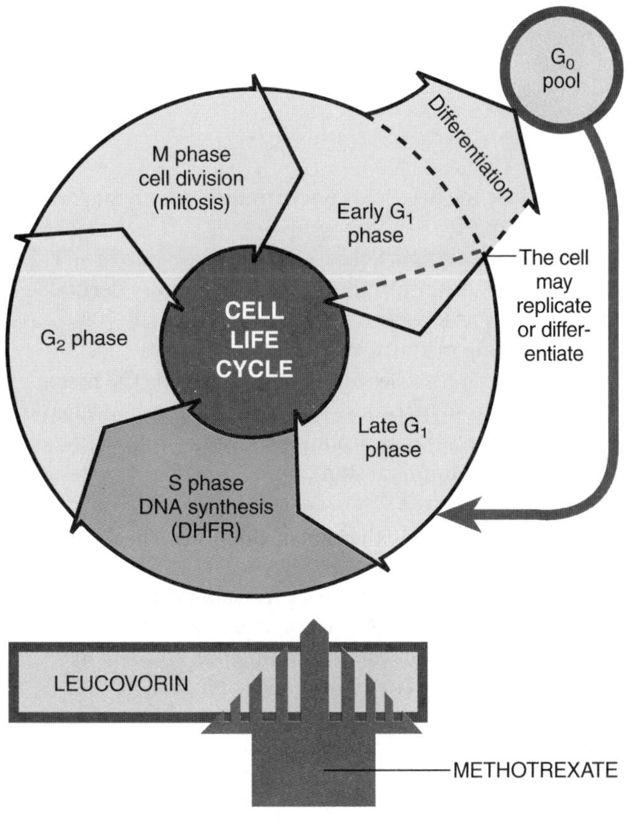

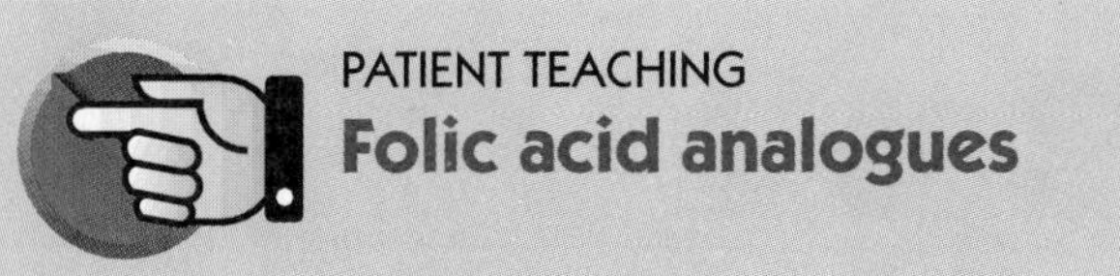

PATIENT TEACHING

Folic acid analogues

- Teach the patient and family the name, dose, frequency, action, and adverse effects of methotrexate.
- Stress the importance of returning for blood and pulmonary function studies.
- Instruct the patient to notify the physician if a fever, nonproductive cough, shortness of breath, or other respiratory change occurs.
- Teach the patient to recognize the signs of liver dysfunction, such as yellowed skin or sclera, darkened urine, and clay-colored stools.
- Advise the patient to drink at least eight 8-oz (240-ml) glasses of fluid daily to increase urine output and prevent methotrexate from precipitating in the renal tubules. Also, instruct the patient to keep a record of fluid intake and output and to test the urine pH regularly.
- Teach the patient to use infection control measures, bleeding precautions, and energy conservation measures, as needed.
- Teach the patient how to manage stomatitis at home.
- Advise the patient to avoid sun exposure when possible or to use a sunscreen, hat, and sunglasses when sun exposure is unavoidable. Inform the patient that a sunburnlike rash may occur even if these precautions are observed.
- Inform the patient that nausea and vomiting are most likely to occur up to 1 hour after methotrexate administration, if at all.
- Inform the patient that alopecia occurs in about 10% of all patients receiving methotrexate.
- Teach the patient receiving intrathecal methotrexate to report immediately any of the following adverse neurologic reactions: paresis, seizures, loss of motor control, headache, stiff neck, fever, confusion, and irritability.
- Instruct the patient to notify the physician if other adverse reactions occur.

NURSING PROCESS APPLICATION

The following information assists the nurse in caring for a patient receiving methotrexate. It includes an overview of assessment activities as well as examples of appropriate nursing diagnoses and related interventions (see "Planning and implementation"). It also highlights the importance of evaluation.

Assessment

Before drug therapy begins, review the patient's history for conditions that contraindicate or require cautious use of methotrexate. Also, review the patient's medication history to identify use of drugs that may interact with it. During therapy, assess the patient for adverse drug reactions and signs of drug interactions. Also, periodically assess the effectiveness of methotrexate therapy. Finally, evaluate the patient's and family's knowledge about the prescribed drug.

Nursing diagnoses

- Risk for injury related to a preexisting condition that contraindicates or requires cautious use of methotrexate
- Risk for injury related to adverse drug reactions or drug interactions
- Knowledge deficit related to methotrexate

Planning and implementation

- Do not administer methotrexate to a patient with a condition that contraindicates its use.
- Administer methotrexate cautiously to a patient at risk because of a preexisting condition.
- Monitor the patient for adverse reactions and drug interactions during methotrexate therapy.

* ***Monitor the patient's BUN and creatinine values before each treatment to detect signs of nephrotoxicity. If values are abnormal, consult the physician for therapy modification.***

- Encourage fluid intake and administer intravenous (I.V.) fluids and sodium bicarbonate, as prescribed, to increase urine alkalinity and volume and prevent nephrotoxicity in a patient receiving high-dose therapy. (See Patient Teaching: *Folic acid analogues.*)
- Document fluid intake and output accurately, and monitor urine pH in a patient receiving high-dose therapy.

* ***Monitor liver function test results regularly during methotrexate therapy to detect early changes in liver function that suggest cirrhosis or acute liver atrophy.***
* Monitor the patient for signs of liver dysfunction, such as jaundice, darkened urine, or clay-colored stools.
* ***Monitor the patient's complete blood count (CBC) and platelet count regularly during methotrexate therapy to detect bone marrow suppression.***

- Monitor the patient for signs of infection if leukopenia occurs. Also take infection control measures until the white blood cell (WBC) count returns to normal.
- Observe the patient for signs and symptoms of bleeding if thrombocytopenia occurs. Take bleeding precautions until the platelet count returns to normal.
- Monitor the serum methotrexate level, especially during high-dose therapy.
- Administer leucovorin with high doses of methotrexate, as prescribed.
- Use only preservative-free methotrexate and diluents for intrathecal drug administration.
- Use other appropriate nursing interventions for a patient with bone marrow suppression, nausea, vomiting, stomatitis, or alopecia. (For details, see the introduction to this unit.)
- Notify the physician if adverse reactions or drug interactions occur.

Evaluation

For each nursing diagnosis, prepare an evaluation statement that describes the patient's or family's response to nursing interventions.

Pyrimidine analogues

The pyrimidine analogues include 5-azacytidine, cytarabine, floxuridine, fluorouracil, and gemcitabine — a diverse group of drugs that inhibit the biosynthesis of pyrimidine nucleotides by mimicry.

PHARMACOKINETICS

Because the pyrimidine analogues are absorbed poorly when given orally, they are usually administered via other routes. With the exception of 5-azacytidine, the pyrimidine analogues are distributed well throughout the body, including cerebrospinal fluid. They are metabolized extensively in the liver and are excreted in the urine.

After subcutaneous administration, 5-azacytidine reaches a peak plasma concentration in 0.5 hour. It has a half-life of 3.5 to 4.5 hours. Continuous I.V. infusion of cytarabine produces a relatively constant plasma concentration level of the drug in 8 to 24 hours. Cytarabine has a plasma half-life of 1 to 3 hours. After intrathecal administration, cytarabine has a half-life of 2 to 11 hours. The peak concentration time and half-life of floxuridine have not been quantified well. However, floxuridine's high hepatic extraction results in low systemic levels and a short half-life. Fluorouracil has a rapid clearance, with a plasma half-life of only 10 to 20 minutes. Gemcitabine should be administered by I.V. infusion over 30 minutes. This produces a rapid onset of effects with peak plasma concentrations occurring within 30 minutes to 1.5 hours. Gemcitabine is excreted mainly through the kidneys.

Route	Onset	Peak	Duration
S.C., I.V.	Rapid	0.2-3 hr	3-24 hr

PHARMACODYNAMICS

The pyrimidine analogues exhibit their **cytotoxic** effects by interfering with the natural function of pyrimidine nucleotides. They interfere with the biosynthesis of natural pyrimidines or mimic the natural pyrimidines to the point where they interfere with cellular functions. The pyrimidine analogues are cell cycle–, S phase–specific.

PHARMACOTHERAPEUTICS

The pyrimidine analogues are used to treat many tumors. However, they are used mostly to treat acute leukemias, **adenocarcinomas** of the GI tract, carcinomas of the breast and ovaries, and malignant lymphomas.

Drug interactions

No significant drug interactions occur with the pyrimidine analogues. Drug-specific incompatibilities exist: 5-

fluorouracil is incompatible with daunorubicin, doxorubicin, idarubicin, cisplatin, cytarabine, and diazepam.

ADVERSE DRUG REACTIONS

Bone marrow suppression evidenced by neutropenia and thrombocytopenia is the major dose-limiting adverse reaction to the pyrimidine analogues. This reaction is noticeable 7 to 14 days after drug administration, with bone marrow recovery occurring 21 to 28 days after the drug is discontinued.

Stomatitis and esophagopharyngitis may occur 5 to 10 days after therapy begins. This adverse reaction can be particularly distressing to the patient because the oral cavity ulcerations and sloughing may be extremely painful and prevent eating.

Like most antineoplastic agents, the pyrimidine analogues can cause fatigue. Lack of energy can limit activities severely as well as the patient's involvement in therapy.

With the exception of 5-azacytidine, the pyrimidine analogues do not cause severe nausea and vomiting. About 70% of patients receiving 5-azacytidine experience moderate to severe nausea and vomiting 1.5 to 3 hours after I.V. administration. Nausea and anorexia may occur with fluorouracil or floxuridine therapy. Diarrhea may occur with fluorouracil administration and may be severe enough to limit or discontinue therapy.

In most cases, fluorouracil is relatively well tolerated. However, it can produce several hypersensitivity reactions, including mild to severe skin reactions. Such reactions may take the form of a pruritic rash on the extremities or less commonly on the trunk, photosensitivity with erythema or increased skin pigmentation, darkening of the veins with prolonged drug administration, or a rash on the hands and feet with prolonged high-dose infusions. Other hypersensitivity reactions may include increased lacrimation, nasal discharge, or epistaxis; these reactions disappear after therapy is discontinued. Alopecia commonly occurs with fluorouracil. Hepatic arterial infusion of floxuridine has been associated with bile duct sclerosis and liver cirrhosis.

Cytarabine and 5-azacytidine may produce fever and flulike symptoms within 24 hours after therapy begins. Cytarabine produces a rash in 4% of patients. Intrathecal cytarabine usually does not cause systemic toxicity. It is more likely to cause nausea, vomiting, fever, and transient headaches.

NURSING PROCESS APPLICATION

The following information assists the nurse in caring for a patient receiving a pyrimidine analogue. It includes an overview of assessment activities as well as examples of appropriate nursing diagnoses and related interventions (see "Planning and implementation"). It also highlights the importance of evaluation.

Assessment

Before drug therapy begins, review the patient's history for conditions that contraindicate or require cautious use of the prescribed pyrimidine analogue. During therapy, assess the patient for adverse drug reactions. Also, periodically assess the effectiveness of therapy with the pyrimidine analogue. Finally, evaluate the patient's and family's knowledge about the prescribed drug.

Nursing diagnoses

• Risk for injury related to a preexisting condition that contraindicates or requires cautious use of a pyrimidine analogue
• Risk for injury related to adverse drug reactions
• Knowledge deficit related to the prescribed pyrimidine analogue

Planning and implementation

• Do not administer a pyrimidine analogue to a patient with a condition that contraindicates its use.
• Administer a pyrimidine analogue cautiously to a patient at risk because of a preexisting condition.
• Monitor the patient for adverse reactions during therapy with the prescribed pyrimidine analogue.
*∗ **Monitor the patient's CBC to detect bone marrow suppression. If neutropenia occurs, monitor the patient for signs of infection. Also take infection control measures until the neutrophil count returns to normal. If thrombocytopenia occurs, monitor the patient for signs and symptoms of bleeding. Also take bleeding precautions until the thrombocyte count returns to normal. Limit the pyrimidine analogue dosage, as prescribed, if hematologic abnormalities occur.***
• Review the results of the patient's liver function studies regularly throughout intra-arterial floxuridine therapy.
• Monitor for fever and flulike symptoms in a patient who is receiving cytarabine or 5-azacytidine. Administer a mild analgesic and antipyretic, as prescribed, to reduce the fever and ease the patient's discomfort. (See Patient Teaching: *Pyrimidine analogues.*)
• Store fluorouracil at room temperature and protect it from light.
*∗ **Do not use a cloudy fluorouracil solution. If crystals form, redissolve the solution by warming.***
• Use plastic I.V. containers to administer continuous fluorouracil infusions because the solution is more stable in plastic I.V. bags than in glass bottles.
• Reconstitute floxuridine with sterile water for injection. For the actual infusion, dilute further in dextrose 5% in water or 0.9% sodium chloride (normal saline) solution.
• Discard refrigerated floxuridine solution after 2 weeks because it becomes unstable after this time.
*∗ **Use preservative-free normal saline solution for intrathecal cytarabine administration.***
• Discard reconstituted cytarabine solution 48 hours after reconstitution because it becomes unstable after that time.

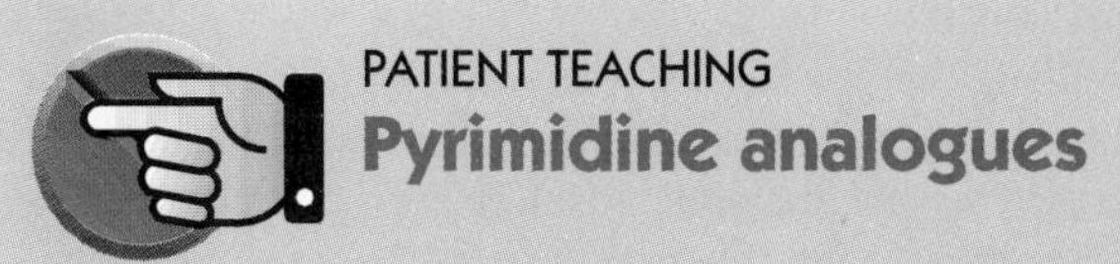

PATIENT TEACHING
Pyrimidine analogues

- Teach the patient and family the name, dose, frequency, action, and adverse effects of the prescribed pyrimidine analogue.
- Stress the importance of returning for follow-up blood tests.
- Teach the patient how to manage stomatitis and esophagopharyngitis at home.
- Review energy conservation measures that the patient can use at home if fatigue occurs.
- Teach the patient to use infection control measures and bleeding precautions as needed.
- Teach the patient how to manage troublesome adverse gastrointestinal reactions.
- Advise the patient receiving fluorouracil that photosensitivity may occur. Instruct the patient to avoid sun exposure or to wear a sunscreen, hat, and sunglasses when sun exposure is unavoidable.
- Inform the patient that fluorouracil may cause increased lacrimation, nasal discharge, or epistaxis. Provide reassurance that these reactions disappear after therapy is discontinued.
- Inform the patient that cytarabine or 5-azacytidine may precipitate fever and flulike symptoms up to 24 hours after the drug is administered. Advise the patient to take an antipyretic and an analgesic, as prescribed.
- Inform the patient that reversible alopecia may occur during fluorouracil therapy.
- Instruct the patient to notify the physician if adverse reactions occur.

• Infuse 5-azacytidine using lactated Ringer's solution because the drug is unstable in other solutions.
• Discard reconstituted 5-azacytidine after 8 hours.
• Use other appropriate nursing interventions for a patient who develops bone marrow suppression, stomatitis, nausea, vomiting, or alopecia.
• Notify the physician if adverse reactions occur.

Evaluation

For each nursing diagnosis, prepare an evaluation statement that describes the patient's or family's response to nursing interventions.

Purine analogues

The purine analogues, fludarabine phosphate, cladribine, mercaptopurine, and thioguanine, are analogues of natural purine bases that must undergo enzymatic conversion to the nucleotide level before they become cytotoxic.

PHARMACOKINETICS

The pharmacokinetics of fludarabine are not defined clearly. The absorption of mercaptopurine and thioguanine are variable and incomplete. They are metabolized in the liver and excreted in the urine.

The peak serum concentration level of fludarabine is not known. After oral administration, mercaptopurine achieves a peak serum concentration level within 2 hours. An oral dose of thioguanine reaches a peak concentration in 6 to 8 hours. Due to cellular uptake, renal excretion, and metabolic degradation, mercaptopurine has a short plasma half-life of 90 minutes. Fludarabine's active metabolite and thioguanine, however, have a plasma half-life of 10 hours and 11 hours, respectively.

Cladribine is administered by I.V. infusion. Onset, peak, and duration information is unknown at present.

Route	Onset	Peak	Duration
P.O.	Unknown	2-8 hr	Unknown
I.V.	Rapid	Immediate-5 hr	1.5-22 hr

PHARMACODYNAMICS

Like the other antimetabolites, fludarabine, mercaptopurine, and thioguanine first must undergo conversion to the nucleotide level to be active. The resulting nucleotides then are incorporated into DNA, where they may inhibit DNA and RNA synthesis as well as other metabolic reactions necessary for proper cell growth. The purine analogues are cell cycle–, S phase–specific.

PHARMACOTHERAPEUTICS

The purine analogues are used to treat acute and chronic leukemias. The purine analogues may also be useful in the treatment of lymphomas.

Drug interactions

Concomitant administration of fludarabine and pentostatin may cause severe pulmonary toxicity that can be fatal. Concomitant administration of mercaptopurine and allopurinol may increase bone marrow suppression by decreasing mercaptopurine metabolism. No significant interactions occur with thioguanine.

ADVERSE DRUG REACTIONS

Purine analogues produce bone marrow suppression, which may not begin for 1 to 6 weeks after therapy is initiated. Leukopenia usually occurs first, followed by thrombocytopenia and **anemia.**

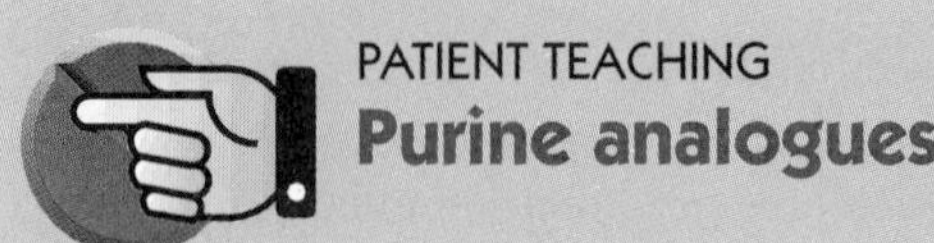

PATIENT TEACHING
Purine analogues

- Teach the patient and family the name, dose, frequency, action, and adverse effects of the prescribed purine analogue.
- Stress the importance of returning regularly for follow-up blood tests.
- Review infection control measures, bleeding precautions, and energy conservation measures that the patient may use as needed.
- Instruct the patient taking mercaptopurine or thioguanine to report any of the following to the physician immediately: yellowed skin or sclera, right upper quadrant pain, darkened urine, or clay-colored stools.
- Also instruct the patient taking fludarabine to report flank pain or hematuria as well as neurologic abnormalities to the physician immediately.
- Teach the patient how to manage troublesome adverse reactions, such as gastrointestinal distress and stomatitis.
- Advise the patient to drink at least thirteen 8-oz (240-ml) glasses of fluid daily to prevent renal damage.
- Instruct the patient to report other adverse reactions to the physician.

Fludarabine, when used at high doses, may cause severe neurologic effects, including blindness, coma, and death. It may also cause tumor lysis syndrome, which may include hyperuricemia, hyperphosphatemia, hypocalcemia, metabolic acidosis, hyperkalemia, hematuria, urate crystalluria, and renal failure. The onset of this syndrome may be heralded by flank pain and hematuria.

Many patients receiving mercaptopurine develop cholestatic jaundice after 1 to 2 months of therapy. This adverse reaction usually is associated with doses that exceed 2.5 mg/kg/day. The patient should report this reaction immediately because the jaundice may be reversible if the drug is discontinued. If the drug is not discontinued, the reaction may be fatal. Jaundice has also been reported with thioguanine use.

Nausea, vomiting, anorexia, mild diarrhea, and stomatitis occur in patients receiving purine analogues. Uric acid levels may also rise as a result of purine catabolism from cellular destruction.

NURSING PROCESS APPLICATION

The following information assists the nurse in caring for a patient receiving a purine analogue. It includes an overview of assessment activities as well as examples of appropriate nursing diagnoses and related interventions (see "Planning and implementation"). It also highlights the importance of evaluation.

Assessment

Before drug therapy begins, review the patient's history for conditions that contraindicate or require cautious use of the prescribed purine analogue. Also review the patient's medication history to identify use of drugs that may interact with it. During therapy, assess the patient for adverse drug reactions and signs of drug interactions. Also, periodically assess the effectiveness of therapy with the purine analogue. Finally, evaluate the patient's and family's knowledge about the prescribed drug.

Nursing diagnoses

- Risk for injury related to a preexisting condition that contraindicates or requires cautious use of a purine analogue
- Risk for injury related to adverse drug reactions or drug interactions
- Altered health maintenance related to bone marrow suppression
- Knowledge deficit related to the prescribed purine analogue

Planning and implementation

- Do not administer a purine analogue to a patient with a condition that contraindicates its use.
- Administer a purine analogue cautiously to a patient at risk because of a preexisting condition.
- Monitor the patient for adverse reactions and drug interactions during therapy with the purine analogue.
- Monitor the CBC weekly or as prescribed, watching for a precipitous decrease.

✱ ***Observe the patient for signs of bleeding and infection. Take infection control measures and bleeding precautions if bone marrow suppression occurs.***

- Monitor the patient taking mercaptopurine or thioguanine for signs of cholestatic jaundice, such as pain in the right upper quadrant and elevated liver function enzymes. Cholestatic jaundice may progress to hepatic necrosis, which may reverse if the drug is stopped promptly. (See Patient Teaching: *Purine analogues.)*

✱ ***Monitor the patient taking high doses of fludarabine for severe neurologic abnormalities.***

- Use other appropriate nursing interventions for a patient who develops bone marrow suppression, nausea, vomiting, or stomatitis.
- Notify the physician if adverse reactions or drug interactions occur.
- Periodically monitor the patient's serum uric acid level.
- Document the patient's fluid intake and output accurately. To minimize the effects of uric acid level elevations, encourage the patient to drink at least thirteen 8-oz (240-ml) glasses of fluids daily, and administer allopurinol as prescribed.
- Notify the physician if the uric acid level remains elevated.

Evaluation

For each nursing diagnosis, prepare an evaluation statement that describes the patient's or family's response to nursing interventions.

CHAPTER SUMMARY

Chapter 54 discussed the antimetabolite agents. Here are the chapter highlights.

The antimetabolites are antineoplastic drugs that can interfere with the synthesis of nucleic acids and proteins. The three major classes of antimetabolite agents are folic acid analogues, pyrimidine analogues, and purine analogues.

Antimetabolites are used to treat acute and chronic leukemias, breast cancer, adenocarcinomas of the GI tract, malignant lymphoma, and squamous cell carcinomas of the head, neck, and cervix.

By applying the nursing process, the nurse helps the patient cope with chemotherapy. Specific interventions include monitoring the patient for signs and symptoms of adverse reactions and providing information about the drug and the patient's role in the therapy.

Questions to consider

See Appendix 1 for answers.

1. Andy Hopkins, age 52, has malignant lymphoma and is receiving chemotherapy with methotrexate. How does this drug produce its therapeutic effects?
   (a) It disrupts the DNA structure.
   (b) It inhibits DNA and RNA synthesis.
   (c) It inhibits hormone-mediated tumor cell growth.
   (d) It intercalates between adjacent pairs of DNA molecules.

2. Which of the following agents is likely to be administered with methotrexate to minimize its adverse reactions?
   (a) fluorouracil
   (b) leucovorin
   (c) cladribine
   (d) cyclophosphamide

3. Larry Madison, age 66, has colon cancer and is admitted to the oncology unit for a course of chemotherapy with fluorouracil. The nurse monitors Mr. Madison for adverse reactions. In addition to stomatitis, which of the following other adverse reactions is Mr. Madison likely to experience?
   (a) Pulmonary infiltrates
   (b) Severe renal dysfunction
   (c) Heart failure
   (d) Bone marrow suppression

4. Katie Crumb, age 7, has acute leukemia. She is receiving methotrexate with mercaptopurine for maintenance therapy. Which of the following instructions should the nurse give Katie's parents regarding mercaptopurine therapy?
   (a) Provide high-acid foods to acidify the urine.
   (b) Protect Katie from exposure to the sun.
   (c) Encourage Katie to drink thirteen 8-oz (240-ml) glasses of fluid daily.
   (d) Encourage Katie to limit her activity.

5. When a patient is receiving mercaptopurine, the nurse should assess her for which adverse reaction?
   (a) Tumor lysis syndrome
   (b) Cholestatic jaundice
   (c) Flulike symptoms
   (d) Pulmonary fibrosis

6. Frances Lorin, age 44, is receiving intrathecal cytarabine for the management of meningeal leukemia. Which of the following adverse effects are associated with intrathecal administration of cytarabine?
   (a) Nausea and vomiting
   (b) Fever
   (c) Transient headaches
   (d) All of the above

55 Antibiotic antineoplastic agents

OBJECTIVES

After reading and studying this chapter, the student should be able to:

1. describe the mechanisms of action of the antibiotic antineoplastic agents.
2. explain why maximum lifetime doses have been established for bleomycin, daunorubicin, doxorubicin, and mitoxantrone.
3. identify the major adverse reactions to the antibiotic antineoplastic agents.
4. describe how to apply the nursing process when caring for a patient who is receiving an antibiotic antineoplastic agent.

INTRODUCTION

Antibiotic antineoplastic agents are antimicrobial products that produce tumoricidal effects by binding with deoxyribonucleic acid (DNA). These agents inhibit the cellular processes of normal and malignant cells. (See *Selected major antibiotic antineoplastic agents.*)

Drugs covered in this chapter include:

- bleomycin sulfate
- dactinomycin
- daunorubicin hydrochloride
- doxorubicin hydrochloride
- idarubicin hydrochloride
- mitomycin
- mitoxantrone hydrochloride
- pentostatin
- plicamycin.

Microbial tumoricidal agents

The antibiotic antineoplastics (bleomycin sulfate, dactinomycin, daunorubicin hydrochloride, doxorubicin hydrochloride, idarubicin hydrochloride, mitomycin, mitoxantrone hydrochloride, pentostatin, and plicamycin) are prescribed to treat many malignant **neoplasms.**

PHARMACOKINETICS

Because the antibiotic antineoplastic agents are usually administered intravenously (I.V.), no absorption occurs. They are considered 100% bioavailable. Some of the drugs are also administered via intracavitary routes. Bleomycin, doxorubicin, and mitomycin are sometimes given as topical bladder instillations. Significant systemic absorption, as assessed by blood concentration levels or systemic toxicity, does not occur. Bleomycin has also been injected into the pleural space for malignant effusions, with up to 50% of the dose absorbed via this route. Distribution throughout the body for the antibiotic antineoplastic agents varies as does their metabolism and elimination.

Bleomycin reaches a peak plasma concentration about 30 to 60 minutes after administration. After an I.V. bolus, the drug has a half-life of about 2 hours, which extends to 9 hours with a continuous infusion. Dactinomycin concentration peaks immediately after I.V. injection, with very little active drug remaining in the circulation after 2 minutes. The plasma half-life of dactinomycin is 36 hours because of the slow release from tissue-binding sites. Daunorubicin has a half-life of 18.5 hours, and its active metabolite has a half-life of about 27 hours. Its analogue, idarubicin, has an estimated mean terminal half-life that exceeds 45 hours. Doxorubicin has a multiphasic elimination pattern, with a half-life of 15 hours. Its active metabolite has a half-life of about 30 hours. Mitomycin reaches a peak plasma concentration of 1.5 mcg/ml after a dose of 20 mg. Its plasma half-life is 17 minutes. The terminal half-life of mitoxantrone is about 5.8 days. The average plasma half-life of pentostatin is 5.7 hours. The peak concentration and half-life of plicamycin have not been determined.

Route	Onset	Peak	Duration
I.V.	Immediate	≤ 1 hr	2 hr-5.8 days

PHARMACODYNAMICS

With the exception of mitomycin and pentostatin, the antibiotic antineoplastic agents intercalate, or insert themselves, between adjacent base pairs of a DNA molecule, physically separating them. When the DNA chain replicates, an extra base is inserted opposite the intercalated antibiotic,

Selected major antibiotic antineoplastic agents

This chart summarizes the major antibiotic antineoplastic agents currently in clinical use.

DRUG	MAJOR INDICATIONS AND USUAL DOSAGES	CONTRAINDICATIONS AND PRECAUTIONS
bleomycin (Blenoxane)	*Testicular carcinoma; squamous cell carcinomas of the head, neck, esophagus, skin, and genitourinary tract; lung cancer; Hodgkin's disease and malignant lymphoma* ADULT: 10 to 20 units/m² I.V., I.M., or S.C. one to two times weekly	• Bleomycin is contraindicated in a patient with known hypersensitivity or idiosyncratic reactions to the drug. • This drug requires cautious use in a patient with significant renal impairment or compromised pulmonary function. • Safety and efficacy in pregnant patients have not been established.
daunorubicin (Cerubidine)	*Adjunct therapy for inducing remission in acute nonlymphocytic leukemia (ANLL)* ADULT: 30 to 45 mg/m² I.V. for 1 to 3 days *Adjunct therapy for inducing remission in acute lymphocytic leukemia* ADULT: 45 mg/m² I.V. daily for 3 days PEDIATRIC: 25 mg/m² I.V. on day 1 in a 7-day cycle	• Daunorubicin is contraindicated in a pregnant patient or one with drug-induced bone marrow suppression (unless the potential benefits outweigh the risks). • This drug requires cautious use in a patient with heart disease.
doxorubicin (Adriamycin PFS)	*Solid tumors, such as breast, lung, ovarian, bladder, and thyroid carcinomas; acute leukemias; Hodgkin's disease and malignant lymphomas* ADULT: 60 to 75 mg/m² I.V. every 3 weeks; or 20 to 30 mg/m² I.V. for 2 to 3 days repeated every 4 weeks; or 20 mg/m² I.V. weekly	• Doxorubicin is contraindicated in a pregnant patient, one with marked myelosuppression or heart disease, or one who has previously received a lifetime dose of daunorubicin, doxorubicin, or both. • This drug requires cautious use in a patient receiving concomitant antineoplastic therapy.
idarubicin (Idamycin)	*Acute myelogenous leukemia* ADULT: 12 mg/m² I.V. slowly (over 10 to 15 minutes) daily for 3 days in combination with cytarabine.	• Idarubicin is contraindicated in a pregnant or breast-feeding patient or one with preexisting bone marrow suppression induced by previous drug therapy or radiotherapy (unless the potential benefits outweigh the risks). • This drug requires cautious use in a patient with heart disease. • Safety and efficacy in children have not been established.
mitoxantrone (Novantrone)	*Acute nonlymphocytic leukemia (ANLL)* ADULT: 12 mg/m² I.V. daily on days 1 through 3 for ANLL induction; 12 mg/m² I.V. daily for days 1 and 2 for ANLL consolidation	• Mitoxantrone is contraindicated in a pregnant patient, one with myelosuppression or known hypersensitivity, or one who has previously received treatment with daunorubicin or doxorubicin (unless the potential benefits outweigh the risks). • This drug requires cautious use in a patient with cardiovascular disease or one who is receiving mediastinal radiation therapy. • Safety and efficacy in children have not been established.
pentostatin (Nipent)	*Interferon-alpha-refractory hairy-cell leukemia* ADULT: 4 mg/m² I.V. every other week	• Pentostatin is contraindicated in a pregnant or breast-feeding patient or one with known hypersensitivity. • This drug requires cautious use in a patient with an existing infection. • Safety and efficacy in children have not been established.
plicamycin (Mithracin)	*Hypercalcemia* ADULT: 25 mcg/kg I.V. daily for 3 to 4 days, repeated weekly as needed *Testicular cancer* ADULT: 25 to 30 mcg/kg I.V. daily for 8 to 10 days	• Plicamycin is contraindicated in a pregnant or breast-feeding patient or one with thrombocytopenia, thrombocytopathy, coagulation disorder, increased susceptibility to bleeding resulting from other causes, or impaired bone marrow function. • This drug requires cautious use in a patient with significant renal or hepatic impairment.

resulting in a mutant DNA molecule. The overall effect is cell death.

Although the exact mechanism of pentostatin's antitumor effect is unknown, it inhibits the enzyme adenosine deaminase, blocking DNA synthesis and inhibiting ribonucleic acid (RNA) synthesis. Mitomycin is activated intracellularly to a bifunctional or even trifunctional alkylating agent. Mitomycin produces single-strand breakage of DNA. It also cross-links DNA and inhibits DNA synthesis.

PHARMACOTHERAPEUTICS

The antibiotic antineoplastic agents are products of microbial fermentation that exhibit antimicrobial activity. Their **cytotoxic** effects, however, preclude their antimicrobial use. These agents act against many **tumors** (including **Hodgkin's disease** and malignant **lymphomas;** testicular **carcinoma;** squamous cell carcinoma of the head, neck, and cervix; **Wilms' tumor,** osteogenic **sarcoma,** and **rhabdomyosarcoma;** Ewing's sarcoma and other soft-tissue sarcomas; breast, ovarian, bladder, and bronchogenic carcinomas; melanoma; carcinomas of the gastrointestinal [GI] tract; and choriocarcinoma), acute **leukemias,** and hypercalcemia.

Drug interactions

Except for idarubicin and pentostatin, no clinically significant drug interactions occur with the antibiotic antineoplastic agents. Idarubicin and pentostatin enhance the effects of vidarabine with concomitant use, thereby increasing the possibility of adverse reactions to vidarabine and pentostatin or idarubicin. Also concurrent therapy with fludarabine and pentostatin or idarubicin is not recommended because of the risk of fatal pulmonary toxicity.

ADVERSE DRUG REACTIONS

Antibiotic antineoplastic agents produce many of the same reactions as other drugs used to treat malignant neoplasms. The primary reaction is bone marrow suppression. All of these agents except bleomycin produce moderate to severe **leukopenia** and **thrombocytopenia.** Mitomycin causes delayed myelosuppression that requires 6 to 8 weeks for the bone marrow to recover.

Bone marrow suppression, **stomatitis,** and **alopecia** are produced by the effect of the antibiotic antineoplastics on rapidly proliferating tissues. Because bone marrow, epithelial tissue, and hair follicles have faster growth rates compared to many other body tissues, these cells are more vulnerable to antineoplastic agents.

Nausea and vomiting may result from the chemical irritation of the emetic center in the brain. Vomiting may also result from psychogenic factors and can be triggered by sights, sounds, and smells experienced during chemotherapy. This is known as anticipatory emesis. (For more information, see the introduction to this unit.)

All antibiotic antineoplastic agents except bleomycin and pentostatin produce severe tissue damage if extravasated. Yet **extravasation** can occur with even the most careful administration.

Bleomycin may produce fever and chills. If these effects become intense, the patient should receive immediate treatment with antihistamines and antipyretics. Patients who develop fever and chills with bleomycin therapy must receive premedication with antihistamines and antipyretics before each bleomycin administration. Bleomycin can result in irreversible pulmonary fibrosis, but this effect is rare, usually affecting patients over age 70 who have received more than the recommended lifetime dosage of 400 units. About 50% of patients receiving bleomycin develop a skin toxicity after receiving 150 to 200 units. Toxicity begins with urticaria and may also produce hyperpigmentation. Anaphylactic reactions have been reported in 1% of patients receiving bleomycin for lymphoma. Therefore, test doses should be given.

The anthracycline antibiotic antineoplastics (daunorubicin, doxorubicin, idarubicin, and mitoxantrone) may cause irreversible cardiomyopathy. These effects are cumulative, dose-related, and irreversible. The potential for cardiomyopathy increases as the patient approaches the lifetime dosage of 550 mg/m^2 or 450 mg/m^2 if previous history of radiation therapy to the chest. Therefore, total lifetime dosages are limited to prevent these effects. These drugs may also produce acute electrocardiogram (ECG) changes.

Dactinomycin and doxorubicin may potentiate the effects of radiation therapy and cause hyperpigmentation of the irradiated area or increased stomatitis or enteritis. Doxorubicin may color the urine red; mitoxantrone may color it blue-green.

Although uncommon, mitomycin may cause renal or pulmonary toxicity. Pain (such as abdominal, back, eye, or ear pain) has been reported in at least 11% of patients receiving pentostatin during clinical trials.

Plicamycin may produce bleeding diathesis, which may be dose-related. Bleeding diathesis may include epistaxis, hematemesis, hemoptysis, ecchymoses, and prolonged clotting and bleeding times. Plicamycin may also produce hypotension and nephrotoxicity.

NURSING PROCESS APPLICATION

The following information assists the nurse in caring for a patient receiving an antibiotic antineoplastic agent. It includes an overview of assessment activities as well as examples of appropriate nursing diagnoses and related interventions (see "Planning and implementation"). It also highlights the importance of evaluation.

Assessment

Before drug therapy begins, review the patient's history for conditions that contraindicate or require cautious use of the prescribed antibiotic antineoplastic agent. Also review the patient's medication history to identify use of drugs that may interact with pentostatin or idarubicin, if prescribed. During therapy, assess the patient for adverse drug reactions and signs of drug interactions. Also, periodically assess the effectiveness of therapy with the antibiotic antineoplastic agent. Finally, evaluate the patient's and family's knowledge about the prescribed drug. (See Patient Teaching: *Microbial tumoricidal agents.*)

Nursing diagnoses

- Risk for injury related to a preexisting condition that contraindicates or requires the cautious use of an antibiotic antineoplastic agent
- Risk for injury related to adverse drug reactions or drug interactions
- Knowledge deficit related to the prescribed antibiotic antineoplastic agent

Planning and implementation

- Do not administer an antibiotic antineoplastic agent to a patient with a condition that contraindicates its use.
- Administer an antibiotic antineoplastic agent cautiously to a patient at risk because of a preexisting condition.
- Monitor the patient for adverse reactions and drug interactions during antibiotic antineoplastic therapy.

* ***Monitor the patient for bone marrow suppression during treatment with any antibiotic antineoplastic except bleomycin.*** Expect acute complications when the absolute **granulocyte** count is below 1,000/mm^3. As the count declines, encourage the patient to maintain adequate nutritional and fluid intake. During the **nadir,** the patient should avoid crowds and anyone with an active contagious infection.

* ***Monitor the hematocrit and the platelet count to detect anemia or thrombocytopenia from bone marrow suppression.*** Because red blood cells (RBCs) have a longer life than white blood cells (WBCs) and platelets, anemia usually does not occur unless the patient has an occult or overt blood loss. When the platelet count is lower than 50,000 mm^3, take additional safety precautions such as avoiding intramuscular injections to prevent trauma. Supportive platelet transfusions and packed RBCs may be administered as prescribed.

- Use extreme caution when administering dactinomycin, daunorubicin, doxorubicin, idarubicin, mitomycin, mitoxantrone, and plicamycin because they are powerful **vesicants.** Vesicants are given most safely via I.V. push into the side port of a freely infusing I.V. line, which enables close supervision of the site throughout administration.
- Stop the infusion immediately and notify the physician if infiltration or extravasation is suspected. Apply cold compresses and elevate the affected extremity. To decrease tissue damage, instill hydrocortisone as prescribed into the affected site via an I.V. catheter, subcutaneous injection, or as indicated by health care facility protocol.
- Consult the physician before initiating scalp hypothermia to decrease alopecia because the procedure is not appropriate for every patient. If appropriate, cool the scalp for 15 to 30 minutes before drug administration, and continue to cool it for 15 to 30 minutes after administration. The use of scalp hypothermia is indicated for a patient receiving a drug with an immediate onset of action, peak concentration, and short duration of action.
- Controversy exists over the use of scalp hypothermia because it may create a sanctuary for micrometastasis of the scalp.

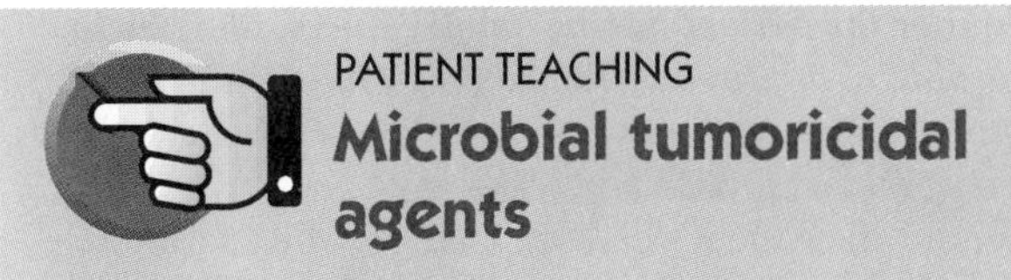

PATIENT TEACHING

Microbial tumoricidal agents

- Teach the patient and family the name, dose, frequency, action, and adverse effects of the prescribed antibiotic antineoplastic agent.
- Instruct the patient to watch for, recognize, and immediately report signs or symptoms of infection, such as fever or sore throat. Also teach this to the hospitalized patient who is at risk for contracting an infection from altered skin integrity, such hospital procedures as venipunctures, or urinary drainage devices.
- Teach the patient to use bleeding precautions and energy conservation measures if needed.
- Instruct the patient to alert the nurse if pain or discomfort occurs at the infusion site during drug administration.
- Teach the patient how to manage troublesome adverse reactions, such as nausea, vomiting, and stomatitis.
- Provide information and support for the patient with alopecia. Inform the patient that the hair loss is temporary, but that hair regrowth may be a different color or texture.
- Teach the patient to recognize the signs and symptoms of pulmonary fibrosis and interstitial pneumonia, such as dry, unproductive cough and dyspnea.
- Instruct the patient receiving bleomycin to take a temperature at home. Stress the importance of reporting fever and chills to the physician.
- Advise the patient receiving bleomycin to report urticaria or hyperpigmentation — possible signs of skin toxicity.
- Teach the patient receiving daunorubicin, doxorubicin, idarubicin, or mitoxantrone to recognize and report the signs and symptoms of heart failure.
- Inform the patient that localized hyperpigmentation and increased stomatitis or enteritis may occur during concomitant therapy with dactinomycin or doxorubicin and radiation therapy.
- Advise the patient to alert the physician if pain occurs during pentostatin therapy.
- Teach the patient receiving plicamycin to watch for — and immediately report — epistaxis, hematemesis, hemoptysis, or ecchymoses.
- Stress the importance of returning for follow-up blood tests.
- Inform the patient that doxorubicin may cause a temporary red coloration of urine; mitoxantrone, a temporary blue-green coloration.
- Give the patient printed information about the prescribed antibiotic antineoplastic agent for home reference.
- Instruct the patient to notify the physician if adverse reactions occur.

**** Monitor the patient during daunorubicin, idarubicin, doxorubicin, or mitoxantrone therapy for signs of heart failure. If the patient exhibits any of these signs, withhold the drug and notify the physician.***

- Monitor the patient's ECG for changes when administering daunorubicin, doxorubicin, idarubicin, or mitoxantrone.
- Monitor the results of pulmonary function studies and chest X-rays for evidence of pulmonary fibrosis in a patient receiving bleomycin (especially if the patient is over age 70 or has received more than 400 units) or mitomycin.
- Monitor the results of baseline and periodic multiple-gated acquisition scans, especially in patients with known cardiac history.

**** Ensure that the patient with lymphoma receives two test doses of 2 to 5 units before the initial dose of bleomycin to identify drug hypersensitivity, which can help prevent an anaphylactic reaction.***

- Ensure that a patient receiving pentostatin receives 500 to 1,000 ml of dextrose 5% in water (D_5W) and 0.9% sodium chloride (normal saline) solution or an equivalent before pentostatin administration and an additional 500 ml of D_5W or equivalent after pentostatin administration to ensure adequate hydration.
- Use other appropriate nursing interventions for a patient with bone marrow suppression, nausea, or vomiting.
- Notify the physician if other adverse reactions occur.

Evaluation

For each nursing diagnosis, prepare an evaluation statement that describes the patient's or family's response to nursing interventions.

CHAPTER SUMMARY

Chapter 55 presented the antibiotic antineoplastic agents. Here are the chapter highlights.

The antibiotic antineoplastic agents include bleomycin, dactinomycin, daunorubicin, doxorubicin, idarubicin, mitomycin, mitoxantrone, pentostatin, and plicamycin.

These drugs are used alone or in combination with other antineoplastic drugs to treat various malignant neoplasms, including Hodgkin's disease, malignant lymphoma, testicular carcinoma, Wilms' tumor, rhabdomyosarcoma, Ewing's sarcoma, acute leukemias, and breast, bladder, lung, and GI tract carcinomas.

The most common adverse reactions to the antibiotic antineoplastic agents include bone marrow suppression, alopecia, nausea, and vomiting.

Except for bleomycin and pentostatin, all antibiotic antineoplastics can cause severe tissue damage if extravasated.

Daunorubicin, doxorubicin, idarubicin, and mitoxantrone may cause cardiomyopathy; bleomycin may produce pulmonary fibrosis. These effects are cumulative, dose-related, and irreversible. Therefore, total lifetime dosages of these drugs are limited to prevent these effects.

Using the nursing process, the nurse helps the patient cope with chemotherapy through careful drug administration, patient teaching, and interventions to minimize adverse reactions.

Questions to consider

See Appendix 1 for answers.

1. Martha Franklin, age 48, has squamous cell carcinoma of the esophagus and is receiving bleomycin. Before administering bleomycin to Ms. Franklin, the nurse administers an antihistamine and an antipyretic, as prescribed. Why?
   (a) To prevent anaphylactic shock
   (b) To prevent bone marrow suppression
   (c) To sedate the patient
   (d) To prevent fever and chills

2. Gerald Holmes, age 68, has a malignant lymphoma and is receiving combination chemotherapy with doxorubicin (Adramycin PFS), cyclophosphamide (Cytoxan), and cisplatin (Platinol). How does doxorubicin exert its cytotoxic effects?
   (a) It prevents DNA synthesis.
   (b) It prevents RNA synthesis.
   (c) It disrupts protein synthesis.
   (d) It intercalates between DNA molecules.

3. Shortly after beginning doxorubicin administration, the nurse notices a slight puffiness near the I.V. insertion site. Which of the following steps should the nurse take *immediately?*
   (a) Stop the infusion.
   (b) Apply a heat pack.
   (c) Administer the antidote.
   (d) Remove the I.V. catheter.

4. Martin Magee, age 63, is receiving idarubicin for the treatment of his acute myeloid leukemia. Which of the following organ specific toxicities is associated with the drug?
   (a) Cardiotoxicity
   (b) Pulmonary fibrosis
   (c) Nephrotoxicity
   (d) Skin toxicity

56 Hormonal antineoplastic agents

OBJECTIVES

After reading and studying this chapter, the student should be able to:
1. describe how each group of hormonal antineoplastic agents works to inhibit malignant growth.
2. differentiate among the specific indications for each group of hormonal antineoplastic agents.
3. identify the major adverse reactions to each group of hormonal antineoplastic agents.
4. describe how to apply the nursing process when caring for a patient who is receiving a hormonal antineoplastic agent.

INTRODUCTION

Hormonal antineoplastic agents are prescribed to alter the growth of malignant **neoplasms** or to manage and treat their physiologic effects. Hormonal therapies prove effective against hormone-dependent **tumors,** such as **cancers** of the prostate, breast, and endometrium. **Lymphomas** and **leukemias** are usually treated with therapies that include corticosteroids because of their potential for affecting lymphocytes. (See *Selected major hormonal antineoplastic agents,* pages 672 and 673.)

Drugs covered in this chapter include:

- aminoglutethimide
- anastrozole
- bicalutamide
- chlorotrianisene
- conjugated estrogens
- dexamethasone
- diethylstilbestrol (DES)
- diethylstilbestrol diphosphate
- ethinyl estradiol
- fluoxymesterone
- flutamide
- goserelin acetate
- hydrocortisone
- hydroxyprogesterone caproate
- leuprolide acetate
- medroxyprogesterone acetate
- megestrol acetate
- methylprednisolone
- nilutamide
- prednisone
- prednisolone
- tamoxifen citrate
- testolactone
- testosterone enantrate
- testosterone propionate.

Estrogens

Estrogens used to treat neoplastic disease include chlorotrianisene, conjugated estrogens, diethylstilbestrol, diethylstilbestrol diphosphate, and ethinyl estradiol.

PHARMACOKINETICS

The estrogens are absorbed readily and rapidly after oral and topical administration. They are distributed well throughout the body. Metabolized in the liver, estrogens undergo enterohepatic recirculation. After conjugation, the estrogens are primarily excreted in the urine. Because estrogens have a slow onset of action, they must be administered for 2 to 3 months before they achieve maximum therapeutic effect.

Route	Onset	Peak	Duration
P.O., I.M., I.V.	Unknown	Unknown	Unknown

PHARMACODYNAMICS

The estrogens act on tumor cells to inhibit hormone-mediated growth. However, their antitumor mechanism of action is not understood completely. The estrogen binds to a receptor on the cell membrane; then this complex is translocated to the nucleus, where it may modulate cell growth. In postmenopausal women with breast cancer, exogenous estrogens may displace endogenous growth-enhancing estrogens from their receptors. Researchers have not discovered how high dosages of estrogens paradoxically inhibit estrogen production. In men with prostate cancer, estrogens act on the pituitary to suppress secretion of luteinizing hormone (LH), which in turn decreases testicular androgen secretion.

PHARMACOTHERAPEUTICS

Estrogen therapy is used as a **palliative** treatment for metastatic breast cancer in postmenopausal women and for metastatic prostate cancer in men. Breast cancer tumor cells that are estrogen receptor–positive respond more to hormonal therapy than those that are not. The average duration of **remission** induced by hormonal therapy is 6 to 12 months.

Selected major hormonal antineoplastic agents

This chart summarizes the major hormonal antineoplastic agents currently in clinical use.

DRUG	MAJOR INDICATIONS AND USUAL DOSAGES	CONTRAINDICATIONS AND PRECAUTIONS
Estrogens		
diethylstilbestrol (DES)	*Metastatic breast cancer in postmenopausal women* ADULT: 5 to 15 mg P.O. daily *Prostate cancer* ADULT: 1 to 3 mg P.O. daily	• DES is contraindicated in a pregnant patient or one with known or suspected breast cancer (except in selected patients being treated for metastatic disease), estrogen-dependent neoplasia, undiagnosed abnormal genital bleeding, active thrombophlebitis or thromboembolic disorder, or history of thrombophlebitis, thrombosis, or thromboembolic disorder associated with previous use of estrogen (except when used to treat breast or prostate cancer). • This drug requires cautious use in a depressed patient or one with epilepsy, migraine headache, cardiac or renal dysfunction, impaired liver function, or metabolic bone disease associated with hypercalcemia.
Antiestrogens		
tamoxifen (Nolvadex)	*Metastatic breast cancer that is estrogen receptor–positive, especially in postmenopausal women; adjunct to surgery in postmenopausal women with axillary lymph nodes that harbor cancer cells and estrogen receptor–positive tumors* ADULT: 10 to 20 mg P.O. b.i.d.	• Tamoxifen is contraindicated in a pregnant or breast-feeding patient or one with known hypersensitivity. • This drug requires cautious use in a patient with leukopenia or thrombocytopenia.
Androgens		
fluoxymesterone (Halotestin)	*Metastatic breast cancer* ADULT: 10 to 40 mg P.O. daily in divided doses	• Fluoxymesterone is contraindicated in a pregnant or breast-feeding patient, a male patient with breast or prostate cancer, or one with known hypersensitivity or serious cardiac, hepatic, or renal disease. • This drug requires cautious use in a patient with benign prostatic hyperplasia.
Antiandrogens		
flutamide (Eulexin)	*Adjunct therapy in managing metastatic prostate cancer* ADULT: 250 mg P.O. every 8 hours	• Flutamide is contraindicated in a pregnant patient or one with known hypersensitivity. • This drug requires cautious use in a patient with impaired liver function.
Adrenocortical suppressants		
aminoglutethimide (Cytadren)	*Hormonally responsive skin, soft-tissue, and bone lesions; metastatic breast and prostate cancer* ADULT: 250 mg P.O. t.i.d., may be increased up to a maximum of 2 g daily	• Aminoglutethimide is contraindicated in a pregnant or breast-feeding patient or one with known hypersensitivity to the drug or glutethimide. • This drug has no known precautions. • Safety and efficacy in children have not been established.
Progestins		
medroxyprogesterone (Depo-Provera)	*Advanced endometrial or renal cancer* ADULT: 400 to 1,000 mg I.M. weekly	• Medroxyprogesterone is contraindicated in a patient with known hypersensitivity, thrombophlebitis, thromboembolic disorder, cerebral apoplexy, breast cancer (except for palliative therapy), undiagnosed vaginal bleeding, or missed abortion. • This drug requires cautious use in a depressed patient or one with epilepsy, migraine headache, asthma, cardiac dysfunction, renal dysfunction (except for palliative therapy for renal cancer), or diabetes mellitus.

Selected major hormonal antineoplastic agents *(continued)*

DRUG	MAJOR INDICATIONS AND USUAL DOSAGES	CONTRAINDICATIONS AND PRECAUTIONS
Corticosteroids		
hydrocortisone (Cortef)	*Adjunct therapy with aminoglutethimide, replacement therapy after adrenalectomy* ADULT: 20 to 30 mg P.O. daily	• Hydrocortisone is contraindicated in a patient with a systemic fungal infection or known hypersensitivity. • This drug requires cautious use in an emotionally unstable or psychotic patient or one with gastrointestinal ulceration, renal disease, hypertension, osteoporosis, varicella infections, vaccinia, exanthema, diabetes mellitus, hypothyroidism, thromboembolic disorder, seizures, myasthenia gravis, heart failure, tuberculosis, ocular herpes simplex, or hypoalbuminemia.
Gonadotropin-releasing hormone analogues		
leuprolide (Lupron)	*Advanced prostate cancer* ADULT: 7.5 mg I.M. monthly	• Leuprolide is contraindicated in a patient with known hypersensitivity or in a female patient who is or may become pregnant while receiving the drug. • This drug requires cautious use in a patient with hypersensitivity to benzyl alcohol (a preservative used in some formulations), one with metastatic vertebral lesions, or urinary tract obstruction.

Drug interactions

Few significant drug interactions occur with the estrogens.

ADVERSE DRUG REACTIONS

Most adverse reactions to estrogens are extensions of their natural hormonal activities. They may cause mild nausea, which is more pronounced in women, who usually receive higher dosages. Abdominal cramps, irritability, and frequent urination may also occur.

Estrogen therapy causes feminization in men, primarily manifested by mammary gland development (gynecomastia) and impotence. Women may experience decreased libido and breast tenderness. Almost all patients display increased pigmentation of the nipples and areolae.

Estrogens may produce some adverse cardiovascular reactions, such as hypertension. High dosages of estrogens predispose patients to an increased risk of thromboembolic complications, including pulmonary embolus, myocardial infarction, and cerebrovascular accident. Estrogens may also alter liver function tests.

Several endocrine and metabolic complications can develop during estrogen therapy. Patients may develop decreased glucose tolerance, increased serum triglyceride level, or both. Sodium retention and resulting fluid retention can occur as dose-dependent adverse reactions. Fluid retention can prove extremely serious for patients with heart failure. Patients, especially those with metastatic bone disease, may also develop hypercalcemia. Uterine breakthrough bleeding can occur in postmenopausal women. Patients with metastatic breast cancer may experience a flare of metastatic lesions, manifested by increased skin nodules or worsening bone pain.

NURSING PROCESS APPLICATION

The following information assists the nurse in caring for a patient receiving an estrogen. It includes an overview of assessment activities as well as examples of appropriate nursing diagnoses and related interventions (see "Planning and implementation"). It also highlights the importance of evaluation.

Assessment

Before drug therapy begins, review the patient's history for conditions that contraindicate or require cautious use of the prescribed estrogen. During therapy, assess the patient for adverse drug reactions. Also, periodically assess the effectiveness of estrogen therapy. Finally, evaluate the patient's and family's knowledge about the prescribed drug.

Nursing diagnoses

- Risk for injury related to a preexisting condition that contraindicates or requires cautious use of an estrogen
- Risk for injury related to adverse drug reactions
- Fluid volume excess related to sodium and fluid retention caused by an estrogen
- Knowledge deficit related to the prescribed estrogen

Planning and implementation

- Do not administer an estrogen to a patient with a condition that contraindicates its use.

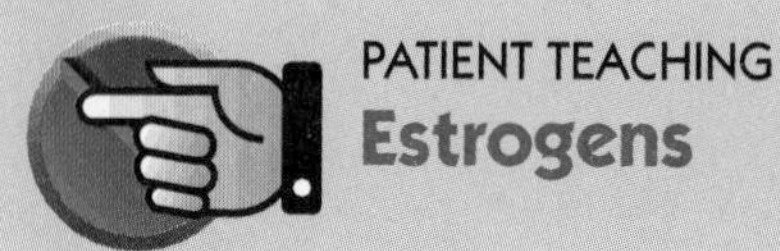

PATIENT TEACHING
Estrogens

- Teach the patient and family the name, dose, frequency, action, and adverse effects of the prescribed estrogen.
- Inform the patient of the possibility of fluid retention and explain how to observe for edema, especially of the hands, ankles, tibia, and sacrum. Advise the patient to restrict sodium intake and measure body weight daily. Instruct the patient to report sudden weight gain or signs of fluid retention.
- Inform a female patient that breakthrough uterine bleeding is not normal, and instruct her to report uterine bleeding to the physician. Also explain that she may notice breast tenderness during therapy.
- Provide emotional support for a male patient undergoing estrogen therapy, especially if it affects sexual characteristics. Reassure the patient that estrogen may cause temporary gynecomastia and impotence, which disappear after therapy ends.
- Inform a female patient that decreased libido may occur during estrogen therapy.
- Instruct the patient to report nausea so that symptomatic treatment may begin. Encourage the patient to eat frequent small meals and increase carbohydrate intake. Reassure the patient that nausea usually disappears after 2 to 3 weeks of therapy.
- Teach the patient and family to recognize the signs and symptoms of hypercalcemia, such as anorexia, nausea, vomiting, lethargy, and polyuria, because the combined effect of estrogen therapy and bone metastasis may produce this imbalance.
- Advise the patient that thromboembolism may occur with long-term use of high-dose estrogens. Instruct the patient to avoid wearing restrictive clothing and sitting for long periods with the legs crossed.
- Reassure the patient that increased pigmentation of the nipples and areolae may occur, but that it is harmless.
- Inform the patient with breast cancer that metastatic lesions may experience flare, causing increased skin nodules or bone pain. If this occurs, advise the patient to request additional analgesics to ease the pain.
- Instruct the patient to notify the physician if adverse reactions occur.

• Administer an estrogen cautiously to a patient at risk because of a preexisting condition.
• Monitor the patient for adverse reactions during estrogen therapy.
• Monitor hydration if the patient experiences nausea or frequent urination. Administer an antiemetic as prescribed. If nausea persists, expect a change in therapy.
• Monitor the patient's serum calcium level monthly, as prescribed. Mobilize the patient and maintain adequate hydration.
• Monitor the patient's liver function studies and blood glucose and triglyceride levels. Note abnormalities that suggest an endocrine or metabolic disorder.
• Administer an analgesic as prescribed if bone pain worsens during estrogen therapy.
Monitor the patient for symptoms of thromboembolism, such as sudden onset of shortness of breath, partial or complete vision loss, headache, and local pain, tenderness, and swelling in the extremities.
• Notify the physician if adverse reactions occur.
Monitor the patient for signs and symptoms of fluid retention, especially if the patient has heart failure. Assess the patient's vital signs frequently.
• Weigh the patient daily at the same time with the same scale and wearing the same amount of clothing to detect sudden weight gain. (See Patient Teaching: *Estrogens.*)
• Document the patient's fluid intake and output.
• Restrict the patient's sodium intake as prescribed.
• Report fluid retention to the physician.

Evaluation

For each nursing diagnosis, prepare an evaluation statement that describes the patient's or family's response to nursing interventions.

Antiestrogens

The antiestrogen tamoxifen citrate is the drug of choice for advanced breast cancer involving estrogen receptor–positive tumors in postmenopausal women.

PHARMACOKINETICS

After oral administration, tamoxifen is absorbed well and undergoes extensive hepatic metabolism before fecal excretion. The peak serum concentration level of tamoxifen occurs in 3 to 6 hours after an oral dose. The half-life of the drug is approximately 7 days. A steady state blood concentration is achieved in 4 weeks. Clinical responses usually occur in 1 to 2 months after therapy is initiated.

Route	Onset	Peak	Duration
P.O.	Rapid	3-6 hr	7 days

PHARMACODYNAMICS

Estrogen receptors, found in the cancer cells of 50% of premenopausal and 75% of postmenopausal women with breast cancer, respond to estrogen to induce tumor growth. The antiestrogen tamoxifen binds to the estrogen receptors and inhibits estrogen-mediated tumor growth. The inhibition may result because tamoxifen binds to receptors at the nuclear level or because the binding reduces the number of free receptors in the cytoplasm. Ultimately, deoxyribonucleic acid (DNA) synthesis and cell growth are inhibited.

PHARMACOTHERAPEUTICS

The antiestrogen tamoxifen is used in the palliative treatment of metastatic breast cancer that is estrogen receptor–positive. Tumors in postmenopausal women are more responsive to tamoxifen than those in premenopausal women. Tamoxifen may also be used as an adjunct to surgery in postmenopausal women with axillary lymph nodes that contain cancer cells and estrogen receptor–positive tumors. The drug should not be used concomitantly with other **cytotoxic** drugs due to a reduction in the efficacy of tamoxifen when this is done.

Drug interactions

Tamoxifen increases the effects of warfarin sodium. Bromocriptine increases the effects of tamoxifen.

ADVERSE DRUG REACTIONS

Tamoxifen is a relatively nontoxic drug. The most common adverse reactions include hot flashes, nausea, and vomiting. Transient mild **leukopenia** or **thrombocytopenia** occurs in about 4% of patients. In patients with bone metastasis, hypercalcemia may occur.

About 1% of patients treated with tamoxifen may experience tumor flare, which may increase the number and size of lesions or increase bone pain; however, this reaction subsides quickly. Patients receiving high dosages of tamoxifen have experienced ocular lesions, retinopathy, and superficial corneal opacity — all reduce visual acuity.

NURSING PROCESS APPLICATION

The following information assists the nurse in caring for a patient receiving tamoxifen. It includes an overview of assessment activities as well as examples of appropriate nursing diagnoses and related interventions (see "Planning and implementation"). It also highlights the importance of evaluation.

Assessment

Before drug therapy begins, review the patient's history for conditions that contraindicate or require cautious use of tamoxifen. During therapy, assess the patient for adverse drug reactions. Also, periodically assess the effectiveness of tamoxifen therapy. Finally, evaluate the patient's and family's knowledge about the prescribed drug.

Nursing diagnoses

- Risk for injury related to a preexisting condition that contraindicates or requires cautious use of tamoxifen
- Risk for injury related to adverse drug reactions
- Sensory or perceptual alterations (visual) related to vision disturbances caused by tamoxifen
- Knowledge deficit related to tamoxifen
- Pain related to tumor flare caused by tamoxifen

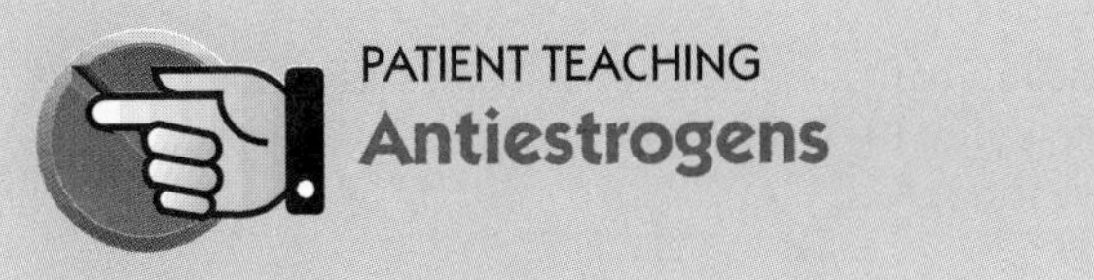

PATIENT TEACHING

Antiestrogens

- Teach the patient and family the name, dose, frequency, action, and adverse effects of tamoxifen.
- Inform the patient that hot flashes, nausea, and occasional vomiting are the most common adverse reactions to tamoxifen, and teach the patient how to manage them at home. Explain that tolerance to these symptoms usually develops rapidly.
- Instruct the patient to report immediately to the physician decreased visual acuity; it may be irreversible. Inform the patient of the need for routine eye examinations by an ophthalmologist, who should be informed about the tamoxifen therapy.
- Assure the patient and family that tumor flare is an expected adverse reaction that will subside. Advise the patient to request increased analgesics in the meantime.
- Instruct the patient to store tamoxifen at room temperature and protect it from light.
- Stress the importance of having follow-up blood tests done.
- Instruct the patient to inform the physician if adverse reactions occur.

Planning and implementation

- Do not administer tamoxifen to a patient with a condition that contraindicates its use.
- Administer tamoxifen cautiously to a patient at risk because of a preexisting condition.
- Monitor the patient for adverse reactions during tamoxifen therapy.
- Monitor hydration if the patient experiences nausea and vomiting during tamoxifen therapy. Administer an antiemetic as prescribed.
- Monitor the patient's white blood cell (WBC) and platelet counts regularly for mild leukopenia or thrombocytopenia. For a patient with bone metastasis, monitor the serum calcium level to detect hypercalcemia.

* ***Observe the patient for signs of tamoxifen-induced tumor flare, such as increased number and size of lesions or increased bone pain. Administer additional analgesics as prescribed.***

- Store tamoxifen tablets at room temperature and protect them from light.
- Notify the physician if adverse reactions occur.

* ***Monitor the patient for decreased visual acuity. High dosages of tamoxifen may produce ocular lesions, retinopathy, and superficial corneal opacity.***

- Schedule the patient for regular eye examinations by an ophthalmologist during tamoxifen therapy. (See Patient Teaching: *Antiestrogens.*)
- Report vision changes to the physician because the drug may need to be discontinued.
- Schedule the patient for yearly gynecological examinations and pap smears.

Evaluation

For each nursing diagnosis, prepare an evaluation statement that describes the patient's or family's response to nursing interventions.

Androgens

The therapeutically useful androgens are synthetic derivatives of naturally occurring testosterone. They include fluoxymesterone, testolactone, testosterone enanthate, and testosterone propionate.

PHARMACOKINETICS

The pharmacokinetic properties of therapeutic androgens resemble those of naturally occurring testosterone. The oral androgens, fluoxymesterone and testolactone, are absorbed well. The parenteral ones, testosterone enanthate and testosterone propionate, are designed specifically for slow absorption. Androgens are distributed well throughout the body and metabolized extensively in the liver, where they are conjugated primarily to the glucuronide. They are excreted in the urine.

The onsets of action of androgens are slow. The oral agents have a short duration of action and require daily dosing. The duration of the parenteral forms is longer because the oil suspension is absorbed slowly. Parenteral androgens are administered one to three times weekly.

Route	Onset	Peak	Duration
P.O., I.M.	Variable	Unknown	Unknown

PHARMACODYNAMICS

Androgens probably act via one or more mechanisms. They may reduce the number of prolactin receptors or may bind competitively to those that are available. Also, androgens may inhibit estrogen synthesis or competitively bind at estrogen receptors. These actions prevent estrogen from affecting estrogen-sensitive tumors.

PHARMACOTHERAPEUTICS

Androgens are indicated for the palliative treatment of advanced breast cancer, particularly in postmenopausal women with bone metastasis. Because of their easy administration, the oral agents are used more commonly than the parenteral agents.

Drug interactions

No drug interactions have been identified for the androgens.

ADVERSE DRUG REACTIONS

Dose-related nausea and vomiting are the most common adverse reactions to androgens. Fluid retention caused by sodium retention may also occur. A female patient may develop masculine characteristics, including increased facial hair, acne, clitoral hypertrophy, increased libido, and a deeper voice.

Prolonged high dosages of androgens have produced jaundice, which may limit the use of these drugs in patients with liver dysfunction. Also, patients with bone metastasis are at greater risk for developing hypercalcemia during prolonged androgen therapy.

NURSING PROCESS APPLICATION

The following information assists the nurse in caring for a patient receiving an androgen. It includes an overview of assessment activities as well as examples of appropriate nursing diagnoses and related interventions (see "Planning and implementation"). It also highlights the importance of evaluation.

Assessment

Before drug therapy begins, review the patient's history for conditions that contraindicate or require cautious use of the prescribed androgen. During therapy, assess the patient for adverse drug reactions. Also, periodically assess the effectiveness of androgen therapy. Finally, evaluate the patient's and family's knowledge about the prescribed drug.

Nursing diagnoses

- Risk for injury related to a preexisting condition that contraindicates or requires cautious use of an androgen
- Risk for injury related to adverse drug reactions
- Altered health maintenance related to hypercalcemia caused by prolonged androgen therapy
- Knowledge deficit related to the prescribed androgen

Planning and implementation

- Do not administer an androgen to a patient with a condition that contraindicates its use.
- Administer an androgen cautiously to a patient at risk because of a preexisting condition.
- Monitor the patient for adverse reactions during androgen therapy.
- Monitor hydration if the patient experiences nausea and vomiting during androgen therapy. Administer an antiemetic before meals as prescribed.

∗ ***Monitor the patient for signs and symptoms of fluid retention. Be especially alert for these signs in a patient with a history of heart failure. If fluid retention occurs, restrict the patient's fluid intake to about six 8-oz (240-ml) glasses daily and the sodium intake to 2 g as prescribed.***

- Monitor the results of liver function studies for a patient receiving prolonged high dosages of an androgen. Also monitor the patient for signs and symptoms of jaundice.

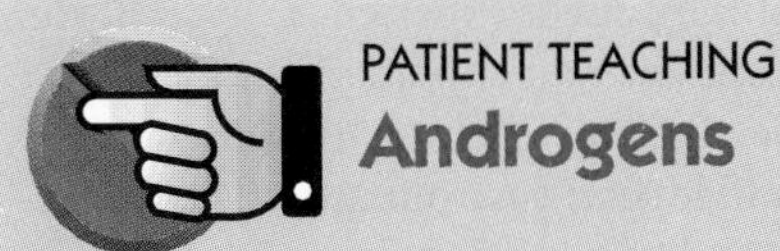

PATIENT TEACHING
Androgens

- Teach the patient and family the name, dose, frequency, action, and adverse effects of the prescribed androgen.
- Inform the patient that systemic reactions to the androgen include fluid retention, nausea, and vomiting. Teach the patient to recognize signs and symptoms and to report them to the physician. Instruct the patient to measure body weight daily and to restrict sodium and fluid intake if fluid retention occurs. If nausea and vomiting occur, advise the patient to request an antiemetic and take it before meals as prescribed.
- Inform the female patient well in advance about potential virilization and provide emotional support. Prolonged androgen therapy can cause hirsutism, mild scalp hair loss, a deeper voice, facial acne, clitoral enlargement, increased libido, and breast regression. If therapy is discontinued at the onset of virilization, the conditions may disappear. If therapy is continued, the conditions may become irreversible.
- Teach the patient to recognize the signs and symptoms of jaundice, including yellowed skin or sclera, darkened urine, clay-colored stools, and pruritus, and to report any of these signs and symptoms immediately to the physician.
- Teach the patient and family members to recognize and report the signs and symptoms of hypercalcemia, including anorexia, nausea, vomiting, lethargy, and polyuria. Explain that these signs and symptoms may be caused by a treatable complication.
- Instruct the patient to notify the physician if adverse reactions occur.

***** ***Use extreme caution with intramuscular (I.M.) injections to avoid inadvertent intravenous (I.V.) or subcutaneous (S.C.) injection. Because I.M. preparations are oil suspensions, a serious oil embolism can occur if an I.M. androgen is administered into a vein.***

***** ***Use a 1″ needle to administer an androgen intramuscularly, and inject the drug deeply into muscle tissue. If irritation or inflammation develops, apply ice for comfort.***

- Notify the physician immediately if adverse reactions occur.
- Monitor the patient's serum calcium level monthly, as prescribed, for hypercalcemia. This adverse reaction is more common in patients with bone metastasis receiving prolonged androgen therapy.
- Prevent hypercalcemia by mobilizing the patient as much as possible and maintaining adequate hydration. Limiting dietary calcium intake does not have a significant effect on the serum calcium level. (See Patient Teaching: *Androgens.*)
- Notify the physician if hypercalcemia occurs.

Evaluation

For each nursing diagnosis, prepare an evaluation statement that describes the patient's or family's response to nursing interventions.

Antiandrogens

The antiandrogens flutamide, nilutamide and bicalutamide are used as an adjunct therapy with gonadotropin-releasing hormone analogues in treating advanced prostate cancer.

PHARMACOKINETICS

After oral administration, the antiandrogens are absorbed rapidly and completely. They are metabolized rapidly and extensively and excreted primarily in the urine. The active metabolite of flutamide reaches a peak plasma concentration level in 2 hours and has a half-life of 6 hours. The availability of nilutamide and bicalutamide is inconclusive at this time.

Route	Onset	Peak	Duration
P.O.	Rapid	2 hr	6 hr

PHARMACODYNAMICS

Flutamide, nilutamide and bicalutamide exert their antiandrogenic action by inhibiting androgen uptake or nuclear binding of androgen in target tissues. Prostate cancer cells are androgen-sensitive and respond to treatments that block androgen stimulation.

PHARMACOTHERAPEUTICS

The antiandrogens are used with a gonadotropin-releasing hormone analogue, such as leuprolide, to treat metastatic prostate cancer. Concomitant administration of antiandrogens and a gonadotropin-releasing hormone analogue may help prevent the disease flare that occurs when the gonadotropin-releasing hormone analogue is used alone.

Drug interactions

The antiandrogens do not interact significantly with other drugs.

ADVERSE DRUG REACTIONS

When the antiandrogens are used with a gonadotropin-releasing hormone analogue, the most common adverse reactions are hot flashes, decreased libido, impotence, diarrhea, nausea, vomiting, and gynecomastia. Other adverse reactions include drowsiness, confusion, depression, anxiety, nervousness, photosensitivity, neuromuscular dysfunction, and elevated liver enzyme and serum creatinine levels.

NURSING PROCESS APPLICATION

The following information assists the nurse in caring for a patient receiving antiandrogens. It includes an overview of assessment activities as well as examples of appropriate

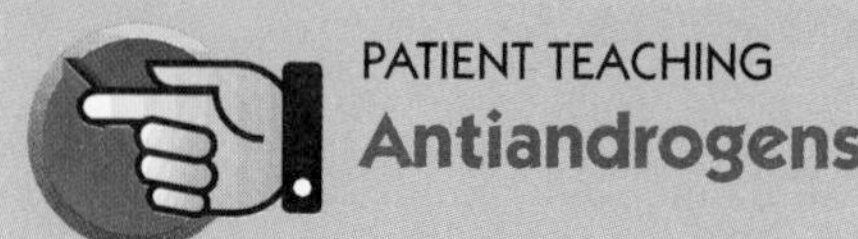

PATIENT TEACHING
Antiandrogens

- Teach the patient and family the name, dose, frequency, action, and adverse effects of flutamide.
- Inform the patient that flutamide and the gonadotropin-releasing hormone analogue are taken together.
- Inform the patient of the potential for hot flashes and sexual dysfunction.
- Advise the patient that gynecomastia may occur.
- Caution the patient not to perform activities that require mental alertness if drowsiness or confusion occurs.
- Inform the patient that anxiety and nervousness can occur and are drug-related.
- Advise the patient to avoid sun exposure whenever possible and to use a sunscreen, hat, and sunglasses if sun exposure cannot be avoided.
- Stress the importance of returning for follow-up blood tests.
- Instruct the patient to notify the physician if adverse reactions occur.

nursing diagnoses and related interventions (see "Planning and implementation"). It also highlights the importance of evaluation.

Assessment
Before drug therapy begins, review the patient's history for conditions that contraindicate or require cautious use of antiandrogens. During therapy, assess the patient for adverse drug reactions. Also, periodically assess the effectiveness of antiandrogen therapy. Finally, evaluate the patient's and family's knowledge about the prescribed drug.

Nursing diagnoses
• Risk for injury related to a preexisting condition that contraindicates or requires cautious use of antiandrogen therapy
• Risk for injury related to adverse drug reactions
• Knowledge deficit related to the antiandrogen therapy

Planning and implementation
• Do not administer antiandrogens to a patient with a condition that contraindicates its use.
• Administer the antiandrogens cautiously to a patient at risk because of a preexisting condition.
• Monitor the patient for adverse reactions during antiandrogen therapy.
*** *Administer an antiandrogen concomitantly with a gonadotropin-releasing hormone analogue as prescribed for maximum effectiveness.***
*** *Monitor the patient's liver enzyme and serum creatinine levels frequently during flutamide and nilutamide therapy. If levels exceed safe ranges, the medications may need to be discontinued.***
• Notify the physician if adverse reactions occur.
• Monitor hydration if the patient experiences nausea, vomiting, and diarrhea. Administer an antiemetic or antidiarrheal as prescribed. (See Patient Teaching: *Antiandrogens.*)
• Notify the physician if adverse gastrointestinal (GI) reactions prevent flutamide administration.

Evaluation
For each nursing diagnosis, prepare an evaluation statement that describes the patient's or family's response to nursing interventions.

Adrenocortical suppressants

The adrenocortical suppressant aminoglutethimide has been proven to be as effective as surgical adrenalectomy in treating advanced breast cancer. Anastrozole has been proven to lower serum estradiol levels.

PHARMACOKINETICS
After oral administration, aminoglutethimide is absorbed adequately and distributed widely into body tissues. About 20% to 25% of the drug binds to plasma proteins. Aminoglutethimide is metabolized in the liver. Approximately 50% of a dose is excreted unchanged in the urine, and 20% to 50% is excreted as metabolites. After oral administration of anastrozole, it is well absorbed systemically. It is chiefly eliminated through the liver.

Data on the onset of action, peak concentration level, and duration of action of aminoglutethimide and anastrozole remain incomplete. The initial plasma half-life of aminoglutethimide is 13 hours, decreasing to 7 hours within 1 to 2 weeks after administration.

Route	Onset	Peak	Duration
P.O.	Unknown	Unknown	Unknown

PHARMACODYNAMICS
Aminoglutethimide acts in the adrenal gland to block the production of cortisol, androgens, and estrogens. In extra-adrenal tissues, it also inhibits the conversion of androgens to estrogens. These actions produce a reversible, chemical adrenalectomy. Anastrozole acts to inhibit aromatase activity, which is a product of breast carcinomas, and thereby reduces estradiole levels.

PHARMACOTHERAPEUTICS
The adrenocortical suppressant aminoglutethimide is used for the palliative treatment of hormonally responsive advanced breast and prostate cancers and Cushing's disease. Because of the compensatory increase in adrenocortico-

tropic hormone release after aminoglutethimide administration, a pituitary-suppressive glucocorticoid such as hydrocortisone must be administered concurrently.
Anastrozole is indicated in the treatment of advanced breast cancer in postmenopausal women with progression following tamoxifen therapy.

Drug interactions

Aminoglutethimide may decrease the efficacy of dexamethasone by inducing its metabolism. Aminoglutethimide may also increase the metabolism of warfarin and thereby reduce its effect. Anastrozole has no significant drug interaction effects.

ADVERSE DRUG REACTIONS

About 50% of patients taking aminoglutethimide experience an adverse reaction that is usually transient. The most common reaction is a rash that appears in the first weeks of treatment and usually disappears after 5 to 8 days. If the rash persists beyond 8 days, the drug should be discontinued. Fatigue, hypotension, drowsiness, and dizziness also may occur.

Rare reactions include leukopenia, thrombocytopenia, nausea, vomiting, and anorexia.

The adverse reactions most closely associated with anastrozole are nausea, vomiting, and anorexia. Hot flashes and headaches are also common. Between 7% and 10% of patients developed peripheral edema.

NURSING PROCESS APPLICATION

The following information assists the nurse in caring for a patient receiving the adrenocortical suppressants. It includes an overview of assessment activities as well as examples of appropriate nursing diagnoses and related interventions (see "Planning and implementation"). It also highlights the importance of evaluation.

Assessment

Before drug therapy begins, review the patient's history for conditions that contraindicate the use of adrenocortical suppressants. Also, review the patient's medication history to identify drugs that may interact with it. During therapy, assess the patient for adverse drug reactions and signs of drug interactions. Also, periodically assess the effectiveness of aminoglutethimide or anastrozole therapy. Finally, evaluate the patient's and family's knowledge about the prescribed drug.

Nursing diagnoses

- Risk for injury related to a preexisting condition that contraindicates the use of aminoglutethimide or anastrozole
- Risk for injury related to adverse drug reactions or drug interactions
- Fatigue related to the adverse effects of aminoglutethimide

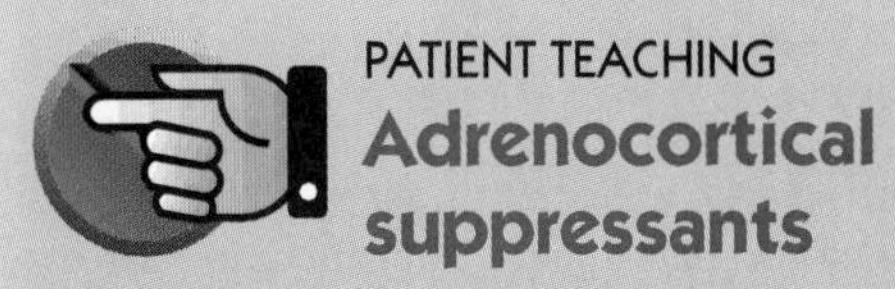

PATIENT TEACHING
Adrenocortical suppressants

- Teach the patient and family the name, dose, frequency, action, and adverse effects of aminoglutethimide.
- Inform the patient that a rash will occur in the first weeks of aminoglutethimide therapy. Advise the patient to notify the physician if it does not disappear or begin to clear within 8 days.
- Teach the patient how to manage troublesome adverse reactions, such as gastrointestinal distress and fatigue.
- Caution the patient to avoid activities that require mental alertness if drowsiness or dizziness occurs.
- Instruct the patient to return for follow-up blood tests. Review infection control measures and bleeding precautions as needed.
- Instruct the patient to notify the physician if adverse reactions occur.

- Knowledge deficit related to aminoglutethimide or anastrozole

Planning and implementation

- Do not administer aminoglutethimide or anastrozole to a patient with a condition that contraindicates its use.
- Monitor the patient for adverse reactions and drug interactions during aminoglutethimide therapy.
- Inspect the patient's skin for a rash, which may appear in the first weeks of therapy. Notify the physician if the rash does not clear after 8 days; the drug should be discontinued. (See Patient Teaching: *Adrenocortical suppressants.*)
- ***Monitor the patient's blood pressure regularly to detect hypotension.***
- ***Monitor the patient's WBC count regularly to detect leukopenia. If leukopenia occurs, monitor the patient for signs of infection. Also, take infection control measures until the WBC count returns to normal.***
- Monitor the patient's platelet count regularly to detect thrombocytopenia. If thrombocytopenia occurs, observe the patient for signs and symptoms of bleeding. Also, take bleeding precautions until the platelet count returns to normal.
- Notify the physician if adverse reactions or drug interactions occur.
- Monitor the patient for fatigue. If fatigue occurs, stagger the patient's activities and encourage frequent rest periods.
- Notify the physician if fatigue becomes severe.

Evaluation

For each nursing diagnosis, prepare an evaluation statement that describes the patient's or family's response to nursing interventions.

Progestins

Progestins are used as palliative treatment of advanced endometrial, breast, and renal cancers. They include hydroxyprogesterone caproate, medroxyprogesterone acetate, and megestrol acetate.

PHARMACOKINETICS

After oral administration, megestrol acetate is absorbed well. After I.M. injection in an aqueous or oil suspension, hydroxyprogesterone caproate and medroxyprogesterone are absorbed slowly from their deposit sites. These drugs are distributed well throughout the body and may sequester in fatty tissue. Progestins are metabolized in the liver and excreted as metabolites in the urine.

Two to three months of progestin therapy may pass before objective responses are observed. These drugs provide varying durations of action, ranging from 1 to 3 days for megestrol, 8 to 14 days for hydroxyprogesterone, and 4 to 6 weeks for medroxyprogesterone.

Route	Onset	Peak	Duration
P.O.	Unknown	Unknown	Variable
I.M.	Unknown	3 wk	Variable

PHARMACODYNAMICS

The antitumor mechanisms of action of the progestins are not understood completely. Researchers believe the drugs bind to a specific receptor to act on hormonally sensitive cells. Because the progestins do not exhibit a cytotoxic activity, they are considered **cytostatic.**

PHARMACOTHERAPEUTICS

The progestins are used for the palliative treatment of advanced endometrial, breast, and renal cancers. Of these agents, megestrol is used most often.

Drug interactions

No drug interactions have been identified for the progestins.

ADVERSE DRUG REACTIONS

Mild fluid retention with accompanying weight gain is probably the most common reaction to progestins. Thromboemboli can develop with the use of progestins and may cause a cerebrovascular accident, pulmonary dysfunction, blocked blood flow to an extremity, and local, superficial tenderness or swelling. Breakthrough bleeding, spotting, changes in menstrual flow, and breast tenderness may also occur with progestins. Liver function abnormalities may also occur.

Oil in the injectable forms can cause oil embolus if the agent is inadvertently injected I.V. With high doses of injected progestins, gluteal abscesses can also occur. Patients who are hypersensitive to the oil carrier used for injection (usually sesame or castor oil) may have a local or systemic hypersensitivity reaction.

NURSING PROCESS APPLICATION

The following information assists the nurse in caring for a patient receiving a progestin. It includes an overview of assessment activities as well as examples of appropriate nursing diagnoses and related interventions (see "Planning and implementation"). It also highlights the importance of evaluation.

Assessment

Before drug therapy begins, review the patient's history for conditions that contraindicate or require cautious use of the prescribed progestin. During therapy, assess the patient for adverse drug reactions. Also, periodically assess the effectiveness of progestin therapy. Finally, evaluate the patient's and family's knowledge about the prescribed drug.

Nursing diagnoses

- Risk for injury related to a preexisting condition that contraindicates or requires cautious use of a progestin
- Risk for injury related to adverse drug reactions
- Altered protection related to a local or systemic hypersensitivity reaction to an oil-based progestin injection
- Knowledge deficit related to the prescribed progestin

Planning and implementation

- Do not administer a progestin to a patient with a condition that contraindicates its use.
- Administer a progestin cautiously to a patient at risk because of a preexisting condition.
- Monitor the patient for adverse reactions during progestin therapy.

∗ ***Do not administer an injectable progestin I.V. The oil in the formulation can cause an oil embolus.***

- Inspect the gluteal injection sites of a parenteral progestin regularly for signs and symptoms of abscess, such as swelling, a fluid-filled sac, and localized pain. If an abscess occurs, avoid injecting the drug into the area, provide such symptomatic relief as the frequent application of warm compresses, and encourage the patient not to put pressure on the site. (See Patient Teaching: *Progestins.*)
- Monitor liver function studies regularly and observe the patient for signs and symptoms of hepatotoxicity.
- Monitor the patient for signs and symptoms of thromboembolism. Notify the physician immediately if thromboembolism is suspected. Expect to begin emergency treatment and anticoagulation therapy as prescribed.
- Notify the physician if other adverse reactions occur.

∗ ***Monitor the patient for local and systemic hypersensitivity reactions regularly. Have standard emergency equip-***

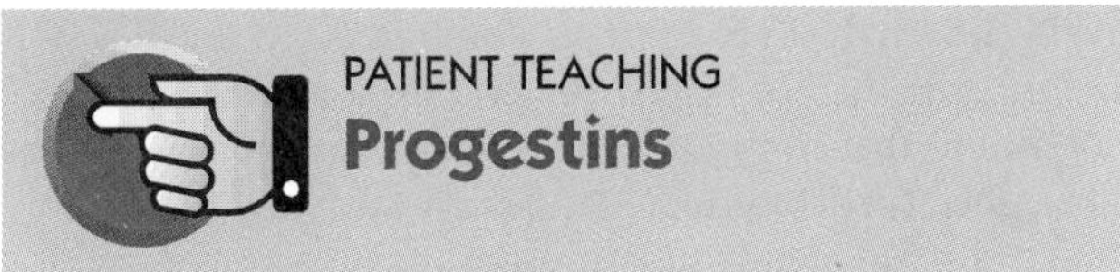

- ➤ Teach the patient and family the name, dose, frequency, action, and adverse effects of the prescribed progestin.
- ➤ Explain the probability of fluid retention to the patient and how to recognize it. Inform the patient that fluid retention from progestin therapy usually is mild and not clinically significant.
- ➤ Teach the patient to recognize and immediately report the signs and symptoms of thromboembolism.
- ➤ Explain that jaundice may indicate hepatotoxicity. Instruct the patient to immediately report yellowed skin or sclera, dark-colored urine, clay-colored stools, or pruritus.
- ➤ Inform the female patient that menstrual irregularities and breast tenderness may occur with progestin therapy.
- ➤ Teach the patient to recognize the signs and symptoms of a local or systemic hypersensitivity reaction and to notify the physician promptly if they occur.
- ➤ Advise the patient that the injections will be painful. Provide reassurance that measures will be taken to make injections less painful.
- ➤ Instruct the patient to notify the physician if adverse reactions occur.

ment nearby. Notify the physician immediately if such reactions occur.

- Avoid local adverse reactions to I.M. progestin by injecting the drug deeply and applying pressure and ice after the injection to lessen pain and irritation.

Evaluation

For each nursing diagnosis, prepare an evaluation statement that describes the patient's or family's response to nursing interventions.

Corticosteroids

Corticosteroids are naturally occurring hormones secreted by the adrenal cortex or synthetic analogues of these hormones. They include dexamethasone, hydrocortisone, methylprednisolone, prednisolone, and prednisone.

PHARMACOKINETICS

When administered orally, the corticosteroids are absorbed rapidly and distributed throughout the body. These drugs are metabolized extensively in the liver and then excreted as conjugated metabolites in the urine. The corticosteroids have rapid onsets of action and reach peak concentration levels within 1 hour after administration. They provide varying durations of action: hydrocortisone, 8 to 12 hours; prednisone, prednisolone, and methylprednisolone, 24 to 36 hours; and dexamethasone, 3 days.

Route	Onset	Peak	Duration
P.O.	Rapid	1 hr	Variable
I.M.	Rapid	Variable	Variable
I.V.	Rapid	Variable	Varaible

PHARMACODYNAMICS

The antitumor mechanisms of action of the corticosteroids are not fully understood. The drugs may inhibit glucose transportation and phosphorylation, two processes that supply cell energy. Without appropriate energy supplies, lymphoid proliferation is inhibited, lymphocyte **mitosis** is impaired, and cell lysis soon results. Leukemic lymphocyte cells may have specific receptors that selectively bind the corticosteroids, thereby drawing the drugs to the tumor cells.

PHARMACOTHERAPEUTICS

The corticosteroids have a lympholytic action that makes them useful in treating **lymphocytic** leukemias, **myelomas,** and malignant lymphomas. For these indications, these drugs are usually used with cytotoxic agents to induce remissions.

Drug interactions

Many clinically significant drug interactions are identified with the corticosteroids.

ADVERSE DRUG REACTIONS

Most adverse reactions to synthetic corticosteroids are similar to those of natural corticosteroids. The large dosages required for cancer therapy account for the possible enhanced toxicities.

Patients with cardiovascular disease, peptic ulcer disease, diabetes mellitus, and psychological disturbances are more likely to have adverse reactions to the corticosteroids, which include fluid and sodium retention and increased potassium and calcium excretion. The corticosteroids can also disturb glucose metabolism and promote gluconeogenesis and anti-insulin effects that cause hyperglycemia. Epigastric distress may occur.

Behavioral changes commonly caused by the corticosteroids include mood swings, insomnia, nervousness, euphoria, sense of well-being, and psychosis. Increased appetite is also common.

Corticosteroids can cause immunosuppression. They may also mask signs of infection, such as fever and inflammation. During prolonged therapy, patients may develop cataracts, glaucoma, or ocular infections.

Patients risk the complete suppression of the adrenal hormones. Many patients on long-term therapy develop some cushingoid symptoms, such as moon face, truncal obesity, purpura, buffalo hump (cervicodorsal fat), and acne. Patients may develop depression after long-term corticosteroid therapy is discontinued.

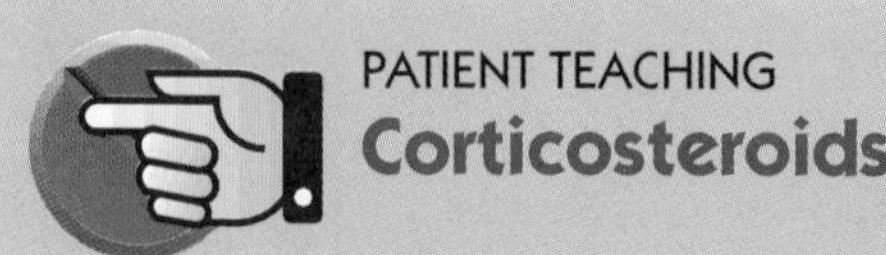

PATIENT TEACHING
Corticosteroids

- Teach the patient and family the name, dose, frequency, action, and adverse effects of the prescribed corticosteroid.
- Instruct the patient to measure body weight daily and to observe for edema and notify the physician if it occurs.
- Teach the patient to recognize the signs and symptoms of hypocalcemia and hypokalemia. Advise the patient to consume more potassium-rich and calcium-rich foods.
- Instruct the patient to recognize the signs and symptoms of hyperglycemia, such as polyuria and polydipsia. Advise the diabetic patient to test blood glucose regularly and adjust the usual treatment according to the glucose level as prescribed.
- Teach the patient when and how to take an oral corticosteroid to minimize gastrointestinal distress.
- Instruct the patient to contact the physician about missed doses.
- Be aware that the behavioral changes associated with corticosteroid therapy may benefit the cancer patient initially. Euphoria and a sense of well-being combined with increased appetite temporarily may improve the patient's lifestyle. Advise the patient and family that such effects may change negatively to mood swings, nervousness, or psychosis. These negative behavioral changes are reversible with drug discontinuation.
- Stress the importance of having routine blood studies done throughout corticosteroid therapy to detect adverse reactions.
- Teach the patient to use infection control measures during corticosteroid therapy.
- Advise the patient to report vision changes or eye discomfort immediately and to have regular eye examinations by an ophthalmologist.
- Inform the patient that corticosteroid therapy may increase the appetite. Encourage the use of nutritious snacks to meet appetite demands.
- Advise the patient who is taking the drug for more than 1 week not to discontinue it abruptly. Explain that the dosage must be decreased gradually.
- Inform the patient that cushingoid symptoms may change the appearance. Reassure the patient that these changes are drug-related.
- Teach the patient to recognize and immediately report the signs and symptoms of adrenal insufficiency. These effects may require a dosage increase. Also advise the patient to notify the physician if illness, injury, or other stress occurs because a dosage increase may be needed.
- Advise the patient to carry medical identification at all times and to notify health care professionals about corticosteroid therapy before undergoing other treatments.
- Instruct the patient to notify the physician if adverse reactions occur.

NURSING PROCESS APPLICATION

The following information assists the nurse in caring for a patient receiving a corticosteroid. It includes an overview of assessment activities as well as examples of appropriate nursing diagnoses and related interventions (see "Planning and implementation"). It also highlights the importance of evaluation.

Assessment

Before drug therapy begins, review the patient's history for conditions that contraindicate or require cautious use of the prescribed corticosteroid. Also review the patient's medication history to identify use of drugs that may interact with it. During therapy, assess the patient for adverse drug reactions and signs of drug interactions. Also, periodically assess the effectiveness of corticosteroid therapy. Finally, evaluate the patient's and family's knowledge about the prescribed drug.

Nursing diagnoses

- Risk for injury related to a preexisting condition that contraindicates or requires cautious use of a corticosteroid
- Risk for injury related to adverse drug reactions or drug interactions
- Risk for infection related to immunosuppression caused by a corticosteroid
- Knowledge deficit related to the prescribed corticosteroid

Planning and implementation

- Do not administer a corticosteroid to a patient with a condition that contraindicates its use.
- Administer a corticosteroid cautiously to a patient at risk because of a preexisting condition.
- Monitor the patient for adverse reactions and drug interactions during corticosteroid therapy, especially if the patient has cardiovascular disease, peptic ulcer disease, diabetes mellitus, or a psychological disturbance.

* ***Monitor the patient for signs of fluid retention.*** Weigh the patient daily at the same time with the same scale and wearing the same amount of clothing to detect sudden weight gain; auscultate the lungs for crackles; and observe for ankle swelling, puffy eyelids, swollen fingers, and other signs of edema. If fluid retention occurs, notify the physician.
* ***Monitor the patient's serum sodium, potassium, and calcium levels for abnormalities (hypernatremia, hypokalemia, or hypocalcemia).***
* ***Monitor the fasting blood glucose level periodically to detect steroid-induced diabetes, which may occur in a patient on long-term therapy, or loss of blood glucose control in a diabetic patient.***

- Minimize GI distress by administering an oral agent with meals and avoiding concomitant use of aspirin or any other nonsteroidal anti-inflammatory drug.
- Monitor the patient for signs of adrenal hormone suppression during and after corticosteroid therapy. Administer additional corticosteroids as prescribed during times of stress.
- Monitor the patient for cushingoid symptoms, such as moon face, truncal obesity, purpura, buffalo hump (cervicodorsal fat), and acne. (See Patient Teaching: *Corticosteroids.*)
- Assess the patient for depression when tapering off the corticosteroid dosage after prolonged therapy.

• Administer parenteral dexamethasone or methylprednisolone by slow I.V. push, or give methylprednisolone by I.M. injection, as prescribed.
• Notify the physician if adverse reactions or drug interactions occur.
• Monitor the patient's WBC count for leukopenia, which indicates immunosuppression. If leukopenia occurs, monitor the patient for signs of infection. Corticosteroids may mask other signs of infection, such as fever and inflammation.
• Use aseptic technique when handling or dressing all wounds, injection sites, tubes, and catheters.
• Take infection control measures. For example, keep the patient away from others with infections, promote adequate rest for the patient, and ensure that the patient remains well hydrated.
• Notify the physician if leukopenia or signs of infection occur. Expect to administer an antibiotic as prescribed.

Evaluation

For each nursing diagnosis, prepare an evaluation statement that describes the patient's or family's response to nursing interventions.

Gonadotropin-releasing hormone analogues

The gonadotropin-releasing hormone analogues goserelin acetate and leuprolide acetate are indicated for advanced prostate cancer.

PHARMACOKINETICS

Goserelin is absorbed slowly for the first 8 days of therapy, and rapidly and continuously thereafter. Its distribution, metabolism, and excretion are not defined clearly. Goserelin achieves a peak concentration level after 12 to 15 days of therapy. Its serum half-life is about 4.2 hours.

After S.C. injection, leuprolide is absorbed well, but its distribution, metabolism, and excretion have not been determined. After I.M. administration of leuprolide suspension, the drug is released slowly and gradually, providing a prolonged duration of action and allowing monthly administration. With daily leuprolide injections, the patient's testosterone level initially rises but falls to castration level in 2 to 4 weeks. The plasma half-life of leuprolide is about 3 hours.

Route	Onset	Peak	Duration
S.C.	2-4 wk	12 days-2 mo	4-12 wk
I.M.	Unknown	2 wk-2 mo	4-12 wk

PHARMACODYNAMICS

Goserelin and leuprolide act on the male's pituitary gland to increase LH secretion, which stimulates testosterone production. The peak testosterone level is reached about 72 hours after daily administration. However, with long-term administration, goserelin and leuprolide inhibit LH release from the pituitary and subsequently inhibit testicular release of testosterone. Because prostate tumor cells are stimulated by testosterone, the reduced testosterone level inhibits tumor growth.

PHARMACOTHERAPEUTICS

Goserelin and leuprolide are used for the palliative treatment of metastatic prostate cancer. The drugs lower the testosterone level without the adverse psychological effects of castration or the adverse cardiovascular effects of DES.

Drug interactions

No drug interactions have been identified with goserelin or leuprolide.

ADVERSE DRUG REACTIONS

Hot flashes are the most commonly reported reactions to goserelin and leuprolide. Impotence and decreased libido are also common. Disease symptoms and pain may worsen or flare during the first 2 weeks of goserelin or leuprolide therapy. The flare can be fatal in patients with bony vertebral metastasis.

Peripheral edema occurs in about 8% of patients. Nausea, vomiting, constipation, and anorexia occur in about 2% of patients. Thromboembolic complications are uncommon; gynecomastia and breast tenderness are rare.

NURSING PROCESS APPLICATION

The following information assists the nurse in caring for a patient receiving a gonadotropin-releasing hormone analogue. It includes an overview of assessment activities as well as examples of appropriate nursing diagnoses and related interventions (see "Planning and implementation"). It also highlights the importance of evaluation.

Assessment

Before drug therapy begins, review the patient's history for conditions that require cautious use of the prescribed gonadotropin-releasing hormone analogue. During therapy, assess the patient for adverse drug reactions. Also, periodically assess the effectiveness of therapy with the gonadotropin-releasing hormone analogue. Finally, evaluate the patient's and family's knowledge about the prescribed drug.

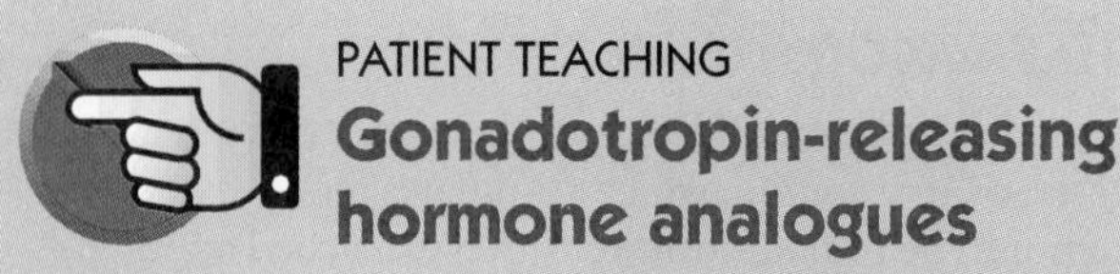

PATIENT TEACHING
Gonadotropin-releasing hormone analogues

- Teach the patient and family the name, dose, frequency, action, and adverse effects of the prescribed gonadotropin-releasing hormone analogue.
- Teach the patient and family how to prepare and administer subcutaneous injections of goserelin or leuprolide and how to rotate injection sites. The manufacturer provides the syringes and needles for injection.
- Instruct the patient to keep an accurate record of the doses administered and the injection sites.
- Inform the patient of the risk of hot flashes, impotence, decreased libido, and tumor flare.
- Encourage the patient to consult with the physician about increasing the analgesic dosage to control pain.
- Teach the patient how to manage troublesome adverse gastrointestinal reactions. For example, advise a patient with anorexia to eat smaller but more frequent meals or counsel a patient with constipation to increase fluid and dietary fiber intake.
- Review the signs and symptoms of thromboembolic complications and instruct the patient to notify the physician immediately if any occur.
- Inform the patient that gynecomastia and breast tenderness may occur.
- Instruct the patient to notify the physician if other adverse reactions occur.

Nursing diagnoses

- Risk for injury related to a preexisting condition that contraindicates or requires cautious use of a gonadotropin-releasing hormone analogue
- Risk for injury related to adverse drug reactions
- Pain related to tumor flare caused by a gonadotropin-releasing hormone analogue
- Knowledge deficit related to the prescribed gonadotropin-releasing hormone analogue

Planning and implementation

- Administer leuprolide cautiously to a patient at risk because of a preexisting condition.
- Monitor the patient for adverse reactions during therapy.

*** *Monitor the patient for signs of thromboembolic complications. If signs occur, notify the physician immediately and prepare to administer emergency treatment.***

- Notify the physician if other adverse reactions occur.
- Monitor the patient for tumor flare, which is exhibited by an increase in disease symptoms and pain during the first 2 weeks of gonadotropin-releasing hormone analogue therapy. (See Patient Teaching: *Gonadotropin-releasing hormone analogues.*)
- Increase the analgesic dosage as prescribed to control pain.

*** *Notify the physician immediately at the first sign of tumor flare. This reaction can be fatal in a patient with bony vertebral metastasis.***

Evaluation

For each nursing diagnosis, prepare an evaluation statement that describes the patient's or family's response to nursing interventions.

CHAPTER SUMMARY

Chapter 56 discussed the hormonal agents used to treat malignant tumors. Here are the chapter highlights.

Estrogen therapy is used as a palliative treatment for metastatic breast cancer in postmenopausal women and for metastatic prostate cancer. Male patients may experience feminization, and female patients may experience decreased libido and breast tenderness with estrogen therapy.

The antiestrogen tamoxifen is used to treat advanced breast cancer with estrogen receptor–positive tumors in postmenopausal women. The drug may cause tumor flare.

Androgens prove effective in treating breast cancer in men and advanced breast cancer in women. Androgen therapy causes virilization and fluid retention.

The antiandrogens are used in combination with a gonadotropin-releasing hormone analogue to treat advanced prostate cancer.

The adrenocortical suppressants aminoglutethemide and anastrozole are used to treat hormonally responsive advanced breast and prostate cancer and Cushing's disease. About 50% of patients taking the drug experience rash, hypotension, fatigue, drowsiness, and dizziness.

The progestins are used as palliative treatment of advanced endometrial, breast, and renal cancers. When giving an I.M. progestin injection, the nurse must be careful to avoid inadvertent I.V. injection.

The corticosteroids are indicated for lymphocytic leukemias, myelomas, and malignant lymphomas. Patients taking corticosteroids may experience fluid and sodium retention, behavioral changes, immunosuppression, and cushingoid symptoms.

The gonadotropin-releasing hormone analogues goserelin and leuprolide treat advanced prostate cancer by decreasing testosterone levels.

By applying the nursing process, the nurse can help the patient cope with hormonal antineoplastic treatment. Nursing care includes teaching about potential adverse reactions and using specific interventions to minimize them.

Questions to consider

See Appendix 1 for answers.

1. Sylvia Potter, age 60, develops an increase in lesion number and size during the first 2 weeks of starting tamoxifen 10 mg P.O. b.i.d. for metastatic breast cancer. What may account for this reaction?
   (a) Metastasis to bone
   (b) Tumor flare
   (c) Resistance to therapy
   (d) Tamoxifen hypersensitivity

2. Rodney Miller, age 68, has advanced prostate cancer. His physician prescribes flutamide 250 mg P.O. every 8 hours. The physician should also prescribe which of the following drugs for Mr. Miller?
   (a) An anabolic steroid
   (b) A synthetic progesterone derivative
   (c) A pituitary-suppressive glucocorticoid
   (d) A gonadotropin-releasing hormone analogue

3. Candy French, age 46, takes megestrol acetate 40 mg P.O. q.i.d. for advanced breast cancer. Which of the following is the most common adverse reaction associated with this drug?
   (a) Blurred vision
   (b) Constipation
   (c) Mild fluid retention
   (d) Dizziness

4. Geraldine Sabolt, age 78, has been diagnosed with breast cancer that has metastasized to the bone. Halotestin 15 mg P.O. b.i.d. has been prescribed. Which of the following is the most common electrolyte imbalance seen in patients with bone metastasis who receive prolonged androgen therapy?
   (a) Hypocalcemia
   (b) Hypercalcemia
   (c) Hypokalemia
   (d) Hyperkalemia

5. The nurse tells a patient about to start treatment with aminoglutethimide about the drug's adverse reactions. Which of the following is the most common adverse reaction to aminoglutethimide?
   (a) Nausea and vomiting
   (b) Rash
   (c) Anorexia
   (d) Leukopenia

57 Other antineoplastic agents

OBJECTIVES

After reading and studying this chapter, the student should be able to:

1. describe the mechanisms of action of the vinca alkaloids, the podophyllotoxins, asparaginase, procarbazine, hydroxyurea, interferons, aldesleukin, altretamine, and paclitaxel.
2. identify the indications for the vinca alkaloids, the podophyllotoxins, asparaginase, procarbazine, hydroxyurea, interferons, aldesleukin, altretamine, and paclitaxel.
3. compare the major adverse reactions to the vinca alkaloids, podophyllotoxins, and interferons.
4. identify the major adverse reactions associated with asparaginase, procarbazine, hydroxyurea, aldesleukin, altretamine, and paclitaxel.
5. describe how to apply the nursing process when caring for a patient receiving an antineoplastic agent.

INTRODUCTION

This chapter presents a subclass of antineoplastic agents, known as natural products, that includes the vinca alkaloids (vinblastine, vincristine, and vinorelbine) and the podophyllotoxins (etoposide and teniposide). It also discusses other antineoplastic agents that cannot be included in existing classifications, including asparaginase, procarbazine, hydroxyurea, interferon, aldesleukin, altretamine, paclitaxel, and docetaxel. (See *Selected major antineoplastic agents.*)

Drugs covered in this chapter include:

- aldesleukin
- alfa interferon
- altretamine
- asparaginase
- docetaxel
- etoposide
- hydroxyurea
- paclitaxel
- pegaspargase
- procarbazine hydrochloride
- teniposide
- vinblastine sulfate
- vincristine sulfate
- vinorelbine.

Vinca alkaloids

The vinca alkaloids (vinblastine sulfate, vincristine sulfate, and vinorelbine) are nitrogenous bases derived from the periwinkle plant. These drugs are **cell cycle–specific** for the M phase.

PHARMACOKINETICS

After intravenous (I.V.) administration, the vinca alkaloids are distributed well throughout the body. They undergo moderate hepatic metabolism before being eliminated, primarily in the feces with a small percentage eliminated in the urine. The vinca alkaloids have multiphasic elimination rates. The terminal half-life is about 25 hours for vinblastine, 85 hours for vincristine, and 24 hours for vindesine.

Route	Onset	Peak	Duration
I.V.	Rapid	1-3.5 days	6-9 days

PHARMACODYNAMICS

The vinca alkaloids may disrupt the normal function of the microtubules by binding to the protein tubulin in the microtubules. With the microtubules unable to separate chromosomes properly, the chromosomes are dispersed throughout the cytoplasm or arranged in unusual groupings. As a result, formation of the mitotic spindle is prevented, and the cells cannot complete **mitosis.** Cell division is arrested in metaphase, causing cell death. Therefore, vinca alkaloids are cell cycle-, M phase-specific. Interruption of the microtubule function may also impair some types of cellular movement, **phagocytosis,** and central nervous system (CNS) functions.

PHARMACOTHERAPEUTICS

Vinblastine is used to treat metastatic testicular **carcinoma, lymphomas,** Kaposi's **sarcoma, neuroblastoma,** breast carcinoma, and choriocarcinoma. Vincristine is used in combination therapy to treat **Hodgkin's disease,** malignant lymphoma, **Wilms' tumor, rhabdomyosarcoma,** and acute **lymphocytic leukemia.** Vinorelbine is used to treat non-small-cell lung cancer. It may also be used in the treatment

Selected major antineoplastic agents

This table summarizes some of the other antineoplastic agents currently in clinical use.

DRUG	MAJOR INDICATIONS AND USUAL DOSAGES	CONTRAINDICATIONS AND PRECAUTIONS
Vinca alkaloids		
vinblastine (Velban)	*Breast carcinoma, neuroblastoma, metastatic testicular cancer, lymphoma, Hodgkin's disease, malignant lymphoma, Kaposi's sarcoma, choriocarcinoma* ADULT: 0.1 mg/kg or 3.7 mg/m^2 I.V. increased weekly by increments of 0.05 mg/kg or 1.8 mg/m^2 up to a maximum of 0.5 mg or 18.5 mg/m^2; maintenance therapy, 0.05 mg/kg or 1.8 mg/m^2 I.V. less than the final dosage every 7 to 14 days. Maintenance dose also based on 6 to 10 mg/m^2 every 2 to 4 weeks in combination with other drugs. PEDIATRIC: 2.5 mg/m^2 I.V. increased weekly by increments of 1.25 mg/m^2 to a maximum of 12.5 mg/m^2; maintenance therapy, 1.25 mg/m^2 I.V. less than the final dosage every 7 to 14 days	• Vinblastine is contraindicated in a pregnant or breast-feeding patient or one with significant granulocytopenia (unless it results from the disease being treated) or bacterial infection. • This drug requires cautious use in a patient with cachexia or ulcerated areas of the skin.
vincristine (Oncovin)	*Hodgkin's disease, non-Hodgkin's disease, acute lymphocytic leukemia* ADULT: 0.5 to 1.4 mg/m^2 I.V. in a single dose, up to a maximum of 2 mg, not more than once weekly; or, continuous I.V. infusion of 0.5 mg/m^2/day for 4 days PEDIATRIC: for children who weigh 10 kg (22 lb) or less or have a body surface area less (BSA) than 1 m^2, 0.05 mg/kg I.V. once weekly; for children who weigh more than 10 kg or have a BSA of 1 m^2 or more, 2 mg/m^2 I.V. once weekly	• Vincristine is contraindicated in a pregnant or breast-feeding patient or one with the demyelinating form of Charcot-Marie-Tooth disease. • This drug requires cautious use in a patient with acute uric acid nephropathy or neuromuscular disease.
vinorelbine (Navelbine)	*Non-small–cell lung cancer* ADULT: 30 mg/m^2 I.V. over 6 to 10 minutes administered alone or in combination with other chemotherapeutic medications every week until progression or dose-toxicity occur	• Vinorelbine is contraindicated in a patient who has a pretreatment granulocyte count of fewer than 1,000 cells/mm^3. • Use with caution in a patient with hepatic impairment and one whose bone marrow has been compromised by radiation or chemotherapy.
Podophyllotoxins		
etoposide (VePesid)	*Testicular cancer* ADULT: 100 mg/m^2 I.V. daily for 5 days,repeated every 3 to 4 weeks *Small-cell lung cancer* ADULT: 35 mg/m^2 I.V. daily for 4 days or 50 mg/m^2 I.V. daily for 5 days, repeated every 3 to 4 weeks	• Etoposide is contraindicated in a pregnant or breast-feeding patient or one with known hypersensitivity. • This drug has no known precautions.
Asparaginases		
asparaginase [L-asparaginase] (Elspar)	*Acute lymphocytic leukemia* ADULT: 200 IU/kg I.V. daily for 28 days or 1,000 IU/kg I.V. daily for 10 days PEDIATRIC: 200 IU/kg I.V. daily for 28 days	• Asparaginase is contraindicated in a breast-feeding patient or one with pancreatitis, a history of pancreatitis, or known hypersensitivity. • This drug requires cautious use in a pregnant patient.
pegaspargase (Oncaspar)	*Acute lymphocytic leukemia in patients allergic to the native form of asparaginase.* ADULT: 2500 IU/m^2 I.V. every 14 days PEDIATRIC: for children who have a BSA less than 0.6 m^2, 82.5 IU/kg I.V. every 14 days	• Pegaspargase is contraindicated in patients with pancreatitis or prior hemorrhagic event. • Use cautiously in a pregnant patient and one with liver disease.

(continued)

Selected major antineoplastic agents *(continued)*

DRUG	MAJOR INDICATIONS AND USUAL DOSAGES	CONTRAINDICATIONS AND PRECAUTIONS
Procarbazine		
procarbazine (Matulane)	*Hodgkin's disease, small-cell lung cancer, non-Hodgkin's lymphoma, myeloma, melanoma, central nervous system tumors* ADULT: 2 to 4 mg/kg P.O. daily for 1 week, then increased to 4 to 6 mg/kg P.O. daily until a maximum response is achieved; maintenance therapy, 1 to 2 mg/kg P.O. daily ADULT: MOPP regimen: 100 mg/m^2/day P.O. for 14 days and repeated every 4 weeks PEDIATRIC: 50 mg/m^2 daily P.O. for 1 week, then increased to 100 mg/m^2 daily until maximum response is achieved; maintenance therapy, 50 mg/m^2 P.O. daily	• Procarbazine is contraindicated in a pregnant or breast-feeding patient or one with inadequate bone marrow reserve or known hypersensitivity. • This drug requires cautious use in a patient with impaired renal or hepatic function.
Hydroxyurea		
hydroxyurea (Hydrea)	*Selected myeloproliferative disorders, melanoma, chronic myelogenous leukemia, and certain carcinomas of the ovary* ADULT: 80 mg/kg P.O. every 3 days or 20 to 30 mg/kg P.O. daily	• Hydroxyurea is contraindicated in a pregnant patient or one with marked bone marrow suppression or severe anemia. • This drug requires cautious use in a patient with marked renal dysfunction or one who has received radiation therapy or cytotoxic cancer chemotherapy. • Pediatric dosages have not been established.
Alfa interferons		
alfa interferon-2A (Roferon-A)	*Hairy-cell leukemia* ADULT: 3 million IU S.C. or I.M. daily for 16 to 24 weeks followed by 3 million IU S.C. or I.M. three times a week *Acquired immunodeficiency syndrome–related to Kaposi's sarcoma* ADULT: 36 million IU I.M. or S.C. daily for 10 to 12 weeks followed by 36 million IU I.M. or S.C. three times a week	• Alfa interferon is contraindicated in a breast-feeding patient or one with known hypersensitivity. • This drug requires cautious use in a pregnant patient or one with a recent myocardial infarction (MI) or a previous or recurrent arrhythmic disorder. • Safety and efficacy in children have not been established.
Aldesleukin		
aldesleukin (Proleukin)	*Metastatic renal cell carcinoma* ADULT: initially, 600,000 IU/kg (0.037 mg/kg) I.V. infused over 15 minutes every 8 hours for 14 doses; after a 9-day rest period, dosage is repeated for another 14 doses for a total of 28 doses per course of therapy	• Aldesleukin is contraindicated in a breast-feeding patient, one with known hypersensitivity, one who has received an organ allograft, or one with abnormal thallium stress test or pulmonary function test results. It also is contraindicated in a patient who has experienced any of the following during an earlier course of therapy: sustained ventricular tachycardia, cardiac arrhythmias unresponsive to conventional management, recurrent chest pain and electrocardiogram changes consistent with angina or MI, intubation for more than 72 hours, pericardial tamponade, renal dysfunction requiring dialysis for more than 72 hours, coma or toxic psychosis lasting more than 48 hours, repeated or difficult-to-control seizures, bowel ischemia or perforation, or gastrointestinal bleeding that required surgery. • This drug requires cautious use in a pregnant patient or one receiving nephrotoxic or hepatotoxic drugs. • Safety and efficacy in children have not been established.

Selected major antineoplastic agents *(continued)*

DRUG	MAJOR INDICATIONS AND USUAL DOSAGES	CONTRAINDICATIONS AND PRECAUTIONS
Altretamine		
altretamine (Hexalen)	*Palliative treatment of persistent or recurrent ovarian cancer after first-line therapy with cisplatin or an alkylating agent–based combination* ADULT: 260 mg/m^2 P.O. daily in four divided doses after meals and at bedtime for 14 or 21 consecutive days in a 28-day cycle	• Altretamine is contraindicated in a pregnant or breast-feeding patient or one with known hypersensitivity; preexisting, severe bone marrow suppression; or neurologic toxicity. • This drug requires cautious use in a patient receiving cimetidine or a monoamine oxidase inhibitor. • Safety and efficacy in children have not been established.
Paclitaxel		
paclitaxel (Taxol)	*Metastatic breast and ovarian carcinoma after failure of first-line or subsequent chemotherapy* ADULT: 135 mg/m^2 I.V. over 24 hours every three weeks (subsequent courses should not be repeated until neutrophil count is equal to or greater than 1,500 cells/mm^3 and the platelet count is equal to or greater than 100,000 cells/mm^3)	• Paclitaxel is contraindicated in a pregnant or breast-feeding patient or one with known hypersensitivity, a history of severe hypersensitivity reaction to other drugs formulated in polyoxyethylated castor oil, or a severe baseline neutropenia of less than 1,500 cells/mm^3. • This drug has no known precautions. • Safety and efficacy in children have not been established.
docetaxel (Taxotere)	*Metastatic breast and ovarian carcinoma after failure of first-line or subsequent chemotherapy* ADULT: 60 to 100 mg/m^2 I.V, over 1 hour every three weeks (subsequent courses should not be repeated until neutrophil count is equal to or greater than 1,500 cells/mm^3 and the platelet count is equal to or greater than 100,000 cells/mm^3)	• Docetaxel is contraindicated in a patient with known hypersensitivity to the drug.

of metastatic breast carcinoma, cisplatin-resistant ovarian carcinoma and Hodgkin's disease.

Drug interactions

Researchers have identified that vinorelbine causes acute pulmonary reactions when administered with mitomycin and therefore recommend not combining the two drugs. Vinblastine is incompatible with furosemide and heparin. Vincristine is incompatible with furosemide and idarubicin. (See Geriatric Considerations: *Vincristine,* page 690.)

ADVERSE DRUG REACTIONS

Minor differences in the chemical structure of the vinca alkaloids cause significant differences in toxicity. Vinblastine and vinorelbine toxicities occur primarily as bone marrow suppression, which is manifested by **leukopenia** and slight **thrombocytopenia.** Leukopenia increases the patient's risk of infection, especially if the absolute **granulocyte** count is less than 1,000/mm^3. Dose adjustments may need to be made based on the degree of neutropenia.

Alopecia occurs in up to 50% of patients receiving vinca alkaloids, although hair loss is more likely with vincristine than vinblastine. Many patients experience partial alopecia; others, total. Men are equally as affected as women by alopecia of the scalp, eyebrows, eyelashes, and body. Alopecia is reversible when the drugs are discontinued, and hair may begin to regrow during therapy.

Neuromuscular abnormalities frequently occur with vincristine and vinorelbine and occasionally with vinblastine therapy. Peripheral neuropathies, which usually are dose-limiting for vincristine and vinorelbine, may include loss of deep tendon reflexes, paresthesia, numbness, pain, and tingling. Other vincristine-induced neurotoxicities include encephalopathies and cranial nerve dysfunction, such as vocal cord paralysis, ptosis (upper eyelid drooping), and jaw pain. Constipation is common with vinorelbine because it causes neuropathy.

Vinca alkaloids, which are **vesicants,** may cause severe local necrosis if **extravasation** occurs.

Stomatitis may occur with the vinca alkaloids. Nausea and vomiting that may occur can be controlled with

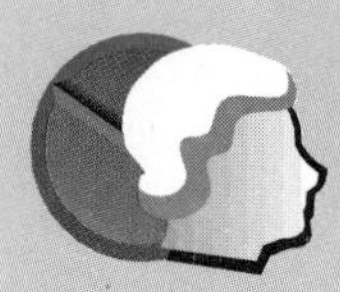

GERIATRIC CONSIDERATIONS

Vincristine

Vincristine may cause bladder atony and therefore may enhance the effects of other medications that cause urinary hesitancy, especially in elderly men who may already have bladder control problems. If a patient is receiving a medication that can cause urine retention, that medication should be discontinued for the first few days of vincristine therapy. Discontinuing the first medication will help determine whether vincristine alone will cause urine retention. If appropriate, the first medication may be added back to the patient's medication regimen. Close monitoring for urine retention symptoms will be necessary.

antiemetics. Prophylactic laxative use sometimes can prevent constipation resulting from vincristine administration.

Vinblastine may produce **tumor** pain described as an intense stinging or burning in the tumor bed, with an abrupt onset 1 to 3 minutes after drug administration. The pain usually lasts 20 minutes to 3 hours. Vincristine may induce the syndrome of inappropriate antidiuretic hormone (SIADH).

NURSING PROCESS APPLICATION

The following information assists the nurse in caring for a patient receiving a vinca alkaloid. It includes an overview of assessment activities as well as examples of appropriate nursing diagnoses and related interventions (see "Planning and implementation"). It also highlights the importance of evaluation.

Assessment

Before drug therapy begins, review the patient's history for conditions that contraindicate or require cautious use of the prescribed vinca alkaloid. During therapy, assess the patient for adverse drug reactions. Also, periodically assess the effectiveness of therapy with the vinca alkaloid. Finally, evaluate the patient's and family's knowledge about the prescribed drug.

Nursing diagnoses

- Risk for injury related to a preexisting condition that contraindicates or requires cautious use of a vinca alkaloid
- Risk for injury related to adverse drug reactions
- Pain at the tumor site related to vinblastine administration
- Knowledge deficit related to the prescribed vinca alkaloid

Planning and implementation

- Do not administer a vinca alkaloid to a patient with a condition that contraindicates its use.
- Administer a vinca alkaloid cautiously to a patient at risk because of a preexisting condition.
- Monitor the patient regularly for adverse reactions during therapy with the vinca alkaloid.

∗ ***Monitor the patient's complete blood count (CBC) and platelet count regularly.*** Note the CBC **nadir** when caring for a patient with bone marrow suppression. At the nadir, which usually occurs 4 to 10 days after drug administration, the patient is at the greatest risk for problems associated with leukopenia and thrombocytopenia.

- Monitor the patient for signs and symptoms of infection if leukopenia occurs. Also take infection control measures until the white blood cell (WBC) count returns to normal.
- Monitor the patient with leukopenia for thrombocytopenia because the two occur sequentially. When the platelet count is under 50,000/mm^3, the patient is at risk for bleeding. When the count drops below 20,000/mm^3, the patient is at severe risk and probably will need a platelet transfusion. Monitor the patient with thrombocytopenia for bleeding. Take bleeding precautions until the platelet count returns to normal. Rectal temperatures and intramuscular (I.M.) injections are contraindicated in a patient with thrombocytopenia or leukopenia.
- Monitor laboratory values that would indicate **anemia.** A patient who is dehydrated from nausea, vomiting, or anorexia may have a normal hematocrit. Once the patient is rehydrated, the hematocrit will fall, thus revealing anemia.
- Monitor the serum uric acid level periodically throughout therapy to detect rapid cell lysis. If the level becomes elevated, administer allopurinol as prescribed. This drug prevents the rapid accumulation of uric acid.
- Monitor the patient for neuromuscular abnormalities when administering vinblastine or vincristine. To detect peripheral neuropathies, assess deep tendon reflexes and ask the patient about paresthesia, numbness, pain, and tingling. During vincristine therapy, observe for signs of other neurotoxicities, such as encephalopathy (drowsiness or decreased level of consciousness) and cranial nerve dysfunction (vocal cord paralysis, jaw pain, or ptosis). Notify the physician if neuromuscular abnormalities occur.

∗ ***Examine the I.V. infusion site for evidence of extravasation, such as redness, swelling, or pain on touch, before administering a vinca alkaloid. If extravasation is suspected, change the infusion site to prevent severe local necrosis. Because vindesine may produce pain and phlebitis without infiltration, use a different infusion site for each dose.***

- Consider the time of drug administration when encouraging patient compliance. Some patients prefer treatments in the evening; patients who are employed may prefer treatments on their days off.

∗ ***Handle vinca alkaloids carefully. Administer the prescribed drug directly into the vein or into the injection port in the tubing of a freely infusing I.V. solution. These methods allow for direct observation of the injection site.***

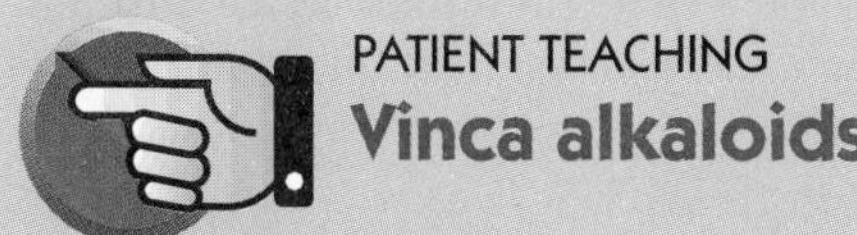

PATIENT TEACHING
Vinca alkaloids

- Teach the patient and family the name, dose, frequency, action, and adverse effects of the prescribed vinca alkaloid.
- Prepare the patient for alopecia by explaining when hair loss usually begins and noting that it is gradual and reversible once treatment ends.
- Explain to the patient that burning or stinging pain commonly occurs at the tumor site after intravenous administration of vinblastine. Reassure the patient that this pain is not caused by a worsening of the tumor, but by cellular destruction that causes tissue swelling.
- Teach the patient and family the signs and symptoms of neurotoxicity.
- Plan an effective teaching program about bone marrow suppression that includes the patient's blood counts, potential sites of infection, and personal habits.
- Advise the patient with leukopenia to maintain proper hygiene and report signs and symptoms of infection, including fever, cough, sore throat, and a burning sensation during urination.
- Instruct the patient at risk for developing leukopenia and thrombocytopenia to avoid cuts and bruises and to use a sponge toothbrush and an electric razor.
- Instruct the patient to report a sudden headache, which may indicate potentially lethal intracranial bleeding.
- Prevent colonic irritation and bleeding that result from vincristine-induced constipation by recommending a bowel program that includes prophylactic stool softeners as prescribed.
- Stress the importance of returning for follow-up blood tests.
- Caution the patient not to engage in activities that require mental alertness if neurotoxicity occurs.
- Teach the patient how to manage troublesome adverse gastrointestinal reactions.
- Advise the patient to alert the nurse immediately if discomfort occurs at the infusion site during drug administration.
- Instruct the patient to report adverse reactions to the physician.
- Give the patient written materials about the prescribed vinca alkaloid for home reference.

- Use other appropriate nursing interventions for a patient who experiences bone marrow suppression, nausea, vomiting, stomatitis, or alopecia.
- Notify the physician if adverse reactions occur.

✱ Monitor the patient for intense stinging or burning in the tumor bed that begins abruptly 1 to 3 minutes after vinblastine administration. Relieve pain with an analgesic as prescribed, because the pain may last up to 3 hours.

- Avoid splashing vinorelbine solution in the eyes. Severe eye irritation will result.
- Observe for signs and symptoms of hypersensitivity such as acute shortness of breath and/or bronchospasm when administering vinorelbine.
- Patients may require stimulant laxatives while on vincristine. (See Patient Teaching: *Vinca alkaloids.*)

Evaluation

For each nursing diagnosis, prepare an evaluation statement that describes the patient's or family's response to nursing interventions.

Podophyllotoxins

The podophyllotoxins etoposide and teniposide are semisynthetic glycosides that are cell cycle–specific. Teniposide has demonstrated some activity in treating Hodgkin's disease, lymphomas, and brain tumors.

PHARMACOKINETICS

With oral administration, the podophyllotoxins are absorbed incompletely. Although the drugs are distributed widely throughout the body, they achieve poor cerebrospinal fluid (CSF) levels. The podophyllotoxins undergo hepatic metabolism and are excreted primarily in the urine.

After oral administration, etoposide typically reaches a peak plasma concentration level in 1 to 1½ hours. The peak plasma concentration after oral administration is usually 50% of that achieved after I.V. administration. The terminal half-life of etoposide ranges from 5 to 11 hours.

After an I.V. dose of 30 mg/m^2, teniposide attains a peak plasma concentration of 10 mcg/ml. Its half-life ranges from 10 to 40 hours.

Route	Onset	Peak	Duration
P.O.	Unknown	1-1.5 hr	Unknown
I.V.	Rapid	4-11 hr	Unknown

PHARMACODYNAMICS

Although their mechanism of action is understood incompletely, the podophyllotoxins produce several biochemical changes in tumor cells. At low concentrations, these drugs block cells at the late S or G_2 phase. At higher concentrations, they arrest the cells in the G_2 phase. Etoposide and teniposide can cause single-strand breaks of deoxyribonucleic acid (DNA), possibly by inhibiting topoisomerase II. These drugs can also inhibit nucleoside transport and incorporation into nucleic acids.

PHARMACOTHERAPEUTICS

Podophyllotoxins are prescribed to treat various tumors. Etoposide is used to treat testicular **cancer** and small-cell lung cancer. It may also be used to treat various lymphomas and leukemias, although these indications have not been approved by the Food and Drug Administration yet. Teniposide is used to treat acute **lymphoblastic** leukemia.

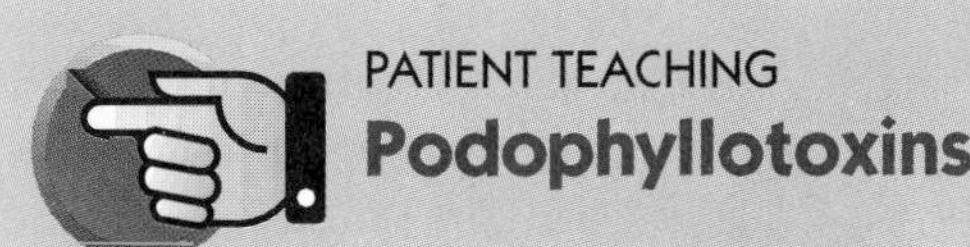

PATIENT TEACHING
Podophyllotoxins

- Teach the patient and family the name, dose, frequency, action, and adverse effects of the prescribed podophyllotoxin.
- Inform the patient that burning or pain may be felt at the infusion site during podophyllotoxin administration.
- Advise the patient to avoid people with active contagious infections, to watch for signs of infection, and to report them immediately to the physician.
- Explain to the patient that acute hypersensitivity reactions may occur with podophyllotoxin therapy. Instruct the patient to report signs or symptoms promptly.
- Prepare the patient for possible alopecia by explaining the timing and speed of hair loss and noting that it may affect the scalp, eyebrows, eyelashes, or other body hair.
- Teach the patient how to manage troublesome adverse reactions, such as nausea and stomatitis, at home.
- Give the patient written materials about the possible effects of the prescribed podophyllotoxin for home reference.
- Instruct the patient to notify the physician if adverse reactions persist or worsen.

Drug interactions

Etoposide and idarubicin are not compatible in solution. No other significant drug interaction has been found.

ADVERSE DRUG REACTIONS

The podophyllotoxins suppress bone marrow with nadirs occurring in 7 to 14 days. These drugs can cause leukopenia and, less commonly, thrombocytopenia; leukopenia resolves in about 3 weeks. About 90% of patients receiving podophyllotoxins experience alopecia, which may resolve as the treatment continues.

About one-third of patients receiving podophyllotoxins develop nausea and vomiting, which last 2 to 6 hours. Anorexia is another common reaction. Stomatitis occurs in 5% of patients.

Acute hypotension may result if a podophyllotoxin is infused too rapidly. Pain and burning at the injection site also have been reported.

Several rare reactions can also occur during podophyllotoxin therapy: acute hypersensitivity, which may be signaled by chills, fever, generalized erythema, pruritus, wheezing, bronchospasm, or tachycardia; transient liver function abnormalities; an elevated alkaline phosphatase level, which indicates impending **hepatotoxicity;** and peripheral neuropathy.

NURSING PROCESS APPLICATION

The following information assists the nurse in caring for a patient receiving a podophyllotoxin. It includes an overview of assessment activities as well as examples of appropriate nursing diagnoses and related interventions (see "Planning and implementation"). It also highlights the importance of evaluation.

Assessment

Before drug therapy begins, review the patient's history for conditions that contraindicate the use of the prescribed podophyllotoxin. During therapy, assess the patient for adverse drug reactions. Also, periodically assess the effectiveness of podophyllotoxin therapy. Finally, evaluate the patient's and family's knowledge about the prescribed drug. (See Patient Teaching: *Podophyllotoxins.*)

Nursing diagnoses

• Risk for injury related to a preexisting condition that contraindicates the use of a podophyllotoxin
• Risk for injury related to adverse drug reactions
• Knowledge deficit related to the prescribed podophyllotoxin

Planning and implementation

• Do not administer a podophyllotoxin to a patient with a condition that contraindicates its use.
• Monitor the patient regularly for adverse reactions during podophyllotoxin therapy.
• Monitor the patient's WBC and platelet counts frequently during therapy, especially during the expected nadir (days 7 to 14 for the WBC count and days 9 to 16 for the platelet count). At the nadir, the patient is at the greatest risk for problems associated with leukopenia and thrombocytopenia. Acute complications occur when the absolute granulocyte count is less than 1,000/mm^3 and the platelet count is less than 20,000/mm^3.
• Monitor the patient with leukopenia for signs of infection. Take infection control measures until the WBC count returns to normal.
• Monitor the patient with thrombocytopenia for signs of bleeding. Take bleeding precautions until the platelet count has returned to normal.
• Administer an antiemetic as prescribed before podophyllotoxin administration and every 2 to 4 hours thereafter, as needed, to prevent or control nausea and vomiting.
* ***Administer I.V. etoposide or teniposide slowly over 30 to 60 minutes to prevent hypotension. Monitor the patient's blood pressure before the infusion and during treatment.***
* ***Monitor the patient for signs of an acute hypersensitivity reaction. If a hypersensitivity reaction occurs, stop the infusion and notify the physician immediately. During podophyllotoxin therapy, have standard emergency equipment, diphenhydramine hydrochloride, and epinephrine nearby.***
• Monitor the patient's liver function studies and alkaline phosphatase level, as prescribed. Abnormalities may indicate impending hepatotoxicity.
• Use other appropriate nursing interventions for a patient with bone marrow suppression, nausea, vomiting, or stomatitis.

• Notify the physician if adverse reactions occur.
• Inspect the patient's mouth regularly for signs of stomatitis, which is temporary. Prophylactic mouth care before chemotherapy may decrease stomatitis severity and provide patient comfort. Therapeutic mouth care, including topical antibiotics and analgesics, may be required, depending on the degree of stomatitis.
• Notify the physician if stomatitis persists or worsens.

Evaluation

For each nursing diagnosis, prepare an evaluation statement that describes the patient's or family's response to nursing interventions.

Asparaginases

Asparaginase, a cell cycle-specific enzyme, exerts its effect by hydrolyzing exogenous asparagine, which leukemic cells need for survival. Pegaspargase is a modified version of asparaginase. Pegaspargase exerts the same effect as its parent drug, asparaginase.

PHARMACOKINETICS

Asparaginase is administered parenterally; it is considered 100% bioavailable when administered I.V. and about 50% bioavailable when administered I.M. After administration, it remains in the vascular compartment, with minimal distribution elsewhere. The metabolic route of asparaginase is unknown. Only trace amounts appear in urine. Its peak plasma concentration level relates to the dose and administration route. The half-life varies from 8 to 30 hours. A cumulative plasma concentration may occur with daily dosing, and active enzymes may appear in the blood up to 3 weeks after administration. Pegaspargase is also administered parenterally. The plasma half-life varies from 1 to 5 days after initial treatment and has been detectable in the plasma up to 15 days after infusion.

Route	Onset	Peak	Duration
I.V.	Unknown	8 hr-5 days	≤15 days

PHARMACODYNAMICS

Asparaginase and pegaspargase capitalize on the biochemical differences between normal cells and tumor cells; most normal cells can synthesize asparagine, but some tumor cells depend on exogenous sources. Asparaginase and pegaspargase act as catalysts in the degradation of asparagine to aspartic acid and ammonia. Deprived of their supply of asparagine, the tumor cells die. Asparaginase and pegaspargase are cell cycle–specific in the G_1 phase.

PHARMACOTHERAPEUTICS

Asparaginase has not proved effective against solid tumors. It is used primarily to induce **remission** in patients with acute lymphocytic leukemia. Pegaspargase is used for the treatment of acute lymphocytic leukemia for patients who are allergic to the native form of asparaginase.

Drug interactions

Researchers have identified no significant drug interactions with asparaginase.

ADVERSE DRUG REACTIONS

Asparaginase and pegaspargase can cause several potentially serious toxicities, which are more severe in adults than in children. Anaphylaxis, the most serious reaction, is more likely to occur with intermittent I.V. dosing than with daily I.V. dosing or I.M. injections.

Many patients receiving asparaginase and pegaspargase develop nausea and vomiting shortly after drug administration. Fever, headache, and abdominal pain may also occur. Hepatotoxicity commonly occurs and is manifested by transient and mild liver enzyme elevations, which peak in the second week of therapy.

Hypersensitivity reactions occur in 20% to 35% of patients receiving asparaginase and pegaspargase. Anaphylaxis also occurs, and the risk of a reaction rises with each successive treatment. Pancreatitis, evidenced by epigastric pain, vomiting, and a high serum amylase level, has appeared in 5% of patients receiving asparaginase. Patients may also become hyperglycemic due to decreased insulin production. CNS toxicity may also occur in 25% of patients. Personality changes, seizures, and abnormal electroencephalogram (EEG) tracings have been reported. Renal impairment and coagulation abnormalities, such as hypofibrinogenemia and depression of other coagulation factors, may also occur.

NURSING PROCESS APPLICATION

The following information assists the nurse in caring for a patient receiving asparaginase and pegaspargase. It includes an overview of assessment activities as well as examples of appropriate nursing diagnoses and related interventions (see "Planning and implementation"). It also highlights the importance of evaluation.

Assessment

Before drug therapy begins, review the patient's history for conditions that contraindicate or require cautious use of asparaginase. During therapy, assess the patient for adverse drug reactions. Also, periodically assess the effectiveness of therapy with asparaginase and pegaspargase. Finally, evaluate the patient's and family's knowledge about the prescribed drug.

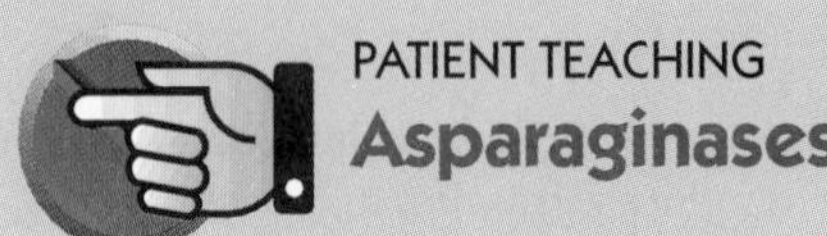

PATIENT TEACHING
Asparaginases

- Teach the patient and family the name, dose, frequency, action, and adverse effects of the asparaginase.
- Inform the patient of the risk of cardiac arrest, and provide support and reassurance. Instruct the patient to immediately report signs or symptoms of hypersensitivity, including restlessness, wheezing, facial flushing or edema, urticaria, pruritus, tachycardia, hypotension, fever, and dyspnea.
- Teach the patient to recognize the signs and symptoms of central nervous system (CNS) toxicity (such as personality changes and seizures) and of pancreatitis (such as abdominal tenderness, midepigastric pain, and vomiting). The CNS changes usually disappear when asparaginase is discontinued, but may persist. Inform the patient that CNS toxicity or pancreatitis may necessitate discontinuation of the asparaginases.
- Teach the patient to recognize and report the signs and symptoms of liver damage, such as yellowed skin or sclera, dark-colored urine, clay-colored stools, and pruritus.
- Advise the patient to take a mild antipyretic and analgesic, as prescribed, if a fever or headache occurs after asparaginase administration.
- Teach the patient to use bleeding precautions if coagulation abnormalities occur.
- Give the patient written materials about the possible effects of asparaginase for home reference.
- Instruct the patient to notify the physician if adverse reactions persist or worsen.

Nursing diagnoses

- Risk for injury related to a preexisting condition that contraindicates or requires cautious use of asparaginase and pegaspargase
- Risk for injury related to adverse drug reactions
- Altered protection related to an acute hypersensitivity reaction to asparaginase and pegaspargase
- Knowledge deficit related to asparaginase and pegaspargase

Planning and implementation

- Do not administer asparaginase or pegaspargase to a patient with a condition that contraindicates its use.
- Administer cautiously to a patient at risk because of a preexisting condition.
- Monitor the patient regularly for adverse reactions during asparaginase and pegaspargase therapy.
- Administer an antiemetic as prescribed because nausea and vomiting are particularly noxious adverse reactions to asparaginase and pegaspargase therapy. If an antiemetic is not prescribed, consult with the physician. Use other appropriate nursing interventions for a patient with nausea or vomiting.
- Monitor the patient's liver and renal function studies and amylase and blood glucose levels. Notify the physician of any abnormal results.

*** *Take seizure precautions during asparaginase therapy. Stop the infusion immediately and notify the physician if seizures occur.***

- Report personality changes to the physician. Such changes may indicate CNS toxicity from asparaginase.
- Note asparaginase treatment on any EEG request slip because it can cause abnormal EEG tracings.
- Pegaspargase is often administered with other chemotherapeutic agents such as vincristine, methotrexate, cytarabine, daunorubicin, and doxorubicin. Be aware of the adverse effects these agents may produce.
- Monitor the patient's plasma coagulation factors. Withhold asparaginase and administer fresh frozen plasma, as prescribed. Take bleeding precautions until the patient's plasma coagulation factor levels return to normal.

*** *Handle I.V. preparations of asparaginase and pegaspargase cautiously.***

- Refrigerate reconstituted asparaginase if the preparation is not used immediately. Use the solution only if it is clear.
- Notify the physician if adverse reactions persist or worsen.
- Administer asparaginase and pegaspargase with a physician present because of the potential for anaphylaxis. Keep available any drugs and equipment necessary to treat cardiac arrest. (See Patient Teaching: *Asparaginases.*)
- Monitor the patient's baseline vital signs before and during asparaginase administration.

*** *Stop the asparaginase or pegaspargase infusion immediately if a hypersensitivity reaction occurs and be prepared to begin emergency treatment. Keep in mind that the risk of anaphylaxis increases with each successive treatment and is more likely to occur with intermittent therapy.***

Evaluation

For each nursing diagnosis, prepare an evaluation statement that describes the patient's or family's response to nursing interventions.

Procarbazine

Procarbazine hydrochloride, a methylhydrazine derivative with monoamine oxidase (MAO) inhibiting properties, is used to treat Hodgkin's disease and primary and metastatic brain tumors.

PHARMACOKINETICS

After oral administration, procarbazine is absorbed well. As a lipophilic molecule, it readily crosses the blood-brain barrier and is distributed well into the CSF. It is metabolized rapidly in the liver and must be activated metabolically by microsomal enzymes. Procarbazine is excreted in urine, primarily as metabolites. Respiratory excretion of the drug occurs as methane and carbon dioxide. Procarbazine achieves a peak plasma concentration level within 1 hour; its half-life is 7 minutes.

Route	Onset	Peak	Duration
P.O.	Rapid	1 hr	24 hr
I.V.	Rapid	10 min	24 hr

PHARMACODYNAMICS

An inert drug, procarbazine must be activated metabolically in the liver and then it can produce various cell changes. It can cause chromosomal damage (including chromatid breaks and translocation), produce antimitotic activity, and inhibit DNA, ribonucleic acid, and protein synthesis. Cancer cells can develop resistance to procarbazine quickly, but that mechanism is not understood completely.

PHARMACOTHERAPEUTICS

Used with other antineoplastic agents, procarbazine is most effective in the MOPP (mechlorethamine, Oncovin (vincristine), procarbazine, and prednisone) regimen for Hodgkin's disease. It is used to treat primary and metastatic brain tumors. The drug may also be useful against small-cell lung cancer, malignant lymphoma, **myeloma, melanoma,** and CNS tumors.

Drug interactions

Concurrent use of alcohol and procarbazine may produce a disulfiram-like reaction (headache, nausea, vomiting, and sweating). Procarbazine produces an additive effect when administered with CNS depressants. Because of procarbazine's MAO inhibiting properties, hypertensive reactions, including hypertensive crisis, may occur when procarbazine is administered concurrently with sympathomimetics, antidepressants, and tyramine-rich foods. (See Drug Interactions: *Food interactions with procarbazine.*)

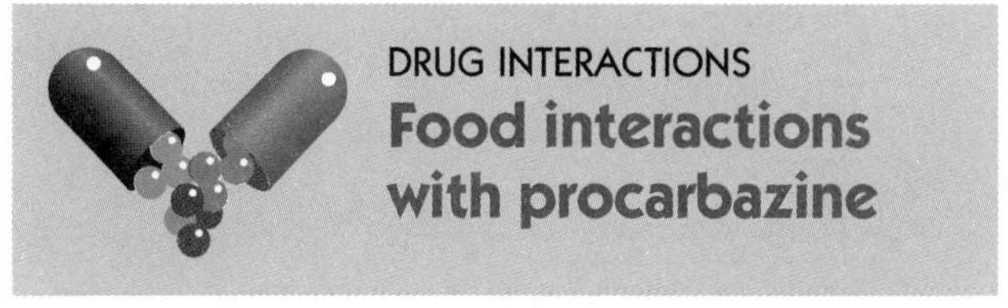

DRUG INTERACTIONS
Food interactions with procarbazine

Foods containing the amino acid tyramine can cause a patient taking procarbazine to develop extreme hypertension, which could develop into a hypertensive crisis. Foods to avoid include:

- yogurt
- bananas
- chicken or beef liver
- chianti wine
- coffee and cola drinks
- ripe or aged cheese
- pickled herring
- beer
- chocolate.

ADVERSE DRUG REACTIONS

Late-onset bone marrow suppression is the most common dose-limiting toxicity associated with procarbazine. The platelet count nadir occurs after about 4 weeks of therapy, followed by the leukocyte count nadir. Complete recovery occurs at about 6 weeks.

Nausea and vomiting occur in 50% of patients. Stomatitis and diarrhea may also occur. Initial procarbazine therapy may induce a flulike syndrome, including fever, chills, sweating, lethargy, and myalgia. High-dose procarbazine therapy can induce azoospermia or cessation of menses. Procarbazine may be teratogenic.

Adverse dermatologic reactions have occurred in about 3% of patients. These reactions include pruritus, acneiform rash, and hyperpigmentation.

Procarbazine may produce CNS toxicity marked by such varied reactions as confusion, depression, psychosis, neuropathies, fingertip paresthesia, footdrop, and lack of muscle coordination. Interstitial pneumonitis and pulmonary fibrosis may occur. Orthostatic hypotension occurs rarely.

NURSING PROCESS APPLICATION

The following information assists the nurse in caring for a patient receiving procarbazine. It includes an overview of assessment activities as well as examples of appropriate nursing diagnoses and related interventions (see "Planning and implementation"). It also highlights the importance of evaluation.

Assessment

Before drug therapy begins, review the patient's history for conditions that contraindicate or require cautious use of procarbazine. Also review the patient's medication history to identify use of drugs that may interact with it. During therapy, assess the patient for adverse drug reactions and signs of drug interactions. Also, periodically assess the effectiveness of procarbazine therapy. Finally, evaluate the patient's and family's knowledge about the prescribed drug.

Nursing diagnoses

- Risk for injury related to a preexisting condition that contraindicates or requires cautious use of procarbazine
- Risk for injury related to adverse drug reactions or drug interactions
- Altered health maintenance related to procarbazine-induced hypertensive crisis
- Knowledge deficit related to procarbazine

Planning and implementation

- Do not administer procarbazine to a patient with a condition that contraindicates its use.
- Administer procarbazine cautiously to a patient at risk because of a preexisting condition.

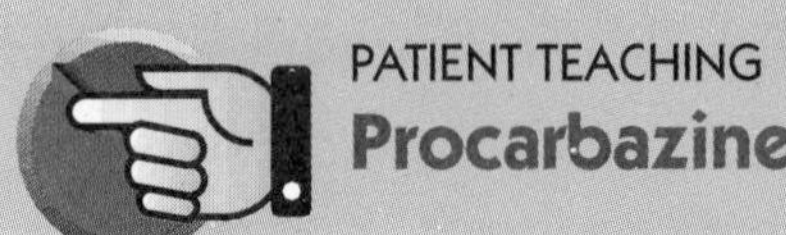

PATIENT TEACHING
Procarbazine

- Teach the patient and family the name, dose, frequency, action, and adverse effects of procarbazine.
- Stress the importance of returning for follow-up blood tests.
- Teach the patient to consume a tyramine-free diet to help prevent a drug and food interaction. The patient should avoid such foods as pickled herring, chicken or beef liver, ripe or aged cheeses, beer, chianti, chocolate, coffee, and cola drinks.
- Instruct the patient to consult the pharmacist or physician before using over-the-counter medication. Such a medication may contain alcohol or a central nervous system (CNS) depressant, which can interact with procarbazine.
- Advise the patient to stagger activities and rest frequently if anemia occurs.
- Advise the patient with leukopenia to avoid people with active contagious infections. Also instruct the patient to watch for signs and symptoms of infection and to report them immediately to the physician.
- Teach the patient with thrombocytopenia to take bleeding precautions.
- Inform the patient and family about the potential for CNS toxicity.
- Advise the female patient to avoid pregnancy during procarbazine therapy because the drug may be teratogenic. This is particularly important because procarbazine is commonly used to treat Hodgkin's disease, which predominantly affects young adults.
- Inform the female patient receiving high dosages of procarbazine that cessation of menses may occur and is drug-related.
- Instruct the patient to avoid activities that require mental alertness if adverse CNS reactions occur.
- Teach the patient how to manage troublesome adverse reactions, such as gastrointestinal distress, stomatitis, and flulike syndrome.
- Give the patient written materials about the possible effects of procarbazine for home reference.
- Instruct the patient to notify the physician if adverse reactions occur.

• Monitor the patient regularly for adverse reactions and drug interactions during procarbazine therapy.
• Monitor the patient's CBC and platelet count for evidence of leukopenia, thrombocytopenia, or anemia. (See Patient Teaching: *Procarbazine*.) Typically, the nadir of bone marrow suppression occurs about 4 weeks after therapy begins; recovery, 6 weeks. Because red blood cells (RBCs) have a longer life than WBCs and platelets, anemia is less of a problem than thrombocytopenia or leukopenia unless the patient has occult or overt blood loss.
• Monitor the patient with leukopenia for signs of infection. Also take infection control measures until the patient's WBC count returns to normal.
• Take bleeding precautions when the platelet count is below 50,000/mm^3. Expect to administer platelet transfusions and packed RBCs as prescribed during times of severe bleeding.
• Minimize procarbazine-induced nausea and vomiting by administering the drug in divided doses and at bedtime.
∗ Monitor the patient for signs of CNS toxicity, such as fingertip paresthesia, footdrop, lack of muscle coordination, confusion, and depression. Immediately report any of these signs and symptoms to the physician.
• Use other appropriate nursing interventions for a patient with bone marrow suppression, nausea, vomiting, or stomatitis.
• Notify the physician if adverse reactions or drug interactions occur.
∗ Place the patient on a tyramine-free diet as prescribed because procarbazine can interact with tyramine, producing hypertension.
∗ Monitor the patient's blood pressure regularly during procarbazine therapy to detect an impending acute hypertensive episode. If the patient displays a sudden elevation in blood pressure, stop the infusion and notify the physician. Have standard emergency equipment nearby and be prepared to begin emergency measures to manage hypertensive crisis.
• Reevaluate compliance with the tyramine-free diet if the patient experiences hypertensive crisis.

Evaluation

For each nursing diagnosis, prepare an evaluation statement that describes the patient's or family's response to nursing interventions.

Hydroxyurea

Hydroxyurea is used most commonly for patients with chronic **myelogenous** leukemia. It is also used for melanoma and certain carcinomas of the ovary.

PHARMACOKINETICS

Hydroxyurea is absorbed readily and distributed well into the CSF after oral administration. It reaches a peak CSF concentration level 3 hours after administration. About 50% of a dose is metabolized by the liver to carbon dioxide, which is excreted by the lungs, or urea, which is excreted by the kidneys. The remaining 50% is excreted unchanged in the urine. Hydroxyurea achieves a peak plasma concentration 1 to 2 hours after administration. Its plasma half-life is 2 hours. Treatment should continue for at least 6 weeks before assessing the drug's clinical effectiveness.

Route	Onset	Peak	Duration
P.O.	Unknown	1-2 hr	24 hr

PHARMACODYNAMICS

Hydroxyurea may act as a DNA-selective antimetabolite. The drug exerts its **cytotoxic** effect by inhibiting the enzyme ribonucleotide reductase, which causes ribonucleotides to convert to deoxyribonucleotides. Without deoxyribonucleotides, DNA synthesis cannot occur. In vitro, hydroxyurea kills cells in the S phase of the **cell cycle** and holds other cells in the G_1 phase, where they are most susceptible to irradiation.

PHARMACOTHERAPEUTICS

Hydroxyurea is used to treat selected **myeloproliferative** disorders. It also is used in combination therapy with radiation to treat carcinomas of the head, neck, and lung. It may produce temporary remissions in some patients with metastatic malignant melanomas.

Drug interactions

Researchers have identified no significant drug interactions with hydroxyurea.

ADVERSE DRUG REACTIONS

Hydroxyurea causes dose-related bone marrow suppression characterized primarily by leukopenia. Patients may also experience drowsiness, headache, nausea, vomiting, and anorexia. These adverse reactions are usually dose-related. Mild dermatologic reactions may include pruritus, facial erythema, and a maculopapular rash.

Rarely, a patient receiving radiation will experience exacerbated radiation erythema when taking hydroxyurea. Stomatitis and alopecia may also occur but are rare. Patients taking hydroxyurea may need to take allopurinol to prevent uric acid nephropathy and its resultant renal damage.

NURSING PROCESS APPLICATION

The following information assists the nurse in caring for a patient receiving hydroxyurea. It includes an overview of assessment activities as well as examples of appropriate nursing diagnoses and related interventions (see "Planning and implementation"). It also highlights the importance of evaluation.

Assessment

Before drug therapy begins, review the patient's history for conditions that contraindicate or require cautious use of hydroxyurea. During therapy, assess the patient for adverse drug reactions. Also, periodically assess the effectiveness of hydroxyurea therapy. Finally, evaluate the patient's and family's knowledge about the prescribed drug. (See Patient Teaching: *Hydroxyurea.)*

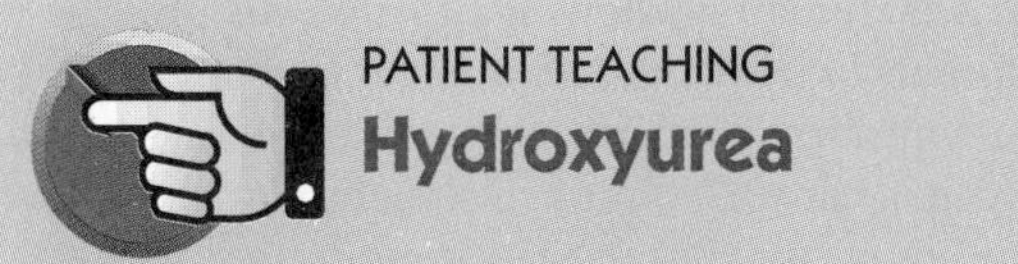

PATIENT TEACHING

Hydroxyurea

- Teach the patient and family the name, dose, frequency, action, and adverse effects of hydroxyurea.
- Stress the importance of returning for follow-up blood tests.
- Instruct the patient to watch for signs and symptoms of infection and to report them immediately to the physician.
- Advise the patient to avoid people with contagious infections.
- Teach the patient about using an oral or suppository antiemetic, as prescribed, if nausea and vomiting occur during hydroxyurea therapy.
- Explain to the patient that mild, reversible dermatologic reactions, such as pruritus, maculopapular rash, and facial erythema, may occur. Instruct the patient to keep previously irradiated skin clean, dry, and protected from sunlight. Also instruct the patient to report exacerbation of erythema at an irradiated site to the physician.
- Caution the patient to avoid activities that require mental alertness if drowsiness occurs.
- Teach the patient how to manage stomatitis at home.
- Prepare the patient for possible alopecia by explaining the timing and speed of hair loss and noting that it may affect the scalp, eyebrows, eyelashes, or other body hair.
- Stress the importance of taking hydroxyurea exactly as prescribed to maximize therapeutic effects and minimize adverse ones.
- Instruct the patient to drink at least eight 8-oz (240-ml) glasses of fluid daily during hydroxyurea therapy.
- Give the patient written materials about hydroxyurea therapy for home reference.
- Instruct the patient to notify the physician if adverse reactions occur.

Nursing diagnoses

- Risk for injury related to a preexisting condition that contraindicates or requires cautious use of hydroxyurea
- Risk for injury related to adverse drug reactions
- Risk for trauma related to hydroxyurea-induced uric acid nephropathy
- Knowledge deficit related to hydroxyurea

Planning and implementation

- Do not administer hydroxyurea to a patient with a condition that contraindicates its use.
- Administer hydroxyurea cautiously to a patient at risk because of a preexisting condition.
- Monitor the patient regularly for adverse reactions during hydroxyurea therapy.
- Monitor the patient's WBC count regularly for leukopenia. If leukopenia occurs, monitor the patient for signs of infection. Also take infection control measures until the WBC count returns to normal.

* ***Administer oral hydroxyurea on a daily or every-third-day schedule, as prescribed, giving a large single dose rather than divided doses to attain higher blood levels. If***

the patient has trouble swallowing capsules, dissolve the capsule contents in water and administer immediately.
• Use other appropriate nursing interventions for a patient with leukopenia, nausea, vomiting, stomatitis, or alopecia.
• Notify the physician if adverse reactions occur.
**** Monitor uric acid, blood urea nitrogen (BUN), and creatinine levels during therapy to detect signs of uric acid nephropathy, such as rising uric acid, BUN, and creatinine levels.***
• Encourage the patient who exhibits signs of nephropathy to drink at least eight 8-oz (240-ml) glasses of fluid daily. Also expect to administer allopurinol as prescribed.
• Notify the physician if uric acid nephropathy occurs.

Evaluation

For each nursing diagnosis, prepare an evaluation statement that describes the patient's or family's response to nursing interventions.

Interferons

A family of naturally occurring glycoproteins, interferons are so named because of their ability to interfere with viral replication. These drugs have anticancer activity as well as activity against condylomata acuminata (soft, wartlike growths on the skin and mucous membrane of the genitalia caused by a virus).

Three types of interferons exist: alfa interferons, which are derived from leukocytes; beta interferons, from fibroblasts; and gamma interferons, from fibroblasts and lymphocytes. Currently, only alfa interferons (alfa-2A, alfa-2B, and alfa-n3) are available commercially. The beta and gamma interferons are limited to investigational use.

PHARMACOKINETICS

After I.M. or subcutaneous (S.C.) administration, alfa interferons are usually absorbed well. They achieve a peak concentration level about 4 hours after I.M. administration or 7 hours after S.C. administration. Information about their distribution is unavailable. Alfa interferons are filtered by the kidneys, where they are degraded. Hepatic metabolism and biliary excretion of interferons are negligible. The half-life of these agents ranges from 2 to 8.5 hours.

Route	Onset	Peak	Duration
I.M.	Unknown	4 hr	Unknown
S.C.	Unknown	7 hr	Unknown

PHARMACODYNAMICS

Interferons are naturally occurring molecules that are produced and secreted by human cells in response to viral infection. Although their exact mechanism of action is unknown, they have been shown to bind to specific membrane receptors on the cell surface. Once bound, they initiate a sequence of intracellular events that includes the induction of certain enzymes. This process may account for the ability of interferons to inhibit viral replication, suppress cell proliferation, enhance macrophage activity, and increase lymphocyte cytotoxicity.

PHARMACOTHERAPEUTICS

Alfa interferons have shown their most promising activity in treating hematologic malignancies, especially hairy cell leukemia. Their approved indications currently include hairy cell leukemia, acquired immunodeficiency syndrome (AIDS)-related Kaposi's sarcoma, and condylomata acuminata. However, alfa interferons also demonstrate some activity against chronic myelogenous leukemia, malignant lymphoma, multiple myeloma, melanoma, and renal cell carcinoma.

Drug interactions

Interferons may enhance the CNS effects of CNS depressants and substantially increase the half-life of methylxanthines (including theophylline and aminophylline), perhaps by interfering with the cytochrome P-450 drug metabolizing enzymes.

Concurrent use of an interferon with a live virus vaccine may potentiate replication of the virus, increasing the adverse effects of the vaccine and decreasing the patient's antibody response.

Bone marrow suppression may be increased when an interferon is used concomitantly with radiation therapy or a drug that causes blood dyscrasias or bone marrow suppression. A dosage reduction for both drugs may be required.

ADVERSE DRUG REACTIONS

The most common adverse reaction to alfa interferons is a flulike syndrome that may produce fever, fatigue, myalgia, headache, chills, and arthralgia.

Hematologic toxicity occurs in up to 50% of patients and may produce leukopenia, neutropenia, thrombocytopenia, and anemia. Adverse gastrointestinal (GI) reactions, such as anorexia, nausea, and diarrhea, occur in 30% to 50% of patients receiving an alfa interferon. CNS disturbances can occur in 10% to 20% of patients and may include dizziness, confusion, paresthesia, numbness, lethargy, and depression.

Coughing and dyspnea have also been associated with interferon therapy, as well as hypotension, edema, chest pain, and heart failure. Adverse dermatologic reactions may include alopecia, rash, and dry skin. Interferons may also cause an elevation in the liver transaminase level and abnormalities in renal function tests.

NURSING PROCESS APPLICATION

The following information assists the nurse in caring for a patient receiving an interferon. It includes an overview of assessment activities as well as examples of appropriate nursing diagnoses and related interventions (see "Planning and implementation"). It also highlights the importance of evaluation.

Assessment

Before drug therapy begins, review the patient's history for conditions that contraindicate or require cautious use of the prescribed interferon. Also review the patient's medication history to identify use of drugs that may interact with it. During therapy, assess the patient for adverse drug reactions and signs of drug interactions. Also, periodically assess the effectiveness of interferon therapy. Finally, evaluate the patient's and family's knowledge about the prescribed drug.

Nursing diagnoses

- Risk for injury related to a preexisting condition that contraindicates or requires cautious use of an interferon
- Risk for injury related to adverse drug reactions or drug interactions
- Altered health maintenance related to flulike syndrome caused by an interferon
- Knowledge deficit related to the prescribed interferon

Planning and implementation

- Do not administer an interferon to a patient with a condition that contraindicates its use.
- Administer an interferon cautiously to a patient at risk because of a preexisting condition.
- Monitor the patient regularly for adverse reactions and drug interactions during interferon therapy.

*** *Monitor the patient's blood pressure to detect hypotension. Regularly inquire about chest pain. Monitor for signs and symptoms of heart failure. Notify the physician if assessments reveal hypotension or signs of heart failure.***

- Monitor the patient's CBC and platelet count for evidence of leukopenia, neutropenia, thrombocytopenia, or anemia. Observe the patient with leukopenia for signs of infection. Take infection control measures until the WBC count returns to normal. Observe the patient with thrombocytopenia for signs of bleeding. Also take bleeding precautions until the platelet count returns to normal. If anemia occurs, encourage the patient to take energy conservation measures until the RBC count returns to normal.
- Monitor for elevations in the patient's liver transaminase level and renal function studies. Abnormal results may require a dosage reduction.
- Use other appropriate nursing interventions for a patient with leukopenia, thrombocytopenia, anemia, nausea, or alopecia.
- Notify the physician if adverse reactions or drug interactions occur.
- Monitor the patient for flulike symptoms, such as fever, headache, fatigue, myalgia, chills, and arthralgia.
- Administer the interferon in the evening as prescribed to minimize troublesome flulike symptoms during the day.

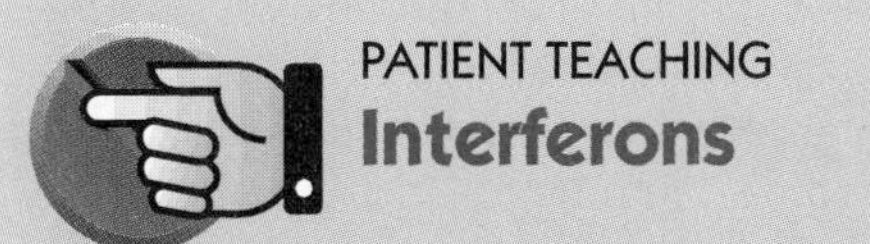

PATIENT TEACHING
Interferons

- Teach the patient and family the name, dose, frequency, action, and adverse effects of the prescribed interferon.
- Instruct the patient not to change to a different brand of interferon because this may result in an unintended dosage change.
- Inform the patient about the likelihood and management of flulike symptoms. Reassure the patient that most people develop a tolerance to these symptoms, which tend to diminish with continued therapy.
- Teach the patient or family member how to administer the drug properly.
- Teach the patient how to manage troublesome gastrointestinal reactions.
- Caution the patient not to perform activities that require mental alertness if central nervous system disturbances occur.
- Instruct the patient to report cough, dyspnea, chest pain, light-headedness, and ankle swelling because these signs and symptoms may suggest heart failure, hypotension, or a respiratory disturbance.
- Teach the patient to use infection control measures, bleeding precautions, and energy conservation measures as needed.
- Stress the importance of returning for follow-up blood tests.
- Give the patient written materials about the possible effects of interferons for home reference.
- Instruct the patient to report other adverse reactions.

- Monitor the patient for CNS disturbances, including dizziness, confusion, paresthesia, numbness, lethargy and depression. Notify physician immediately if these symptoms occur.
- Consult with the physician about premedicating the patient with acetaminophen to help relieve flulike symptoms. (See Patient Teaching: *Interferons.)*
- Notify the physician if flulike symptoms become intolerable.

Evaluation

For each nursing diagnosis, prepare an evaluation statement that describes the patient's or family's response to nursing interventions.

Aldesleukin

Aldesleukin is a human recombinant interleukin-2 derivative that is used to treat metastatic renal cell carcinoma.

PHARMACOKINETICS

After I.V. administration of aldesleukin, about 30% is absorbed into the plasma and about 70% is absorbed rapidly by the liver, kidneys, and lungs. The drug is excreted primarily by the kidneys. Its plasma half-life after a 5-minute infusion is approximately 85 minutes.

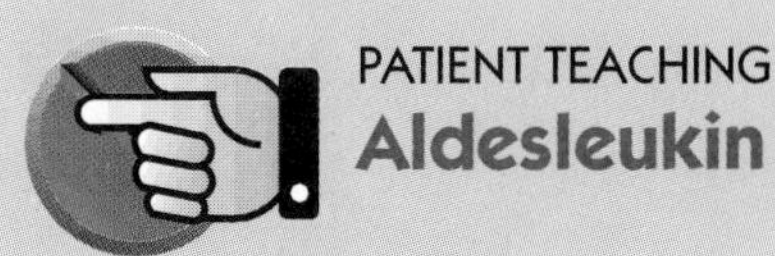

PATIENT TEACHING
Aldesleukin

- Teach the patient and family the name, dose, frequency, action, and adverse effects of aldesleukin.
- Stress the importance of returning for follow-up blood tests.
- Instruct the patient to consult the pharmacist or physician before using over-the-counter medications. They may contain ingredients that may produce additive central nervous system effects when administered concomitantly with aldesleukin.
- Advise the patient to stagger activities and to rest frequently if anemia occurs.
- Advise the patient with leukopenia to avoid people with active contagious infections. Also instruct the patient to watch for signs and symptoms of infection and to report them immediately to the physician.
- Teach the patient with thrombocytopenia to take bleeding precautions.
- Teach the patient how to manage troublesome adverse reactions, such as gastrointestinal distress, stomatitis, and flulike syndrome.
- Give the patient written materials about the possible effects of aldesleukin for home reference.
- Instruct the patient to notify the physician if adverse reactions occur.
- Prepare the patient for possible alopecia by explaining the timing and speed of hair loss and noting that it may affect the scalp, eyebrows, eyelashes, or other body hair.

Route	Onset	Peak	Duration
I.V.	Rapid	0.1-1.5 hr	Unknown

PHARMACODYNAMICS

A human recombinant interleukin-2 derivative, aldesleukin exhibits antitumor activity. Its exact mechanism of action is unknown.

PHARMACOTHERAPEUTICS

Aldesleukin is used to treat metastatic renal cell carcinoma. Aldesleukin may also be used in the treatment of Kaposi's sarcoma and metastatic melanoma.

Drug interactions

Concomitant administration of drugs with psychotropic properties, such as narcotics, analgesics, antiemetics, sedatives, and tranquilizers, may produce additive CNS effects. Because glucocorticoids may reduce aldesleukin's antitumor effects, these two drugs should not be used together. Antihypertensive agents may potentiate aldesleukin's hypotensive effects. Concurrent therapy with nephrotoxic, myelotoxic, cardiotoxic, or hepatotoxic drugs has not been studied.

ADVERSE DRUG REACTIONS

During clinical trials, more than 15% of patients developed these adverse reactions to aldesleukin: pulmonary congestion, dyspnea, anemia, thrombocytopenia, leukopenia, hypomagnesemia, acidosis, oliguria, anuria, stomatitis, nausea, vomiting, pruritus, erythema, rash, dry skin, fever, chills, fatigue, malaise, weakness, edema, infection, pain, weight gain, and elevated bilirubin, transaminase, alkaline phosphate, or serum creatinine level.

NURSING PROCESS APPLICATION

The following information assists the nurse in caring for a patient receiving aldesleukin. It includes an overview of assessment activities as well as examples of appropriate nursing diagnoses and related interventions (see "Planning and implementation"). It also highlights the importance of evaluation.

Assessment

Before drug therapy begins, review the patient's history for conditions that contraindicate or require cautious use of aldesleukin. Also review the patient's medication history to identify use of drugs that may interact with it. During therapy, assess the patient for adverse drug reactions and signs of drug interactions. Also, periodically assess the effectiveness of aldesleukin therapy. Finally, evaluate the patient's and family's knowledge about the prescribed drug. (See Patient Teaching: *Aldesleukin.*)

Nursing diagnoses

- Risk for injury related to a preexisting condition that contraindicates or requires cautious use of aldesleukin
- Risk for injury related to adverse drug reactions or drug interactions
- Altered protection related to aldesleukin-induced thrombocytopenia or leukopenia
- Knowledge deficit related to aldesleukin

Planning and implementation

- Do not administer aldesleukin to a patient with a condition that contraindicates its use.
- Administer aldesleukin cautiously to a patient at risk because of a preexisting condition.
- Monitor the patient regularly for adverse reactions and drug interactions during aldesleukin therapy.

***** *Verify that cardiac, pulmonary, hepatic, and CNS functions are normal before beginning therapy. Hematologic tests, pulmonary and cardiac function tests, blood chemistries, and chest X-rays should be obtained before therapy starts and then daily during therapy.***

- Monitor the patient's CBC and platelet count for evidence of leukopenia, thrombocytopenia, or anemia. Because RBCs have a longer life than WBCs and platelets, anemia is less of a problem than thrombocytopenia or leukopenia unless the patient has occult or overt blood loss.

• Monitor the patient with leukopenia for signs of infection, such as fever, sore throat, chills, and malaise. Also take infection control measures until the patient's WBC count returns to normal.
• Take bleeding precautions when the platelet count is below 50,000/mm^3. Expect to administer platelet transfusions and packed RBCs as prescribed during times of severe bleeding.
• Take energy conservation measures for a patient with anemia. For example, stagger the patient's activities, help with tasks, and arrange for frequent rest periods.
• Monitor the patient for flulike syndrome, characterized by fever, chills, malaise, and myalgia. Administer a mild antipyretic and analgesic as prescribed.
• Monitor the patient closely for signs of impaired thyroid function after aldesleukin therapy.
• Use other appropriate nursing interventions for a patient with thrombocytopenia, leukopenia, nausea, vomiting, or stomatitis.
• Notify the physician if adverse reactions or drug interactions occur.

Evaluation

For each nursing diagnosis, prepare an evaluation statement that describes the patient's or family's response to nursing interventions.

Altretamine

Altretamine is a synthetic cytotoxic antineoplastic agent that is used as **palliative** treatment for patients with ovarian cancer.

PHARMACOKINETICS

Altretamine is absorbed well after oral administration. It is metabolized extensively in the liver and excreted by the liver and kidneys. The parent compound is approximately 6% bound to plasma proteins. Altretamine and its metabolites have an average half-life of 7.4 hours.

Route	Onset	Peak	Duration
P.O.	Unknown	0.5-3 hr	Unknown

PHARMACODYNAMICS

The exact mechanism of action of altretamine is unknown.

PHARMACOTHERAPEUTICS

Altretamine is used as palliative treatment of persistent or recurring ovarian cancer after first-line therapy with cisplatin or an alkylating agent–based combination.

Drug interactions

Concomitant therapy with cimetidine may increase altretamine's half-life, requiring frequent monitoring for altretamine toxicity. Use with an MAO inhibitor may cause severe orthostatic hypotension.

ADVERSE DRUG REACTIONS

More than 10% of patients in clinical trials exhibited these adverse reactions to altretamine: nausea, vomiting, neurotoxicity, peripheral neuropathy, and anemia. Bone marrow suppression is common and can cause leukopenia, thrombocytopenia, and anemia.

NURSING PROCESS APPLICATION

The following information assists the nurse in caring for a patient receiving altretamine. It includes an overview of assessment activities as well as examples of appropriate nursing diagnoses and related interventions (see "Planning and implementation"). It also highlights the importance of evaluation.

Assessment

Before drug therapy begins, review the patient's history for conditions that contraindicate or require cautious use of altretamine. Also review the patient's medication history to identify use of drugs that may interact with it. During therapy, assess the patient for adverse drug reactions and signs of drug interactions. Also, periodically assess the effectiveness of altretamine therapy. Finally, evaluate the patient's and family's knowledge about the prescribed drug.

Nursing diagnoses

• Risk for injury related to a preexisting condition that contraindicates or requires cautious use of altretamine
• Risk for injury related to adverse drug reactions or drug interactions
• Altered health maintenance related to concomitant use of altretamine and an MAO inhibitor
• Knowledge deficit related to altretamine

Planning and implementation

• Do not administer altretamine to a patient with a condition that contraindicates its use.
• Administer altretamine cautiously to a patient at risk because of a preexisting condition.
• Monitor the patient regularly for adverse reactions and drug interactions during altretamine therapy.
*** *Monitor the patient's CBC and platelet count for evidence of leukopenia, thrombocytopenia, or anemia. Typically, the nadir of bone marrow suppression occurs about 4 weeks after therapy begins; recovery, at 6 weeks. Because RBCs have a longer life than WBCs and platelets, anemia is less of a problem than thrombocytopenia or leukopenia unless the patient has occult or overt blood loss.***

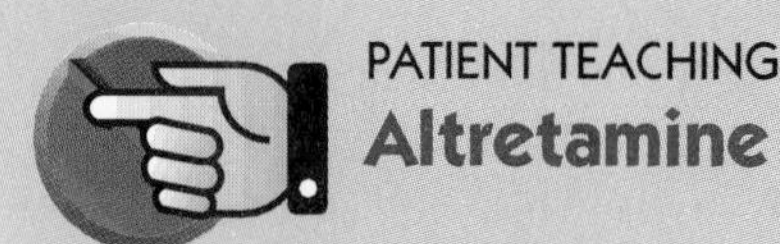

PATIENT TEACHING
Altretamine

- Teach the patient and family the name, dose, frequency, action, and adverse effects of altretamine.
- Stress the importance of returning for follow-up blood tests.
- Advise the patient to stagger activities and to rest frequently if anemia occurs.
- Advise the patient with leukopenia to avoid people with active contagious infections. Also instruct the patient to watch for signs and symptoms of infection and to report them immediately to the physician.
- Teach the patient with thrombocytopenia to take bleeding precautions.
- Inform the patient and family about the potential for central nervous system (CNS) toxicity.
- Advise the female patient to avoid pregnancy during altretamine therapy because the drug may be teratogenic.
- Instruct the patient to avoid activities that require mental alertness if adverse CNS reactions occur.
- Teach the patient how to manage troublesome adverse reactions, such as gastrointestinal distress and immunosuppression.
- Give the patient written materials about the possible effects of altretamine for home reference.
- Instruct the patient to notify the physician if adverse reactions occur.

• Monitor the patient with leukopenia for signs of infection. Also take infection control measures until the patient's WBC count returns to normal.
• Take bleeding precautions when the platelet count is below 50,000/mm^3. Expect to administer platelet transfusions and packed RBCs as prescribed during times of severe bleeding.
• Expect to discontinue altretamine for at least 14 days if the patient develops GI intolerance unresponsive to conventional measures, WBC count less than 2,000/mm^3 or granulocyte count less than 1,000/mm^3, platelet count less than 75,000/mm^3, or progressive neurotoxicity. Restart the dosage at 200 mg/m^2 daily, as prescribed. If neurologic symptoms persist despite the dosage reduction, expect to discontinue altretamine therapy.
• Take energy conservation measures for a patient with anemia. For example, stagger the patient's activities, help with tasks, and arrange for frequent rest periods.
*∗ **Monitor the patient for signs and symptoms of neurotoxicity and peripheral neuropathy. Perform a neurologic examination before each course of therapy. Immediately report any signs and symptoms to the physician.***
• Use other appropriate nursing interventions for a patient with bone marrow suppression, nausea, or vomiting.
• Notify the physician if adverse reactions or drug interactions occur.
*∗ **Monitor the patient for signs and symptoms of orthostatic hypotension, such as light-headedness or dizziness upon arising during concomitant therapy with an MAO inhibitor. Advise the patient to avoid sudden position changes.*** (See Patient Teaching: *Altretamine.*)
• Monitor the patient's blood pressure regularly to detect acute changes during concomitant therapy with an MAO inhibitor. Notify the physician if the patient displays severe orthostatic hypotension.

Evaluation

For each nursing diagnosis, prepare an evaluation statement that describes the patient's or family's response to nursing interventions.

Taxines

Paclitaxel and docetaxel are antimicrotubule agents used to treat metastatic ovarian and breast carcinoma after chemotherapy has failed. They are also used to treat non-small-cell lung cancer, cancer of the head and neck, and prostate cancer.

PHARMACOKINETICS

After I.V. administration, paclitaxel is 89% to 98% bound to plasma proteins. The drug is metabolized primarily in the liver and a small amount excreted unchanged in the urine. Paclitaxel demonstrates a biphasic decline in plasma concentration; its plasma elimination half-life ranges from 5.3 to 17.4 hours. Docetaxel is administered I.V. with a rapid onset of action. Its half-life is up to 11 hours. It is excreted primarily through feces.

Route	Onset	Peak	Duration
I.V.	Rapid	11 hr-8 wk	Unknown

PHARMACODYNAMICS

Paclitaxel and docetaxel exert their chemotherapeutic effect by preventing the depolymerization of microtubules. This inhibits the normal reorganization of the microtubule network, which is essential for mitosis and other vital cellular functions.

PHARMACOTHERAPEUTICS

Paclitaxel is used when first-line or subsequent chemotherapy has failed in treating metastatic ovarian carcinoma as well as metastatic breast cancer. The taxines may also be used for the treatment of head and neck cancer, prostate cancer, and non-small-cell lung cancer.

Drug interactions

Concomitant use of paclitaxel and cisplatin may cause additive myelosuppressive effects. Ketoconazole may inhibit paclitaxel metabolism.

ADVERSE DRUG REACTIONS

During clinical trials, 25% or more patients experienced these adverse reactions to paclitaxel: bone marrow suppression resulting in neutropenia, leukopenia, thrombocytopenia, or anemia; hypersensitivity reactions; abnormal EEG tracings; peripheral neuropathy; myalgia; arthralgia; nausea, vomiting, and diarrhea; **mucositis** and alopecia.

Hypersensitivity reactions occur in 30% of the patients who are given docetaxel. Fluid retention, leukopenia, neutropenia, thrombocytopenia, alopecia, stomatitis, paresthesia, pain, fatigue, and weakness are other adverse effects. Studies of American and Japanese patients show that adverse reactions vary from culture to culture. (See Cultural Considerations: *Docetaxel.*)

CULTURAL CONSIDERATIONS

Docetaxel

Clinical trials of docetaxel conducted in Japanese and American patients with breast cancer revealed significant differences in the incidence of adverse effects between the two cultures.

The Japanese women were more likely to develop thrombocytopenia — 14.4% vs. 5.5%.

However, the Japanese women in this study were less likely to develop many of the other adverse effects, such as hypersensitivity reactions — 0.6% vs. the 29.1% seen in the American patients. Other results showed fewer incidences of fluid retention, neurosensory effects, myalgia, infection, and development of anemia. The study also indicated that Japanese patients are more likely to develop fatigue and weakness than American women.

These results are important to consider when caring for patients receiving docetaxel. The information can provide clues for developing a plan of care and for knowing what adverse effects to expect.

NURSING PROCESS APPLICATION

The following information assists the nurse in caring for a patient receiving a taxine. It includes an overview of assessment activities as well as examples of appropriate nursing diagnoses and related interventions (see "Planning and implementation"). It also highlights the importance of evaluation.

Assessment

Before drug therapy begins, review the patient's history for conditions that contraindicate the use of a taxine. Also review the patient's medication history to identify use of drugs that may interact with it. During therapy, assess the patient for adverse drug reactions and signs of drug interactions. Also, periodically assess the effectiveness of taxine therapy. Finally, evaluate the patient's and family's knowledge about the prescribed drug.

Nursing diagnoses

- Risk for injury related to a preexisting condition that contraindicates the use of taxines
- Risk for injury related to adverse drug reactions or drug interactions
- Knowledge deficit related to paclitaxel or docetaxel

Planning and implementation

- Do not administer paclitaxel to a patient with a condition that contraindicates its use.
- Monitor the patient regularly for adverse reactions and drug interactions during paclitaxel or docetaxel therapy.

∗ ***Premedicate a patient with corticosteroids, diphenhydramine, or histamine$_2$-receptor antagonists, as prescribed, to reduce the incidence of severe hypersensitivity reactions and fluid retention.***

- Administer an antiemetic as prescribed. Use other appropriate nursing interventions for a patient with nausea or vomiting.
- Note paclitaxel treatment on any EEG request slip because it can cause abnormal EEG tracings. Also be aware that if a patient develops significant cardiac conduction abnormalities while receiving paclitaxel, appropriate therapy should be administered and continuous cardiac monitoring should be performed during subsequent infusions.
- Monitor the patient's CBC and platelet counts for evidence of leukopenia, thrombocytopenia, or anemia. Typically, the nadir of bone marrow suppression occurs about 4 weeks after therapy begins; recovery, at 6 weeks. Because RBCs have a longer life than WBCs and platelets, anemia is less of a problem than thrombocytopenia or leukopenia unless the patient has occult or overt blood loss.

∗ ***Monitor the patient with leukopenia for signs of infection, such as fever, sore throat, chills, and malaise. Also take infection control measures until the patient's WBC count returns to normal.***

- Take bleeding precautions when the platelet count is below 50,000/mm^3. Expect to administer platelet transfusions and packed RBCs as prescribed during times of severe bleeding.
- Take energy conservation measures for a patient with anemia. For example, stagger the patient's activities, help with tasks, and arrange for frequent rest periods. (See Patient Teaching: *Taxines,* page 704.)
- Administer I.V. paclitaxel through an in-line filter. Prepare and store the drug in glass containers.
- Notify the physician if adverse reactions or drug interactions persist or worsen.

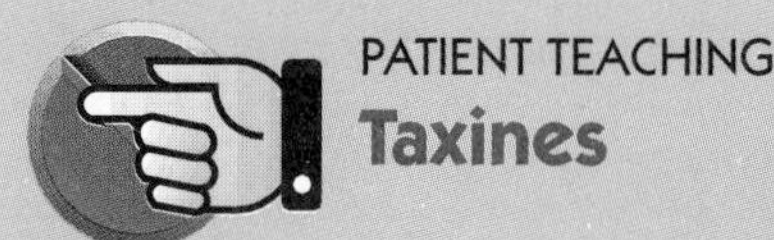

PATIENT TEACHING
Taxines

- Teach the patient and family the name, dose, frequency, action, and adverse effects of the taxines.
- Stress the importance of returning for follow-up blood tests.
- Advise the patient to stagger activities and take frequent rests if anemia occurs.
- Advise the patient with leukopenia to avoid people with active contagious infections. Also instruct the patient to watch for signs and symptoms of infection and to report them immediately to the physician.
- Teach the patient with thrombocytopenia to take bleeding precautions.
- Teach the patient how to manage troublesome adverse reactions, such as gastrointestinal distress.
- Give the patient written materials about the possible effects of taxines for home reference.
- Instruct the patient to notify the physician if adverse reactions occur.
- Prepare the patient for alopecia by explaining the timing and speed of hair loss and noting that it may affect the scalp, eyebrows, eyelashes, or other body hair.
- Stress the importance of taking premedications before taking the taxine to alleviate noxious adverse effects.

Evaluation

For each nursing diagnosis, prepare an evaluation statement that describes the patient's or family's response to nursing interventions.

CHAPTER SUMMARY

Chapter 57 discussed various antineoplastic agents, including the vinca alkaloids, podophyllotoxins, asparaginase, pegaspargase, procarbazine, hydroxyurea, interferons, aldesleukin, altretamine, and taxines. Here are the chapter highlights.

The vinca alkaloids and podophyllotoxins are cell cycle-specific drugs.

The vinca alkaloids, which are vesicants that must be administered carefully to prevent extravasation, are used to treat Hodgkin's disease, malignant lymphoma, testicular cancer, Kaposi's sarcoma, neuroblastoma, choriocarcinoma, breast cancer, acute lymphocytic leukemia, rhabdomyosarcoma, and Wilms' tumor. The podophyllotoxins are used to treat various tumors, including lymphomas, small-cell lung carcinoma, and testicular carcinoma, as well as leukemias.

Asparaginase is a cell cycle–specific enzyme used primarily to induce remission in acute lymphocytic leukemia. Because asparaginase increases the patient's risk of anaphylaxis, it must be administered with a physician present.

Procarbazine is used to treat Hodgkin's disease and primary and metastatic brain tumors. Because procarbazine has MAO-inhibiting properties, it interacts with tyramine-rich foods, which can cause severe hypertension. Therefore, a patient taking procarbazine should avoid eating tyramine-rich foods.

Hydroxyurea is used primarily to treat chronic myelogenous leukemia and blast crisis.

Interferons are naturally occurring molecules that inhibit viral replication, suppress cell proliferation, enhance macrophage activity, and increase lymphocyte cytotoxicity. They are used to treat hairy cell leukemia, AIDS-related Kaposi's sarcoma, and condylomata acuminata.

Aldesleukin, a human recombinant interleukin-2 derivative, is used to treat metastatic renal cell carcinoma.

Altretamine is used for palliative treatment of persistent or recurring ovarian cancer after first-line therapy has been tried. Concomitant administration with an MAO inhibitor may cause severe orthostatic hypotension.

Taxines are antimicrotubule agents used to treat metastatic ovarian and breast cancers after first-line or subsequent chemotherapy has failed.

The nurse should administer antineoplastic agents with extreme caution because they can produce many serious adverse reactions. For a patient receiving one of these agents, the nurse follows the steps of the nursing process to provide care that helps minimize such reactions.

Questions to consider

See Appendix 1 for answers.

1. Sharon Harris, age 36, is diagnosed with Hodgkin's disease. The physician prescribes vincristine as part of her therapy. Vincristine commonly produces which of the following adverse reactions?
   (a) Fever
   (b) Hypotension
   (c) Alopecia
   (d) Photophobia

2. Emily Kilmer, age 25, is receiving procarbazine. Which of the following drug-related dietary instructions should the nurse give her?
   (a) Avoid tyramine-rich foods, such as coffee, chocolate, and aged cheese.
   (b) Avoid calcium-rich foods, such as milk, yogurt, and other dairy products.
   (c) Increase fluid consumption to thirteen 8-oz (240-ml) glasses daily, unless contraindicated.
   (d) Increase vitamin and mineral intake by taking supplements.

3. Nelson Rockford, age 22, is diagnosed with acute lymphocytic leukemia. His physician prescribes asparaginase as part of his chemotherapy. When administering the drug, the nurse observes Mr. Rockford closely for anaphylaxis. Which of the following administration methods increases the risk of anaphylaxis?
   (a) Daily I.M. administration
   (b) Daily I.V. administration
   (c) Intermittent I.M. administration
   (d) Intermittent I.V. administration

4. Tyler Hampton, age 28, has developed AIDS-related Kaposi's sarcoma and must receive interferon alfa-2A. During interferon therapy, he is *most* likely to develop which of the following adverse reactions?
   (a) Flulike syndrome
   (b) Rash
   (c) Dry skin
   (d) Alopecia

5. Marie Carter, age 56, is receiving her fourth course of treatment with a regimen that includes vinblastine. Prior to the start of the infusion, she complains of intermittent numbness and tingling in her extremities. What should the nurse do?
   (a) Document this complaint and proceed with administration of the drug.
   (b) Perform a complete neurologic assessment and then proceed with the infusion.
   (c) Perform a complete neurologic assessment and notify the attending physician.
   (d) Proceed with the infusion.

6. Michael Martin, age 60, is receiving hydroxyurea for the treatment of his chronic myelogenous leukemia. Which of the following drugs is most commonly administered to prevent uric acid nephropathy and its resultant kidney damage in patients receiving hydroxyurea?
   (a) allopurinol
   (b) furosemide
   (c) mesna
   (d) dexamethasone

UNIT XVI

Other major drugs

Although oral and parenteral agents may be used to treat certain sensory system disorders, this unit emphasizes topical agents used to treat disorders of the eyes, ears, and skin. (See *Structures of the eyes and ears.*) In addition, it includes uncategorized agents and new agents used to treat rare diseases and other disorders.

In ophthalmology, eyedrops and ointments are used to relieve inflammation, reduce intraocular pressure and corneal edema, remove opacified corneal epithelium, and provide anesthesia during surgery. They are also used for diagnostic procedures.

Disorders of the external ear include fungal infections, impacted **cerumen,** and external **otitis** (swimmer's ear). These disorders usually require treatment with topical otic agents — the same agents used to manage dermatitis. Therapy also involves thorough cleaning, restoring an acidic surface pH, reducing swelling, eliminating infection, and controlling predisposing factors.

Disorders of the middle ear include acute and chronic otitis media. Both disorders usually require a systemic agent to control the infection and possibly a systemic decongestant.

Dermatologic agents are used to treat various skin disorders, including bacterial, fungal, and viral infections; parasitic infestations; and acne and other dermatologic inflammatory conditions. They may also be used to treat hair loss, keratoses (overgrowths of the epidermal horny layer), and superficial basal cell carcinomas.

A group of uncategorized agents, which do not fall into any pharmacologic classification in this text, and a number of other agents are used to treat rare disorders or disorders that differ from those treated by the other drugs in the classification. Some are used to treat uncommon conditions, such as severe homozygous cystinuria and urea cycle enzymopathies. Others are indicated for more familiar conditions, such as **strabismus,** gallstones, and cancer.

Structures of the eyes and ears

Ophthalmic and otic agents affect different structures of the eyes and ears, as detailed below.

Eye

Topical ophthalmic agents are absorbed through the cornea, conjunctiva, and sclera. Because the cornea is extremely sensitive, these agents must be applied to or instilled in the lower conjunctival sac to avoid direct corneal contact. If an ophthalmic agent, such as atropine, can be absorbed systemically, pressure should be applied to the inner (medial) canthus to help prevent the agent from flowing into the tear duct and entering the systemic circulation.

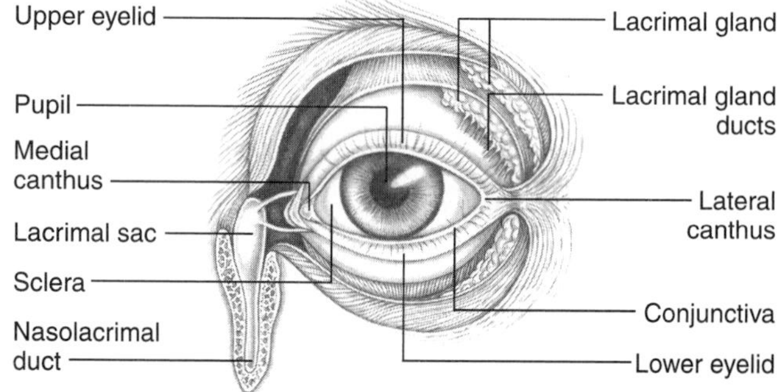

Ear

Topical otic agents primarily affect external ear structures. Systemic agents must be used to treat middle and inner ear disorders.

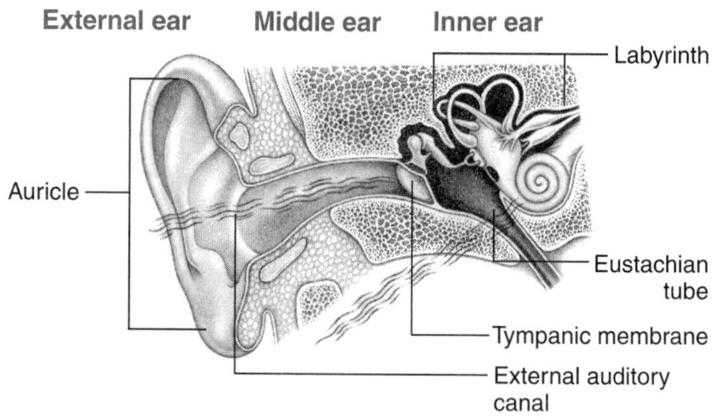

58 Ophthalmic agents

OBJECTIVES

After reading and studying this chapter, the student should be able to:

1. identify the clinical indications for mydriatic, cycloplegic, and miotic agents.
2. describe the mechanism of action of ophthalmic drugs used to lower intraocular pressure.
3. describe the adverse reactions to ophthalmic anesthetic agents and how to prevent them.
4. discuss the clinical indications for ophthalmic anti-inflammatory agents.
5. differentiate the ophthalmic conditions that are treated with topical anti-infectives from those that are treated with systemic anti-infectives.
6. explain how to instill eyedrops and apply eye ointments.
7. describe how to apply the nursing process when caring for a patient receiving an ophthalmic agent.

INTRODUCTION

The ophthalmic agents discussed in this chapter are instilled primarily as drops or applied as ointments. Mydriatics, cycloplegics, and miotics are the three groups of ophthalmic agents most commonly used. Besides these three groups, ophthalmic agents that lower intraocular pressure, anesthetic agents, anti-inflammatory agents, and anti-infective preparations are also discussed in this chapter. (See *Selected major ophthalmic agents,* pages 708 to 710.)

Drugs discussed in this chapter include:

- acetazolamide
- acetazolamide sodium
- apruclonidine
- atropine sulfate
- bacitracin
- betaxolol hydrochloride
- boric acid
- carbachol
- chloramphenicol
- chlortetracycline hydrochloride
- cyclopentolate hydrochloride
- demecarium bromide
- dexamethasone
- dipivefrine
- epinephrine bitartrate
- epinephrine hydrochloride
- epinephryl borate
- erythromycin
- ethothiophate iodide
- fluorometholone
- flurbiprofen sodium
- gentamicin sulfate
- glycerin
- homatropine hydrobromide
- idoxuridine
- isoflurophate
- isosorbide
- levobunolol hydrochloride
- mannitol
- medrysone
- methazolamide
- natamycin
- phenylephrine hydrochloride
- phenylephrine hydrochloride
- physostigmine salicylate
- physostigmine sulfate
- pilocarpine hydrochloride
- pilocarpine nitrate
- polymyxin B sulfate
- prednisolone acetate
- prednisolone sodium phosphate
- proparacaine hydrochloride
- scopolamine hydrobromide
- silver nitrate 1%
- sulfacetamide sodium
- tetracaine
- tetracycline hydrochloride
- timolol maleate
- ttobramycin
- trifluridine
- tropicamide
- urea
- vidarabine.

Mydriatics and cycloplegics

Mydriatics and **cycloplegics** include atropine sulfate, cyclopentolate hydrochloride, dipivefrin, epinephrine bitartrate, epinephrine hydrochloride, epinephryl borate, homatropine hydrobromide, phenylephrine hydrochloride, scopolamine hydrobromide, and tropicamide. Of these, dipivefrin, epinephrine bitartrate, epinephrine hydrochloride, epinephryl borate, and phenylephrine hydrochloride act only as mydriatics, and the rest have combined mydriatic-cycloplegic effects. Dipivefrin, epinephrine bitartrate, epinephrine hydrochloride, and epinephryl borate also lower intraocular pressure.

PHARMACOKINETICS

Atropine, cyclopentolate, epinephrine, phenylephrine, and scopolamine may be absorbed systemically, which may cause adverse reactions, especially in pediatric and geriatric patients. Systemic absorption may occur through the conjunctiva or through the gastrointestinal tract after a drug drains into the nasal sinuses and is swallowed. Absorption is

Selected major ophthalmic agents

The following chart summarizes the major ophthalmic agents currently in clinical use.

DRUG	MAJOR INDICATIONS AND USUAL DOSAGES	CONTRAINDICATIONS AND PRECAUTIONS
Mydriatics and cycloplegics		
atropine (Atropisol, Isopto Atropine)	*Acute iritis* ADULT: 1 to 2 drops of 0.5% to 2% solution b.i.d. or t.i.d. PEDIATRIC: 1 to 2 drops of 0.5% solution b.i.d. or t.i.d. *Refraction* ADULT: 1 to 2 drops of 1% solution 1 hour before examination PEDIATRIC: for children under age 5, 1 to 2 drops of 0.5% solution instilled in each eye for 1 to 3 days before eye examination and again 1 hour before examination	• Atropine is contraindicated in a patient with known or suspected angle-closure glaucoma or known hypersensitivity. • This drug requires cautious use in an infant, a young child, or a child with spastic paralysis or brain damage.
cyclopentolate (Cyclogyl)	*Mydriasis and cycloplegia* ADULT: 1 drop of 1% or 2% solution followed by 1 drop of 1% solution 5 minutes later; use 2% solution in patients with heavily pigmented irises PEDIATRIC: for children age 1 and over, 1 drop of 0.5%, 1%, or 2% solution followed by 1 drop of 0.5% or 1% solution 5 minutes later if needed; for children under age 1, 1 drop of 0.5% solution followed by 1 drop of 0.5% solution 5 minutes later if needed	• Cyclopentolate is contraindicated in a patient with angle-closure glaucoma. • This drug requires cautious use in a geriatric patient or one who is predisposed to increased intraocular pressure.
tropicamide (Mydriacyl)	*Refraction* ADULT: 1 to 2 drops of 1% solution 20 minutes before examination; repeat in 5 minutes. Instill another drop if patient is not seen in 20 to 30 minutes PEDIATRIC: same as adult dosage *Ophthalmoscopic examination* ADULT: 1 to 2 drops of 0.5% solution 15 to 20 minutes before examination; repeat in 20 to 30 minutes if necessary PEDIATRIC: same as adult dosage	• Tropicamide is contraindicated in a patient with known or suspected angle-closure glaucoma or known hypersensitivity. • This drug requires cautious use in a pregnant patient.
Miotics		
carbachol (Isopto Carbachol)	*Miosis* ADULT: 0.5 ml of 0.01% solution into the anterior chamber of the eye before or after securing sutures *Open-angle or angle-closure glaucoma* ADULT: 1 to 2 drops of 0.75% to 3% solution instilled into the conjunctival sac every 4 to 8 hours	• Carbachol has no contraindications when applied intraocularly. • This drug requires cautious use in a patient with corneal abrasions.
pilocarpine hydrochloride (Isopto Carpine, Pilocar)	*Chronic open-angle glaucoma* ADULT: 1 to 2 drops of 1% to 2% solution every 4 to 8 hours PEDIATRIC: same as adult dosage *Treatment of acute angle-closure glaucoma before surgery* ADULT: 1 drop of 2% solution instilled three to six times over a 30-minute period before surgery, followed by 1 drop every 1 to 3 hours until pressure is controlled PEDIATRIC: same as adult dosage	• Pilocarpine is contraindicated in a patient with a history of or predisposition to retinal detachment, glaucoma associated with acute inflammation, or known hypersensitivity. • This drug requires cautious use in a patient with corneal abrasions.

Selected major ophthalmic agents *(continued)*

DRUG	MAJOR INDICATIONS AND USUAL DOSAGES	CONTRAINDICATIONS AND PRECAUTIONS
Other drugs that lower intraocular pressure		
betaxolol (Betoptic)	*Chronic open-angle glaucoma* ADULT: 1 to 2 drops of 0.25% resin-formulated suspension or 0.5% solution b.i.d.	• Betaxolol is contraindicated in a patient with sinus bradycardia; first-, second-, or third-degree atrioventricular block; cardiogenic shock; overt cardiac failure; or known hypersensitivity. • This drug requires cautious use in a pregnant or breast-feeding patient or one with diabetes, hyperthyroidism, or pulmonary dysfunction. • Safety and efficacy in children have not been established.
glycerin [anhydrous] (Ophthalgan)	*Reduction of superficial corneal edema* ADULT: 1 or 2 drops of glycerin ophthalmic solution every 3 or 4 hours *Preparation for ophthalmoscopic or gonioscopic examination* ADULT: 1 or 2 drops instilled into the eye before the examination	• Glycerin (anhydrous) is contraindicated in a patient with known hypersensitivity. • This drug has no major precautions. • Safety and efficacy in children have not been established.
timolol (Timoptic)	*Chronic open-angle glaucoma, aphakic glaucoma, increased intraocular pressure* ADULT: initially, 1 drop of 0.25% solution b.i.d.; increased to 1 drop of 0.5% solution b.i.d., if needed	• Timolol is contraindicated in a breast-feeding patient or one with bronchial asthma, a history of bronchial asthma, or severe chronic obstructive pulmonary disease. • This drug requires cautious use in a pregnant patient or one with diabetes mellitus, hyperthyroidism, or cerebral vascular insufficiency. • Safety and efficacy in children have not been established.
Ophthalmic anesthetic agents		
tetracaine (Pontocaine Eye)	*Tonometry, gonioscopy, removal of foreign bodies from the cornea, corneal suture removal, other diagnostic and minor surgical procedures* ADULT: 1 or 2 drops of 0.5% solution or ½" to 1" (1- to 2.5-cm) ribbon of 0.5% ointment just before the procedure PEDIATRIC: same as adult dosage	• Tetracaine is contraindicated in a patient with known hypersensitivity. • This drug requires cautious use in a patient with allergies, cardiac disease, or hyperthyroidism.
Ophthalmic anti-inflammatory agents		
medrysone (HMS Liquifilm Ophthalmic)	*Allergic conjunctivitis, vernal conjunctivitis, episcleritis, ophthalmic epinephrine reaction* ADULT: 1 drop of 1% solution instilled in the conjunctival sac b.i.d. to q.i.d.; may be used every hour during the first 1 to 2 days, as needed PEDIATRIC: same as adult dosage	• Medrysone is contraindicated in a patient with an acute, untreated, purulent bacterial, viral, or fungal eye infection; acute, superficial herpes simplex keratitis; vaccinia, varicella, or other viral disease of the cornea or conjunctiva; or known hypersensitivity. • This drug requires cautious use in a pregnant or breast-feeding patient or one with corneal abrasions.
flurbiprofen sodium (Ocufen)	*Inhibition of intraoperative miosis* ADULT: 1 drop of 0.03% solution instilled in the affected eye every 30 minutes beginning 2 hours before surgery for a total of 4 drops	• Flurbiprofen sodium is contraindicated in a patient with known hypersensitivity to the drug or its components. • This drug requires cautious use in a patient with known bleeding tendencies, in a patient taking a drug known to cause bleeding, in a patient with herpes simplex keratitis, and in a pregnant or breast-feeding patient.

(continued)

Selected major ophthalmic agents *(continued)*

DRUG	MAJOR INDICATIONS AND USUAL DOSAGES	CONTRAINDICATIONS AND PRECAUTIONS
Ophthalmic anti-infective agents *(continued)*		
polymyxin B sulfate (Neosporin Ophthalmic)	*Corneal ulcers from infections with* Pseudomonas *or other gram-negative organisms* ADULT: 1 to 3 drops of 0.1% to 0.25% solution every hour or 0.5% ointment placed in the conjunctival sac every 3 to 4 hours PEDIATRIC: same as adult dosage	• Polymyxin B sulfate is contraindicated in a patient with known hypersensitivity. • This drug requires cautious use in a patient with neuromuscular disease.

enhanced during surgical procedures and treatment of traumatized eyes.

The onset of action of dipivefrin, epinephrine, epinephryl, and phenylephrine occurs within 10 to 15 minutes. The drugs achieve a peak concentration level 20 to 40 minutes after instillation, and have a duration of action (pupil dilation) of 2 to 3 hours. When used to lower intraocular pressure, dipivefrin and epinephrine have a duration of about 12 hours.

Atropine, cyclopentolate, homatropine, scopolamine, and tropicamide have an onset of action of 10 to 30 minutes for mydriatic effects and of 15 minutes to several hours for cycloplegic effects. Their duration of action is longer than that of the sympathomimetic drugs. The action of atropine, for example, may last for days.

Route	Onset	Peak	Duration
Ophthalmic	10 min-hours	20 min-1 hr	50 min-days

PHARMACODYNAMICS

Mydriatic drops act on the iris to dilate the pupil. Cycloplegic drops act on the ciliary body to paralyze the fine-focusing muscles, thereby preventing **accommodation** for near vision.

PHARMACOTHERAPEUTICS

Mydriatics are used primarily to dilate the pupils for intraocular examinations. Cycloplegics are essential for performing refraction in children; they are also used before and after ophthalmic surgery and as an adjunct treatment for conditions involving the iris.

Pupil dilation in diabetic patients or in those with darkly pigmented irides requires stronger concentrations and repeated instillations of both types of drugs.

Drug interactions

Mydriatics and cycloplegics do not interact significantly with other drugs.

ADVERSE DRUG REACTIONS

Many local adverse reactions occur with the mydriatics and cycloplegics, including irritation, blurred vision, and transient burning sensations and stinging. With prolonged use, some of these drugs can increase intraocular pressure and cause ocular congestion, **conjunctivitis,** contact dermatitis, and eye dryness.

Systemic reactions include tachycardia, palpitations, flushing, dry skin, ataxia, and confusion. Dry mouth and tachycardia commonly occur after instillation of atropine, cyclopentolate, or scopolamine. Atropine, cyclopentolate, homatropine, and scopolamine may cause photophobia.

NURSING PROCESS APPLICATION

The following information assists the nurse in caring for a patient receiving a mydriatic or cycloplegic. It includes an overview of assessment activities as well as examples of appropriate nursing diagnoses and related interventions (under "Planning and implementation"). It also highlights the importance of evaluation.

Assessment

Before drug therapy begins, review the patient's history for conditions that contraindicate or require cautious use of the prescribed mydriatic or cycloplegic. During therapy, assess the patient for adverse drug reactions. Also, periodically assess the effectiveness of therapy with the mydriatic or cycloplegic. Finally, evaluate the patient's and family's knowledge about the prescribed drug. (See Patient Teaching: *Mydriatics and cycloplegics.*)

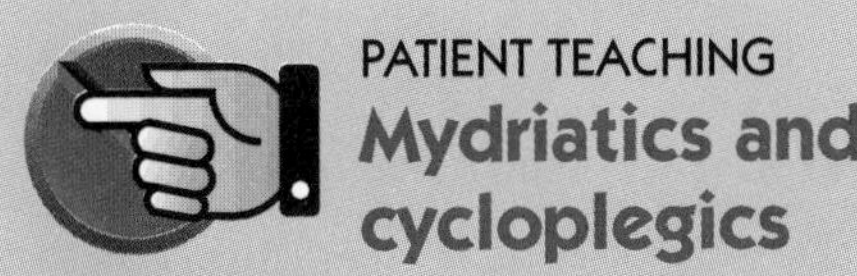

PATIENT TEACHING
Mydriatics and cycloplegics

- Teach the patient and family the name, dose, frequency, action, and adverse effects of the prescribed mydriatic or cycloplegic.
- Warn the patient that eye irritation, blurred vision, and transient burning and stinging sensations may occur with mydriatic or cycloplegic administration.
- Instruct the patient to wear dark glasses after administration and to avoid operating machinery until blurred vision disappears. Also advise the patient receiving atropine, cyclopentolate, homatropine, or scopolamine to wear dark glasses if photophobia occurs.
- Teach the patient the proper method of instillation, including hand washing before and after administering the drops. Also remind the patient not to touch the dropper to the eye or surrounding tissue.
- Advise the patient to discard any discolored epinephrine solution.
- Stress the importance of regular follow-up visits and ophthalmic examinations.
- Teach the patient to recognize and report systemic adverse reactions.
- Instruct the patient to report sudden visual changes or eye pain or drainage to the physician immediately.

Nursing diagnoses

- Risk for injury related to a preexisting condition that contraindicates or requires cautious use of a mydriatic or cycloplegic
- Risk for injury related to adverse drug reactions
- Sensory/perceptual alterations (visual) related to the adverse ocular effects of a mydriatic or cycloplegic
- Knowledge deficit related to the prescribed mydriatic or cycloplegic

Planning and implementation

- Do not administer a mydriatic or cycloplegic to a patient with a condition that contraindicates its use. (See Geriatric Considerations: *Use of cycloplegic mydriatics in an older patient.*)
- Administer a mydriatic or cycloplegic cautiously to a patient at risk because of a preexisting condition.
- Monitor the patient for adverse reactions during mydriatic or cycloplegic therapy.
- Instill the drops properly. (See *Administering ophthalmic agents,* page 712.)

*** *Minimize systemic absorption by applying digital pressure over the punctum at the inner canthus for 2 to 3 minutes after instilling the drops.***

- Ask the patient about photophobia during atropine, cyclopentolate, homatropine, or scopolamine therapy.
- Notify the physician if systemic adverse reactions occur.

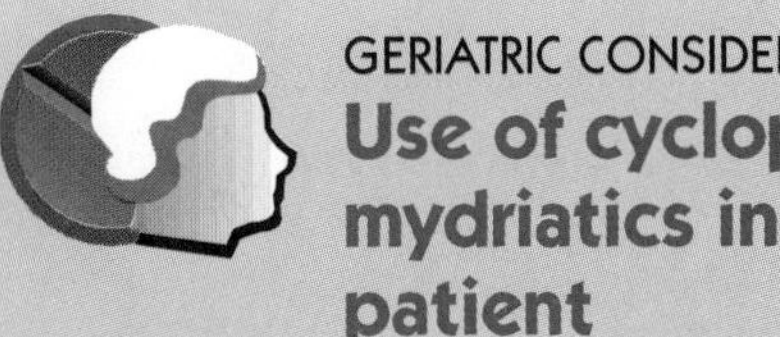

GERIATRIC CONSIDERATIONS
Use of cycloplegic mydriatics in an older patient

Cycloplegic mydriatics should be used with caution in an older person who may be predisposed to increased intraocular pressure. Signs and symptoms of increased intraocular pressure may include a pressure greater than 23 mm Hg and decreased eye function due to aqueous humor build-up.

*** *Inspect the patient's eyes regularly for signs of irritation (redness), dryness, conjunctivitis (drainage), or contact dermatitis (redness and tearing).***

- Ask the patient about ocular disturbances, such as blurred vision and eye pain or itching.
- Encourage the patient to have regular eye examinations, including **tonometric** readings.
- Notify the physician if adverse ocular reactions occur.

Evaluation

For each nursing diagnosis, prepare an evaluation statement that describes the patient's or family's response to nursing interventions.

Miotics

Miotics constrict the pupils and include direct-acting cholinergic drugs (carbachol, pilocarpine hydrochloride, and pilocarpine nitrate), short-acting anticholinesterases (physostigmine salicylate and physostigmine sulfate), and long-acting anticholinesterases (demecarium bromide, echothiophate iodide, and isoflurophate).

PHARMACOKINETICS

Some systemic absorption is possible with all miotics, but this seldom occurs. Pilocarpine, available in hydrochloride and nitrate forms, has an onset of action of 15 to 30 minutes, reaches a peak concentration level in 2 hours, and has a duration of action of 4 to 8 hours. Carbachol has a similar duration — 4 to 8 hours. However, carbachol is absorbed poorly through the cornea and is used only if pilocarpine is ineffective or if the patient is hypersensitive to pilocarpine. Physostigmine, the short-acting anticholinesterase available in salicylate and sulfate forms, has an onset of action of 10 minutes, reaches a peak concentration level in 3 to 4 hours, and has a duration of action of 12 to 36 hours. The long-acting anticholinesterases, demecarium, echothiophate, and isoflurophate, are potent miotics with a duration of action ranging from days to weeks.

Administering ophthalmic agents

Many ophthalmic agents come in two forms: eyedrops for instillation and ointments for application. The form of an agent determines how it is administered, as shown below. With either form, hand washing is essential before and after administration.

Applying eye ointment

Place the patient in a supine position or in a seated position with the neck hyperextended. Clean the eyelashes with saline solution and swabs to remove any secretions. Have the patient look upward; then pull down the lower lid with a finger. As the patient continues to look up, apply a thin ribbon of ointment directly into the conjunctival sac, beginning at the inner canthus.

To avoid contamination, do not let the tube touch the eye or conjunctiva. At the outer canthus, rotate the tube to detach the ointment.

Instruct the patient to close the eye gently, but not to squeeze it closed.

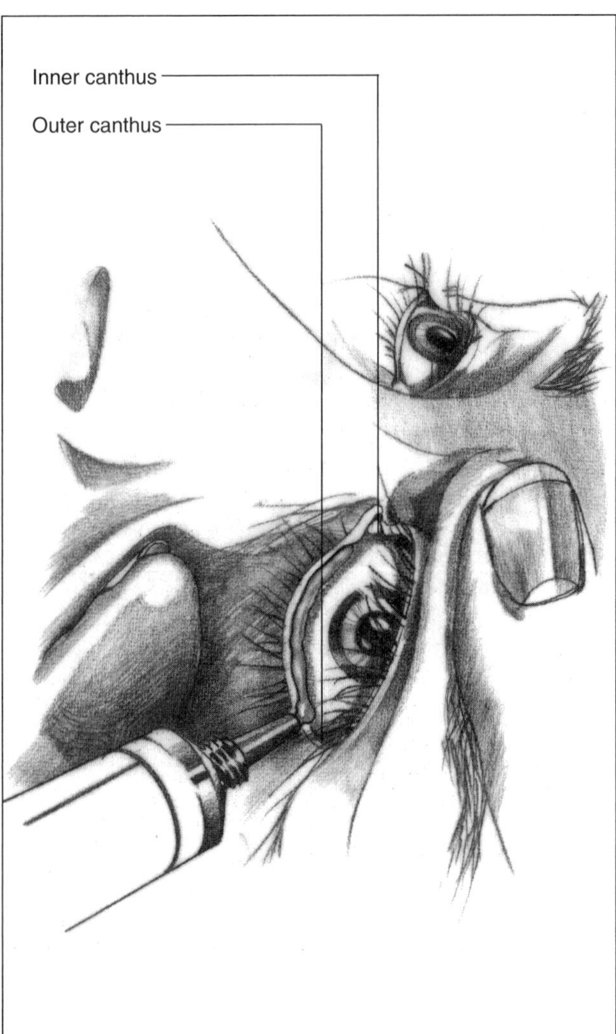

Instilling eyedrops

Place the patient in a supine position or in a seated position with the neck hyperextended, looking toward the ceiling. With a finger, pull down firmly on the lower lid while the patient continues to look upward. This movement exposes the lower conjunctival sac by relaxing the upper tarsal plate as it is retracted into the orbit.

Instill 1 drop of medication into the lower conjunctival sac. Instruct the patient to close the eye gently, but not to squeeze it closed. Wipe away excess tears with a cotton ball or tissue.

The eye can hold only 1 drop. When instilling more than 1 drop, wait 2 to 3 minutes between drops to avoid losing a drop from tearing or blinking.

After instilling drops, apply digital pressure over the punctum at the inner canthus for 2 to 3 minutes, and have the patient close the eyelids gently for 2 to 3 minutes to prevent drainage through the nasolacrimal duct. Stopping drainage through the nasolacrimal duct when instilling eyedrops helps prevent systemic absorption. It also prevents the patient from tasting the drops.

To avoid contamination, do not allow the tip of the dropper to touch the lid or eyelashes.

Discard discolored solutions or solutions with floating particles.

When instilling a mydriatic or cycloplegic, pay special attention during administration to prevent accidental instillation into the unaffected eye.

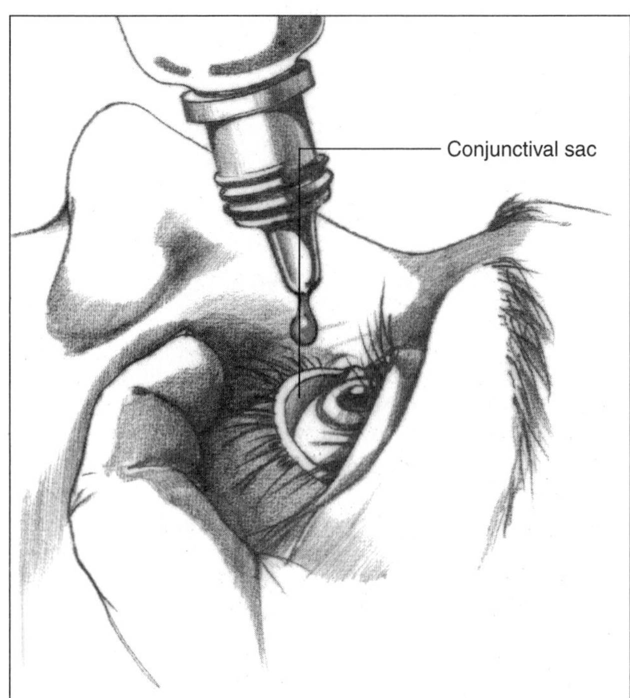

Route	Onset	Peak	Duration
Ophthalmic	10-30 min	2-4 hr	4 hr-several weeks

PHARMACODYNAMICS

Miotics stimulate and contract the sphincter muscle of the iris, thereby constricting the pupil. This action is called **miosis.** Miotics also improve aqueous outflow from the anterior chamber of the eye by decreasing resistance.

PHARMACOTHERAPEUTICS

The miotics are used to treat chronic open-angle **glaucoma,** acute and chronic angle-closure glaucoma, and certain cases of secondary glaucoma resulting from disease-induced or injury-induced increases in intraocular pressure. However, if inflammation (such as **iritis**) is present, miotics should not be used because they may exacerbate the inflammation.

Controlling intraocular pressure is the cornerstone of glaucoma therapy, and direct-acting miotics, such as pilocarpine, are usually the drugs of choice. Long-acting miotics (such as isoflurophate), which can be toxic, are used only in patients refractory to direct- or short-acting agents.

Drug interactions

Echothiophate, isoflurophate, and physostigmine may interact with succinylcholine, resulting in respiratory or cardiovascular collapse. Therefore, these agents should not be administered concomitantly. Pilocarpine interacts with carbachol, causing additive effects, and with phenylephrine, decreasing phenylephrine-induced **mydriasis.** These interactions prohibit concomitant use of these drugs.

ADVERSE DRUG REACTIONS

Miotics commonly cause blurred vision and eye and eyebrow pain. Reversible iris cysts, eyelid pain, photosensitivity, and cataract formation may also occur. Although uncommon, systemic absorption can lead to abdominal cramps, diarrhea, and increased salivation. The miotics can also cause bronchial constriction and spasm as well as pulmonary edema. In dark-skinned patients, hypersensitivity reactions to physostigmine can lead to reversible depigmentation of eyelid skin.

NURSING PROCESS APPLICATION

The following information assists the nurse in caring for a patient receiving a miotic. It includes an overview of assessment activities as well as examples of appropriate nursing diagnoses and related interventions (under "Planning and implementation"). It also highlights the importance of evaluation.

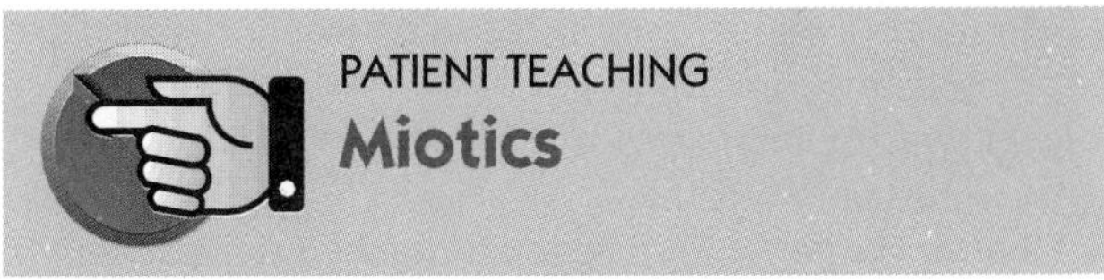

PATIENT TEACHING

Miotics

- Teach the patient and family the name, dose, frequency, action, and adverse effects of the prescribed miotic.
- Explain to the patient that blurred vision will occur after administration; instruct the patient to instill drops at bedtime, if possible, to minimize problems resulting from blurred vision.
- Inform the patient that eye, eyebrow, or eyelid pain commonly occurs with miotic therapy. If pain persists or worsens, advise the patient to notify the physician.
- Advise the patient to wear dark glasses if photosensitivity occurs.
- Stress the importance of regular follow-up visits and ophthalmologic examinations to detect adverse ocular reactions and assess the drug's effectiveness.
- Teach the patient or a family member how to administer the prescribed miotic correctly.
- Teach the patient how to reconstitute echothiophate with the enclosed diluent. Reconstituted echothiophate solution will remain stable for 1 month at room temperature or 6 months under refrigeration.
- Instruct the patient to notify the physician if adverse ocular reactions occur.
- Reassure the dark-skinned patient that depigmentation of eyelid skin is reversible.
- Teach the patient to recognize the signs and symptoms of pulmonary edema and bronchoconstriction and to seek emergency care if they occur.
- Advise the patient that abdominal cramps, diarrhea, and increased salivation may occur during miotic therapy.
- Instruct the patient to notify the physician if any systemic adverse reactions occur.

Assessment

Before drug therapy begins, review the patient's history for conditions that contraindicate or require cautious use of the prescribed miotic. Also review the patient's medication history to identify use of drugs that may interact with it. During therapy, assess the patient for adverse drug reactions and signs of drug interactions. Also, periodically assess the effectiveness of miotic therapy. Finally, evaluate the patient's and family's knowledge about the prescribed drug. (See Patient Teaching: *Miotics.*)

Nursing diagnoses

- Risk for injury related to a preexisting condition that contraindicates or requires cautious use of a miotic
- Risk for injury related to adverse drug reactions or drug interactions
- Sensory/perceptual alterations (visual) related to the adverse ocular effects of the miotic
- Knowledge deficit related to the prescribed miotic

Planning and implementation

- Do not administer a miotic to a patient with a condition that contraindicates its use.

- Administer a miotic cautiously to a patient at risk because of a preexisting condition.
- Monitor the patient for adverse reactions and drug interactions during miotic therapy.

∗ ***Monitor the patient for signs of bronchial constriction or spasm and pulmonary edema, such as wheezing, crackles, jugular vein distention, and shortness of breath. Notify the physician if respiratory dysfunction occurs. Expect to administer a bronchodilator, diuretic, or other emergency treatment as prescribed.***

- Observe the dark-skinned patient for depigmentation of eyelid skin, which indicates a hypersensitivity reaction to physostigmine.
- Administer the prescribed miotic properly.

∗ ***Minimize systemic absorption of the miotic by applying digital pressure over the punctum at the inner canthus for 2 to 3 minutes after instilling eyedrops.***

- Notify the physician if systemic adverse reactions occur.
- Ask the patient about blurred vision during miotic therapy. Take safety precautions until the patient's vision returns to normal. For example, keep the bed rails raised and supervise the patient's ambulation.
- Ask the patient about eye, eyebrow, or eyelid pain and photosensitivity.
- Encourage the patient to have routine ophthalmic examinations to detect iris cysts or cataracts.
- Notify the physician if adverse ocular effects or drug interactions occur.

Evaluation

For each nursing diagnosis, prepare an evaluation statement that describes the patient's or family's response to nursing interventions.

Other drugs that lower intraocular pressure

Topical adrenergic-blocking agents, hyperosmotic agents, and carbonic anhydrase inhibitors are used to lower intraocular pressure. Topical adrenergic-blocking agents include apraclonidine hydrochloride (a selective alpha-adrenergic blocker), betaxolol hydrochloride (a cardioselective receptor blocker), levobunolol hydrochloride (a nonselective beta-adrenergic blocker), and timolol maleate (a nonselective adrenergic blocker). Hyperosmotic agents include glycerin, glycerin (anhydrous), isosorbide, mannitol, and urea. The carbonic anhydrase inhibitors are acetazolamide, acetazolamide sodium, dichlorphenamide, and methazolamide.

PHARMACOKINETICS

The extent of ocular and systemic absorption of apraclonidine and betaxolol has not been elucidated. Levobunolol and timolol are absorbed systemically. After oral administration, glycerin and isosorbide are absorbed rapidly; their onsets of action begin within 30 minutes. Both drugs are distributed widely and excreted unchanged in the kidneys. The distribution, metabolism, and excretion of the adrenergic blockers vary. The hyperosmotic agents, mannitol and urea, are administered intravenously (I.V.) and distributed immediately. The carbonic anhydrase inhibitors are administered by various routes, so their pharmacokinetics differ accordingly.

The onset of action of the topical adrenergic-blockers occurs 20 minutes after administration, with a peak concentration level usually occurring within 1 to 2 hours. The duration of action of these drugs can range up to 24 hours.

The hyperosmotic agents' onsets of action occur within 15 minutes of administration and have a duration of 5 to 8 hours.

The onset of action for the carbonic anhydrase inhibitors varies. The effects of acetazolamide sodium appear within 2 minutes after an injection, whereas the onset of oral acetazolamide is 60 to 90 minutes. Oral dichlorphenamide produces effects within 30 to 60 minutes. The effects of methazolamide do not appear until 2 hours after administration. The duration of the carbonic anhydrase inhibitors varies — from 4 to 5 hours for I.V. acetazolamide to 18 to 24 hours for sustained-release acetazolamide.

Route	Onset	Peak	Duration
P.O.	10 min-2 hr	30 min-2 hr	4-24 hr
I.V.	2-60 min	1-2 hr	4-6 hr
Topical	20 min	1-2 hr	≤ 24 hr

PHARMACODYNAMICS

Each group of drugs lowers intraocular pressure by a different mechanism of action. The adrenergic blocker timolol's action is not understood well. It may primarily reduce aqueous humor formation and slightly increase aqueous humor outflow. The mechanism of action for apraclonidine, betaxolol, and levobunolol in reducing intraocular pressure has not been established. However, it may be similar to that of timolol.

Hyperosmotic agents increase water absorption from the eye into the general circulation, thus lowering intraocular pressure.

The enzyme carbonic anhydrase is involved in aqueous humor production in the eye, so drugs that inhibit the action of carbonic anhydrase decrease aqueous production — by 30% to 60% — without affecting aqueous outflow. As less aqueous fluid enters the eye, intraocular pressure decreases.

PHARMACOTHERAPEUTICS

The indications for topical adrenergic blockers vary. Apraclonidine is used to prevent or control elevated intraocular pressure after argon laser trabeculoplasty or iridotomy. Betaxolol, levobunolol, and timolol are used to treat chronic open-angle glaucoma.

The hyperosmotic agents are reserved for emergencies and are used to treat acute angle-closure glaucoma; they are also used before and after ocular surgery.

The carbonic anhydrase inhibitors are used to treat chronic open-angle glaucoma, episodes of acute angle-closure glaucoma, and secondary glaucomas.

Drug interactions

No significant interactions occur between hyperosmotic agents and other drugs. Interactions between timolol and such oral beta-adrenergic blockers as propranolol increase ocular and systemic effects; caution is required with concomitant use of these drugs. The adrenergic blockers should also be used cautiously with monoamine oxidase inhibitors. Patients using acetazolamide with a salicylate may need a reduction in the salicylate dosage.

ADVERSE DRUG REACTIONS

Adverse reactions vary among the topical adrenergic agents, hyperosmotic agents, and carbonic anhydrase inhibitors. The adrenergic blockers can reduce the heart rate, causing headaches and fatigue, and the beta blockade effects resulting from systemic timolol absorption may lead to bradycardia and bronchospasm. Apraclonidine may cause upper eyelid elevation, conjunctival blanching, and mydriasis.

The hyperosmotic agents can cause stinging when administered. Use of a topical anesthetic is recommended with glycerin administration.

Carbonic anhydrase inhibitors, such as acetazolamide, can cause drowsiness, hypokalemia, nausea, vomiting, leukopenia, hemolytic anemia, and aplastic anemia.

NURSING PROCESS APPLICATION

The following information assists the nurse in caring for a patient receiving a drug that lowers intraocular pressure. It includes an overview of assessment activities as well as examples of appropriate nursing diagnoses and related interventions (under "Planning and implementation"). It also highlights the importance of evaluation.

Assessment

Before drug therapy begins, review the patient's history for conditions that contraindicate or require cautious use of the prescribed drug that lowers intraocular pressure. Also, review the patient's medication history to identify use of drugs that may interact with it. During therapy, assess the patient for adverse drug reactions and signs of drug interactions. Also, periodically assess the effectiveness of drug therapy. Finally, evaluate the patient's and family's knowledge about the prescribed drug. (See Patient Teaching: *Selected drugs that lower intraocular pressure.*)

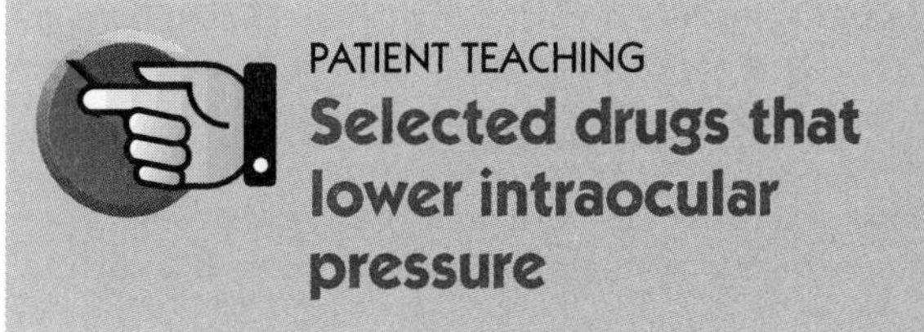

PATIENT TEACHING

Selected drugs that lower intraocular pressure

- Teach the patient and family the name, dose, frequency, action, and adverse effects of the prescribed drug that lowers intraocular pressure.
- Instruct the patient in self-instillation of eyedrops, as appropriate. Explain the importance of not touching the eyedropper to the eye and of hand washing before and after self-instillation.
- Inform the patient that apraclonidine may cause upper eyelid elevation, conjunctival blanching, and mydriasis. Teach the patient how to manage these adverse reactions.
- Advise the patient that administration of a hyperosmotic agent may cause stinging, but that an ophthalmic anesthetic agent can be used concomitantly to promote comfort.
- Instruct the patient to report to the physician a pulse rate below 60 beats/minute or wheezing.
- Advise the patient to take a mild analgesic if headache occurs.
- Warn the patient not to perform activities that require mental alertness if drowsiness occurs.
- Teach the patient to use energy conservation measures if fatigue or anemia occurs, and to take infection control measures if leukopenia occurs.
- Stress the importance of returning for blood tests, such as complete blood count and serum potassium determination, to detect adverse reactions.
- Instruct the patient to notify the physician if adverse reactions occur.

Nursing diagnoses

- Risk for injury related to a preexisting condition that contraindicates or requires cautious use of a drug that lowers intraocular pressure
- Risk for injury related to adverse drug reactions or drug interactions
- Risk for injury related to the adverse ocular effects of a drug that lowers intraocular pressure
- Knowledge deficit related to the prescribed drug that lowers intraocular pressure

Planning and implementation

- Do not administer a drug that lowers intraocular pressure to a patient with a condition that contraindicates its use.
- Administer a drug that lowers intraocular pressure cautiously to a patient at risk because of a preexisting condition.
- Monitor the patient for adverse reactions and drug interactions during therapy.

*✱ **Monitor the heart rate to detect bradycardia in a patient receiving an adrenergic blocker. If the heart rate falls below 60 beats/minute, notify the physician and expect to administer a different drug as prescribed.***

* ***Auscultate the patient's lungs frequently during timolol therapy to detect bronchospasm. If bronchospasm occurs, notify the physician and expect to administer a bronchodilator and discontinue timolol as prescribed.***
- Monitor the patient's serum potassium level for hypokalemia during treatment with a carbonic anhydrase inhibitor.
- Monitor the complete blood count regularly to detect leukopenia or anemia in a patient taking a carbonic anhydrase inhibitor. If leukopenia occurs, monitor the patient for signs of infection, such as sore throat, malaise, and fever, and take infection control measures until the white blood count returns to normal. If anemia occurs, institute energy conservation measures.
- Instill the prescribed drops properly.
- Notify the physician if systemic adverse reactions or drug interactions occur.
- Observe for upper eyelid elevation, conjunctival blanching, and mydriasis in a patient receiving apraclonidine after laser surgery.
- Administer a topical anesthetic with glycerin to help prevent stinging during administration.
- Notify the physician if adverse ocular reactions occur.

Evaluation
For each nursing diagnosis, prepare an evaluation statement that describes the patient's or family's response to nursing interventions.

Ophthalmic anesthetic agents

Because the cornea and the conjunctiva contain delicate sensory nerves, surgical (and some diagnostic) procedures involving the eye would be impossible without anesthetics. This section discusses the topical ophthalmic anesthetics proparacaine hydrochloride and tetracaine.

Topical cocaine is a natural compound. Because of its corneal toxicity and adverse central nervous system reactions, it has been replaced by synthetic anesthetics and is not covered here.

PHARMACOKINETICS
Most of these anesthetics have an onset of action of 1 minute.

Route	Onset	Peak	Duration
Ophthalmic	20 sec-1 min	Variable	≥15 min

PHARMACODYNAMICS
Proparacaine and tetracaine act by interfering with cell activity; more drops may be required to anesthetize an inflamed eye because the blood vessels carry the anesthetic away.

PHARMACOTHERAPEUTICS
Besides anesthetizing the cornea to allow application of instruments for measuring intraocular pressure or removing foreign bodies, topical ophthalmic anesthetics are used for suture removal, for conjunctival or corneal scraping, and for lacrimal canal manipulation.

Drug interactions
The only significant interaction involving the topical ophthalmic anesthetics occurs with tetracaine, which interferes with the antibacterial action of sulfonamides. They should be administered at least 30 minutes apart to prevent this interaction.

ADVERSE DRUG REACTIONS
All three topical ophthalmic anesthetics can cause transient eye pain and redness. Prolonged use can cause **keratitis,** corneal opacities, scarring, loss of visual acuity, and delayed corneal healing.

NURSING PROCESS APPLICATION
The following information assists the nurse in caring for a patient receiving an ophthalmic anesthetic agent. It includes an overview of assessment activities as well as examples of appropriate nursing diagnoses and related interventions (under "Planning and implementation"). It also highlights the importance of evaluation.

Assessment
Before drug therapy begins, review the patient's history for conditions that contraindicate or require cautious use of the prescribed ophthalmic anesthetic. Also review the patient's medication history to identify use of sulfonamides that may interact with tetracaine. During therapy, assess the patient for adverse drug reactions and signs of drug interactions. Also, periodically assess the effectiveness of ophthalmic anesthetic therapy. Finally, evaluate the patient's and family's knowledge about the prescribed drug. (See Patient Teaching: *Ophthalmic anesthetic agents.*)

Nursing diagnoses
- Risk for injury related to a preexisting condition that contraindicates or requires cautious use of an ophthalmic anesthetic
- Risk for injury related to adverse drug reactions or drug interactions
- Sensory/perceptual alterations (visual) related to the adverse ocular effects of the ophthalmic anesthetic
- Knowledge deficit related to the prescribed ophthalmic anesthetic

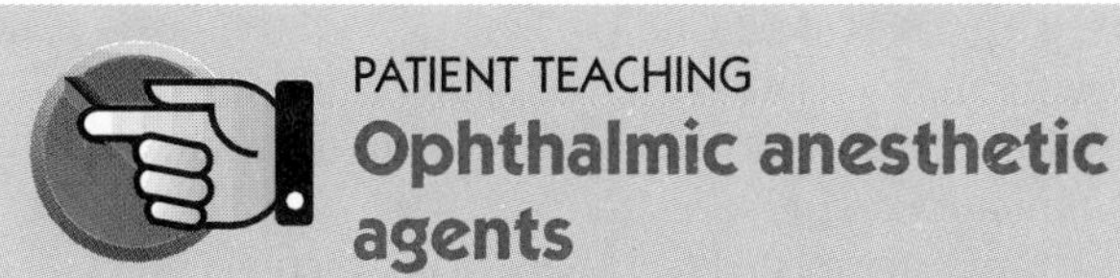

PATIENT TEACHING
Ophthalmic anesthetic agents

- Teach the patient and family the name, dose, frequency, action, and adverse effects of the prescribed ophthalmic anesthetic.
- Advise the patient receiving a topical anesthetic not to rub the eyes; explain that corneal abrasion may occur because the usual pain signal is absent. Also explain that the anesthetic will cause transient blurred vision.
- Stress the importance of regular follow-up visits and ophthalmic examinations during prolonged therapy with an ophthalmic anesthetic.
- Instruct the patient to report any vision disturbances or eye discomfort to the physician.

Planning and implementation

- Do not administer an ophthalmic anesthetic to a patient with a condition that contraindicates its use.
- Administer an ophthalmic anesthetic cautiously to a patient at risk because of a preexisting condition.
- Monitor the patient for adverse reactions and drug interactions to the ophthalmic anesthetic.
- Administer the ophthalmic anesthetic properly.

***** ***Apply digital pressure over the punctum at the inner canthus for 2 to 3 minutes after administering the anesthetic to prevent systemic absorption.***

- Observe the patient for eye redness during ophthalmic anesthetic use. Ask the patient about eye pain.

***** ***Encourage regular ophthalmic examinations to detect keratitis, corneal opacities, scarring, or delayed corneal healing in a patient receiving an ophthalmic anesthetic agent over a prolonged time.***

- Monitor the patient's visual acuity regularly.
- Provide the patient with a protective eye patch, if necessary, while the anesthetic effects of the drug last.
- Notify the physician if adverse ocular reactions or drug interactions occur.

Evaluation

For each nursing diagnosis, prepare an evaluation statement that describes the patient's or family's response to nursing interventions.

Ophthalmic anti-inflammatory agents

The corticosteroids — hormones secreted by the adrenal glands — are produced synthetically for pharmacologic, including ophthalmic, use. Ophthalmic anti-inflammatory agents are corticosteroid solutions or suspensions that decrease leukocyte infiltration at the site of ocular inflammation. The topical agents include dexamethasone, fluorometholone, medrysone, prednisolone acetate, and prednisolone sodium phosphate.

PHARMACOKINETICS

Absorption of topical anti-inflammatory agents through the intact cornea is minimal. Suspensions such as dexamethasone are usually absorbed more completely than solutions such as prednisolone sodium phosphate. The onset of action and duration of action vary among these anti-inflammatory agents; specific information is unavailable.

Route	Onset	Peak	Duration
Ophthalmic	Variable	Variable	Variable

PHARMACODYNAMICS

The ophthalmic anti-inflammatory agents decrease leukocyte infiltration at inflammation sites. This reduces the exudative reaction of diseased tissue, leading to reduced edema, redness, and scarring.

PHARMACOTHERAPEUTICS

Corticosteroids are used to treat inflammatory disorders and hypersensitivity-related conditions of the cornea, iris, conjunctiva, sclera, and anterior uvea.

Drug interactions

Ophthalmic corticosteroid anti-inflammatory agents do not interact significantly with other drugs.

ADVERSE DRUG REACTIONS

These drugs may increase intraocular pressure. Corneal thinning or ulceration, interference with corneal wound healing, and increased susceptibility to viral or fungal corneal **infection** can also occur. Long-term or excessive use of these drugs can lead to exacerbation of glaucoma, cataracts, reduced visual acuity, and optic nerve damage. Excessive or long-term use of suspensions, which are absorbed more readily, can lead to adrenal suppression.

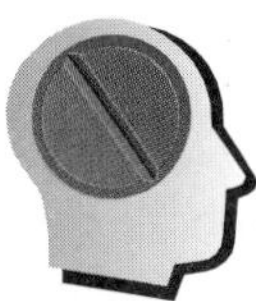

CRITICAL THINKING: To enhance your critical thinking skills about ophthalmic agents, consider the following situation and its analysis. **Situation:** Albert Fine, age 58, has been admitted to your unit with dehydration and weakness. His serum sodium level is 130 mg/ml, and his serum potassium level is 5.3 mEq/L. He has no significant findings from his medical history other than being treated for allergic conjunctivitis 2 months ago with medrysone ophthalmic suspension. He says he continued the medrysone past the prescribed time because he didn't want

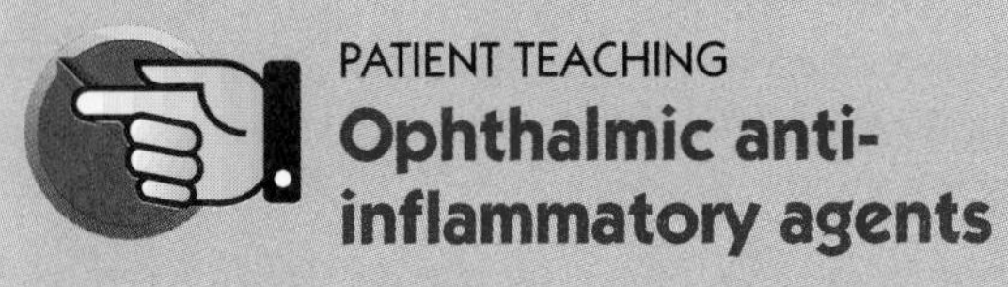

PATIENT TEACHING

Ophthalmic anti-inflammatory agents

- Teach the patient and family the name, dose, frequency, action, and adverse effects of the prescribed ophthalmic anti-inflammatory agent.
- Instruct the patient to notify the physician if eye discomfort or any change in visual acuity occurs.
- Teach the patient how to instill the drug. Instruct the patient to shake the suspension well before instillation. Also advise the patient to apply digital pressure over the punctum at the inner canthus for 2 to 3 minutes after instillation to minimize systemic absorption.
- Stress the importance of regular ophthalmic examinations.
- Review the signs and symptoms of adrenal suppression with a patient who must receive high-dosage or long-term therapy with an anti-inflammatory suspension. Instruct the patient to report such signs and symptoms to the physician at once.
- Advise the patient to wear or carry medical identification describing the patient's use of an ophthalmic anti-inflammatory agent that may suppress adrenal function.
- Instruct the patient to notify the physician if adverse reactions occur.

the allergic conjunctivitis to return. What could be causing Mr. Fine's symptoms now?

Analysis: Patients receiving high-dose or long-term therapy with an anti-inflammatory ophthalmic agent are at risk for adrenal suppression. Dehydration, weakness, hyponatremia, and hyperkalemia are signs and symptoms of adrenal suppression. Mr. Fine should be instructed to discontinue use of medrysone and be prepared for adrenal function tests.

NURSING PROCESS APPLICATION

The following information assists the nurse in caring for a patient receiving an ophthalmic anti-inflammatory agent. It includes an overview of assessment activities as well as examples of appropriate nursing diagnoses and related interventions (under "Planning and implementation"). It also highlights the importance of evaluation.

Assessment

Before drug therapy begins, review the patient's history for conditions that contraindicate or require cautious use of the prescribed ophthalmic anti-inflammatory agent. During therapy, assess the patient for adverse drug reactions. Also, periodically assess the effectiveness of therapy with the ophthalmic anti-inflammatory agent. Finally, evaluate the patient's and family's knowledge about the prescribed drug. (See Patient Teaching: *Ophthalmic anti-inflammatory agents.*)

Nursing diagnoses

- Risk for injury related to a preexisting condition that contraindicates or requires cautious use of an ophthalmic anti-inflammatory agent
- Risk for injury related to adverse drug reactions
- Altered protection related to adrenal suppression caused by excessive or long-term use of an ophthalmic anti-inflammatory suspension
- Knowledge deficit related to the prescribed ophthalmic anti-inflammatory agent

Planning and implementation

- Do not administer an ophthalmic anti-inflammatory agent to a patient with a condition that contraindicates its use.
- Administer an ophthalmic anti-inflammatory agent cautiously to a patient at risk because of a preexisting condition.
- Monitor the patient for adverse reactions during therapy.
- Ask the patient frequently about vision disturbances or eye discomfort.

* ***Inspect the patient's eyes regularly for signs of infection (such as purulent drainage, redness, and swelling), corneal ulceration, and delayed corneal wound healing.***
* ***Encourage the patient to have regular ophthalmic examinations to detect adverse ocular reactions, such as exacerbation of glaucoma, cataracts, reduced visual acuity, and optic nerve damage.***

- Instill the prescribed drug properly.
- Notify the physician if adverse reactions occur.
- Monitor for signs of adrenal suppression, such as dehydration and weakness, in a patient receiving high-dosage or long-term therapy with an ophthalmic anti-inflammatory suspension. Monitor the patient's electrolyte levels regularly to detect other signs of adrenal suppression, such as hyponatremia and hyperkalemia. If adrenal suppression is suspected, prepare the patient for adrenal function tests.
- Notify the physician if adrenal suppression is suspected. Expect to provide oral steroids and discontinue the anti-inflammatory suspension as prescribed.

Evaluation

For each nursing diagnosis, prepare an evaluation statement that describes the patient's or family's response to nursing interventions.

Ophthalmic anti-infective agents

Ophthalmic anti-infective agents include antibacterial, antiseptic, and antiviral agents. To treat eye diseases, anti-infective agents may be injected beneath the conjunctiva, administered orally, or instilled into the eye. However, this section presents only the topical anti-infective agents.

Applied as solution or ointment, topical anti-infective agents include bacitracin, boric acid, chloramphenicol, chlortetracycline hydrochloride, erythromycin, gentamicin sulfate, idoxuridine, natamycin, polymyxin B sulfate, silver nitrate 1%, sulfacetamide sodium, tetracycline hydrochloride, tobramycin, trifluridine, and vidarabine.

Systemic antibacterials may be used along with topical anti-infective agents to treat some patients with conjunctivitis, endophthalmitis, or infections of the **adnexa oculi** (eyelids and lacrimal apparatus).

PHARMACOKINETICS

Bacitracin, chloramphenicol, polymyxin B sulfate, and tobramycin penetrate the cornea and conjunctiva; chloramphenicol and tobramycin also penetrate aqueous humor. Silver nitrate 1% does not penetrate the eye. Topical boric acid and idoxuridine are absorbed poorly. Erythromycin, gentamicin sulfate, polymyxin B sulfate, and the tetracyclines penetrate poorly through an intact cornea but well through corneal abrasions. Natamycin does not reach measurable levels in the deeper corneal layers unless a defect in the epithelium is present. Sulfacetamide's intraocular penetration varies. Trifluridine and vidarabine are found in trace amounts in the aqueous humor after topical application to a cornea with an epithelial defect or inflammation, but neither drug displays significant systemic absorption.

Bacitracin, chloramphenicol, gentamicin, and polymyxin B sulfate are excreted via the nasolacrimal system. Excretion of the other anti-infective agents is unknown.

As a rule, ophthalmic anti-infective agents are administered in frequent doses — as often as every 2 hours. The onset and duration of action vary according to the patient's disorder and response.

Route	Onset	Peak	Duration
Ophthalmic	Variable	Variable	Variable

PHARMACODYNAMICS

Bacitracin, chloramphenicol, chlortetracycline, erythromycin, gentamicin, polymyxin B sulfate, and the tetracyclines inhibit protein synthesis in susceptible microorganisms. Boric acid's mechanism of action is unknown. Idoxuridine, trifluridine, and vidarabine interfere with deoxyribonucleic acid synthesis in susceptible organisms. Natamycin increases fungal cell membrane permeability. Silver nitrate 1%, instilled in the eyes of neonates, causes protein denaturation that prevents gonorrheal ophthalmia neonatorum. Sulfacetamide prevents uptake of para-aminobenzoic acid, a metabolite of bacterial folic acid synthesis. Tobramycin's mechanism of action is unknown, but it may inhibit protein synthesis.

PHARMACOTHERAPEUTICS

Bacitracin is effective against infections with gram-positive organisms. An antiseptic agent, boric acid is used to irrigate the eye after ocular procedures and to soothe and clean the eye, especially in connection with contact lens use. Chloramphenicol and gentamicin are used to treat gram-positive and gram-negative bacterial infections. Chlortetracycline is prescribed for superficial ocular infections. Erythromycin is used to fight infections caused by gram-positive cocci and gram-positive bacilli. The earliest developed antiviral agent, idoxuridine is invaluable in treating herpes simplex of the cornea, because it prevents the herpes virus from feeding off of the cells of the corneal epithelium. Natamycin is used to treat fungal infections. Polymyxin B sulfate is effective against infections with gram-negative organisms.

Silver nitrate 1% is an antiseptic agent used to prevent gonorrheal ophthalmia neonatorum. Sulfacetamide provides a wide spectrum of activity and effectiveness against some gram-positive and gram-negative bacterial infections. Tetracycline is used to treat superficial ocular infections, inclusion conjunctivitis, and **trachoma.** Tobramycin is used to treat external ocular infections caused by susceptible gram-negative bacteria. Trifluridine, an antiviral solution, is also used to treat herpes simplex infections, primary keratoconjunctivitis, and recurrent epithelial keratitis. The antiviral ophthalmic ointment vidarabine is also used to treat corneal herpes simplex, particularly in the early stages.

Drug interactions

No significant interactions occur between most anti-infectives and other drugs. However, combined use of bacitracin and silver nitrate 1% inactivates bacitracin. Sulfacetamide action will be decreased if it is used with a local anesthetic, such as procaine, tetracaine, or a para-aminobenzoic acid derivative. This interaction can be prevented by waiting 30 to 60 minutes after anesthetic instillation before instilling sulfacetamide.

ADVERSE DRUG REACTIONS

Hypersensitivity reactions to sulfonamides may occur; reactions may be severe. Secondary eye infections may occur with prolonged use of an ophthalmic anti-infective agent.

NURSING PROCESS APPLICATION

The following information assists the nurse in caring for a patient receiving an ophthalmic anti-infective agent. It includes an overview of assessment activities as well as examples of appropriate nursing diagnoses and related interventions (under "Planning and implementation"). It also highlights the importance of evaluation.

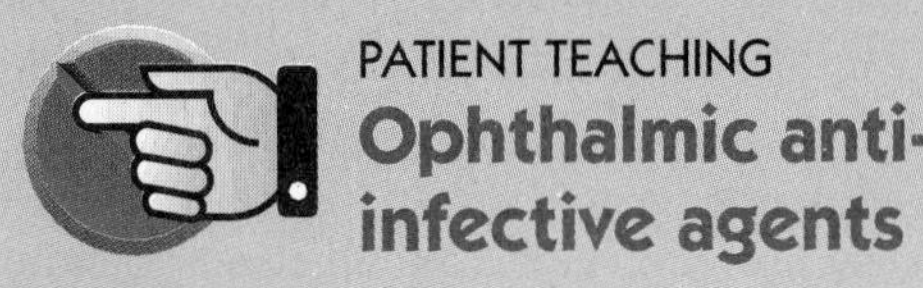

PATIENT TEACHING

Ophthalmic anti-infective agents

- Teach the patient and family the name, dose, frequency, action, and adverse effects of the prescribed anti-infective agent.
- Advise the patient against indiscriminate or prolonged use of ophthalmic anti-infectives; hypersensitivity or bacterial resistance may develop.
- Encourage the patient to see an ophthalmologist if a secondary eye infection occurs and to notify the ophthalmologist if the condition does not improve within 48 hours of initial treatment.
- Teach the patient with herpes simplex infection about the course of this disease. Explain that herpes will recur and that, at the first sign of recurrence, the patient should contact the ophthalmologist and start the prescribed medication.
- Teach the patient how to administer the prescribed ophthalmic anti-infective agent.
- Instruct the patient to withhold the drug and notify the physician if a hypersensitivity reaction occurs.

Assessment

Before drug therapy begins, review the patient's history for conditions that contraindicate or require cautious use of the prescribed ophthalmic anti-infective agent. Also review the patient's medication history to identify use of drugs that may interact with it. During therapy, assess the patient for adverse drug reactions and signs of drug interactions. Also, periodically assess the effectiveness of therapy with the ophthalmic anti-infective agent. Finally, evaluate the patient's and family's knowledge about the prescribed drug. (See Patient Teaching: *Ophthalmic anti-infective agents.*)

Nursing diagnoses

- Risk for injury related to a preexisting condition that contraindicates or requires cautious use of an ophthalmic anti-infective agent
- Risk for injury related to adverse reactions or drug interactions.
- Risk for injury related to a hypersensitivity reaction to a sulfonamide ophthalmic anti-infective agent
- Knowledge deficit related to the prescribed ophthalmic anti-infective agent

Planning and implementation

- Do not administer an ophthalmic anti-infective agent to a patient with a condition that contraindicates its use.
- Administer an ophthalmic anti-infective agent cautiously to a patient at risk because of a preexisting condition.
- Document the patient's history of allergy if sulfacetamide is prescribed. Hypersensitivity reactions to sulfonamides can be severe.

***** ***Monitor for hypersensitivity reactions in a patient receiving a sulfonamide ophthalmic anti-infective agent. Have standard emergency equipment nearby.***
- Administer the anti-infective agent properly.
- Notify the physician immediately if a hypersensitivity reaction occurs and withhold the prescribed ophthalmic anti-infective agent. Also notify the physician if other adverse reactions or drug interactions occur.

Evaluation

For each nursing diagnosis, prepare an evaluation statement that describes the patient's or family's response to nursing interventions.

CHAPTER SUMMARY

Chapter 58 discussed ophthalmic agents used to achieve mydriasis, cycloplegia, miosis, and anesthesia; lower intraocular pressure; and treat ocular inflammation and infection. Here are the chapter highlights.

Mydriatics dilate the pupil; cycloplegics paralyze the accommodative muscle of the ciliary body of the eye. Mydriatics and cycloplegics are used primarily for intraocular examinations and refractions. Some mydriatics are also used to treat open-angle glaucoma.

Miotics — including direct-acting cholinergic drugs, short-acting anticholinesterases, and long-acting anticholinesterases — are used primarily to treat glaucoma.

Other drugs that lower intraocular pressure include topical adrenergic blockers, hyperosmotic agents, and carbonic anhydrase inhibitors.

Topical anesthetics anesthetize the corneal surface so that instruments can be applied to measure intraocular pressure or to remove foreign bodies.

Corticosteroid ophthalmic anti-inflammatory agents reduce ocular edema, redness, and scarring.

Ophthalmic anti-infective agents include antibacterial, antiseptic, and antiviral agents.

The nurse should teach the patient or family how to administer the prescribed ophthalmic agent and should teach the patient to recognize and report systemic and ocular adverse reactions.

Questions to consider

See Appendix 1 for answers.

1. Sophie Green, age 48, is given cyclopentolate (Cyclogyl) eyedrops to produce mydriatic and cycloplegic effects before her eye examination. Which of the following adverse reactions commonly occurs after instillation of the drug?
   (a) Bradycardia
   (b) Tachycardia
   (c) Headache
   (d) Abdominal pain

2. Larry Wilcox, age 42, develops chronic open-angle glaucoma. The physician prescribes pilocarpine eyedrops. When teaching Mr. Wilcox how to administer them, the nurse should instruct him to instill the drops in which of the following locations?

(a) On the iris
(b) On the sclera
(c) On the cornea
(d) In the lower conjunctival sac

3. After a car accident, Terri Baker age 19, needs to have a foreign body removed from her cornea. The physician orders the topical anesthetic proparacaine before removing it. After the foreign body is removed, the nurse advises Ms. Baker not to rub her eyes. Why shouldn't she?

(a) This action may result in eye redness.
(b) This action may increase systemic absorption of the drug.
(c) This action may cause excessive tearing, which would wash away the anesthetic.
(d) This action may cause corneal abrasion.

4. Ruth Carpenter, age 72, takes betaxolol (Betoptic), as prescribed to lower intraocular pressure caused by chronic open-angle glaucoma. This drug belongs to which of the following groups of drugs?

(a) Corticosteroids
(b) Adrenergic blockers
(c) Hyperosmotic agents
(d) Carbonic anhydrase inhibitors

5. Andy Mellon, age 33, develops a corneal ulcer caused by a *Pseudomonas* infection. The physician prescribes polymyxin B sulfate ophthalmic ointment. Which of the following other drugs might be effective against this infection?

(a) idoxuridine
(b) natamycin
(c) bacitracin
(d) gentamicin sulfate

59 Otic agents

OBJECTIVES

After reading and studying this chapter, the student should be able to:

1. identify the indications for the different classes of otic agents, including anti-infective, anti-inflammatory, local anesthetic, and ceruminolytic agents.
2. describe the administration techniques for the various types of otic agents.
3. identify the possible adverse reactions to the otic anti-infective and anti-inflammatory agents.
4. describe the mechanism of action for the otic anesthetic agent benzocaine, and the ceruminolytic agent carbamide peroxide.
5. describe how to apply the nursing process when caring for a patient receiving an otic agent.

INTRODUCTION

Otic agents are prescribed to treat ear **infection,** inflammation, and pain, and to soften **cerumen** (earwax). These drugs are categorized as anti-infective, anti-inflammatory, local anesthetic, and ceruminolytic agents. Otic agents are administered via eardrops, ear irrigations, or ear wicks. Several combination products that contain anti-infective and anti-inflammatory agents are available. (See *Selected major otic agents.*)

Drugs to be covered in this chapter include:

- acetic acid
- benzocaine
- boric acid
- carbamide peroxide
- chloramphenicol
- colistin sulfate
- dexamethasone sodium phosphate
- hydrocortisone (or hydrocortisone acetate)
- polymyxin B sulfate
- triethanolamine polypeptide oleate-condensate.

Otic anti-infective agents

The otic anti-infective agents represent natural antibiotics or synthetic antibiotic derivatives. Used to treat ear infections, these agents may also be combined with systemic anti-infective therapy. This section discusses the following anti-infective agents: acetic acid, boric acid, chloramphenicol, colistin sulfate, and polymyxin B sulfate.

PHARMACOKINETICS

These agents have a varying peak but relatively constant duration.

Route	Onset	Peak	Duration
Topical	<1 hr	Variable	4 hr

PHARMACODYNAMICS

Otic anti-infective agents are bactericidal (kill bacteria) or bacteriostatic (inhibit bacterial growth). Boric acid and acetic acid possess weak bacteriostatic properties and also are fungistatic (inhibit fungal growth).

PHARMACOTHERAPEUTICS

Otic anti-infective agents are prescribed for **otitis externa** caused by various **bacteria.** Colistin and polymyxin B sulfate also prove effective in treating **otitis media.** Many combination products treat a wide range of microorganisms as well as ear pain and inflammation.

Drug interactions

When administered concomitantly with an otic anti-infective agent, a topical steroid may mask the clinical signs of bacterial, fungal, or viral infections and may suppress hypersensitivity.

Boric acid is incompatible with alkali carbonates, hydroxides, and benzalkonium chloride. It precipitates when combined with salicylic acid. Cumulative nephrotoxicity and neurotoxicity can occur if polymyxin B sulfate is administered topically along with systemic polymyxin B sulfate therapy.

ADVERSE DRUG REACTIONS

Superinfections sometimes occur when use of otic anti-infective agents results in overgrowth of nonsusceptible organisms. Hypersensitivity reactions, such as ear pruritus or burning, urticaria, and vesicular or maculopapular dermatitis, may occur with use of any otic anti-infective agent.

Selected major otic agents

The following chart summarizes the major otic agents currently in clinical use.

DRUG	MAJOR INDICATIONS AND USUAL DOSAGES	CONTRAINDICATIONS AND PRECAUTIONS
Otic anti-infective agents		
boric acid (Ear-Dry, Swim-Ear)	*Otitis externa* ADULT: 4 to 6 drops in each ear, plugged with cotton, t.i.d. or q.i.d. PEDIATRIC: same as adult dosage	• Boric acid is contraindicated as the sole treatment for earache in any patient. • This drug has no precautions.
chloramphenicol (Chloromycetin Otic)	*Otitis externa* ADULT: 2 to 3 drops t.i.d. PEDIATRIC: same as adult dosage	• Chloramphenicol is contraindicated in a patient with a perforated tympanic membrane or known hypersensitivity. • This drug requires cautious use in a patient who has received the drug for a prolonged time.
Otic anti-inflammatory agents		
dexamethasone sodium phosphate (Decadron Phosphate cream)	*External auditory canal inflammation* ADULT: 3 to 4 drops b.i.d. or t.i.d. PEDIATRIC: same as adult dosage	• Dexamethasone sodium phosphate is contraindicated in a patient with acute purulent bacterial, viral, or fungal otic infection; a perforated tympanic membrane; or known hypersensitivity. • This drug has no precautions.
hydrocortisone (VoSol HC Otic, Acetasol HC)	*External auditory canal inflammation* ADULT: 4 to 5 drops b.i.d. or t.i.d. PEDIATRIC: 3 drops t.i.d or q.i.d.	• Hydrocortisone is contraindicated in a patient with acute purulent bacterial, viral, or fungal otic infection; a perforated tympanic membrane; or known hypersensitivity. • This drug has no precautions.
Otic local anesthetic agents		
benzocaine (Americaine Otic, Auralgan Otic, Tympagesic)	*Ear pain resulting from ear infection or other ear conditions* ADULT: 4 to 5 drops t.i.d. or q.i.d. every 1 to 2 hours, as needed PEDIATRIC: same as adult dosage	• Benzocaine is contraindicated in a patient with a perforated tympanic membrane or known hypersensitivity. • This drug has no precautions.
Ceruminolytic agents		
carbamide peroxide (Debrox, Murine Ear)	*Removal of hardened or impacted cerumen, prevention of ceruminosis* ADULT: 5 to 10 drops b.i.d. in ear, then irrigated gently after a few minutes, for 4 days PEDIATRIC: for children under age 12, dosage individualized by physician	• Carbamide peroxide is contraindicated in a patient with perforated tympanic membrane; ear drainage, pain, irritation, or rash; dizziness; or known hypersensitivity. • This drug has no precautions.
triethanolamine polypeptide oleate-condensate (Cerumenex)	*Removal of hardened or impacted cerumen; ear canal clearance before examination, otologic therapy, or audiometry* ADULT: ear canal filled with solution and plugged with cotton for 15 to 30 minutes, then irrigated gently	• Triethanolamine is contraindicated in a patient with a perforated tympanic membrane, a history of otitis media, or known hypersensitivity. • This drug requires cautious use in a patient with dermatologic disorders or a history of allergic reactions.

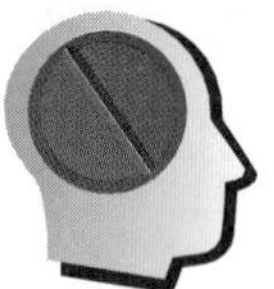

CRITICAL THINKING: To enhance your critical thinking skills about otic agents, consider the following situation and its analysis.
Situation: Karen White, age 17, is being treated for bacterial otitis externa. Her physician prescribes topical otic boric acid, 6 drops t.i.d., and topical otic hydrocortisone, 5 drops q.i.d. Five days after treatment has begun, Ms. White feels worse, even though she has been taking the medications exactly as instructed. What may be causing this worsening of symptoms?
Analysis: One possibility is that the anti-infective ordered is not appropriate for Ms. White's infection. Boric acid is a weak bacteriostatic anti-infective and may not provide sufficient coverage. Another possibility is that the use of an anti-inflammatory agent such as hydrocortisone may exacerbate an infection. The patient's medications may need to be changed in order to treat this infection effectively.

NURSING PROCESS APPLICATION

The following information assists the nurse in caring for a patient receiving an otic anti-infective agent. It includes an overview of assessment activities as well as examples of appropriate nursing diagnoses and related interventions (under "Planning and implementation"). It also highlights the importance of evaluation.

Assessment

Before drug therapy begins, review the patient's history for conditions that contraindicate or require cautious use of the prescribed otic anti-infective agent. Also review the patient's medication history to identify use of drugs that may interact with it. During therapy, assess the patient for adverse drug reactions and signs of drug interactions. Also, periodically assess the effectiveness of therapy with the otic anti-infective agent. Finally, evaluate the patient's and family's knowledge about the prescribed drug.

Nursing diagnoses

- Risk for injury related to a preexisting condition that contraindicates or requires cautious use of an otic anti-infective agent
- Risk for injury related to adverse drug reactions or drug interactions
- Knowledge deficit related to the prescribed otic anti-infective agent

Planning and implementation

- Do not administer an otic anti-infective agent to a patient with a condition that contraindicates its use. (See *Administering eardrops.*)
- Administer an otic anti-infective agent cautiously to a patient at risk because of a preexisting condition.
- Monitor the patient for adverse reactions and drug interactions during therapy with an otic anti-infective agent.

Administering eardrops

The nurse should administer eardrops appropriately for an adult or pediatric patient, as described below.

Adult patient

- Shake the bottle, as directed, and open it. Fill the dropper and place the bottle within reach.
- Tilt the patient's head so that the affected ear is up. Gently pull the top of the ear up and back to straighten the ear canal.
- Position the dropper above but not touching the ear, and release the prescribed number of drops.
- Keep the patient's head tilted for 10 minutes. If desired, plug the ear with cotton moistened with the eardrops. Do not use dry cotton, because it will absorb the drops.
- Repeat the procedure for the other ear, if prescribed.

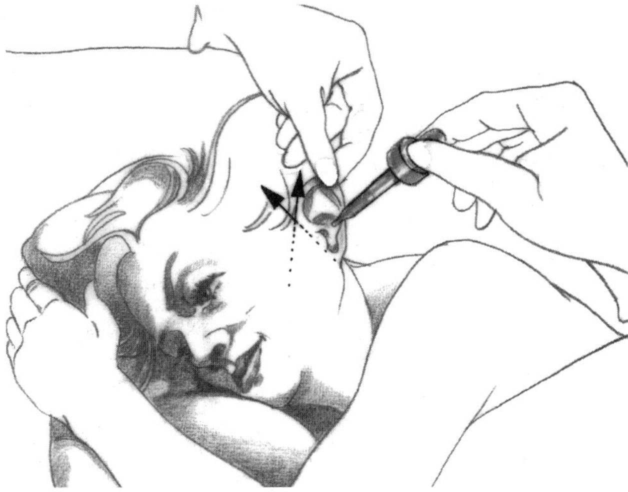

Pediatric patient

- Lay the child on his side so that the affected ear is turned up.
- Gently pull the ear down and back to straighten the ear canal.
- Position the dropper above but not touching the ear, and release the prescribed number of drops. (Note the difference in the direction the ear is moved for a child. This is because the child's ear cartilage is immature.)
- Notify the physician if the child experiences pain after instillation.

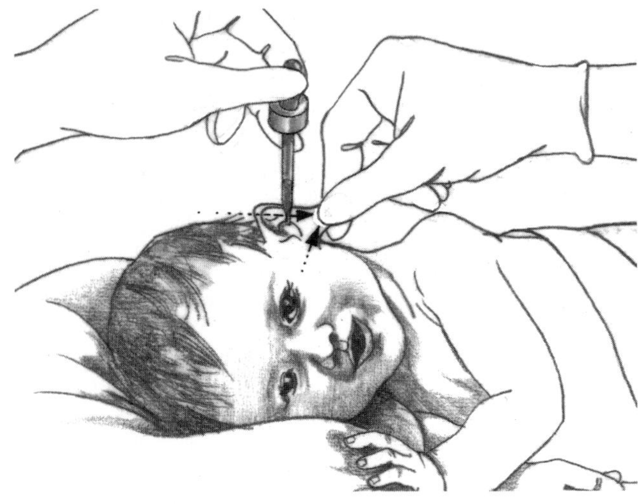

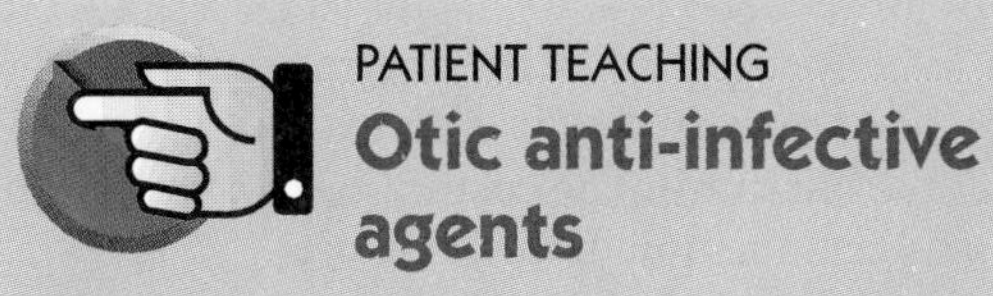

PATIENT TEACHING
Otic anti-infective agents

- Teach the patient and family the name, dose, frequency, action, and adverse effects of the prescribed otic anti-infective agent.
- Instruct the patient to contact the physician immediately upon experiencing tinnitus, decreased hearing acuity, dizziness, or unsteady gait.
- Advise the patient to discontinue the otic anti-infective agent and contact the physician if an allergic reaction occurs.
- Teach the patient (or parent of the pediatric patient) how to instill eardrops.
- Instruct the patient not to wash the dropper after use.
- Demonstrate how to gently insert cotton moistened with the eardrops into the ear canal. Inform the patient that the placement of the cotton may impair hearing.
- Instruct the patient or parent to notify the physician if adverse reactions occur.

• Monitor the patient for evidence of superinfection, such as continued ear pain, inflammation, and fever. If superinfection is suspected, notify the physician.
• Monitor the patient for signs of nephrotoxicity and neurotoxicity when topical polymyxin B sulfate is administered with systemic polymyxin B sulfate therapy. If neurotoxicity or nephrotoxocity is suspected, withhold the drug and notify the physician.
• Perform a patch test to assess for allergic contact dermatitis before administering an otic anti-infective agent to a patient who is sensitive to other topical agents. To perform this test, apply the otic agent onto the flexor surface of the patient's arm. Cover the area with a small sterile bandage and wait 24 hours before observing for erythema and urticaria. (See Patient Teaching: *Otic anti-infective agents.*)
• Monitor the patient for signs and symptoms of a hypersensitivity reaction to the otic anti-infective agent, such as ear pruritus or burning, urticaria, and vesicular or maculopapular dermatitis. If such findings are detected, notify the physician because a different drug may be needed.
• Clean and dry the ear canal before administering an otic anti-infective solution or suspension.
• Warm the otic anti-infective agent to room temperature before instillation. To do this, roll the bottle between the hands or allow it to stand at room temperature for about 30 minutes. A solution that is too hot or cold may stimulate the central nervous system, possibly causing vertigo or nausea.
• Administer an otic anti-infective agent properly.
• Only use the prescribed amount of drops of the otic infective agent to prevent accumulation of debris in the ear.
• Notify the physician if adverse reactions or drug interactions occur.

Evaluation

For each nursing diagnosis, prepare an evaluation statement that describes the patient's or family's response to nursing interventions.

Otic anti-inflammatory agents

Otic anti-inflammatory agents are administered to the ear canal to produce anti-inflammatory, antipruritic, and vasoconstrictor effects. These agents include hydrocortisone (or hydrocortisone acetate) and its synthetic derivative dexamethasone sodium phosphate.

PHARMACOKINETICS

Long-term use of otic anti-inflammatory agents may cause some systemic absorption, although no clinical effects of the absorption have been noted.

Route	Onset	Peak	Duration
Topical	<1 hr	Variable	4 hr

PHARMACODYNAMICS

In an acute inflammatory reaction, otic anti-inflammatory agents inhibit edema, capillary dilatation, fibrin deposition, and phagocyte and leukocyte migration. These drugs also reduce capillary and fibroblast proliferation, collagen deposition, and scar formation. Researchers have not determined the exact mechanisms of action for these responses. Some anti-inflammatory agents are fluorinated, which enhances their anti-inflammatory action.

PHARMACOTHERAPEUTICS

Otic anti-inflammatory agents are used for inflammatory conditions of the external ear canal and are administered with a dropper, via an ear wick, or as a cream or ointment.

Drug interactions

Otic anti-inflammatory agents do not interact significantly with other drugs.

ADVERSE DRUG REACTIONS

Common adverse reactions to otic anti-inflammatory agents are transient, local, stinging, or burning sensations. These agents may also mask or exacerbate an underlying otic infection. Although rare, a hypersensitivity reaction can occur, producing such effects as ear itching or burning, urticaria, and vesicular or maculopapular dermatitis.

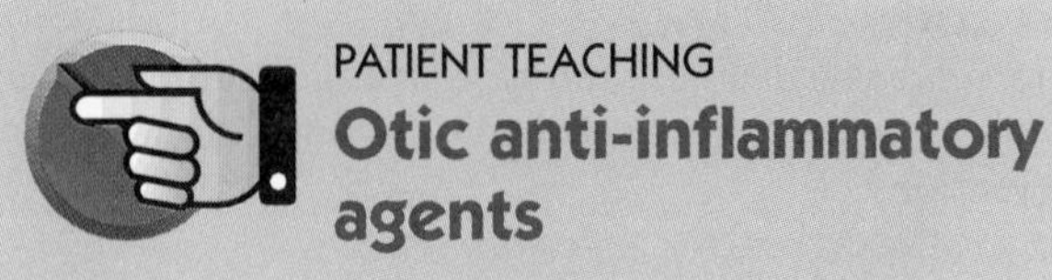

PATIENT TEACHING
Otic anti-inflammatory agents

- Teach the patient and family the name, dose, frequency, action, and adverse effects of the prescribed otic anti-inflammatory agent.
- Instruct the patient to discontinue the medication and contact the physician if signs of an allergic reaction occur.
- Teach the patient (or parent of the pediatric patient) how to instill eardrops.
- Show the patient how to insert a gauze wick into the ear canal, allowing the loose end of the wick to hang out of the ear canal.
- Instruct the patient or parent to notify the physician if other adverse reactions occur or if the ear infection persists or worsens.

NURSING PROCESS APPLICATION

The following information assists the nurse in caring for a patient receiving an otic anti-inflammatory agent. It includes an overview of assessment activities as well as examples of appropriate nursing diagnoses and related interventions (under "Planning and implementation"). It also highlights the importance of evaluation.

Assessment

Before drug therapy begins, review the patient's history for conditions that contraindicate or require cautious use of the prescribed otic anti-inflammatory agent. During therapy, assess the patient for adverse drug reactions. Also, periodically assess the effectiveness of therapy with the otic anti-inflammatory agent. Finally, evaluate the patient's and family's knowledge about the prescribed drug. (See Patient Teaching: *Otic anti-inflammatory agents.*)

Nursing diagnoses

- Risk for injury related to a preexisting condition that contraindicates the use of an otic anti-inflammatory agent
- Risk for injury related to adverse drug reactions
- Knowledge deficit related to the prescribed otic anti-inflammatory agent

Planning and implementation

- Do not administer an otic anti-inflammatory agent to a patient with a condition that contraindicates its use.
- Monitor the patient for adverse reactions during therapy with an otic anti-inflammatory agent.
- Observe the patient for signs and symptoms of a hypersensitivity reaction, such as ear pruritus or burning, urticaria, and vesicular or maculopapular dermatitis. If a hypersensitivity reaction occurs, notify the physician.
- Clean and dry the ear canal before administering an otic anti-inflammatory agent.
- Do not administer the otic anti-inflammatory agent with an otic anti-infective agent when the otic anti-inflammatory agent is prescribed to treat allergic otitis externa.
- Administer the otic anti-inflammatory agent sparingly to prevent debris accumulation in the ear canal.
- Expect to administer the otic anti-inflammatory agent with an otic anti-infective agent as prescribed to treat bacterial otitis externa.

**** Monitor the patient for worsening of symptoms, which may indicate exacerbation of the infection. Notify the physician if the patient's ear infection persists or worsens during otic anti-inflammatory agent therapy.***

- Notify the physician if there is no improvement in symptoms after 5 to 7 days of therapy.

Evaluation

For each nursing diagnosis, prepare an evaluation statement that describes the patient's or family's response to nursing interventions.

Otic local anesthetic agents

Local anesthetic agents block nerve conduction at and around the application site to produce an analgesic effect. The only local anesthetic approved for otic use is benzocaine. It is administered topically as a solution or a gel.

PHARMACOKINETICS

Benzocaine is not absorbed systemically.

Route	Onset	Peak	Duration
Topical	Within minutes	Variable	1 hr

PHARMACODYNAMICS

Local anesthetic agents temporarily interrupt the conduction of nerve impulses. In an area of mixed nerve fibers, local anesthetics initially affect autonomic nerve fibers, first blocking the small, nonmyelinated C fibers that mediate pain and produce vasoconstrictor responses, then the myelinated A-delta fibers that mediate pain and temperature. Then the local anesthetics block the large fibers that carry sensory impulses, thereby blocking impulse conduction in the motor nerves.

PHARMACOTHERAPEUTICS

Benzocaine is used for temporary relief of ear pain. It may be used with an otic anti-infective agent if an ear infection is present.

Drug interactions

Benzocaine does not interact significantly with other drugs.

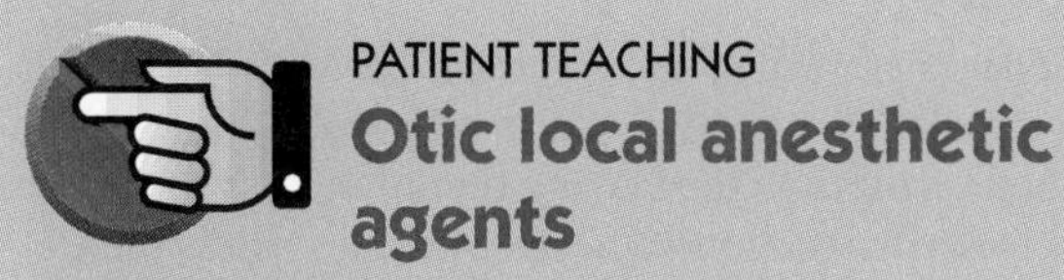

PATIENT TEACHING

Otic local anesthetic agents

- ➤ Teach the patient and family the name, dose, frequency, action, and adverse effects of benzocaine.
- ➤ Instruct the patient to avoid prolonged use of benzocaine and to contact the physician if the ear problem persists or worsens.
- ➤ Teach the patient (or parent of a pediatric patient) how to instill eardrops.
- ➤ Instruct the patient to report hearing loss, dizziness, or ear irritation, pruritus, or sense of fullness in the ear to the physician.
- ➤ Instruct the patient to stop the drug and notify the physician if urticaria occurs.

ADVERSE DRUG REACTIONS

Benzocaine may cause ear irritation, pruritus, and edema. It may mask the symptoms of a fulminating middle ear infection, although hearing loss, dizziness, or a sensation of fullness in the ear may remain. It also may cause urticaria, a hypersensitivity reaction.

NURSING PROCESS APPLICATION

The following information assists the nurse in caring for a patient receiving benzocaine. It includes an overview of assessment activities as well as examples of appropriate nursing diagnoses and related interventions (under "Planning and implementation"). It also highlights the importance of evaluation.

Assessment

Before drug therapy begins, review the patient's history for conditions that contraindicate the use of benzocaine. During therapy, assess the patient for adverse drug reactions. Also, periodically assess the effectiveness of benzocaine therapy. Finally, evaluate the patient's and family's knowledge about the prescribed drug. (See Patient Teaching: *Otic local anesthetic agents.*)

Nursing diagnoses

- Risk for injury related to a preexisting condition that contraindicates the use of benzocaine
- Risk for injury related to adverse drug reactions
- Knowledge deficit related to benzocaine

Planning and implementation

- Do not administer benzocaine to a patient with a condition that contraindicates its use.
- Monitor the patient for adverse reactions to benzocaine.
- Inspect the patient's ear canal for signs of irritation or edema before each benzocaine application. If inspection reveals either reaction, withhold benzocaine and notify the physician.
- Irrigate the ear gently before administration to clear it of debris and impacted cerumen.
- Monitor the patient for early signs of an allergic reaction, such as urticaria. Discontinue the drug immediately and notify the physician if an allergic reaction is suspected.
- Monitor the patient for signs of middle ear infection, such as hearing loss and dizziness. Notify the physician if either occurs.
- Instill the drops properly. Avoid touching the patient's ear with the dropper; do not rinse the dropper.
- Notify the physician if ear pain persists or worsens.

Evaluation

For each nursing diagnosis, prepare an evaluation statement that describes the patient's or family's response to nursing interventions.

Ceruminolytic agents

Ceruminolytic agents emulsify hardened or impacted cerumen (or earwax). They also prevent excessive cerumen accumulation. Ceruminolytic agents discussed in this section include carbamide peroxide and triethanolamine polypeptide oleate-condensate.

PHARMACOKINETICS

Ceruminolytics are not absorbed systemically.

Route	Onset	Peak	Duration
Topical	2-4 days	Variable	Variable

PHARMACODYNAMICS

Ceruminolytics reduce hardened cerumen by emulsifying and mechanically loosening it. Carbamide peroxide is combined with anhydrous glycerin to soften cerumen. Exposing the carbamide peroxide to moisture releases oxygen and hydrogen peroxide, which produces an effervescence that mechanically removes cerumen. Carbamide peroxide also acts to deodorize odor-causing bacteria in the ear.

PHARMACOTHERAPEUTICS

Carbamide peroxide is used to loosen hardened or impacted cerumen and to prevent ceruminosis (excessive cerumen). Triethanolamine may be used to remove excess or impacted cerumen and to clear the ear canal before an ear examination or procedure. Nonetheless, the patient's ear should be irrigated after therapy to remove debris.

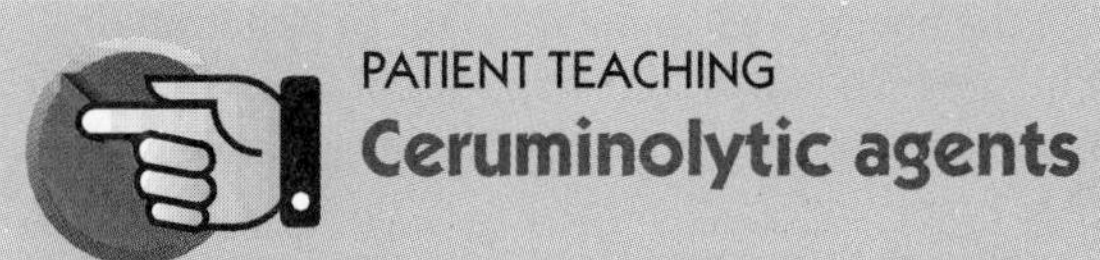

PATIENT TEACHING
Ceruminolytic agents

- Teach the patient and family the name, dose, frequency, action, and adverse effects of the prescribed ceruminolytic agent.
- Instruct the patient to contact the physician if an allergic reaction occurs.
- Instruct the patient not to use carbamide peroxide for more than 4 days, unless supervised by a physician, and not to use triethanolamine for more than 15 to 30 minutes unless instructed otherwise by the physician.
- Instruct the patient to allow the ceruminolytic solution to remain in the ear canal for at least 15 minutes.
- Instruct the patient to store the ceruminolytic agent in a light-resistant container, away from heat.
- Teach the patient (or parent of a pediatric patient) how to administer eardrops.
- Teach the patient how to irrigate the ear. Show how to tilt the head with the affected ear upward. Explain that the tip of the irrigating device is placed inside the meatus and directed toward the roof of the ear canal. Then warm water is allowed to flow into the ear canal. Explain that a basin should be positioned below the ear to collect the irrigating fluid as it flows out of the ear. Instruct the patient to lie on the affected side after irrigation to allow the irrigating solution to flow out.
- Inform the patient that a fizzing sound is normal during application of the ceruminolytic agent.
- Instruct the patient not to use cotton swabs in an attempt to remove cerumen because accidental perforation of the tympanic membrane could occur.
- Instruct the patient to notify the physician if adverse reactions occur.

Drug interactions
Ceruminolytics do not interact significantly with other drugs.

ADVERSE DRUG REACTIONS
Adverse reactions to ceruminolytics are usually insignificant. Mild, localized erythema and pruritus may occur with carbamide peroxide or triethanolamine. Some patients using triethanolamine experience hypersensitivity reactions, such as severe eczema.

NURSING PROCESS APPLICATION
The following information assists the nurse in caring for a patient receiving a ceruminolytic. It includes an overview of assessment activities as well as examples of appropriate nursing diagnoses and related interventions (under "Planning and implementation"). It also highlights the importance of evaluation.

Assessment
Before drug therapy begins, review the patient's history for conditions that contraindicate or require cautious use of the prescribed ceruminolytic. During therapy, assess the patient for adverse drug reactions. Also, periodically assess the effectiveness of ceruminolytic therapy. Finally, evaluate the patient's and family's knowledge about the prescribed drug. (See Patient Teaching: *Ceruminolytic agents.*)

Nursing diagnoses
- Risk for injury related to a preexisting condition that contraindicates or requires cautious use of a ceruminolytic
- Risk for injury related to adverse drug reactions
- Knowledge deficit related to the prescribed ceruminolytic

Planning and implementation
- Do not administer a ceruminolytic to a patient with a condition that contraindicates its use.
- Administer triethanolamine cautiously to a patient at risk because of a preexisting condition.
- Perform a patch test before administering triethanolamine to determine the possibility of an allergic reaction. To do this, put a drop of the ceruminolytic on the flexor surface of the arm. Then cover the area with a small sterile bandage, and observe it, usually after 24 hours, for erythema and swelling.
- Monitor the patient for adverse reactions during ceruminolytic therapy.
- Inspect the patient's skin for eczema (patchy, scaly, red blotches) when administering triethanolamine. If eczema is present, withhold the drug and notify the physician because this may be a hypersensitivity reaction.
- Inspect the ear canal for erythema before administering each dose of the ceruminolytic. Ask the patient about pruritus. Notify the physician if erythema or pruritus occurs.
- Instill the prescribed ceruminolytic properly. Do not touch the patient's ear with the dropper.
- Keep the medication in a tightly closed, light-resistant container and away from heat.
- Irrigate the affected ear gently with warm water after administering the ceruminolytic agent. Avoid excessive pressure. Irrigation will help remove the cerumen loosened by the ceruminolytic agent.
- Wash skin surfaces with soap and water if they come in contact with the ceruminolytic agent.
- Notify the physician if adverse reactions occur or if the ceruminolytic is ineffective.

Evaluation
For each nursing diagnosis, prepare an evaluation statement that describes the patient's or family's response to nursing interventions.

CHAPTER SUMMARY

Chapter 59 presented information on four classes of otic drugs: anti-infective, anti-inflammatory, local anesthetic, and ceruminolytic agents. Here are the chapter highlights.

Otic anti-infective agents include acetic acid, boric acid, chloramphenicol, colistin sulfate, and polymyxin B sulfate. Adverse reactions to these otic agents include hypersensitivity reactions and superinfection.

Otic anti-inflammatory agents produce anti-inflammatory, antipruritic, and vasoconstrictor effects. These agents include dexamethasone sodium phosphate and hydrocortisone. Otic anti-inflammatory agents may precipitate a hypersensitivity reaction and may mask or exacerbate an underlying otic infection.

Local anesthetics produce analgesia by blocking nerve impulse transmission in a given area. Benzocaine is the local anesthetic approved for otic use.

Ceruminolytic agents emulsify hardened or impacted cerumen. They also deodorize odor-causing bacteria in the ear.

As needed, the nurse should teach the patient or parent how to instill eardrops, irrigate the ear (when a ceruminolytic is used), or use an ear wick for drug administration. The nurse should also teach the patient and family member to recognize and report important adverse reactions.

Questions to consider

See Appendix 1 for answers.

1. William Spencer, age 51, develops otitis externa. The physician prescribes the otic anti-infective agent chloramphenicol, 2 to 3 drops in the external auditory canal t.i.d. How should Mr. Spencer straighten the ear canal for instilling the drops?

(a) Pull the ear up and back
(b) Pull the ear down and back
(c) Pull the ear up and forward
(d) Pull the ear down and forward

2. Kelly Hernandez, age 25, is prescribed the otic anti-inflammatory agent hydrocortisone, 4 drops t.i.d., for external auditory canal inflammation. Which of the following conditions would contraindicate otic hydrocortisone administration?

(a) Vertigo
(b) Tinnitus
(c) Otitis externa
(d) Perforated tympanic membrane

3. Harry Althorp, age 31, is being treated for ceruminosis. Carbamide peroxide is prescribed. Which of the following instructions should the nurse give Mr. Althorp about administering ceruminolytic agents?

(a) Instill the solution and irrigate the ear canal immediately.
(b) Let the solution remain in the ear canal for at least 15 minutes.
(c) Instill the solution and insert a dry cotton plug.
(d) Instill the solution and use a cotton swab to remove cerumen.

4. Soo Kim, age 4, is prescribed benzocaine 4 drops t.i.d. to relieve ear pain related to otitis media. The patient's mother is instructed that pain relief should occur within how long after benzocaine administration?

(a) Minutes
(b) 1 to 2 hours
(c) 4 to 6 hours
(d) 24 hours

60 Dermatologic agents

OBJECTIVES

After reading and studying this chapter, the student should be able to:

1. describe how topical dermatologic agents are affected by various factors.
2. list the major classes of dermatologic agents, and identify their mechanisms of action and indications.
3. explain how to apply specific dermatologic agents.
4. compare the therapeutic and adverse effects of the most commonly used dermatologic agents.
5. describe how to apply the nursing process when caring for a patient who is receiving a dermatologic agent.

INTRODUCTION

Skin disorders are common and may go unnoticed, except by the patient. They are seldom life-threatening, but can cause discomfort, pain, occupational disability, body image disturbance, and embarrassment. Common disorders include allergic skin reactions, **acne,** moles, neoplasms, parasitic infestations, and bacterial, fungal, or viral infections.

To provide effective care for a patient with a skin disorder, the nurse must understand that the skin's functions can affect topical dermatologic agents. (See *Effects of normal skin functions on topical drugs.*) Those drugs are many and varied and are used to treat a wide variety of conditions. (See *Selected major dermatologic agents,* pages 732 and 733.)

Drugs covered in this chapter include:

- aclometasone dipropionate
- acyclovir
- amphotericin B
- bacitracin
- benzoyl peroxide
- betamethasone dipropromate
- betamethasone valerate
- clindamycin
- clotrimazole
- crotamiton
- erythromycin
- flucinolone acetonide
- flucinonide
- fluorouracil
- fluticasone propionate
- gentamicin sulfate
- halobetasol propionate
- hydrocortisone
- ketoconazole
- lindane
- mafenide acetate
- malathion
- miconazole nitrate
- minoxidil
- mupirocin
- nystatin
- permethrin
- salicylic acid
- silver sulfadiazine
- terconazole
- tetracycline hydrochloride
- tolnaftate
- tretinoin
- triamcinolone acetonide.

Dermatologic anti-infective agents

For the skin to function optimally, it must remain intact. Dermal integrity can be disrupted by such factors as trauma, disease, poor hygiene, or aging. This disruption creates a portal of entry for invasion by pathogens that cause dermatologic infections, which may be treated by dermatologic anti-infective agents.

This section discusses three types of topical dermatologic anti-infective agents: antibacterial, antifungal, and antiviral agents. Antibacterial agents include bacitracin, gentamicin sulfate, mafenide acetate, mupirocin, and silver sulfadiazine. Antifungal agents include amphotericin B, clotrimazole, ketoconazole, miconazole nitrate, nystatin, terconazole, and tolnaftate. Acyclovir is the only dermatologic antiviral agent discussed.

Topical anti-infective agents can be applied as a cream, ointment, gel, powder, aerosol, lotion, or solution. They are used for their local effects at the application site, when systemic absorption is undesirable or unnecessary (such as in an isolated wound infection). If the topical agent cannot control the infection, a systemic antibiotic is needed. If a dermatologic infection is severe, topical and systemic agents may be used concomitantly.

PHARMACOKINETICS

The absorption of dermatologic anti-infective agents is affected by the site and frequency of application, dose applied, drug preparation, and the skin's overall health and integrity.

When topical anti-infectives are applied directly to the infected area, absorption is usually limited to the application site. However, systemic absorption may occur if the drug is applied to a denuded area that covers 20% or more of the body surface (as in a second- or third-degree burn).

Effects of normal skin functions on topical drugs

Several normal functions of the skin can affect topical drug absorption and other effects — as well as those of some systemic drugs.

SKIN FUNCTION	EFFECT ON DRUG
Barrier	Prevents topical drug penetration into underlying tissue and systemic circulation
Excretory (cell migration and shedding)	Allows systemic drug absorption through dermal layers to epidermal surface
Reservoir	Increases topical drug absorption when the stratum corneum is occluded, which increases water content and tissue permeability
Metabolic	Increases the time of tissue exposure — and increases absorption — for agents structured to compete with enzymatic action during synthesis and metabolism
Sensory	Can be altered by topical anesthetics to allow application of irritating therapeutic agents
Temperature regulation	May enhance or retard topical drug delivery
Vasoconstriction (during cold exposure)	Decreases blood flow to the dermis, slowing drug delivery.
Vasodilation (during heat exposure)	Increases blood flow to the dermis, enhancing drug delivery.
Sweat production (during heat exposure)	Could retard drug delivery because sweat contains metabolites that may alter drug properties.

If this occurs, anti-infective agents are distributed, metabolized, and excreted in different ways, depending on the type.

Absorption of the topical agent can be enhanced by increased dermal blood flow or skin temperature, or slowed by decreased skin temperature or topical application of a vasoconstrictor. No evidence suggests active transport of topical drugs in the skin itself. The onset, peak, and duration of action vary based on the patient and disorder being treated.

PHARMACODYNAMICS

Bacitracin may be bactericidal or bacteriostatic, depending on its concentration and the organism's susceptibility. It acts by inhibiting cell wall synthesis. Gentamicin sulfate, which is bacteriostatic, also acts by inhibiting cell wall synthesis. Mafenide acetate is a bacteriostatic agent that interferes with cell wall synthesis and metabolism. Mupirocin inhibits bacterial protein synthesis; it is usually bacteriostatic, but can be bactericidal at high concentrations. Silver sulfadiazine is bacteriostatic, acting to inhibit bacterial growth by inhibiting essential enzyme synthesis.

The antifungal agents act by disrupting the fungal cell membrane, permitting the loss of valuable elements from the cell. These agents can be fungistatic or fungicidal, depending on the infecting organism and their concentration (for example, terconazole is available as a 0.4% and 0.8% cream.)

The antiviral acyclovir, which is available as a 5% ointment, acts against the herpes virus by inhibiting deoxyribonucleic acid (DNA) synthesis.

PHARMACOTHERAPEUTICS

Bacitracin is effective against skin infections caused by gram-positive organisms. Gentamicin sulfate is used to treat primary and secondary skin infections caused by aerobic gram-negative bacteria. Mafenide acetate and silver sulfadiazine are used to prevent infections in leg ulcers, abrasions, second- and third-degree burns, and skin grafts. They are effective against *Pseudomonas aeruginosa* and other strains or anaerobes. Mupirocin is used to treat impetigo and primary or secondary skin infections caused by certain strains of aerobic gram-positive and gram-negative bacteria.

The antifungal agents are used to treat *Candida albicans* infections of the outer layers of the skin, mucous membranes, vagina, uncircumcised penis, and anorectal area. They are also used to treat dermatophyte infections of the hair, skin, and nails. These fungal infections, known as mycoses or tinea, are classified by their location on the body.

Acyclovir is used to treat Type 1 herpes lesions on the lips and Type 2 herpes lesions on the genitals.

Drug interactions

Dermatologic anti-infective agents have no reported drug interactions.

ADVERSE DRUG REACTIONS

The most common adverse reactions to dermatologic anti-infectives affect the skin. These reactions include stinging, rash, contact dermatitis, skin dryness, burning, pruritus, tenderness,

Select major dermatologic agents

The following chart summarizes the major dermatologic agents in current use. All doses given are appropriate for adults and children except where specified.

DRUG	MAJOR INDICATIONS AND USUAL DOSAGES	CONTRAINDICATIONS AND PRECAUTIONS
Dermatologic anti-infective agents		
acyclovir (Zovirax)	*Primary herpes genitalis, limited non-life-threatening mucocutaneous herpes simplex virus infections in immunocompromised patients* Apply in sufficient quantities to cover all lesions every 3 hours, six times daily for 7 days	• Acyclovir is contraindicated in a patient with hypersensitivity or chemical intolerance to the drug.
bacitracin (Baciguent)	*Gram-positive bacterial skin infections* Apply a thin film q.d. to t.i.d. to affected area	• Bacitracin is contraindicated in a patient with hypersensitivity to the drug or one who is atopic.
terconazole (Terazol 3, Terazol 7)	*Vulvovaginal candidiasis* Apply 1 applicatorful (5 g) intravaginally once daily h.s. for 3 consecutive days with 0.8% cream or suppositories; or 1 applicatorful for 7 consecutive days with 0.4% cream	• Terconazole is contraindicated in a patient with hypersensitivity to the drug or any inactive ingredient in it.
Dermatologic anti-inflammatory agents		
betamethasone dipropionate (Diprolene, Diprolene AF)	*Psoriasis, contact dermatitis, eczema, pruritus* Apply sparingly q.d. or b.i.d. to affected area	• Betamethasone dipropionate is contraindicated in a patient with hypersensitivity to corticosteroids. • This drug requires cautious use in an infant or a child, in a pregnant or breast-feeding patient, or in a patient with a bacterial, fungal, or viral infection.
hydrocortisone (Cetacort, Cortaid, Cort-Dome, Hytone)	*Psoriasis, contact dermatitis, eczema, pruritus* ADULTS: Apply a thin film b.i.d. to q.i.d. to affected area	• Hydrocortisone is contraindicated in a patient with hypersensitivity to corticosteroids. • This drug requires cautious use in an infant or a child, in a breast-feeding patient, or in a patient with a bacterial, fungal, or viral infection.
Topical anti-acne agents		
tetracycline hydrochloride (Topicycline)	*Inflammatory acne vulgaris* ADULTS: Apply generously b.i.d. to affected area	• Tetracycline hydrochloride is contraindicated in a patient with hypersensitivity to the drug. • This drug requires cautious use in a patient with hepatic or renal impairment.
tretinoin (Retin-A)	*Acne vulgaris* ADULTS: Apply nightly to affected area	• Tretinoin is contraindicated in a patient with hypersensitivity to any tretinoin component. • This drug requires cautious use in a patient with eczema.
Scabicides and pediculicides		
lindane (Kwell, Scabene)	*Scabies and pediculosis* Apply cream or lotion to dry skin in a thin layer over the entire body from the neck down, rub it in thoroughly, leave it on for 8 to 12 hours, then remove it thoroughly by bathing; alternatively, shampoo the affected area for 4 to 5 minutes, rinse and dry hair, and then comb hair with a fine-tooth comb to remove remaining nits	• Lindane is contraindicated in a patient with hypersensitivity to the drug, raw or inflamed skin, or a seizure disorder. The lotion form is contraindicated in a premature infant. • This drug requires cautious use in an infant or young child because of the increased risk of central nervous system toxicity.

Select major dermatologic agents *(continued)*

DRUG	MAJOR INDICATIONS AND USUAL DOSAGES	CONTRAINDICATIONS AND PRECAUTIONS
Scabicides and pediculicides *(continued)*		
permethrin (Elimite, Nix)	*Scabies* ADULTS and CHILDREN > 2 months: Apply in sufficient quantities to cover or saturate the hair and scalp; leave on hair for 10 minutes before rinsing	• Permethrin is contraindicated in a patient with hypersensitivity to pyrethrins or chrysanthemums.
Topical minoxidil		
minoxidil (Rogaine)	*Alopecia androgenetica* ADULTS: Apply 1 ml to affected area b.i.d.	• Topical minoxidil is contraindicated in a patient with hypersensitivity to the drug or any component of the solution. • This drug requires cautious use in a patient over age 50 or one with cardiac, renal, or hepatic disease.
Topical fluorouracil		
fluorouracil (Efudex, Fluoroplex)	*Multiple actinic (solar) keratoses* ADULTS: Apply 1% to 5% cream or solution b.i.d. for 2 to 6 weeks or until erosion occurs *Superficial basal cell carcinoma* Apply 5% cream or solution to lesion b.i.d. for 3 to 6 weeks or until erosion occurs	• Topical fluorouracil is contraindicated in a patient with hypersensitivity to the drug, poor nutrition, bone marrow suppression, or a potentially serious infection or one who has had major surgery in the past month. • This drug requires cautious use in a patient with impaired hepatic or renal function or widespread neoplastic infiltration of bone marrow or in one who has received high-dose pelvic radiation or alkylating agent therapy.
Topical salicylic acid		
salicylic acid (Occlusal, Sal-Acid)	*Hyperkeratotic skin disorders, such as verrucae and various ichthyoses, keratosis palmaris and plantaris, keratosis pilaris, pityriasis rubra pilaris, and psoriasis* Apply thoroughly to affected skin that has been hydrated for 5 minutes, occlude overnight, and wash off the medication in the morning	• Salicylic acid is contraindicated in a patient with hypersensitivity to the drug or any components of the solution.

erythema, peeling, and an increase in normal hair loss. Use of antifungal vaginal suppositories can cause pelvic cramping.

Hypersensitivity reactions can occur. If the agent is absorbed systemically, the patient may develop ototoxicity, nephrotoxicity, eosinophilia, tachypnea, metabolic acidosis, and facial edema.

NURSING PROCESS APPLICATION

The following information assists the nurse in caring for a patient who is receiving a dermatologic anti-infective agent. It includes an overview of assessment activities, as well as examples of appropriate nursing diagnoses and related interventions. It also highlights the importance of evaluation.

Assessment

Before drug therapy begins, review the patient's history for conditions that contraindicate or require cautious use of the prescribed dermatologic anti-infective agent. During therapy, assess the patient for adverse drug reactions. Also, periodically assess the effectiveness of therapy. Finally, evaluate the patient's and family's knowledge about the prescribed dermatologic anti-infective agent. (See Patient Teaching: *Dermatologic anti-infective agents,* page 734.)

Nursing diagnoses

- Risk for injury related to a preexisting condition that contraindicates use of a dermatologic anti-infective agent
- Risk for injury related to adverse drug reactions
- Body image disturbance related to a skin disorder
- Knowledge deficit related to the prescribed dermatologic anti-infective agent

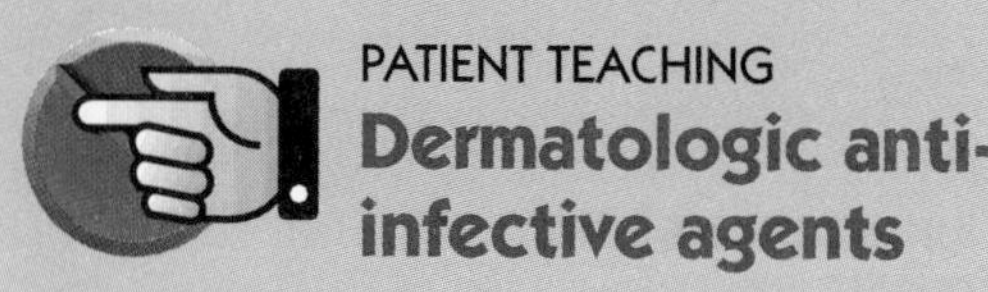

PATIENT TEACHING

Dermatologic anti-infective agents

- Teach the patient and family the name, dose, frequency, action, and adverse effects of the prescribed dermatologic anti-infective agent.
- Instruct the patient to cover the affected area thoroughly with the drug.
- Inform the patient that acyclovir is not a cure for herpes and that it should be applied as soon as symptoms begin.
- Teach the patient to clean the affected area before applying the drug.
- Instruct the patient to recognize and report systemic adverse reactions.
- Advise the patient to continue the drug for the prescribed amount of time and not to miss any doses.
- Instruct the patient to contact the physician if the infection worsens or does not improve within 1 week.
- Advise the patient to withhold the drug and notify the physician if a hypersensitivity reaction occurs.
- Instruct the patient against indiscriminate or prolonged use of a dermatologic anti-infective agent; hypersensitivity or superinfection may occur.

Planning and implementation

- Do not administer a dermatologic anti-infective agent to a patient with a condition that contraindicates its use.
- Administer a dermatologic anti-infective agent cautiously to a patient at risk because of a pre-existing condition.
- Monitor the patient for adverse reactions during dermatologic anti-infective therapy.

* ***Monitor for hypersensitivity reactions in a patient receiving a sulfonamide dermatologic agent, such as mafenide acetate or silver sulfadiazine. Keep standard emergency equipment nearby.***

- Notify the physician immediately and withhold the prescribed agent if a hypersensitivity reaction occurs. Also notify the physician if other adverse reactions occur.
- Provide emotional support to a patient whose body image is affected by the skin disorder.
- Clean the affected area before applying the prescribed agent.
- Depending on the size and location of the wound, apply the agent with a glove, applicator, or tongue blade and maintain standard precautions.

* ***Do not apply the agent to a wide area or large lesion; otherwise, toxic systemic effects may occur. Monitor fluid intake and output to detect early signs of nephrotoxicity.***

- Do not use an occlusive dressing because it may alter the action of the dermatologic agent.
- Advise the patient to return for reevaluation if the site shows no improvement after 3 to 5 days of treatment.

Evaluation

For each nursing diagnosis, prepare an evaluation statement that describes the patient's or family's response to nursing interventions.

Dermatologic anti-inflammatory agents

As dermatologic anti-inflammatory agents, corticosteroids are widely use for topical treatment of local inflammatory and pruritic skin disorders caused by mechanical, chemical, microbiologic, and immunologic factors. These drugs include alclometasone dipropionate, betamethasone dipropionate, betamethasone valerate, flucinonide, fluocinolone acetonide, fluticasone propionate, halobetasol propionate, hydrocortisone, and triamcinolone acetonide.

PHARMACOKINETICS

When applied to small areas of intact skin, topical corticosteroids are primarily absorbed locally. Small amounts are absorbed into the circulation, metabolized by the liver, and excreted by the kidneys. The onset, peak, and duration of these drugs vary based on the patient and disorder being treated.

PHARMACODYNAMICS

Topical corticosteroids suppress inflammation by binding to intracellular corticosteroid receptors, which initiates a cascade of anti-inflammatory mediators. These agents also cause vasoconstriction in inflamed tissue and prevent macrophages and leukocytes from moving into the area; this decreases swelling, redness, and itching. The drugs can slow the rate of cell division, which helps treat skin conditions that increase epidermal cell proliferation, such as psoriasis.

PHARMACOTHERAPEUTICS

Dermatologic anti-inflammatory agents are used to relieve inflammation and itching in topical steroid–responsive disorders, including eczema, psoriasis, angioedema, contact dermatitis, seborrheic dermatitis, atopic dermatitis, and urticaria.

Lotions work best on weeping eruptions in areas prone to chafing, such as the axillae, feet, or groin. Ointments are preferred for dry, scaly lesions. Creams and gels are suitable for most inflammations. Topical corticosteroids come in different potencies. For example, betamethasone dipropionate products are considered high-potency; hydrocortisone products are considered low-potency.

Drug interactions

No significant interactions occur between topical corticosteroids and other drugs. However, chemicals used in their formulation may interact with the corticosteroids and cause urticaria or contact dermatitis. If topical corticosteroids formulated in a base are combined with other drugs or a different base, their potency may be reduced.

ADVERSE DRUG REACTIONS

When applied to small areas of intact skin, dermatologic anti-inflammatory agents seldom cause adverse drug reactions. When used in high concentrations, in large areas, or on broken skin, they can cause adverse reactions. When used for 3 to 4 weeks, they may produce striae and epidermal atrophy in areas of sweating, occlusion, or high permeability. Prolonged or improper use can produce acneform eruptions; perioral dermatitis with red, papular eruptions; purpura in areas of thin skin; and allergic contact dermatitis.

Occasionally, topical corticosteroids cause hypersensitivity reactions. Systemic absorption may rapidly lead to adrenal hormone suppression, producing such signs and symptoms as edema, muscle pain, lack of energy, depression, hypotension, and weight loss. Most adverse reactions are easily reversed if recognized and treated early.

NURSING PROCESS APPLICATION

The following information assists the nurse in caring for a patient who is receiving a dermatologic anti-inflammatory agent. It includes an overview of assessment activities as well as examples of appropriate nursing diagnoses and related interventions. It also highlights the importance of evaluation.

Assessment

Before drug therapy begins, review the patient's history for conditions that contraindicate or require cautious use of the prescribed dermatologic anti-inflammatory agent. During therapy, assess the patient for adverse drug reactions. Also, periodically assess the effectiveness of therapy with the dermatologic anti-inflammatory agent. Finally, evaluate the patient's and family's knowledge about the prescribed drug. (See Patient Teaching: *Dermatologic anti-inflammatory agents.*)

Nursing diagnoses

- Risk for injury related to a preexisting condition that contraindicates or requires cautious use of a dermatologic anti-inflammatory agent
- Risk for injury related to adverse drug reactions
- Knowledge deficit related to the prescribed dermatologic anti-inflammatory agent

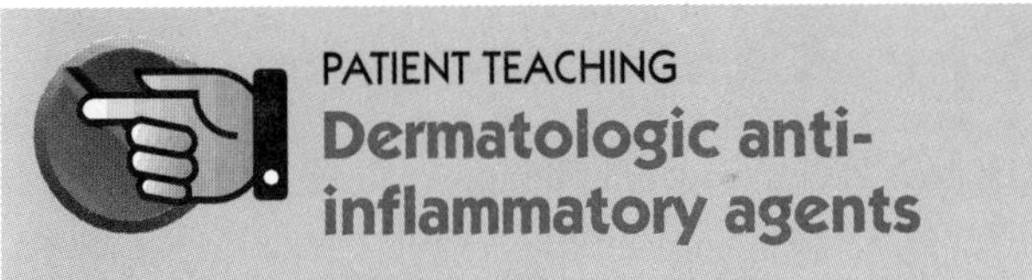

PATIENT TEACHING

Dermatologic anti-inflammatory agents

- ➤ Teach the patient and family the name, dose, frequency, action, and adverse effects of the prescribed dermatologic anti-inflammatory agent.
- ➤ Review the signs and symptoms of adrenal suppression with a patient who must receive high-dose or long-term therapy with the drug. Tell the patient to report such signs and symptoms to the physician at once.
- ➤ Instruct the patient to notify the physician if other adverse reactions occur.
- ➤ Teach the patient to clean the affected area, apply a light film of the drug, and rub it in gently.
- ➤ Advise the patient to avoid using the drug around the eyes, on the face, or in the axillae, skin creases, or genital or rectal areas, unless directed by the physician.
- ➤ Instruct the patient not to put bandages, dressings, cosmetics, or other skin products over the affected area, unless directed by the physician.
- ➤ Advise the patient to notify the physician if the condition worsens or does not improve in 1 week.

Planning and implementation

- Do not administer a dermatologic anti-inflammatory agent to a patient with a condition that contraindicates its use.
- Administer a dermatologic anti-inflammatory agent cautiously to a patient at risk because of a preexisting condition.
- Monitor the patient for adverse reactions during therapy.
- Wash the area before applying the agent to increase its penetration.
- Apply ointment, lotion, or cream in the smallest amount and lowest concentration possible.
- Avoid prolonged use of the agent in the anogenital area and skin creases, near the eyes, or on the face, unless prescribed. Do not use on denuded, infected, or weeping skin, unless prescribed.
- Provide appropriate wound care if lesions are present.
- Offer pain-relief measures if application causes discomfort.
- Do not use an occlusive dressing over the anti-inflammatory agent. Such dressings increase the risk of systemic absorption.

✱ ***Assess the patient routinely for signs and symptoms of systemic absorption and adrenal suppression, such as edema, depression, and weight loss.***

- Teach the patient about the prescribed agent.

Evaluation

For each nursing diagnosis, prepare an evaluation statement that describes the patient's or family's response to nursing interventions.

Topical anti-acne agents

Acne is a self-limiting inflammation caused by androgenic hormones, which are common in both sexes during adolescence. These hormones stimulate the sebaceous glands to grow and increase their sebum output.

Topical anti-acne agents may be classified as **keratolytics** (agents that desquamate) such as tretinoin, counterirritants such as benzoyl peroxide, and antimicrobials, such as clindamycin, erythromycin, and tetracycline hydrochloride. Salicylic acid, which may be used to treat acne and other skin disorders, is discussed later in this chapter.

PHARMACOKINETICS

Because topical anti-acne agents act locally, they are usually not absorbed through the skin. However, after multiple applications, scant levels may be detected in the serum and urine. The metabolism of these agents is unknown; their onset, peak, and duration vary with the patient and the agent used.

PHARMACODYNAMICS

The mechanisms of action of the topical anti-acne agents have not been determined fully. Benzoyl peroxide combats acne-causing bacteria by slowly liberating active oxygen, which produces antibacterial, antiseptic, drying, and keratolytic effects. Antimicrobials, such as clindamycin, erythromycin, and tetracycline hydrochloride, reduce inflammation by halting the growth of acne-causing bacteria. Tretinoin stimulates epithelial cell turnover, resulting in skin peeling. This reduces the free fatty acids to which cells must adhere in order to form a comedo (pimple).

PHARMACOTHERAPEUTICS

Topical anti-acne agents are used to treat mild acne, oily skin, and acne vulgaris.

Drug interactions

Although topical anti-acne agents have no known drug interactions, the use of more than one anti-acne agent at a time may cause increased skin irritation.

ADVERSE DRUG REACTIONS

Common adverse reactions include local skin irritation, rash, urticaria, skin dryness, burning, scaling, inflammation, blistering, and peeling. With prolonged use of an antimicrobial anti-acne agent, superinfection may occur.

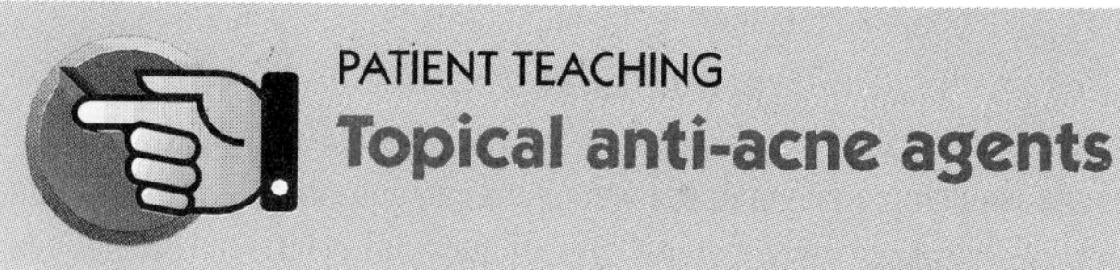

- Teach the patient and family the name, dose, frequency, action, and adverse effects of the prescribed topical anti-acne agent.
- Advise the patient to keep the drug away from the eyes and mucous membranes. If contact occurs, rinse with water.
- Inform the patient that the drug may cause a temporary feeling of warmth or stinging.
- Warn the patient to avoid skin irritants, such as abrasive soap, sunlight, sunlamps, and other topical anti-acne agents, unless directed by the physician.
- Inform the patient that normal use of water-based cosmetics is permissible.
- Instruct the patient to apply tetracycline hydrochloride solution generously until the skin is thoroughly wet. Teach the patient who uses a different anti-acne agent to clean the affected area and then apply a light film of cream or ointment.
- Inform the patient that tetracycline hydrochloride may cause skin yellowing, which may be removed with washing.
- Instruct the patient to notify the physician if adverse reactions occur.

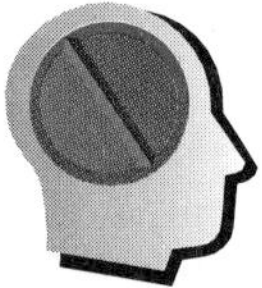

CRITICAL THINKING To enhance your critical thinking about dermatologic agents, consider the following situation and its analysis.

Situation: Two weeks ago, Julie Gonzalez, age 19, received a prescription for tretinoin to treat her acne vulgaris. At that time, her physician instructed her to apply the agent once a day before bed, 15 minutes after cleaning her skin. Ms. Gonzalez later seeks care because of excessive skin redness and peeling. She reports that she has not changed her skin care routine; she washes twice a day (in the morning and at bedtime) with a soap that contains crushed almonds. She also states that she applies tretinoin, as directed, after each cleaning. What may be causing her skin to redden and peel, and how can this be managed?

Analysis: Skin irritation and peeling are adverse reactions to tretinoin. However, tretinoin application more than once a day can exacerbate these reactions. So can exposure to sunlight and the use of an abrasive soap, such as the one Ms. Gonzalez uses. To manage this health concern, the nurse should reteach Ms. Gonzalez about tretinoin application and precautions.

NURSING PROCESS APPLICATION

The following information assists the nurse in caring for a patient receiving a topical anti-acne agent. It includes an overview of assessment activities as well as examples of appropriate nursing diagnoses and related interventions. It also highlights the importance of evaluation.

Assessment
Before drug therapy begins, review the patient's history for conditions that contraindicate or require cautious use of the prescribed topical anti-acne agent use. During therapy, assess the patient for adverse drug reactions. Also, periodically assess the effectiveness of therapy with the topical anti-acne agent. Finally, evaluate the patient's and family's knowledge about the prescribed drug. (See Patient Teaching: *Topical anti-acne agents.*)

Nursing diagnoses
- Risk for injury related to a preexisting condition that contraindicates or requires cautious use of a topical anti-acne agent
- Risk for injury related to adverse drug reactions
- Body image disturbance related to acne
- Knowledge deficit related to the prescribed topical anti-acne agent

Planning and implementation
- Do not administer a topical anti-acne agent to a patient with a condition that contraindicates its use.
- Administer a topical anti-acne agent cautiously to a patient at risk because of a preexisting condition.
- Monitor the patient for adverse reactions during anti-acne therapy.
- Provide emotional support to the patient whose body image is affected by acne.
- Clean the area before applying the anti-acne agent. Be sure to rinse well and pat dry. If tretinoin is used, let the skin dry for 15 to 30 minutes before application.
- Notify the physician if adverse reactions occur.

Evaluation
For each nursing diagnosis, prepare an evaluation statement that describes the patient's or family's response to nursing interventions.

Scabicides and pediculicides

Scabies is a pruritic skin eruption caused by burrowing of *Sarcoptes scabiei* (itch mites) into the skin. Pediculosis is a skin condition caused by parasitic lice that live in the hair and feed on blood. Scabicides and pediculicides are applied topically to eradicate these parasitic infestations. They include crotamiton, lindane, malathion, and permethrin.

PHARMACOKINETICS
Because scabicides and pediculicides can penetrate the skin, they may be absorbed systemically. However, the amount absorbed after a single application has not been determined precisely. They are rapidly metabolized by ester hydrolysis to inactive metabolites, which are excreted primarily in the urine.

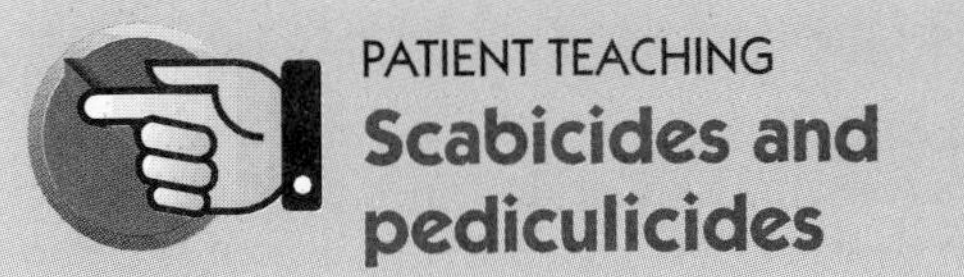

PATIENT TEACHING
Scabicides and pediculicides

- Teach the patient and the family the name, dose, frequency, action, and adverse effects of the prescribed scabicide or pediculicide.
- Instruct the patient that the drug is for external use only.
- Warn the patient to avoid open cuts, extensive excoriations, eyes, mucous membranes, and unaffected skin areas.
- Inform the patient that contaminated clothing and bed linens must be dry cleaned or washed in hot water.
- Instruct the patient to notify the physician if adverse reactions occur.
- Advise the patient to read thoroughly and follow the instructions for applying the prescribed scabicide or pediculicide because application varies with the product used.

PHARMACODYNAMICS
Scabicides and pediculicides act on the parasites' nerve cell membranes to disrupt the sodium channel current. This delays repolarization and paralyzes the pests. Beside being scabicidal and pediculicidal, some agents are ovicidal.

PHARMACOTHERAPEUTICS
Scabicides and pediculicides are used to treat scabies as well as pediculosis, which may affect the head, body, or pubic area. Most are available in cream or lotion form; lindane is also available as a shampoo.

Drug interactions
Oils may enhance the absorption of topical scabicides; therefore, concomitant use of creams, ointments, or oils should be avoided. Pentobarbital, phenobarbital, or diazepam can worsen the adverse central nervous system (CNS) effects in children.

Topical pediculicides do not interact significantly with other drugs.

ADVERSE DRUG REACTIONS
Adverse reactions to scabicides and pediculicides include eczema; irritation of the eyes, ears, throat, and nose; numbness at the application site; and rash, redness, itching, burning, and tingling. (See Patient Teaching: *Scabicides and pediculicides.*)

Contact dermatitis and respiratory allergy symptoms may occur, especially in patients sensitive to ragweed pollen. Sensitivity to pyrethrins or any other component of the product may cause a hypersensitivity reaction. Misuse of scabicides can cause CNS stimulation, producing effects that range from dizziness to convulsions.

NURSING PROCESS APPLICATION

The following information assists the nurse in caring for a patient who is receiving a scabicide or pediculicide. It includes an overview of assessment activities as well as examples of appropriate nursing diagnoses and related interventions. It also highlights the importance of evaluation.

Assessment

Before drug therapy begins, review the patient's history for conditions that contraindicate or require cautious use of the prescribed scabicide or pediculicide. Also review the patient's medication history to identify use of drugs that may interact with it. During therapy, assess the patient for adverse drug reactions and signs of drug interactions. Also, periodically assess the effectiveness of therapy with the scabicide or pediculicide. Finally, evaluate the patient's and family's knowledge about the prescribed drug.

Nursing diagnoses

- Risk for injury related to a preexisting condition that contraindicates or requires cautious use of a scabicide or pediculicide
- Risk for injury related to adverse drug reactions
- Body image disturbance related to skin disorder
- Knowledge deficit related to the prescribed scabicide or pediculicide

Planning and implementation

- Do not administer a scabicide or pediculicide to a patient with any condition that contraindicates its use.
- Administer a scabicide or pediculicide cautiously to a patient at risk because of a preexisting condition.
- Monitor the patient for adverse reactions during scabicide or pediculicide therapy.

∗ *Monitor closely for hypersensitivity reactions.*

- Notify the physician if hypersensitivity or other adverse reactions occur.
- Provide emotional support for the patient whose body image is affected by a skin disorder.
- Bathe the patient with soap and water, rinse well, and dry thoroughly before applying the medication.
- Prepare the agent for application by shaking it well.
- Do not apply the agent to inflamed skin, raw or weeping areas, or near the eyes or mouth.
- Follow standard precautions because scabies and pediculosis are extremely contagious.

Evaluation

For each nursing diagnosis, prepare an evaluation statement that describes the patient's or family's response to nursing interventions.

Topical minoxidil

As a topical agent, minoxidil is used to treat hair loss.

PHARMACOKINETICS

Systemic absorption of topical minoxidil is possible. After topical application ceases, 95% of the systemically absorbed drug is eliminated within 4 days. Therapeutic effects occur in approximately 4 months.

PHARMACODYNAMICS

Topical minoxidil stimulates hair growth at the top (or crown) of the head by causing vasodilation, which increases cutaneous blood flow. The drug's exact mechanism of action is not known.

PHARMACOTHERAPEUTICS

Topical minoxidil is used to treat male and female pattern hair loss. It is available as a 2% solution.

Drug interactions

Use of topical minoxidil with other topical agents may increase systemic drug absorption.

ADVERSE DRUG REACTIONS

Adverse reactions to topical minoxidil include tachycardia, fluid retention, and weight gain. The risk of adverse reactions increases if topical minoxidil is used on nonintact scalp (because of increased systemic absorption), if misused, or if the patient is hypersensitive to the drug. Adverse reactions may be especially serious in a patient with heart disease. (See Patient Teaching: *Topical minoxidil.*)

NURSING PROCESS APPLICATION

The following information assists the nurse in caring for a patient receiving topical minoxidil. It includes an overview of assessment activities as well as examples of appropriate nursing diagnoses and related interventions. It also highlights the importance of evaluation.

Assessment

Before drug therapy begins, review the patient's history for conditions that contraindicate or require cautious use of topical minoxidil. During therapy, assess the patient for adverse drug reactions. Also, periodically assess the effectiveness of therapy with topical minoxidil. Finally, evaluate the patient's and family's knowledge about the prescribed drug.

Nursing diagnoses

- Risk for injury related to a preexisting condition that contraindicates or requires cautious use of topical minoxidil

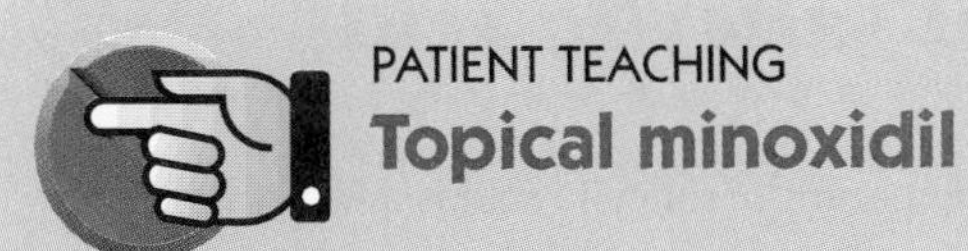

PATIENT TEACHING
Topical minoxidil

- Teach the patient and family the dose, frequency, action, and adverse effects of topical minoxidil.
- Inform the patient that hair growth usually takes 4 months or longer.
- Warn the patient that more frequent or larger doses will not speed hair growth and may increase the risk of adverse reactions.
- Advise the patient to avoid contact with topical minoxidil in the eyes, mucous membranes, or sensitive skin areas; contact can cause burning and irritation.
- Instruct the patient to notify the physician if adverse reactions occur.
- Advise the patient to use topical minoxidil only on the scalp and not to use it if the scalp becomes irritated or sunburned.

- Risk for injury related to adverse drug reactions
- Body image disturbance related to hair loss
- Knowledge deficit related to topical minoxidil

Planning and implementation

- Do not administer topical minoxidil to a patient with a condition that contraindicates its use.
- Administer topical minoxidil cautiously to a patient at risk because of a preexisting condition.
- Monitor the patient for adverse reactions during topical minoxidil therapy.
- Monitor the patient at least 1 month after starting therapy and at least once every 6 months thereafter.
- Notify the physician if adverse reactions occur.
- Provide emotional support to the patient concerned about hair loss.
- Ensure that the hair and scalp are dry before application.
- Apply topical minoxidil only to the scalp — and no other body part — using your fingertips.
- Wash your hands after applying the drug.

*** *Do not use topical minoxidil with any other medication on scalp.***

Evaluation

For each nursing diagnosis, prepare an evaluation statement that describes the patient's or family's response to nursing interventions.

Topical fluorouracil

The topical antineoplastic agent fluorouracil is used to treat certain types of skin cancer.

PHARMACOKINETICS

For each 100-mg dose of topical fluorouracil, about 5 to 6 mg are absorbed systemically. Negligible amounts of the drug have been found in plasma, urine, and expired carbon dioxide after 3 days of topical treatment. Complete healing occurs within 1 to 2 months.

PHARMACODYNAMICS

Fluorouracil inhibits thymidylate synthetase, which inhibits DNA synthesis. This halts the development and proliferation of malignant cells and leads to inflammation and disintegration of malignant tissue.

PHARMACOTHERAPEUTICS

Topical fluorouracil is used to treat multiple actinic (solar) keratoses and superficial basal cell carcinoma. It also is undergoing clinical trials for treating condylomata acuminata (genital warts).

Drug interactions

Topical fluorouracil produces no significant drug interactions.

ADVERSE DRUG REACTIONS

Local reactions to topical fluorouracil include several days of erythema, followed by severe inflammation, burning, stinging, and vesicle formation. Then the patient may experience skin erosion, ulceration, necrosis, pain, crusting, and reepithelialization. After therapy ends, the patient may have some residual redness and temporary hyperpigmentation.

Other adverse reactions include insomnia, irritability, dermatitis, nail changes, alopecia, weakness, malaise, photosensitivity, and toxic granulation (See Patient Teaching: *Topical fluorouracil*, page 740.)

NURSING PROCESS APPLICATION

The following information assists the nurse in caring for a patient receiving topical fluorouracil. It includes an overview of assessment activities as well as examples of appropriate nursing diagnoses and related interventions. It also highlights the importance of evaluation.

Assessment

Before drug therapy begins, review the patient's history for conditions that contraindicate or require cautious use of topical fluorouracil. During therapy, assess the patient for adverse drug reactions. Also, periodically assess the effectiveness of therapy with topical fluorouracil. Finally, evaluate the patient's and family's knowledge about the prescribed drug.

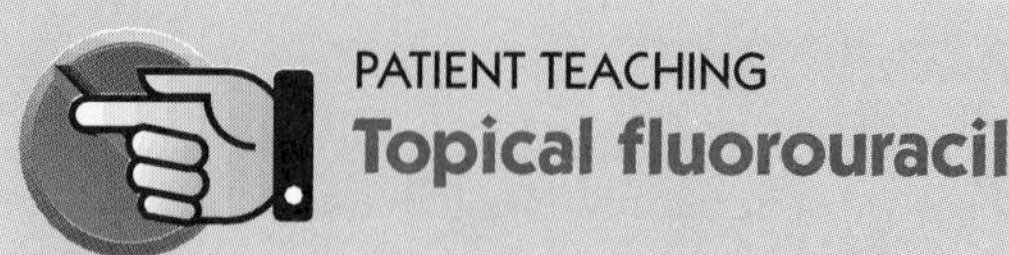

PATIENT TEACHING
Topical fluorouracil

- Teach the patient and family the dose, frequency, action, and adverse effects of topical fluorouracil.
- Instruct the patient to avoid prolonged exposure to sunlight, ultraviolet rays, or irradiation while using this drug.
- Advise the patient to wear gloves or apply the drug with a nonmetal applicator.
- Instruct the patient to apply the drug carefully around the eyes, nose, or mouth.
- Caution the patient that the treated area may appear unsightly during therapy, and possibly for several weeks after therapy ends.
- Advise the female patient not to use this drug if she is pregnant or breast-feeding.
- Inform the patient that complete healing may take 1 to 2 months.
- Instruct the patient to notify the physician if adverse reactions occur.

Nursing diagnoses

- Risk for injury related to a preexisting condition that contraindicates or requires cautious use of topical fluorouracil
- Risk for injury related to adverse drug reactions
- Knowledge deficit related to topical fluorouracil

Planning and implementation

- Do not administer topical fluorouracil to a patient with a condition that contraindicates its use.
- Administer topical fluorouracil cautiously to a patient at risk because of a preexisting condition.
- Monitor the patient for adverse reactions during topical fluorouracil therapy.

**** Prevent exposure to strong sunlight and other sources of ultraviolet light because they can intensify dermatologic reactions to the drug.***

- Notify the physician if systemic adverse effects occur.
- Apply the drug with gloved fingertips or a nonmetallic applicator, avoiding the surrounding normal skin.
- Wash your hands before and immediately after application.
- Teach the patient about the prescribed drug.

Evaluation

For each nursing diagnosis, prepare an evaluation statement that describes the patient's or family's response to nursing interventions.

Topical salicylic acid

As a topical preparation, salicylic acid is a keratolytic agent.

PHARMACOKINETICS

Topical salicylic acid is absorbed in the serum, and excreted in the urine as metabolites. The serum level peaks in 5 hours.

PHARMACODYNAMICS

When applied topically, salicylic acid produces desquamation of the skin's horny layer by dissolving an intercellular cement substance; it does not affect the epidermal structures. The drug's keratolytic action causes the cornified epithelium to swell by increasing water binding; this hydrates the keratin, causing it to soften, mature, and then desquamate.

PHARMACOTHERAPEUTICS

Salicylic acid is used topically to safely remove corns, calluses, and warts. It may also be used alone or in combination to treat dandruff, seborrheic dermatitis, acne, tinea infections, and psoriasis.

Drug interactions

When used together, salicylic acid and sulfur may produce synergistic keratolytic effects.

ADVERSE DRUG REACTIONS

Topical salicylic acid may cause contact dermatitis. With prolonged use over large areas, it may cause salicylate toxicity, which produces such effects as dizziness, tinnitus, nausea, vomiting, diarrhea, confusion, headache, sweating, and hyperventilation.

NURSING PROCESS APPLICATION

The following information assists the nurse in caring for a patient receiving salicylic acid. It includes an overview of assessment activities as well as examples of appropriate nursing diagnoses and related interventions. It also highlights the importance of evaluation.

Assessment

Before drug therapy begins, review the patient's history for conditions that contraindicate or require cautious use of salicylic acid. Also review the patient's medication history to identify use of drugs that may interact with it. During therapy, assess the patient for adverse drug reactions and signs of drug interactions. Also, periodically assess the effective-

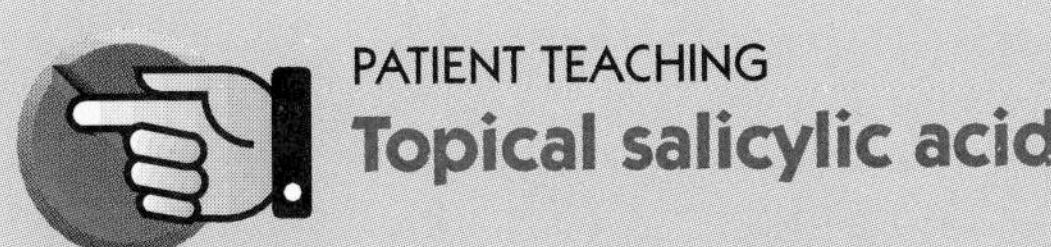

PATIENT TEACHING
Topical salicylic acid

- Teach the patient and family the dose, frequency, action, and adverse effects of salicylic acid.
- Instruct the patient to avoid contact of the drug with the eyes, face, genitals, mucous membranes, and unaffected areas.
- Inform the patient that salicylic acid may cause skin reddening or scaling when used on open skin lesions.
- Warn the patient that overuse or prolonged use of this drug increases the risk of systemic absorption — and salicylate toxicity.
- Instruct the patient not to use salicylic acid on warts with hair growth, moles, or birthmarks; doing so can severely irritate the affected area.
- Teach the patient to avoid exposure to strong sunlight or other ultraviolet light because such exposure can intensify adverse dermatologic reactions.
- Advise the patient to notify the physician if adverse reactions occur.

ness of salicylic acid therapy. Finally, evaluate the patient's and family's knowledge about the prescribed drug. (See Patient Teaching: *Topical salicylic acid.*)

Nursing diagnoses

- Risk for injury related to a preexisting condition that contraindicates or requires cautious use of salicylic acid
- Risk for injury related to adverse drug reactions or drug interactions
- Knowledge deficit related to salicylic acid

Planning and implementation

- Do not administer salicylic acid to a patient with a condition that contraindicates its use.
- Administer salicylic acid cautiously to a patient at risk because of a preexisting condition.
- Monitor the patient for adverse reactions and drug interactions during salicylic acid therapy.

* ***Be alert for signs of salicylate toxicity, which may occur with prolonged use of salicylic acid over large areas.***

- Notify the physician if adverse reactions or drug interactions occur.
- Apply salicylic acid more frequently to areas that cannot be occluded.
- Teach the patient about salicylic acid.

Evaluation

For each nursing diagnosis, prepare an evaluation statement that describes the patient's or family's response to nursing interventions.

CHAPTER SUMMARY

Chapter 60 discussed dermatologic agents used to treat infections caused by bacteria, fungi, and viruses; inflammatory skin conditions; acne; parasite infestations; and other skin disorders. Here are the chapter highlights.

Dermatologic anti-infective agents are used to treat primary and secondary skin infections caused by various bacteria, fungi, and the herpes virus.

Dermatologic anti-inflammatory agents reduce local inflammation in pruritic skin disorders caused by various conditions.

Drugs from several classes are used to treat oily skin, mild acne, and acne vulgaris.

Scabicides and pediculicides are used in treating the parasitic infestations scabies and pediculosis.

As a topical agent, minoxidil may be used to treat hair loss in men and women.

Topical fluorouracil is used to treat certain types of skin cancer.

The keratolytic agent salicylic acid is used to remove corns, calluses, and warts and to manage other dermatologic conditions.

Questions to consider

See Appendix 1 for answers.

1. Theresa White, age 79, sustained a third-degree burn on her forearm during a kitchen accident. Her physician prescribes mafenide acetate to prevent infection of the burn. Which of the following dermatologic agents may be used for this purpose?
   (a) silver sulfadiazine
   (b) amphotericin B
   (c) acyclovir
   (d) lindane

2. To treat her eczema, Kelly Wilson, age 32, has received a prescription for halobetasol propionate. To which of the following classes does this drug belong?
   (a) Scabicides
   (b) Keratolytics
   (c) Anti-infective agents
   (d) Anti-inflammatory agents

(continued)

3. Daniel Wheeler, age 6, has pediculosis (head lice). His mother purchases permethrin liquid and administers it according to the instructions on the package. What else should Daniel's mother do to treat this condition?
(a) Take no other actions.
(b) Administer 1 tsp of the drug orally.
(c) Apply a second dose with another pediculicide.
(d) Dry clean contaminated clothing and bed linens or wash them in hot water.

4. Patrick Cogan, age 36, uses topical minoxidil for male-pattern hair loss. Which of the following adverse reactions is he *most* likely to develop?
(a) Abdominal pain
(b) Hypertension
(c) Tachycardia
(d) Bradycardia

5. The physician prescribes topical fluorouracil for Robert Johnson, age 53, to treat a superficial basal cell carcinoma on his ear. What should the nurse teach him about self-administering this drug?
(a) Scrub the affected area before administering the drug.
(b) Apply the drug to the affected area and surrounding skin.
(c) Use ungloved hands to apply the drug; then wash the hands thoroughly.
(d) Use gloved fingertips or a nonmetallic applicator to apply the drug.

61 Uncategorized and other agents

OBJECTIVES

After reading and studying this chapter, the student should be able to:

1. identify drugs that are used as miscellaneous respiratory, gastrointestinal (GI), endocrine, metabolic, and hematologic agents.
2. identify the anti-infective agents used to treat Hansen's disease.
3. explain how gallium nitrate, pamidronate, and sodium polystyrene sulfonate modify electrolyte balance.
4. discuss the clinical indications for the immune-system modulating agents interferon gamma-1b and levamisole hydrochloride.
5. discuss the therapeutic uses of botulinum toxin type A, ethanolamine oleate, levocarnitine, mesna, nimodipine, octreotide acetate, and ursodiol.
6. describe the nursing implications of the uncategorized and other agents.

INTRODUCTION

For discussion purposes, the uncategorized and other agents in chapter 61 have been grouped into 10 categories:

Miscellaneous respiratory agents
- alpha$_1$-proteinase inhibitor
- beractant
- colfosceril palmitate

Miscellaneous GI agents
- lactulose
- mesalamine
- olsalazine sodium
- sulfasalazine

Miscellaneous endocrine agents
- clomiphene citrate
- histrelin acetate
- human chorionic gonadotropin
- menotropins
- nafarelin acetate

Miscellaneous anti-infective agents
- clofazimine
- dapsone

Miscellaneous metabolic agents
- pegademase bovine
- sodium benzoate 10% and sodium phenylacetate 10%
- tiopronin

Electrolyte modifying agents
- gallium nitrate
- pamidronate
- sodium polysstyrene sulfonate

Miscellaneous hematologic agents
- filgrastim
- pentoxifylline
- sargramostim

Miscellaneous immune-system modulating agents
- interferon gamma-1b
- levamisole hydrochloride

Miscellaneous drugs
- botulinum toxin type A
- ethanolamine oleateA
- levocarnitine
- mesna
- nimodipine
- octreotide acetat
- ursodiol.

For each drug, chapter 61 discusses its pharmacologic properties (including its pharmacokinetics, pharmacodynamics, pharmacotherapeutics, drug interactions, and adverse drug reactions, if known) as well as related nursing implications.

Miscellaneous respiratory agents

These respiratory agents include alpha$_1$-proteinase inhibitor, beractant, and colfosceril palmitate.

ALPHA$_1$-PROTEINASE INHIBITOR

An orphan drug, purified human alpha$_1$-proteinase inhibitor is classified as an enzyme inhibitor.

Pharmacology

Information on the pharmacokinetics of alpha$_1$-proteinase inhibitor is unavailable. This proteinase inhibitor inactivates several proteases, including trypsin, chymotrypsin, plasmin, thrombin, and neutrophil elastase. Without such inactivation, a person with congenital alpha$_1$-antitrypsin deficiency develops emphysema resulting from chronic degradation of elastin tissue.

This drug is used for long-term replacement therapy in patients with congenital deficiency of alpha$_1$-antitrypsin and clinically demonstrable chronic degradation of elastin tissue (panacinar emphysema). The usual adult dosage is 60 mg/kg intravenously (I.V.) once weekly.

No known drug interactions exist. $Alpha_1$-proteinase inhibitor may cause delayed fever, light-headedness, dizziness, and mild leukocytosis.

Nursing implications

When caring for a patient receiving $alpha_1$-proteinase inhibitor, the nurse should be aware of the following implications.

• Do not administer $alpha_1$-proteinase inhibitor to a patient with an immunoglobulin A (IgA) deficiency who has antibodies against IgA (anti-IgA antibodies) because severe reactions, including anaphylaxis, may occur.

• Administer this drug cautiously to a pregnant or breast-feeding patient or one who is at risk for circulatory overload. Be aware that the safety and efficacy of $alpha_1$-proteinase inhibitor in children have not been established.

* ***Recommend immunization against hepatitis B before the patient begins $alpha_1$-proteinase inhibitor therapy. This drug is made from human plasma and may contain the hepatitis virus.***

• Reconstitute the drug with sterile water. Do not mix it with other agents or diluting solutions. Administer I.V. only within 3 hours.

BERACTANT

Beractant is a respiratory **surfactant** produced from bovine lung extract.

Pharmacology

The pharmacokinetics of beractant are unknown. The drug lowers surface tension on alveolar surfaces during respiration and stabilizes the alveoli against collapse at resting transpulmonary pressures. In premature infants, respiratory distress syndrome (RDS) results from a deficiency of pulmonary surfactant. This drug replenishes surfactant and allows normal lung activity in these infants.

Beractant is used to prevent and treat neonatal RDS. The recommended dosage is 100 mg/kg of birth weight (4 ml/kg) given endotracheally every 6 hours, up to a maximum of four doses in the first 48 hours after birth.

No drugs are known to interact with beractant. During clinical trials, adverse reactions to beractant have included transient bradycardia, oxygen desaturation, endotracheal tube reflux or blockage, pallor, vasoconstriction, hypotension or hypertension, hypocapnia or hypercapnia, and apnea.

Nursing implications

When caring for a patient receiving beractant, the nurse should be aware of the following implications.

• Avoid the use of beractant in neonates who weigh less than 600 g (1 lb, 5 oz) or more than 1,750 g (5 lb, 11 oz) at birth. Although no known contraindications or precautions are associated with beractant, use in these patients has not been evaluated in controlled trials.

• Monitor the neonate's pulmonary status frequently after beractant administration. Crackles and moist breath sounds can occur transiently after administration. However, endotracheal suctioning and similar actions are not necessary unless signs of airway obstruction are present.

• Monitor the neonate's electrocardiogram (ECG) and arterial or transcutaneous oxygen saturation results continuously.

* ***Withhold the drug and notify the physician if transient bradycardia or decreased oxygen saturation occurs during therapy.***

• Expect trained medical personnel to administer this drug directly into the trachea.

• Inspect beractant solution for discoloration before administration. Normally, the solution appears off-white to light brown. If settling occurs during storage, swirl the vial gently but do not shake it to disperse its contents. Surface foaming may occur during handling, but is considered harmless.

COLFOSCERIL PALMITATE

Colfosceril palmitate is an artificial respiratory surfactant.

Pharmacology

Absorbed from the alveoli into lung tissue after endotracheal administration, colfosceril is metabolized extensively. Its by-products are incorporated into alveolar phospholipid synthesis and secretion.

As an artificial surfactant, colfosceril reduces the surface tension of alveolar tissue. By replacing insufficient respiratory surfactant, it may reduce the risk and severity of RDS.

Colfosceril is indicated for the prophylaxis and rescue treatment of neonatal RDS. The usual dosage is 5 ml/kg administered through the side port of an endotracheal tube adaptor; each dose is divided in half and given over 1 to 2 minutes with the neonate in the midline position. After the first half-dose is administered, the neonate is held for 30 seconds at a 45-degree angle to the right; after the second half-dose, at a 45-degree angle to the left. For prophylaxis against RDS, the drug is administered as soon as possible after delivery, with the second and third doses given at 12 and 24 hours if the neonate remains on mechanical ventilation. For rescue treatment, the first dose is administered as soon as RDS is identified; the second dose, at 12 hours if the neonate remains on mechanical ventilation. Colfosceril has no known contraindications or precautions.

No known drug interactions exist. During clinical trials, neonates who received colfosceril had a higher incidence of pulmonary hemorrhage and apnea than those who received a placebo.

Nursing implications

When caring for a patient receiving colfosceril, the nurse should be aware of the following implications.

• Expect trained medical personnel to administer this drug directly into the trachea.

• Obtain an accurate birth weight to calculate the dosage.
• Reconstitute colfosceril with the accompanying diluent just before administration.
*** *Suction the neonate before drug administration to decrease the risk of mucus plug formation in the endotracheal tube. Do not suction for 2 hours after administration unless physiologically necessary.***
• Monitor the neonate's pulmonary function frequently during colfosceril administration because the drug can affect oxygenation and lung compliance.
*** *Observe for signs of pulmonary hemorrhage, such as bloody sputum or secretions.***
• Monitor the neonate's ECG and transcutaneous oxygen saturation results continuously during drug administration.

Miscellaneous gastrointestinal agents

The miscellaneous GI agents include lactulose, mesalamine, olsalazine sodium, and sulfasalazine.

LACTULOSE

Lactulose is an ammonium-detoxicating agent used primarily to treat systemic portal encephalopathy.

Pharmacology

After oral administration, lactulose is absorbed slightly from the GI tract. It is distributed only in the intestine, metabolized by the intestinal microflora into lactate and other organic acids, and excreted in the feces.

Lactulose decreases the blood ammonia concentration and reduces the degree of systemic portal encephalopathy. Lactulose is metabolized by intestinal **bacteria** to lactic, acetic, and formic acids, thereby acidifying the colon contents. As the colon contents become more acidic, ammonia diffuses from the blood into the colon. There, the ammonia becomes trapped in the stool as ammonium ions. Then, the laxative action of lactulose expels the trapped ammonium ions from the colon.

Lactulose is used primarily to reduce ammonia levels in patients with systemic portal encephalopathy. It may also be used to manage chronic constipation. For systemic portal encephalopathy, the usual adult dosage is 20 to 30 g (30 to 45 ml) orally three or four times daily, until two or three soft stools are produced daily; or 200 g (300 ml) diluted in 700 ml of water or normal saline solution, given via rectal balloon catheter and retained 30 to 60 minutes, every 4 to 6 hours. For constipation, the usual adult dosage is 10 to 20 g (15 to 30 ml) by mouth daily.

No drugs produce significant interactions when administered concomitantly with lactulose. Common adverse reactions to lactulose include abdominal distention, flatulence, and abdominal cramps. Other adverse reactions include nausea, vomiting, diarrhea, hypokalemia, hypovolemia, increased blood glucose level in patients with impaired glucose tolerance, and increased systemic portal encephalopathy in patients with severe hepatic dysfunction.

Nursing implications

When caring for a patient receiving lactulose, the nurse should be aware of the following implications.
• Do not administer lactulose to a patient who requires a low-galactose diet.
• Administer lactulose cautiously to a pregnant or breast-feeding patient or one with diabetes mellitus. Be aware that the safety and efficacy of lactulose in children have not been established.
• Monitor the blood glucose level once every shift or as prescribed for a patient with impaired glucose tolerance. Also, observe for signs of hyperglycemia, such as polyuria, polydipsia, polyphagia, and weakness.
• Teach the patient with impaired glucose tolerance to be alert for signs of hyperglycemia and to monitor blood glucose levels regularly during lactulose therapy.
• Dilute lactulose with water, milk, or unsweetened juice before administration to reduce the sweetness and prevent nausea.
• Store lactulose below 86° F (30° C), but do not allow the drug to freeze.
• Teach the patient how to prepare and store lactulose properly.

MESALAMINE

Mesalamine is an anti-inflammatory agent used to treat inflammatory disorders that affect the GI tract.

Pharmacology

Administered as a rectal enema, mesalamine is absorbed poorly through the bowel wall. Unabsorbed mesalamine is excreted primarily in the feces. Absorbed mesalamine is metabolized at an unknown site and excreted in the urine. The plasma half-life of mesalamine ranges from 0.5 to 1.5 hours.

Although the exact mechanism of action is unknown, mesalamine may act locally to decrease inflammation by blocking cyclooxygenase and inhibiting prostaglandin in the colon.

As a suspension enema, mesalamine is prescribed to treat mild to moderate distal ulcerative colitis, proctosigmoiditis, or proctitis. The usual adult dosage is 60 ml (4 g) given rectally once a day (preferably at bedtime) and retained for about 8 hours.

Concomitant administration with sulfasalazine and other oral products that also release mesalamine may result in renal dysfunction. Mesalamine primarily causes adverse GI reactions, such as abdominal pain, cramps, and discomfort; flatulence; nausea; diarrhea or constipation; and hemorrhoids. Other adverse reactions include leg and joint pain, headache, dizziness, insomnia, weakness, malaise, fatigue, fever, rash, sore throat, flulike symptoms, back pain, hair loss, peripheral edema, urinary tract **infection,** and burning sensation upon urination.

Nursing implications

When caring for a patient receiving mesalamine, the nurse should be aware of the following implications.

- Do not administer mesalamine to a patient with known hypersensitivity to mesalamine, any of its components, or sulfites.
- Administer mesalamine cautiously to a pregnant patient, one with renal disease, or one receiving an oral product that liberates mesalamine, such as sulfasalazine. Be aware that the safety and efficacy of mesalamine in children have not been established.
- Monitor urinalysis results and blood urea nitrogen (BUN) and serum creatinine levels during mesalamine therapy for a patient with renal dysfunction.
- Discontinue mesalamine and notify the physician if rash or fever develops.

OLSALAZINE SODIUM

Olsalazine sodium is a salicylate derivative used to treat ulcerative colitis.

Pharmacology

After oral administration, olsalazine exhibits minimal absorption. However, the drug is more than 99% bound to plasma proteins. About 0.1% of an oral dose is metabolized in the liver to olsalazine-0-sulfate, which has a half-life of 7 days. The drug is excreted primarily in the feces.

The mechanism of action of olsalazine is unknown, but appears to be topical rather than systemic. Converted to 5-amino salicylic acid, olsalazine may reduce colonic inflammation by blocking cyclooxygenase and inhibiting prostaglandin production in the bowel mucosa.

For patients who cannot tolerate sulfasalazine, olsalazine is used to maintain remission of ulcerative colitis. The usual adult dosage is 1 g by mouth daily in two divided doses with food.

No known drug interactions exist. The most common adverse reaction to olsalazine is diarrhea. Other common adverse reactions include abdominal pain and cramps, headache, and arthralgia. Less common reactions include fatigue, drowsiness, lethargy, depression, vertigo, nausea, dyspepsia, bloating, anorexia, vomiting, stomatitis, rash, and pruritus.

Nursing implications

When caring for a patient receiving olsalazine, the nurse should be aware of the following implications.

- Do not administer olsalazine to a patient with known hypersensitivity to salicylates.
- Administer olsalazine cautiously to a pregnant or breast-feeding patient or one with renal dysfunction. Be aware that the safety and efficacy of olsalazine in children have not been established.
- Monitor urinalysis results and BUN and creatinine levels regularly during olsalazine therapy — especially in a patient with renal dysfunction — because olsalazine may damage the renal tubules. (However, this effect has not been reported in clinical trials.)
- Inform the patient that diarrhea is the most common adverse reaction to olsalazine; instruct the patient to notify the physician if diarrhea occurs.
- Teach the patient to take this drug in evenly divided doses with food.
- The incidence of inflammatory GI disorders is higher in Whites than in Blacks and Asians. The incidence is significantly increased (four to five times the normal rate) among Ashkenazi Jews. If your patient is from one of these susceptible groups, be sure to investigate any patient or family history of inflammatory GI disorders as part of your initial assessment.

SULFASALAZINE

Sulfasalazine is a sulfonamide used to treat ulcerative colitis.

Pharmacology

Sulfasalazine is absorbed poorly from the GI tract after oral administration. Intestinal flora metabolize the drug to its active ingredients, which exert their effects locally. Sulfasalazine is excreted primarily in the urine. Its plasma half-life is approximately 6 to 8 hours.

The exact mechanism of action of sulfasalazine in ulcerative colitis is unknown.

Sulfasalazine is used to treat mild to moderate ulcerative colitis and, as adjunct therapy, to treat severe ulcerative colitis. For adults, the usual initial dosage is 3 to 4 g by mouth daily in evenly divided doses; the usual maintenance dosage, 1.5 to 2 g by mouth daily in divided doses every 6 hours. To minimize adverse reactions, the dosage may start at 1 to 2 g and be increased gradually. For children over age 2, the usual initial dosage is 40 to 60 mg/kg by mouth daily in three to six divided doses, then 30 mg/kg daily in four doses. If GI intolerance occurs, a lower dosage may be used initially.

Sulfasalazine may inhibit hepatic metabolism of oral anticoagulants, enhancing anticoagulant effects. Concomitant use with oral hypoglycemic agents enhances hypoglycemic effects. Sulfasalazine may reduce GI absorption of digoxin and folic acid. Concomitant use of urinary acidifiers, such as ammonium chloride and ascorbic acid, decreases urine **pH** and sulfonamide solubility, thereby increasing the risk of crystalluria. Concomitant use with antibiotics that alter intestinal flora may decrease the drug's effectiveness. Concomitant antacid use may cause premature dissolution of enteric-coated tablets, enhancing their systemic absorption and increasing the risk of toxicity.

Adverse central nervous system (CNS) reactions to sulfasalazine include headache, depression, seizures, hallucinations, and tinnitus. In the GI system, adverse reactions include nausea, vomiting, diarrhea, abdominal pain, anorexia, and stomatitis. Adverse genitourinary reactions include general toxic nephrosis with oliguria and anuria, crystalluria, hematuria, oligospermia, and infertility. Hematologic reactions include aplastic anemia, megaloblastic anemia, thrombocytopenia, leukopenia, and hemolytic anemia. Other adverse reactions include jaundice, hypersensitivity, serum sickness, drug fever, anaphylaxis, and bacterial and fungal superinfections. The drug may also cause skin and urine discoloration.

Nursing implications

When caring for a patient receiving sulfasalazine, the nurse should be aware of the following implications.

- Do not administer sulfasalazine to a pregnant patient who is at term; a breast-feeding patient; one with known hypersensitivity to salicylates, sulfonamides, or other sulfa-containing drug (such as thiazides, furosemide, or oral sulfonylureas); or one with porphyria or severe renal or hepatic dysfunction.
- Administer sulfasalazine cautiously to a patient with mild to moderate renal or hepatic impairment, severe allergies, asthma, blood dyscrasias, or glucose-6-phosphate dehydrogenase (G6PD) deficiency.
- Monitor the patient for adverse drug reactions and signs of drug interactions.
- Space the doses evenly and administer the drug after meals to minimize adverse reactions and aid drug absorption.
- Do not administer antacids concomitantly with enteric-coated sulfasalazine tablets because antacids may alter drug absorption.
- Teach the patient to take this drug after meals and to avoid taking antacids concomitantly.
- Inform the patient that sulfasalazine normally discolors the urine orange-yellow and may discolor the skin orange-yellow.

Miscellaneous endocrine agents

Miscellaneous endocrine agents include the antiestrogenic agent clomiphene citrate; the infertility agents human chorionic gonadotropin (hCG) and menotropins; and the gonadotropin-releasing hormone (GnRH) agonists histrelin acetate and nafarelin acetate.

CLOMIPHENE CITRATE

Clomiphene citrate is an antiestrogen agent used to stimulate ovulation in females.

Pharmacology

After oral administration, clomiphene is absorbed readily from the GI tract. Its distribution is not clear. The drug may undergo enterohepatic recirculation or may be stored in body fat. Clomiphene is metabolized in the liver and excreted primarily in the feces via bile elimination. Its half-life is 5 days; however, the drug can be found in the feces up to 6 weeks after administration.

Clomiphene occupies estrogen receptor sites in the hypothalamus, preventing estrogen from binding to these sites. In turn, the hypothalamus stimulates the pituitary gland to release greater amounts of follicle-stimulating hormone (FSH) and luteinizing hormone (LH); these hormones then initiate and enhance the growth of ovarian follicles in females.

Clomiphene is prescribed to treat anovulation and oligo-ovulation and to regulate ovulatory cycles that are shorter than 23 days or longer than 37 days. The usual adult dosage is 50 mg orally daily from day 5 to day 9 of the cycle. If the patient has not had recent uterine bleeding, the drug can be started at any time after a negative pregnancy test. If ovulation does not occur, the dosage may be increased by 50-mg increments each cycle until ovulation occurs or a daily dosage of 200 mg is reached.

No significant drug interactions are associated with clomiphene. Adverse reactions to clomiphene include insomnia, hypertension, blurred vision, nausea, vomiting, bloating, photophobia, urinary frequency, polyuria, and ovarian enlargement and cyst formation (both of which regress spontaneously when the drug is discontinued). Occasionally, hyperglycemia occurs. Other adverse reactions include hot flashes, reversible alopecia, breast discomfort, and multiple fetuses. Hypersensitivity reactions to clomiphene include urticaria, rash, and dermatitis.

Nursing implications

When caring for a patient receiving clomiphene, the nurse should be aware of the following implications.

- Do not administer clomiphene to a pregnant patient or one with liver disease, abnormal uterine bleeding, or cancer of the breast or reproductive organs.
- Administer clomiphene cautiously to a patient with polycystic ovary syndrome.
- Teach the patient how to calculate the length of her menstrual cycle, using the first day of menstrual blood flow as the first day of the cycle. Also teach the patient how and when to take her basal body temperature to identify the period of maximum fertility (usually 10 to 12 days after taking the last clomiphene tablet.)
- Inform the patient that maximum fertility usually occurs 10 to 12 days after taking the last clomiphene tablet.
- Encourage the patient to have sexual intercourse every 36 to 40 hours during the maximum fertility period.
- Stress the importance of obtaining a pregnancy test if menstruation does not occur 16 days after the patient takes the last clomiphene tablet.

• Instruct the patient to stop taking clomiphene and call the physician immediately if abdominal pain occurs. This may indicate ovarian enlargement or ovarian cyst.
• Understand that among most Mexican-Americans, the family is the strongest traditional value, and fertility is seen as a crucial sign of a Mexican-American male being a man. Therefore, when caring for an infertile Mexican-American couple, the nurse should address issues related to infertility with great tact and sensitivity.

HISTRELIN ACETATE

Histrelin acetate is a GnRH agonist.

Pharmacology

The pharmacokinetics of histrelin are unknown. When administered daily in therapeutic dosages, histrelin inhibits pituitary gonadotropin secretion. Because of this action, long-term administration of this drug decreases steroid levels and reverses the development of secondary sexual characteristics.

Histrelin is used to control the manifestations of precocious puberty. The recommended dosage is 10 mcg/kg subcutaneously (S.C.) once daily.

No drugs reportedly interact with histrelin. During clinical trials, the drug produced the following adverse reactions in more than 10% of patients: headache; redness, swelling, and itching at the injection site; and vaginal bleeding. In some patients, histrelin caused angioedema.

Nursing implications

When caring for a patient receiving histrelin, the nurse should be aware of the following implications.
• Do not administer histrelin to a pregnant or breast-feeding patient or one with known hypersensitivity to any of the drug's components.
• Be aware that this drug has no specific precautions. Its safety and efficacy in children under age 2 have not been established.
• Instruct the patient and family to discontinue the drug and notify the physician immediately if rash, urticaria, rapid heartbeat, difficulty in swallowing and breathing, or swelling occurs — these may be signs of angioedema.
• Teach the patient or a family member to administer the injection around the same time each day. Also instruct them to rotate the injection sites in the upper arms, thighs, and abdomen.

HUMAN CHORIONIC GONADOTROPIN

Human chorionic gonadotropin, or hCG, is a fertility agent used to treat male and female infertility.

Pharmacology

Because hCG is destroyed by the GI tract, it is administered parenterally. After intramuscular (I.M.) administration, the drug is distributed primarily to the ovaries and testes and excreted by the kidneys. HCG reaches a peak concentration level 5 to 6 hours after administration; its half-life is 12 hours.

In females, hCG mimics the action of LH and allows ovarian follicle rupture. It also stimulates the corpus luteum to produce progesterone, which is needed to sustain the fertilized ovum. In males, hCG stimulates secretion of testosterone (a hormone needed for spermatogenesis) by Leydig's cells in the testes, development of secondary sex characteristics, and possibly testicular descent when no anatomical obstruction is present.

When used to treat hypogonadotropic **hypogonadism** due to pituitary deficiency or prepubertal cryptorchidism not due to anatomical obstruction, hCG may induce testicular descent in patients for whom descent would have occurred at puberty. In some patients, testicular descent is permanent; in most patients, it is temporary. HCG may help predict whether orchiopexy will be needed in the future. Treatment usually begins between ages 4 and 9.

HCG is also used to treat infertility disorders by inducing ovulation in females and stimulating spermatogenesis in males. When used to treat infertility, hCG is used with menotropins. The dosage varies with the indication, the patient's age and weight, and physician preference. The usual adult dosage for males with hypogonadotropic hypogonadism is 500 to 1,000 IU I.M. three times weekly for 3 weeks, or 4,000 IU I.M. three times weekly for 3 months. The usual dosage for boys with prepubertal cryptorchidism is 4,000 IU I.M. three times weekly for 3 weeks, 5,000 IU I.M. every other day for four doses, or 15 doses of 500 to 1,000 IU I.M. over 6 weeks; if this course of therapy is unsuccessful, a subsequent course may begin 1 month later with a dosage of 1,000 IU I.M. three times weekly for 4 to 6 weeks. The usual adult dosage for stimulation of spermatogenesis in males is 5,000 IU I.M. three times weekly until the serum testosterone level is normal. Treatment may require 4 to 6 months. Once the serum testosterone level is normal, menotropins therapy begins and the hCG dosage is reduced to 2,000 IU I.M. twice weekly for at least 4 months. The usual adult dosage for females is 5,000 to 10,000 IU I.M. at the time of ovulation or on the day after discontinuing menotropins.

No significant drug interactions exist. Dose-related adverse reactions associated with hCG include headache, irritability, fatigue, depression, weight gain (from fluid retention), and gynecomastia. HCG may also cause ovarian hyperstimulation and multiple fetuses. Pain may occur at the injection site.

Nursing implications

When caring for a patient receiving hCG, the nurse should be aware of the following implications.
• Do not administer hCG to a patient with precocious puberty, prostatic cancer or other androgen-dependent cancer, or known hypersensitivity.

• Administer hCG cautiously to a patient with asthma, seizure disorder, migraine headache, or cardiac or renal disease.
• Teach the patient about hCG administration and explain when to engage in sexual intercourse relative to administration (usually 24 to 36 hours after injection).

MENOTROPINS

Menotropins is a fertility agent used to treat male and female infertility.

Pharmacology

Because menotropins is destroyed by the GI tract, it is administered I.M. The drug is distributed to the ovaries and testes. Its metabolism is unknown; however, about 8% of the dose is excreted unchanged in the urine. Menotropins has a half-life of several hours.

Menotropins produces the physiologic effects of FSH by stimulating development and maturation of the ovarian follicles. Menotropins also mimics LH, causing ovulation and stimulating development of the corpus luteum in females. In males, menotropins stimulates spermatogenesis.

In females, menotropins is prescribed mainly to initiate ovulation; it is also used to stimulate ovulation for special procedures (such as in vitro fertilization, gamete intrafallopian transfer, or egg donation). In males, menotropins is prescribed for hypogonadotropic hypogonadism. For females, the dosage depends on the indication. The usual initial dosage is one ampule of menotropins (containing 75 IU of FSH and 75 IU of LH) I.M. once daily for 9 to 12 days, followed by 5,000 to 10,000 IU I.M. of menotropins on the day after the last menotropins dose. For males, pretreatment consists of 5,000 IU of hCG three times weekly until the testosterone level is normal; then, one ampule of HMG (containing 75 IU of FSH and 75 IU of LH) I.M. three times weekly with 2,000 IU I.M. of hCG twice weekly for 4 months. If spermatogenesis is not increased after 4 months of therapy, treatment can continue with the same dosage or a dosage increase to 150 IU of FSH and 150 IU of LH I.M. three times weekly; the hCG dosage should not be changed.

Menotropins produces no significant drug interactions. The most common adverse reaction to menotropins is ovarian enlargement, which may be accompanied by lower abdominal pain and distention. Ovarian hyperstimulation syndrome (OHSS), a life-threatening disorder, is much less common — and occurs only when menotropins is administered with hCG. In severe cases, OHSS may involve ovarian enlargement, ascites, and pleural effusion. Electrolyte imbalance, increased capillary permeability, and hypercoagulability sometimes accompany the syndrome. Other adverse reactions to menotropins include hemoperitoneum (from ruptured ovarian cyst) and arterial thromboembolism.

Nursing implications

When caring for a patient receiving menotropins, the nurse should be aware of the following implications.
• Do not administer menotropins to a pregnant patient; a female patient with primary ovarian failure, uncontrolled thyroid and adrenal dysfunction, organic intracranial lesion, abnormal uterine bleeding, ovarian cysts or enlargement not due to polycystic ovary syndrome; or a male patient with normal gonadotropin levels, primary testicular failure, infertility disorder other than hypogonadotropic hypogonadism, or known hypersensitivity.
• Administer menotropins cautiously to a breast-feeding patient or one with polycystic ovary syndrome.
• Advise the patient that menotropins therapy is expensive, requires close monitoring by an infertility specialist, and commonly requires travel to a special facility that offers the treatment. Also explain that hCG injections are needed to initiate ovulation.
• Instruct the patient when and how to administer menotropins and hCG, as prescribed, and teach the patient when to engage in sexual intercourse relative to hCG administration (usually 24 to 36 hours after injection).

NAFARELIN ACETATE

Nafarelin acetate is a GnRH agonist used to treat endometriosis.

Pharmacology

After intranasal administration, nafarelin is absorbed rapidly into the bloodstream and reaches a peak plasma concentration level in 10 to 40 minutes. The drug is approximately 80% plasma protein-bound; its half-life is about 3 hours. After extensive metabolism, the drug is eliminated in the urine and feces.

A GnRH agonist, nafarelin decreases the secretion of gonadal steroids and suppresses their physiologic effects during long-term administration.

Nafarelin is prescribed to reduce endometrial lesions and to relieve pain in the management of endometriosis. The usual adult dosage is 400 mcg daily as one spray (200 mcg) into one nostril in the morning and one spray into the other nostril in the evening, beginning between days 2 and 4 of the menstrual cycle. For persistent regular menstruation after 2 months of treatment, the dosage should be 800 mcg daily as one spray into each nostril in the morning and evening. Therapy should not exceed 6 months.

No significant drug interactions have been reported. However, use of a nasal decongestant may interfere with nafarelin absorption. During clinical trials, nafarelin caused the following adverse reactions in more than 5% of patients: hot flashes, decreased libido, vaginal dryness, headache, emotional lability, acne, myalgia, reduced breast size, edema, seborrhea, weight gain, and nasal irritation. In some patients, nafarelin caused bone density loss.

Nursing implications
When caring for a patient receiving nafarelin, the nurse should be aware of the following implications.

- Do not administer nafarelin to a pregnant or breast-feeding patient, one with known hypersensitivity to GnRH or GnRH-agonist analogues, or one with undiagnosed abnormal vaginal bleeding.
- Administer nafarelin cautiously to a patient with polycystic ovary syndrome. Be aware that safety and efficacy of this drug in children have not been established.
- Inform a patient receiving long-term therapy that nafarelin may cause a slight loss of bone density, some of which may be irreversible. Advise the patient that this increases the risk of fracture.
- Instruct the patient to notify her physician if regular menstruation persists during therapy; the dosage may have to be increased.
- Instruct the patient to consult her physician if she uses a nasal decongestant. To prevent altered drug absorption, teach the patient to use the decongestant at least 2 hours after taking nafarelin.
- Inform the patient that the maximum duration of nafarelin treatment is 6 months.

Miscellaneous anti-infective agents

Miscellaneous anti-infective agents include the antileprotic agents clofazimine and dapsone.

CLOFAZIMINE
Clofazimine is used to treat **Hansen's disease** (leprosy).

Pharmacology
After oral administration, clofazimine is absorbed incompletely, distributed primarily to fatty tissues and the reticuloendothelial system, and excreted primarily unchanged in the urine and feces. The drug reaches a peak plasma concentration level 4 to 12 hours after administration. The half-life after repeated doses is about 70 days.

Clofazimine is a phenazine dye whose mechanism of action against mycobacteria is not understood completely. It appears to bind to mycobacterial deoxyribonucleic acid and inhibit replication and growth. It also has anti-inflammatory and immunosuppressant properties, although the mechanisms of action for these properties remain unknown.

Clofazimine is used to treat lepromatous Hansen's disease, including the type that does not respond to dapsone therapy and the type that is complicated by erythema nodosum leprosum. Combination therapy is recommended for initial treatment of multibacillary Hansen's disease to prevent the development of drug resistance. For lepromatous Hansen's disease, the usual adult dosage is 50 to 100 mg by mouth once daily or 50 mg once daily plus an additional 300-mg dose given once monthly with other antileprotic drugs. For dapsone-resistant Hansen's disease, the usual adult dosage is 50 to 100 mg by mouth once daily given with other antileprotic drugs for 2 years, followed by 50 to 100 mg by mouth once daily for 10 or more years. For erythema nodosum leprosum, the dosage depends on the severity of the symptoms and must be individualized.

No clinically significant drug interactions have been reported with clofazimine. The drug is usually tolerated well. Discoloration, such as changes in skin pigmentation, is the most common adverse reaction to clofazimine and occurs in 75% to 100% of patients. Other adverse reactions include ichthyosis, skin dryness, rash, pruritus, epigastric pain, diarrhea, nausea, and vomiting.

Nursing implications
When caring for a patient receiving clofazimine, the nurse should be aware of the following implications.

- Administer clofazimine cautiously to a pregnant or breast-feeding patient or one with GI problems, such as abdominal pain or diarrhea. Although clofazimine has no known contraindications, be aware that its safety and efficacy in children have not been established.
- Inspect the patient for dermatologic reactions, such as changes in skin pigmentation, ichthyosis, skin dryness, rash, or pruritus, during clofazimine therapy.
- Stress the importance of compliance with clofazimine therapy.
- Instruct the patient to take clofazimine with meals to minimize adverse GI reactions.
- Warn the patient that clofazimine may discolor the skin, conjunctivae, tears, sweat, sputum, urine, and feces. Also explain that this discoloration may take months or years to disappear.

DAPSONE
Like clofazimine, dapsone is an antileprotic agent.

Pharmacology
After oral administration, dapsone is absorbed slowly but completely from the GI tract, distributed throughout the body, metabolized in the liver, and excreted in the urine. Dapsone reaches a peak serum concentration 2 to 8 hours after administration. The drug's half-life averages 20 to 30 hours.

Dapsone is bacteriostatic for *Mycobacterium leprae.* Although its antibacterial action is not understood fully, it may resemble that of the sulfonamides. Like those drugs, dapsone inhibits folic acid synthesis by bacteria.

Dapsone is used to treat all forms of Hansen's disease and dermatitis herpetiformis. To treat Hansen's disease, the usual adult dosage is 50 to 100 mg by mouth once daily; the usual pediatric dosage, 1 to 1.5 mg/kg by mouth daily. To treat dermatitis herpetiformis, the usual adult dosage is 25 to 400 mg by mouth daily.

Probenecid may decrease urinary excretion of dapsone metabolites, thus increasing the drug's serum concentration. Rifampin may increase dapsone metabolism, thus lowering its serum concentration. Concurrent use of folic acid antagonists, such as pyrimethamine, may cause additive adverse hematologic effects.

Hemolytic anemia and methemoglobinemia are the most common dose-related reactions to dapsone. Other adverse reactions include granulocytopenia and a syndrome that resembles infectious mononucleosis. Hypersensitivity reactions rarely occur, but may cause cutaneous reactions, such as exfoliative dermatitis, toxic erythema, erythema multiforme, urticaria, and erythema nodosum.

Nursing implications

When caring for a patient receiving dapsone, the nurse should be aware of the following implications.

- Do not administer dapsone to a breast-feeding patient or one with known hypersensitivity to the drug or any of its derivatives.
- Administer dapsone cautiously to a pregnant patient or one with G6PD deficiency, methemoglobin reductase deficiency, or a condition (or exposure to an agent) that can produce hemolysis, such as diabetic ketosis.
- Monitor the patient who receives 200 to 300 mg of dapsone daily or who has G6PD deficiency for signs and symptoms of hemolytic anemia (pallor, fatigue, dyspnea) or methemoglobinemia (cyanosis).
- Monitor the patient's complete blood count (CBC) weekly during the first 6 months of dapsone therapy and monthly thereafter. Notify the physician if any abnormality occurs.
- Monitor the patient for granulocytopenia and dapsone syndrome, exhibited by fever, sore throat, swollen lymph glands, and easy bruising.
- Stress the importance of compliance with dapsone therapy.
- Instruct the patient to report adverse reactions.

Miscellaneous metabolic agents

Agents used to treat metabolic abnormalities include pegademase bovine, sodium benzoate 10% and sodium phenylacetate 10%, and tiopronin.

PEGADEMASE BOVINE

Pegademase bovine is a modified form of the enzyme adenosine deaminase (ADA) used for replacement therapy in patients with ADA deficiency.

Pharmacology

Little information on the pharmacokinetics of pegademase bovine is known. In 2 to 3 days after I.M. injection, plasma levels of ADA peak. The plasma elimination half-life of ADA varies — even in the same patient — and ranges from 3 days to more than 6 days.

Pegademase bovine specifically replaces the deficient enzyme ADA. When ADA is absent, the purine substrates adenosine and 2'-deoxyadenosine accumulate, causing metabolic abnormalities that are toxic to lymphocytes. Pegademase bovine acts directly to correct these metabolic abnormalities. The interval between correction of metabolic abnormalities and improved immune function varies from a few weeks to 6 months.

As enzyme replacement therapy for ADA deficiency, pegademase bovine is prescribed for patients with severe combined immunodeficiency diseases who are not suitable candidates for bone marrow transplantation or for whom that procedure has failed. It is recommended for use in neonates and children of any age. The usual pediatric dosage is 10 U/kg I.M. as a single dose followed by a second dose of 15 U/kg I.M. after 7 days and a third dose of 20 U/kg I.M. after 7 more days; for maintenance, 20 U/kg I.M. once a week. Further increases of 5 U/kg/week may be necessary. However, the maximum single dose should not exceed 30 U/kg. Preferably, the dosage is tailored according to plasma ADA activity levels.

Clinical experience with pegademase bovine is limited; one patient reported headache and two patients reported pain at the injection site.

Nursing implications

When caring for a patient receiving pegademase bovine, the nurse should be aware of the following implications.

- Do not administer pegademase bovine to a patient with severe thrombocytopenia.
- Administer pegademase bovine cautiously to a pregnant or breast-feeding patient or one with mild to moderate thrombocytopenia. Be aware that the safety and efficacy of pegademase bovine used as preparatory or support therapy for bone marrow transplantation has not been established.
- Do not dilute or mix pegademase bovine with any other drug before administration.
- Continue to provide care that protects an immunologically compromised patient until immune function improves.
- Monitor plasma ADA activity before treatment begins and regularly during treatment.
- Refrigerate but do not freeze this drug. Do not use pegademase bovine if it may have been frozen.

SODIUM BENZOATE 10% AND SODIUM PHENYLACETATE 10%

A combination drug, sodium benzoate 10% and sodium phenylacetate 10% reduces the amount of ammonia in blood.

Pharmacology

Pharmacokinetic data on sodium benzoate and sodium phenylacetate and their metabolites are limited. After oral administration of a single dose, the plasma concentration level peaks within 1 hour. Distribution is unknown. Most of the compound is metabolized by the liver and kidneys. Within 24 hours of administration, 80% to 100% of the compound is excreted via the kidneys.

Sodium benzoate and sodium phenylacetate are metabolically active substances that decrease elevated serum ammonia concentrations in patients with abnormalities related to ureagenesis. Their action results from acylation of amino acids, which decreases ammonia production. Benzoate and phenylacetate first activate enzymatic pathways, then act as a substitute in the defective ureagenetic pathways in patients with urea cycle enzymopathies (UCEs), thereby preventing ammonia accumulation.

Sodium benzoate 10% and sodium phenylacetate 10% is prescribed as adjunct therapy to prevent or treat hyperammonemia in the long-term management of UCE in infants. The usual pediatric dosage is 2.5 ml/kg by mouth daily (250 mg sodium benzoate and 250 mg sodium phenylacetate) in three to six equally divided doses, up to a maximum of 100 ml daily.

Concomitant administration of sodium benzoate and sodium phenylacetate with penicillin should be avoided because both drugs may compete for active secretion by the renal tubules, altering the renal excretion rate. Probenecid inhibits renal transport of many organic compounds and may alter renal elimination of sodium benzoate and sodium phenylacetate.

Reported adverse reactions to sodium benzoate and sodium phenylacetate include nausea and vomiting. Certain adverse reactions associated with salicylate administration (such as exacerbation of peptic ulcers, mild hyperventilation, and mild respiratory alkalosis) may also occur because of similarities between benzoate and salicylates.

Nursing implications

When caring for a patient receiving sodium benzoate and sodium phenylacetate, the nurse should be aware of the following implications.

- Do not administer sodium benzoate 10% and sodium phenylacetate 10% to a patient with known hypersensitivity to either agent.
- Administer this drug cautiously to a patient with heart failure, renal insufficiency, or other condition that may increase the risk of sodium retention and edema. Administer it cautiously to a neonate with hyperbilirubinemia because benzoate may compete with bilirubin for albumin-binding sites.
- Dilute the solution before administering.
- Avoid concomitant administration with penicillin or probenecid.
- Discontinue sodium benzoate and sodium phenylacetate therapy and notify the physician if adverse reactions occur.

TIOPRONIN

A urinary cystine reducing agent, tiopronin is used prophylactically in selected patients.

Pharmacology

After oral administration, tiopronin is absorbed rapidly. Its distribution and metabolism are not fully known. The drug is excreted in the urine.

Tiopronin forms a water-soluble chemical complex with cystine in the urine. This decreases cystine concentration and prevents formation of urinary cystine calculi in patients with severe homozygous cystinuria.

Tiopronin is prescribed to prevent urinary cystine calculi formation in patients with severe homozygous cystinuria (defined as urinary cystine excretion exceeding 500 mg daily) that has not responded to other therapies. The usual adult dosage begins with 800 mg by mouth daily in three divided doses; then it is adjusted to control urinary cystine levels. The usual pediatric dosage is 15 mg/kg by mouth daily in three divided doses.

No drug interactions have been reported during tiopronin therapy. Fatal complications from aplastic anemia, granulocytopenia, thrombocytopenia, or myasthenia gravis are possible, although these reactions have not been reported. Granulocytic leukopenia without eosinophilia and immunologic thrombocytopenia may occur. Membranous glomerulopathy may lead to severe proteinuria and nephrotic syndrome. A systemic lupus erythematous–like reaction may occur; this may be associated with a positive antinuclear antibody test. Fever, arthralgia, and lymphadenopathy may be accompanied by nephropathy.

Drug fever may develop, especially during the first month of therapy. A generalized rash with mild pruritus may arise during the first few months of therapy. A less common rash may occur after at least 6 months of therapy. This rash appears on the trunk, is accompanied by intense pruritus, and disappears slowly after drug discontinuation.

The effects of tiopronin on collagen may cause skin wrinkling and friability. Chelation of trace metals by the drug can cause hypogeusia (diminished taste sensitivity).

Rare reactions to tiopronin include Goodpasture's syndrome (indicated by abnormal urinary findings, pulmonary infiltrates, and hemoptysis), myasthenic syndrome (indicated by severe muscle weakness), and pemphigus-like reactions (indicated by bullous skin eruptions).

Nursing implications

When caring for a patient receiving tiopronin, the nurse should be aware of the following implications.

- Do not administer tiopronin to a patient with a history of granulocytopenia, aplastic anemia, or thrombocytopenia.

• Expect to adjust the dosage to keep the urine cystine level below 250 mg/liter.
• Administer tiopronin at least 1 hour before or 2 hours after a meal.
• Schedule the patient for laboratory tests every 3 to 6 months or as prescribed during tiopronin therapy. These tests typically include CBC, platelet count, hemoglobin and serum albumin levels, liver function tests, 24-hour urine protein assay, and urinalysis.
• Monitor the patient's urinary cystine level frequently during the first 6 months of therapy to assess therapeutic response. Then monitor it at least once every 6 months.
• Teach the patient to recognize and report signs of hematologic abnormalities, such as infection or abnormal bleeding or bruising.

Electrolyte modifying agents

Three drugs may be used to alter a patient's electrolyte balance: gallium nitrate, pamidronate, and sodium polystyrene sulfonate.

GALLIUM NITRATE

Gallium nitrate is a nitrate salt of the element gallium that may be used to alter the calcium concentration in the body.

Pharmacology

Little information is available about the pharmacokinetics of gallium. After I.V. administration, gallium is not metabolized and is excreted primarily by the kidneys. The drug's precise mechanism of action in inhibiting calcium resorption has not been determined.

Gallium is used to manage symptomatic cancer-related **hypercalcemia** that does not respond to adequate hydration. The usual adult dosage is 200 mg/m^2 I.V. daily for 5 days. (In a patient with mild hypercalcemia, 100 mg/m^2 for 5 days may be sufficient.) The daily dosage must be administered by continuous I.V. infusion over 24 hours.

Concomitant use of highly nephrotoxic drugs with gallium may increase the risk of renal insufficiency. During clinical trials, the most common adverse reactions to gallium have included transient hypophosphatemia, decreased serum bicarbonate levels, and renal toxicity. Other adverse reactions may include hypocalcemia, anemia, mild hypotension, and vision and hearing disturbances.

Nursing implications

When caring for a patient receiving gallium, the nurse should be aware of the following implications.
• Do not administer gallium to a breast-feeding patient or one with severe renal impairment.
• Administer gallium cautiously to a pregnant patient. Be aware that the drug's safety and efficacy in children have not been established.
• Monitor the patient's serum creatinine level frequently during therapy. Withhold the drug and notify the physician if the patient's serum creatinine level exceeds 2.5 mg/dl.
• Provide adequate hydration with oral or I.V. fluids (preferably saline), as prescribed, and ensure that urine output is satisfactory (2 L daily) before beginning gallium therapy. Maintain adequate hydration throughout the course of therapy.
• Monitor the patient's serum calcium level to evaluate the effectiveness of therapy and to detect hypocalcemia. If hypocalcemia occurs, withhold the gallium and notify the physician.

PAMIDRONATE

The biphosphonate pamidronate is an antihypercalcemic agent that inhibits bone resorption.

Pharmacology

Little pharmacokinetic information is available about pamidronate. After I.V administration, it is absorbed by the bone and slowly eliminated by the kidneys. Its elimination half-life in bone is estimated at 300 days. Pamidronate's antiresorptive mechanism of action is not understood completely.

Pamidronate is prescribed to treat moderate to severe hypercalcemia associated with cancer, with or without bone metastasis. The usual adult dosage for moderate hypercalcemia is 60 mg given as a single I.V. infusion over at least 4 hours. For severe hypercalcemia, the dosage may be 90 mg as a single I.V. infusion given over 24 hours. Treatment may be repeated if hypercalcemia recurs; a minimum of 7 days between treatments is recommended.

When mixed with pamidronate, calcium-containing solutions form a precipitate. No other drugs reportedly interact with pamidronate. During clinical trials, the most common adverse reactions have included fatigue, anorexia, nausea, and redness, swelling, and pain at the infusion site.

Nursing implications

When caring for a patient receiving pamidronate, the nurse should be aware of the following implications.
• Do not administer pamidronate to a patient with known hypersensitivity to the drug or other biphosphonates.
• Administer pamidronate cautiously to a pregnant or breast-feeding patient. Be aware that safety and efficacy of this drug in children have not been established.
• Monitor standard metabolic parameters related to hypercalcemia, such as serum calcium, phosphate, magnesium, and potassium levels, during pamidronate therapy.
• Reconstitute the drug by adding 10 ml of sterile water to each vial. Dissolve the pamidronate completely before withdrawing the solution for injection.

• Do not administer pamidronate with calcium-containing infusion solutions, such as lactated Ringer's solution.

SODIUM POLYSTYRENE SULFONATE

A synthetic **cation**-exchange resin, sodium polystyrene sulfonate exchanges sodium ions for potassium ions. That is why it is known as a potassium-removing resin.

Pharmacology

Sodium polystyrene sulfonate is not absorbed from the GI tract. Therefore, resin distribution is limited to the GI tract. The drug is not metabolized to any extent and is excreted in the feces, primarily as potassium polystyrene sulfonate. After oral administration of sodium polystyrene sulfonate, the onset of action may not occur for 2 to 24 hours; after rectal administration, it may be somewhat shorter. The drug's duration of action is about 4 to 6 hours.

After oral administration of sodium polystyrene sulfonate, sodium ions are exchanged with hydrogen ions found in the stomach's acidic environment. As the resin passes through the GI tract, hydrogen ions are released in exchange for other cations present in higher concentrations. Because of the high concentration of potassium in the large intestine, potassium readily exchanges with hydrogen ions. Then the modified resin is eliminated in the feces. After rectal administration of sodium polystyrene sulfonate, sodium ions are released directly in exchange for potassium ions.

Sodium polystyrene sulfonate is used to treat **hyperkalemia** when urgent reduction of the serum potassium level is not necessary. The dosage and duration of therapy must be individualized based on the daily assessment of total body potassium. For oral therapy, the usual adult dosage is 15 g orally one to four times daily, with each dose given as a suspension in 20 to 100 ml of water or a syrup (such as 70% sorbitol). For rectal therapy, the usual adult dosage is 30 to 50 g administered as a retention enema every 1 to 2 hours initially, then every 6 hours or as needed. The agent should be retained at least 20 to 30 minutes to be effective. The usual pediatric dosage is 1 g for each mEq of potassium to be removed.

Antacids that contain certain cations (such as calcium or magnesium) tend to interfere with the effectiveness of sodium polystyrene sulfonate and may cause systemic alkalosis. Foods or liquids that contain potassium may also reduce the drug's effectiveness. Concurrent administration of an aluminum hydroxide-containing antacid with sodium polystyrene sulfonate may result in intestinal obstruction.

Serious hypokalemia may result from sodium polystyrene sulfonate therapy. Hypokalemia may cause disturbances of muscle function, cardiac rhythm, acid-base balance, and deep tendon reflexes, as well as potential digitalis toxicity. Calcium and magnesium deficiencies have also been noted during therapy with sodium polystyrene sulfonate. GI disturbances commonly occur and may include nausea, vomiting, anorexia, and constipation.

Nursing implications

When caring for a patient receiving sodium polystyrene sulfonate, the nurse should be aware of the following implications.

• Do not administer sodium polystyrene sulfonate to a patient with hypokalemia or known hypersensitivity.
• Administer this drug cautiously to a pregnant or breast-feeding patient or one who cannot tolerate sodium, such as a patient with heart failure.
• Monitor the patient's serum potassium level at least once daily and observe for signs of hypokalemia. Also monitor the patient's ECG and clinical condition because the serum potassium level may not reflect an intracellular potassium deficiency.
• Identify and eliminate, if possible, any exogenous sources of potassium the patient may be receiving.
• Administer a sodium polystyrene sulfonate enema by placing the tip of the rectal catheter at least 8"(20 cm) into the colon. Encourage the patient to retain the enema for 20 to 30 minutes or as prescribed. If the patient has difficulty retaining the enema, elevate the patient's hips on pillows, have the patient assume a knee-chest position, or instill the enema through a catheter held in place with an inflatable balloon.
• Mix sodium polystyrene sulfonate with 20 to 100 ml of fruit juice, water, syrup, or a soft drink to increase its palatability for oral administration. However, avoid fluids with a high potassium content. Administer the drug as a suspension because it is much more effective than in paste form.
• Monitor the patient's bowel function frequently to ensure that the resin is being eliminated. If the patient becomes constipated, mix the drug in 70% sorbitol solution, as prescribed, to produce one or two soft stools daily.
• Notify the physician if adverse reactions occur or if the drug is ineffective.
• Teach the patient to recognize and report sodium and potassium imbalances.
• Instruct the patient to take the drug mixed with sorbitol early in the day to prevent sorbitol-induced diarrhea at night.

Miscellaneous hematologic agents

Miscellaneous hematologic agents include filgrastim, pentoxifylline, and sargramostim.

FILGRASTIM

Also known as granulocyte colony–stimulating factor (G-CSF), filgrastim is a hematopoietic growth factor agent.

Pharmacology

Little is known about the pharmacokinetics of filgrastim. Its half-life is approximately 3.5 hours. Filgrastim regulates neutrophil production in the bone marrow by binding to specific cell surface receptors.

Filgrastim is used to decrease the incidence of infection in patients with nonmyeloid malignancies who receive myelosuppressive antineoplastic agents that commonly cause severe neutropenia and fever. The usual dosage for adults and children is 5 mcg/kg S.C. or I.V. daily as a single injection.

No drug interactions with filgrastim have been reported. In clinical trials, the most common adverse reaction was bone pain. Other adverse reactions reported in more than 10% of patients included nausea, vomiting, alopecia, diarrhea, fever, mucositis, and fatigue.

Nursing implications

When caring for a patient receiving filgrastim, the nurse should be aware of the following implications.

- Do not administer filgrastim to a patient with known hypersensitivity to proteins derived from *Escherichia coli.* Also, do not administer the drug 24 hours before to 24 hours after administration of a cytotoxic chemotherapeutic agent.
- Administer filgrastim cautiously to a pregnant or breast-feeding patient or one with a myeloid-type malignancy.
- Obtain a CBC twice a week, as prescribed, to detect excessive leukocytosis.
- Store filgrastim solution in the refrigerator. Let it come to room temperature before using it for injection. However, if the vial has been at room temperature for more than 6 hours, discard it. Avoid shaking the filgrastim solution.

PENTOXIFYLLINE

A xanthine derivative, pentoxifylline is a hemorrheologic agent that decreases blood viscosity.

Pharmacology

After oral administration, pentoxifylline is absorbed extensively from the GI tract. However, its distribution is unknown. The drug is metabolized extensively by red blood cells (RBCs) and the liver during first-pass hepatic metabolism. Pentoxifylline and its metabolites are excreted primarily in the urine. The half-life of the unchanged drug is approximately 30 to 45 minutes; the half-life of its metabolites is approximately 1 to 1.5 hours. The peak concentration level occurs in 2 to 4 hours; however, clinical effect requires 2 to 4 weeks of continuous therapy.

Pentoxifylline and its metabolites improve capillary blood flow by increasing RBC flexibility and reducing blood viscosity. The drug is used to treat chronic occlusive peripheral vascular disease in the management of intermittent claudication. The usual adult dosage is 400 mg orally three times daily with meals.

Concomitant use of pentoxifylline and antihypertensives may cause an increased hypotensive response. Bleeding abnormalities may occur in patients taking pentoxifylline concomitantly with oral anticoagulants or drugs that inhibit platelet aggregation.

The most common adverse reactions to pentoxifylline include GI complaints, such as dyspepsia, nausea, vomiting, belching, flatus, and bloating, and CNS reactions, such as dizziness, headache, and tremor. Adverse cardiovascular reactions rarely occur, but may include chest pain, arrhythmias, tachycardia, palpitations, flushing, dyspnea, edema, and hypotension.

CRITICAL THINKING. To enhance your critical thinking about the agents in this chapter, consider the following situation and its analysis.

Situation: Jean Martin, age 54, is receiving pentoxifylline as prescribed for intermittent claudication. While obtaining a medication history, the nurse learns that Ms. Martin has been taking 650 mg of aspirin three to four times a day for arthritis. When assessing the patient, the nurse notices bruises on her legs. Ms. Martin says the bruises are painless, but cannot recall what caused them. Based on this information, what nursing interventions are appropriate?

Analysis: First, the nurse should suspect that the bruises are signs of bleeding abnormalities, which can occur when pentoxifylline is used with another drug that inhibits platelet aggregation, such as aspirin. Then the nurse should consult with the physician about ordering coagulation tests. When the test results are known, the nurse should take appropriate measures. For example, if the results indicate a bleeding abnormality, the nurse should place Ms. Martin on bed rest, take bleeding precautions, and teach her not to take any over-the-counter drug without the physician's approval.

Nursing implications

When caring for a patient receiving pentoxifylline, the nurse should be aware of the following implications.

- Do not administer pentoxifylline to a breast-feeding patient or one with known intolerance to the drug or methylxanthines.
- Administer pentoxifylline cautiously to a pregnant patient. Be aware that safety and efficacy of this drug in children have not been established.
- Notify the physician and expect to reduce the pentoxifylline dosage if the patient develops adverse GI or CNS reactions. If adverse reactions persist after the dosage is reduced, expect to discontinue the drug.
- Frequently monitor for other signs of arteriosclerotic disease, such as angina, hypotension, and arrhythmias, in a patient with chronic occlusive peripheral vascular disease.

• Monitor the patient's blood pressure when starting pentoxifylline therapy, especially during concomitant antihypertensive therapy.
• Do not split or crush pentoxifylline tablets because this destroys their sustained-release properties.
• Advise the patient to take pentoxifylline with meals to minimize GI distress.
• Inform the patient that therapy must continue for at least 8 weeks and that the drug must not be discontinued without medical approval.

SARGRAMOSTIM

Also known as granulocyte-macrophage–colony stimulating factor (GM-CSF), sargramostim is a hematopoietic growth factor agent.

Pharmacology

Little information is known about the pharmacokinetics of sargramostim. After administration, the drug's onset of action may occur within 5 minutes; its peak plasma concentration, within 2 hours.

Sargramostim stimulates the proliferation and differentiation of hematopoietic progenitor cells by inducing these cells to divide and differentiate in the granulocyte-macrophage pathways. The drug can also activate mature granulocytes and macrophages by binding to specific receptors on their cell surfaces.

Sargramostim is used to accelerate myeloid recovery in patients with non-Hodgkin's lymphoma or acute lymphoblastic leukemia and in patients undergoing autologous bone marrow transplantation. The recommended adult dosage is 250 mcg/m^2 I.V. daily as a 2-hour infusion for 21 days, beginning 2 to 4 hours after bone marrow transplantation, no less than 24 hours after the last dose of chemotherapy, and 12 hours after the first dose of radiotherapy.

Drugs, such as lithium and corticosteroids, may potentiate sargramostim's myeloproliferative effects. During clinical trials, the most common adverse reactions included fever, mucous membrane disorders, asthenia, malaise, nausea, vomiting, diarrhea, anorexia, and alopecia. Rarely, serious hypersensitivity reactions occurred. In some patients, sargramostim caused transient rashes, local reactions at the injection site, and dyspnea.

Nursing implications

When caring for a patient receiving sargramostim, the nurse should be aware of the following implications.
• Do not administer sargramostim to a patient with excessive leukemic myeloid blasts in the bone marrow or peripheral blood or with known hypersensitivity to any components of the drug or to yeast-derived products.
• Administer sargramostim cautiously to a pregnant or breast-feeding patient or one with cardiac disease, fluid retention, pulmonary infiltrates, heart failure, respiratory disease (especially hypoxia), renal or hepatic dysfunction, or malignancy with myeloid characteristics. Be aware that the drug's safety and efficacy in children have not been established.
• Monitor the patient's respiratory status during sargramostim therapy. If respiratory abnormalities occur, reduce the infusion rate by half. If symptoms worsen despite this reduction, discontinue the infusion, as prescribed.
• Obtain a CBC with differential (including examination for blast cells) twice weekly, as prescribed. Also, frequently monitor renal or hepatic function test results in a patient with renal or hepatic dysfunction.

Miscellaneous immune-system modulating agents

Immune-system modulating agents include interferon gamma-1b and levamisole hydrochloride.

INTERFERON GAMMA 1B

Interferon gamma-1b is a biological response modifier.

Pharmacology

Little is known about the pharmacokinetics of interferon gamma-1b. With I.V., I.M., and S.C. administration of this drug, the mean elimination half-lives are about 38 minutes, 2.9 hours, and 5.9 hours, respectively. Plasma concentration levels peak about 4 hours after I.M. administration and 7 hours after S.C. administration.

Interferon gamma-1b has potent phagocyte-activating properties that act against such organisms as *Staphylococcus aureus, Toxoplasma gondii, Leishmania donovani, Listeria monocytogenes,* and *Mycobacterium avium-intracellulare.*

This **immunomodulator** is used to reduce the frequency and severity of serious infections associated with chronic granulomatous disease. For adults and children, the usual dosage is 50 mcg/m^2 S.C. three times weekly for patients whose body surface area (BSA) exceeds 0.5 m^2; for patients whose BSA equals or is less than 0.5 m^2, the dosage is 1.5 mcg/m^2 S.C. three times weekly.

Interferon gamma-1b may decrease the metabolism of drugs that are metabolized in the liver. During clinical trials, patients commonly reported flulike symptoms, such as fever, headache, chills, myalgia, and fatigue. They also commonly reported rash.

Nursing implications

When caring for a patient receiving interferon gamma-1b, the nurse should be aware of the following implications.
• Do not administer interferon gamma-1b to a breast-feeding patient or one with known hypersensitivity to the drug, any of its components, or products derived from *Escherichia coli.*

• Administer interferon gamma-1b cautiously to a pregnant patient or one with cardiac disease, seizure disorder, compromised CNS function, or myelosuppression. Be aware that safety and efficacy of this drug in children under age 1 has not been established.
• Administer interferon gamma-1b at bedtime to minimize flulike symptoms. Also administer acetaminophen, as prescribed, to prevent or help relieve fever and headache.

LEVAMISOLE HYDROCHLORIDE

The immunomodulator levamisole hydrochloride is an antineoplastic agent used to treat a specific type of colon cancer.

Pharmacology

After oral administration, levamisole is absorbed well and achieves a peak plasma concentration level within 2 hours. The drug undergoes extensive metabolism in the liver and is excreted primarily in the urine. Its plasma half-life is approximately 3.5 hours.

Levamisole restores depressed immune function rather than stimulates the immune response. Its mechanism of action in combination with fluorouracil, with which it is administered, is unknown.

After surgical resection of Dukes' stage C colon cancer, levamisole is prescribed as adjuvant therapy with fluorouracil. The usual adult dosage for initial therapy is 50 mg by mouth. every 8 hours for 3 days starting 7 to 30 days after surgery; for maintenance, 50 mg by mouth every 8 hours for 3 days, administered every 2 weeks.

Levamisole may increase the plasma phenytoin level. If taken with alcohol, it may cause a disulfiram-like reaction. Adverse reactions reported in more than 5% of patients during clinical trials include nausea, vomiting, diarrhea, taste changes, dermatitis, fatigue, arthralgia, and infection. Adverse reactions reported in more than 2% of patients include leukopenia, alopecia, fever, rigidity, stomatitis, myalgia, dizziness, headache, and somnolence. Combination therapy with fluorouracil increases the frequency or severity of adverse reactions, especially hematologic ones.

Nursing implications

When caring for a patient receiving levamisole, the nurse should be aware of the following implications.
• Do not administer levamisole to a pregnant or breast-feeding patient or one with known hypersensitivity.
• Be aware that the safety and efficacy of levamisole in children have not been established.
∗ Monitor the patient for anemia, neutropenia, and thrombocytopenia because combination therapy with fluorouracil is associated with a high incidence of these disorders.
• Ensure that the patient has a complete laboratory workup (including a CBC with differential, platelet count, electrolyte levels, and liver function tests) on the first day of combination therapy, as prescribed. Expect to repeat the CBC with differential and platelet counts weekly and the electrolyte levels and liver function tests every 3 months for 1 year.
• Advise the patient to avoid alcohol to prevent disulfiram-like reactions.
• Instruct the patient to report sore throat, fever, and other signs of infection because levamisole may cause leukopenia, which increases the risk of infection.

Miscellaneous agents

Other miscellaneous agents include botulinum toxin type A, a neurotoxin; ethanolamine oleate, a sclerosing agent; levocarnitine, a nutritional agent; mesna, a detoxifying agent; nimodipine, a calcium channel blocker; octreotide acetate, a long-acting octapeptide; and ursodiol, a gallstone-solubilizing agent.

BOTULINUM TOXIN TYPE A

Botulinum toxin type A is a neurotoxin used to treat eye muscle disorders.

Pharmacology

The pharmacokinetics of botulinum toxin type A are unknown. The drug causes neuromuscular paralysis by binding to acetylcholine receptors on the motor end plate. It also may inhibit the release of acetylcholine from presynaptic nerve endings.

Botulinum toxin type A is a muscle relaxant used to treat **strabismus** and blepharospasm. For strabismus, the usual adult dosage varies with the degree of deviation (lower dosages are used for milder deviations). For vertical muscles and for horizontal strabismus of less than 20 prism diopters, the adult dosage is 1.25 to 2.5 units injected into any one muscle; for horizontal strabismus of 20 to 50 prism diopters, 2.5 to 5 units injected into any one muscle. For persistent palsy of the seventh cranial nerve lasting more than 1 month, 1.25 to 2.5 units injected into the medial rectus muscle. The maximum single dosage for any one muscle is 25 units. For blepharospasm, the initial adult dosage is usually 1.25 to 2.5 units injected into the medial and lateral pretarsal orbicularis oculi of the upper and lower lids. In subsequent treatments, the dosage may be doubled if inadequate paralysis is achieved. However, exceeding 5 units per site has no apparent benefit. The effects of each treatment last about 3 months. Treatment can be repeated indefinitely.

No drug interactions with botulinum toxin type A have been reported. Adverse reactions are limited primarily to the ocular area. They include double vision, blurred vision, spatial disorientation, ptosis, vertical deviation (after treatment of strabismus), irritation (after treatment of blepharospasm), a local diffuse rash, eyelid swelling, and ecchymosis. Because botulinum toxin type A is a protein, it can cause anaphylaxis.

Nursing implications

When caring for a patient receiving botulinum toxin type A, the nurse should be aware of the following implications.

• Do not administer botulinum toxin type A to a patient with known hypersensitivity to any ingredient in the formulation.

• Administer this drug cautiously to a breast-feeding or pregnant patient.

*** *Have emergency equipment nearby because the patient may develop an anaphylactic reaction to this drug.***

• Administer several drops of a local anesthetic and an ocular decongestant, as prescribed, several minutes before injection.

• Reconstitute botulinum toxin type A using normal saline solution as the diluent. Inject the diluent into the vial gently because the drug is denatured by bubbling or similarly violent agitation.

• Administer the drug up to 4 hours after reconstitution; during those 4 hours, keep the drug refrigerated.

ETHANOLAMINE OLEATE

The sclerosing agent ethanolamine oleate is used to treat esophageal varices.

Pharmacology

When injected locally, ethanolamine is cleared via the portal vein within 5 minutes. Other information on the pharmacokinetics of ethanolamine is unknown.

A mild sclerosing agent, ethanolamine irritates the intimal endothelium of the vein, causing a sterile inflammatory response that leads to fibrosis and occlusion.

Ethanolamine is used to prevent further bleeding in patients who have had a recent bleeding episode caused by esophageal varices. It should be administered by a gastroenterologist or other specialist because it must be instilled via gastroscope or endoscope directly into the esophageal area. The usual adult dosage is 1.5 to 5 ml injected locally into each varix. The maximum dosage per treatment should not exceed 20 ml or 0.4 ml/kg. Subsequent injections usually follow at intervals of 1 week, 6 weeks, 3 months, and 6 months.

No known drug interactions exist. Adverse reactions to ethanolamine include GI reactions, such as esophagitis, local mucosal sloughing or necrosis, and esophageal ulcer, stricture, or tearing; genitourinary reactions, such as acute renal failure; and respiratory reactions, such as pleural effusion or infiltration, pneumonia, and aspiration pneumonia. Other adverse reactions include pyrexia, retrosternal pain, and anaphylaxis.

Nursing implications

When caring for a patient receiving ethanolamine, the nurse should be aware of the following implications.

• Do not administer ethanolamine to a patient with known hypersensitivity or one with esophageal varices that have not bled.

• Expect to administer smaller doses to a patient with cardiopulmonary disease to minimize adverse reactions.

• Avoid submucosal injection because this is more likely to cause mucosal ulceration.

• Explain the administration technique to the patient and stress the need to return for follow-up visits, as prescribed, to ensure successful therapy.

*** *Instruct the patient to immediately report chest pain, shortness of breath, or bleeding.***

*** *Have emergency drugs and equipment nearby in case the patient develops ethanolamine-induced anaphylaxis; make sure that epinephrine 1:1,000 and antihistamines are readily available.***

*** *Monitor the serum potassium level frequently, particularly in a patient also receiving a diuretic. If hypokalemia occurs, notify the physician and observe for signs of digitalis toxicity in a patient receiving a cardiac glycoside.***

LEVOCARNITINE

The nutritional agent levocarnitine is used to treat deficiency of the amino acid carnitine.

Pharmacology

The pharmacokinetics of levocarnitine have not yet been determined. A naturally occurring substance composed of amino acids that are required for mammalian energy metabolism, levocarnitine produces energy by facilitating long-chain fatty acid entry into cell mitochondria.

Levocarnitine is used to treat primary systemic carnitine deficiency. The usual adult dosage is 990 mg in tablet form by mouth two or three times daily, (available as a 330-mg tablet), or 1 to 3 g enteral liquid form by mouth daily in evenly divided doses for a patient weighing 110 lb (50 kg). For the enteral liquid form, the intial dosage is 1 g daily; it is increased, as needed, to reflect the patient's tolerance and clinical response. The usual pediatric dosage of the enteral liquid form is 50 to 100 mg/kg by mouth daily in divided doses, up to a maximum of 3 g daily. Begin the dosage with 50 mg/kg by mouth daily, and increase it according to the patient's tolerance and clinical response. For treatment of acute and chronic secondary levocarnitine deficiency, the usual adult dosage is 50 mg/kg I.V. slowly over 2 to 3 minutes every 3 to 4 hours.

Levocarnitine causes no known drug interactions. Its most common adverse reactions include nausea, vomiting, abdominal cramps, diarrhea, and drug-related body odor.

Nursing implications

When caring for a patient receiving levocarnitine, the nurse should be aware of the following implications.

- Administer levocarnitine cautiously to a pregnant patient. Be aware that this drug has no known contraindications.
- Closely monitor the patient's ability to tolerate the drug during the first week of therapy and after each dosage increase.
- Monitor periodic blood chemistries, vital signs, and plasma carnitine concentrations, as prescribed. Also monitor the patient's general nutritional condition.
- Use the entire or partial contents of each container immediately after opening. Discard unused contents of open containers.
- Advise the patient that GI symptoms may be decreased by taking the drug slowly or by diluting the liquid form.
- Inform the patient that drug-related body odor may occur with levocarnitine use. If the odor becomes offensive, tell the patient to discuss dosage reduction with the physician.

MESNA

A thiol derivative, mesna is used as a detoxifying agent in conjunction with ifosfamide therapy.

Pharmacology

After I.V. administration, mesna remains in the vascular compartment and is metabolized to mesna disulfide. It is eliminated by the kidneys. After an 800-mg I.V. dose, the half-lives of mesna and mesna disulfide are 0.36 hours and 1.17 hours, respectively.

In the kidneys, mesna disulfide is reduced to a free thiol compound that reacts chemically with urotoxic ifosfamide metabolites to detoxify them, preventing ifosfamide-induced hemorrhagic cystitis.

Mesna is prescribed prophylactically to reduce the risk of ifosfamide-induced hemorrhagic cystitis. The usual adult dosage is equivalent to 20% of each ifosfamide dosage on a weight-per-weight basis, given by I.V. bolus injection three times daily. The first dose is given with ifosfamide; the next two doses are given 4 and 8 hours after each ifosfamide dose, for a daily dosage equivalent to 60% of the ifosfamide dosage.

Drug interactions with mesna have not been identified. Because mesna is administered with ifosfamide and other antineoplastic agents, its adverse reactions are difficult to isolate. The following reactions were reported during clinical trials in a limited number of patients: bad taste in the mouth, soft stools, diarrhea, limb pain, headache, fatigue, nausea, vomiting, hypotension, and allergy.

Nursing implications

When caring for a patient receiving mesna, the nurse should be aware of the following implications.

- Do not administer mesna to a breast-feeding patient or one with known hypersensitivity to mesna or other thiol compounds.
- Administer mesna cautiously to a pregnant patient.
- Expect to administer mesna concurrently with ifosfamide, as prescribed, for maximum effectiveness.
- Inform the patient that mesna does not prevent ifosfamide-induced hemorrhagic cystitis in every case and cannot reduce other toxicities associated with ifosfamide.

NIMODIPINE

The calcium channel blocker nimodipine is used to induce cerebral vasodilation in certain patients.

Pharmacology

After oral administration, nimodipine is absorbed rapidly, with the peak concentration level usually occurring within 1 hour. Approximately 95% protein-bound, the drug is metabolized in the liver and eliminated by the kidneys. Its half-life is 1 to 2 hours.

Nimodipine inhibits contraction of vascular smooth muscle. This action makes it useful in treating neurologic deficits caused by cerebral spasms resulting from a ruptured congenital aneurysm in patients who are otherwise neurologically healthy. Therapy should begin within 96 hours of the hemorrhage and continue for 21 days. The usual adult dosage is 60 mg by mouth every 4 hours for 21 days. For patients with severe liver disease, the usual dosage is 30 mg by mouth every 4 hours.

Concomitant administration of nimodipine with another calcium channel blocker may cause additive cardiovascular effects. During clinical trials, adverse reactions to nimodipine included hypotension, abnormal liver function test results, edema, diarrhea, rash, headache, nausea and other GI symptoms, dyspnea, ECG abnormalities, tachycardia or bradycardia, muscle pain or cramps, acne, and depression.

Nursing implications

When caring for a patient receiving nimodipine, the nurse should be aware of the following implications.

- Do not administer nimodipine to a breast-feeding patient.
- Administer nimodipine cautiously to a pregnant patient. Be aware that safety and efficacy of this drug in children have not been established.

∗ ***Monitor the patient's blood pressure and pulse frequently because calcium channel blockers have cardiovascular effects.***

- Expect to decrease the nimodipine dosage in a patient with severe liver disease.
- Assist the patient who cannot swallow the nimodipine capsule by extracting its contents with an 18G needle and administering them through a nasogastric tube. Follow this with 30 ml of normal saline solution.

OCTREOTIDE ACETATE

Octreotide acetate , a long-acting octapeptide, is used to treat selected metastatic tumors.

Pharmacology

Octreotide is absorbed rapidly and completely after S.C. injection. It achieves a peak concentration level 24 minutes after a 100-mcg dose. The drug is bound approximately 65% to lipoproteins and albumin; its duration of action varies and may be as long as 12 hours under certain conditions. Octreotide is excreted unchanged in the urine. Its elimination half-life is approximately 1.5 hours.

The pharmacologic properties of octreotide resemble those of the natural hormone somatostatin. Normally, somatostatin suppresses secretion of serotonin, gastrin, vasoactive intestinal peptide, insulin, glucagon, secretin, motilin, and pancreatic polypeptide. Octreotide may also suppress growth hormone and decrease splanchnic blood flow.

Octreotide is used to relieve symptoms of metastatic carcinoma and vasoactive intestinal polypeptide secreting tumors (VIPomas). For carcinoid tumors, the usual adult dosage is 100 to 600 mcg S.C. daily in two, three, or four divided doses for the first 2 weeks of therapy. For VIPomas, the usual adult dosage is 200 to 300 mcg S.C. daily in two, three, or four divided doses during the first 2 weeks of therapy; it is adjusted according to patient response and symptom control. Daily maintenance dosages above 450 mcg are rarely required.

Octreotide may decrease the plasma level of cyclosporine. Concomitant use with insulin, an oral hypoglycemic agent, or oral diazoxide may require dosage adjustment. Octreotide therapy may necessitate dosage adjustment of other drugs used to control disease symptoms, such as beta blockers.

From 3% to 10% of patients experienced the following adverse reactions to octreotide during clinical trials: nausea, pain at the injection site, diarrhea, abdominal pain or discomfort, and vomiting. From 1% to 2% of patients reported headache, fat malabsorption, dizziness, light-headedness, fatigue, flushing, hypoglycemia or hyperglycemia, edema, weakness, and wheal or erythema at the injection site.

Nursing implications

When caring for a patient receiving octreotide, the nurse should be aware of the following implications.

• Do not administer octreotide to a patient with known hypersensitivity to the drug or any of its components.

• Administer octreotide cautiously to a breast-feeding patient.

✱ Monitor the patient closely for signs and symptoms of hypoglycemia or hyperglycemia because octreotide may alter the ratio among insulin, glucagon, and growth hormone. Also advise the patient taking insulin that insulin dosage changes may be required during octreotide therapy.

• Arrange for periodic measurements of fecal fat and serum carotene levels, as prescribed, because octreotide may cause fat malabsorption.

• Do not administer octreotide if the vial contains particulate matter or if its contents are discolored.

URSODIOL

Ursodiol is a gallstone-solubilizing agent used to manage gallstones in selected patients.

Pharmacology

After oral administration, approximately 90% of the dose is absorbed in the small intestine. After absorption, most of the drug is extracted by the liver, where it is conjugated and secreted into the hepatic bile ducts. It is then metabolized by the liver and excreted primarily in the feces.

A naturally occurring bile acid, ursodiol apparently suppresses cholesterol synthesis and secretion and inhibits intestinal resorption of cholesterol.

The drug is used to dissolve radiolucent, noncalcified gallstones less than 20 mm in diameter in patients for whom elective cholecystectomy carries an increased surgical risk (because of systemic disease, advanced age, or idiosyncratic reaction to general anesthesia) and in patients who refuse surgery. Gallstone dissolution with ursodiol requires months of therapy. The usual adult dosage is 8 to 10 mg/kg by mouth daily in two or three divided doses.

Concomitant administration of bile-sequestering agents, such as cholestyramine and colestipol, or aluminum-containing antacids may decrease ursodiol absorption. Drugs that increase hepatic cholesterol secretion, such as estrogen, oral contraceptives, and clofibrate, may encourage gallstone formation, counteracting the effects of ursodiol.

During clinical trials, adverse reactions to ursodiol included pruritus, urticaria, dry skin, diaphoresis, thinning hair, nausea, vomiting, dyspepsia, metallic taste, abdominal pain, biliary pain, cholecystitis, diarrhea or constipation, stomatitis, flatulence, headache, fatigue, anxiety, depression, sleep disorders, arthralgia, myalgia, back pain, cough, and rhinitis.

Nursing implications

When caring for a patient receiving ursodiol, the nurse should be aware of the following implications.

• Do not administer ursodiol to a patient with known hypersensitivity to bile salts, one with chronic liver disease, or one who requires cholecystectomy because of unremitting acute cholecystitis, cholangitis, biliary obstruction, gallstones, pancreatitis, or biliary-GI fistula. Also, do not administer ursodiol to a patient with calcified cholesterol or radiopaque or radiolucent bile pigment stones; the drug does not dissolve these stones.

• Administer ursodiol cautiously to a patient taking a bile-sequestering agent, aluminum-containing antacid, estrogen, oral contraceptive, or clofibrate.

• Ensure that the patient has liver function tests as prescribed, typically at the beginning of ursodiol therapy, after 1 month and 3 months of therapy, and at 6-month intervals thereafter.

CHAPTER SUMMARY

Chapter 61 discussed uncategorized and other agents. Here are the chapter highlights.

Miscellaneous respiratory agents include alpha$_1$-proteinase inhibitor and the pulmonary surfactant agents, beractant and colfosceril palmitate. The pulmonary surfactant agents must be administered directly into the trachea by trained personnel only.

Miscellaneous GI agents include lactulose, which reduces ammonia levels in patients with portal encephalopathy, and mesalamine, olsalazine sodium, and sulfasalazine, which are used to treat ulcerative colitis.

Miscellaneous endocrine agents include the antiestrogen clomiphene citrate, the fertility agents hCG and menotropins, and the GnRH agonists histrelin acetate and nafarelin acetate.

Miscellaneous anti-infective agents include the antileprotic agents clofazimine and dapsone. These drugs usually require prolonged therapy to treat Hansen's disease.

Miscellaneous metabolic agents include pegademase bovine, which is used as enzyme replacement therapy in patients with ADA deficiency; sodium benzoate 10% and sodium phenylacetate 10%, which is used to treat or prevent hyperammonemia in infants; and tiopronin, which is used to prevent urinary cystine calculi formation in severe homozygous cystinuria.

The electrolyte modifying agents include gallium nitrate, pamidronate, and sodium polystyrene sulfonate. The first two of these agents reduce calcium levels associated with cancer; the third one reduces the potassium level in blood.

Miscellaneous hematologic agents include the hematopoietic growth factor agents filgrastim (G-CSF) and sargramostim (GM-CSF), and the hemorrheologic agent pentoxifylline.

Immune-system modulating agents include interferon gamma-1b, which reduces the frequency of infection associated with chronic granulomatous disease, and levamisole hydrochloride, which is used in the treatment of Dukes' stage C colon cancer.

Other agents discussed in the chapter include botulinum toxin type A, a neurotoxin used to treat selected eye muscle disorders; ethanolamine oleate, a sclerosing agent used to prevent bleeding from esophageal varices; levocarnitine, a nutritional agent used to treat an amino acid deficiency; mesna, a detoxifying agent used to prevent ifosfamide-induced hemorrhagic cystitis; nimodipine, a calcium channel blocker used to induce cerebral vasodilation in certain patients; octreotide acetate, an agent used to treat selected metastatic tumors; and ursodiol, a gallstone-solubilizing agent used to manage gallstones in selected patients.

Because the adverse reactions and drug interactions of many of the drugs discussed in chapter 61 may not be known fully, the nurse should monitor the patient closely when administering these agents.

Questions to consider

See Appendix 1 for answers.

1. Charles Nash, age 27, has a congenital deficiency of alpha$_1$ antitrypsin. Recently, he developed panacinar emphysema and now must take alpha$_1$-proteinase inhibitor. What is the usual adult dosage for this agent?
- (a) 20 mg/kg by mouth b.i.d.
- (b) 40 mg/kg S.C. once daily
- (c) 60 mg/kg I.V. once weekly
- (d) 80 I.M. every other week

2. One hour after birth, Kelly Minton develops RDS. Which of the following drugs is used to treat neonatal RDS?
- (a) mesalamine
- (b) colfosceril
- (c) histrelin
- (d) mesna

3. John Waters, age 55, has cirrhosis of the liver. His physician prescribes lactulose to treat systemic portal encephalopathy. Which of the following drugs may interact with lactulose if administered concurrently?
- (a) erythromycin
- (b) mesalamine
- (c) bactrim
- (d) No drug

4. Brian Ferguson, age 52, is receiving chemotherapy for cancer. He is also receiving gallium nitrate for an electrolyte imbalance. Gallium corrects an imbalance of which of the following electrolytes?
- (a) sodium
- (b) calcium
- (c) potassium
- (d) magnesium

5. Diana Earl, age 63, has Dukes' stage C colon cancer. One week after surgery, the physician prescribes levamisole 50 mg by mouth every 8 hours for 3 days. Which of the following drugs may interact with levamisole if administered concurrently?
   (a) ursodiol
   (b) phenytoin
   (c) fluorouracil
   (d) pentoxifylline

6. John Benson, age 68, is hospitalized with bleeding esophageal varices. The physician prescribes ethanolamine oleate to prevent new bleeding. Which of the following types of agents is ethanolamine oleate?
   (a) Sclerosing agent
   (b) Neurotoxic agent
   (c) Anticoagulant agent
   (d) Hematorrheologic agent

Appendices, Glossary, Selected References, and Index

Appendices

Appendix 1

Answers to Questions to Consider

Unit 1: Overview of Pharmacology

Chapter 1 Introduction to Pharmacology

1. b, **2.** c, **3.** b, **4.** c, **5.** b, **6.** a

Chapter 2 Fundamental Principles of Pharmacology

1. c, **2.** d, **3.** d, **4.** c, **5.** a, **6.** d, **7.** a

Unit 2: The Nursing Process and Drug Administration

Chapter 3 Responsibilities in Drug Administration

1. b, **2.** c, **3.** b, **4.** b, **5.** c, **6.** c

Chapter 4 Dosage Measurements and Calculations

1. a, **2.** c, **3.** c, **4.** b, **5.** a, **6.** c, **7.** d

Chapter 5 Routes and Techniques of Administration

1. c, **2.** a, **3.** b, **4.** d, **5.** c, **6.** a, **7.** b

Unit 3: Drugs Affecting the Autonomic Nervous System

Chapter 6 Cholinergic Agents

1. c, **2.** a, **3.** c, **4.** a, **5.** d

Chapter 7 Cholinergic Blocking Agents

1. d, **2.** c, **3.** b, **4.** b

Chapter 8 Adrenergic Agents

1. a, **2.** a, **3.** d, **4.** d, **5.** b, **6.** b

Chapter 9 Adrenergic Blocking Agents

1. b, **2.** d, **3.** c, **4.** a, **5.** b, **6.** a, **7.** d

Chapter 10 Neuromuscular Blocking Agents

1. d, **2.** b, **3.** a, **4.** b, **5.** c

Unit 4: Drugs to Treat Neurologic and Neuromuscular System Disorders

Chapter 11 Skeletal Muscle Relaxing Agents

1. d, **2.** a, **3.** d, **4.** b, **5.** c

Chapter 12 Antiparkinsonian Agents

1. a, **2.** b, **3.** b, **4.** d, **5.** c, **6.** c, **7.** d

Chapter 13 Anticonvulsant Agents

1. b, **2.** b, **3.** a, **4.** c, **5.** d, **6.** a, **7.** b, **8.** c

Unit 5: Drugs to Prevent and Treat Pain

Chapter 14 Nonnarcotic Analgesic, Antipyretic, and Nonsteroidal Anti-Inflammatory Agents

1. b, **2.** d, **3.** a, **4.** d, **5.** c

Chapter 15 Narcotic Agonist and Antagonist Agents

1. a, **2.** b, **3.** a, **4.** d, **5.** c

Chapter 16 Anesthetic Agents

1. a, **2.** b, **3.** a, **4.** d, **5.** b, **6.** a, **7.** d, **8.** c

Unit 6: Drugs to Improve Cardiovascular Function

Chapter 17 Cardiac Glycoside Agents and Phosphodiesterase Inhibitors

1. b, **2.** b, **3.** a, **4.** d, **5.** b, **6.** b

Chapter 18 Antiarrhythmic Agents

1. a, **2.** c, **3.** b, **4.** d, **5.** a, **6.** b

Chapter 19 Antianginal Agents

1. b, **2.** c, **3.** c, **4.** d, **5.** a, **6.** d

Chapter 20 Antihypertensive Agents

1. c, **2.** d, **3.** a, **4.** b, **5.** b, **6.** a

Chapter 21 Diuretic Agents

1. a, **2.** d, **3.** c, **4.** d, **5.** d, **6.** a

Chapter 22 Antilipemic Agents

1. c, **2.** d, **3.** a, **4.** a, **5.** b, **6.** d

Unit 7: Drugs Affecting the Hematologic System

Chapter 23 Hematinic Agents

1. c, **2.** a, **3.** b, **4.** d, **5.** c, **6.** b

Chapter 24 Anticoagulant and Thrombolytic Agents

1. c, **2.** c, **3.** a, **4.** a, **5.** d

Unit 8: Drugs to Improve Respiratory Function

Chapter 25 Methylxanthine Agents

1. b, **2.** b, **3.** c, **4.** d, **5.** a

Chapter 26 Expectorant, Antitussive, Mucolytic, and Decongestant Agents

1. b, **2.** b, **3.** d, **4.** c, **5.** a, **6.** d

Unit 9: Drugs to Improve Gastrointestinal Function

Chapter 27 Peptic Ulcer Agents

1. a, **2.** c, **3.** d, **4.** b

Chapter 28 Adsorbent, Antiflatulent, and Digestive Agents

1. a, **2.** c, **3.** d, **4.** b

Chapter 29 Antidiarrheal and Laxative Agents

1. d, **2.** a, **3.** b, **4.** a

Chapter 30 Antiemetic and Emetic Agents

1. b, **2.** d, **3.** c, **4.** a

Unit 10: Drugs to Prevent or Treat Infection

Chapter 31 Antibacterial Agents
1. a, **2.** b, **3.** d, **4.** d, **5.** c, **6.** c

Chapter 32 Antiviral Agents
1. d, **2.** c, **3.** d, **4.** b

Chapter 33 Antitubercular Agents
1. d, **2.** c, **3.** d, **4.** a

Chapter 34 Antimycotic (Antifungal) Agents
1. b, **2.** c, **3.** d, **4.** d

Chapter 35 Anthelmintic Agents
1. b, **2.** a, **3.** d

Chapter 36 Antimalarial and Other Antiprotozoal Agents
1. a, **2.** c, **3.** b, **4.** d

Chapter 37 Urinary Antiseptic Agents
1. b, **2.** c, **3.** d, **4.** a

Unit 11: Drugs to Control Inflammation, Allergy, and Organ Rejection

Chapter 38 Antihistaminic Agents
1. b, **2.** c, **3.** b, **4.** d, **5.** c

Chapter 39 Corticosteroid and Other Immunosuppressant Agents
1. b, **2.** d, **3.** a, **4.** d

Chapter 40 Uricosurics, Other Antigout Agents, and Gold Salts
1. d, **2.** b, **3.** a, **4.** c, **5.** c, **6.** d, **7.** d

Unit 12: Drugs to Alter Psychogenic Behavior and Promote Sleep

Chapter 41 Sedative and Hypnotic Agents
1. b, **2.** c, **3.** d, **4.** d, **5.** d, **6.** c, **7.** b

Chapter 42 Antidepressant and Antimanic Agents
1. d, **2.** d, **3.** c, **4.** d, **5.** c, **6.** c, **7.** d

Chapter 43 Antianxiety Agents
1. d, **2.** b, **3.** c, **4.** d

Chapter 44 Antipsychotic Agents
1. b, **2.** b, **3.** a, **4.** c, **5.** d

Unit 13: Drugs to Treat Endocrine System Disorders

Chapter 45 Antidiabetic Agents and Glucagon
1. c, **2.** d, **3.** d, **4.** c

Chapter 46 Thyroid, Antithyroid, and Parathyroid Agents
1. a, **2.** a, **3.** b

Chapter 47 Pituitary Agents
1. a, **2.** d, **3.** d, **4.** a

Chapter 48 Estrogens, Progestins, and Oral Contraceptive Agents
1. b, **2.** a, **3.** d, **4.** c, **5.** c, **6.** b

Chapter 49 Androgenic and Anabolic Steroid Agents
1. a, **2.** b, **3.** c, **4.** b

Unit 14: Drugs for Fluid, Electrolyte, and Nutritional Balance

Chapter 50 Vitamin and Mineral Agents
1. a, **2.** d, **3.** c, **4.** c, **5.** b, **6.** c

Chapter 51 Electrolyte Replacement Agents
1. a, **2.** c, **3.** b, **4.** d, **5.** c

Chapter 52 Alkalinizing and Acidifying Agents
1. a, **2.** b, **3.** c, **4.** a, **5.** b

Unit 15: Drugs to Treat Malignant Neoplasms

Chapter 53 Alkylating Agents
1. a, **2.** d, **3.** c, **4.** c, **5.** c, **6.** a

Chapter 54 Antimetabolite Agents
1. b, **2.** b, **3.** d, **4.** c, **5.** b, **6.** d

Chapter 55 Antibiotic Antineoplastic Agents
1. d, **2.** d, **3.** a, **4.** a

Chapter 56 Hormonal Antineoplastic Agents
1. b, **2.** d, **3.** c, **4.** b, **5.** b

Chapter 57 Other Antineoplastic Agents
1. c, **2.** a, **3.** d, **4.** a, **5.** c, **6.** a

Unit 16: Other Major Drugs

Chapter 58 Ophthalmic Agents
1. b, **2.** d, **3.** b, **4.** d

Chapter 59 Otic Agents
1. a, **2.** d, **3.** b, **4.** a

Chapter 60 Dermatologic Agents
1. a, **2.** d, **3.** d, **4.** c, **5.** d

Chapter 61 Uncategorized and Other Agents
1. c, **2.** b, **3.** d, **4.** b, **5.** b, **6.** a

Appendix 2

Complementary therapies

Complementary therapies, such as environmental medicine, herbal remedies, holistic medicine, naturopathy, and traditional Chinese medicine, are used by some patients to replace or augment drug therapy in treating various disorders. A recent study estimated that Americans made about 425 million visits to providers of complementary therapy during a 1-year survey period — far more than the number of visits to all U.S. primary care doctors during the same period (388 million). The most common medical conditions reported by respondents were back problems, allergies, arthritis, insomnia, sprains or strains, headache, high blood pressure, digestive problems, anxiety, and depression.

Because more people are turning to complementary therapies, more health care professionals are learning about them and applying them in their practice. In addition, the federal government recently established an Office for the Study of Unconventional Medical Practices at the National Institutes of Health to promote scholarly research and education about complementary therapies.

This concise guide presents selected complementary therapies, some of which may be familiar to you. Be aware, however, that some methods may not be officially approved for use in the United States. This guide is solely informational and does not imply endorsement of the therapies listed.

ACUPUNCTURE

This ancient Chinese practice involves puncturing the body with special needles at specific points called acupoints. The needles stimulate deep nerve endings to cure disease or relieve pain.

Acupuncture is based on the theory that life energy (qi or chi) circulates throughout the body along 12 to 14 major energy pathways called meridians. The qi is thought to concentrate at some 500 to 1,000 acupoints along these meridians. Stimulation of acupoints with needles, heat (as in moxibustion), or hand pressure (as in shiatsu) is thought to release trapped life energy, thereby readjusting the energy balance of the body.

Acupuncture is used to treat a wide range of physical illnesses as well as mental illnesses and drug addiction. It has also been successfully used to provide anesthesia during complex surgical procedures such as open-heart surgery.

AROMATHERAPY

A form of herbal medicine, aromatherapy uses essential oils (concentrated plant extracts) that are believed to exert tranquilizing and antimicrobial effects. The oils are inhaled, added to a bath, or applied during massage to treat headaches, sleep problems, chronic pain, and anxiety and to stimulate the immune system to fight infections.

BACH FLOWER REMEDIES

A combination of homeopathic and herbal medicine, this alternative therapy employs extracts from certain flowers, trees, and grasses to treat emotional and psychological problems that predispose a person to mental and organic illnesses. The extracts are taken with liquids or placed under the tongue. They're used for 1 to 12 weeks until symptoms disappear.

BEE VENOM THERAPY

In homeopathy, an extreme dilution of honeybee extract may be used to treat a disorder whose symptoms mimic those produced by the remedy. Conventional medicine uses bee venom to desensitize susceptible persons to bee stings. This immunotherapy uses whole-venom antigens with maintenance doses for up to 5 years.

CELL THERAPY

This therapy involves injection of living or freeze-dried cellular material prepared from embryos, fetuses, or adult organ tissues into the body to stimulate the immune system and treat certain degenerative diseases. For example, human fetal cell transplants are being tested as treatments for Parkinson's and Alzheimer's diseases. The technique is also used in an attempt to slow the aging process and to treat various cancers.

CHELATION THERAPY

A form of detoxification, chelation therapy involves an injection or oral administration of ethylene diamine tetra-acetic acid (EDTA). A synthetic amino acid, EDTA attaches to toxic substances (such as lead, cadmium, aluminum, and other metals) in the blood to facilitate their removal from the body in urine.

Because EDTA is also believed to remove excess calcium from the body, it's used by some practitioners to treat hardening of the arteries (atherosclerosis), heart attack, stroke, other blood vessel diseases, arthritis, and gangrene.

CHINESE HERBAL THERAPY

An important part of traditional Chinese medicine, herbs are classified according to their taste, which signifies their medicinal action and, in many cases, their natural affinity to particular body organs. Herbs are used to enhance immune function and treat stress as well as to treat skin, intestinal, joint, and menstrual problems.

COBRA VENOM THERAPY

In homeopathy, an extremely diluted form of snake venom may be used to treat a disorder whose symptoms mimic those produced by the remedy. Cobra venom is claimed to be effective against arthritis.

COLONIC THERAPY

In this type of hydrotherapy, filtered water is passed through a tube into a person's colon under light pressure; the colon's contents are gently flushed out to remove toxins. A variant of this, colonic ozone therapy, maintains that the body needs pure oxygen to thrive.

Colonic therapy is used to treat headache and backache as well as indigestion, constipation, and other stomach and intestinal conditions.

COLORED LIGHT THERAPY

This form of light therapy uses intermittent or steady beams of red, blue, or white light, which are thought to stimulate parts of the nervous system and influence production of certain chemicals in the brain. Also called photostimulation, colored light therapy has been used for sleep disorders, chronic pain, anxiety, allergies, diabetes, and wound healing.

CUPPING

Used in Ayurvedic and traditional Chinese medicine, heated suction cups are placed over wounds and abscesses to improve local circulation. Cupping also may be used with bloodletting at the cupping sites. Its proponents claim that the practice treats high blood pressure, abdominal pain, or arthritis.

DETOXIFICATION THERAPY

A form of naturopathy, this therapy hinges on the claim that the body is a "bioaccumulator." As a result, the body becomes contaminated with a wide variety of toxic chemicals and pollutants (such as pesticides, food additives, and drug residues) that ultimately impair the immune system and lead to disease.

Detoxification therapies include juice and water fasting, chelation, and nutritional, herbal, and homeopathic methods to assist the body's natural cleaning processes. The therapy may be used to treat headaches, joint or back pain, arthritis, insomnia, allergies, and mood disorders.

ECLECTICISM

In the early 1800s, eclecticism took root in the United States. It employs herbal medicine, purgatives, enemas, and steam baths. It's based on the theory that illness results from imbalances among the four elements: earth, air, fire, and water. Eclecticism encouraged people to treat themselves from a special medical manual.

ENEMAS

In this form of hydrotherapy, the large intestine (called the colon) is irrigated with water or other solutions to aid defecation. Enemas differ from colonic therapy primarily in that they clean only the last 8" to 12" (20 to 30 cm) of the large intestine. Enemas are used to relieve constipation and remove toxic substances.

ENVIRONMENTAL MEDICINE

Here, environmental factors are considered to contribute to a person's illness. These factors include diet, airborne pollutants, molds, pollen, harmful radiation from the earth, and the many chemicals used in everyday products.

Environmental medicine approaches are used to treat food and other allergies, chemical sensitivity, and rheumatoid arthritis.

ENZYME THERAPY

This form of nutritional therapy prescribes dietary supplements containing plant enzymes or pancreatic enzymes to aid the body's natural digestion. Raw vegetables also are prescribed for their enzyme content as well as their obvious nutritional benefits. The therapy is used to treat inflammation and various intestinal disorders.

FISH OIL THERAPY

Cold water fish, such as herring, salmon, or sardines, are rich in omega-3 fatty acids — polyunsaturated fats that are believed to have some beneficial effect in treating breast cancer and reducing the inflammation of arthritis.

HERBAL REMEDIES

The use of plants, plant parts, and plant extracts to treat diseases is an important part of folk medicine worldwide. Herbal remedies also are employed in traditional Chinese medicine, homeopathy, and Ayurvedic medicine.

Many of today's prescription drugs have an herbal origin. For instance, the widely used cardiac glycoside digoxin comes from the foxglove flower. Reserpine, an antihypertensive agent, comes from Indian snakeroot. The narcotic analgesic morphine comes from the opium poppy.

Herbs are used to cure (garlic to kill germs), to prevent problems (rosemary as an insect repellent), and to relieve pain and discomfort (aloe vera for arthritis pain and for minor burns).

HOLISTIC MEDICINE

This system of medicine focuses on the entire person, not just the illness. It's based on three principles: recognition of the psychological, environmental, and social contributions to the patient's illness; involvement of the patient in treatment; and emphasis on preventive medicine and lifestyles that reduce the risk of developing an illness.

Holistic medicine includes acupuncture, shiatsu (acupressure), chiropractic, herbal medicine, spiritual healing, and other complementary therapies.

HOMEOPATHY

This system of medicine hinges on the belief that the symptoms of an illness are evidence of a curative process going on within the body in response to the disease. The homeopathic practitioner attempts to promote the further development of these symptoms to accelerate the body's self-cure; this is the principle of "like cures like." For example, diarrhea might be treated by giving the person a tiny dose of a laxative. Other disorders treated by homeopathy include colds and flu, headaches, respiratory infections, allergies, and intestinal disorders.

HYDROGEN PEROXIDE THERAPY

In this form of oxidation therapy, hydrogen peroxide is injected to treat a wide variety of diseases. Treatment aims to use oxygen's antiseptic effect.

IMMUNO-AUGMENTATIVE THERAPY (IAT)

This treatment rests on the theory that cancer results from imbalances among four blood protein components: tumor antibody, tumor complement, blocking protein, and deblocking protein. Treatment involves injections of various amounts of the four components.

LIVINGSTON-WHEELER THERAPY

This cancer treatment assumes that a type of bacteria, called Progenitor cryptocides is found in all cancers. Treatment aims to restore the immune system through a combination of vaccines derived from cultures of the person's own bacteria, or from bacillus Calmette-Guérin, a mild tuberculin vaccine; antibiotics; megavitamins, nutritional supplements, and digestive enzymes; enemas; and a whole-foods diet that excludes eggs and poultry.

MEGAVITAMIN THERAPY

Proponents of this therapy contend that governmental Recommended Daily Allowances (RDAs) for nutrients in foods are inadequate to provide optimum health and that certain vitamins are required by the body in amounts far beyond the RDA. For example, megadoses of vitamin C have been used to treat colds, flu, infections, allergies, autoimmune diseases, burns, and viral pneumonia and to assist wound healing.

MIND-BODY MEDICINE

This therapy recognizes the role of the mind and the emotions in health, the body's innate healing capabilities, and the role of self-responsibility in the healing process. The so-called mind-body connection is being revealed as the complex interplay of the brain and the endocrine and immune systems along nerve pathways.

Knowledge gained in the new field of psychoneuroimmunology lends support to many mental healing methods such as biofeedback, meditation, guided imagery, hypnotherapy, and yoga.

NATUROPATHY

This system of holistic medicine relies on using natural agents and forces to bring about a cure. The naturopath makes use of herbs and vitamins, rather than synthetic drugs and surgery, and may also employ diet therapy, hydrotherapy, exercise, chiropractic therapy, bodywork, homeopathy, electrical treatments, and counseling on preventive medicine and lifestyle modification.

NEURAL THERAPY

In this form of energy medicine, small amounts of anesthetics are injected into various acupuncture points to restore normal flow to the body's electrical force fields in tissues that lie in the area of injury. Neural therapy is used to treat many kinds of disorders.

OXYGEN THERAPY

Use of various forms of oxygen (ozone, peroxide, or as gas under pressure) purportedly promotes healing and destroys toxins in the body. It's based on the theory that the body's normal oxidation processes (in which electrons are donated from one molecular substance to another in normal chemical reactions) may be imbalanced due to environmental stress or disease. By supplying additional oxygen, the treatment restores this balance.

Oxygen may be used with other therapies to treat lung disorders, multiple sclerosis, infections, and arthritis.

OZONE THERAPY

This form of oxygen therapy employs ozone, a less stable but more reactive form of oxygen. It's used to treat infections, arthritis, hepatitis, allergies, and various pain disorders and to assist wound healing.

PLACEBO EFFECT

A placebo is an inert substance made to appear indistinguishable from an authentic drug. It may be prescribed when there's no apparent physical cause of an illness. The placebo effect is attributed to psychological factors that influence the body at some chemical level.

In conditions involving the nervous system, such as pain or anxiety, placebo effects commonly mimic the effects of an active drug. Placebos have been used to treat arthritis, chest pain (angina), and other chronic pain problems.

RECONSTRUCTIVE THERAPY

A nonsurgical method, reconstructive therapy attempts to repair torn ligaments and other damaged joint structures with injections of mild irritating solutions. The injections stimulate the body to generate new connective tissue and enhance healing. The therapy is used for arthritis, carpal tunnel syndrome, migraine headaches, degenerative bone disorders, herniated discs, and bursitis.

REJUVENATION

A part of the Ayurvedic medical regimen, this isn't a treatment all by itself. Rejuvenation follows a program of cleaning and detoxification procedures and is a "physiological tuneup" involving administration of herbal and mineral preparations as well as use of certain yoga and breathing exercises.

SHARK CARTILAGE THERAPY

This treatment of cancer hinges on the idea that cartilage, a type of connective tissue, contains compounds that prevent formation of blood vessels. Treating tumors with cartilage cuts off their blood supply, thereby stopping tumor growth and killing tumor cells. The cartilage, derived from sharks, is applied using a retention enema or injection.

TRADITIONAL CHINESE MEDICINE

This complete system of medicine emphasizes lifestyle modification, diet, and exercise to prevent illness. Health is believed to result from a person's ability to adjust successfully to changes within the body and within the natural world and to maintain a balance between opposing physical forces — the yin and yang. These forces flow along specific pathways (meridians) that form a complex energy network in the body.

Medicinal herbs, acupuncture, diet therapy, massage, and therapeutic exercise are used to correct yin-yang imbalances that cause disease.

Appendix 3

Drugs that should not be crushed

Each time a nurse prepares to administer a solid drug for a patient who can't swallow a tablet or capsule whole, care must be taken not to crush or dissolve the drug if doing so impairs its effectiveness or absorption. Many drug forms, such as slow release, enteric coated, encapsulated beads, wax matrix, sublingual, or buccal preparations, are made to release their active ingredients over a certain period of time or at preset points after administration. The disruptions caused by crushing those formulations can dramatically affect absorption rate and increase the risk of adverse reactions.

Other reasons not to crush a drug form involve such considerations as taste, tissue irritation, and unusual formulation—for example, a capsule within a capsule, a liquid within a capsule, or a multiple compressed tablet. Avoid crushing the following drugs, listed here by brand name, for the reasons noted beside them.

Accutane (mucous membrane irritant)
Acutrim (slow release)
Adipost capsules (slow release)
Aerolate SR, JR, III (slow release)
Aller-Chlor (slow release)
Allerest 12-Hour (slow release)
Ammonium Chloride Enseals (enteric coated)
Artane Sequels (slow release)
Asbron G INLAY (multiple compressed tablet)
Atrohist LA, Sprinkle (slow release)
Azulfidine EN-Tabs (enteric coated)
Bellergal-S (slow release)
Betachron E-R (slow release)
Betapen-VK (taste)
Bisacodyl (enteric coated)
Bisco-Lax (enteric coated)
Bontril Slow-Release (slow release)
Breonesin (liquid filled)
Brexin LA (slow release)
Bromfed (slow release)
Bromfed-PD (slow release)
Bromphen (slow release)
Bromphen TD (slow release)
Calan SR (slow release)
Carbiset-TR (slow release)
Cardizem CD, SR (slow release)
Carter's Little Pills (enteric coated)
Ceftin (taste)
Cerespan (slow release)
Charcoal Plus (enteric coated)
Chloral Hydrate (liquid within a capsule, taste)
Chlor-Trimeton Decongestant Repetabs (slow release)
Chlor-Trimeton Repetabs(slow release)
Choledyl (enteric coated)
Choledyl SA (slow release)
Cipro (taste)
Codimal-LA (slow release)
Colace (liquid within a capsule, taste)
Comhist LA (slow release)
Compazine Spansules (slow release)
Congess SR, JR (slow release)
Constant-T (slow release)
Contac 12-Hour, Maximum
Strength 12-Hour (slow release)
Control (slow release)
Cotazym-S (enteric coated)
Creon (enteric coated)
Cystospaz-M (slow release)
Dallergy (slow release)
Dallergy D, JR (slow release)
Deconamine SR (slow release)
Deconsal, Sprinkle Capsules (slow release)
Dehist (slow release)
Demazin Repetabs (slow release)
Depakene (slow release, mucous membrane irritant)
Depakote (enteric coated)
Desoxyn Gradumet (slow release)
Desyrel (taste)
Dexatrim (slow release)
Dexedrine Spansules (slow release)
Diamox Sequels (slow release)
Dilatrate-SR (slow release)
Dimetane Extentabs (slow release)
Dimetapp Extentabs (slow release)
Disobrom (slow release)
Donnatal Extentabs (slow release)

Donnazyme (slow release)
Drisdol (liquid filled)
Drixoral (slow release)
Drixoral Sinus (slow release)
Drize (slow release)
Dulcolax (enteric coated)
Duotrate (slow release)
Duraquin (slow release)
Easprin (enteric coated)
Ecotrin (enteric coated)
Ecotrin Maximum Strength (enteric coated)
E.E.S. 400 Filmtab (enteric coated)
Elixophyllin SR (slow release)
E-Mycin (enteric coated)
Endafed (slow release)
Entex LA (slow release)
Entozyme (enteric coated)
Equanil (taste)
Ergostat (sublingual)
Eryc (enteric coated)
Ery-Tab (enteric coated)
Erythrocin Stearate (enteric coated)
Erythromycin Base (enteric coated)
Eskalith CR (slow release)
Extendryl SR, JR (slow release)
Fedahist Gyrocaps, Timecaps (slow release)
Feldene (mucous membrane irritant)
Feocyte (slow release)
Feosol (enteric coated)
Feratab (enteric coated)
Fergon (slow release)
Fero-Grad-500 (slow release)
Fero-Gradumet (slow release)
Ferralet SR (slow release)
Ferralyn Lanacap (slow release)
Ferro-Sequel (slow release)
Feverall Children's Capsules, Sprinkle (taste)
Fumatinic (slow release)
Genabid (slow release)
Geocillin (taste)
Gris-PEG (crushing may cause precipitation of larger particles)
Guaifed (slow release)
Guaifed-PD (slow release)
Humibid Sprinkle, DM, DM Sprinkle, LA (slow release)
Hydergine LC (liquid within a capsule)
Hytakerol (liquid filled)
Iberet (slow release)
Iberet-500 (slow release)
ICaps Plus (slow release)
ICaps Time Release (slow release)
Ilotycin (enteric coated)
Inderal LA (slow release)
Inderide LA (slow release)
Indocin SR (slow release)
Ionamin (slow release)
Iso-Bid (slow release)
Isoclor Timesules (slow release)
Isoptin SR (slow release)
Isordil Sublingual (sublingual)
Isordil Tembids (slow release)
Isosorbide Dinitrate Sublingual (sublingual)
Isuprel Glossets (sublingual)
Kaon Cl (slow release)
K-Dur (slow release)
Klor-Con (slow release)
Klotrix (slow release)
K-Tab (slow release)
Levsinex Timecaps (slow release)
Lithobid (slow release)
Lodrane LD (slow release)
Meprospan (slow release)
Mestinon Timespans (slow release)
Micro-K (slow release)
Micro-K Extencaps (slow release)
Motrin (taste)
MS Contin (slow release)
Naldecon (slow release)
Niac (slow release)
Nico-400 (slow release)
Nicobid (slow release)
Nicobid Tempules (slow release)
Nitro-Bid (slow release)
Nitroglyn (slow release)

Nitrong (sublingual)
Nitrospan (slow release)
Nitrostat (sublingual)
Noctec (liquid within a capsule)
Nolamine (slow release)
Nolex LA (slow release)
Norflex (slow release)
Norpace CR (slow release)
Novafed (slow release)
Novafed A (slow release)
Oramorph SR (slow release)
Ornade Spansules (slow release)
Pabalate (enteric coated)
Pancrease (enteric coated)
Pancrease MT (enteric coated)
PBZ-SR (slow release)
PCE (slow release)
Perdiem (wax coated)
Peritrate SA (slow release)
Phazyme (slow release)
Phazyme 95 (slow release)
Phenergan (taste)
Phyllocontin (slow release)
Plendil (slow release)
Polaramine Repetabs (slow release)
Poly-Histine D (slow release)
Prelu-2 (slow release)
Prevacid (delayed release)
Prilosec (slow release)
Pro-Banthine (taste)
Procainamide HCL SR (slow release)
Procan SR (slow release)
Procardia (delayed absorption)
Procardia XL (slow release)
Pronestyl-SR (slow release)
Proventil Repetabs (slow release)
Prozac (slow release)
Quadra Hist (slow release)
Quibron-T/SR (slow release)
Quinaglute Dura-Tabs (slow release)
Quinidex Extentabs (slow release)
Respaire SR (slow release)
Respbid (slow release)
Ritalin SR (slow release)
Rondec TR (slow release)
Ru-Tuss (slow release)
Ru-Tuss DE, II (slow release)
Sinemet CR (slow release)
Singlet (slow release)
Slo-bid Gyrocaps (slow release)
Slo-Niacin (slow release)
Slo-Phyllin GG, Gyrocaps (slow release)
Slow-Fe (slow release)
Slow-K (slow release)
Slow-Mag (slow release)
Sorbitrate SA (slow release)
Span-FF (slow release)
Sparine (taste)
S-P-T (liquid gelatin suspension)
Sudafed 12-Hour (slow release)
Sustaire (slow release)
Tamine SR (slow release)
Tavist-D (multiple compressed tablet)
Teldrin (slow release)
Teldrin Spansules (slow release)
Ten-K (slow release)
Tenuate Dospan (slow release)
Tepanil Ten-Tab (slow release)
Tessalon Perles (slow release)
Theobid Duracap, JR Duracap (slow release)
Theochron (slow release)
Theoclear LA (slow release)
Theo-Dur (slow release)
Theo-Dur Sprinkle (slow release)
Theolair-SR (slow release)
Theo-Sav (slow release)
Theospan-SR (slow release)
Theo-Time (slow release)
Theo-24 (slow release)
TheOvent (slow release)
Theo-x (slow release)
Thorazine Spansule (slow release)
Toprol XL (slow release)
T-Phyl (slow release)
Tranxene-SD (slow release)
Trental (slow release)

Triaminic (slow release)
Triaminic TR (slow release)
Triaminic-12 (slow release)
Trilafon Repetabs (slow release)
Trinalin Repetabs (slow release)
Triptone Caplets (slow release)
Tuss-LA (slow release)
Tuss-Ornade Spansules (slow release)
Tylenol Extended Relief (slow release)
ULR-LA (slow release)
Uniphyl (slow release)
Valrelease (slow release)
Verelan (slow release)
Verin (slow release)
Voltaren-XR (enteric coated)
Wellbutrin (mucous-membrane anesthetic)
Wyamycin S (slow release)
Wygesic (taste)
ZORprin (slow release)
Zymase (enteric coated)

Appendix 4

Active immunity agents

Vaccines and toxoids provide active immunity. This chart presents indications, usual dosages, and nursing implications for the major active immunity agents.

DRUG	MAJOR INDICATIONS AND USUAL DOSAGES	NURSING IMPLICATIONS
diphtheria and tetanus toxoids and pertussis vaccine (DTP)	*Immunity to diphtheria, tetanus, and pertussis* PEDIATRIC: 0.5 ml I.M. at ages 2, 4, 6, and 15 to 18 months, followed by a booster before school entry (ages 4 to 6)	• Do not administer a live attenuated virus to an immunocompromised patient because the virus can cause the disease; wait until immunotherapy has been discontinued for 3 months. • Withhold DTP in a patient with an acute febrile illness to avoid the problem of differentiating signs and symptoms of illness from those of reaction; children should return for DTP as soon as they are well.
***haemophilus influenzae* and type b conjugate vaccine (HbOC and PRP-OMP)**	*Prevention of* Haemophilus influenzae *infections* PEDIATRIC: ages 2 to 6 months, 0.5 mg I.M.; the HbOC vaccine is given in three doses at 2-month intervals followed by a fourth dose at age 15 months; the PRP-OMP vaccine is given in two doses at 2-month intervals followed by a third dose at age 15 to 18 months	• Administer in the outer aspect area of the vastus lateralis or deltoid muscle. • Do not administer I.V. • Follow the initial dose of HbOC with two doses of HbOC. • Follow the initial dose of PRP-OMP with two doses of PRP-OMP; do not substitute HbOC.
hepatitis B vaccine, recombinant (Engerix-B, Recombivax HB)	*Immunity to hepatitis B and subtypes of hepatitis B* ADULT: 1 ml I.M., followed by another 1-ml dose 1 month later, and a third 1-ml dose 6 months after the first dose; for an immunocompromised patient or one receiving dialysis, 2 ml I.M., followed by another 2-ml dose 1 month later, and a third 2-ml dose 6 months after the first dose (the 2-ml doses should be divided into two 1-ml doses and administered at different sites) PEDIATRIC: over age 10, same as adult; neonates and children up to age 10, 0.5 ml I.M., followed by another 0.5-ml dose 1 month later, and a third 0.5-ml dose 6 months after the first dose	• Administer cautiously to a patient with a serious, active infection or compromised cardiac or pulmonary status or one for whom a febrile or systemic reaction could pose a serious risk. • Administer the hepatitis B vaccine in the arm rather than the buttock. The Centers for Disease Control and Prevention reports that administration in the arm produces a significantly better response to the vaccine. • Administer the vaccine subcutaneously *only* to patients who are at risk for hemorrhage such as hemophiliacs. • Agitate the vial thoroughly just before administration to restore suspension. • Store opened and unopened vials in the refrigerator. Do not freeze the vaccine. • Be aware that the recommended dosages in micrograms for Engerix-B and Recombivax HB are different. Select the correct preparation and dosage for each.
influenza virus vaccine, trivalent types A and B (whole or split virus)	*Prevention of influenza virus infection* ADULT: 0.5 ml of whole or split virus vaccine I.M. in the deltoid PEDIATRIC: over age 12, same as adult; ages 9 to 12, 0.5 ml of split virus vaccine I.M.; ages 3 to 8, 0.5 ml of split virus vaccine I.M. repeated in 4 weeks; ages 6 to 35 months, 0.25 ml of split virus vaccine I.M. repeated in 4 weeks	• Do not administer to a patient who is allergic to eggs. • Defer or delay immunization if the patient has an acute respiratory illness. • Be aware that influenza and pneumococcal vaccines can be administered to children at the same time in different sites without increased adverse effects.
measles, mumps, and rubella virus vaccine, live (M-M-RII)	*Prevention of measles, mumps, and rubella* PEDIATRIC: 0.5 ml S.C. at age 12 to 15 months, followed by a second at age 4 to 6 years or 11 to 12 years	• Be aware that M-M-RII is contraindicated in a patient with severe febrile illness and after the administration of antimetabolites, steroids, or steroidlike medications. • Do not administer M-M-RII to a patient who is allergic to eggs or neomycin. • Do not administer to an immunocompromised patient; M-M-RII may be given after chemotherapy has been discontinued for 3 months. • Do not administer to a woman of childbearing age; if the vaccine is given, the woman must not become pregnant for 3 months.

Active immunity agents *(continued)*

DRUG	MAJOR INDICATIONS AND USUAL DOSAGES	NURSING IMPLICATIONS
measles, mumps, and rubella virus vaccine, live (M-M-RII) *(continued)*		• Know that children age 6 months and over can be immunized during a measles outbreak but must be reimmunized at age 15 months. • Administer live-virus vaccines on the same day. If this is not possible, wait at least 1 month before administering another live-virus vaccine. • Have epinephrine (1:1,000) readily available to treat anaphylactic reactions should they occur. • Do not administer M-M-RII I.V. • Refrigerate M-M-RII vaccine at 36° to 46° F (2° to 8° C). • Protect the vaccine from heat and light.
pneumococcal vaccine, polyvalent	*Prevention of pneumococcal diseases, such as pneumonia and meningitis* ADULT: 0.5 ml I.M. or S.C. PEDIATRIC: age 2 and over, same as adult	• Do not administer to a patient with known hypersensitivity to a portion of the vaccine or to a patient receiving immunosuppressive therapy. • Know that influenza and pneumococcal vaccines can be administered to children at the same time in different sites without increased adverse effects. • Consider a booster dose or routine revaccination after 3 to 5 years for a child with nephrotic syndrome, asplenia, or sickle cell anemia or one with a rapid decline in antibody levels who would be age 10 or younger at revaccination. • Do not administer this vaccine I.V.
poliovirus vaccine, live, oral, trivalent (TOPV)	*Immunity to poliovirus* ADULT: 0.5 ml P.O.; primary series is administered in three doses—the first two doses are given 6 to 8 weeks apart, and a third dose is given 12 months later PEDIATRIC: same as adult; if given to infants, the first dose is given at age 2 months, the second dose at 4 months, the third dose at 15 to 18 months, and the fourth dose at 4 to 6 years	• Be aware that TOPV is contraindicated in an immunocompromised patient; administer the inactivated form. • Avoid administering TOPV to a pregnant patient or one with diarrhea, vomiting, or an acute illness. • Administer by mouth only. • Administer live-virus vaccines on the same day. If this is not possible, wait at least 1 month before administering another live-virus vaccine. • Store frozen TOPV at 7° F (–13° C). Once thawed, store it at 36° to 46° F (2° to 8° C) and use within 30 days.
varicella virus vaccine	*Prevention of varicella infection* ADULT: 0.5 ml S.C., followed by 0.5 ml S.C. 4 to 8 weeks after the first dose PEDIATRIC: 0.5 ml S.C. as a single dose between age 12 months and 12 years	• Be aware that varicella virus vaccine is contraindicated in a pregnant or immunocompromised patient or one with hypersensitivity to any component of the drug, a history of anaphylactic reaction to neomycin, or blood dyscrasias. • Avoid administering the vaccine to a patient with a fever. • Instruct the patient to avoid salicylates for 6 weeks after vaccination because Reye's syndrome has been reported after salicylate use during varicella infection. • Administer the vaccine subcutaneously in the deltoid muscle. • Store unreconstituted vaccine frozen at 5° F (–15° C). After reconstitution, store it at 36° to 46° F (2° to 8° C) for up to 72 hours.

Appendix 5

Passive immunity agents

This chart presents indications, usual dosages, and nursing implications for the major passive immunity agents.

DRUG	MAJOR INDICATIONS AND USUAL DOSAGES	NURSING IMPLICATIONS
hepatitis B immune globulin (HBIG)	*Exposure to hepatitis B; posthepatitis exposure prophylaxis* ADULT: 0.06 ml/kg I.M. (most adults will receive a dose of 3 to 5 ml) within 7 days after exposure; a second injection is given 28 to 30 days later PEDIATRIC: same as adult; for neonates whose mothers are HBsAg-positive, 0.5 ml I.M. as soon as possible after birth and no later than 24 hours after birth; this dose is repeated at ages 3 months and 6 months	• Be aware that HBIG requires cautious use in a patient who has experienced systemic allergic reactions to other human immunoglobulins. • Administer HBIG to a pregnant patient only when clearly indicated and ordered. • Administer HBIG I.M., preferably into the deltoid in adults and older children and into the vastus lateralis in infants and young children; always aspirate to be sure the injection is not inadvertently administered I.V. • Store HBIG at 36° to 46° F (2° to 8° C); do not freeze. • Teach an adult patient the importance of receiving the second dose. Inform parents about the importance of obtaining the second and third doses for their child.
rabies immune globulin (RIG)	*Exposure to rabies, postrabies prophylaxis* ADULT: 20 IU/kg; about half the dose should be used to infiltrate the wound and the remainder administered I.M. PEDIATRIC: same as adult	• Be aware that RIG requires cautious use in a patient with a history of systemic hypersensitivity reactions to immunoglobulins or known allergy to thimerosal. • Know the risks and benefits of RIG for patients with isolated immunoglobulin A (IgA) deficiency because hypersensitivity can develop from increased antibodies to IgA. Anaphylaxis can occur with subsequent administration of products that contain IgA. • Teach the patient about the predictable adverse reactions. • Administer the medication I.M. in the deltoid in adults and older children; inject it into the vastus lateralis in infants and young children. • Store RIG at 36° to 46° F; do not freeze. • Expect RIG and human diploid cell rabies vaccine to be administered if treatment against rabies is necessary. Do not administer these medications at the same site or in the same syringe.
tetanus immune globulin (TIG)	*Susceptible wounds in nonimmunized patients, posttetanus prophylaxis* ADULT: 250 to 500 U I.M. PEDIATRIC: same as adult *Treatment of tetanus* ADULT: 3,000 to 6,000 U I.M. PEDIATRIC: same as adult	• Be aware that TIG is contraindicated in a patient with known hypersensitivity to immune globulin (IG) or thimerosal. • Do not perform a skin test with TIG because an area of inflammation after the injection may be interpreted as a positive skin reaction when actually it is a chemical irritation of the tissues. • Administer TIG I.M. to decrease the risk of anaphylaxis. • Monitor closely for anaphylaxis and a sharp decrease in blood pressure if TIG must be administered I.V. • Store TIG at 36° to 46° F. If the TIG has been frozen, do not use it. • Encourage the patient to schedule follow-up visits if the wound does not heal.
varicella-zoster immune globulin (VZIG)	*Exposure to chickenpox of immunocompromised children* PEDIATRIC: children weighing up to 22 lb (10 kg), 125 U I.M.; 22 to 44 lb (20 kg), 250 U I.M.; 44 to 66 lb (30 kg), 375 U I.M.; 66 to 88 lb (40 kg), 500 U I.M.; over 88 lb, 625 U I.M.	• Be aware that VZIG is contraindicated in a patient with a history of severe hypersensitivity reactions to IG and in patients with severe thrombocytopenia. • Know that VZIG is not recommended during pregnancy. The pregnant patient and her physician should determine if the benefits outweigh the risks. • Administer VZIG I.M. to avoid anaphylaxis, which may occur with I.V. injection. • Do not administer fractional doses. • Help the family plan a bland diet if the child experiences GI distress.

Appendix 6

Uterine motility agents

This table summarizes the major uterine motility agents currently in clinical use.

DRUG	MAJOR INDICATIONS AND USUAL ADULT DOSAGES	NURSING IMPLICATIONS
Prostaglandins		
carboprost tromethamine (Hemabate, Prostin/15 M)	*Termination of pregnancy between weeks 13 and 20 of gestation* 250 mcg deep I.M., followed by 250 to 500 mcg I.M. every 1½ to 3½ hours as needed *Postpartal hemorrhage* 250 mcg deep I.M., repeated every 15 to 90 minutes, as needed	• Be aware that carboprost tromethamine is contraindicated in a patient with known hypersensitivity or a history of pelvic inflammatory disease. • Know that this drug requires cautious use in a patient with cervical lacerations or uterine rupture. • Monitor uterine contractions and cervical dilation frequently. • Monitor the patient's vital signs regularly, particularly noting hypotension or fever. • Do not administer the drug repeatedly for more than 48 hours. • Store the drug in a refrigerator at 36° to 46° F (2° to 8° C).
dinoprostone (Prostin E_2)	*Termination of pregnancy between weeks 12 and 20 of gestation* One 20-mg suppository inserted high into the vagina; additional suppositories may be administered every 3 to 5 hours as needed	• Be aware that dinoprostone is contraindicated in a patient with known hypersensitivity, acute pelvic inflammatory disease, or active cardiac, pulmonary, renal, or hepatic disease. • Know that this drug requires cautious use in a patient with cervicitis; infected endocervical lesions; acute vaginitis; compromised (scarred) uterus; history of asthma, hypertension, or hypotension; epilepsy; diabetes mellitus; anemia; jaundice; or cardiovascular, renal, or hepatic disease. • Monitor uterine contractions and cervical dilation frequently. • Monitor the patient's vital signs regularly, particularly noting hypotension or fever. • Instruct the patient to remain supine for at least 10 minutes after insertion of vaginal suppository, to allow adequate absorption. • Store the suppositories in a freezer at temperatures below –4° F (–20° C), but bring them to room temperature before use.
Ergot alkaloids		
ergonovine maleate (Ergotrate maleate)	*Postpartal and postabortion hemorrhage* 0.2 mg I.M. every 2 to 4 hours to a maximum of five doses *Severe vaginal bleeding* 2 mg I.V. over at least 1 minute; after initial I.M. or I.V. dose, 0.2 to 0.4 mg P.O. every 6 to 12 hours for 2 to 7 days	• Be aware that ergonovine maleate is contraindicated in a patient with threatened spontaneous abortion, hypertension, heart disease, venoatrial shunts, mitral valve stenosis, obliterative vascular disease, or known hypersensitivity or idiosyncratic reaction to the drug. • Know that this drug requires cautious use in a patient with sepsis or hepatic or renal impairment. • Monitor the patient frequently for nausea, vomiting, hypertension, ergot poisoning, and other adverse reactions. • Dilute an I.V. preparation to a volume of 5 ml with normal saline solution. • Monitor blood pressure and uterine contractions continuously when administering the I.V. form of the drug.
methylergonovine maleate (Methergine)	*Postpartal and postabortion hemorrhage* 0.2 mg I.M. every 2 to 4 hours to a maximum of five doses *Severe vaginal bleeding* 0.2 mg I.V. over at least 1 minute; after initial I.M. or I.V. dose, 0.2 to 0.4 mg P.O. every 6 to 12 hours for 2 to 7 days	• Be aware that methylergonovine maleate is contraindicated in a patient with threatened spontaneous abortion, hypertension, heart disease, venoatrial shunts, mitral valve stenosis, obliterative vascular disease, or known hypersensitivity or idiosyncratic reaction to the drug. • Know that this drug requires cautious use in a patient with sepsis or hepatic or renal impairment. • Monitor the patient frequently for nausea, vomiting, hypertension, ergot poisoning, and other adverse reactions. • Dilute an I.V. preparation to a volume of 5 ml with 0.9% sodium chloride (normal saline) solution. • Monitor blood pressure and uterine contractions continuously when administering the I.V. form of the drug.

(continued)

Uterine motility agents *(continued)*

DRUG	MAJOR INDICATIONS AND USUAL DOSAGES	NURSING IMPLICATIONS
Tocolytic agents		
magnesium sulfate	*Prevention or treatment of seizures in preeclampsia or eclampsia* Initially, 4 g I.V. in 250 ml dextrose 5% in water (not to exceed 3 ml per minute) and 4 g deep I.M. into each buttock, followed by 4 g deep I.M. into alternate buttock every 4 hours as needed; alternatively, 4 g I.V. as a loading dose followed by 1 to 2 g hourly as an infusion *Treatment of premature labor* Initially, 4 to 6 g I.V. infused over 20 minutes, then 2 to 4 g per hour for 12 to 24 hours as tolerated after contractions cease *Hypomagnesemia* 1 g I.M. every 6 hours for four doses	• Be aware that parenteral magnesium sulfate is contraindicated in a patient with heart block or myocardial damage. • Know that this drug requires cautious use in a patient with impaired renal function. • Monitor the patient closely for adverse reactions, which typically depend on the drug dosage, the rapidity of administration, and the patient's serum magnesium level. • Be aware that a mother who receives magnesium sulfate may give birth to a neonate with hypermagnesemia, hypotonia, or central nervous system or respiratory depression. • Administer a bolus dose of the drug slowly, at a rate of 150 mg/minute, to prevent nausea, vomiting, headache, palpitations, and flushing.
ritodrine hydrochloride (Yutopar)	*Treatment of premature labor* Initially, 50 to 100 mcg/minute I.V., increased every 10 minutes by 50 mcg/minute up to a maximum of 350 mcg/minute until contractions stop or adverse reactions occur; for maintenance, 10 mg P.O. 30 minutes before stopping the I.V. infusion, repeated every 2 hours for the first 24 hours, then 10 to 20 mg P.O. every 4 to 6 hours, up to a maximum of 120 mg daily	• Be aware that ritodrine hydrochloride is contraindicated before the 20th week of pregnancy, in a patient with known hypersensitivity, or one with a condition that makes continuation of pregnancy hazardous, such as antepartal hemorrhage that demands immediate delivery, eclampsia, severe preeclampsia, intrauterine fetal death, chorioamnionitis, maternal cardiac disease, pulmonary hypertension, maternal hyperthyroidism, or uncontrolled maternal diabetes mellitus. • Know that this drug has no known precautions. • Monitor maternal vital signs and a 20- to 30-minute fetal monitor strip before initiating therapy. Also assess the maternal heart rate and blood pressure before increasing the infusion rate. • Monitor uterine activity and fetal heart rate continuously during therapy. • Prevent hypervolemia by ensuring that the I.V. infusion rate does not exceed 150 ml/hour. • Dilute drug in dextrose 5% solution rather than 0.9% sodium chloride solution to decrease risk of pulmonary edema.
terbutaline sulfate (Brethine, Bricanyl)	*Treatment of preterm labor* Initially, 2.5 mcg/minute I.V. increasing every 20 minutes by 2.5 mcg/minute to a maximum of 17.5 mcg/minute until contractions stop or adverse reactions occur; once contractions cease, continue I.V. infusion for 60 minutes to determine the lowest effective dosage; continue lowest effective dosage for at least 12 hours, then begin 15 mg P.O./day maintenance therapy	• Be aware that terbutaline sulfate is contraindicated in a patient with known hypersensitivity to any of its ingredients or to other sympathomimetic agents. • Administer with caution to a patient with diabetes mellitus, hypertension, hyperthyroidism, or a history of seizures or cardiac disease. • Know that this drug is not approved or labeled for use as a tocolytic although it is commonly used to treat preterm labor. • Monitor maternal vital signs and a 20- to 30-minute fetal monitor strip before initiating therapy. Also assess the maternal heart rate and blood pressure before increasing the infusion rate. • Monitor uterine activity and fetal heart rate continuously during therapy. • Prevent hypervolemia by ensuring that the I.V. infusion rate does not exceed 150 ml/hour • If therapy is continued beyond 1 week, periodic monitoring of oral glucose tolerance levels is recommended.

Appendix 7

Drugs used to treat poisoning

Despite an extensive campaign against it, poisoning remains a serious problem in the United States. Somewhere in the vicinity of 2 to 3 million poisonings occur annually, resulting in more than 700 deaths.

Although some poisonings result from the intentional ingestion of toxic substances and others from homicidal actions, most incidents are accidental. Drug ingestion, in many cases in conjunction with alcohol, commonly causes accidental poisoning as does the ingestion of household substances used for cleaning and maintenance. Industrial poisonings from environmental pollutants, pesticides, and radioactive substances pose a growing threat.

Treating acute poisoning usually is complex because specific systemic antidotes are available for only a small number of drugs and toxic substances as shown in the chart below. To treat acute poisoning most effectively, the physician or nurse should obtain the following information as soon as possible: the drug or substance ingested, the amount and time of ingestion, and any significant medical problem that the patient had before the poisoning. If this information is not available, the physician or nurse must assume that the patient might have ingested multiple substances.

Treatment goals for a poisoned patient include:

- administering the appropriate antidote, if available
- supporting vital functions
- decreasing further absorption of the toxic substance
- promoting excretion of the toxin
- managing complications.

The most common complications of poisoning are central nervous system (CNS) depression and coma. Other complications include toxic delirium, seizures, blood pressure alterations, arrhythmias, and tissue damage.

Antidotes to selected poisons

This chart outlines potential poisons, their antidotes, and how each antidote works to remove or neutralize the poison.

POISON	ANTIDOTE	TYPE AND EFFECT OF ANTIDOTE
acetaminophen	acetylcysteine	Dispositional antagonist: hastens detoxification
anticholinergics	physostigmine	Receptor antidote: blocks receptors
anticholinesterases (organophosphates)	atropine	Receptor antidote: blocks muscarinic receptors
	pralidoxime	Dispositional antagonist: reactivates cholinesterase
benzodiazepines	flumazenil	Receptor antagonist: inhibits benzodiazepine-receptor activity
carbon monoxide	oxygen	Dispositional antagonist: hastens carboxyhemoglobin breakdown
fluoride	calcium	Chemical antidote: precipitates fluoride
iron	sodium bicarbonate (before absorption)	Chemical antidote: forms insoluble iron carbonate
	deferoxamine mesylate	Chemical antidote: forms iron chelate that is excreted in urine
lead	succimer	Chemical antidote: forms water-soluble lead chelate that is excreted in urine
	edetate calcium disodium (Calcium EDTA)	Chemical antidote: is displaced by lead to form stable complexes that are excreted in urine
methanol	ethanol	Dispositional antidote: slows formation of toxic products
	sodium bicarbonate	Physiologic antagonist: offsets acidosis
narcotics and narcotic derivatives	naloxone, nalmefene, naltrexone	Receptor antidotes: displace narcotic from receptor
strychnine	diazepam, barbiturates	Physiologic antagonists: offset CNS stimulation

Appendix 8

Substance abuse

Substance abuse is a maladaptive pattern of continuing substance use despite knowledge of impaired social, occupational, psychological, or physical functioning caused or exacerbated by that use. The abused substance may be nicotine, alcohol, or an over-the-counter, prescription, or illegal drug.

BEHAVIORS THAT INDICATE ABUSE

According to the American Psychiatric Association, any three or more of the following behaviors indicate abuse:

- ingesting the substance more frequently or in larger amounts than prescribed
- persistently desiring to quit or reduce use or unsuccessfully attempting to quit or reduce use
- spending an inordinate amount of time seeking, taking, or recovering from the substance
- neglecting obligations because of intoxication or withdrawal symptoms
- reducing important occupational or social activities because of substance use
- continuing substance use despite knowledge of adverse effects
- developing a tolerance to the effects of the substance
- manifesting characteristic withdrawal symptoms when not taking the substance
- taking the substance to relieve or prevent withdrawal symptoms.

ADDICTION

The nurse who cares for a substance abuser should keep the following points in mind:

- Addictive substances act on the brain, engaging brain circuits related to emotion, motivation, and behavior.
- Addictive behavior is motivated by the pleasure or reward the substance gives.
- Susceptibility to addictive drugs and the capacity to recover from addiction vary greatly among individuals.
- No single addictive personality exists, although personality traits may play a role in addiction.

Addictive drugs include alcohol, cocaine, marijuana, opiates, barbiturates, amphetamines, hallucinogens, tranquilizers, and sedatives. (See *Commonly abused substances.*)

DEFENSE MECHANISMS IN SUBSTANCE ABUSE

A substance abuser typically uses two key defense mechanisms: denial and isolation. With denial, the abuser rejects the notion that the abused substance is causing a problem, thus impeding treatment and recovery. With isolation, the abuser separates himself or herself from people, situations, information, or feelings that challenge the denial. Use of denial may prevent recovery or promote a relapse in a former substance abuser.

The denial-isolation pattern that enables the user to continue substance abuse also may induce guilt, shame, low self-esteem, and loneliness. The abuser may rationalize the dependence or project emotions onto others, resulting in dependence on others, lying about or making excuses for continued substance abuse, extreme withdrawal symptoms, social isolation, or loss of responsibility.

NURSING IMPLICATIONS

When obtaining a drug history, the nurse should ask the patient about all drug use and should be aware that a substance abuse problem may be complicated by polypharmacy (simultaneous use of several drugs). Polypharmacy is a major cause of drug-related deaths.

During the drug history, the nurse should ask about illegal drug use. When providing this information, the patient may use street names to refer to particular drugs or drug classes, rather than the correct pharmacologic names. Therefore, the nurse should be familiar with commonly used names for street drugs. (See *Glossary of street drug names,* page 783.)

After identifying a substance abuse problem, the nurse can intervene by teaching the patient about treatment and rehabilitation measures, making referrals for substance abuse programs, and helping family members identify and cope with their feelings about the problem.

Commonly abused substances

When caring for a patient who abuses alcohol or drugs, the nurse should be familiar with the incidence, signs and symptoms, and treatment of abuse for each substance.

SUBSTANCE AND INCIDENCE	SIGNS AND SYMPTOMS OF ABUSE	TREATMENT
Alcohol		
More than 174 million people in the United States admit to having used alcohol at least once in their lives. More than 110 million use it at least once a month.*	• Depressed brain activity and respirations • Blood vessel dilation resulting in flushed skin, sweating, and clammy palms • Alcohol-related medical complications, such as cirrhosis, gastritis, pancreatitis, polyneuropathy, cardiac muscle disease, heart failure, and coronary artery disease • Alcoholic blackouts (amnesia of the time period when drinking) • Drinking bouts of 48 hours or more • Alcohol-related problems, such as arrests for drunken driving, work problems, drinking before breakfast, or controlling the alcohol craving by drinking mouthwash, antifreeze, or other forms of nonbeverage alcohol *Withdrawal signs and symptoms* • Mild signs or symptoms: agitation, tremulousness, anorexia, disturbed sleep, and occasional hallucinations and seizures • Severe signs or symptoms: seizures, hallucinations, and delirium tremens (acute psychotic reaction to alcohol withdrawal)	• Detoxification (process of freeing the patient from alcohol dependence by lowering the blood alcohol level and controlling withdrawal symptoms) • Withdrawal over 3 days or more • Treatment of withdrawal symptoms with medications and support from a health care professional, friend, or family member • Total avoidance of alcohol and reliance on a supportive network after detoxification • Referral to an alcoholic rehabilitation program such as Alcoholics Anonymous • Referral to a family support group
Cocaine		
Nearly 22 million people in the United States admit to having used cocaine at least once in their lives. Nearly 1.5 million use it monthly.*	• Vasoconstriction, tachycardia, increased blood pressure • Euphoria, hallucinations, feelings of increased mental and physical prowess • Gaunt appearance • Maladaptive behavior, impaired judgment and social or occupational functioning • Postcocaine crash lasting several hours or days after drug binge, producing severe depression, anxiety, irritability, and migrainelike headaches *Withdrawal signs and symptoms* • Drug craving, irritability, shaking • Anorexia or hunger and nausea • Irregular sleep patterns • Lack of motivation, intense subjective feelings, depression, suicidal urges	• Detoxification • Withdrawal over 3 or more days • Treatment of withdrawal symptoms with medications and support from a health care professional, friend, or family member • Strict control over or total avoidance of cocaine use • Replacement of the cocaine addiction with activities that support positive human relationships and increase self-esteem • Referral to a drug rehabilitation program
Marijuana (cannabis sativa)		
Approximately 65.5 million people in the United States admit to using marijuana at least once in their lives. Nearly 10 million use it at least once a month.*	• Dreamlike state, sense of contentment, improved social interaction, loss of inhibitions • Damage to nasal mucosa, alveolar cells, bronchioles, and airways *Acute panic reactions* • Flashback phenomenon, acute psychosis, paranoia • Abdominal discomfort, headache *Acute toxicity* • Impaired reflexes, short-term memory, and depth perception	• Treatment to improve disturbed interpersonal relationships (particularly helpful in adolescents, who may use marijuana to defy authority) • Time to outgrow the habit • Establishment of permanent relationships with nondrug users to help decrease drug use

(continued)

Commonly abused substances *(continued)*

SUBSTANCE AND INCIDENCE	SIGNS AND SYMPTOMS OF ABUSE	TREATMENT
Opiates		
Use is high, probably because opiates are readily available on the street.	• Lethargy, nodding, warm, flushed skin • Lower abdominal sensation of intense pleasure • Sensation of pleasure lasting 2 or more hours *Withdrawal signs 8 to 12 hours after the last dose of heroin or morphine* • Dilated pupils, rhinorrhea, lacrimation • Sweating, slight temperature elevation *Withdrawal signs and symptoms 2 to 14 days after the last dose of heroin or morphine* • Insomnia • Nausea, vomiting, diarrhea • Tachycardia, hypertension • Muscle weakness, twitches, joint pain, piloerection	• Correction of opiate overdose with naloxone or naltrexone • Detoxification with methadone • Referral to a specific drug treatment center
Barbiturates		
Use is unknown because barbiturates are obtained easily by prescription.	• Slurred speech, unsteady gait • Vertical or horizontal nystagmus *Overdose* • Respiratory depression, death *Withdrawal signs and symptoms* • Seizures	• Detoxification with decreasing doses of pentobarbital until the drug is metabolized to prevent seizures associated with a rapid drop in barbiturate blood level
Amphetamines		
Amphetamine use is estimated to be higher than opiate use in the United States.	• Rapid speech • Headache, anorexia, nausea • Elevated pulse and blood pressure • Fine tremor of the extremities • Dilated pupils with decreased light reactivity *Withdrawal signs and symptoms* • Lethargy, severe depression	• Detoxification with the benzodiazepine diazepam (Valium) to promote sedation and propranolol (Inderal) to counteract severe adrenergic hyperactivity • Hospitalization to control suicidal impulses if postamphetamine depression persists
Hallucinogens		
Use is high, probably because hallucinogens are the easiest and least expensive illicit drugs to manufacture.	• Kaleidoscopic hallucinations • Tactile, visual, and auditory images • Strong feelings of introspection and disengagement • Feelings of superhuman powers • Extreme excitement, unpredictable destructive behavior, frightening hallucinations	• Supportive management for undesirable adverse reactions • Hospitalization for severe panic reactions or prolonged psychotic episodes
Tranquilizers and sedatives		
Use is high, probably because tranquilizers, especially diazepam (Valium) and sedatives are obtained easily by prescription.	• Drowsiness, fatigue, dizziness, slurred speech • Impaired motor coordination, reaction time, and cognitive reasoning *Overdose* • Confusion, coma, diminished reflexes • Hypotension, depression *Withdrawal signs and symptoms* • Hyperreflexia, seizures, hallucinations	• Gradual withdrawal under medical supervision • Rehabilitation to prevent recurrence of drug abuse

*National Institute on Drug Abuse. *National Household Survey on Drug Abuse: Population Estimate 1995.* Rockville, Md., 1996.

Appendix 9

Glossary of street drug names

Central nervous system (CNS) stimulants*

Bennies
Blue angels
Blue beauties
Chris
Christine
Christmas trees
Coast to coast
Coke (cocaine)
Copilot
Crack (cocaine)
Crisscross
Crossroads
Crystal (I.V. methamphetamine)**
Double cross
Flake (cocaine)
Footballs
Gold dust (cocaine)
Green and clears
Greenies
Hearts
LA turnaround
Lid poppers
Meth
Oranges
Peaches
Pep pills
Pink and green
Pinks
Rock (cocaine)
Roses
Snow (cocaine)
Speed
Speedball (heroin plus cocaine)
Toot (cocaine)
Truck drivers
Turnarounds
Uppers
Ups
Wake-ups
Whites
Yellow jackets

Phencyclidine (PCP)

Angel dust
Aurora
Bust bee
Cheap cocaine
Cosmos
Criptal
Dummy mist
Goon
Green
Guerilla
Hog
Jet
K
Lovely
Mauve
Mist
Mumm dust
Peace pill
Purple
Rocket fuel
Shermans
Sherms
Special L.A. coke
Superacid
Supercoke
Supergrass
Superjoint
Trangs
Tranq**
Whack

Heroin

Black tar
Brown
Chinese white
H
H and stuff
Horse
Junk
Mexican mud
Scat
Shit
Skag
Smack
Snow
Stuff
Tango and Cash

Other analgesics

Black (opium)
Blue velvet (paregoric plus amphetamine)
Dollies (methadone)
M (morphine)
Microdots (morphine)
PG or PO (paregoric)
Pinks and grays (propoxyphene hydrochloride)
Poppy (opium)
Tar (opium)
Terp (terpin hydrate or cough syrup with codeine)

CNS depressants***

Blue birds
Blue devil
Blue heaven
Blues
Bullets
Dolls
Double trouble
Downs
Goofballs
Green and whites (chlordiazepoxide)
Greenies
Ludes
Nembies
Peanuts
Peter (chloral hydrate)
Rainbows
Red devils
Roaches (chlordiazepoxide)**
Seccy
Seggy
T-birds
Toolies
Tranqs**
Wallbangers
Yellow jackets
Yellows

(continued)

Hallucinogens

Acid (LSD)
Blue dots (LSD)
Cactus (mescaline)
Crystal**
Cube (LSD)
D (LSD)
Mesc (mescaline)
Mexican mushroom (psilocybin)
Owsleys (LSD)
Pearly gates (morning glory seeds)

Cannabinols

Acapulco gold
Bhang
Brick
Charas
Colombian
Gage
Ganja
Grass
Hash
Hay
Hemp
J
Jane
Jive
Joint
Key or kee
Lid
Locoweed
Mary Jane
Mexican
MJ
Muggles
Pot
Reefer
Roach**
Rope
Sativa
Stick
Sweet Lucy
Tea
Texas tea
Weed
Yesca

Solvents and inhalants

Huffing
Jac aroma
Kicks
Locker room
Poppers
Rush
Snappers
Sniffers

* A form of amphetamine unless otherwise stated.
** Many drugs have the same name.
*** Moderate length of action, like secobarbital, unless otherwise noted.

Source: Schuckit, M.A. (1995). *Drug and alcohol abuse* (4th ed.). New York: Plenum Publishing Corp. Reprinted with permission of the publisher.

Glossary

Absence seizure: generalized seizure characterized by an abrupt loss of consciousness or unawareness accompanied by staring; also called petit mal seizure.

Absorption: process by which a drug leaves an administration site, passes through or across tissue into the general circulation, and becomes biologically available.

Accommodation: adjustment of the eyes for vision at various distances.

Acetylcholine: choline acetic acid ester, present in many parts of the body, that facilitates impulse transmission from one nerve fiber to another or from a nerve to a muscle.

Acetylcholinesterase: enzyme that breaks down acetylcholine into acetic acid and choline.

Acid-fast: describing an organism that retains carbolfuchsin stain after being decolorized with 95% ethyl alcohol and 3% hydrochloric acid; a unique characteristic of mycobacteria.

Acne: dermatologic inflammatory disorder that affects the sebaceous glands and produces comedos; also called acne vulgaris.

Activated partial thromboplastin time (APTT): screening test to evaluate the intrinsic coagulation pathway (except factor VII and factor XIII) and the common pathway and to monitor heparin therapy.

Active transport: use of cellular energy to move a drug from an area of low concentration to one of higher concentration.

Adenocarcinoma: malignant tumor that forms in a gland, infiltrates surrounding tissues, and leads to metastases.

Adnexa oculi: lacrimal apparatus, eyelids, and related structures of the eye.

Adrenergic: activated or transmitted by epinephrine, norepinephrine, or a similar substance.

Adrenocorticotropin: anterior pituitary hormone that stimulates the adrenal cortex.

Adsorbent: agent that attracts molecules of a liquid, gas, or dissolved substance to its surface.

Adverse drug reaction: undesirable patient response ranging from mild effects to severe, life-threatening hypersensitivity reactions; these reactions can be dose-related or patient-sensitivity–related.

Aerobe: microorganism that can live and grow only in the presence of molecular oxygen.

Affective disorder: mood disturbance in the presence of an elated or depressive state.

Afterload: pressure in the arteries leading from the ventricle that must be overcome for ejection (of blood) to occur.

Agonist: drug that has an affinity for a receptor and enhances or stimulates the receptor's functional properties.

Akinesia: abnormal absence of movement.

Alkylation: linkage between a substance and deoxyribonucleic acid (DNA) that causes irreversible inhibition of the DNA molecule by enzyme modification.

Allergen: substance capable of producing a hypersensitivity reaction.

Allograft, allogenic graft, or homograft: tissue transplanted between genetically different individuals of the same species.

Alopecia: loss of hair.

Alpha$_1$-proteinase inhibitor: agent that inactivates several proteinases, including trypsin, chymotrypsin, factor XI, plasmin, thrombin, and neutrophil elastase.

Alpha-adrenergic receptor: adrenergic receptor of the sympathetic nervous system that responds to norepinephrine and various blocking agents.

Amebicidal: pertaining to an agent that destroys amoebas.

Ampule: small, sterile, sealed glass or plastic container that holds a single drug dose.

Anabolic: promoting general body growth.

Anaerobe: microorganism that can live and grow only in the complete, or almost complete, absence of molecular oxygen.

Analgesia: absence of sensitivity to pain.

Androgenic: producing masculine characteristics.

Anemia: blood disorder characterized by a decreased number of erythrocytes, amount of hemoglobin, or volume of packed red cells.

Anesthesia: loss of feeling or sensation.

Anion: negatively charged ion.

Antacid: drug that neutralizes gastric acids.

Antagonist: . drug that occupies a receptor and inhibits the receptor's functional properties.

Antibacterial: substance (can be derived from cultures or semi-synthetically produced) that inhibits bacterial growth or kills bacteria.

Antibiotic: substance (can be derived from cultures or semi-synthetically produced) that inhibits growth of or kills other organisms, such as parasites.

Antibody: immunoglobulin synthesized by lymphoid tissue in response to an antigenic stimulus.

Anticholinesterase: substance that inhibits the breakdown of acetylcholine by acetylcholinesterase.

Anticoagulant: substance that suppresses, delays, or negates blood coagulation.

Antidepressant: agent that prevents or relieves depression.

Antidiarrheal: drug that decreases the frequency of defecation and water content of the stools.

Antiemetic: drug that relieves nausea and vomiting.

Antiflatulent: drug that decreases gastrointestinal (GI) gas.
Antigen: high-molecular-weight foreign protein or protein-polysaccharide complex that can stimulate the synthesis of a specific antibody.
Antimalarial: drug that is therapeutically effective against malaria.
Antimanic: agent that prevents or diminishes mania.
Antimicrobial: substance used to treat infection caused by pathogenic microorganisms.
Antimuscarinic: agent that inhibits stimulation of muscarinic receptors; also called anticholinergic or parasympatholytic.
Antiplatelet: substance that interferes with activity of blood platelets.
Antiprotozoal: substance that kills or inhibits the growth of protozoa.
Antipsychotic: agent that prevents or diminishes psychosis.
Antithrombin III: alpha globulin that neutralizes the thrombin action and thus inhibits blood coagulation.
Antitussive: agent that suppresses or inhibits cough.
Antiviral: substance that destroys viruses or suppresses their replication.
Anxiety: feeling of apprehension, uncertainty, and fear.
Anxiety disorder: primary medical condition or disorder secondary to another medical or social problem characterized by excessive anxiety.
Anxiolytic: agent that prevents or diminishes anxiety.
Apothecaries' system: old system of drug weights and measures that uses Roman numerals and places the unit of measurement before the Roman numeral.
Arrhythmia: abnormal variation in cardiac conduction, rhythm, or rate.
Assessment: part of the nursing process in which the nurse gathers information about the patient's condition.
Ataxia: impaired ability to coordinate movement.
Atonic seizure: generalized seizure accompanied by akinesia and, usually, loss of consciousness.
Atony: relaxation or lack of tone, usually associated with muscles or muscle groups.
Atrioventricular (AV) block: obstructed transmission of electrical impulses from the atria to the ventricles caused by AV node damage or depression.
Autoimmune: pertaining to abnormal reactivity of the body to its own tissue.
Automaticity: ability to independently generate an electrical impulse.
Autonomic nervous system: portion of the nervous system that controls the involuntary visceral functions of the body.
Avoirdupois system: system of weights and measures commonly used for ordering and purchasing pharmaceutical products and for weighing patients.
Axon: cylindrical extension of a nerve cell that carries impulses away from the neuron cell body.
B cell: bursal lymphocyte responsible for humoral immunity.
Bacillus: any rod-shaped, gram-positive, spore-forming microorganism.
Bacteremia: presence of bacteria in the blood.
Bacteria: group of single-cell organisms, usually possessing a rigid cell wall, dividing by binary fission, and exhibiting either round, rodlike, or spiral forms.
Bactericidal: pertaining to an agent that destroys bacteria.
Bacteriostatic: pertaining to an agent that inhibits growth or multiplication of bacteria.
Bacteriuria: presence of bacteria in the urine.
Beriberi: polyneuritis caused by a thiamine deficiency and characterized by spasmodic rigidity of the lower limbs, muscular atrophy, paralysis, anemia, and neuralgia.
Beta-adrenergic receptor: adrenergic receptor of the sympathetic nervous system that responds to epinephrine and various blocking agents.
Bioavailability: extent to which a drug's active ingredient is absorbed and transported to its site of action.
Bipolar disorder: mood disorder in which manic and depressive episodes occur.
Bronchodilator: substance that relaxes bronchiolar smooth-muscle cells, resulting in a widened lumen of the bronchi and bronchioles.
Bronchorrhea: excessive secretions from the bronchial mucous membrane.
Bronchospasm: paroxysmal bronchoconstriction resulting from smooth-muscle constriction.
Buccal route: oral medication administration in tablet form, which then is placed on the inside of the cheek.
Buffer: any substance in a solution that offsets a change in pH when an acid or base is added.
Calcitonin: thyroid hormone that decreases the serum calcium level.
Cancer: general term for the many malignant neoplasms associated with infiltration, metastasis, and death.
Capsule: gelatin shell that dissolves in the stomach and contains drug in a powder, sustained-release bead, or liquid form.
Carbonic anhydrase: enzyme that catalyzes the breakdown of carbonic acid to carbon dioxide and water, or the formation of carbonic acid from carbon dioxide and water.
Carcinogenesis: cancer cell production.

Carcinoma: malignant neoplasm composed of epithelial cells, which tends to infiltrate surrounding tissues and lead to metastasis.

Cardiac output: amount of blood pumped by the heart per unit of time, normally about 5 L/minute.

Catecholamine: class of sympathomimetic neuroregulators that includes dobutamine, dopamine, isoproterenol, norepinephrine, and epinephrine.

Catechol-O-methyltransferase: enzyme found in all body tissues that breaks down catecholamines.

Cathartic: agent that promotes evacuation of the bowels.

Cation: positively charged ion.

Cell cycle: pattern of cell division characterized by five phases: nonproliferation, G_0; presynthesis, G_1; DNA synthesis, S; RNA production, G_2; and mitosis (cell division), M.

Cell cycle–nonspecific: capable of acting during several or all stages of the cell cycle.

Cell cycle–specific: capable of acting only during particular stages of the cell cycle.

Cerumen: waxlike secretion found in the external opening of the ear; earwax.

Cestode: tapeworm or platyhelminth that has a head, or scolex, and segmented joints, or proglottids.

Chemical name: name that precisely describes a drug's atomic and molecular structure.

Chemotaxis: movement of an organism in response to a chemical stimulus.

Cholinergic: having the property of being stimulated, activated, or transmitted by acetylcholine or a similar substance.

Chronotropic: altering the rate of cardiac muscle contraction; a drug with a negative chronotropic effect slows the heart rate.

Chvostek's sign: facial muscle spasm elicited by tapping the muscles or facial nerve in a hypocalcemic patient.

Cilia: minute, vibrating, hairlike projections attached to the free surface of cells.

Clonic seizure: generalized seizure characterized by rhythmic contraction and relaxation of muscles, loss of consciousness, and marked autonomic signs and symptoms.

Coagulation: conversion of blood from a free-flowing liquid state to a semisolid gel through clotting, a process that can occur within an intact vessel, but usually begins with tissue damage and exposure of the blood to air.

Coccus: a spherical bacterial cell, usually slightly less than 1 micron in diameter.

Competitive inhibition: displacement of an agent from an opiate receptor site by an antagonist.

Complement: serum substance that combines with an antibody-antigen complex, thereby producing antigen lysis.

Compliance: degree to which a patient follows the advice of a health care professional.

Conductivity: capacity of cells to conduct electric current.

Conjunctivitis: inflammation of the conjunctiva, the mucous membrane lining the eyelids and covering the exposed surface of the eyeball.

Constipation: decreased movement of fecal matter through the large intestine.

Contractility: capacity for shortening or contracting in response to a stimulus.

Controlled drug: pharmacologic agent or medication that may lead to drug abuse or dependence; its use is controlled by federal, state, and local laws.

Coryza: profuse discharge from the nasal mucosa.

Cough (tussis): sudden noisy expulsion of air from the lungs.

Cream: thick emollient (substance that softens tissue) containing a paste-drug mixture of oil and water; designed for topical use.

Cryptorchidism: failure of the testicles to descend into the scrotum.

Cycloplegic: agent that causes ciliary muscle paralysis.

Cytostatic: capable of halting cell growth and multiplication.

Cytotoxic: capable of destroying or poisoning cells.

Decongestant: agent that reduces swelling of mucous membranes and relieves congestion.

Dementia: progressive mental or intellectual decline.

Dendrite: branching process that extends from the nerve cell and carries impulses to the cell body.

Depolarization: neutralization of electrical polarity in cardiac cells caused by an influx of sodium ions.

Depression: emotional dejection characterized by an absence of cheerfulness and hope disproportionate to circumstances.

Dermal route: medication administration by topical application to the skin.

Diabetes insipidus: metabolic disorder characterized by extreme polyuria and polydipsia resulting from deficient secretion of antidiuretic hormone (ADH) or the inability of kidney tubules to respond to ADH.

Diabetes mellitus: metabolic disorder in which the ability to metabolize carbohydrates is lost because of decreased insulin secretion; characterized by hyperglycemia, glycosuria, polyuria, polydipsia, polyphagia, emaciation, and weakness.

Diarrhea: increased frequency or weight and liquidity of stools produced by the rapid movement of fecal matter through the large intestine.

Diastole: period of ventricular dilation that occurs between the second and first heart sounds.
Diastolic blood pressure: pressure exerted in the vessels when the ventricles are at rest.
Digestant: drug that enhances digestion in the GI tract; also called digestive agent.
Distribution: degree to which an absorbed or I.V. drug is delivered to various body fluids and tissues.
Dopamine: neurotransmitter produced by the decarboxylation of dopa, an intermediate product in norepinephrine synthesis.
Dopaminergic: having the property of being stimulated, activated, or transmitted by dopamine.
Dromotropic: influencing conduction in cardiac muscle; a drug with a negative dromotropic effect slows conduction through the atrioventricular node.
Drop: medical administration of a minute sphere of medicated liquid.
Drug: pharmacologic agent or medication capable of interacting with living organisms to produce biological effects.
Drug abuse: self-directed use of drugs for nontherapeutic purposes.
Drug action: interaction between a drug and cellular components.
Drug dependence: physiologic or psychological reliance on drugs that limits a person's ability to control drug intake.
Drug effect: response resulting from a drug's action.
Drug efficacy: maximal response or effect achieved when the dose-response curve reaches its plateau.
Drug holiday: discontinuation of an antipsychotic agent for 4 weeks or more to detect tardive dyskinesia, which may be masked by the drug's effects.
Drug interactions: relationships between concurrently administered drugs that result in alterations in the therapeutic effects of any or all of the drugs.
Drug misuse: improper use of common drugs, which can lead to acute and chronic toxicity.
Drug potency: relative amount of a drug required to produce the desired response.
Dyspepsia: impaired digestion; usually referring to epigastric discomfort after eating.
Eclampsia: severe complication of pregnancy characterized by seizures, coma, hypertension, edema, and proteinuria.
Ectopy: generation of electrical impulses by cardiac cells outside the normal conduction pathways.
Electroencephalogram: graphic recording of electrical currents produced in the brain.
Electrolyte: ion that can conduct electricity when dissolved in solution.
Elixir: flavored, sweetened hydroalcoholic (water and alcohol) liquid that contains a medicinal agent.
Embolus: clot or other plug (composed of fat, bone, or another substance foreign to blood) that is totally or partially dislodged from its site of origin and moved by blood flow to a more distant, narrower site in the circulatory system, where it may obstruct flow.
Emesis: vomiting.
Emetic: drug that induces vomiting.
Emollient: drug that softens the stool by increasing the water content of fecal material through a reduction in surface tension of bowel contents.
Encephalitis: inflammation of the brain.
Endorphin: endogenous opiate present in the hypothalamus and pituitary.
Enkephalin: endogenous opiate present throughout the central and peripheral nervous systems.
Enteric-coated tablet: tablet with a thin coating that prevents release and absorption of its contents until it reaches the small intestine.
Epidural block: loss of feeling or sensation produced by injecting an anesthetic agent between the vertebrae and beneath the ligaments into the space surrounding the dura mater of the spinal column.
Epidural route: medication administration through a catheter inserted into the space surrounding the dura mater of the spinal column.
Epigastric pain: pain originating in the upper central area of the abdomen.
Epilepsy: disorder characterized by one or more of the following signs and symptoms: paroxysmally recurring impairment or loss of consciousness, involuntary excess or cessation of muscle movements, psychic or sensory disturbances, and derangement of the autonomic nervous system.
Equianalgesic dose: amount of an analgesic drug that will produce the same level of pain relief as a standard agent used for comparison.
Erythropoiesis: production of red blood cells (RBCs).
Ethical responsibility: duty to use fundamental moral values when making nursing decisions.
Euphoria: exaggerated sense of well-being.
Euthyroid: having a normal thyroid gland.
Evaluation: part of the nursing process in which the nurse judges the effectiveness of care based on preestablished criteria.

Excretion: process of drug elimination from the body.
Exocrine gland: gland that secretes externally through a duct to the skin.
Expectorant: agent that promotes the expulsion of respiratory secretions.
Extracellular fluid: fluid outside the cells that accounts for about 40% of total body water and includes functional plasma and interstitial fluid; representative components of extracellular fluid include protein, magnesium, potassium, chloride, calcium, and certain sulfates.
Extravasation: escape of blood or solution from a vessel into surrounding tissues.
Ferritin: one of the complexes in which iron is stored in the body.
Fibrillation: twitching movements of cardiac muscle resulting from a transmission of independent impulses so rapid that coordinated contractions cannot occur.
Fibrin: insoluble protein formed from fibrinogen by thrombin action; fibrin is the major element of a blood clot.
Fibrinogen: high-molecular-weight plasma protein that is converted to fibrin through thrombin action; also called factor I.
Fibroblast: connective tissue cell.
Field block: regional loss of feeling or sensation produced by using several injections of an anesthetic agent to create a pain-free area around an operative site.
First-pass effect: process by which orally administered drugs progress from the intestinal lumen to the hepatic system and undergo partial metabolism before entering the general circulation.
Flatulence: presence of excessive air or gas in the stomach or intestine.
Fungicidal: pertaining to an agent that destroys fungi.
Fungistatic: pertaining to an agent that inhibits fungal growth.
Gamma-aminobutyric acid (GABA): inhibitory neurotransmitter secreted by nerve terminals in the spinal cord, the cerebellum, the basal ganglia, and many areas of the cerebral cortex.
Ganglia: group of nerve cell bodies located outside the central nervous system.
Generalized seizure: bilaterally symmetrical, violent, involuntary contractions of voluntary muscles involving loss of consciousness; more specifically classified as absence, myoclonic, clonic, tonic, tonic-clonic, or atonic seizure.
Generic name: drug name selected by the United States Adopted Names Council; usually a shortened form of the chemical name.
Gilles de la Tourette's syndrome: disease characterized by motor incoordination, the meaningless repetition of words, and the use of obscene language.
Glaucoma: eye disorder characterized by increased intraocular pressure.
Globulin: class of proteins characterized by solubility in saline solutions but not in water.
Glucocorticoid: adrenocortical hormone that increases gluconeogenesis (thus raising the concentration of liver glycogen and blood glucose) and inhibits the inflammatory response.
Gluconeogenesis: carbohydrate formation from protein molecules.
Glycogenolysis: breakdown of the polysaccharide glycogen in body tissues.
Goal: objective or aim of directed nursing care efforts.
Goblet cells:
unicellular mucous glands found especially in respiratory and GI epithelium.
Gonadotropic: stimulating the ovaries or testes.
Gout: condition caused by abnormal purine metabolism, characterized by an increased serum uric acid level, acute arthritic episodes, and formation of chalky urate deposits in the joints.
Gram stain: laboratory dye used to differentiate organisms. An organism that retains the dye is classified as gram-positive; otherwise, the organism is gram-negative.
Granulocyte: leukocyte with granules in its cytoplasm; basophils, neutrophils, and eosinophils are granulocytes.
Gynecomastia: excessive development of male mammary glands.
Half-life: time required to metabolize or inactivate the total amount of a drug in a person's body by 50%.
Hansen's disease: chronic communicable disease caused by *Mycobacterium leprae,* characterized by granulomatous lesions in the skin, mucous membranes, and peripheral nervous system; also called leprosy.
Helminth: worm or wormlike parasite.
Helper T cell: cell released by T lymphocytes in response to an antigen that activates other T cells, B cells, and macrophages.
Hematinic: agent capable of improving blood quality by increasing the hemoglobin level and the number of RBCs.
Hemoglobin: oxygen-carrying pigment of RBCs.
Hemolytic anemia: disorder characterized by the premature destruction of RBCs; anemia may be minimal if the bone marrow can increase RBC production.
Hepatotoxic: capable of destroying or poisoning liver cells.

Histamine: powerful tissue substance released during an allergic reaction that dilates capillaries, contracts most smooth muscles, increases heart rate, and stimulates gastric secretions.

Histamine$_2$ (H_2)- receptor antagonist: drug that decreases gastric acid secretion by blocking gastric histamine$_2$ (H_2) receptors.

Hodgkin's disease: malignant disorder that causes painless, progressive enlargement of the lymph nodes, spleen, and lymphoid tissues; also called malignant granuloma or Hodgkin's lymphoma.

Household system: system of weights and measures commonly used in recipes, over-the-counter drugs, and home remedies.

Huntington's disease: hereditary disease characterized by chronic, progressive motor disturbances and mental deterioration.

Hypercalcemia: excess calcium in the blood.

Hypercoagulability: state of abnormally increased coagulation.

Hyperglycemia: excess glucose in the blood.

Hyperkalemia: excess potassium in the blood.

Hyperkinesia: abnormally increased motor function or activity.

Hyperlipoproteinemia: excess lipoproteins in the blood.

Hyperpyrexia: highly elevated body temperature.

Hypersensitivity: exaggerated immune system reaction, with characteristic symptoms, to contact with certain substances (allergens) that are innocuous to nonsensitized individuals.

Hypersomnia: disorder of excessive somnolence such as narcolepsy (sleep attacks).

Hypertension: systolic blood pressure of 140 mm Hg or higher and diastolic blood pressure of 90 mm Hg or higher on two or more occasions.

Hyperuricemia: excess uric acid in the blood.

Hypervitaminosis: condition resulting from excessive intake of one or more vitamins.

Hypnotic: agent that induces sleep.

Hypocalcemia: insufficient calcium in the blood.

Hypoglycemia: insufficient glucose in the blood.

Hypogonadism: condition resulting from abnormally decreased functioning of the ovaries or testes, characterized by retarded growth and retarded sexual development.

Hypokalemia: insufficient potassium in the blood.

Hypotension: systolic blood pressure of 90 mm Hg or lower and diastolic blood pressure of 60 mm Hg or a drop of 30 mm Hg below normal baseline.

Hypotonia: abnormally decreased muscle tone, tension, or activity.

Immunomodulator: substance that alters the immune response by augmenting or reducing the ability of the immune system to produce antibodies or sensitized cells that recognize and react with antigens.

Immunosuppression: inhibition of the body's immune response to foreign substances.

Implementation: part of the nursing process in which the nurse puts interventions into action and carries out the nursing care plan.

Infarction: formation of a localized area of tissue necrosis caused by hypoxia resulting from inadequate blood flow to the area.

Infection: tissue reaction to invading pathogenic microorganisms and the toxins they generate.

Inflammation: tissue reaction to injury characterized by pain, heat, redness, edema, and, sometimes, loss of function.

Inhalant: medicinal vapors administered through the nose, trachea, or respiratory system.

Injection: introduction of a liquid into the body using a syringe; a solution of a medication suitable for injection.

Inotropic: altering the force of cardiac muscle contraction; a drug with a positive inotropic effect increases the strength of the muscle contraction.

Insomnia: inability to sleep; abnormal wakefulness.

Inspissated: thickened or dried out; used to describe mucus.

Interneuron: any neuron in a chain of neurons that is situated between the primary afferent neuron and the final motor neuron.

Intra-articular route: medication administration by instillation or injection into a joint.

Intracellular fluid: fluid inside the cells that accounts for 60% of total body water, and includes intracellular and RBC fluid.

Intradermal route: medication administration by injection of small amounts of solution, usually antigens, between the epidermal and dermal (skin) layers.

Intramuscular route: medication administration by injection of a solution into a muscle.

Intrathecal: within a sheath, as in the cerebrospinal fluid within the subarachnoid space.

Intrathecal route: medication administration by direct injection through the theca (enclosing sheath) of the spinal cord into the subarachnoid space.

Intravenous route: medication administration by injection or infusion into a vein.

Iodism: toxicity resulting from excessive ingestion of iodine, characterized by glandular atrophy, coryza, frontal headache, emaciation, weakness, and skin eruptions.

Iritis: inflammation of the iris.

Irritant: agent that produces undue sensitivity or tenderness.

Ischemia: decreased blood supply to an area caused by vascular constriction or obstruction.

Keratitis: inflammation of the cornea.

Keratolytic: agent that produces softening and peeling of the horny layer of the epidermis.

Labyrinthitis: inner ear inflammation.

Lactic acidosis: decreased serum pH caused by the anaerobic metabolism of pyruvic acid to lactic acid.

Laxative: drug that stimulates defecation by adding bulk to stools, stimulating peristalsis, or providing lubrication or chemical irritation.

Legal responsibility: duty to abide by nursing practice acts and court decisions.

Leukemia: malignant disorder of the blood-forming organs marked by increased leukocytes and leukocyte precursors in the blood and bone marrow.

Leukopenia: decreased leukocytes in the blood, usually under 5,000/mm^3.

Lipid: fatty substance in the blood.

Lipoatrophy: wasting of the body's fatty tissues.

Lipodystrophy: disturbance of fat metabolism involving regional loss of subcutaneous fat.

Lipohypertrophy: excessive enlargement of fatty tissues.

Lipolysis: fat breakdown.

Lipoprotein: combination of different lipids with proteins.

Local infiltration: loss of feeling or sensation in a confined area produced by injecting an anesthetic agent.

Lotion: medicated liquid applied topically to protect the skin or treat a dermatologic disorder.

Lozenge: tablet containing a drug, flavoring, sweetener, and mucilage that is made to dissolve in the mouth.

Lymphoblastic: pertaining to lymphoblasts (immature nucleolated lymphocytes).

Lymphocyte: white blood cell with a single nucleus and nongranular protoplasm that arises from the reticular tissue of the lymph gland.

Lymphocytic: pertaining to lymphocytes.

Lymphokine: soluble substance released by a lymphocyte when stimulated by an antigen.

Lymphoma: neoplastic disorder of lymphoid tissue.

Lysosome: minute cellular body containing hydrolytic enzymes that are released upon injury to the cell.

Macrocytic anemia: disorder characterized by abnormally large, fragile RBCs; usually caused by vitamin B_{12} or folic acid deficiency.

Macrophage: large mononuclear cell that ingests microorganisms, other cells, or foreign particles.

Malabsorption: impaired absorption of nutrients.

Malaria: infectious febrile disease caused by protozoa and transmitted by the bites of infected mosquitoes; characterized by periodic attacks of chills, fever, and diaphoresis.

Malpractice: wrongful conduct, improper discharge of duties, or failure of a professional to meet standards of care that causes harm to another; negligence is a form of malpractice.

Mania: mood disorder characterized by an expansive emotional state, elation, hyperirritability, over-talkativeness, flight of ideas, and increased motor activity.

Manic-depressive disorder: bipolar mental disorder characterized by fluctuations between mania and depression.

Megaloblastic anemia: disorder characterized by immature, large, dysfunctional RBCs.

Melanoma: malignant neoplasm composed of melanin-pigmented cells.

Meningitis: inflammation of the membranes that envelop the brain and spinal cord.

Metabolic acidosis: decreased serum pH caused by excess hydrogen ions in the extracellular fluid.

Metabolic alkalosis: increased serum pH caused by excess bicarbonate in the extracellular fluid.

Metabolism: biological process of altering or converting a drug from its present form to an inactive substance; also called biotransformation.

Metastasis: disease transfer from one organ or part to distant parts of the body.

Methylxanthine: classification of a group of drugs (which includes caffeine and theophylline) whose actions include central nervous system stimulation, smooth-muscle relaxation, vasodilation, diuresis, and cardiac stimulation.

Metric system: system of weights and measures in which units are based on multiples of ten.

Microcytic anemia: disorder characterized by abnormally small, incompletely hemoglobinized RBCs in the bone marrow.

Microorganism: microscopic organism, including bacteria, spiral organisms, viruses, molds, yeasts, and protozoa.

Milliequivalent: number of grams of a solute in one milliliter of a normal solution.

Mineral: naturally occurring inorganic substance with a distinctive chemical composition.

Mineralocorticoid: adrenocortical hormone that increases sodium retention and potassium excretion.
Miosis: contraction of the pupil.
Mitosis: type of cell division that results in two morphologically identical cells.
Monoamine oxidase (MAO): enzyme in the nerve endings that breaks down catecholamines.
Monoamine oxidase (MAO) inhibitor: substance that opposes the action of monoamine oxidase.
Motor end plate: branching nerve terminals of a motor neuron of the voluntary muscles.
Mucokinesis: movement of mucus in the respiratory tract.
Mucolytic: having the ability to break down the composition of mucus.
Mucositis: inflammation of the mucous membrane.
Mucus: coating of the mucous membranes that contains glandular secretions, various inorganic salts, desquamated cells, and leukocytes.
Muscarinic receptor: receptor located in effector cells that is stimulated by acetylcholine, muscarine, or a similar substance.
Mycobacteria: slender, gram-positive, acid-fast, rod-shaped microorganisms.
Mycosis: disease caused by fungi.
Mydriasis: extreme dilation of the pupil.
Mydriatic: agent that causes extreme dilation of the pupil.
Myelogenous: pertaining to cells produced in the bone marrow.
Myeloma: neoplasm composed of cells that normally appear in the bone marrow.
Myeloproliferative: pertaining to or characterized by extramedullary and medullary proliferation of bone marrow constituents.
Myelosuppression: inhibition of blood cell production by the bone marrow.
Myoclonic seizure: generalized seizure characterized by bilaterally symmetrical, involuntary lightning jerks of voluntary muscles lasting from seconds to minutes; consciousness is maintained.
Myxedema: condition resulting from hypothyroidism and characterized by dry, waxy, nonpitting edema; abnormal mucin deposits in the skin; swollen lips; and a thickened nose.
Nadir: lowest point on a scale or curve, commonly related to blood counts.
Narcotic: drug derived from opium or produced synthetically that alters pain perception, induces mental changes, promotes deep sleep, depresses respirations, constricts pupils, and decreases GI motility.
Nausea: unpleasant epigastric or abdominal sensation that, in many cases, leads to vomiting.
Negligence: failure to do something that could reasonably be expected to be done by an individual in a given situation or the performance of an act that a reasonable and prudent person would not do.
Nematode: multicellular parasite, such as a roundworm or threadworm.
Neoplasm: new abnormal growth of tissue; may be benign or malignant.
Neuroblastoma: malignant tumor of the nervous system composed primarily of immature nerve cells (neuroblasts).
Neuroleptic: drug that reduces body movements produced by mental disturbances; an antipsychotic agent.
Neurolysis: destruction or dissolution of nerve tissue.
Neuromuscular junction: joining of a nerve ending and a muscle fiber.
Neuron: nerve cell; the structural unit of the nervous system.
Neurotransmitter: chemical substance secreted by the neuron at the synapse that acts on receptor proteins in the membrane of the adjacent neuron to stimulate, inhibit, or modify the other neuron's activity.
Nicotinic receptor: receptor located in effector cells that is stimulated by acetylcholine and nicotine.
Nociceptor: free nerve ending that transmits pain impulses when stimulated by chemical mediators or chemical, mechanical, or thermal stimuli.
Nonprescription drug: drug considered safe and effective when used according to proper direction by consumers without a physician's supervision; also called an over-the-counter drug.
Normocytic anemia: disorder characterized by too few RBCs in the blood.
Nosocomial: originating in or pertaining to a hospital; used to describe infections acquired during hospitalization.
Nurse practice act: state (or Canadian province) legislation that describes the educational requirements for professional licensure and the professional scope of nursing practice.
Nursing care plan: written plan that includes prioritized goals, nursing interventions, and outcome criteria for a specific patient.
Nursing diagnosis: part of the nursing process in which the nurse uses a standard nomenclature to describe actual and potential patient care problems, their etiologies, and their signs and symptoms.
Nursing intervention: actions by the nurse to help the patient reach the desired behavior or response goals.

Nursing process: framework for nursing care that includes assessment, diagnosis, planning, implementation, and evaluation.

Obsessive-compulsive disorder: mental disorder characterized by the need to perform certain acts repetitively or to carry out certain rituals.

Official name: drug name as listed in the United States Pharmacopeia and in the National Formulary.

Ointment: semisolid, oil-based preparation that contains a medication for topical application.

Orphan drug: drug useful for treating disease but undeveloped by a company, usually because of a limited market (such as a drug for a rare disease) or risk of serious adverse reactions.

Orthostatic hypotension: decrease in blood pressure that occurs when a person stands erect; also called postural hypotension.

Osmotic pump tablet: tablet that releases drug through a tiny hole; movement of the drug into tissue is driven by moisture and concentration (osmosis).

Otitis: inflammation of the ear.

Otitis externa: inflammation of the external ear.

Otitis media: inflammation of the middle ear.

Ototoxicity: quality or property of exerting a destructive or poisonous effect on cranial nerve VIII or the organs of hearing and balance.

Outcome criteria: statement of desired results that contains a content area, an action verb, a time frame, and criterion modifiers.

Paget's disease: progressive metabolic bone disease characterized by enlargement, bowing, destruction, or deformity of the bones; tenderness; and dull, aching pain.

Palliative: providing relief but not cure.

Pancreatitis: inflammation of the pancreas.

Pancytopenia: deficiency of all cellular elements in the blood.

Panic: extreme, irrational anxiety or fear.

Parasite: plant or animal that lives upon or within another living organism, at whose expense it obtains some advantage without return compensation.

Parasomnia: dysfunction associated with sleep, the sleep cycle, or partial arousals.

Parasympathetic nervous system: cholinergic division of the autonomic nervous system.

Parasympatholytic: agent that opposes the effects of impulses conveyed by the parasympathetic nervous system; also called anticholinergic or antimuscarinic.

Parasympathomimetic: agent that produces effects similar to those from stimulation of the parasympathetic nerves; also called cholinergic or muscarinic.

Parenteral route: medication administration by injection, such as intradermal, I.M., or I.V. injection.

Parkinson's disease: disorder characterized by muscular rigidity, immobile facies, tremors that disappear upon volitional movement, and loss of associated autonomic movement and salivation.

Partial seizure: focal or local violent, involuntary contractions of voluntary muscles; more specifically classified as simple or complex.

Partial thromboplastin time (PTT): screening test to evaluate the intrinsic coagulation pathway (except for factor VII and factor XIII) and the common pathway and to monitor heparin therapy; less sensitive than APTT.

Passive transport: movement of a drug from an area of high concentration to one of lower concentration without expending cellular energy.

Patch: thin membrane or gel base applied to the skin that releases a measured dose of medication over an extended period.

Pathogen: disease-producing microorganism or material.

Peak concentration level: point at which drug absorption and elimination are equal.

Pepsin: proteolytic enzyme in gastric secretions that acts as a catalyst in protein hydrolysis.

Peptic ulcer agent: drug used to treat peptic ulcers.

Percentage solution: solution in which the solute (solid) represents a percentage of the solution's total weight; for example, *0.9% sodium chloride solution* means that every 100 ml of solution contains 0.9 g of sodium chloride (or every liter of solution contains 9 g of sodium chloride).

Peripheral nerve block: regional loss of feeling or sensation produced by injecting an anesthetic agent around or near a nerve to interrupt its conductivity.

Peripheral vascular resistance: pressure that blood must overcome as it flows in a vessel.

Peristalsis: movement of the intestines or other tubular structure characterized by waves of alternating muscle contraction and relaxation.

pH: abbreviation for the relative hydrogen ion concentration (acidity or alkalinity) of a solution; a pH of 7 is neutral, below 7 is acidic, and above 7 is alkaline.

Phagocytosis: engulfment of microorganisms, cells, or foreign particles by reticuloendothelial cells, polymorphonuclear leukocytes, monocytes, or macrophages.

Pharmacodynamics: study of the biochemical and physical effects and mechanisms of action of drugs in living organisms.

Pharmacognosy: study of the natural sources of drugs, such as plants, animals, and minerals, and their products.

Pharmacokinetics: study of a drug's alterations as it is absorbed into, distributed through, metabolized in, and excreted from a living organism.

Pharmacology: scientific study of the origin, nature, chemistry, effects, and uses of drugs.

Pharmacotherapeutics: study of the uses of drugs to prevent, diagnose, and treat disease in living organisms.

Phobia: persistent, abnormal dread or fear.

Pinocytosis: movement of a drug by cellular engulfment.

Placebo: inactive substance such as normal saline solution or a less-than-effective dose of a substance such as a vitamin prescribed as if it were an effective medication dose.

Planning: part of the nursing process in which the nurse determines the nursing plan of care for the patient.

Plasmin: highly specific proteolytic enzyme that dissolves fibrin clots.

Plasminogen: inactive precursor of plasmin.

Polycythemia vera: myeloproliferative disease characterized by increased RBCs and total blood volume and often accompanied by splenomegaly, leukocytosis, thrombocytosis, and bone marrow hyperactivity.

Polymorphonuclear leukocyte: white blood cell with a lobed nucleus that responds to allergic and inflammatory stimuli.

Powder: small particles of medication obtained by grinding a solid drug.

Preeclampsia: complication of the third trimester of pregnancy characterized by hypertension, proteinuria, and edema.

Preload: blood volume in the ventricle at the end of diastole.

Prescription: order for medication, therapy, or a therapeutic device given by a properly authorized person to a person properly authorized to dispense or perform the order.

Prescription drug: drug safely used only under the supervision of a person licensed to prescribe and dispense in accordance with a state's laws.

Proarrhythmia: arrhythmia that occurs when another already is present.

Prophylaxis: disease prevention.

Prostaglandins: naturally occurring fatty acids abundant in cells that affect many different cellular functions.

Prothrombin: glycoprotein converted to thrombin by extrinsic thromboplastin during the second stage of blood coagulation; also called factor II.

Prothrombin time (PT): screening test to evaluate the extrinsic coagulation and common pathways, and to monitor oral anticoagulant therapy.

Protozoa: unicellular organisms constituting the lowest division of the animal kingdom.

Pseudoparkinsonism: state resembling Parkinson's disease and characterized by muscle rigidity, tremors, shuffling gait, drooling, and decreased arm swing and associative movements when walking; a common adverse reaction to antipsychotic agents.

Psychosis: mental disorder characterized by loss of contact with reality and derangement of personality.

Pyrogen: fever-producing substance such as the secretions of toxic bacteria.

Rapid eye movement (REM) sleep: fifth and last stage of sleep characterized by rapid eye movements; REM sleep is essential for physiologic and mental restoration.

Receptor: specialized reactive substance or large group of molecules that interlocks with a drug molecule; the interaction of a drug and its receptor should result in a drug effect, or pharmacologic response.

Recreational drug: drug used for its pleasant psychological or physical effects with no therapeutic intent.

Rectal route: medication administration by insertion or infusion into the rectum.

Reentry or circus movement: abnormal transmission of an electrical impulse around and around in cardiac muscle without stopping.

Refractory period: period of depolarization after excitation, during which cardiac muscle cannot respond to another normal cardiac impulse.

Regional anesthesia: loss of feeling or sensation produced by interrupting the sensory nerve conductivity from a specific body area.

Relaxant: agent that reduces or lessens muscle tension.

Remission: partial or complete disappearance of the clinical or subjective characteristics of a chronic or malignant disease.

Resistance: natural ability of an organism to ward off deleterious effects of noxious agents, such as drugs, toxins, poisons, irritants, or pathogenic microorganisms.

Rhabdomyosarcoma: malignant neoplasm composed of striated muscle cells.

Rheumatoid arthritis: autoimmune disease characterized by connective tissue inflammation, especially in the muscles and the joints.

Rhinitis: inflammation of the nasal mucosa.

Ribosome: minute granule composed of nucleic acid attached to the membranes of the endoplasmic reticulum of a cell where cellular protein synthesis occurs.

Rigidity: abnormal muscle stiffness or inflexibility.

Salicylism: toxic effects of excessive salicylic acid ingestion.

Sarcoma: malignant neoplasm composed of a substance similar to embryonic connective tissue.

Schistosome: a type of trematode parasite; also called blood fluke because it is found in the blood.

Schizophrenia: group of severe emotional disorders characterized by delusions, hallucinations, loss of contact with reality, and bizarre or regressive behavior.

Sedative: agent that allays excitement and produces drowsiness.

Sepsis: poisoning from pathogenic organisms or their toxins.

Serotonin: neurotransmitter and powerful vasoconstrictor synthesized in intestinal cells and neurons; it inhibits pain pathways, helps control an individual's mood, and may induce sleep.

Serum sickness: type of immunologic, complex, hypersensitivity reaction occurring 6 to 14 days after injection with foreign serum; characterized by edema, fever, inflammation of the blood vessels and joints, and urticaria.

Spasm: sudden, violent, involuntary contraction of a muscle or group of muscles, accompanied by pain, dysfunction, involuntary movement, and distortion.

Spasticity: increased muscle tension resulting in continually increased resistance to stretching.

Spectrum: range of bacteria affected by an antibacterial agent.

Spinal block: loss of feeling or sensation produced by injecting an anesthetic agent into the cerebrospinal fluid in the subarachnoid space around the spinal cord.

Status epilepticus: series of rapidly repeated epileptic seizures without periods of consciousness separating them.

Steatorrhea: passage of large amounts of fat in the feces, resulting from failure to digest and absorb fat; steatorrhea primarily occurs in pancreatic disease and other malabsorption syndromes.

Sterol: monohydroxyl alcohol of high molecular weight, commonly classified as a lipid.

Stomatitis: inflammation of the mouth that may affect the buccal mucosa, palate, tongue, floor of the mouth, and gingivae.

Strabismus: misalignment of the optic axis of each eye.

Subcutaneous route: medication administration by injection of a substance under the skin into the layer of loose connective tissue.

Sublingual route: medication administration by placement of a tablet on the floor of the mouth under the tongue.

Superinfection: condition produced by the sudden overgrowth of resistant bacteria or fungi, which can occur in a patient receiving antibiotics.

Suppository: medicated semisolid substance, usually cone-shaped, that melts or dissolves after insertion into a body cavity.

Suppressor T cell: cell released by T lymphocytes in response to an antigen that prevents other T cells from producing an excessive immune response that might severely damage the body.

Surfactant: mixture of phospholipids secreted by alveolar cells that reduces the surface tension of pulmonary fluids and increases the elasticity of pulmonary tissue.

Suspension: preparation in which small particles of a solid drug are dispersed — but not dissolved — in a liquid for administration; stirring or shaking the mixture maintains dispersal.

Sympathetic block: loss of feeling or sensation produced by the paravertebral injection of an anesthetic agent to block the sympathetic trunk.

Sympathetic nervous system: adrenergic division of the autonomic nervous system.

Sympatholytic: agent that opposes the impulses conveyed by the adrenergic postganglionic fibers of the sympathetic nervous system.

Sympathomimetic: agent that produces effects similar to those of impulses conveyed by the adrenergic postganglionic fibers of the sympathetic nervous system.

Synapse: area surrounding the point of contact between the processes of two adjacent neurons or between a neuron and effector organ where an impulse is transmitted through the action of a neurotransmitter.

Synechia: adhesion of the iris to the cornea or lens.

Syrup: concentrated solution that contains a medication, flavoring, sugar, and water.

Systole: period of ventricular contraction that occurs between the first and second heart sounds.

Systolic blood pressure: pressure exerted in the vessels when the ventricles contract.

T cell: thymus-dependent lymphocyte responsible for cell-mediated immunity.

Tablet: solid preparation in which medication is combined with inert ingredients and compressed into a shape.

Tardive dyskinesia: neurologic syndrome characterized by abnormal muscle movement, particularly around the mouth (such as lip smacking, rhythmic darting of the tongue, and constant chewing movements), and slow, aimless involuntary movements of the arms and legs; a common adverse reaction to antipsychotic agents.

Tetany: manifestation of abnormal calcium metabolism by sharp flexion of the wrist and ankle joints (carpopedal spasms), muscle twitching, muscle cramps, seizures, and stridor.

Therapeutic index: relationship between a drug's therapeutic effects and adverse effects; also called margin of safety.

Thrombin: enzyme derived from prothrombin that converts fibrinogen to fibrin.

Thrombin time: qualitative test used to measure the functional fibrinogen level.

Thrombocytopenia: decrease in the number of platelets in the blood.

Thromboembolism: blood vessel obstruction caused by a thrombus dislodged from its site of origin.

Thrombosis: process of forming or developing a thrombus.

Thrombus: solid mass, clot, or plug formed in the circulatory system from the coagulation of blood constituents.

Thrush: fungal infection characterized by whitish spots and shallow ulcers in the oral cavity, fever, and GI irritation; usually resulting from superinfection.

Thyroglobulin: iodine-containing protein in the colloid of thyroid gland follicles, which stores thyroid hormones.

Thyroiditis: inflammation of the thyroid gland.

Thyrotoxicosis: disorder caused by thyroid gland hyperactivity; also called hyperthyroidism.

Thyrotropin: anterior pituitary hormone that stimulates the thyroid gland.

Tincture: liquid preparation that contains a medication and alcohol (alcoholic solution) or a medication, water, and alcohol (hydroalcoholic solution).

Tolerance: decreased response or sensitivity of a receptor to a drug at the same dose over time.

Tonic seizure: generalized seizure characterized by an abrupt increase in muscle tone, resulting in contraction, loss of consciousness, and marked autonomic signs and symptoms.

Tonic-clonic seizure: generalized seizure characterized by contraction of all skeletal muscles in rhythmic alternating tonic and clonic patterns, followed by depression of all central functions; also known as grand mal seizure.

Tonometric: relating to the indirect measurement of intraocular pressure by determining the resistance of the eyeball to indentation by an applied force.

Tophi: chalky urate deposits in the tissue around joints; they typically are found in individuals who have gout.

Topical anesthesia: loss of feeling or sensation produced by direct application of a local anesthetic agent to a specific area.

Toxicity: quality of being poisonous; also the condition caused by excess drug in the body.

Toxicology: study of poisons, including the adverse effects of drugs, on living organisms.

Trachoma: infectious disease of the conjunctiva and cornea characterized by redness, inflammation, photophobia, and lacrimation.

Trade name: brand name or proprietary name of a drug, which is chosen by the manufacturer.

Trematode: parasitic worm; also known as a fluke; infection can result from ingestion of fluke-contaminated uncooked fish, crustaceans, or vegetation.

Tremor: involuntary trembling or quivering.

Troche: see Lozenge.

Trough level: lowest serum therapeutic concentration of a drug.

Trousseau's sign: carpopedal spasm elicited by putting pressure on large nerves in a hypocalcemic patient.

Tuberculosis: infectious disease caused by a species of *Mycobacterium,* characterized by small rounded nodules in the tissues, as well as fever, emaciation, and night sweats.

Tumor: new tissue growth marked by progressive, uncontrolled cell multiplication; neoplasm.

Tumoricidal: destructive to tumors.

Ulcer: cutaneous or mucosal lesion caused by gradual erosion, disintegration, and necrosis of underlying tissue.

Uricosuric: agent that promotes uric acid excretion.

Urinary acidifier: agent that decreases urine pH level.

Urinary alkalinizer: agent that increases urine pH level.

Urticaria: skin reaction characterized by transient wheals that are paler or redder than the surrounding skin and commonly are accompanied by severe itching; also called hives.

Vaginal route: medication administration by insertion or injection into the vagina.

Valsalva's maneuver: forced expiratory effort against a closed airway.

Vasoconstrictor: agent that constricts or narrows the lumen of blood vessels.

Vesicant: agent that produces blisters.

Vial: small, glass, multidose medication container sealed with a rubber diaphragm.

Virus: group of minute infectious agents characterized by a lack of independent metabolism and by the ability to replicate within living host cells only.

Viscid: sticky; adhesive.

Vitamin: organic substance in food that is necessary for normal metabolism; classified as fat-soluble or water-soluble.

Vomiting: forcible expulsion of gastric contents through the mouth.

Wax matrix tablet: wax, honeycomb structure containing medication that is slowly released as the comb dissolves.

Wilms' tumor: rapidly developing, malignant kidney tumor composed of embryonic elements, which usually affects children under age 5.

Zollinger-Ellison syndrome: triad of effects: peptic ulceration, gastric hyperacidity, and non–beta cell tumors of the pancreatic islets.

Selected references

GENERAL REFERENCES

AHFS drug information 97. (1997). Bethesda, MD: American Society of Health-System Pharmacists.

American Nurses' Association. (1997). *Facts and comparisons: Drug facts,* St. Louis: Wolters Kluwer.

Billups, N.F. and Billups, S.M. (1997). *American drug index: Facts and comparisons.* St. Louis: Wolters Kluwer.

Copstead, L. (1995). *Perspectives on pathophysiology.* Philadelphia: W.B. Saunders.

Drug information for the health care professional. (17th ed., 1997). Rockville, MD: U.S. Government Printing Office.

Ganong, W. (1995). *Review of medical physiology.* (17th ed.). East Norwalk, CT: Appleton & Lange.

Hussar, D. (Ed.). (1997). *Modell's drugs in current use and new drugs, 1997.* New York: Springer Publishing..

Mosby's complete drug reference-Physician GenRx. (7th ed., 1997). St. Louis: Mosby–Year Book.

Nursing 98 drug handbook. (1998). Springhouse, PA: Springhouse.

Physicians' desk reference. (51st ed., 1997). Montvale, NJ: Medical Economics.

UNIT REFERENCES

Unit I: Overview of pharmacology

Clark, et al. (1996). *Pharmacologic basis of nursing practice.* (5th ed.). St. Louis: Mosby–YearBook.

Dipiro, J., et al. (1997). *Pharmacology: A pathophysiologic approach.* (3rd ed.). East Norwalk, CT: Appleton & Lange.

Hardiman, J., et al. (Eds.). (1997). *Goodman and Gilman's The pharmacological basis of therapeutics.* (9th ed.). New York: McGraw-Hill.

Jaffe, M. (1996). *Medical-surgical nursing care plans.* East Norwalk, CT: Appleton & Lange.

Katzung, B. (1997). *Basic and clinical pharmacology.* (7th ed.). East Norwalk, CT: Appleton & Lange.

Lehne, R. (1997). *Pharmacology for nursing care.* (3rd ed.). Philadelphia: W.B. Saunders.

NANDA Nursing diagnoses: Definitions and classification, 1997-1998. (1996). Philadelphia: North American Nursing Diagnosis Association.

Unit II: The nursing process and drug administration

Black, J. and Matassarin-Jacobs, E. (1997). *Medical-surgical nursing: Clinical management for continuity of care.* (5th ed.). Philadelphia: W.B. Saunders.

Cheek, J. (1997). Nursing and the administration of medications: Broadening the focus. *Nursing Research,* 6(3):253-74.

Gray, D. (1997). *Calculate with confidence.* (2nd ed.). St. Louis: Mosby–Year Book.

Hays, G., et al. (1997). *Current pediatric diagnosis and treatment.* (13th ed.). East Norwalk, CT: Appleton & Lange.

Nursing photobooks: Giving medications. (1996). Springhouse, PA: Springhouse.

Nursing Procedures. (2nd ed., 1996). Springhouse, PA: Springhouse.

Polaski, A. and Tatro, S. (1996). *Luckman's core principles and practice of medical-surgical nursing.* Philadelphia: W.B. Saunders.

Todd, C. and Erickson, B. (1997). *Dosage calculations manual.* (3rd ed.). Springhouse, PA: Springhouse.

Wilson, B. and Shannon, M. (1996). *Dosage calculation: A simplified approach.* (3rd ed.). East Norwalk, CT: Appleton & Lange.

Wong, D. and Wilson, D. (Eds.). (1995). *Nursing care of infants and children.* (5th ed.). St. Louis: Mosby–Year Book.

Unit III: Drugs affecting the autonomic nervous system

Alexander, R., et al. (1997). *Hurst's The heart.* New York: McGraw-Hill.

Burns, L.S. (Mar., 1997). Advances in pediatric anesthesia. *Nursing Clinics of North America,* 32(1):45-71.

Harrison, T. and Fauci, A. (1997). *Harrison's principles of internal medicine.* (14th ed.). New York: McGraw-Hill.

Hickey, J. (1996). *The clinical practice of neurological and neuroscience nursing.* (4th ed.). Philadelphia: Lippincott-Raven.

Hooper, V. (Nov.-Dec., 1996). Applied pharmacology. Reversal agents to counteract muscle relaxation: Nursing considerations. *Dimensions of Critical Care Nursing,* 15(6):284-95.

Huddleston, S. and Ferguson, S. (1997). *Critical care and emergency nursing.* (3rd. ed.). Springhouse, PA.: Springhouse.

Kernich, C. and Kaminski, H. (Aug., 1995). Myasthenia gravis: Pathophysiology, diagnosis, and collaborative care. *Journal of Neuroscience Nursing,* 27(4):207-18.

Kleinpell R., et al. (Nov., 1996). Use of peripheral nerve stimulators to monitor patients with neuromuscular blockade in the ICU. *American Journal of Critical Care,* 5(6):449-54.

Lilly, L. and Guanci, R. (Feb., 1997). Med errors: Neuromuscular blocking agents. *American Journal of Nursing,* 97:12, 14.

Matthews, L. (1996). *Cardiopulmonary anatomy and physiology.* Philadelphia: Lippincott-Raven.

McAuliffe, M. and Hartshorn E. (May, 1997). Anesthetic drug interactions. *CRNA, The Clinical Forum for Nurse Anesthetists,* 8(2):84-7.

National Heart, Lung, and Blood Institute. (1995). *Global initiative for asthma.* (Pub. No. 95-3659). Bethesda, MD: National Institutes of Health.

Professional quick reference: Cardiovascular drug therapy. (1995). Springhouse, PA.: Springhouse.

Providing respiratory care. (1996). Springhouse, PA.: Springhouse.

Rennard, S. (May, 1995). Combination bronchodilator therapy in COPD. *Chest,* 107(5): Suppl.: 171S-75S.

Urden, L., et al. (1996). *Priorities in critical care nursing.* (2nd ed.). St. Louis: Mosby–Year Book.

Unit IV: Drugs to treat neurologic and neuromuscular system disorders

Anonymous. (Mar.-Apr., 1997). Parkinson's disease. CE article: part II of III. *PMA,* 30(2):15-24.

Calne, D. (Jan. 15, 1995). Diagnosis and treatment of Parkinson's disease. *Hospital Practice,* 30(1):83-6.

Casale, R., et al. (July, 1995). Reduction of spastic hypertonia in patients with spinal cord injury: A double-blind comparison of intravenous orphenadrine citrate and placebo. *Archives of Physical Medicine & Rehabilitation,* 76(7):660-5.

Childs, N., et al. (May, 1996). Sinemet in locked-in syndrome. *Archives of Physical Medicine & Rehabilitation,* 77(5):523-4.

Cutson, T., et al. (May, 1995). Pharmacological and nonpharmacological interventions in the treatment of Parkinson's disease. *Physical Therapy,* 75(5):363-73.

Hartshorn, J. (1996). Seizures and the elderly. *Critical Care Nursing Clinics of North America,* 8(8):71-8.

Joseph, C., et al. (Jan., 1995). Adverse reactions to controlled release levodopa/carbidopa in older persons: Case reports. *Journal of the American Geriatrics Society,* 43(1):47-50.

Schachter, S. (1996). Update in the treatment of epilepsy. *Comprehensive Therapy,* 22(3):152-5.

Spiekermann, B., et al. (June, 1995). Nonsurgical airway management: General considerations and specific considerations in patients with coexisting disease. *Respiratory Care,* 40(6):644-54.

Spoltore, T. and O'Brien, A. (May-June, 1995). Rehabilitation of the spinal cord-injured patient. *Orthopëdic Nursing,* 14(3):7-16.

Wilder, B., et al. (1996). Safety and tolerance of multiple doses of intramuscular fosphenytoin substituted for oral phenytoin in epilepsy or neurosurgery. *Archives of Neurology,* 53(8):764-8.

Unit V: Drugs to treat and prevent pain

Clochesy, J. et al. (1996). *Critical care nursing.* (2nd ed.). Philadelphia: W.B. Saunders.

Dunn, D. (1997). Home study program: Malignant hyperthermia. *AORN,* 65(4):726+.

GoldFrank's Toxicologic emergencies. (5th ed., 1994). East Norwalk, CT: Appleton & Lange.

Nagelhout, J. and Zaglanickny, K. (Eds.). (1997). *Nurse anesthesia.* Philadelphia: W.B. Saunders.

Portenoy, R. and Kanner, R. (Eds.). (1996). *Pain management: Theory and practice.* Philadelphia: F.A. Davis.

Safety and control of long-acting local anesthetic agent. (1997). *AANA,* 65(1), 2-page insert.

Salerno, E. and Willens, J. (1996). *Pain management handbook: An interdisciplinary approach.* St. Louis: Mosby–Year Book.

Stimme, B. (1997). *Pain and its relief without addiction: Clinical issues in the use of opioids and other analgesics.* New York: Haworth.

Weiner, R. (1997). *Pain management.* Boca Raton, FL: St. Lucie.

Unit VI: Drugs to improve cardiovascular function

Adroque, H. and Wesson, D. (1995). *Heart failure.* Cambridge, MA: Blackwell Scientific.

Advanced cardiac life support. (1997). Dallas, TX: American Heart Association.

Anonymous. (Oct., 1995). What's new in drugs. Cholesterol fighter saves lives, says the FDA. Simvastatin. *RN,* 58(10):72.

Cardiovascular drugs and sudden death. (Nov., 1995). *Nurses Drug Alert,* 19(11):81-2.

Clark, J. (March, 1995). Lipid-lowering drugs in heart disease prevention. *Community Nurse,* 1:3-4.

Fulterman, L. and Lemberg, L. (May, 1997). Amiodarone: A late comer. *American Journal of Critical Care,* 6(3):233-9.

Ganda, O. and Simonson, D. (Feb. 15, 1995). Controlling lipids and blood pressure. *Patient Care,* 29(3):61-64, 66, 69-72.

Gurwitz, J., et al. (1997). Optimizing drug therapy in the elderly. *Pharmacy and Therapeutics,* 22(7):331-46.

Keep thiazide dosages low. (March, 1995). *Emergency Medicine,* 27(3):61.

Khan, G. (1996). *Heart disease diagnosis and therapy: A practical approach.* Baltimore: Williams & Wilkins.

Khan, M. (1995). *Cardiac drug therapy.* (4th ed.). Philadelphia: W.B. Saunders.

LaForge, R. and Thomas T. (Oct., 1996). Outpatient management of lipid disorders. *Journal of Cardiovascular Nursing,* 11(1):39-53.

Marwick C. (1996), FDA gives calcium-channel blockers clean bill of health but warns of short-acting nifedipine hazards. *Journal of the American Medical Association,* 275(6):423-4.

Pill, M. (June, 1997). Ibutilide: A new antiarrhythmic agent for the critical care environment. *Critical Care Nurse,* 17(3):19-22.

Scott, A. (1997). *Hypertension in the older adult.* Boston: Arnold.

Smith, T. (1996). *Cardiovascular therapeutics: A companion to Braunwald's Heart disease.* Philadelphia: W.B. Saunders.

Unit VII: Drugs affecting the hematologic system

Blacksher, J., et al. (1996). Management of atrial fibrillation in adults: Prevention of thromboembolism and symptomatic treatment. *Mayo Clinic Proceedings,* (71):150-160.

Dolman, S. and Paradiso-Hardy, F. (Dec., 1996). Intracoronary urokinase for restoring circulation in occluded saphenous vein grafts. *Critical Nurse,* 6(16).

Galloway, R. and McGuire, J. (Oct., 1996). Daily versus weekly: How many iron pills do pregnant women need? *Nutrition Reviews,* 54(10):318-23.

Higgins, C. (May 31-June 6, 1995). Deficiency testing for iron, vitamin B_{12} and folate. *Nursing Times,* 91(22):38-40.

Wurnig, C., et al. (Feb., 1996). Prevention of chemotherapy-induced anemia by the use of erythropoietin in patients with primary malignant bone tumors. *Transfusion,* 36(2):155-9.

Unit VIII: Drugs to improve respiratory function

Connolly, M. (May, 1995). Mucolytics and the critically ill patient: Help or hindrance? *Advanced Practice in Acute & Critical Care,* 6(2):307-15.

Davis, A., et al. (Jan. 15, 1996). Acute bronchitis in adults and children. *Patient Care,* 30(1):102-4, 110.

Mays, M., and Leiner, S. (1996). Primary care for women: Management of common respiratory problems. *Journal of Nurse Midwifery,* 41(2):139-54.

Middleton, A. (Jan., 1997). Managing asthma: It takes teamwork. *American Journal of Nursing,* 97:39-43.

Sherman, C. (Dec., 1995). Late-onset asthma: Making the diagnosis, choosing drug therapy. *Geriatrics,* 50(12):24-6, 29-30, 33.

Silverstone, T. (1997). Clinical practice. Coughs and colds: Advising on what to take. *Professional Care of Mother & Child,* 7(1):13-16.

Whatling, J. (Nov. 15-21, 1995). Managing chronic obstructive disease. *Nursing Standard,* 10(8):34-7.

Unit IX: Drugs to improve gastrointestinal function

Anatazi, J. and Sun, V. (1996). Controlling diarrhea in the HIV patient. *American Journal of Nursing,* 96(8):35-40.

Anonymous. (Oct., 1995). Using activated charcoal: It's no picnic. *Nursing,* 25(10):9.

Brozenec, S. (Sept., 1996). Ulcer therapy update. *RN,* 59(9):48-50, 52-4.

Cave, D. and Hoffman, J. (Jan. 15, 1996). Management of *Helicobacter pylori* infection in ulcer disease. *Hospital Practice,* 31(1):63-4, 67-9.

Diagnosis of diarrhea. (June 21, 1996). *Practice Nurse,* 12(1): 56-7.

Drug combo relieves chemotherapy nausea. (May, 1995). *Case Management Advisor,* 6(5):68-9.

Goebel, C. (Jan., 1996). Prevention and control of nausea and vomiting for patients with cancer. *Home Healthcare Nurse,* 14(1):15-22.

Hellman, M. (June, 1996). Pediatric poisonings. *Emergency Medical Services,* 25(6):21, 23, 25-8.

Heslin, J. (Jan., 1997). Peptic ulcer disease: Making a case against the prime suspect. *Nursing,* 27(1):34-9.

Minton, N. and Henry, J. (Oct., 1996). Treatment of theophylline overdose. *American Journal of Emergency Medicine,* 14(6):606-12.

Podolski, J. (July-Aug., 1996). Recent advances in peptic ulcer disease. *Helicobacter pylori* infection and its treatment. *Gastroenterology Nursing,* 19(4):128-36.

Rhodes, V., et al. (Nov., 1995). Nausea, vomiting and retching: The management of the symptom experience. *Seminars in Oncology Nursing,* 11(4):256-65.

Shuster, J. (Jan., 1996). Adverse drug reactions: Compazine. *Nursing,* 26(1):30.

Unit X: Drugs to prevent or treat infection

Benjamini, E., et al. (1996). *Immunology: A short course* . (3rd ed.). New York: Wiley-Liss.

Calvert, L. (April, 1996). Advice on malaria. *Practical Nurse,* 11(7):445-6, 448-9.

Cohen, F. and Durham, J. (1995). *Tuberculosis: A source book for nursing practice.* New York: Springer Publishing.

Compton, J. (April, 1997). Malaria in the emergency department. *Journal of Emergency Nursing,* 23(2):120-3.

DiMaggio, C. (April, 1996). Primaquine in malaria prophylaxis. *Physician Assistant,* 20(4):15.

Hung, L. (July, 1996). Mycology and indoor air quality. *Laboratory Medicine,* 27(7)454-61.

Immune and infectious disorders. (1994). Springhouse, PA: Springhouse.

Karlowicz, K. (Ed.). (1995). *Urologic nursing principles and practice.* Philadelphia: W.B. Saunders.

Kmietowicz, Z. (July, 1996). Special report: Using antibiotics more selectively. *Community Nurse,* (6):20, 22.

Levine, D. (1997). *Caring for the renal patient.* Philadelphia: W.B. Saunders.

Libman, H. and Witzberg, R. (Eds.). (1996). *HIV infection: A primary care manual.* (3rd ed.). New York: Little-Brown.

Mainous, A. (July, 1996). Overuse of antibiotics. *Healthline,* 15(7):9.

Nayer, R., et al. (June, 1996). Clinical pathology rounds: Early diagnosis of fungemia in children. *Laboratory Medicine,* 26(6):381-3.

Reiss, P. (March, 1996). Battling the superbugs. *RN,* 59(3):36-41.

Soule, B., et al. (1995). *Infections and the nursing practice.* St. Louis: Mosby–Year Book.

Soule, B., et al. (1995). *Infections and nursing practice: Prevention and control.* St. Louis: Mosby–Year Book.

Unit XI: Drugs to control inflammation, allergy, and organ rejection

Bielan, B. (1995). What's your assessment? Urticaria. *Dermatologic Nursing,* 7(4):240-1.

Brown, E. (Aug., 1995). Gout: No longer a rich man's affliction. *Medical Update,* 19(2):2.

Cohen, M. (May, 1996). Medication errors. Claritin-D: Delivering the right drug. *Nursing,* 27(5):26.

Mathewson, H. (March, 1996). Drug Capsule. Antihistamines and asthma. *Respiratory Care,* 41(3):212-4.

Professional care guide: Immune disorders. (1995). Springhouse, PA: Springhouse.

Shaffer, L. and Phillips, M. (Aug., 1997). Successful treatment of acquired hemophilia with oral immunosuppressive therapy. *Annals of Internal Medicine,* 127(3):206-9.

Star, V. (Nov., 1995). Gout: Options for its therapy and prevention. *Hospital Medicine,* 31(11):25+.

Stites, D., et al. (1994). *Basic and clinical immunology.* (8th ed.). East Norwalk, CT: Appleton & Lange.

Unit XII: Drugs to alter psychogenic behavior and promote sleep

Copel, L. (1996). *Nurse's clinical guide: Psychiatric and mental health care.* Springhouse, PA: Springhouse.

DSM IV Diagnostic and statistical manual of mental disorders. (4th ed., 1994). Washington, DC: American Psychiatric Association.

Fortunash, K. and Holoday-Worret, P. (1996). *Psychiatric-mental health nursing.* St. Louis: Mosby–Year Book.

Johnson, B. (1997). *Adaptation and growth: Psychiatric-mental health nursing,* (4th ed.). Philadelphia: Lippincott-Raven.

Keltner, N., et al. (1995). *Psychiatric nursing.* (2nd ed.). St. Louis: Mosby–Year Book.

Loraia, M. and Stuart, G. (1995). *Quick psychopharmacology reference.* St. Louis: Mosby–Year Book.

Kendrick, T,. et al. (1996). *The prevention of mental illness in primary care.* Cambridge, MA: Cambridge University Press.

Skolnick, P. (1997). *Antidepressants: New pharmacological strategies.* Totowa, NJ: Humana Press.

Wilson, H. and Kneisl, C. (1996). *Psychiatric nursing.* (5th ed.). Menlo Park, CA: Addison-Wesley.

Unit XIII: Drugs to treat endocrine disorders

Caldwell, J. (June, 1996). Hyperthyroidism during pregnancy: Nursing care issues. *Journal of Obstetric, Gynecologic, & Neonatal Nursing,* 25(5):395-400.

Jardim, J., et al. (May, 1996). Nutrition, anabolic steroids, and growth hormones. *Physical Medicine Rehabilitation Clinics of North America,* 7(2): 235-75.

Kennedy, J. and Caro, J. (1996, May). The ABCs of managing hyperthyroidism in the older patient. *Geriatrics,* 51(5):22-4, 27, 31-2.

Lowdermilk, D., et al. (1997). *Maternity and women's health care.* (6th ed.). St. Louis: Mosby–Year Book.

Melchert, R., et al. (1995, Sept.). Cardiovascular effects of androgenic-anabolic steroids. *Medicine and Science in Sports Exercise,* 27(a):1252-62.

Nasso, J. (May/June, 1997). Planning for pregnancy. *The American Journal of Maternal Child Nursing,* (22):142-6.

Payton, R.G., et al. (May-June, 1997). Pharmacologic considerations and management of common endocrine disorders in women. *Journal of Nurse Midwifery,* 42(3):186-206.

Potteiger, et al. (March,1994). Anabolic steroid use in the adolescent athlete. *Journal of Athletic Training,* 29(1):60+.

Roberts, A. (Oct. 9-15, 1996). Pancreas: insulin and glucagon. *Nursing Times,* 92(41):42-4.

Romeo, J. (Dec., 1996). Hyperfunction and hypofunction in the anterior pituitary. *Nursing Clinics of North America,* 31(4):769-78.

Strowig, S. (June, 1995). Diabetes 2000 insulin therapy. *RN,* 58(6):30-7.

Tordjman, K., et al. (April, 1995).The role of the low dose adrenocorticotropin test in the evaluation of patients with pituitary diseases. *Journal of Clinical Endocrinology & Metabolism,* 80(4):1301-5.

Torlone, E., et al. (Sept.,1996). Effects of the short-acting insulin analog on postprandial blood glucose control in IDDM. *Diabetes Care,* 19(9):945-52.

What every woman should know about menopause. (Jan., 1996). *AJN,* 25-32.

Unit XIV: Drugs for fluid, electrolyte, and nutritional balance

Fluids and electrolytes made incredibly easy. (1997). Springhouse, PA: Springhouse.

Huddleston, S. and Ferguson, S. (1997). *Springhouse Notes: Critical care and emergency nursing.* (3rd ed.). Springhouse, PA: Springhouse.

Innerarity, S. and Stark, J. (1997). *Springhouse Notes: Fluids and electrolytes.* Springhouse, PA: Springhouse.

Narins, R. (1994). *Maxwell and Kleeman's Clinical disorders of fluid and electrolyte balance.* (5th ed.). New York: McGraw-Hill.

Ooms, M., et al. (1995). Prevention of bone loss by vitamin D supplementation in elderly women. A randomized double-blind trial. *Journal of Clinical Endocrinologic Metabolism,* (80):1052-8.

Packer, L. and Fuch, J. (1997). *Vitamin C in health and disease.* New York: Marcel Dekker.

Unit XV: Drugs to treat malignant neoplasms

Chabner, B. and Longo, D. (1996). *Cancer chemotherapy and biotherapy: Principles and practice* (2nd ed.). Lippincott-Raven: Philadelphia

Groenwald, S., et al. (1997). *Cancer nursing principles and practice.* Boston: Jones & Bartlett.
Liebman, M. and Camp-Sorrell, D. (1996). *Multimodal therapy in oncology nursing.* St. Louis: Mosby–Year Book.
McCorkle, R., et al. (1996). *Cancer nursing: A comprehensive textbook.* Philadelphia: W.B. Saunders.
Miaskowski, C. (1996). *Oncology nursing: An essential guide for patient care.* Philadelphia: W.B. Saunders.
Otto, S. (1997). *Oncology nursing.* (3rd ed.). St. Louis: Mosby–Year Book.
Primo, S. (1994). Infectious and inflammatory diseases. *Optometry clinics,* 3(4):99-127.
Professional care guide to neoplastic disorders. (1995). Springhouse, PA: Springhouse.
Shapiro, T., et al. (March, 1995). Breast cancer: What the primary care provider needs to know. *Nurse Practitioner,* 20(3): 36-53.
Shelton, B., et al. (1997). *Oncology critical care nursing.* Boston: Jones & Bartlett.

Unit XVI: Other major drugs

Bielan, B. (Aug., 1996.). What's your assessment? *Dermatology Nursing,* 8(4):283-4.
Hill, M. (1994). *Skin disorders.* St. Louis: Mosby–Year Book.
Maklebust, J. and Sieggreen, M. (1996). *Pressure ulcers.* (2nd ed.). Springhouse, PA: Springhouse.
Over-the-counter update. Our A-Z guide to OTC medicine: Ear and eye preparations. (July, 1996). *Community Nurse,* 2(6):38.
Papastamelos, A., et al. (Sept., 1995). Antibacterial agents in infections of the central nervous system and eye. *Infectious Disease Clinics of North America,* 9(3).
Poyner, T. (Dec., 1995). The role of infection in skin diseases. *Community Nurse,* 1(11):16, 18.
Quick, G. (May, 1995). Warm weather woes: Stemming the tide of swimmer's ear. *Consultant,* 35(3):629-30.
Riley, T., et al. (1995). Major drug highlight '95. *U.S. Pharmacist,* 20(10):55-100.
Thomas-Hess, C. (1998). *Nurse's clinical guide to wound care.* (2nd ed.). Springhouse, PA: Springhouse.
Thurgood, K., et al. (June 22-July 12, 1995). Ear syringing: A clinical skill. *British Journal of Nursing,* 4(12):682-7.

Index

i refers to an illustration; t, to a table.

i refers to an illustration; t, to a table.

i refers to an illustration; t, to a table.

i refers to an illustration; t, to a table.

i refers to an illustration; t, to a table.

i refers to an illustration; t, to a table.

i refers to an illustration; t, to a table.

i refers to an illustration; t, to a table.

i refers to an illustration; t, to a table.

i refers to an illustration; t, to a table.

K

L

i refers to an illustration; t, to a table.

i refers to an illustration; t, to a table.

i refers to an illustration; t, to a table.

O

i refers to an illustration; t, to a table.

P

i refers to an illustration; t, to a table.

Q

R

i refers to an illustration; t, to a table.

i refers to an illustration; t, to a table.

T

i refers to an illustration; t, to a table.

i refers to an illustration; t, to a table.

About *PharmTest*

PharmTest: Test Bank for Essentials of Clinical Pharmacology in Nursing, Third Edition, lets you test your knowledge of more than 300 drugs in every therapeutic classification. The test items are written in the style of national licensing examinations, a plus when studying for nursing boards.

PREFERRED SYSTEM REQUIREMENTS

- IBM-compatible personal computer with Pentium processor (486/33MHz minimum)
- Windows® 95 (Windows 3.1 minimum)
- High-density 3½" floppy drive
- 8 MB RAM (4 MB minimum)
- SVGA monitor capable of displaying 256 colors or greater (VGA minimum)
- 4 MB of available space on hard drive
- Windows-compatible mouse and word processing program

INSTALLING AND RUNNING THE PROGRAM

Note: Before installing this program, make sure your monitor is set to display 256 colors or greater. If it isn't, consult your user's manual for instructions about changing the display settings.

- Turn on computer, and insert diskette into drive A (or B). From the Program menu, select "File," and then "Run." (For Windows 95, click "Start" and select "Run.")
- Type **a:\setup** (where **a:** is the letter of your floppy drive), and click OK. Follow on-screen instructions.
- For technical support, call 215-628-7736 Monday through Friday, 9 a.m. to 6 p.m. Eastern Standard Time.
- For information about obtaining a network license for *PharmTest,* call 1-800-346-7844, Ext. 790, Monday through Friday, 9 a.m. to 5 p.m. Eastern Standard Time.

The clinical information and tools in *PharmTest: Test Bank for Essentials of Clinical Pharmacology in Nursing,* Third Edition, are based on research and consultation with nursing, medical, and legal authorities. To the best of our knowledge, this program reflects currently accepted practice; nevertheless, it can't be considered absolute and universal. For individual application, all recommendations must be considered in light of your institution's policies and procedures, the patient's clinical condition and, before administration of new or infrequently used drugs, in light of the latest package-insert information. The authors and publisher disclaim responsibility for adverse effects resulting directly or indirectly from the suggested procedures, from undetected errors, or from the reader's misunderstanding of the program.

Springhouse Corporation warrants to the user that the program media on which the software is recorded shall be free from defects in materials and workmanship for a period of ninety (90) days from the date of the user's purchase. Springhouse Corporation's liability shall be limited to correction or replacement of defective media.